ANNALS OF OTOLOGY, RHINOLOGY AND LARYNGOLOGY

FOUNDED IN 1892

VOLUME 84

PUBLISHED BIMONTHLY

BY THE

ANNALS PUBLISHING COMPANY

Before prescribing, please consult complete product information, a summary of which follows:

Indications: Infections due to susceptible strains of the following gram-negative organisms: *H. influenzae, E. coli, P. mirabilis* and *N. gonorrhoeae;* and gram-positive organisms: streptococci (including *Streptococcus faecalis*), *D. pneumoniae* and non-penicillinase-producing staphylococci. Therapy may be instituted prior to obtaining results from bacteriological and susceptibility studies to determine causative organisms and susceptibility to amoxicillin.

Contraindications: In individuals with history of allergic reaction to penicillins.

WARNINGS: SERIOUS AND OCCASIONALLY FATAL HYPERSENSITIVITY (ANAPHYLACTOID) REACTIONS REPORTED IN PATIENTS ON PENICILLIN THERAPY. ALTHOUGH MORE FREQUENT FOLLOWING PARENTERAL THERAPY, ANAPHYLAXIS HAS OCCURRED IN PATIENTS ON ORAL PENICILLINS. MORE LIKELY IN INDIVIDUALS WITH HISTORY OF SENSITIVITY TO MULTIPLE ALLERGENS. BEFORE THERAPY, INQUIRE CONCERNING PREVIOUS HYPERSENSITIVITY REACTIONS TO PENICILLINS, CEPHALOSPORINS OR OTHER ALLERGENS. IF ALLERGIC REACTION OCCURS, INSTITUTE APPROPRIATE THERAPY AND CONSIDER DISCONTINUANCE OF AMOXICILLIN. **SERIOUS ANAPHYLACTOID REACTIONS REQUIRE IMMEDIATE EMERGENCY TREATMENT WITH EPINEPHRINE. ADMINISTER OXYGEN, INTRAVENOUS STEROIDS AND AIRWAY MANAGEMENT, INCLUDING INTUBATION, AS INDICATED.**

Usage in Pregnancy: Safety in pregnancy not established.

Precautions: As with any potent drug, assess renal, hepatic and hematopoietic function periodically during prolonged therapy. Keep in mind possibility of superinfections with mycotic or bacterial pathogens; if they occur, discontinue drug and/or institute appropriate therapy.

Adverse Reactions: As with other penicillins, untoward reactions will likely be essentially limited to sensitivity phenomena and more likely occur in individuals previously demonstrating penicillin hypersensitivity and those with history of allergy, asthma, hay fever or urticaria. Adverse reactions reported as associated with use of penicillins: *Gastrointestinal:* Nausea, vomiting, diarrhea. *Hypersensitivity Reactions:* Erythematous maculopapular rashes, urticaria. *NOTE:* Urticaria, other skin rashes and serum sickness-like reactions may be controlled with antihistamines and, if necessary, systemic corticosteroids. Discontinue amoxicillin unless condition is believed to be life-threatening and amenable only to amoxicillin therapy. *Liver:* Moderate rise in SGOT noted, but significance unknown. *Hemic and Lymphatic Systems:* Anemia, thrombocytopenia, thrombocytopenic purpura, eosinophilia, leukopenia, agranulocytosis. All are usually reversible on discontinuation of therapy and believed to be hypersensitivity phenomena.

Dosage: *Ear, nose, throat, genitourinary tract, skin and soft tissue infections*—Adults: 250 mg every 8 hours. Children: 20 mg/kg/day in divided doses every 8 hours; under 6 kg, 0.5 ml of Pediatric Drops every 8 hours; 6-8 kg, 1 ml of Pediatric Drops every 8 hours. *Lower respiratory tract infections and severe infections or those caused by less susceptible organisms*—Adults: 500 mg every 8 hours. Children: 40 mg/kg/day in divided doses every 8 hours; under 6 kg, 1 ml of Pediatric Drops every 8 hours; 6-8 kg, 2 ml of Pediatric Drops every 8 hours. *Gonorrhea* (acute uncomplicated anogenital and urethral infections)—Males and females: 3 grams as a single oral dose. *NOTE:* Children weighing more than 8 kg should receive appropriate dose of oral suspension 125 mg or 250 mg/5 ml. Children weighing 20 kg or more should be dosed according to adult recommendations.

Note: In gonorrhea with suspected lesion of syphilis, perform dark-field examinations before amoxicillin therapy and monthly serological tests for at least four months. In chronic urinary tract infections, frequent bacteriological and clinical appraisals are necessary. Smaller than recommended doses should not be used. In stubborn infections, several weeks' therapy may be required. Except for gonorrhea, continue treatment for a minimum of 48-72 hours after patient is asymptomatic or bacterial eradication is evidenced. Treat hemolytic streptococcal infections for at least 10 days to prevent acute rheumatic fever or glomerulonephritis.

Supplied: Amoxicillin as the trihydrate: Capsules, 250 mg and 500 mg; oral suspension, 125 mg/5 ml and 250 mg/5 ml; pediatric drops, 50 mg/ml.

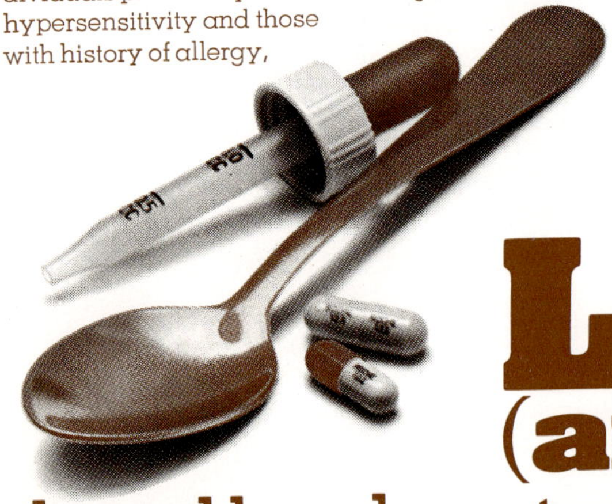

ROCHE

Roche Laboratories
Division of Hoffmann-La Roche Inc.
Nutley, New Jersey 07110

Larotid (amoxicillin)

the oral broad spectrum antibiotic from Roche

ANNALS OF OTOLOGY, RHINOLOGY AND LARYNGOLOGY

VOL. 84 JULY - AUGUST, 1975 NO. 4

CONTENTS

PAGE

Experimental Aural Cholesteatoma Causing Bone Resorption. Maxwell Abramson, M.D., Iowa City, Iowa, Richard G. Asarch, M.D., Denver, Colorado, Ward B. Litton, M.D., Moline, Illinois 425

Idiopathic Facial Paralysis, Pregnancy, and the Menstrual Cycle. Raymond L. Hilsinger, Jr., M.D., Kedar K. Adour, M.D., H. E. Doty, Oakland, California..... 433

Innervation of the Cochlea of the Guinea Pig by Use of the Golgi Stain. Catherine A. Smith, Ph.D., Portland, Oregon 443

Genetic Sensorineural Deafness in Adults. Michael M. Paparella, M.D., David G. Hanson, M.D., K. N. Rao, M.D., Rolf Ulvestad, M.D., Minneapolis, Minnesota 459

Operative Treatment of Surgical Lesions with Objective Tinnitus. Paul H. Ward, M.D., Richard Babin, M.D., Thomas C. Calcaterra, M.D., H. R. Konrad, M.D., Los Angeles, California 473

Eustachian Tube Lymphatics. Jack L. Pulec, M.D., Los Angeles, California, Tomokazu Kamio, M.D., Tokyo, Japan, Malcolm D. Graham, M.D., Los Angeles, California 483

The Cochlear Implant: Current Status. William F. House, M.D., Los Angeles, California. (Abstract) 493

Present Status and Future Development of the Cochlear Prosthesis. Robin P. Michelson, M.D., Robert A. Schindler, M.D., Michael M. Merzenich, Ph.D., David N. Schindler, M.D., San Francisco, California 494

Cochlear Potentials and Oxygen Associated with Hypoxia. Merle Lawrence, Ph.D., Alfred L. Nuttall, Ph.D., Paul A. Burgio, A.B., Ann Arbor, Michigan 499

Conservative Management of Ménière's Disease: Furstenberg Regimen Revisited. Roger Boles, M.D., San Francisco, California, Dale H. Rice, M.D., Roger Hybels, M.D., Walter P. Work, M.D., Ann Arbor, Michigan 513

PAGE

Grafting Materials and Methods in Reconstructive Ear Surgery. Rodney Perkins, M.D., Palo Alto, California 518

Otology and Industrial Hearing Conservation. Joseph Sataloff, M.D., Philadelphia, Pennsylvania 527

Complications in Acoustic Neuroma Surgery. Michael E. Glasscock III, M.D., James W. Hays, M.D., James P. Murphy, M.D., Nashville, Tennessee 530

Electronystagmography: A Review of 17 Years Experience. Wallace Rubin, M.D., Metairie, Louisiana 541

Sensorineural Hearing Loss Due to Cochlear Otospongiosis: Theoretical Considerations of Etiology. Fred H. Linthicum, Jr., M.D., Los Angeles, California, Roberto Filipo, M.D., Rome, Italy, Sidney Brody, P.E., Los Angeles, California 544

Reconstruction of the Open Mastoidectomy Ear: A Six Year Progress Report. Mansfield F. W. Smith, M.D., San Jose, California 552

Temporal Bone Histopathological Findings in Trisomy 13 Syndrome. Isamu Sando, M.D., Alberto Leiberman, M.D., LaVonne Bergstrom, M.D., Denver, Colorado, Soji Izumi, M.D., Yokohama, Japan, Raymond P. Wood II, M.D., Denver, Colorado .... Supplement No. 21

Paget's Disease of the Temporal Bone. George T. Nager, M.D., Baltimore, Maryland .... Supplement No. 22

X-Ray of the Month

James Rhea, M.D., Alfred L. Weber, M.D., Boston, Massachusetts 558

Communications

Conference of Animal Models of Aging in the Auditory System. David E. Crowley, Ph.D., St. Louis, Missouri 560

Book Reviews 561

Program of Research Forum; Committee for Research in Otolaryngology, AAOO, and Association for Research in Otolaryngology 565

Index to Advertisers 567

ANNALS OF OTOLOGY, RHINOLOGY AND LARYNGOLOGY

VOL. 84 SEPT - OCT, 1975 No. 5

CONTENTS

PAGE

Physiology and Pathophysiology of the Lower Esophageal Sphincter. Capt. Donald O. Castell, MC USN, Bethesda, Maryland 569

Surgical Management of Severe Lye Burns of the Esophagus by Colon Interposition. Wallace P. Berkowitz, M.D., Charles L. Roper, M.D., Donald G. Sessions, M.D., Gershon J. Spector, M.D., Joseph H. Ogura, M.D., St. Louis, Missouri 576

Early Lung Cancer Detection and Localization. David R. Sanderson, M.D., Robert S. Fontana, M.D., Rochester, Minnesota 583

Delayed Clearance of Tantalum by Radiologically Occult Cancer. Frederick P. Stitik, M.D., Donald F. Proctor, M.D., Baltimore, Maryland 589

Transbronchial Lung Biopsy Through the Fiberoptic Bronchoscope in Diffuse Lung Disease. Lee Roy Joyner, M.D., David J. Scheinhorn, Washington, D.C. 596

Clinical Experience with Pleuroscopy Utilizing the Bronchofiberscope. Gerald R. Kerby, M.D., George Pierce, M.D., William E. Ruth, M.D., Kansas City, Kansas 602

Treatment of Papillomatosis of the Larynx with Transfer Factor. Cedric A. Quick, M.D., Hans W. Behrens, M.D., Margo Brinton-Darnell, PhD., Minneapolis, Minnesota, Robert A. Good, M.D., New York, New York 607

Carcinoma and Juvenile Papillomatosis. Paul R. Zehnder, Jr., M.D., George D. Lyons, M.D., New Orleans, Louisiana 614

Extraluminal Foreign Bodies (Coins) in the Food and Air Passages. King F. Yee, M.D., Joyce A. Schild, M.D., Paul H. Holinger, M.D., Chicago, Illinois 619

The Problem of the Open Safety Pin. Bernard R. Marsh, M.D., Baltimore, Maryland 624

Unexpected Radiographic Findings Related to Foreign Bodies. Wilfred T. Morioka, M.D., Robert H. Maisel, M.D., Thomas W. Smith, M.D., Robert W. Cantrell, M.D., San Diego, California 627

PAGE

Special New Low Resistance to Flow Tube and Endotracheal Tube Adapter for Use During Fiberoptic Bronchoscopy. Edward Carden, FRCP(C), Phulchand P. Raj, M.D., Los Angeles, California 631

Evaluation of Major Airway Lesions Using the Flow-Volume Loop. Robert E. Hyatt, M.D., Rochester, Minnesota 635

Hyoid Autograft Repair of Chronic Subglottic Stenosis. Douglas A. Finnegan, M.D., Matthew L. Wong, M.D., Haskins K. Kashima, M.D., Baltimore, Maryland 643

Foreign Body Removal: A New Role for the Fiberoptic Bronchoscope. Donald C. Zavala, M.D., Mitchell L. Rhodes, M.D., Iowa City, Iowa 650

Swyer-James Syndrome: A Cause of Hyperlucent Lung. Jacobo Guzowski, M.D., Arndt J. Duvall III, M.D., Minneapolis, Minnesota 657

Objective Evaluation of Vocal Pathology Using Voice Spectrography. Eugene Rontal, M.D., Michael Rontal, M.D., Michael I. Rolnick, Ph.D., Southfield, Michigan 662

Hypogeusia, Dysgeusia, Hyposmia, and Dysosmia Following Influenza-Like Infection. R. I. Henkin, M.D., A. L. Larson, M.D., R. D. Powell, M.D., Bethesda, Maryland 672

New Approach to Caloric Stimulation of the Vestibular Receptor. Leonard R. Proctor, M.D., Rollin C. Dix, Ph.D., Chicago, Illinois 683

Facial Nerve Reconstruction and its Prognosis. J. Sadé, M.D., Kfar Saba, Israel 695

Grand Rounds. Clinical Pathological Conference, Massachusetts Eye and Ear Infirmary. Chairman: Harold F. Schuknecht, M.D., Boston, Massachusets 704

Frequency Responses of Hearing Aids and Their Effects on the Speech Perception of Hearing-Impaired Subjects. David P. Pascoe, Ph.D. ..... Supplement No. 23

X-Ray of the Month
Guillermo F. Carrera, M.D., Alfred Weber, M.D., Boston, Massachusetts 719

Book Reviews 720

Abstracts of Current Articles 722

Roster of Societies 724

Information to Contributors 726

Index to Advertisers 727

ANNALS OF OTOLOGY, RHINOLOGY AND LARYNGOLOGY

VOL. 84 | NOV - DEC, 1975 | NO. 6

CONTENTS

———

PAGE

Some Reflections on our Specialty. John J. Conley, M.D., New York, New York 729

Frey's Syndrome — A Technical Remedy. Roy B. Sessions, M.D., David T. Roark, M.D., Bobby R. Alford, M.D., Houston, Texas 734

Preoperative Embolization of Juvenile Angiofibromas of the Nasopharynx. James D. Pletcher, M.D., Thomas H. Newton, M.D., Herbert H. Dedo, M.D., David Norman, M.D., San Francisco California 740

Cleft Larynx. A Report of Seven Cases. Seymour R. Cohen, M.D., Los Angeles, California 747

Nontraumatic, Nonneoplastic Subglottic Stenosis. Mohsen Djalilian, M.D., Thomas J. McDonald, M.D., Kenneth D. Devine, M.D., Louis H. Weiland, M.D., Rochester, Minnesota 758

Injuries to the Neonatal Larynx from Long-Term Endotracheal Tube Intubation and Suggested Tube Modification for Prevention. Arthur S. Hengerer, M.D., Rochester, New York, Marshall Strome, M.D., Burton F. Jaffe, M.D., Boston, Massachusetts 764

Second Primary Cancer After Irradiation of Laryngeal Cancer. William Lawson, M.D., Max Som, M.D., New York, New York 771

Experimental Granuloma of the Larynx. Fernando R. Kirchner, M.D., Kansas City, Kansas 776

Tracheal Incision as a Contributing Factor to Tracheal Stenosis. An Experimental Study. Gary C. Lulenski, M.D., John G. Batsakis, M.D., Ann Arbor, Michigan 781

Characterization of Tumor Antigen in Epidermoid Carcinoma. Charles J. Krause, M.D., John Nysather, Brian F. McCabe, M.D., Iowa City, Iowa 787

PAGE

Pyriform Sinus Cancer: A Clinical and Laboratory Study. John A. Kirchner, M.D., New Haven, Connecticut ... 793

Radiation Failures in Cancer of the Larynx. Emanuel M. Skolnik, M.D., Lawrence Martin, M.D., King F. Yee, M.D., Michael A. Wheatley, M.D., Chicago, Illinois ... 804

Rehabilitation of the Shoulder after Radical Neck Dissection. W. H. Saunders, M.D., E. W. Johnson, M.D., Columbus, Ohio ... 812

Carcinoma of the Nasopharynx in Children. James B. Snow, Jr., M.D., Philadelphia, Pennsylvania ... 817

Observations on the Primate Hyoepiglottic Complex. Gabriel Tucker, Jr., M.D., John A. Tucker, M.D., Philadelphia, Pennsylvania ... 827

Incidence, Predisposing Factors and Outcome of Pharyngocutaneous Fistulas Complicating Head and Neck Cancer Surgery. Douglas D. Dedo, M.D., William A. Alonso, M.D., Joseph H. Ogura, M.D., St. Louis, Missouri ... 833

Vertigo of Delayed Onset After Sudden Deafness. Joseph B. Nadol, Jr., M.D., Alfred D. Weiss, M.D., Stephen W. Parker, M.D., Boston, Massachusetts ... 841

Rates of Ion Movement from Plasma to Endolymph in the Dogfish. Thomas H. Maren, M.D., Erik R. Swenson, A.B., Albert D. F. Addink, Ph.D., Gainesville, Florida ... 847

Grand Rounds: Paranasal Sinus Infection. The University of Iowa Department of Otolaryngology and Maxillofacial Surgery. Chairman: Brian F. McCabe, M.D., Iowa City, Iowa ... 859

X-Ray of the Month: Lymphoepithelioma of the Nasopharynx. Saadoon Kadir, M.D., Alfred L .Weber, M.D., Boston, Massachusetts ... 865

Communications ... 867

Abstracts of Current Articles ... 867

Calendar of Events ... 870

Author Index ... 872

Subject Index ... 874

Index to Advertisers ... 887

Ann Otol 84: 1975

EXPERIMENTAL AURAL CHOLESTEATOMA CAUSING BONE RESORPTION

MAXWELL ABRAMSON, M.D.

IOWA CITY, IOWA

RICHARD G. ASARCH, M.D.

DENVER, COLORADO

WARD B. LITTON, M.D.

MOLINE, ILLINOIS

SUMMARY – A series of experiments were carried out on 55 guinea pigs in four groups to study the conditions fostering bone resorbing epidermal cysts. The first group had free grafts of canal wall skin applied to the cochlea with and without talc application. The second group had canal skin flaps applied to the cochlea with and without subsequent talc application. The third group had talc applied either to the tympanic membrane or on the cochlea. The fourth group had a canal skin flap inserted into a mucosal pocket in the bulla. The animals were killed three to four months after surgery and the temporal bones were prepared for histology. Epidermal cysts were found at the cochlea in 8 of 55 animals. Cochlear fistulas were found in 6 of 55 animals. The fistulas were associated with epidermal cysts in three cases, otitis media in two cases, and talc granuloma in one case. These experiments show that migrating skin attached to a source of epithelium is capable of inducing bone resorption. Chronic foreign body granulomas and chronic sepsis are also capable of resorbing bone. These three conditions all produce a layer of undifferentiated connective tissue containing chronic inflammatory cells lying against the resorbing bone.

Ever since Berberich began pouring hot tar into the external ears of laboratory animals almost fifty years ago,[1] otologists have been attempting to create an experimental model of middle ear cholesteatoma. A variety of inflammatory agents have been instilled through a defect in the tympanic membrane or bulla in order to induce epidermal cysts in the middle ear. Beginning with hot and cold tar,[1] these agents have included croton oil, olive oil, benzypyrene,[2] oxalic acid,[3] talc,[4] quinine,[5] and methyl cholantholene.[6] Friedmann[7,8] induced otitis media with a variety of bacterial cultures while Milstein[9] and more recently, Walsh and co-workers,[10] transplanted skin into the middle ear in attempts to create experimental cholesteatomas. These methods met with various degrees of success, supporting the hypothesis that cholesteatomas result from migration of canal wall skin into the middle ear and do not arise *de novo* from metaplasia. The likelihood of finding skin in the ears in these animals appears to correlate with the degree of inflammation caused by the agent and the extent of suppuration. Middle ear cholesteatoma in humans, however, occurs without external inflammatory agents and even without a history of antecedent acute suppurative otitis media.

We have defined middle ear cholesteatoma in both histologic and functional terms as an epidermal cyst containing subepithelial granulation tissue, characterized by progressive growth and the ability to induce underlying bone resorption. The mechanism of this

From the Department of Otolaryngology and Maxillofacial Surgery at the University of Iowa, Iowa City, Iowa.

This investigation was supported by PHS grant NS 10608 from the National Institute of Neurological Diseases and Stroke and the Deafness Research Foundation.

Presented at the meeting of the American Otological Society, Inc., Atlanta, Georgia, April 11-12, 1975.

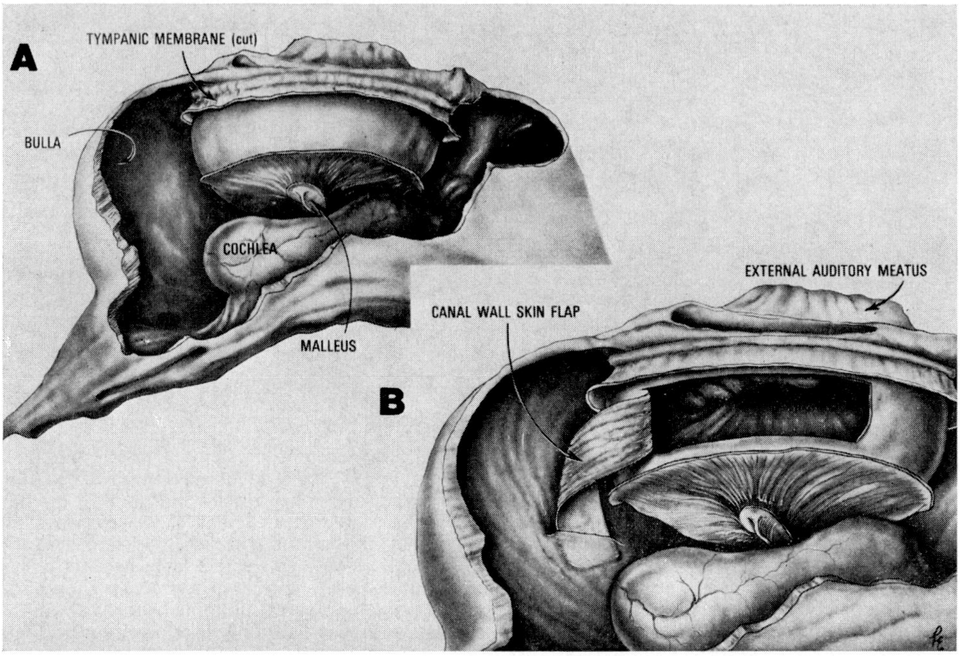

Fig. 1. View of the operative approach used in the experiments. The animal's left ear is shown from a ventral approach through the neck. The nose would be at the left side of the illustration and the left pinna would be at the top. A) The ventral wall of the bulla and the outer tympanic membrane have been removed in preparation for removal of ventral canal wall skin. B) The operation used on Group 4 is shown. A flap of canal skin has been inserted into a mucosal pocket in the bulla dorso-lateral to the cochlea.

bone resorption is perhaps the most important clinical question posed by the disease, since the morbidity of cholesteatoma results from loss of bone causing conductive hearing loss and exposing underlying soft tissues to injury. Our interest in the interaction of cholesteatoma and bone was stimulated by Abramson's finding of a collagen dissolving enzyme produced by cholesteatomas *in vitro.* [1] This enzyme was present in greatest amounts in the cholesteatoma matrix and in the skin of the bony ear canal compared with the cartilaginous ear canal and arm skin. If proteolytic enzymes produced by a cholesteatoma are relevant in the bone resorption process, then skin should be capable of resorbing bone without pressure or perhaps even without sepsis.

In this study we have sought to reproduce the conditions necessary to induce bone resorption in chronic otitis media by using various techniques to introduce skin into the ear of guinea pigs. We have focused our attention on the cochlea for two reasons. First, the peculiar configuration of the guinea pig's middle ear makes determination of the boundary difficult between the middle and external ear on histologic sections. Epidermal cysts at the cochlea would be unquestionably in the middle ear. Second, we needed to define a site where net resorption of bone could be clearly determined. The bone of the cochlea is not only thin but also encloses a delicate and easily altered organ. We used canal wall skin as free grafts, as pedicled grafts on the cochlea, and as pedicled grafts inserted into a mucosal pocket in the bulla. Talc was used to stimulate a granulomatous response either by itself or with skin since it is essentially inert and does not have a direct, injurious effect on bone. We were able to induce epidermal middle

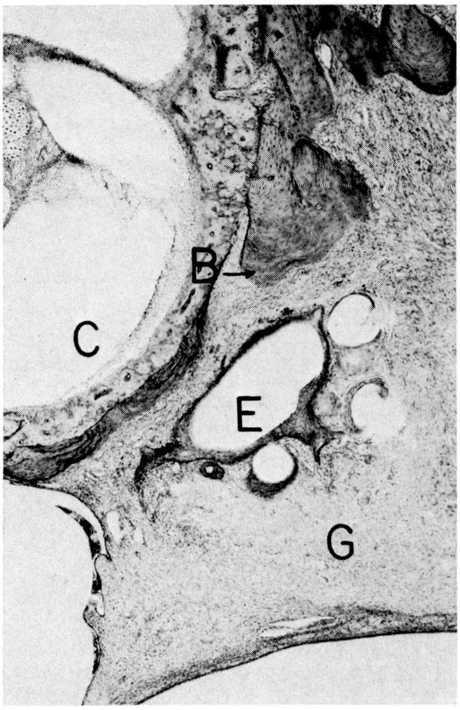

Fig. 2. Animal 4 from Group 1:B shown three months after a free graft of canal wall skin and talc was placed on the cochlea. A granuloma (G) as well as a cyst of hypertrophic squamous epithelium (E) is seen at the cochlea (C). There is new bone (B) at the cochlea. X40.

ear cysts and bone resorption under various conditions but with certain histologic features in common.

METHODS AND MATERIALS

Four groups of young guinea pigs (150 - 200 gm) were operated upon from a ventral approach through the neck exposing the middle ear through the bulla. In group I:A, ventral canal wall skin was removed as a free graft through a defect in the tympanic membrane and placed on the cochlea after removing the mucosa (Fig. 1A). Group I:B had talc placed on the cochlea at the same time as the skin graft. In Group 2:A, the canal wall skin was left attached nasally and rotated onto bare cochlea; shreds of mucosa removed from the cochlea were used to cover the tip of the flap. In Group 2:B, the bulla was reopened two months after the first operation and talc placed in the middle ear. Group 3:A had talc applied to the medial aspect of the intact tympanic membrane following the method described by Ruedi.[4] Group 3:B had talc applied to the bare cochlea. In Group 4, a pedicled flap was fashioned as in Group 2, rotated into the middle ear but placed in a mucosal pocket just dorso-lateral to the cochlea (Fig. 1B).

Animals were killed three to four months after initial surgery. The bullas were removed, fixed in 10% buffered formalin, decalcified, and embedded in celloidin. The bones were sectioned in a coronal plane from nasal to caudal, stained with H. and E., and examined under light microscopy.

RESULTS

Epidermal Cysts at Cochlea. Epi-

TABLE I

RESULTS OF EXPERIMENTAL CHOLESTEATOMA IN GUINEA PIGS

Group	*Method*	*Duration (months)*	*No. of Animals*	*Epidermal Cyst at Cochlea*	*Cochlea Fistula*	*Otitis Media*
1:A	Canal skin graft to cochlea	4	10	0	0	9
1:B	Canal skin graft and talc to cochlea	3	6	2	0	6
2:A	Canal skin flap to cochlea	4.5	11	1	0	0
2:B	Canal skin flap to cochlea then talc in middle ear	4.5	5	2	1	3
3:A	Talc to TM	4.5	7	0	1	0
3:B	Talc to cochlea	3	6	0	0	0
4	Canal skin flap under bulla mucosa	4	10	3	4	7
Total			55	8(15%)	6(11%)	25(45%)

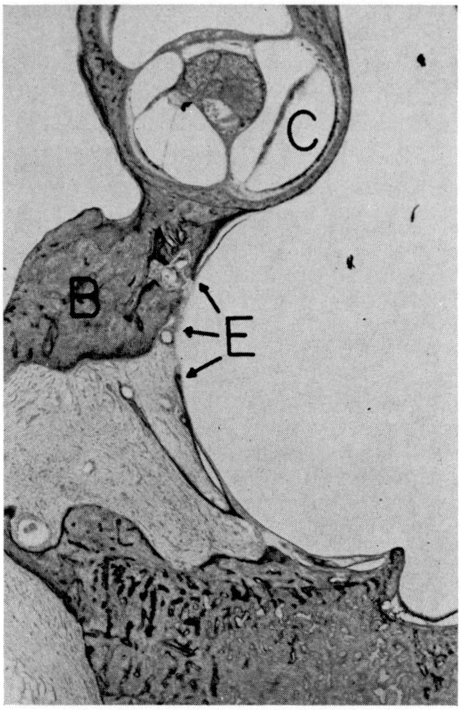

Fig. 3. Animal 4 from Group 2:A with a canal skin flap placed on the cochlea. New bone (B) is seen extending from bulla defect to the cochlea (C). The canal skin flap containing several small epidermal cysts (E) extends to the cochlea (C). X20.

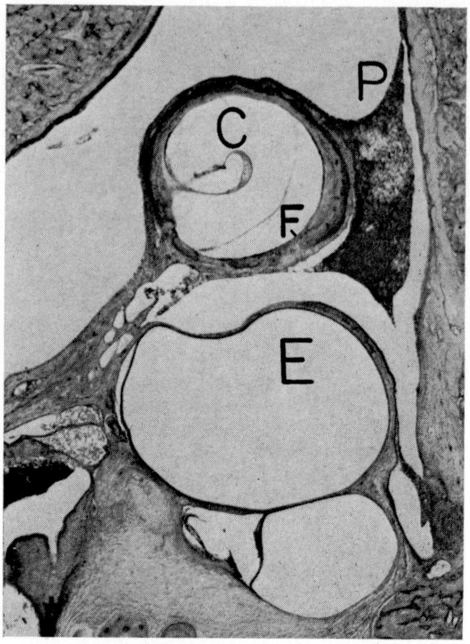

Fig. 4. Animal 5 from Group 2:B, two months after having a canal skin flap on the cochlea and talc instilled into the middle ear. A large epidermal cyst (E) is shown adjacent to a fistula (F) of the cochlea (C) wall as well as a collection of pus cells (P). X20.

dermal cysts at the cochlea were induced in 15% or 8 of 55 animals (Table I). Free grafts of canal wall skin, Group I:A, failed to produce epidermal cysts in ten animals. The addition of talc, Group I:B, resulted in epidermal cysts at the cochlea in two of six animals (Fig. 2).

Small epidermal cysts were found in only 1 of 11 animals with canal wall skin flaps (Fig. 3) but were present in two of five animals having subsequent talc placements (Fig. 4). We were not able to produce epidermal cysts with talc alone in 13 animals, either at the tympanic membrane or on the cochlea. Epidermal cysts were found in three of ten animals having skin placed in the mucosal pocket at the bulla (Figs. 5, 6, and 7). These experiments indicate that free grafts of canal skin do not

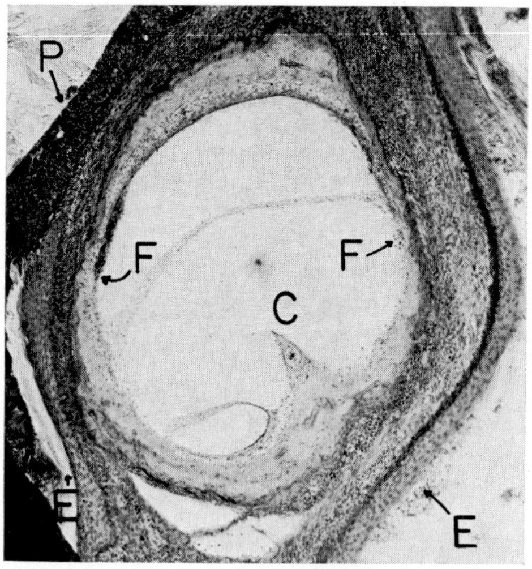

Fig. 5. Animal 6 from Group 4, with a canal skin flap placed under bulla mucosa. Squamous epithelium (E) has migrated around the cochlea (C) producing a cochlear fistula on both sides (F and F). Purulent exudate (P) is also present at the cochlea. X40.

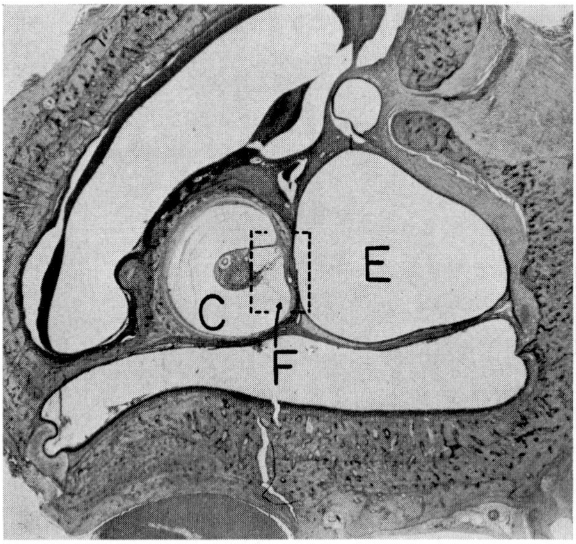

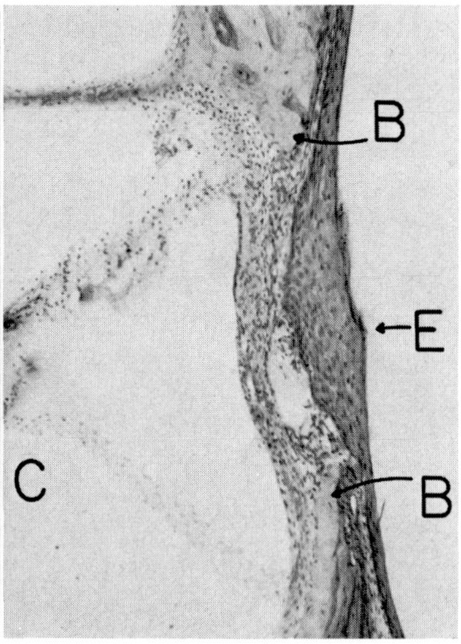

Fig. 6. Animal 3 from Group 4, showing a large epidermal cyst (E) in the middle ear eroding the bony wall of the cochlea (C) at F. There is no retained epithelial debris or sign of sepsis in the area of bone resorption. X15.

Fig 7. Animal 3 showing the area in brackets on Figure 6 in higher magnification. The hypertrophic epidermal layer (E) is shown resorbing the cochlea (C) wall at B. There are no pus cells. Loosely arranged subepithelial connective tissue covers the bony defect. X100.

readily grow on the cochlea. Epidermal proliferation seems to be enhanced, however, by the inflammatory effect of talc. Skin that is well covered by mucosa (Group 4) and is attached to a source of epithelium is most likely to migrate and proliferate into a cyst.

Bone Resorption at the Cochlea. A cochlear fistula or complete resorption of otic capsule at the cochlea was induced in 6 of 55 animals for an incidence of 11% (Table I). Bone resorption was not seen in Group I with free skin grafts on the cochlea despite the presence of otitis media in 15 of the 16 animals.

Otitis media, defined by the presence of purulent exudate in the middle ear cavity, occurred in 21 animals for an incidence of 21% (Table I). The exudate consisted primarily of decomposing neutrophils, as in acute otitis media.

In Group 2:B, a fistula of the cochlea occurred in one animal in which a canal wall flap was made and talc was applied. An epidermal cyst plus purulent exudate is seen adjacent to the defect (Fig. 4).

Cochlear fistula occurred in one animal in which talc only was applied to the tympanic membrane (Fig. 8). Connective tissue could be seen extending from the tympanic membrane to the cochlea. Talc particles were evident at the tympanic membrane but were not seen at the cochlea. The connective tissue at the bony defect contained some inflammatory cells but no exudate was found in the middle ear (Fig. 9).

Four cochlear fistulas occurred in Group 4 with a canal skin flap in the bulla. They occurred in two animals with otitis media alone (Figs. 10 and 11), one animal with skin plus otitis media (Fig. 5), and one animal with skin only (Figs. 6 and 7).

Table II lists the six cases of bone resorption in terms of the tissue adjacent to the cochlea. Cochlear fistulas occurred in three of eight animals with epidermal cysts of the cochlea, including one of three with skin but no otitis

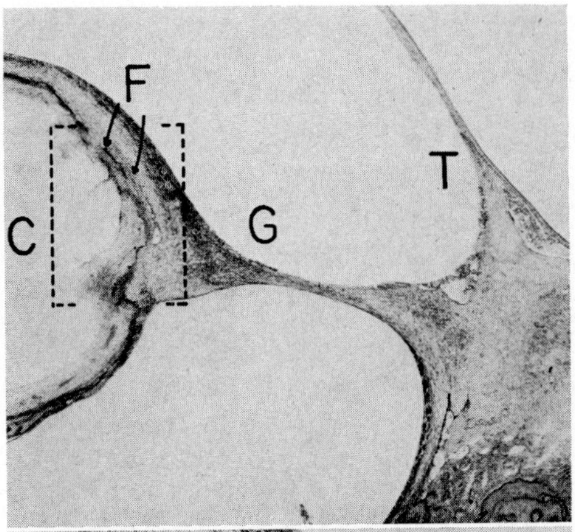

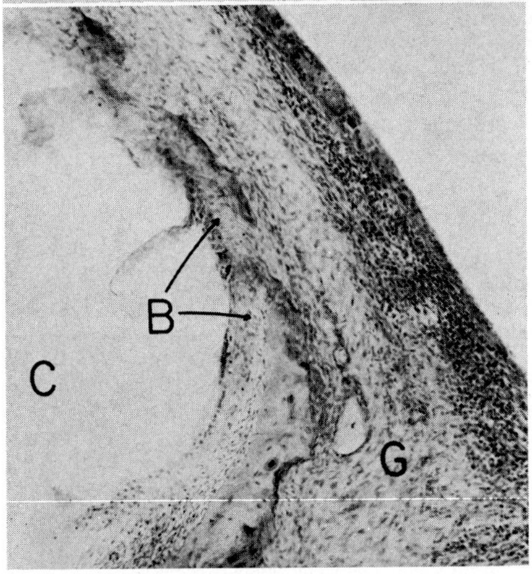

Fig. 8. Animal 7 from Group 3:A, which had talc placed on the medial aspect of the tympanic membrane (T). Granulation tissue (G) can be seen extending from the tympanic membrane (T) to the cochlea (C) producing a fistula at F. There is no evidence of suppurative otitis media. X40.

Fig. 9. Animal 7. The area outlined in brackets on Figure 8 is shown in higher magnification revealing bone resorption (B) of the cochlea (C) wall. The granulation tissue (G) contains numerous inflammatory cells but no foreign body giant cells or talc particles. X100.

media at the cochlea and two of five animals with skin plus otitis media at the cochlea. Bone resorption also occurred in 2 of 21 animals with otitis media without skin and in one animal with a talc granuloma having neither skin nor otitis media.

TABLE II

INCIDENCE OF BONE RESORPTION

Adjacent Tissue	*No. of Animals*	*No. of Cochlea Fistulas*
Total epidermal cyst	8	3 (38%)
With otitis media	5	2
No otitis media	3	1
Total no epidermal cyst	47	3 (6%)
with otitis media	21	2
No otitis media	26	*1
Total	55	6 (11%)

* Talc granuloma

These results show that bone resorption occurs from otitis media alone, from epidermal cysts without adjacent sepsis or pressure, and also from chronic granulomas. Bone resorption is more likely to occur, however, in association with a migrating, proliferating epidermal cyst (Table II). Typical appearing osteoclasts could not be identified at the absorbing margin. Each of the fistulas was covered by a cellular, loosely arranged connective tissue layer containing numerous fibroblasts, lymphocytes, macrophages, and capillary buds (Figs. 7, 9, and 11).

DISCUSSION

This study has not entirely resolved the question of the relative role of sepsis in the bone resorption of chronic otitis media. The absence of exudate at the sites of bone resorption in two animals in our series (Figs. 6 and 8) might be due to sampling error. A histologic study of this type cannot rule out the possibility of a transient episode of sepsis at some time prior to the animal's death.

Otologists are often faced with the problem of if and when to operate on a dry cholesteatoma. Perhaps a dry ear is a safe ear. Histologic evidence from our study suggests that there must be an inflammatory stage at some time in the proliferation of epithelium into a bone resorbing cyst. This would not have to be septic or bacterial in origin and would not necessarily lead to per-

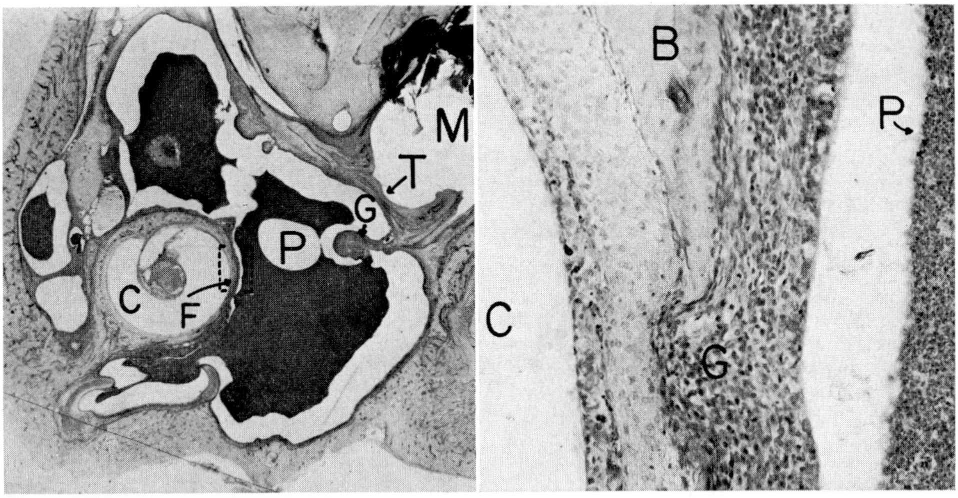

Fig. 10. Animal 7 from Group 4, showing a cochlea (C) fistula (F) secondary to sepsis in the middle ear without adjacent epidermal cysts. The external auditory meatus (M) and healed tympanic membrane (T) are shown as well as a granulomatous polyp (G) at the site of the canal skin flap. The middle ear is filled with purulent exudate (P). The middle ear and cochlea are lined with a thick granulomatous mucosa. X15.

Fig. 11. Animal 7. The area of cochlea fistula outlined in brackets in Figure 10 is shown in higher magnification. The pus cells (P) are separated from the resorbing bone (B) by a layer of cellular connective tissue (G) containing numerous capillary buds, fibroblasts, lymphocytes, and macrophages. X250.

foration at the tympanic membrane and drainage even if it were due to sepsis. The crucial activity occurs at the interface with bone and not at the external aspect of the tympanic membrane.

As otologists, we tend to look at cholesteatomas in the same way that we examine a patient, from the outside in. To study bone resorption, one must look from the bone's point of view, or from the inside out. Resorbing bone is covered by a layer of loosely arranged connective tissue resembling the mesenchyme seen in embryonic development or a healing wound. This inflamed connective tissue has recently been described under bone resorbing cholesteatomas in man by Thomsen and co-workers.[12] As in our study, they were unable to find osteoclasts at the resorbing margin of bone.

The process of bone resorption is not well understood, but it is clearly an active process involving a series of events. Bone resorption can be viewed in terms of two initial stages: first, an inflammatory stage, and second, a proliferative stage. The inflammatory stimulus can be sepsis, a foreign body reaction or a migrating epithelial layer. The organism responds to these various inflammatory stimuli with a single proliferative mesenchymal reaction. This mesenchyme shares histologic features with other destructive processes. It resembles a pannus lying against resorbing articular cartilage in rheumatoid arthritis and is essentially identical with the primitive connective tissue in an invasive epidermoid carcinoma located between tumor and host. These destructive processes differ from a healing wound in the chronicity of the inflammatory stimulus and the persistence of the proliferative response.

Sadé and Halevy[13] recently recorded the effects of chronic otitis media on bone removed surgically. They point out that chronic otitis media without cholesteatoma commonly causes bone resorption. Their data show that ossicles from patients undergoing surgery for chronic otitis media without cholesteatoma had a 42.5% incidence of resorption, while ossicles from patients with cholesteatoma had an 84% incidence of resorption. This coincides with the results of our study in which the incidence of bone resorption with suppurative otitis without cholesteatoma is 10%, or 2 of 21 animals, while the incidence of bone resorption with cholesteatoma is 38%, or three of eight animals. The epidermis of cholesteatoma is not simply passive but appears to play an active and significant role in bone resorption. The intercellular communication that results in bone resorption in the ear is an example of an epithelial-mesenchymal interaction. The biochemistry of this interaction is still obscure, but is the subject of current investigations in our laboratory.

Request for reprints should be sent to Maxwell Abramson, M.D., Dept. of Otolaryngology and Maxillofacial Surgery, University of Iowa Hospitals and Clinics, The University of Iowa, Iowa City, Iowa 52242.

Richard G. Asarch, M.D., is now at the Division of Dermatology, University of Colorado, Denver, Colorado. Ward B. Litton, M.D., is now located in Moline, Illinois.

Acknowledgment—The slides were prepared by Joan K. Schnute and Crystal Smith. The illustration was prepared by Ronald J. Ervin.

REFERENCES

1. Berberich J: Das experimentalle Mittelohrcholesteatom. Z Hals-Nas-Ohrenheilk 10:881, 1927

2. Schroer R: Entwicklungsgeschichtliche und experimentelle Untersuchungen zur genese des Mittelohrcholesteatoms. Arch Klin Exp Ohren Nasen Kehlkopfheilkd 170:265-316, 1957

3. Dota T, Nakamura K, Saheki M, *et al*: Cholesterol granuloma. Experimental observations. Ann Otol Rhinol Laryngol 72:345-356, 1963

4. Ruedi L: Cholesteatoma formation in the middle ear in animal experiments. Acta Otolaryngol 50:233-242, 1959

5. Fernandez C, Lindsay JR: Aural cholesteatoma. Experimental observations. Laryngoscope 70:1119-1141, 1960

6. Nishiura I: Experimental studies on cholesteatoma. J Otolaryngol Jap 72:719-747, 1969

7. Friedmann I: The comparative pathology of otitis media — experimental and human. I. Experimental otitis of the guinea-pig. J Laryngol Otol 69:27-50, 1955

8. Friedmann I: The comparative pathology of otitis media — experimental and human. II. The histopathology of experimental otitis of the guinea-pig with particular reference to experimental cholesteatoma. J Laryngol Otol 69:588-601, 1955

9. Milstein T: Contribution a l'etude experimentale de la genese du cholesteatome. Acta Otolaryngol (Stockh) 25:311-327, 1937

10. Walsh TE, Covell WP, Ogura JH: The effect of cholesteatosis on bone. Ann Otol Rhinol Laryngol 60:1100-1113, 1951

11. Abramson M: Collagenolytic activity in middle ear cholesteatoma. Ann Otol Rhinol Laryngol 78:112-125, 1969

12. Thomsen J, Jorgensen MB, Bretlau P, *et al*: Bone resorption in chronic otitis media. A histological and ultrastructural study. II. Cholesteatoma. J Laryngol Otol 88:983-992, 1974

13. Sadé J, Halevy A: The aetiology of bone destruction in chronic otitis media. J Laryngol Otol 88:139-143, 1974

Ann Otol 84: 1975

IDIOPATHIC FACIAL PARALYSIS, PREGNANCY, AND THE MENSTRUAL CYCLE

RAYMOND L. HILSINGER, JR., M.D.

KEDAR KARIM ADOUR, M.D. H. E. DOTY

OAKLAND, CALIFORNIA

SUMMARY – The records of 42 women with Bell's palsy during pregnancy, and of 91 nonpregnant women, whose dates of onset of Bell's palsy and of the preceding menstrual cycle were precisely known, were studied for factors that might show relation between pregnancy or the menstrual cycle and Bell's palsy. Of the 42 cases in pregnancy, 31 occurred in the third trimester, five in the first two weeks postpartum, and six in the first two trimesters combined. Our calculated frequency of Bell's palsy in pregnant women is 45.1/100,000 births; for nonpregnant women of the same age group the calculated incidence is 17.4/100,000 per year. No causative relation was found between toxemia, hypertension or primigravidity, and Bell's palsy. Over 60% of the cases in nonpregnant women occurred in the first 14 days of the menstrual cycle with peaks on the first and seventh days and near ovulation. No clear evidence for an etiologic relationship was seen with edema or hormonal changes in either pregnancy or the menstrual cycle. A number of factors in pregnancy and the menstrual cycle suggested an etiologic role for herpes simplex virus reactivation in Bell's palsy. There was no evidence that prednisone treatment is contraindicated during pregnancy.

In 1830, Bell alluded to the possible association of pregnancy with paralysis of the facial muscles.[1] Since that time, several unsuccessful attempts have been made to establish or refute a definite relationship between idiopathic facial paralysis (Bell's palsy) and pregnancy.[2-15] Although none of the authors felt that their reports showed a statistically valid association, they hoped that their articles would point out the need for further study in this area.[5-7,10,11,14,15]

Reports of large series of patients with facial paralysis have shown a slightly greater overall incidence in females than in males;[16-20] and between the ages of 10 and 20 years, the female is two to four times more likely to contract Bell's palsy than is her male counterpart.[16,18,20] After age 50, women are less likely than men to have the disease.[16,18,20] In El-Ebiary's patients,[20] recurrence was twice as common in females as in males; he offered the interesting suggestion that premenstrual water retention might be a predisposing factor.

Although these facts suggest a relationship between Bell's palsy, menarche and menopause, and pregnancy, we have seen no published effort to analyze incidence statistics in the light of a potential link between Bell's palsy and the menstrual cycle. This article examines those relationships.

METHODS AND MATERIALS

The patients were members of the Kaiser Foundation Health Plan, a prepaid health care program which has approximately one million subscribers in Northern California. While devoid of the indigent and extremely wealthy, the characteristics of this population, including its age-sex distribution, compare closely to a

From the Facial Paralysis Research Clinic, Department of Otolaryngology, Kaiser Permanente Medical Center, Oakland, Calif.

Supported by the Community Service Program of the Kaiser Foundation Hospitals.

Presented at the meeting of the American Otological Society, Inc., Atlanta, Georgia, April 11-12, 1975.

TABLE I

FACIAL PARALYSIS RECOVERY PROFILE

Site	0	No. of Points Assigned to Each Unit of Recovery* 0%-25%	25%-50%	50%-75%	75%-100%
Forehead	0	+1	+1	+2	+2
Eye	0	+1	+2	+3	+4
Mouth	0	+1	+2	+3	+4

* Return of facial function measured in units of 25%.

cross section of the population of California, and probably of the United States as a whole. All patients with facial paralysis seen in the ten Northern California Kaiser Permanente Medical Centers in the San Francisco Bay area (the center in Sacramento, at a greater distance, is excluded) are evaluated in the Facial Paralysis Research Clinic of the Department of Otolaryngology in the Oakland facility. Each patient receives our standard workup, which has been outlined in previous publications.[17,21]

Pregnancy. To facilitate precise statistical comparison of incidence figures, we selected a three-year period (1969-1972) during which the number, age and sex distribution, the number of births in these medical centers, and the number of cases of idiopathic facial paralysis were known. For the total study, we included the 53 pregnant women, with facial paralysis from any cause, who were seen between 1966 and 1974. Among these 53 cases of facial paralysis, one each resulted from acute otitis media, a central nervous system (CNS) disease (hemiplegic migraine), and mumps; eight resulted from herpes zoster oticus. The remaining 42 cases were considered to be idiopathic. These 42 women ranged in age from 16 to 40 years; their average age was 25.3 years.

Menstruation. In 91 women, the exact dates of onset, both of the idiopathic facial paralysis and of the preceding menstrual period, were known. Any case in which these data were ambiguous, or the menstrual cycle was longer than 40 days, was excluded from this consideration. Because our early records did not routinely include the precise date of onset of menstruation, this is not a consecutive list of cases. We now record the onset, duration, and periodicity of the menstrual cycle and the use and type of birth control pills.

The 91 cases were analyzed as to symptomatology, physical findings, treatment, and recovery from facial paralysis. The final means of assessing outcome was the previously described[17,21] Facial Paralysis Recovery Profile (FPRP) and the Facial Paralysis Recovery Index (FPRI). The FPRP is a simple, accurate, reproducible method of assessing the degree of return of function in the region of forehead, eye, and mouth, and of cosmetic result (Table I). Possible scores range from 0 to +10, equating with 0 to 100% recovery of facial function: a FPRP score of +5 equals 50% recovery of muscle motion; +7 equals 70% recovery. The FPRI takes into consideration the negative effect of complications of the facial paralysis on the final result. Contracture, synkinesis, facial spasm, gustatory tears, and ptosis of the eyebrow are each assigned one minus point and the total is then subtracted from the final FPRP. Consequently, a FPRP of +9 and a FPRI of +7 means 90% return of facial function with two complications.

FINDINGS

Of the 446 cases of idiopathic facial paralysis seen during 1969-1972, 234 (52%) were in women; 138 (31%) of the cases were in women of the childbearing age (15-39 years). Our calculated overall incidence of idiopathic facial paralysis in women is 16.9/100,000 per year; in women of the childbearing age, the incidence is 17.4/100,000 per year.

Pregnancy. During the same three years, 37,655 births occurred in our health plan population, and we saw 17 cases of idiopathic facial paralysis among those pregnant women. Thirteen of the 17 cases occurred during the third trimester or within the first two weeks postpartum. Thus, the frequency of idiopathic facial paralysis in pregnant women was 45.1/100,000 births. Per year of exposure, the risk to pregnant women was 3.3 times the risk to nonpregnant women of the same age group. Assuming 14 weeks for each trimester plus two weeks postpartum, the incidence for the third trimester and early puerperium alone is 118.2/100,000 per year of exposure.

Of the 42 cases of Bell's palsy seen in pregnant women over the longer period 1966-1974, 31 occurred in the third trimester, five in the early puerperium, and only six in the first two trimesters combined. Two of the 42 women had toxemia of pregnancy, described in one instance as a mild case of preeclampsia. There were no instances of hypertension due to other causes.

Statistics from the entire health plan population in this area for 1960-1966 showed that 29.7% of all mothers who delivered were primigravidas. Among the 42 women with Bell's palsy in pregnancy, 15 (35.7%) were primigravidas. Obviously, no statistical comparison can be made between these data from disparate timespans; but the risk of Bell's palsy does not appear to be greater in the first than in subsequent pregnancies.

Twenty-six of the 42 pregnant women with Bell's palsy received prednisone starting with 40-60 mg daily and tapering to zero in 8-10 days. Fourteen of the 16 who did not receive prednisone were seen between 1967 and 1969. All but two of the patients seen since 1970 have been treated with prednisone.

Thirty-one of the overall total had long-term follow-up. Their average FPRP was +9.74; their average FPRI, +9.16. Seven of the eight mothers with herpes zoster facial paralysis had adequate follow-up. Their average FPRP was +8.6; their average FPRI, +7. The average FPRP for the 23 prednisone-treated patients with long-term follow-up was +10; their average FPRI was +9.43. Only six of 12 untreated mothers had significant follow-up; their FPRPs and FPRIs both averaged +9.83. Two patients originally in the untreated group developed partial denervation and underwent decompression of the vertical segment of the facial nerve. Their eventual FPRPs were +10 and +3; their final FPRIs, +8 and 0. Contracture and synkinesis developed in both; facial spasm, in one. None of the other untreated patients had these complications. Five of the prednisone-treated group had contracture and synkinesis; two of these had, in addition, facial spasm. Three of the five with these complications were treated with 40 mg of prednisone on the first day of palsy, rather than the 60 mg we use now. Three of the five cases of contracture and synkinesis were minimal and were unnoticeable to the patient.

Three of the prednisone-treated group without long-term follow-up had an average FPRI of +5 when last seen. One of the three had contracture and synkinesis and an FPRI of 0. Her prednisone had been discontinued by another physician after one day of therapy (40 mg). Severe occipital pain recurred. When she was retested three days later, there was complete loss of nerve excitability (complete denervation), whereupon prednisone was restarted. This was the only pregnant woman with Bell's palsy in this series in whom complete denervation developed. If her score is excluded from the group, the average FPRI of the three prednisone-treated patients with incomplete follow-up, when last seen, was +7.5. The six untreated patients who had inadequate follow-up had an average FPRI of +6.3 when last seen.

Effects on Infants. Twenty of the infants of mothers with Bell's palsy were male, 22 female. In 100 consecutive births at the Oakland facility during January-February 1975, the average one-minute Apgar score of infants was 8.4. The one-minute Apgar scores of 40 infants delivered to mothers with Bell's palsy are known; these averaged 9.0, ranging from 10.0 in 18 infants to 5.0 in two infants. The Apgar scores of infants of the 11 mothers with facial paralysis of demonstrable cause averaged 8.55. The Apgar scores of the infants of 25 of 26 women with Bell's palsy who received prednisone are known; they averaged 8.88. Adding the Apgar scores of six infants of mothers with herpes zoster facial paralysis treated with prednisone, the average for the 31 infants in the prednisone-treated group was 8.7. There were no complications before or during childbirth, or during the neonatal hospitaliza-

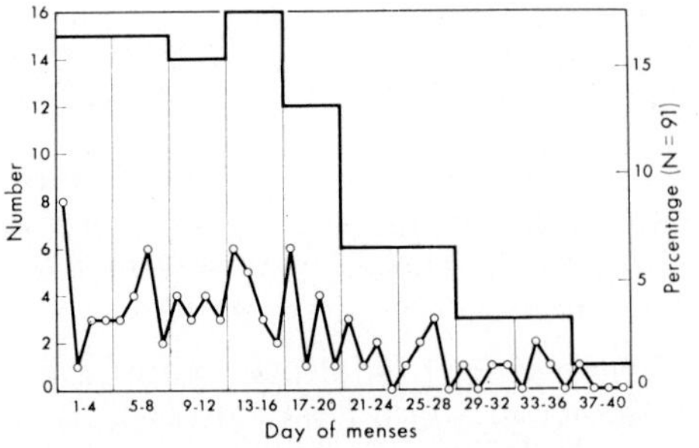

Fig. 1. Number of cases of Bell's palsy occurring each day after onset of menses in 91 women. Bar graph (4-day intervals) shows that the vast majority of cases occur during the first half of the cycle.

tion, that were related to prednisone therapy.

Menstruation. The entire group of 91 menstrual women included seven whose cycles were as long as 37 days; in 84, the cycle was 28 days. The number of cases of Bell's palsy occurring on each day after onset of menstruation in the 91 women is shown in Figure 1. The rate is highest on the first menstrual day; secondary peaks of incidence are seen on the seventh, thirteenth, fourteenth, and seventeenth day of the cycle. Although 60.4% of the cases in the total group occurred within the first 14 days of the menstrual cycle, among the 84 women with a 28-day cycle, 65.5% of the cases occurred within the first half of the cycle.

The presenting signs and symptoms seen in these 91 women — ageusia, epiphora, pain, and subjectively or objectively decreased tearing — were similar in incidence to those in a general population with idiopathic facial paralysis. Except that hyperacusis, which indicates more widespread disease, was somewhat more frequent among these patients than in a general population with Bell's palsy, the eventual FPRPs of the 91 patients were similar to those generally seen.

DISCUSSION

Nerve Disease in Pregnancy. Altered body needs as well as changed hormonal, fluid, and electrolyte levels are among the factors thought to contribute to the presence of neurologic abnormalities during gestation.[22,23] Of the many possible neurologic complications of pregnancy, peripheral mononeuropathy has not been considered common.[10,22,23] Vascular disorders of the brain and spinal cord, chorea, and polyneuritis are linked with pregnancy, as is the tendency to exacerbation or aggravation of chronic neurologic diseases.[10]

The peripheral nerve diseases most commonly associated with pregnancy are brachial neuralgia, disease of the lumbosacral plexus and nerves, or peripheral polyneuritis.[23] A possible complication is the carpal tunnel syndrome. While its cause is not known,[10,22,23] it has been suggested that hormonal alterations of pregnancy[22] lead to an increase in the volume of the content of the carpal tunnel canal. Ischemia of the compressed nerve is believed to cause paresthesias and sensory disturbance, weakness, and atrophy of the abductor pollicis brevis and opponens pollicis muscles. Treatment is conservative, in expectation of complete postpartum recovery. A case of oculomotor palsy in pregnancy, with a similar course, has also been described.[10]

This report adds idiopathic facial paralysis to the list of pregnancy-related diseases. Women are at an increased risk of Bell's palsy when pregnant, particularly in the third trimester. Why this is true and what changes occur in pregnancy that account for this increased risk are not known.

Toxemia and Facial Palsy. While no statistical analysis has appeared of a possible relation between facial paralysis and toxemia of pregnancy, three authors have suggested that toxemia might be an etiologic factor in the development of facial palsy.[5,9,11] Mild elevation of blood pressure or toxemia of pregnancy was observed in 45% and 60% of two series: the 20 patients reported by Pope and Kenan[5] and the 15 reported by Robinson and Pou.[11] Gerber and Collins[9] and Bezjian, Spellacy, and Little[8] noted single cases of preeclampsia with Bell's palsy. A review of Edwards'[3] study shows that three of the 11 pregnant women with facial palsy had hypertension.

The high incidence of toxemia noted by some of these authors[3,5,11] may have been due to a selection factor since their cases were collected in the southeastern United States. Fifteen of the total of 20 cases of Bell's palsy in women with mild to severe toxemia reported by them were in Negroes. The incidence of toxemia has been believed to be related to socioeconomic factors, and has been shown to be comparatively high in the Negro population and in the southeastern United States.[22-25] During 1960-1966, 22.7% of the total deliveries to members of our Health Plan in Northern California were to Negro women; and subscribers to this plan are employed persons and their dependents. Two of the women with Bell's palsy in the present series had toxemia in pregnancy; one was Negro, the other Mexican-American. No statistical relationship exists between toxemia and idiopathic facial paralysis of pregnancy.

Hypertension and Facial Palsy. Hypertension as a cause of isolated facial nerve palsy was first reported in a single patient by Moxon in 1869;[26] no statistical analysis of a possible relation between these entities has appeared. Merwarth[27] published 24 cases of peripheral facial paralysis associated with hypertensive vascular disease: in 16 of the patients the facial paralysis was considered to be a direct result of the hypertensive disease; in the remainder it was believed to be Bell's palsy with coexisting hypertension. Clarke and Murphy[28] saw seven cases of unilateral facial (and one of abducens) nerve palsy among 79 patients with malignant hypertension involving the nervous system. Lloyd, Jewitt, and Still,[29] reviewing 35 cases of severe hypertension in children, noted that six of the patients had had single or multiple episodes of unilateral peripheral facial paralysis. In 1966, an editorial in the *British Medical Journal* on facial paralysis in hypertension called attention to the "well-documented association between lower motor neurone facial paralysis and severe hypertension."[30] Miller[31] commented on the relation between facial paralysis and both severe hypertension and toxemia of pregnancy. Adour and Wingerd[32] noted that hypertension was one of several prognostic indicators in Bell's palsy and that patients with hypertension were therefore overrepresented in series of cases of Bell's palsy from hospital and specialty clinic populations, leading to a false impression of causality. No significant relation was seen between facial paralysis and hypertension in the present series.

Gravidity and Facial Paralysis. No evidence for a significant relation between facial paralysis and the occurrence or nonoccurrence of previous pregnancy was seen in this study: 29.7% of Health Plan members delivering at a given time and 35.7% of mothers with Bell's palsy were primigravidas. It has been suggested[10] that primigravidas tend to contract Bell's palsy in the last week of gestation. In our series, only two of 15 primigravidas contracted the palsy during the last week of pregnancy; in an additional three of the 15, the onset occurred during the penultimate week. In four multiparas, Bell's palsy had its onset during the last week; in five, during the penultimate week.

EDEMA HYPOTHESIS

The first of two widely considered hypotheses for the causation of Bell's palsy is that a vasospastic response leads to edema and mechanical compression of the facial nerve in the fallopian canal resulting in paralysis.[33,34]

Pregnancy. A suggestion which has gained increasing acceptance is that the edema of pregnancy[7,8,10] is a secondary or even the primary factor leading to Bell's palsy in pregnant women. Mair, Elverland, and Johannessen,[15] however, concluded that tissue edema is not the cause of idiopathic facial paralysis, on the grounds that no association had been observed between facial paralysis and tissue edema due to other states, notably the use of oral contraceptives, or second or subsequent pregnancies. They also noted that there had not been

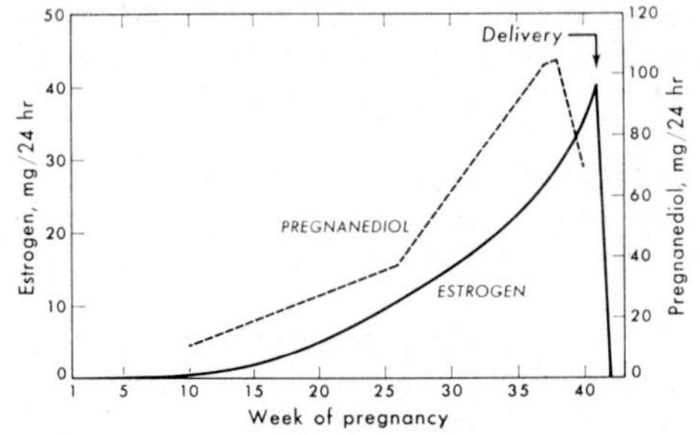

Fig. 2. Urinary excretion of pregnanediol and estrogen during pregnancy.

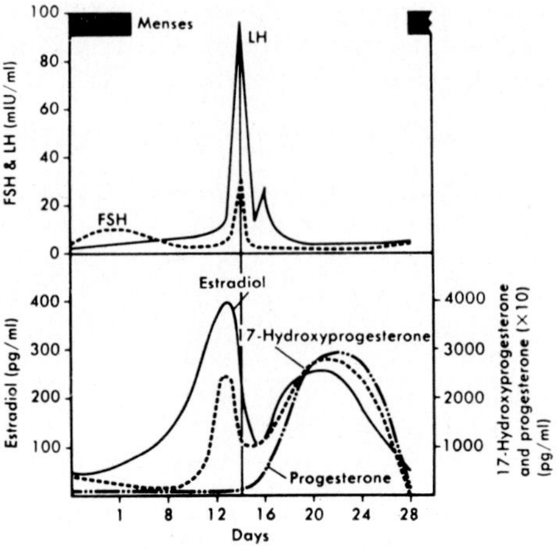

Fig. 3. Schema of the fluctuations in serum luteinizing hormone (LH), follicle stimulating hormone (FSH), progesterone, 17-hydroxyprogesterone, and estradiol during the normal menstrual cycle. (Reproduced by permission from Odell WD, Moyer DL: *Physiology of Reproduction,* St. Louis, The C. V. Mosby Company, 1971, p 66, Fig 5-2.)

an increase in recurrence of facial paralysis in the Melkersson-Rosenthal syndrome with pregnancy.

Water retention is, indeed, an integral part of pregnancy. Early in gestation, plasma volume increases faster than extracellular fluid; this relation reverses about 80 days before labor, when a marked increase in the interstitial fluid volume occurs, augmented by a prelabor decrease in plasma volume. After delivery, plasma volume diminishes rapidly but the interstitial fluid volume returns only slowly to normal. The increased incidence of facial paralysis in pregnancy and the early postpartum period certainly coincides with the curve of interstitial fluid volume, but whether and how the fluid volume might sensitize the facial nerve is not clear.

Menstrual Cycle Edema. It has also been proposed[20] that the edema of the premenstrual period, although considerably less than that of pregnancy, is a primary or secondary cause of Bell's palsy. In the menstrual cycle, edema begins with ovulation and continues until the onset of menses. If edema, related or not to vasospasm, were the primary or secondary cause of Bell's palsy one would expect the incidence of the disease to increase after day 14 of the cycle. Two-thirds of the cases of facial paralysis in the nonpregnant women of the present series occurred during the first 14 days after the onset of menses.

HORMONAL CHANGES

During Pregnancy. Bezjian and coworkers[8] and Korczyn[10] speculated that the rise of incidence of Bell's palsy late in pregnancy reflects hormonal increases with length of gestation. The hormones that increase during pregnancy are predominantly progesterone and estrogen (Fig. 2). These are measured in the urine as pregnanediol, the major known urinary metabolite of progesterone, and as estrogen. Both peak in the last trimester, as does the incidence of Bell's palsy in pregnant women. While estrogen remains high until the end of pregnancy, however, progesterone starts to fall shortly before delivery. To determine whether the levels of these hormones or changes in them are related to the occurrence of Bell's palsy, it would be necessary to make serial hormone determinations in pregnant women with and without idiopathic facial paralysis.

During the Menstrual Cycle. There was no apparent correlation between the hormonal changes that characterize the phases of the menstrual cycle and the observed higher incidence of Bell's palsy during the first half of the cycle of the women in this series (Fig. 3).

Follicle-stimulating hormone (FSH) increases early in the cycle and stimulates release of estradiol and 17-hydroxyprogesterone, which rise to a peak just before ovulation. The estradiol causes release of luteinizing hormone (LH) (Fig. 3) and to a lesser degree, of FSH; these induce ovulation and formation of the corpus luteum. Progesterone is then secreted in progressively larger amounts, peaking in the second half of the cycle together with estradiol and 17-hydroxyprogesterone, which rise after a postovulatory dip to attain a second peak in the midluteal phase. If the ovum is not fertilized, all three diminish and menstruation results.[24,25,35] Although the incidence of Bell's palsy in the women of this series showed peaks around the time of ovulation, no gonadotrophic hormone is at a high level at the onset of menses. These events may also cast doubt on the possible etiologic relation of hormones to facial paralysis in pregnancy.

VIRAL HYPOTHESIS

The second major hypothesis for the causation of Bell's palsy suggests a viral inflammatory reaction with subsequent demyelinization.[36-41] Mumps, rubella, and herpes simplex have been suggested as possible etiologic agents.[36,39,41] Herpes zoster is an accepted cause of facial paralysis;[41] it was the etiologic agent in eight of the pregnant women in our total series.

Naib and coworkers[42] have demonstrated that the incidence of herpes simplex virus in pregnant women is higher than in nonpregnant women. Herpes simplex virus can be reactivated by upper respiratory tract infection, a cold draft, exposure to ultraviolet rays or sunlight, emotional upsets, dental extraction, or menstruation.[41,43] Most recently, this virus has been implicated in Bell's palsy.[39,41] Gestational immunosuppression,[44] induced by the steady rise in cortisol levels through each trimester, is believed to be the stimulus for reactivation of the virus in pregnancy. That herpes simplex is reactivated by menstruation and by body temperature elevation may explain the cluster of cases of Bell's palsy that we noted on the first day of the menstrual cycle, towards the end of menstruation, and at or around the ovulation date when body temperature rises temporarily. Further confirmation of these peaks will be needed with a larger series and a consecutive list of cases.

The consideration that 100% of patients with Bell's palsy have evidence of previous infection with herpes simplex virus[41] lends very believable support to the viral hypothesis for causation of this disease. Furthermore, support for the viral hypothesis comes from factors extraneous to pregnancy and menstruation: Bell's palsy is not a unilateral mononeuropathy of the facial nerve in the fallopian canal; it is a cranial polyneuritis involving the sensory and motor branches of the trigeminal nerve, the acoustic-vestibular nerve, the glossopharyngeal nerve, and often the clinically uninvolved contralateral facial nerve. In some cases, CSF shows increased protein, lymphocytic pleocytosis, or both.[45-48]

Thus, if we were to select a hypothesis for the cause of Bell's palsy that fits the clinical picture, we would have to choose the viral rather than the vasospasm-edema concept.

PREDNISONE THERAPY OF BELL'S PALSY

During Pregnancy. Treatment of idiopathic facial paralysis has varied in pregnant women as it has in the general population. Some authors have advised symptomatic treatment only, since they feel that Bell's palsy in the last month of pregnancy is a relatively innocuous disease, which will resolve shortly after delivery of the infant.[4,10] Surgical decompression under local or general anesthesia has been advised.[5,7,11,49-51] One observer has encouraged induction of delivery early in the last week of pregnancy for women with facial paralysis to allow for facial nerve decompression under general anesthesia.[50]

The use of prednisone in pregnant women has been controversial in view of possible detrimental effects on the embryo and fetus.[4,8] Occasional reports of adrenal insufficiency in infants whose mothers have received steroids has increased the reluctance of many physicians to use these substances.[52] Recent work has shown that the placenta oxidizes the majority of the biologically active glucocorticoids to their corresponding ketones, which are probably inactive.[53] Beitins and coworkers[53] demonstrated that fetal levels of trihydroxyprednisone and trihydroxyprednisolone are nearly equal to one another and are exceeded eight- to tenfold by maternal trihydroxyprednisolone concentration. Consequently, there is very little likelihood that prednisone, even if given in high concentration, will have an adverse effect on the fetus. None of the 31 infants of mothers in our total series who had received prednisone for facial palsy due to any cause had any complications believed to be associated with this agent; the infants' average one-minute Apgar score was 8.7. Recovery of facial function in the vast majority of these women has been excellent: in 93.5% of those who had Bell's palsy while pregnant, the FPRP was +10. Consequently, we believe that in the pregnant woman as in other patients, prednisone is the treatment of choice for Bell's palsy. We have seen no evidence to support surgical intervention for idiopathic facial paralysis whether or not the patient is pregnant.

That the FPRP and FPRI scores for the treated (+10/+9.43) and the untreated (+9.8/+9.8) pregnant women in this series should be so nearly identical is most interesting, since in our general patient population, the average outcomes for untreated Bell's palsy are FPRP 8.96; FPRI 8.02. There may be some selection factor since these groups were from different timespans (the untreated women were seen between 1967 and 1969; the treated, between 1970 and 1974), and six of our 12 untreated pregnant women were lost to follow-up. However, the difference in timespan is also true of the treated and untreated groups in our general population. When last seen, the FPRI scores of four of the six untreated women were +7, +8, +9, and +10; in the other two, these scores were +1 and +3.

In pregnancy, a dichotomous situation exists in which the high levels of circulating cortisol are immunosuppressant, while at the same time they reduce inflammatory response. It is well known that inflammatory reaction in other diseases is reduced during pregnancy; rheumatoid arthritis, severe dermatologic conditions, and allergic states tend to be in remission in the last trimester. It may be that the high levels of cortisol in the pregnant woman give her a better chance for successful recovery from Bell's palsy without prednisone treatment. The fact that all of the pregnant women in our series who had contracture, synkinesis, and facial spasm were in the third trimester at the time they contracted Bell's palsy may, however, negate this hypothesis.

The effects of prednisone on the embryo and fetus during the first trimester are unknown. Four of our patients received prednisone during the first or second trimester; none had complications of pregnancy and each delivered a normal infant. We know that the therapeutic addition of 40-60 mg of prednisone daily affects the natural course of Bell's palsy, even in pregnancy. Occipital (postauricular) pain subsided 12-24 hours after treatment was started in these patients. Abrupt cessation of treatment in one led to recurrence of occipital pain. Because of this known effect, we elect to treat women who have Bell's palsy in the second and third trimester. We are probably overtreating some, even in giving them prednisone. Further work is needed to determine which mothers will and which will not benefit from prednisone. We now give 60 mg in divided doses for the first few days, and taper to 5 mg at the end of ten days. If postauricular pain recurs, or if partial denervation is suggested by a rise in the nerve excitability threshold as determined by comparison with the opposite side, the dose is raised to 60 mg. Since the active disease process seems to be resolved within two weeks, we do not believe prednisone treatment is needed beyond 21 days.

Request for reprints should be sent to Dr. Raymond L. Hilsinger, Jr., Kaiser Permanente Medical Center, 280 West MacArthur Boulevard, Oakland, California 94611.

REFERENCES

1. Bell C: *The Nervous System of the Human Body.* London: Longman, Rees, Orme, Brown, and Green; J. Taylor, 1830, Appendix pp iv-v

2. Faris BD: Facial paralysis during pregnancy. Med Times 83:185, 1955

3. Edwards CE: Bell's palsy in the last trimester of pregnancy and the puerperium. Am J Obstet Gynecol 89:274-276, 1964

4. Smith PN, Newton M: Bell's palsy in pregnancy. Obstet Gynecol 30:134-136, 1967

5. Pope TH, Kenan PD: Bell's palsy in pregnancy. Arch Otolaryngol 89:52-56, 1969

6. Adour KK: Bell's palsy (letter to the Editor). Arch Otolaryngol 91:310, 1970

7. Pope TH, Kenan PD: Reply [to Adour[6]]. Arch Otolaryngol 91:310-311, 1970

8. Bezjian AA, Spellacy WN, Little WA: Idiopathic Bell's palsy in pregnancy. Florida Med Assoc J 57:25-27, 1970

9. Gerber AH, Collins MJ: A case of preeclampsia with Bell's palsy and concomitant fetal anomalies. Med Ann DC 40:317-319, 1971

10. Korczyn AD: Bell's palsy and pregnancy. Acta Neurol Scand 47:603-607, 1971

11. Robinson JD, Pou JN: Bell's palsy; a predisposition of pregnant women. Arch Otolaryngol 95:125-129, 1972

12. Levy AH: Bell's palsy (letter to Editor). Arch Otolaryngol 95:192, 1972

13. Donaldson JA: Reply; Donaldson on Robinson. Arch Otolaryngol 95:192-193, 1972

14. Robinson JR, Pou JW: Reply to Levy and Donaldson. Arch Otolaryngol 95:193, 1972

15. Mair IWS, Elverland HH, Johannessen TA: Idiopathic facial palsy and pregnancy. Ann Otol Rhinol Laryngol 82:235-239, 1973

16. Hauser WA, Karnes WE, Annis J, *et al*: Incidence and prognosis of Bell's palsy in the population of Rochester, Minnesota. Mayo Clin Proc 46:258-264, 1971

17. Adour KK, Swanson PJ Jr: Facial paralysis in 403 consecutive patients. Emphasis on treatment response in patients with Bell's palsy. Trans Am Acad Ophthalmol Otolaryngol 75:1284-1301, 1971

18. Adour KK, Bell DN, Wingerd J: Bell palsy. Dilemma of diabetes mellitus. Arch Otolaryngol 99:114-117, 1974

19. Waterman GA: Facial paralysis: a study of three hundred and thirty-five cases. J Nerv Ment Dis 36:65-76, 1909

20. El-Ebiary HM: Facial paralysis: a clinical study of 580 cases. Rheumatol Phys Med 11:100-110, 1971

21. Manning JJ,, Adour KK: Facial paralysis in children. Pediatrics 49:102-109, 1972

22. Haynes DM: *Medical Complications during Pregnancy.* New York, McGraw-Hill, 1969, pp 225-301

23. Krieger HP: Neurologic complications, in Rovinsky JJ, Guttmacher AF (eds): *Medical, Surgical, and Gynecologic Complications of Pregnancy*, edition 2. Baltimore, The Williams & Wilkins Company, 1965, pp 418-452

24. Wilson JR, Beecham CT, Carrington ER: *Obstetrics and Gynecology.* St. Louis, The C. V. Mosby Company, 1966, pp 59-71, 236-262, 281-288, 349-360

25. Reid DE, Ryan KJ, Benirschke K: *Principles and Management of Human Reproduction.* Philadelphia, W. B. Saunders Company, 1972, pp 7-16, 16-22, 110-123, 221-249, 335-361, 745-769

26. Moxon: Apoplexy into canal of Fallopius in a case of Bright's disease, causing facial paralysis. Trans Pathol Soc London 20:420-421, 1869

27. Merwarth HR: The occurrence of peripheral facial paralysis in hypertensive vascular disease. Ann Intern Med 17:298-307, 1942

28. Clarke E, Murphy EA: Neurological manifestations of malignant hypertension. Br Med J 2:1319-1326, 1956

29. Lloyd AVC, Jewitt DE, Still JDL: Facial paralysis in children with hypertension. Arch Dis Child 41:292-294, 1966

30. Editorial: Facial paralysis in hypertension. Br Med J 2:1547, 1966

31. Miller H: Facial paralysis. Br Med J 3:815-819, 1967

32. Adour KK, Wingerd J: Idiopathic facial paralysis (Bell's palsy): factors affecting severity and outcome in 446 patients. Neurology 24:1112-1116, 1974

33. Hilger JA: The nature of Bell's palsy. Laryngoscope 59: 228-235, 1949

34. Blunt JM: The possible role of vascular changes in the aetiology of Bell's palsy. J Laryngol Otol 70:701-703, 1956

35. Swerdloff RS (moderator), Odell WD, Bray GA, *et al*: Complications of oral contraceptive agents – a symposium. West J Med 122::20-49, 1975

36. Saunders WH, Lippy WH: Sudden deafness and Bell's palsy: a common cause. Ann Otol Rhinol Laryngol 86:830-837, 1959

37. Saunders WH: Viral infections and cranial nerve paralysis. Arch Otolaryngol 78: 101-106, 1963

38. Schuring A, Saunders WH: Facial diplegia, a viral disease? Arch Otolaryngol 80: 103-105, 1964

39. McCormick DP: Herpes-simplex virus as a cause of Bell's palsy. Lancet 2:937-938, 1972

40. Adour KK, Doty HE: Electronystagmographic comparison of acute idiopathic and herpes zoster facial paralysis. Laryngoscope 83:2029-2034, 1973

41. Adour KK, Bell DN, Hilsinger RL Jr: Herpes simplex virus as causative agent in idiopathic facial paralysis (Bell palsy). JAMA. To be published

42. Naib ZM, Nahmias AJ, Josey WE, *et al*: Relation of cytohistopathology of genital herpesvirus infection to cervical anaplasia. Cancer Res 33:1452-1463, 1973

43. Nahmias AJ, Roizman B: Infection with herpes-simplex viruses 1 and 2. N Engl J Med 289:781-789,1973

44. Jewett JF: Herpes simplex encephalitis. N Engl J Med 292:531, 1975

45. Hopf HC: Electromyographic study on so-called mononeuritis. Arch Neurol 9:113-118, 1963

46. Safman BL: Bilateral pathology in Bell's palsy. Arch Otolaryngol 93:55-57, 1971

47. Chaco J: Subclinical peripheral nerve involvement in unilateral Bell's palsy. Am J Phys Med 52:195-197, 1973

48. McNair Scott TF, Tokumaru T: The herpesvirus group, in Horsfall FL Jr, Tamm I (eds): *Viral and Rickettsial Infections of Man*, edition 4. Philadelphia, J. B. Lippincott Company, 1965, pp 892-903

49. Glasscock ME III: [Bell's palsy in pregnancy]. Collected letters. Int Corresp Soc Ophthalmol Otolaryngol 19:42, 1974

50. Pulec JL: Collected letters. Int Corresp Soc Ophthalmol Otolaryngol 19:42-43, 1974

51. Elliott DC: Collected letters. Int Corresp Soc Ophthalmol Otolaryngol 19:43-44, 1974

52. Grimm G (Question), Villee DB (Answer): What risk to fetus from maternal steroid therapy. JAMA 230:1202, 1974

53. Beitins IZ, Bayard F, Anees IG, *et al*: The transplacental passage of prednisone and prednisolone in pregnancy near term. J Pediatr 81:936-945, 1972

SOCIETY FOR EAR, NOSE AND THROAT ADVANCES IN CHILDREN

The third annual meeting of the Society for Ear, Nose and Throat Advances in Children (SENTAC) will be held at the Hospital del Niño IMAN (Institucion Mexicana de Asistencia a la Niñez) in Mexico City November 5-9, 1975. Papers of 10 to 20 minutes' duration are invited; abstracts should be submitted by September 15 either to Ernesto Deutsch, M.D., Servicio de Otorrinolaringologia, Hospital del Niño IMAN, Insurgentes Sur 3700-C, Mexico 22, D.F., or to Sanford E. Gerber, Ph.D., Department of Speech, University of California, Santa Barbara, CA 93106. For information concerning travel and accommodations write to Dr. Deutsch.

Ann Otol 84: 1975

INNERVATION OF THE COCHLEA OF THE GUINEA PIG BY USE OF THE GOLGI STAIN

CATHERINE A. SMITH, PH.D.

PORTLAND, OREGON

SUMMARY – Nerve fibers with distinctive branching patterns have been demonstrated in guinea pigs by use of the Golgi stain. The cochlear nerve fibers in the basal turn tend to supply a limited segment of the basilar membrane and have most endings on a single row of hair cells. The efferent olivocochlear nerve fibers ramify in a manner which varies from base to apex. Some efferents which terminate on outer hair cells also give branches which course in the inner spiral bundle. Other nerve fibers were studied in the spiral lamina which did not penetrate into the organ of Corti.

Our first study on the terminal branching of the cochlear nerve fibers in the guinea pig after use of the Golgi method, reported in 1973,[1] gave preliminary evidence for distinctive branching patterns of both cochlear nerve dendrites and efferent nerve axons. In later studies,[2] we confirmed our assumption that some of the more apical cochlear nerve fibers supply a larger segment of basilar membrane than do the basal fibers, by means of electron microscopy. Since that time, more observations have been made on a larger number of newborn guinea pigs. A résumé of our present results is presented in this study. This is not to be considered the final story, for there is enough variation in terminal ramification to make it necessary that more observations be made before final conclusions can be reached.

METHODS AND MATERIALS

Thirty-six guinea pigs were used in this study. Eighteen of them were adults; 18 were newborns, sacrificed at times ranging from 4-36 hours postpartum. The ears from 34 animals were fixed by intralabyrinthine perfusion and impregnated as previously described.[1] The rapid Golgi method as given by Valverde[3] was used throughout.

The ears from one newborn were fixed with Dalton's 1% OsO_4 while the animal was under anesthesia, by our standard method of labyrinthine perfusion,[4] and embedded in araldite for electron microscopy. The cochleas from another newborn guinea pig were incubated and stained for acetylcholinesterase with the technique given by Karnovsky,[5] and used by Takasaka and Smith[6] for the pigeon's basilar papilla.

After impregnation or staining was complete, in all the animals except those prepared for electron microscopy, the bony otic capsule was removed from each cochlea. The entire organ of Corti was dissected free from the modiolus and mounted on slides for study.

Camera lucida drawings were made either with a 40x high-dry, or 50x or 100x oil-immersion lenses and 10x or 15x eyepieces. Photographs were taken with Panatomic X or Ektachrome X film.* The fibers were studied by either a Wild** or Zeiss*** microscope, the latter being equipped with Nomarski-interference optics.

After the above preparations were completed, some specimens were floated free of the slide and cover-slip by overnight soaking in xylene. They were embedded in araldite, using toluene as an intermediary agent. Serial sections were made of the nerve fibers previ-

* Eastman Kodak Co., Rochester, N.Y.
** Wild Heerbrugg Instruments, Inc., Farmingdale, N.Y.
*** Carl Zeiss, Inc., N.Y., N.Y.

From the Department of Otolaryngology, University of Oregon Health Science Center, Portland.

Supported by PHS Grant No. NS-08813.

Presented at the meeting of the American Otological Society, Atlanta, Ga., April 11-12, 1975.

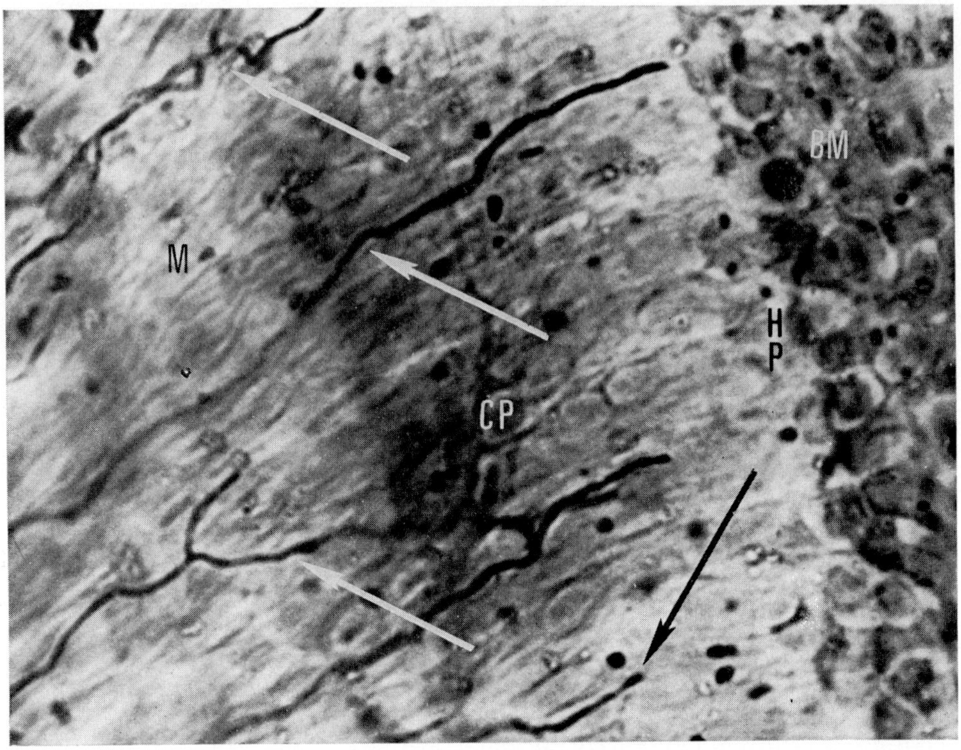

Fig. 1. Photomicrograph of spiral lamina from the apical turn of No. 534R. A number of impregnated nerve fibers cross the field from left to right (white arrows). The fiber at lower center terminates in a small end bulb (black arrow): BM: basilar membrane, CP: capillary, HP: habenula perforata, M: myelinated nerve fibers. X1,000

ously drawn, with either glass or diamond knives. In order to avoid any further precipitate which might be introduced by heavy metal staining, the sections were put into the microscope and photographed without any further treatment. Use of the 40 Kv accelerating voltage in the EMU 300* and a double-strength HRP developing solution** enhanced the contrast.

FINDINGS

Any nerve fibers that are present in the tissue can be stained by the Golgi method. The cochlear nerve fibers, the olivocochlear axons, and some other nerve fibers in the spiral lamina which correspond in location and pattern to the adrenergic fibers described by Spoendlin and Lichtensteiger,[7] Teryama, *et al*,[8] and Spoendlin[9] have been studied.

Nerve Fibers in the Spiral Lamina. Some nerve fibers have been consistently seen in the spiral lamina which do not enter into the membranous cochlear duct. Some of these approach the habenula perforata but before reaching it (0.1 to 0.14 mm distant in three fibers measured) reverse themselves and loop back toward the modiolus. Most give off a few branches in their course through the spiral lamina; some branches also turn back toward the modiolus, whereas others are short and slender, with delicate end bulbs. Other fibers are straight and end within the spiral lamina. Some of the latter reach the neighborhood of the habenula perforata and seem to terminate occasionally by means of small end bulbs (Fig. 1). These nerve fibers have been studied in the apex where, because of the deficient bony shelf, they can be visualized more readily.

* Philips Electron Instruments, Inc., Mt. Vernon, N.Y.
** Eastman Kodak Co., Rochester, N.Y.

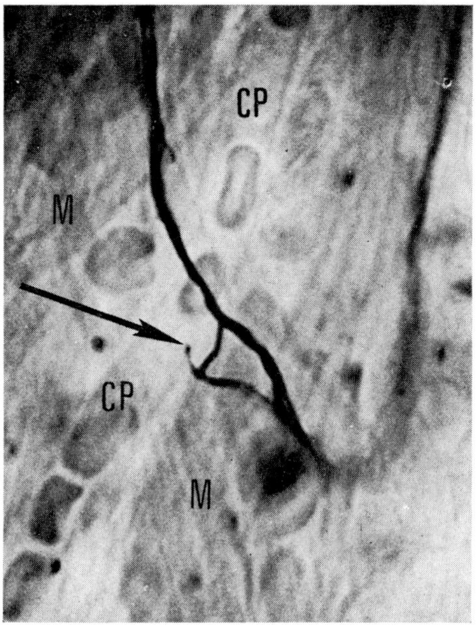

Fig. 2. Photomicrograph of the apical turn of spiral lamina from No. 533L. A looped nerve fiber enters and exists at top. It has a branch whose end bulb (arrow) is situated close to the capillary wall (CP). M: myelinated nerve fibers. X1,250

For the most part, those fibers which end, or seem to do so, send their terminal branches among the myelinated nerve fibers. A smaller number are closely related to the capillaries. Small end bulbs on slender branches have been visualized, under oil immersion and by means of Nomarski optics, which lie between the capillary wall and the myelinated nerve fibers. However, as seen in Figure 2, the nerve fibers do not follow the capillaries, but rather give off branches as they approximate or cross the blood vessels.

Cochlear Nerve Fibers. It was found that the cochlear nerve fibers were more easily impregnated in newborn animals than in adults, and many have been found and studied in the newborn cochleas. Preliminary observations reported in the previous studies[1,2] indicated that the branching pattern of the external spirals varied from basal to apical ends. The present studies are in general agreement, but there are still problems in the absolute identification of some fibers in the apical half of the cochlea. For the most part, the present findings will be confined to the basal external spiral nerve fibers. Table I includes a selection of 15 nerve fibers most of which are in the basal turns of the cochleas. One from the second turn whose identity has been provided by electron microscopy is included, for it illustrates the different apical branching pattern.

The fibers given in the table (except for No. 531L, T_2) are typical of the cochlear fibers in the basal coil (the basal 9 mm of basilar membrane[10]). The complete distance they coursed along the basilar membrane was in many cases indeterminate because the fibers were broken. However, the cochlear nerve fibers appear to cross the tunnel immediately after emerging from their respective foramina in the habenula and to turn toward the basal end of the cochlea in between the Deiters cells (Fig. 3) where they course in a spiral direction for distances ranging up to approximately 0.6 mm before branching. They branch over a shorter segment of basilar membrane, generally not much over 0.1 mm, and often less. The terminal branching length of the fiber from No. 542L (Table I) is only 43 μ. The length of basilar membrane innervated depends to some degree on the number of hair cells supplied, and this varies from 6 to 20. However, if the terminals do not supply consecutive hair cells, the branching length increases. A consecutive versus a nonconsecutive sensory cell innervation accounts for the 63 micron difference in the basilar membrane segments innervated by the first and fourth nerve fibers in No. 531L, T_1, mid (Table I) whose number of nerve endings differs only by one, and number of hair cells innervated only by two.

A second feature of the basal nerve fibers is their tendency to have an innervation preference for a single row. Figure 3 is a photomicrograph of the third nerve fiber in No. 531L, T_1, mid (Table I). A number of nerve endings are visible, all terminating on outer hair cells in the first row. Many nerve fibers

TABLE I

SAMPLES OF COCHLEAR NERVE FIBERS IN THE BASAL TURN (EXCEPT ONE IN THE LOWER SECOND TURN) FROM SIX DIFFERENT EARS (FIVE INDIVIDUALS)

Animal No.	*Cochlear Locus*	*Length of External Spiral (in microns)*	*Length of Terminal Branch (in microns)*	*Number of Nerve Endings*	*Number of Hair Cells Innervated*	*Nerve Endings on Hair Cell Rows*
		500	84	18	12	all on ohc II
370	T_1	430	68	11	6	all on ohc I
L	Lower	706	102	16	12	all on ohc III
531 L	T_1 Mid	336*‡	91	20	13	19 on 12 ohc I 1 on 1 ohc II
		308*	112	20	20	17 on ohc I 3 on ohc II
		235*	117	20	13	all on ohc I
		560*	154	21	15	all on ohc II
		420*‡	126	23		all on ohc II
531 L	T_2 Lower	469‡	284	62		32 on ohc II 30 on ohc III
542 R	T_1 Upper	316	73	20	13	7 on 5 ohc I 8 on 4 ohc II 5 on 4 ohc III
542 L	T_1 Lower	at least 193	43	11	7	10 on 6 ohc I 1 on 1 ohc II
543 L	T_1 Lower	at least 160	73	21	11	20 on 10 ohc I 1 on 1 ohc II
556	T_1	230	90	14	10	all on ohc I
R	Lower	140	73	13	8	7 on ohc I 1 on ohc II
		197	93	16	12	11 on ohc I 1 on ohc II

* - Estimates; ‡ - embedded & sectioned ohc - outer hair cells

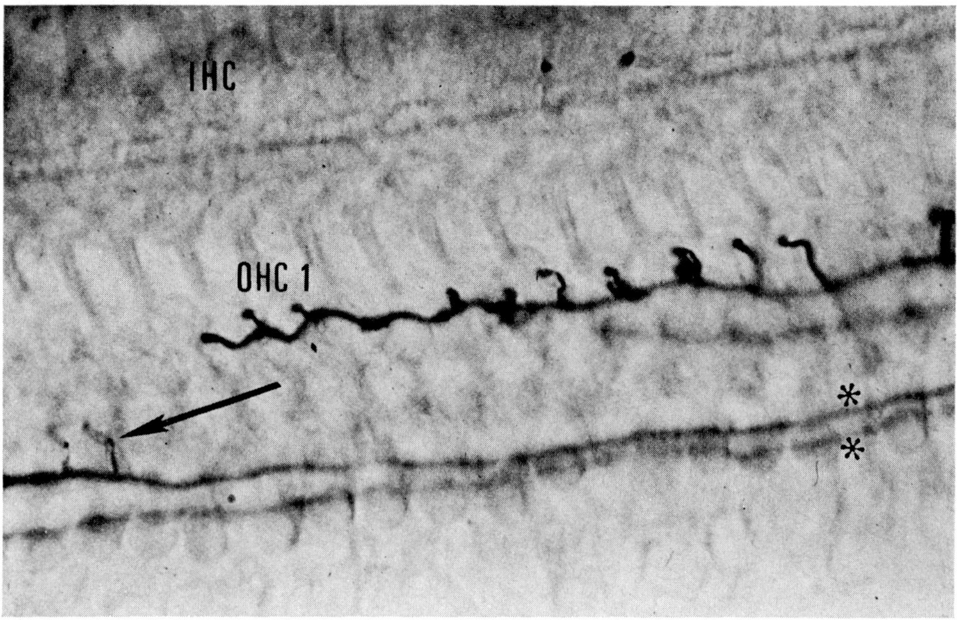

Fig. 3. Photomicrograph of external spirals in basal turn, No. 531L. The upper fiber has many branches on outer hair cells (OHC) in row 1 only. The other fibers are out of the focal field (asterisks); one at extreme left has two nerve endings on row 2 (arrow). X975

do innervate only a single row of outer hair cells; some give a few nerve endings to another row. The only exception to this seen to date is the fiber in No. 542R (Table I), whose nerve endings are rather evenly divided between the three rows; a camera ludica drawing of this fiber is shown in Figure 4.

The latter type of branching pattern is more typical of the upper half of the cochlea. The nerve fiber from the lower second turn of No. 531L (Table I) illustrates the pattern generally seen in the upper turns. A large number of nerve endings, 62 are divided between the hair cells in the second and third rows (Figs. 5 and 6). Not all the nerve fibers in the upper turns which display the afferent branching features supply several rows of outer hair cells, but they are much more frequently found there.

Several of the nerve fibers have been embedded, sectioned in a series, and studied by electron microscopy. A camera lucida drawing and photomicrograph of the first fiber in T_1, mid No. 531L in Table I are shown in Figures 7 and 8. Figure 9 is an electron micrograph from the same fiber, or an outer hair cell in row 1, where all but one nerve ending from that fiber terminated. The parent fiber, the impregnated dendrite, is visible at the lateral edge of the tunnel, in a channel formed by the Deiters cell processes approximately 12 μ below the hair cell. Other nonimpreg-

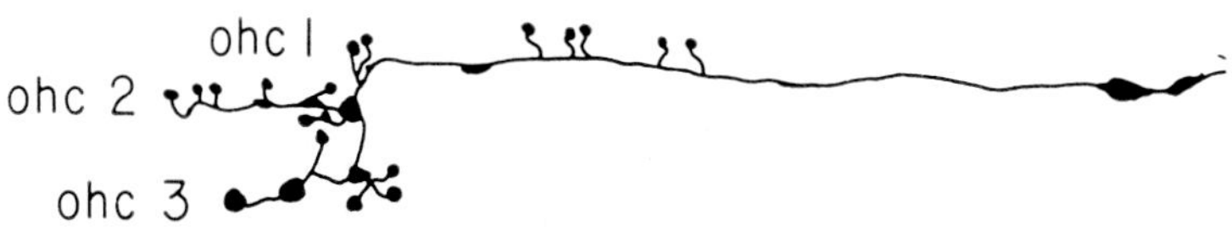

Fig. 4. Camera lucida drawing of nerve fiber from the upper basal turn, No. 542R. This nerve fiber, with nerve endings evenly divided between rows 1, 2, and 3 of outer hair cells is the only one of this type so far found in the basal turn.

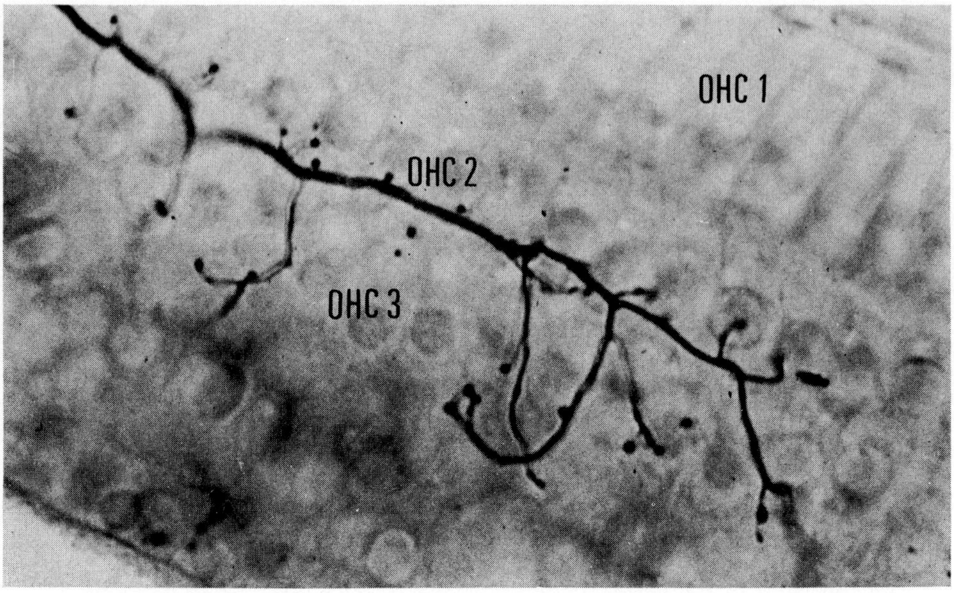

Fig. 5. Photomicrograph of the terminal end of an external spiral fiber in the second turn of No. 531L. Most nerve endings are on row 2 (OHC 2) and row 3 (OHC 3) of outer hair cells. Some branches turn out to Hensen's cells. X975

nated external spirals are visible nearby. In other micrographs the slender preterminal branch could be followed up to the small end bulb at the base of the outer hair cell, visible here. Figure 10 shows another ending from this nerve fiber, on another hair cell at higher magnification. This terminal is heavily impregnated with the dense precipitate; synaptic organelles are either masked or have been destroyed. Some of the precipitate often falls out during sectioning and/or flotation prior to collecting the sections on the grids. Cytoplasmic organelles in the surrounding cells are remarkably well preserved when one considers the long soaking process to which the tissue has been exposed.

Figure 11 is an electron micrograph from the nerve fiber in the second turn, illustrated in Figures 5 and 6. It shows an impregnated, small bulbous nerve ending with attached preterminal at the base of a hair cell in the second row. It is similar in form and size to the adjacent cochlear nerve endings. The nerve endings studied by electron microscopy are identified by their size and shape. Previous experimental studies have shown that in the guinea pig,[11] the chinchilla,[12,13] and the rat,[14] the small, one micron, nerve endings on outer hair cells are those that survive after efferent nerve section and that these are the afferent cochlear nerve terminals. Electron microscopic observations on the newborn cochleas revealed that the nerve fibers and nerve endings were similar to those in adult animals.

The Olivocochlear Efferents. The

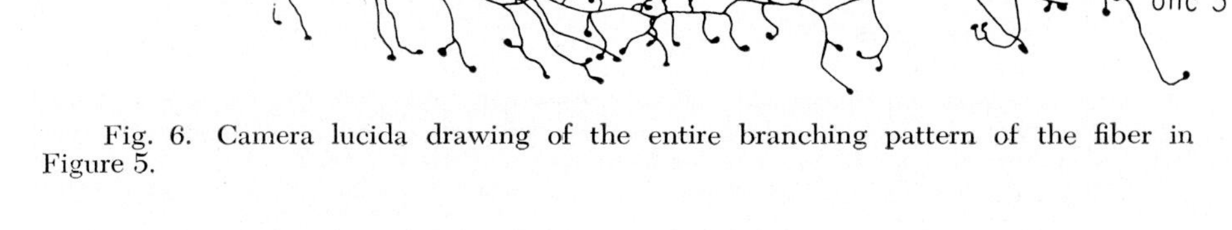

Fig. 6. Camera lucida drawing of the entire branching pattern of the fiber in Figure 5.

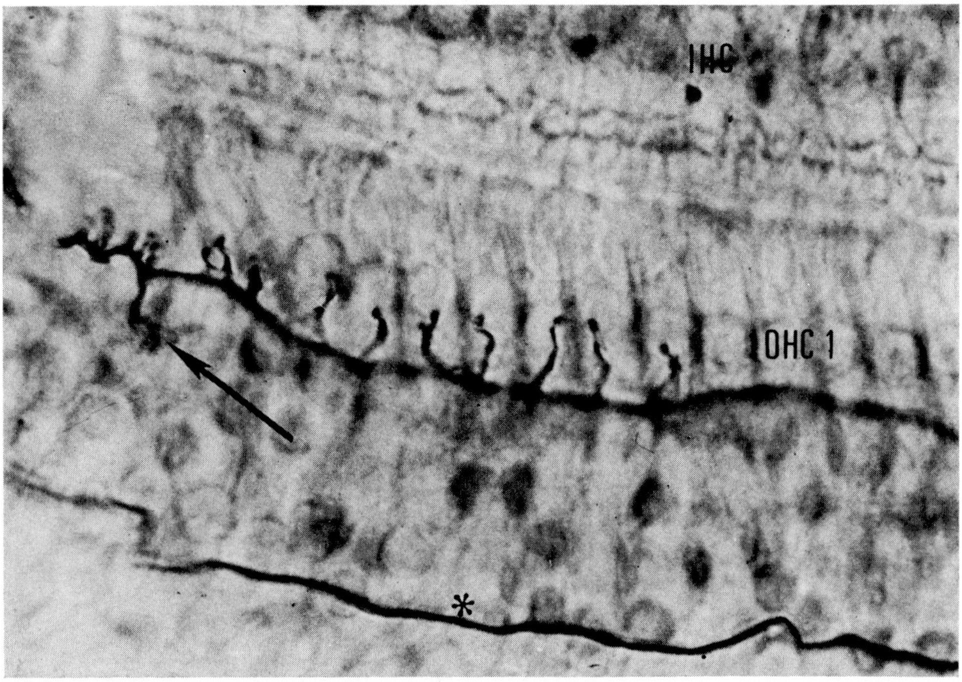

Fig. 7. Photomicrograph of external spirals in basal turn of No. 531L. The upper fiber gives most branches to row 1 (OHC 1) and one to a single hair cell in the second row (arrow). An unbranched fiber is below (asterisk). IHC: inner hair cells. X975

axons and nerve endings which belong to the olivocochlear tract can usually be recognized by the size of the endings (Fig. 12) which are approximately three times as large as the cochlear nerve terminals.[15,16] They can also be recognized by their course which was studied, as a whole by the AChE stains and, in the past, in de-efferented chinchillas.[12,13,16,17]

Experimental studies have previously shown[12] that they form a large part of the inner spiral bundle, the tunnel bundle, and the large nerve endings on the outer hair cells. AChE stains on the newborns also demonstrated a spirally directed network not far distant from the basal ends of the outer hair cells. All of these features, plus some others, are evident in the Golgi-stained fibers.

There are many fibers that course long distances (more than 1 mm) in the inner spiral bundle. One in the basal coil coursed for approximately

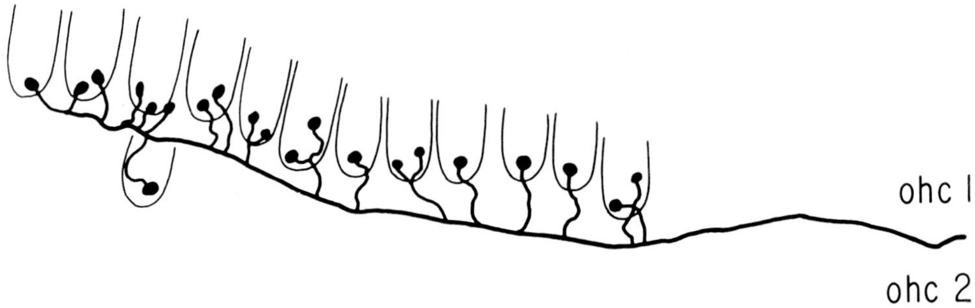

Fig. 8. Camera lucida drawing of the fiber in Figure 7.

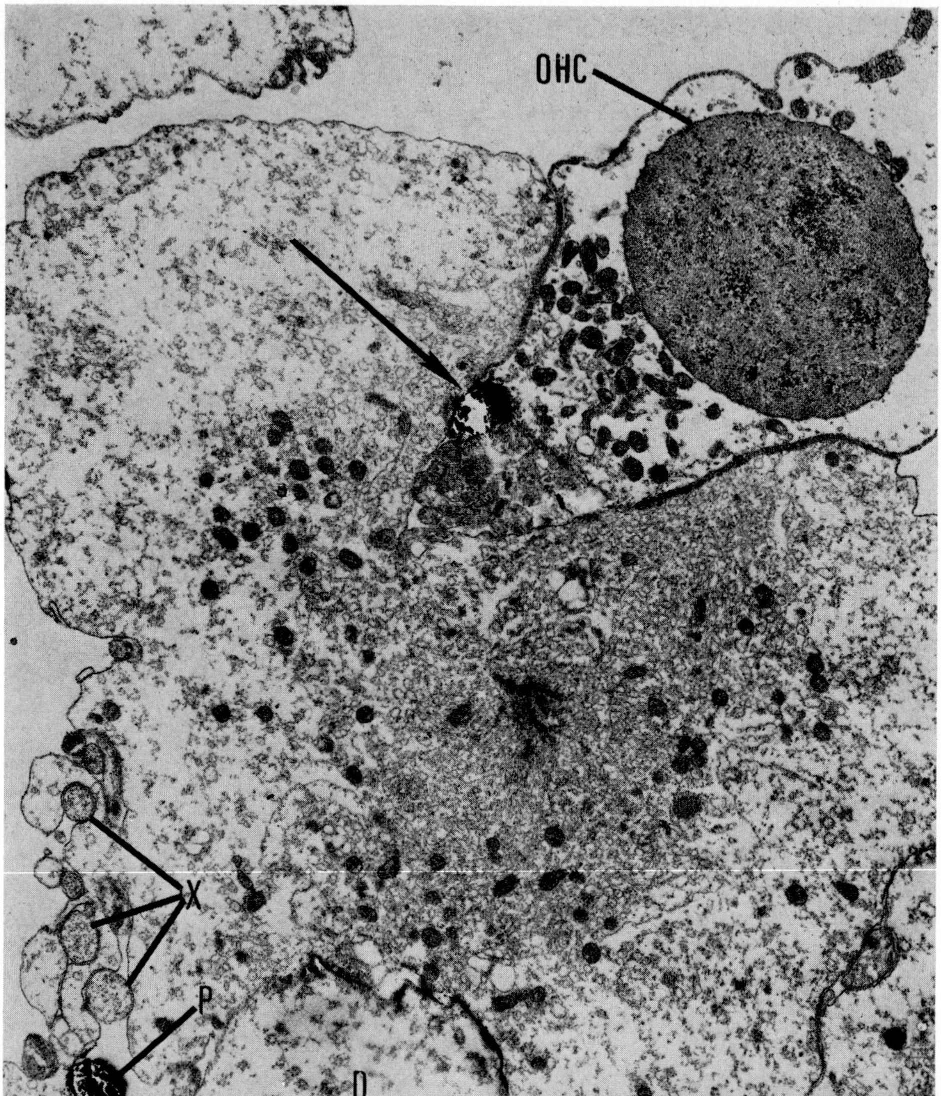

Fig. 9. Electron micrograph of outer hair cell (OHC), with small nerve ending filled with precipitate (arrow), from the nerve fiber in Figures 7 and 8. The parent dendrite (P) is at lower left in a Deiters cell (D) channel. X: other external spirals. X7,600

560 μ, without branching for most of that distance; it finally bifurcated, and one branch appeared to terminate on an inner hair cell. The fibers in the inner spiral bundle have many beaded enlargements. They also have short side branches with end bulbs, but these are infrequent. These latter branches are not generally near the inner hair cells, although some do touch the inner hair cells, as shown by electron micrographs (Fig. 13). Some inner spirals give branches which course in the tunnel bundle, or the main fiber itself may turn out to join the tunnel bundle. In ears where many fibers were stained in

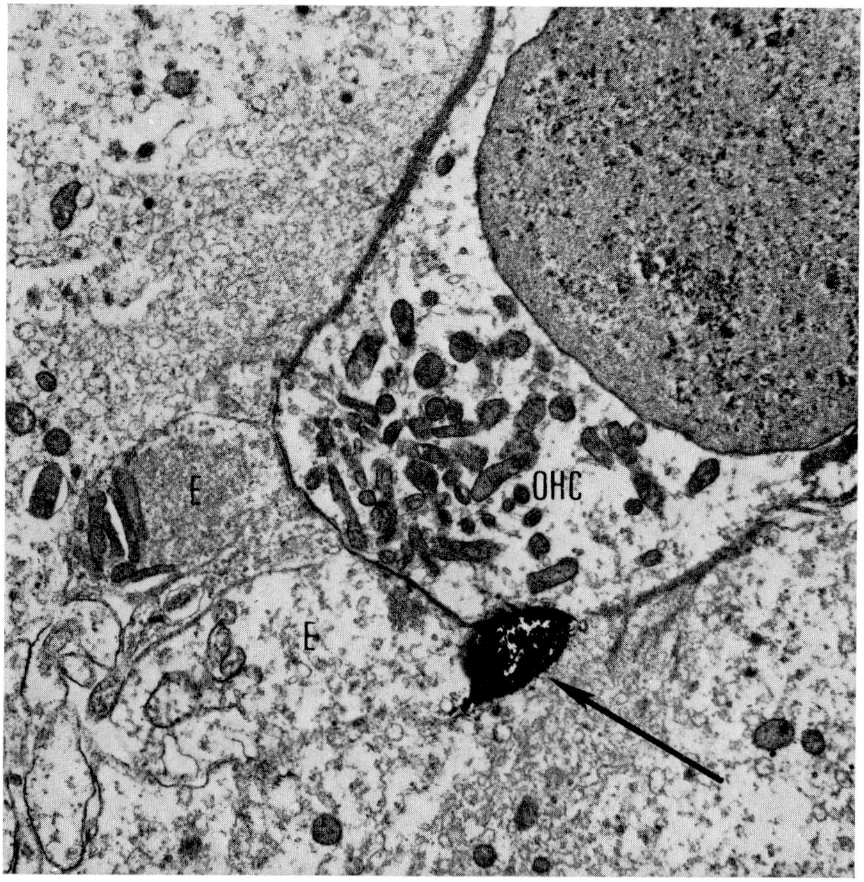

Fig. 10. Electron micrograph of outer hair cell (OHC) with impregnated nerve endings at arrow, from the nerve fiber in Figures 7 and 8. E: efferent nerve endings. X12,000

both inner spiral and tunnel bundles, there were repeated communications crossing between the inner hair cells, indicating a common source of the two bundles. This was also obvious in the AChE-stained cochleas. Wright and Preston[18] have recently demonstrated these communications between tunnel and inner spiral bundles by use of the Maillet stain.

Some of the efferent axons enter the organ of Corti through the foramina nervosa and directly cross the tunnel to the outer hair cells. Here, they ramify among the Deiters cells (between rows 1 and 2 in the lower part of the cochlea). In the basal turn, the nerve endings per terminal axon branch tend to be few in number (3, 5, 8, *etc.*) and to be distributed over a short segment of basilar membrane, to one, two, or three rows (Fig. 14). The large nerve endings on the long slender stalks look much like bunches of grapes hanging from an arbor, and we[1] have called the pattern a "grape arbor" form.

Other efferent terminal axons do not directly cross the tunnel, but course in the inner spiral bundle for some distance before crossing. Or they give off a branch which courses with the inner spiral bundle. One inner spiral fiber (upper third turn) sent a branch to the tunnel bundle where it traveled for 100 μ, finally giving off three branches. Branches one and three crossed the

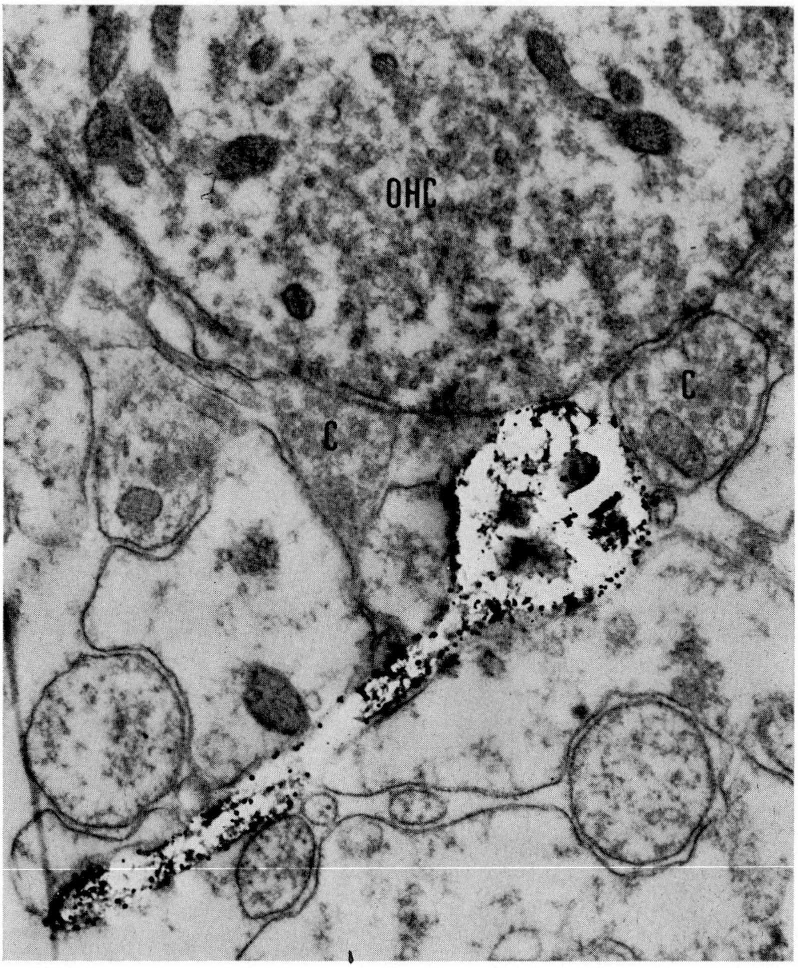

Fig. 11. Electron micrograph of an impregnated nerve ending with slender preterminal, synapsing on an outer hair cell (OHC) in second turn from the nerve fiber in Figures 5 and 6. C: unimpregnated cochlear nerve endings. X27,300

tunnel, ramified, and terminated in approximately eight large nerve endings on the first row, and smaller ones to the second and third rows of hair cells. The middle branch simply made a blind loop in the tunnel.

Figure 15 is a drawing of an efferent axon in the apical coil which bifurcated shortly after emerging from its foramen. Both branches terminated on the outer hair cells, but one coursed for 190 μ in the inner spiral bundle before doing so. There is no evidence in the present study, whether these axons have their source in the homo- or contralateral olivocochlear tracts.

The position of the spirally directed efferent network beneath the outer hair cells in the upper part of the third turn shifts laterally. It is thinner and is located beneath the second row of outer hair cells. The ramification of the axons also changes in the upper part of the cochlea (Fig. 15). Fewer hair cells in the second and third rows have efferent nerve endings, and the segment of basilar membrane innervated by a single axon is broader than in the basal turn. In the apical turn only scattered islands of hair cells in rows two, three,

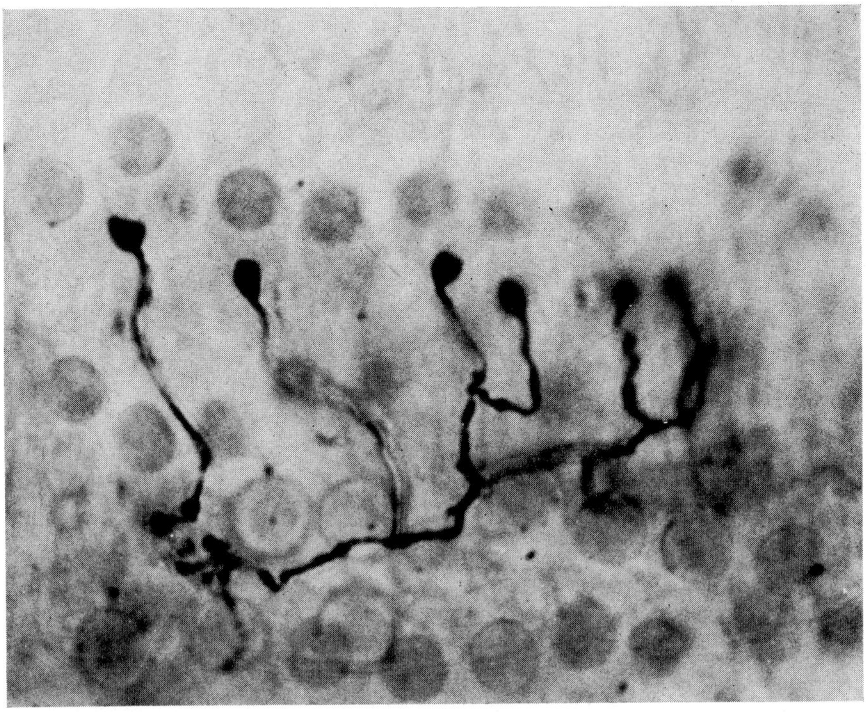

Fig. 12. Photomicrograph of efferent nerve fiber and terminals, from the third turn of No. 556L. X1,250

and four are innervated, mostly by beaded enlargements. Some branches are diverted toward the Hensen's cells.

There are some spiral efferents in the upper turns (also noted by Wright and Preston[18]). One from the fourth turn was studied and drawn. This nerve fiber coursed for a distance of approximately 235 μ toward the apex and then turned and completely reversed its course. When it coursed in the neighborhood of the first row of the outer hair cells, branches with large nerve endings were given off; when it coursed somewhat distant from the hair cells, there were no branches. These efferent spiral fibers, which seem quite rare, are different from the cochlear spiral fibers in that they take a rambling course, and are not "arrow-straight," such as the cochlear nerve fibers tend to be.

DISCUSSION

The results emphasize once more that cochlear innervation is not simple and that information going in to the cochlear nuclei reflects not only neural activity generated by sensory cells in response to the wave form along the basilar membrane, but also possible interaction between different neural systems. First, there are the efferent axons of the olivocochlear tract. The close relationships of these axons to the cochlear nerve fibers beneath the inner hair cells was described in the guinea pig by the present author in 1961,[19] and in the cat by Spoendlin and Gacek.[20] Axodendritic synapses have also been demonstrated beneath outer hair cells in several species.[21] There are close relationships between the efferents in the tunnel and cochlear nerve fibers coming from outer hair cells in the chinchilla.[17] There is also the possibility of influence by sympathetic or parasympathetic fibers.

The presence of adrenergic nerve fibers in the spiral lamina was first demonstrated by Spoendlin and Lichten-

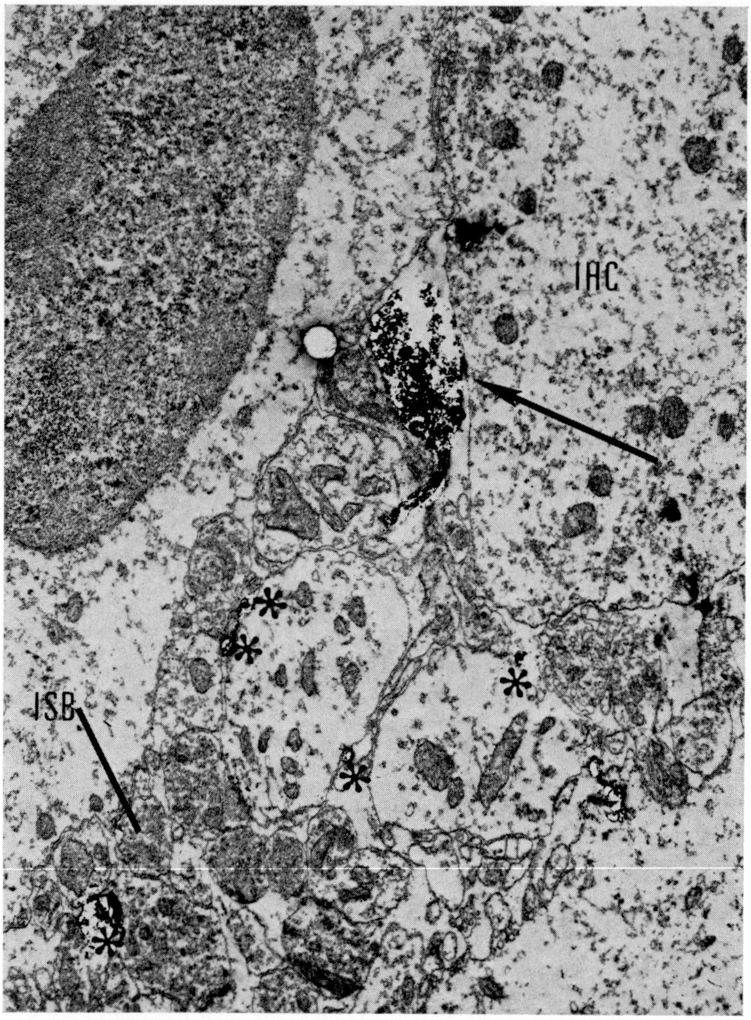

Fig. 13. Photomicrograph of inner hair cell (IHC) from the apical turn of No. 535R. A large impregnated efferent nerve ending with slender preterminal is visible at the hair cell membrane (arrow). A few other stained fibers are seen below (asterisks). The dense material associated with the tear at lower right could be artifact. ISB: inner spiral bundle. X12,000

steiger[7] and Terayama, *et al.*[8] Spoendlin[9] later found that there were two plexuses, one related to blood vessels and one which was independent of the vascular elements. A recent electron microscopic study by Densert and Flock[22] showed that adrenergic nerve fibers reach and apparently terminate at the habenula but do not pass through the foramina into the organ of Corti. The fibers presently described in the spiral lamina could be those fibers. Some appeared to actually end close to the habenula although there is always the possibility these could have been incompletely impregnated fibers. Other nearby fibers made loops and turned back toward the modiolus. The latter gave off small branches, some of which were close to the capillaries, others of which terminated among the myelinated nerve fibers. At present, no nerve fibers have been seen which actually followed the capillaries. Possibly the observations

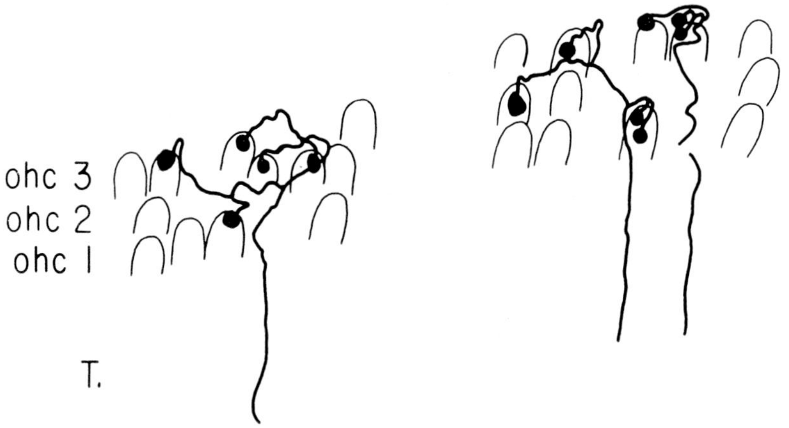

Fig. 14. Camera lucida drawing of three efferent fibers from the lower basal turn of No. 534L, showing the limited branching pattern found in the basal turn. The nerve fiber at right was broken during dissection. T - tunnel.

are biased by the fact that only the apical spiral lamina could be examined in these animals. It seems that the fibers presently studied belong to the adrenergic plexuses previously described[7-9,22] although further study is needed.

There are many basic questions being raised today about cochlear innervation, mostly stimulated by studies of single nerve responses initiated by Tasaki,[23] and so successfully pursued by Kiang.[24] Responses from single nerve fibers can best be correlated with knowledge about single nerve fiber patterns. However, the present studies have yielded data regarding the external spiral cochlear fibers only. Most of the response curves in physiological studies probably would have been obtained from nerve fibers from the inner hair cells, which seem to be in preponderance.[25] Because of the tendency for all fibers to respond in a manner fairly similar, it has been suggested that there may be some bifurcation or branching of a fiber which terminates on the outer hair cells, whereby it supplies both inner and outer hair cells. Perkins[26] found that in young cats and rats, the external spirals formed at least one angular enlargement beneath the inner hair cells. In the present studies, there is no evidence that the external spirals in their course from the habenula to the tunnel give any branches, or even pass close to the inner hair cells. The more completely developed ears of the newborn guinea pigs used here may account for this difference. A recent study by Pfeiffer and Kim[27] has indicated that cochlear nerve fibers might be classed in two groups if one looks at responses to increased sound pressure levels. A small percentage of single fibers from cats produced an increasing number of peaks in response to increased sound pressure level (SPL). This would seem to fit in with the branching pattern of the external spirals, where summation of activity generated by a large number of hair cells innervated by a single fiber could occur. The nerve fiber in No. 531, T_2, with 62 nerve endings would be more likely to respond in this manner than some of the external spirals in the basal turn which innervate only six, seven, or eight hair cells.

The newborn guinea pigs are relatively mature animals at birth. They move about quite freely within an hour postpartum. They have good pinna reflexes, and microscopic examination reveals their middle ears to be free of gelatinous material such as found in newborn rats and cats. Electron microscopic examination showed the innervation of the hair cells to be similar to those of adult animals. In all prob-

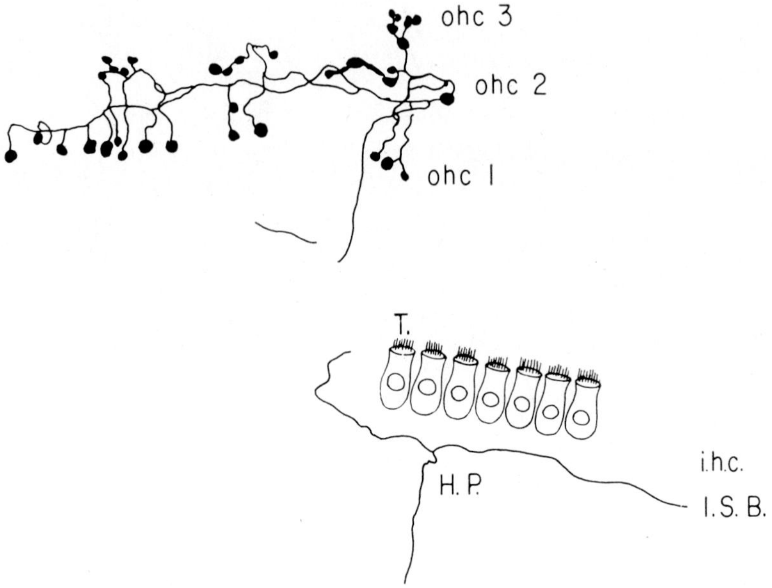

Fig. 15. Camera lucida drawing of an efferent nerve fiber in the third turn of No. 530R. The nerve fiber bifurcates after penetrating the habenula perforata (H.P.) and sends one branch to the inner spiral bundle (I.S.B.). The other branch crosses the tunnel (T.) (broken in dissection) and ramifies under the outer hair cells.

ability, the afferent neural pattern herein described is greatly similar, if not identical, to that of full-grown animals. The efferent axons apparently enter the organ of Corti at a period postdating that of VIII nerve innervation. According to Kikuchi and Hilding,[28] the efferent terminals are not present in the young mouse until the tenth day postpartum. Mice, rats, and cats, however, are quite immature at birth and it is well known that the cochleas of rodents are not fully developed until about two weeks postpartum. Rossi[29] found that colored precipitate did not appear lateral to the tunnel, in the apical turn of the guinea pig cochlea after use of the AChE stain, until the fiftieth day of life. This is not in agreement with the present findings, for an AChE - positive plexus beneath the outer hair cells of the fourth turn was demonstrable in the newborn cochlea. However, we used a later, improved Karnovsky technique[5] with prior fixation of the ear. Rossi did not fix his sections and the smaller amount of enzyme in the apex may have diffused away. At any rate, some of the present data regarding Golgi-stained efferents was obtained from older, adult animals. We have seen no obvious differences between efferent innervation of the newborn and animals of 400-500 g weight.

The efferent pattern presently described does demonstrate an interesting feature, which has also been seen in the cat and rat by Perkins and Morest.[30] That is that some of the axons, after penetration of the habenula, bifurcate with one branch being diverted to the inner spiral bundle, whereas the other crosses the tunnel to terminate on the outer hair cells. The branching is sometimes more complex, but the critical feature is that a single terminal efferent branch with this pattern thus has the possibilities for influencing information coming from both inner and outer hair cells. Of course, one must remember that only the terminal branching is visualized here. According to Rasmussen[31] considerable ramification has already occurred in the spiral lamina before this point so that possibly a single fiber which comes through the habenula and turns into the inner spiral bundle may have the same parent fiber in the spiral lamina, with one that leaves the habenula and directly crosses the tunnel to terminate on the outer hair cells. The studies made by Wiederhold and Kiang,[32] Wiederhold,[33] and Teas, Konishi, and Neilsen,[34] in which stimulation of the crossed olivocochlear bundle caused changes in discharge rates of most of the nerve fibers studied, could best be explained by a pattern whereby at least some crossed efferents were in a position to influence cochlear nerve fibers coming from inner as well as outer hair cells. The present data demonstrates that this could occur, assuming the fibers stained were from the crossed tract. They could also be homolateral fibers, for we[17] have recently found that some of these terminate on outer hair cells.

The present observations are not entirely consistent with Spoendlin's[25] recent schema derived from electron microscopic observations on cats although this may be a species difference. As pointed out before, the fibers in the guinea pig's basal turn only rarely supply all three rows such as he illustrates. Neither is the efferent innervation of outer hair cells a simple radial pattern throughout the cochlea.

Continuing observations, the results of which have been given here, appear to confirm our preliminary assumption that the cochlear innervation pattern in guinea pigs varies from basal to apical turns. The apical external spirals more frequently innervate a longer and wider segment of basilar membrane than in the basal turn. In efferent innervation, also, a limited innervation by a single fiber was more frequently seen in the lower turns, whereas a longer segment of basilar membrane was supplied by single fibers crossing the tunnel in the apical turns. So that again, we appear to have more evidence for the variation in innervation from base to apex, such as we found previously[15] in hair cell innervation. Nevertheless, many more observations are necessary before we can establish a true picture of innervation characteristics from base to apex.

Lastly, this description is based on the assumption that only two kinds of nerve fibers (afferent and olivocochlear) are in the organ of Corti, for we have no good evidence, at this time, for the presence of others.

Request for reprints should be sent to Catherine A. Smith, Ph.D., University of Oregon Medical School, Department of Otolaryngology, 3181 S.W. Sam Jackson Road, Portland, Ore. 97201.

ACKNOWLEDGMENTS—The expert assistance of Susan Cameron, Betty Haglan, Robert Richter, and Ruth Robbins is gratefully acknowledged. The author also appreciates the courtesy of Dr. Kent Morest in supplying a preprint of Perkins and Morest: "A Study of Cochlear Innervation Patterns in Cats and Rats with the Golgi Method and Nomarski Optics."

REFERENCES

1. Smith CA, Haglan BJ: Golgi stains on the guinea pig organ of Corti. Acta Otolaryngol (Stockh) 75:203-210, 1973

2. Smith CA, Haglan BJ: Golgi stains of the cochlear nerve fibers. J Acoust Soc Am 54: 283-284, 1973

3. Valverde F: The Golgi method. A tool for comparative structural analysis, in Nauta W, Ebbesson S (eds) *Contemporary Research Methods in Neuroanatomy.* New York, Springer-Verlag, 1970, pp 12-31

4. Smith CA, Dempsey EW: Electron microscopy of the organ of Corti. Am J Anat 100:337-368, 1957

5. Karnovsky MJ: The localization of cholinesterase activity in rat cardiac muscle by electron microscopy. J Cell Biol 23:217-252, 1964

6. Takasaka T, Smith CA: The structure and innervation of the pigeon's basilar papilla. J Ultrastruct Res 35:20-65, 1971

7. Spoendlin H, Lichtensteiger W: The adrenergic innervation of the labyrinth. Acta Otolaryngol (Stockh) 61:423-434, 1966

8. Terayama Y, Holz E, Beck C: Adrenergic innervation of the cochlea. Ann Otol Rhinol Laryngol 75:69-86, 1966

9. Spoendlin H: Autonomic nerve supply to the inner ear, in de Lorenzo AJ (ed): *Vascular Disorders and Hearing Defects.* Balti-

more, University Park Press, 1972, pp 93-109

10. Fernandez C: Dimensions of the cochlea (guinea pig). J Acoust Soc Am 24:519-523, 1952

11. Kimura RS, Wersall J: Termination of the olivo-cochlear bundle in relation to the outer hair cells of the organ of Corti in the guinea pig. Acta Otolaryngol (Stockh) 55: 1-32, 1962

12. Smith CA, Rasmussen GL: Recent observations on the olivo-cochlear bundle. Ann Otol Rhinol Laryngol 72:489-507, 1963

13. Iurato S, Smith CA, Eldredge DH, *et al*: Electron microscopic observations and cochlear potentials after section of the crossed olivo-cochlear tract in the chinchilla; in *4th Europ Reg Conf on Electron Microscopy*, Rome, 1968, pp 561-562

14. Iurato S: Efferent fibers to the sensory cells of Corti's organ. Exp Cell Res 27:162-164, 1962

15. Smith CA, Sjostrand F: Structure of the nerve endings on the external hair cells of the guinea pig cochlea as studied by serial sections. J Ultrastruct Res 5:523-556, 1961

16. Smith CA, Rasmussen GL: Degeneration in the efferent nerve endings in the cochlea after axonal section. J Cell Biol 26:63-77, 1965

17. Iurato S, Smith CA, Eldredge DH, Henderson D: Distribution of the crossed olivo-cochlear bundle in the chinchilla's cochlea. To be published

18. Wright CG, Preston RE: Degeneration and distribution of efferent nerve fibers in the guinea pig organ of Corti. A light and scanning electron microscopic study. Brain Res 58:37-59, 1973

19. Smith CA: Innervation pattern of the cochlea. Ann Otol Rhinol Laryngol 70:504-527, 1961

20. Spoendlin H, Gacek RR: Electronmicroscopic study of the efferent and afferent innervation of the organ of Corti in the cat. Ann Otol Rhinol Laryngol 72:1-27, 1963

21. Smith CA: Morphological features of axo-dendritic relationships between efferent and cochlear nerves in the cochlea of mammal and pigeon, in von Euler C, Skoglund S, Soderberg U (eds) *Structure and Function of Inhibitory Neuronal Mechanisms.* New York, Pergamon Press, 1968 pp 141-146

22. Densert O, Flock A: An electron-microscopic study of adrenergic innervation in the cochlea. Acta Otolaryngol (Stockh) 77:185-197, 1974

23. Tasaki I: Nerve impulses in individual auditory nerve fibers of guinea pig. J Neurophysiol 17:97-122, 1954

24. Kiang NY-S: *Discharge Patterns of Single Fibers in the Cat's Auditory Nerve.* Boston, MIT Press, 1965

25. Spoendlin H: Neuroanatomy of the cochlea, in Zwicker E, Terhardt E (eds) *Facts and Models of Hearing.* New York, Springer-Verlag, 1974, pp 18-32

26. Perkins RE: Innervation patterns in cochleas of cat and rat: study with rapid Golgi techniques. Anat Rec 175:410, 1973

27. Pfeiffer RR, Kim DO: Response patterns of single cochlear nerve fibers to click stimuli: descriptions for cat. J Acoust Soc Am 52:1669-1677, 1972

28. Kikuchi K, Hilding D: The development of the organ of Corti in the mouse. Acta Otolaryngol (Stockh) 60:207-222, 1965

29. Rossi G: L'acetylcholinesterase au cours du development de l'oreille interne du cobaye. Acta Otolaryngol (Stockh) [Suppl] 170, 1961

30. Perkins RE, Morest DK: A study of cochlear innervation patterns in cats and rats with the Golgi method and Nomarski optics. J Comp Neurol. To be published

31. Rasmussen GL: Efferent fibers of the cochlear nerve and cochlear nucleus, in Rasmussen G, Windle W (eds) *Neural Mechanisms of the Audiotory & Vestibular Systems.* Springfield, Ill., CC Thomas, 1960, pp 105-115

32. Wiederhold ML, Kiang NY-S: Effects of electric stimulation of the crossed olivocochlear bundle on single auditory nerve fibers in the cat. J Acoust Soc Am 48:950-965, 1970

33. Wiederhold ML: Variations in the effects of electric stimulation of the crossed olivocochlear bundle on cat single auditory nerve fiber responses to tone bursts. J Acoust Soc Am 48:966-977, 1970

34. Teas DC, Konishi T, Nielsen DW: Electrophysiological studies on the spatial distribution of the crossed olivocochlear bundle along the guinea pig cochlea. J Acoust Soc Am 51:1256-1263, 1972

GENETIC SENSORINEURAL DEAFNESS IN ADULTS

MICHAEL M. PAPARELLA, M.D.

DAVID G. HANSON, M.D. K. N. RAO, M.D.

ROLF ULVESTAD, M.D.

MINNEAPOLIS, MINNESOTA

SUMMARY — Progressive genetic sensorineural hearing loss is a common problem in adults which is frequently incorrectly diagnosed or escapes diagnosis as to etiology altogether. If the hearing problem becomes manifest in the twilight of the patient's life it is often identified with the nondescriptive term "presbycusis." In all patients with sensorineural hearing loss, extrinsic (environmental) causes should be ruled out after which intrinsic or genetic etiology should strongly be considered, recognizing that extrinsic factors can be superimposed. A group of young adults was studied and diagnosed as having genetic progressive hearing loss. Polytomography ruled out the theoretical possibility of cochlear otosclerosis. The diagnosis of this disorder rests most heavily on the history and audiometric configuration which is characteristically flat or basin shaped with fairly good discrimination. Of further diagnostic significance was the fact that some patients, early in the course of their difficulty, presented with a predominantly low- or high-frequency loss which, over time, assumed a flat audiometric shape. The most important pathological finding from human temporal bone studies was atrophy of the stria vascularis.

The best available statistics estimate that between eight and nine million people (10 to 15% of the adult population) in the United States are affected by significant hearing loss. Yet, in the face of these figures, we know relatively little about many of the causes of this problem. In the 1968 National Center for Vital Health Statistics survey,[1] 20% of patients with significant hearing loss ascribed it to an infectious etiology, and 7% felt their hearing loss was due to trauma. Thirty-five percent listed hearing loss as due to unknown causes. "Other ill-defined conditions" included another 35%. These "ill-defined conditions" included old age, heredity, and noise trauma.

Hearing loss has long been accepted by the general population as an inevitable product of aging. The term "presbycusis" was coined to describe this process by Zwaardemaker in 1893.[2] Unfortunately the term "presbycusis" does not further elucidate the nature of the causes of adult hearing loss. Interest in noise trauma has raised the question of its role in the deafness of aging. Accumulative ototoxic effects may also have a role in aged hearing loss. However, it is clear that the etiology of deafness of aging is not at all well understood. If presbycusis is due only to the aging process, why do some people become deaf at 60 years of age and others have good hearing into their eighties? Environmental factors do not explain the wide range of variability of hearing loss in people who have lived and worked in the same environment all of their lives.

The role of hereditary influence on adult hearing loss is certainly most significant but is still not adequately ap-

From the Department of Otolaryngology, University of Minnesota, Minneapolis, Minn.

This study was supported by NINDS Training Grant 5-T01-NS05349-14 and NINDS Program Project Grant 1 PO1 NS 12125-01.

Presented at the meeting of the American Otological Society, Atlanta, Georgia, April 11-12, 1975.

preciated. It is our purpose here to emphasize the place of adult genetic hearing loss and describe briefly how these patients may be identified in practice. We will also describe briefly some of the genetic characteristics and discuss, with temporal bone evaluation, possible relationships to cochlear otosclerosis and the deafness of aging.

PATTERNS OF INHERITANCE

A brief simple review of single gene inheritance may be in order. The development of the ear is dependent on perhaps thousands of genes controlling anatomy and physiology in the development and maintenance of hearing function. While organ development may be dependent on many genes, an abnormality in any single gene may have profound influences on hearing. Likewise, genetic patterns may be influenced by several factors. When a given gene is present, it may not be apparent clinically. "Penetrance" is the term referring to the frequency with which a genotype is morphologically manifest. "Expressivity" refers to the degree to which a gene is expressed, *i.e.*, some offspring may not show full expression of a phenotype even though the gene is dominant or homozygous recessive.

Autosomal Dominant Inheritance. This pattern is carried vertically from one generation to another. The trait is carried on an autosomal gene, and the trait is inherited in the presence of that gene. The affected parent passes on the trait to approximately 50% of offspring. Males and females are equally affected.

Autosomal Recessive Inheritance. It takes two genes, one from each parent, for the recessive trait to be expressed. Usually the parents are clinically normal and transmit the trait (phenotype) to one-quarter of their children (homozygous). Another one-quarter of the children do not carry the gene or trait, and one-half of the children are heterozygous or have one gene for the trait, as do the parents. Parental consanguinity is not unusual in recessive inheritance patterns, especially in rare disorders. Chung, *et al*,[3] used statistical techniques in studying frequency of consanguinity of parents in relationship to the incidence of deafness in the population. They estimated that there may be 24 to 48 types of recessive hearing loss and felt that there may be one in eight people heterozygous for at least one of the genes which can affect deafness.

X-Linked Inheritance. In x-linked inheritance there is never male-to-male transmission. The trait is carried on the x-gene. One-half of males will receive the affected gene from a carrier mother. The affected heterozygote male will likewise pass on the gene to all of his daughters. Heterozygotic females may be affected by the gene as one chromosome is often suppressed, allowing the affected gene to be expressed (the Lyon hypothesis). Rarely, a homozygous female results from the union of an affected male and a female heterozygote.

TABLE I

SENSORINEURAL HEARING LOSS

- I. Congenital Hearing Loss
  - A. Genetic (intrinsic)
    - 1. Associated with other abnormalities (syndromes)
    - 2. Occurring alone
  - B. Nongenetic (extrinsic)
- II. Progressive or Delayed Hearing Loss
  - A. Genetic (intrinsic)
    - 1. Associated with other abnormalities (syndromes)
    - 2. Occurring alone
  - B. Nongenetic (extrinsic)

ADULT GENETIC HEARING LOSS

Table I suggests a general outline of sensorineural hearing loss. This paper concerns the category of progressive genetic hearing loss not associated with other abnormalities. Hereditary hearing loss occurs in many forms. It can be transmitted in dominant, recessive, or x-linked patterns. The large majority (90%) of genetic congenital deafness is recessive in inheritance patterns. Most adult, progressive, genetic hearing loss is inherited in a dominant manner.

Genetic hearing loss is thought to be responsible for deafness in as many as

50% of congenitally deaf patients. Hereditary deafness may occur as often as one in 650 school children.[4] Approximately one-third of these children have other associated anomalies. Hereditary deafness syndrome associated with other system abnormalities are rather well defined because of the obvious associated anomalies.

Isolated hearing loss without other organ anomalies has been less readily recognized as being genetic in origin. Yet, there are perhaps more than 15 types of hereditary hearing loss with no associated abnormalities.[5] Many can be separated from each other by mode of transmission, age of onset, severity of hearing loss, and audiogram type. Even less frequently recognized has been genetic hearing loss, which may be delayed in onset well into the adult years. This classification has been adapted from Konigsmark and Gorlin.[6] In all probability, these groups will be further fragmented into distinct disorders as they are more carefully identified and studied. Audiometric and vestibular testing is usually rudimentary in even the best-studied genetic groups at present. In the future, further sophisticaiton of testing and the addition of temporal bone tomography, histopathology, and histochemistry with biochemical evaluation of associated enzyme defects (in the case of recessive disorders) will define specific gene disorders.

The recognition and classification of deafness due to dominant inheritance and of delayed onset unassociated with other abnormalities began in the 1920's and is generally credited to Albrecht.[7] Subsequently, several types of adult genetic hearing loss appear to have emerged as separate entities.

Dominant Progressive Early Onset Sensorineural Hearing Loss. A type of early onset progressive hearing loss beginning in early adult life has been described by Stevens and Dolowitz,[8] Johnsen,[9] Huizing, *et al*,[10] Lenzi,[11] and Nance and Sweeney.[12] Teig's study of a family of 25 members showed progression of hearing loss over a 15-year follow-up.[13] Typically the pattern in these families is of high-frequency loss, onset in late childhood or early adulthood years, progressing to a flat audiogram. Positive recruitment tests were characteristic. Heredity appears to be autosomal dominant.

Dominant Low-Frequency Sensorineural Hearing Loss. Hearing loss progressing from low-frequency deafness to a later involvement of all frequencies was described by Konigsmark, *et al*,[14] and by the Vanderbilt study group.[15] Other audiometric testing showed the SISI test positive in about 75% of cases. Tone decay was negative, discrimination was good, and vestibular testing was normal. Temporal bone tomograms were also normal. Each of the kindreds with this syndrome has shown autosomal dominant transmission.

Dominant Midfrequency Sensorineural Hearing Loss. Hearing loss involving the midfrequencies and a basin-shaped curve audiometric pattern in childhood or young adult years has been described by Martensson,[16] Williams and Roblee,[17] and Konigsmark, *et al.*[18] This pattern is progressive, involving all frequencies in later life. Tone decay tests were negative, and SISI tests were usually positive. Caloric testing was normal.

Recessive Early Onset Sensorineural Hearing Loss. The only recessive pattern of progressive hearing loss not present at birth is described in the cases of several kindreds and progresses rapidly to complete deafness at an early age.[6]

X-Linked Progressive Sensorineural Deafness. X-linked early onset sensorineural deafness likewise was described by Mohr and Mayeray.[19] It is transmitted in an x-linked pattern and progresses rapidly during childhood years. Livan described a family with an apparent x-linked pattern of inheritance of a slowly progressive sensorineural hearing loss which was first noted at about the age of ten.[20] The hearing loss progressed to involve high frequencies first, and later, low frequencies.

There are other genetic patterns of

TABLE II

PATIENTS WITH PURE APPARENT PROGRESSIVE HEARING LOSS

Pt. Name	Age	Onset	Type of Loss	Severity (R&L Average) 500	1000	2000	4000	Polytomes
AM	53	13-15	Flat	70	70	75	80	Negative
CM	31	16	Flat	45	55	45	48	Negative
HM	29	15	Low Basin	45	50	38	15	Negative
DLM	20	15	Low Basin	45	40	28	23	
WM	4	Asymp	Low Basin	50	48	13	10	
DKM	25	12	Low Basin	52	52	42	15	Negative
VM	26	5	Flat	55	55	55	40	
MG	66	60	Flat	48	50	45	50	Negative
RS	56	38	Flat → High Tone	33	38	30	65	
MS	51	36	Flat Basin	38	45	55	50	Negative
HR	66	19	Flat	68	78	75	75	Negative
GB	47	38	High Tone	35	50	65	68	Negative
MB	50	18	Flat	55	63	63	58	
JM	42	17	Flat	58	53	45	48	
JK	31	20	Flat → High Tone	30	38	43	55	Negative
EB	78	15	Flat	55	55	55	65	Negative
PS	51	35	Basin	23	40	48	28	Negative
JC	47	21	Flat	50	50	58	75	
PH	58	35	High Tone	33	45	70	75	
LC	24	13	Flat	80	85	75	65	Negative
KP	12	9	Basin	18	40	50	35	
OM			High Tone	40	52	55	70	

hearing loss progressing in adult years which are well described. These are more easily identified because of other associated syndromes. These syndromes will not be discussed here; the interested reader is referred to a textbook by Bruce W. Konigsmark and Robert J. Gorlin, soon to be published.[6]

Diagnosing Genetic Adult Hearing Loss. In the practice of otology, we encounter many patients with progressive sensorineural hearing loss of unknown etiology. If the patients are older, they may be labeled with the nondescriptive term "presbycusis." However, in this study we were especially interested in identifying these problems in young adults, recognizing the problem was not apparent unless the speech reception threshold (SRT) had reached, generally, a level of 40 dB or higher. The audiometric patterns in this group were, in the main, flat or basin shaped with fairly good speech discrimination. Some of these patients were misdiagnosed by others or could easily have been misdiagnosed as having pure cochlear otosclerosis. Polytomography ruled out this theoretical possibility. Some patients had positive family histories of similar auditory involvement; others did not. For those who had an absence of a positive family history, having ruled out all possible extrinsic causes, (*e.g.*, drugs, trauma, noise, infection) we were, by process of exclusion, left with an intrinsic cause, genetic sensorineural hearing loss.

These patients were selected as a random sampling. Thus, no inferences can be drawn as to incidence although such studies are highly worthwhile. Twenty-two patients from 18 families are represented in Table II. All of these patients had completely normal otological examinations with the exception of their abnormal audiograms. No significant history of noise exposure, trauma,

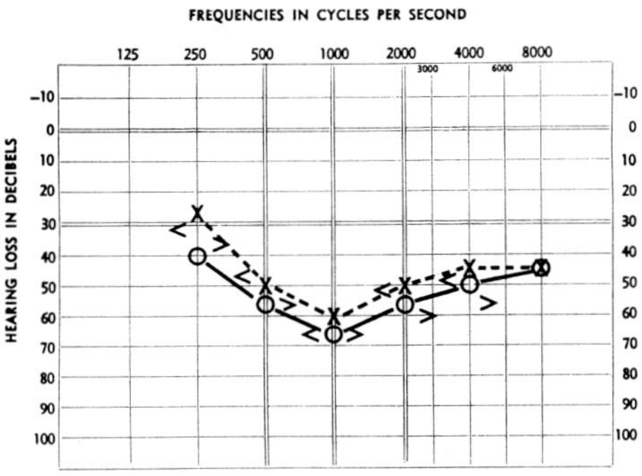

Fig. 1. Audiogram (MB.)

ototoxic drugs, or significant illnesses could be detected by careful history in any of these patients, all of whom were considered reliable historians.

Several variables were found in these patients, including age of onset of symptomatic hearing loss which varied from childhood to the late thirties. Fifty percent of patients had symptomatic onset between the ages of 15 and 30 years of age. These patients also demonstrated a variety of audiometric patterns of loss, but most had a flat or basin-type audiogram. A number of patients, who had hearing loss with similar characteristics, onset in young adult years, often with similar family histories, are not included in this report because of superimposed middle ear or other problems or because of a questionable history of trauma or noise exposure. It is likely, however, that these additional patients also had genetic hearing loss. Further, other patients with probable genetic hearing loss were simply not identified for this study.

CASE REPORTS

The following five patients are representative and characteristic of the different ways in which hearing loss presented in this group.

Case 1. M.B., a 50-year-old female,

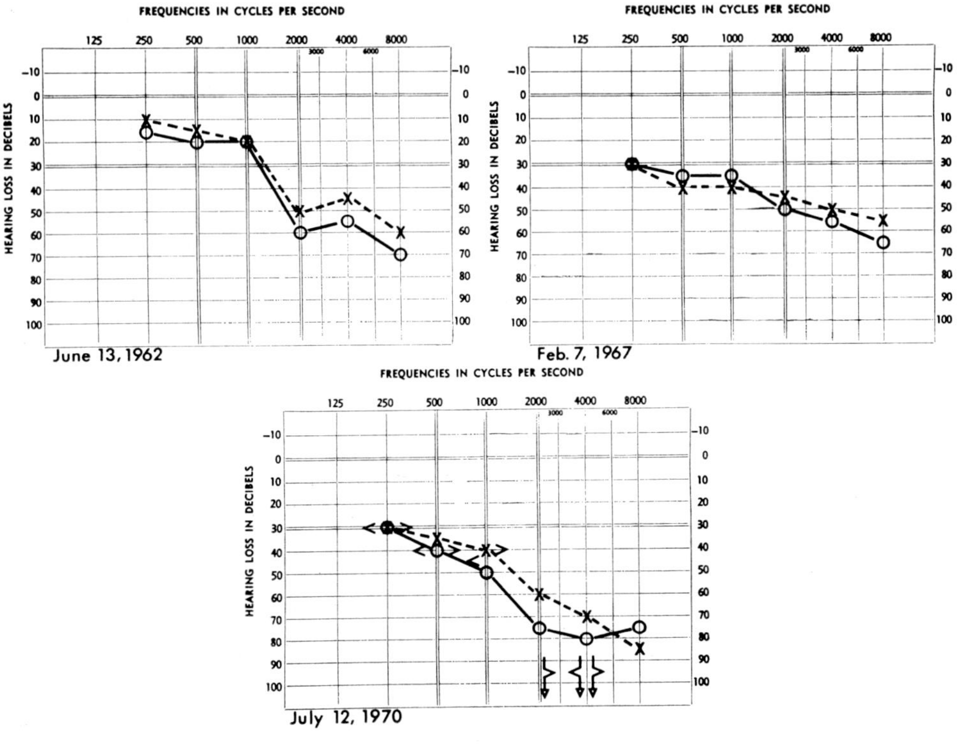

Fig 2. Three successive audiograms, over a period of time, showing progression of loss. (PH)

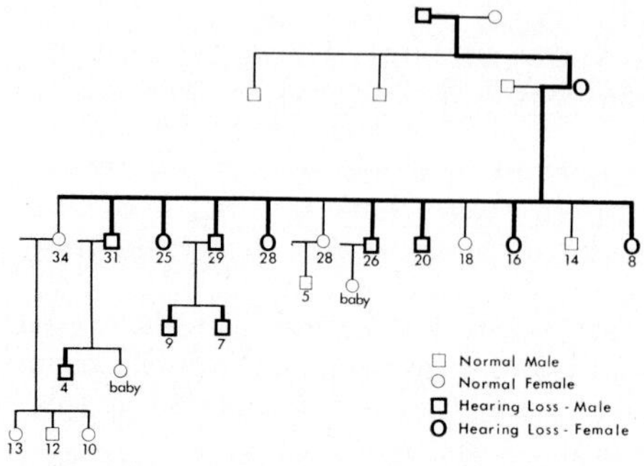

Fig. 3. Family tree of D.K.M. Affected family members (dark lines) show basin-shaped sensorineural losses of moderate to severe degree. Temporal bone tomograms are normal on all family members studied.

the third of 11 children, noted onset of symptomatic hearing loss at age 18. Four of the 11 children in her family developed symptomatic hearing loss before the age of 30. The patient had taken no ototoxic drugs, and there was no history of significant noise trauma or temporal bone trauma (Fig. 1). Temporal bone polytomography was normal, showing no abnormality of the osseous labyrinth.

Case 2. P.H. is a 58-year-old male with hearing loss of symptomatic onset at age 35. Three successive audiograms (Fig. 2) show progressive hearing loss in the high frequencies. It is of interest that the initial high-frequency loss eventually assumes a flatter configuration. The patient's 93-year-old father recalls that his own hearing loss began at about age 40. Again, there is no history of ototoxic drugs, trauma, or noise exposure. Temporal bone polytomography was normal.

Case 3. D.K.M., a 25-year-old female clerical worker, is one of eight siblings with a similar hearing loss in a family of 12. Figure 3 shows a family tree for this patient. This patient's audiogram (Fig. 4) is typical for the family with the greatest loss in the low- to midrange. It is of interest that D.K.M's affected siblings appear to have onset of hearing loss at a younger age than the preceding generation. Temporal bone polytomography of D.K.M. and other members of her family have been normal.

Case 4. P.S. is a 51-year-old male real estate agent with onset of hearing loss at age 35. His audiograms show a basin-shaped loss with more involvement for the midfrequencies. Examination and history were otherwise negative. Temporal bone polytomography was normal (Fig. 5).

Case 5. G.P. was a female patient who died October 13, 1965, at the age of 52. Her case represents, to our knowledge, the first described temporal bone findings in a case of genetic, adult, progressive sensorineural hearing loss.[21]

CLINICAL INFORMATION

This patient had a history of bilateral hearing loss since late childhood. There was a strong history of deafness, and the patient's mother and one sister also

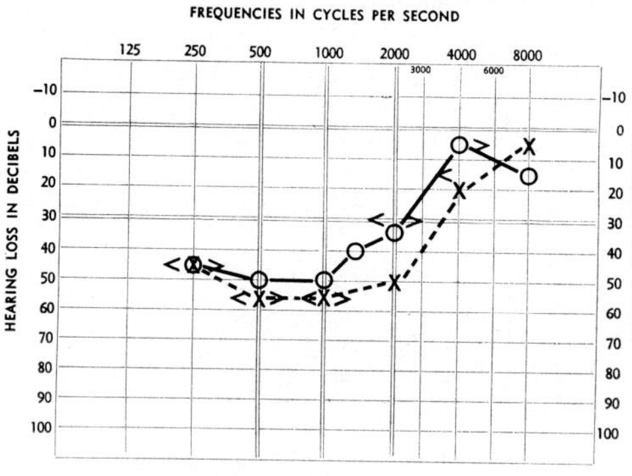

Fig. 4. Audiogram (D.K.M.)

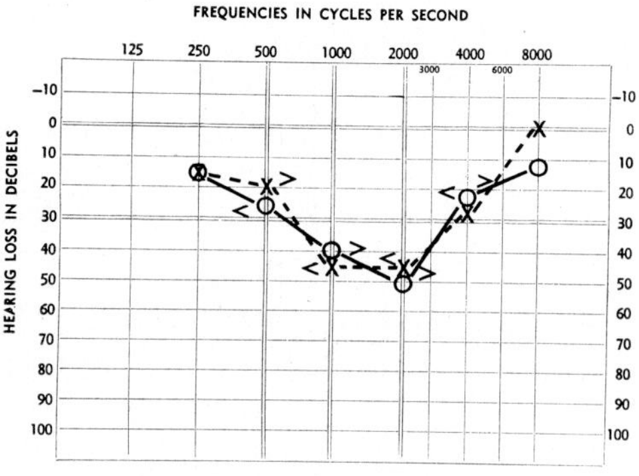

Fig. 5. Audiogram (P.S.)

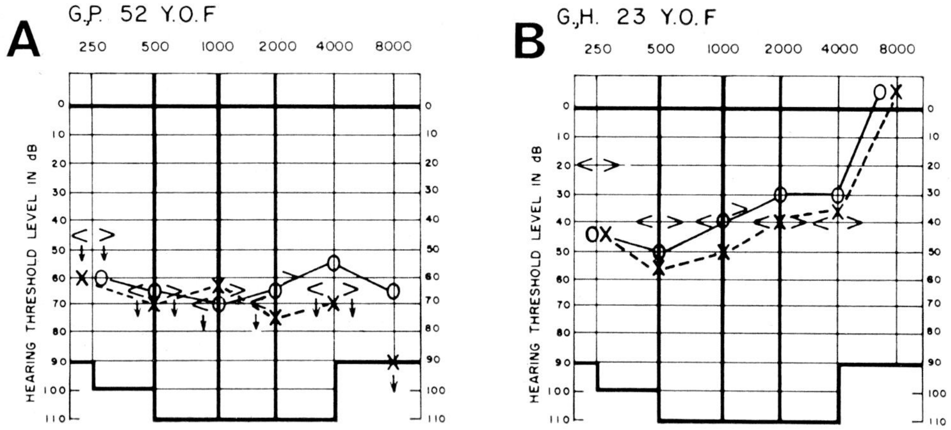

Fig. 6. A) Mother's audiogram (G.P.). B) Daughter's audiogram.

had what was considered to be either congenital deafness or deafness occurring during childhood. This patient had noted bilateral, severe tinnitus, especially over the past many years, decreasing somewhat in recent years. The hearing progressively worsened, and during the past few years she had worn binaural aids with adequate results. There was no history of acoustic trauma, maternal rubella, severe infection, or other causes to suggest other nongenetic types of congenital or acquired deafness. An exploratory tympanotomy was done by another otolaryngologist in an apparent attempt to rule out a diagnosis of stapes fixation and cochlear otosclerosis. None was found. The patient had two daughters, one of whom, at the age of 23 years, has the same difficulty. Otological and audiological information was available for this daughter. The audiogram revealed a bilateral, relatively flat sensorineural hearing loss at approximately a 40-45 dB level, with a rise at 8 kHz (Fig. 6A, B).

Complete physical examination revealed no associated congenital or genetic lesions. The patient received a careful otological and audiometric examination which was negative with the exception of hearing dysfunction. This patient's last audiogram was approximately ten months prior to death (Fig. 6A), demonstrating a severe, flat sensorineural loss around 65 to 70 dB with discrimination scores of 60% and 68% using phonetically balanced maximum words. The patient had developed carcinoma of the breast two years prior to death. She had a mastectomy but developed metastases throughout the body and finally died. There were skull metastases without evidence of temporal bone involvement. She was treated with chemotherapeutic agents and had large doses of irradiation to the brain prior to death.

TEMPORAL BONE HISTOPATHOLOGY

The temporal bones were removed seven hours after death. The same findings were present on both sides and are described together.

Middle Ear and Mastoid. There were some slight chronic changes in the middle ear mucosa in the region of the round window niche, characterized by secretory elements with thickened mucosa. Otherwise, the middle ear and mastoid were normal.

Inner Ear. Osseous Labyrinth: The osseous labyrinth appeared normally developed throughout. There was no evidence of otosclerosis. Membranous Labyrinth: The labyrinth was in a fairly good state of preservation. The vestibular labyrinth was essentially normal in appearance. The saccular wall appeared somewhat collapsed although the macula of the saccule appeared

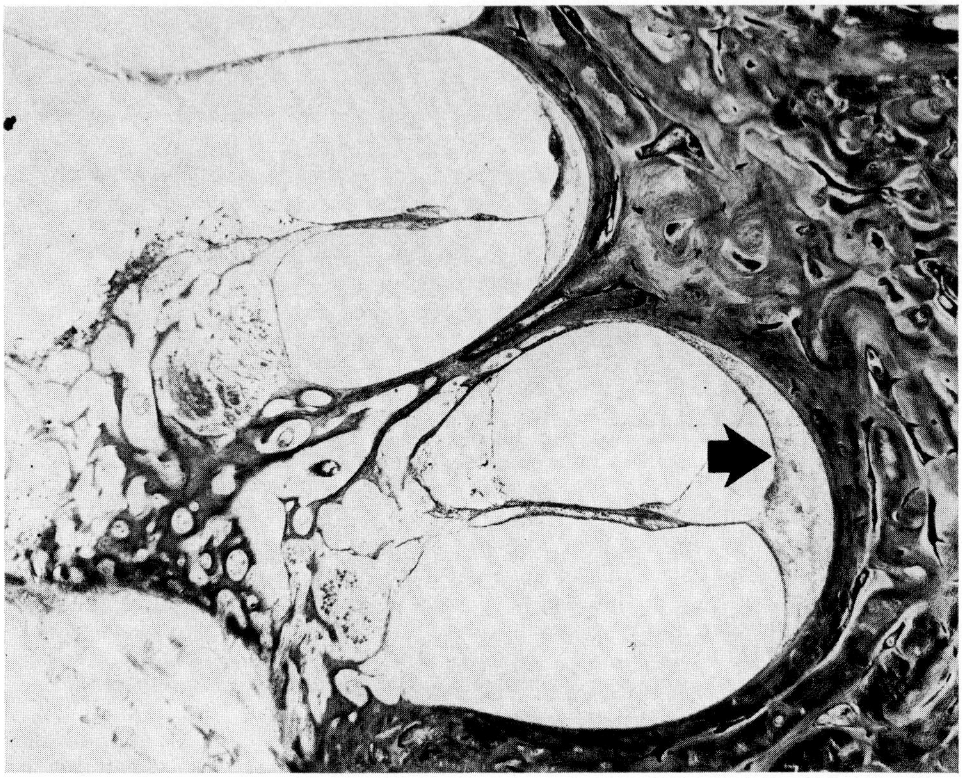

Fig. 7. Temporal bone of mother (G.P.). Note strial atrophy in basal turn (arrow).

normal, as did the utricle. The pathological findings of interest were located primarily in the anterior membranous labyrinth. There was complete loss of the organ of Corti in the basal turn. Corti's organ could be identified in the apex and in certain areas of the middle turn but was seen largely as a clump of cells. Hair cells and other elements could not be distinguised. The tectorial membrane appeared shrunken. Associated with these changes, there was a normal-appearing spiral ligament in all turns. The stria vascularis appeared markedly atrophic or missing in a spotty distribution. The stria was better seen in certain areas of the upper cochlear turns but had severely degenerated in the basal turn. In some areas Reissner's membrane appeared slightly collapsed, as in the upper basal turn. This may have been related to histological preparation. Neural Structures: There was a marked loss of spiral ganglion cells, especially well seen in the upper basal turn area, as well as in the lower basal turn and hook area (Fig. 7). In some places there appeared to be as much as an 80% loss of ganglion cells. The spiral ganglion canal of the apex appeared to contain relatively normal numbers of ganglion cells. The loss of ganglion cells was more marked on the right than on the left ear. Peripheral dendrites appeared missing in proportion to the loss of ganglion cells. Axons and ganglia within the internal auditory canal (IAC) appeared normal.

Summary of Pathological Findings. This patient had many cochlear findings which would account for the sensorineural hearing loss including: loss of the organ of Corti, especially in the basal turn; marked degeneration of the stria vascularis in an irregular distribu-

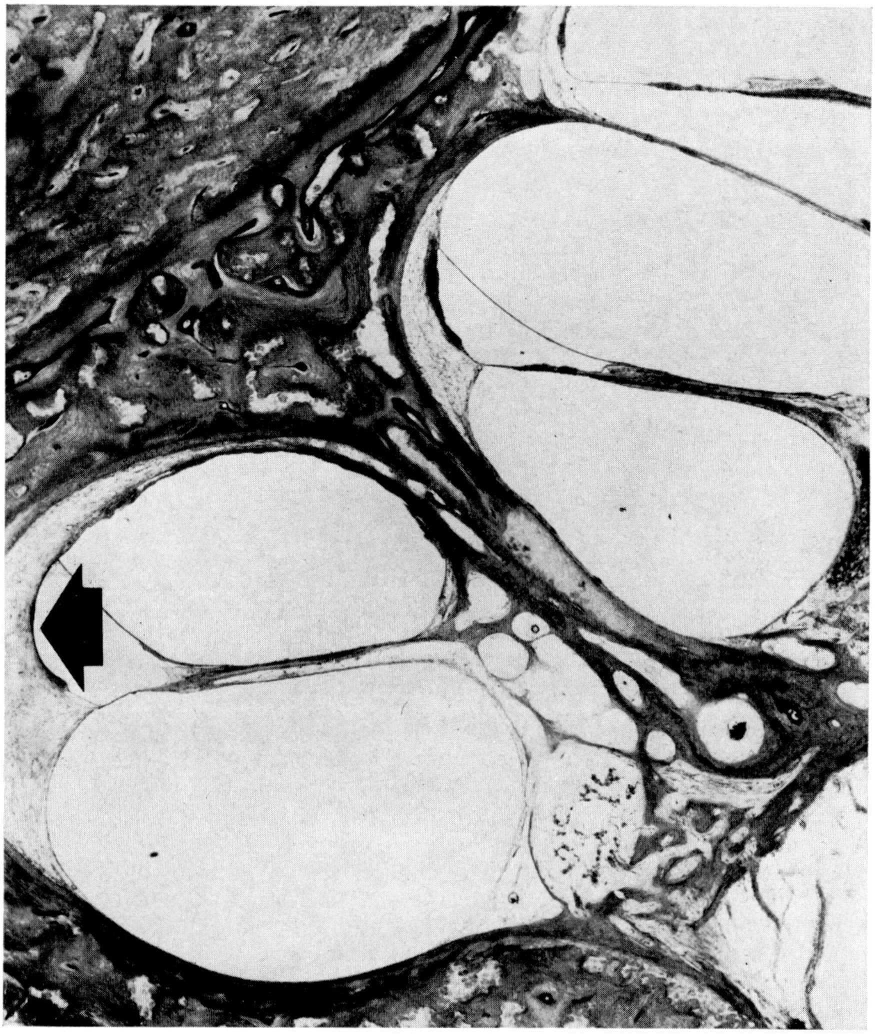

Fig. 8. Temporal bone pathology (PM). Note strial atrophy (arrow).

tion; and loss of ganglion cells more marked in the basal turn.

The pathological correlate of atrophy of the stria vascularis has been described and substantiated by Schuknecht and Ishii[22] in cases of presbycusis. In a study of nine patients with slowly progressive hearing loss and flat audiometric patterns, they established the finding of atrophy of the stria vascularis. They attributed the uniform involvement of all frequencies to biochemical and bioelectrical alterations in endolymph. In 1974, Schuknecht described 160 ears from 101 individuals which showed slowly progressive hearing loss by history or audiograms and had no known cause for loss by history or examination. Strial atrophy was thought to be the principal lesion in 52 ears of 35 individuals.[23]

We analyzed our temporal bone collection for older patients with no hearing loss or with no apparent explanation for their hearing loss, such as infection or trauma. One hundred and thirty-five cases were studied of patients older than 45 years of age, includ-

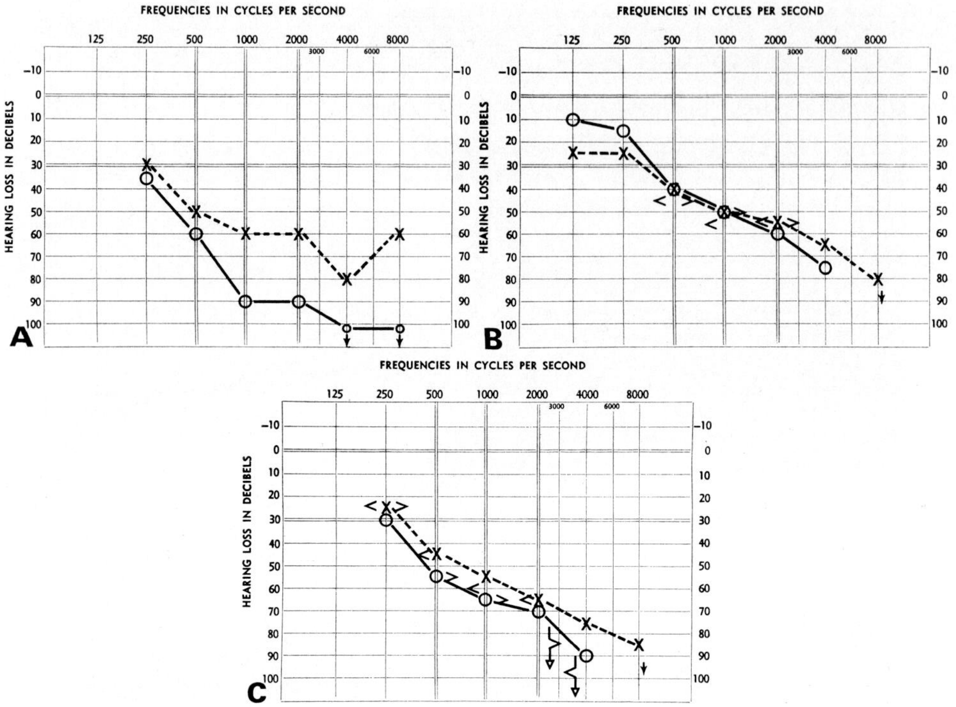

Fig. 9. A) Audiogram (P.M.) B) Audiogram (I.K.) C) Audiogram (C.B.)

ing 115 cases in patients 60 years or older. The pathological features are summarized according to findings in the stria vascularis and other changes (Fig. 8). Temporal bones of 21 cases showed pathological changes including changes of the cochlear duct, organ of Corti, ganglion cells, and stria vascularis. Thirteen cases showed bilateral pathology. Atrophy of the stria vascularis was seen in 18 cases and appeared marked or severe in seven cases. "Severe" refers to complete absence of the three layers of the stria vascularis in one or more cochlear turns. "Moderate" refers to atrophy of the epithelial or middle layer of the stria in one or more turns. In addition to these pathological findings, audiograms were available on some patients (Figs. 9A, B, C, 10, and 11).

DISCUSSION

It is our belief that genetic hearing loss is far more prevalent in adults than is currently realized. In the practice of medicine every attempt should be made to diagnose a disease or disorder according to etiology before steps are taken toward treatment or rehabilitation. It is our firm conviction that too many adult patients with sensorineural hearing loss are not properly diagnosed and are unaware of the nature of their problem or its potential effect on offspring in future generations. In the diagnosis of progressive sensorineural hearing loss, every attempt should be made to identify extrinsic causative factors. Having done so, we are left with the likelihood of an intrinsic problem, and genetic hearing loss should strongly be considered.

Our study indicates that the two most important diagnostic considerations are the history and the audiometric configuration, including audiometric changes over time. The history, with all of its imperfections, is still our most important tool. Genetic hearing loss associated with other abnormalities (syndromes) is more easily identified than

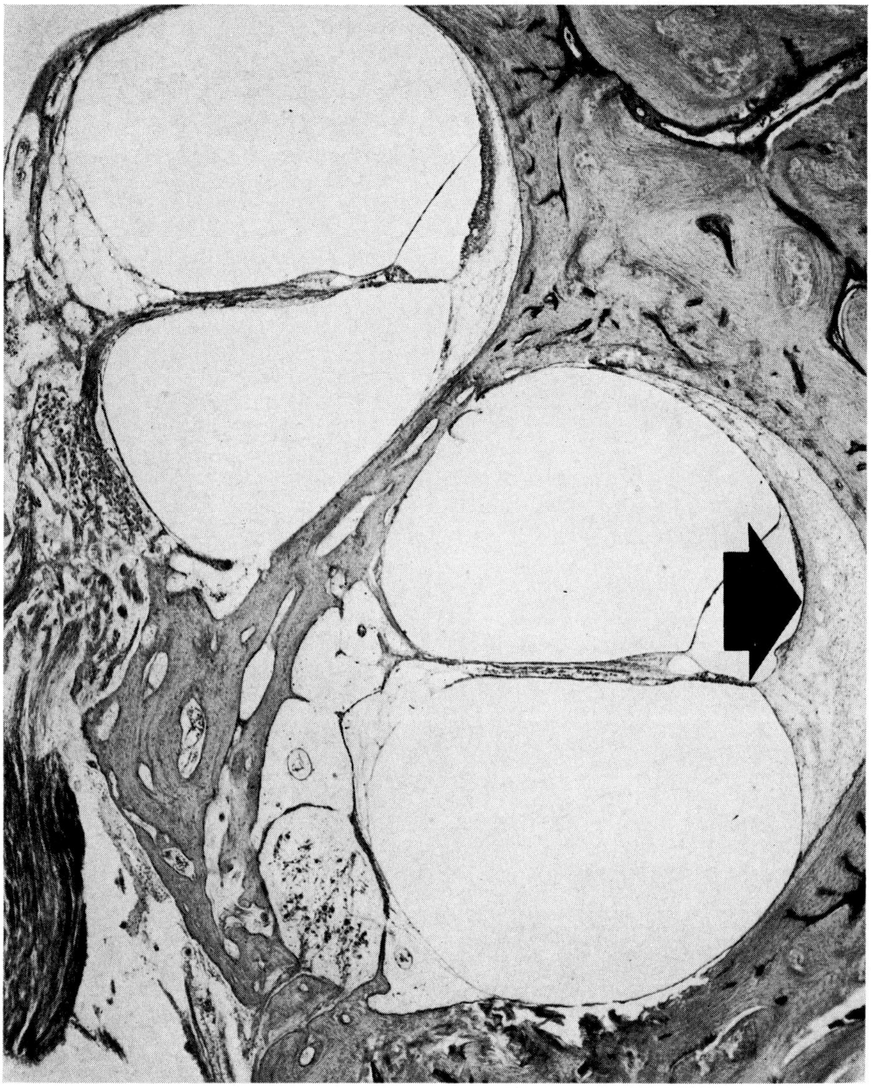

Fig. 10. Temporal bone pathology. Note strial atrophy in basal turn (arrow).

genetic hearing loss occurring alone. This latter category, although more nebulous, represents by far the most common type of genetic adult hearing loss. A positive family history is, of course, helpful, but a negative family history does not preclude the diagnosis of genetic hearing loss because of such considerations as lack of information or forgetfulness on the part of the patient, lack of penetrance, and mutations occurring over generations. Also, although otosclerosis is the best understood example of adult genetic hearing loss, it is not uncommon to have a confirmed diagnosis at the time of surgery with no family history of involvement.

The audiometric picture is a flat or basin-shaped curve with fairly good discrimination. A very interesting and important observation in our patients is that patients in the early course of their problem may demonstrate a predominant low-or high-frequency loss,

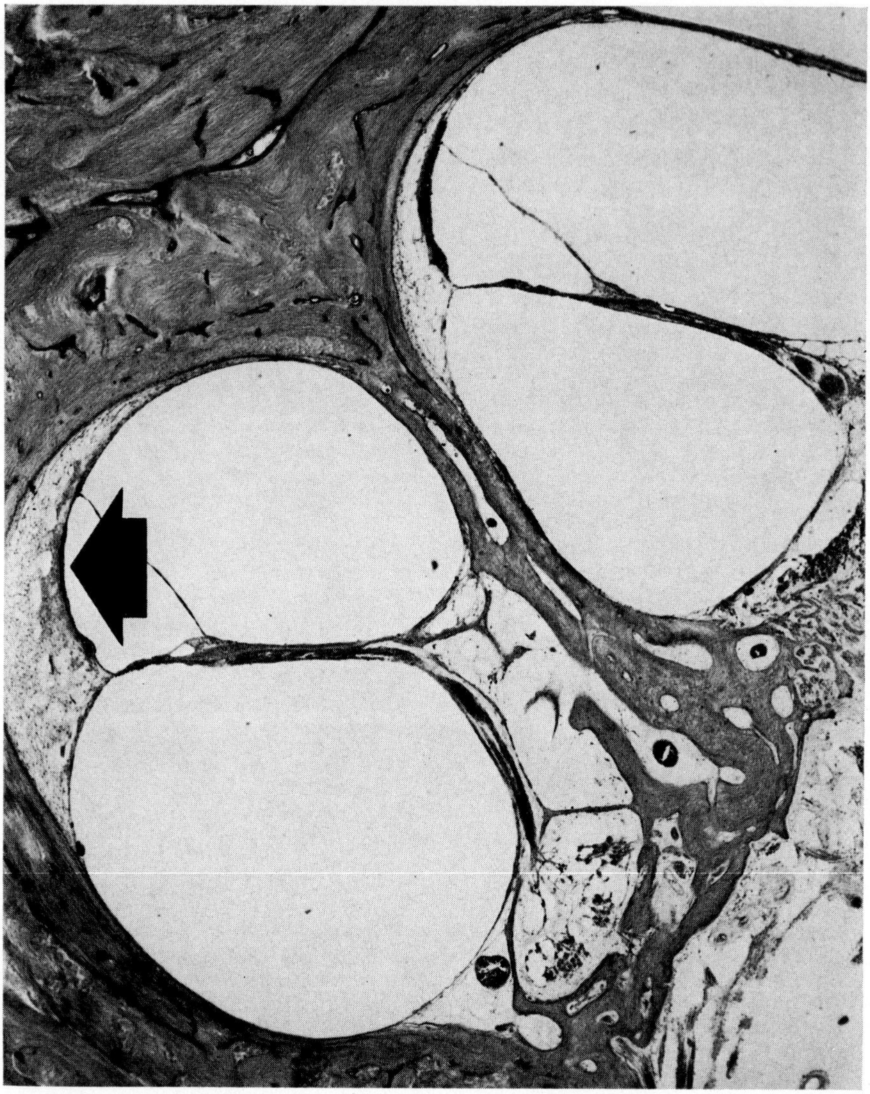

Fig. 11. Temporal bone pathology. Note strial atrophy in basal turn (arrow).

but over a period of time, a flat audiometric pattern evolves. If this finding is confirmed, it has diagnostic significance. It might be added here that patients with genetic hearing loss are subject to all of the environmental factors which affect anyone else. Thus, as the patient grows older, there is no reason, for example, that the effects of environmental noise cannot superimpose themselves on a genetically induced loss, thus altering the audiogram.

Presbycusis is not the specific subject of this discussion, but it relates to it. The term "presbycusis" is a nondescriptive catch all term referring to the vague concept of aging deafness. It is too easy to categorize hearing loss in older patients as "presbycusis," thus negating the need to apply careful, differential diagnostic methods as we are more apt to do for younger patients. Hopefully, some day we will be able to retire the term "presbycusis" with its due dignity, allowing health professionals to properly diagnose sensorineural hearing loss in older adults according to extrinsic or intrinsic etiologies as is done with all other patients. Genetic, adult sensorineural hearing loss can become manifest as a hearing problem at any age; childhood, younger, middle, or old adulthood. In all cases, the initial onset of hearing loss occurs years prior to the patient's complaint because of the insidiously progressive nature of its occurrence. In this study, we concentrate on genetic hearing loss in young adulthood, recognizing that these patients could be identified as having presbycusis later in life. Indeed, Cawthorne and Hinchcliffe employed the term "abiotrophy" referring to premature presbycusis although he fully understood this to be a manifestation of genetic hearing loss.[24]

This study is largely exploratory in nature and suggests the need for more definite studies of genetic sensorineural hearing loss in adults of all ages, including, especially, those currently diagnosed as "presbycusis." Laboratory studies would be beneficial, but there is a more urgent need for clinical, otological, and audiological studies. In the meantime, as diagnosticians concerned with the hearing welfare of our patients, we should consider genetic hearing loss in every patient with progressive sensorineural hearing loss accompanied by a flat or relatively flat audiometric pattern.

Request for reprints should be sent to Michael M. Paparella, M.D., Dept. of Otolaryngology, University of Minnesota Medical School, Minneapolis, Minnesota 55455.

REFERENCES

1. *Characteristics of Persons with Impaired Hearing.* United States Ser 10:No. 48, National Center for Vital and Health Statistics, November, 1968

2. Zwaardemaker: Ueber das presbyakustische Gesitz an der unteren Grenze unseres Gehoers. Arch Klin Exp Ohren Nasen Kehlkopfheilkd: 35:299, 1893

3. Chung CS, Robinson OW, Morton NE: A note on deaf mutism. Ann Hum Genet 23:357-366, 1959

4. Sank D, Kallman FJ: The role of heredity in total deafness. Volta Rev 68:461-470, 1963

5. Konigsmark BW: Hereditary deafness in man. N Engl J Med 281:713-720, 1969

6. Konigsmark BW, Gorlin RJ: *Hereditary Deafness and Deafness Syndromes.* To be published, 1975

7. Albrecht W: Über die Vererbung der konstitutionell sporadischen Taubstummheit der hereditären labyrinthschwer Hörigkeit und der Otoscleroses. Arch Klin Exp Ohren Nasen Kehlkopfheilkd 110:15-48, 1923

8. Stephens FE, Dolowitz DA: Hereditary nerve deafness. Am J Hum Genet 1:37-51, 1949

9. Johnsen S: The heredity of perceptive deafness. Acta Otolaryngol (Stockh) 42:539-552, 1952

10. Huizing EH, van Bolhuis AH, Odenthal DW: Studies on progressive hereditary perceptive deafness in a family of 355 members. Acta Otolaryngol (Stockh) 61:35-41, 161-167, 1966

11. Lenzi P: Sulle sordità ereditarie (studio genetico e clinico di un ceppo familiare). Arch Ital Otol 80:453-485, 1969

12. Nance WE, Sweeney A: Genetic factors in deafness of early life. Otolaryngol Clin North Am 8:1, 19-48, 1975

13. Teig E: Hereditary progressive perceptive deafness. Acta Otolaryngol (Stockh) 65:365-372, 1968

14. Konigsmark BW, Mengal MC, Berlin CI: Familial low frequency hearing loss. Laryngoscope 81:759-771, 1971

15. Vanderbilt University Hereditary Deafness Study Group: Dominantly inherited low-frequency hearing loss. Arch Otolaryngol 88: 242-250, 1968

16. Mårtensson B: Dominant hereditary nerve deafness. Acta Otolaryngol (Stockh) 52:270-274, 1960

17. Williams F, Roblee LA: Hereditary nerve deafness. Arch Otolaryngol 75:69-77, 1962

18. Konigsmark BW, Salman S, Haskins H, *et al*: Dominant midfrequency hearing loss. Ann Otol Rhinol Laryngol 79:42-54, 1970

19. Mohr J, Mayeray K: Sex-linked deafness of a possibly new type. Acta Genet (Basel) 10:54-62, 1960

20. Livan M: Contributo alla conoscenza dula sordità ereditarie. Arch Ital Otol 72:331-339, 1961

21. Paparella MM, Sugiura S, Hoshinot: Familial progressive sensorineural deafness. Arch Otolaryngol 90:44-51, 1969

22. Schuknecht HF, Ishii T: Hearing loss caused by atrophy of the stria vascularis. J Otol Jap 69:1825-1833, 1966

23. Schuknecht HF: Atrophy of the stria vascularis, a common cause for hearing loss. Laryngoscope 84:10, 1777-1821, 1974

24. Cawthrone TE, Hinchcliffe R: Familial perceptive deafness. Pract Otorhinolaryngol (Basel) 19:69-83, 1957

XIII INTERNATIONAL CONGRESS OF AUDIOLOGY

The XIII International Congress of Audiology under the auspices of the International Society of Audiology will be held October 18-21, 1976 in Florence, Italy. For information write: Fondazione Giovanni Lorenzini, Via G. Lorenzini, 2 (ex via Brembo, 65) 20139 - Milano.

COSMETIC SURGERY OF THE NOSE AND FACE

The First Panamerican Course of Cosmetic Surgery of the Nose and Face, sponsored by the Panamerican Association of Otolaryngology will be held February 12-17, 1976 at the Intercontinental Hotel, Medellin, Colombia, South America. For further information write: Dr. Jaime Florez, 4220 Central Ave., St. Petersburg, Florida 33711.

CERVICAL LYMPHONODE METASTASIS

An International Symposium on Cervical Lymphonode Metastasis will be held in Milan, Italy November 24-28, 1975, sponsored by Gruppo Italiano Oncologia Cervico-cefalica della Società Italiana di Cancerologia; Institut "Gustave-Roussy", Villejuif, France; Clinica Otorinolaringologica dell'Università di Milano; Instituto Nazionale per lo Studio e la Cura dei Tumori, Milano.

For information write: Miss Lucia Manfredi, Ufficio Attività Didattiche, Instituto Nazionale per lo Studio e la Cura dei Tumori, Via G. Venezian, 1, 20133, Milan, Italy.

Ann Otol 84: 1975

OPERATIVE TREATMENT OF SURGICAL LESIONS WITH OBJECTIVE TINNITUS

Paul H. Ward, M.D. Richard Babin, M.D.
Thomas C. Calcaterra, M.D. H. R. Konrad, M.D.
Los Angeles, California

SUMMARY – This article discusses the importance of the evaluation and diagnosis of objective tinnitus (tinnitus heard by the patient and the physician). Intracranial arteriovenous communications and vascular anomalies are most frequently responsible for the tinnitus and auscultable bruits and are highly amenable to current surgical treatment. While the otolaryngologists may initially see these patients and be responsible for the diagnosis of their problem, the surgical correction of the intracranial lesions is usually the province of the neurosurgeon. Illustrative cases of extracranial causes are presented. Particular emphasis is placed on the diagnosis and treatment of venous hum. Formerly called cephalic bruit and essential objective tinnitus, venous hum is now a recognized nosological entity that is amenable to treatment by ligation of the internal jugular vein.

Tinnitus at a subliminal level is common to all of us. Ringing, roaring, hissing, or other noise sensations are experienced whenever we listen for them in quiet surroundings or place a seashell over our ear. The etiology of the tinnitus as a chief complaint often defies elucidation even after extensive medical evaluation. The small group of cases of objective tinnitus, that is, where the physician can also appreciate by ascultation the presence of this symptom or sign, is of great importance. Accurate diagnosis in these cases is essential since most objective tinnitus is amenable to therapy, and in some instances, failure to treat the cause appropriately can lead to progression of the disease responsible for the symptom. The successful treatment of the various causes of objective tinnitus depends upon a thorough understanding of the anatomy and physiology involved and may require the cooperative efforts of several disciplines, especially true in the vascular causes.

Objective tinitus in the broadest sense represents all noise produced by an individual's body which is loud enough to impinge on his consciousness. It differs from the more common intrinsic tinnitus in that it represents true sound wave energy, rather than just a sound sensation. Body sounds under normal circumstances are sublimated by many factors, including structural considerations in the middle ear and the skull, cochlear thresholds and adaptation, and the projection of sound energy away from the temporal bone. These mechanisms can break down in several ways: by an increase in the perception of a normal sound, by an increased intensity of normal sounds, or by the production of abnormal sounds. If either of the latter two occurs, a tinnitus results which may be documented by another observer, a phonocardiogram, or a tape recorder. It is amazing how little we are aware of the numerous body vibrations secondary to muscular activity,

----

From The Department of Surgery/Division of Head and Neck Surgery, The University of California School of Medicine, Los Angeles, California.

This work was supported in part by Grant USPHS #NS09823-04

Presented at the meeting of the American Otological Society, Inc., Atlanta, Georgia, April 11-12, 1975.

joint motion, respirations, voice, and vascular pulsations. All of these sounds in the close vicinity of the ear, comprise an ever-present baseline noise level. Remarkably sophisticated mechanisms have evolved in man which attenuate this high level of persisent noise input into the ear. Whether the failure to perceive this noise is due to peripheral factors or to central adaptation is not known.

The generation of objective tinnitus appears to be due either to increase in the loudness of normal sounds or to the production of abnormal sounds. The latter problem will be considered first.

The Production of Abnormal Sounds. The most common cause of objective tinnitus of the vascular type is an arteriovenous (A-V) malformation in the posterior fossa.[1] Usually branches of the occipital artery and transverse sinus are involved since there are numerous communications between these vessels. Frequently no history of trauma precedes their presentation. Branches of the internal carotid artery and vertebral artery may also produce A-V fistulae. Less common causes of arterial objective tinnitus include: vascular abnormalities in the middle fossa between the posterior branches of the middle meningeal artery and the greater petrosal sinus; cervical lesions between the internal maxillary artery and vein and cerebral angiomas; cervical and cerebral angiomas; and giant cell tumors of the mandible. Infrequent, but of serious importance, are the arteriovenous communications between the internal carotid artery and the cavernous sinuses, which almost always follow severe head trauma.

The pulsatile tinnitus in these cases is noted by the patient and physician and palpation often reveals a significant bruit. Headaches are a frequently associated complaint when the lesion is intracranial. Approximately 50% of the patients will have nonlocalizing neurologic signs, such as papilledema. In a small percentage of patients with pulsatile mass behind the ear, the tinnitus may be reduced by pressure over the lesion or by compression of the carotid artery. If the left to right shunt is sufficiently large, a high output failure syndrome may result. In such cases, pressure over the lesion may dramatically reduce the tachycardia that is part of the syndrome.

Elucidation of the underlying lesion responsible for the tinnitus and the planning of definitive therapy is dependent upon good selective angiography. If a single branch of the external carotid system is involved, ligation of this vessel and excision of the lesion should eradicate the symptoms. If the internal carotid also contributes to the tinnitus, the symptoms may be expected to return as the secondary system dilates and flow increases. If the vertebral system is involved as well, only extensive ligation of feeding vessels and excision of the communicating vessels can be expected to eliminate the problem. As a general rule, the vascular malformation at surgery is considerably more extensive than it appeared to be on arteriography. Complications of these lesions include high output cardiac failure, neurological defects, intracranial hemorrhage and bleeding diathesis secondary to intercapillary coagulopathy, and fibrinolysis.

Other less common causes of an objective tinnitus are atheroscleromatous plaque in the carotid arteries and Eagle's syndrome (elongated styloid process or calcified styloid-hyoid ligament). This latter condition was first implicated in a cephalofacial pain syndrome involving the distribution of either the external or internal carotids frequently following tonsillectomy.[2] More recently it has been described as a cause of a bruit in the same distribution and objective tinnitus, relieved by excision of the styloid process.[3]

In 1872 Polizer described a patient with pulsatile objective tinnitus associated with rhythmic contractions of the soft palate.[4] Since that time, objective tinnitus has been documented from myoclonic contractions of the tensor vili palatini, the levator vili palatini; the tensor tympani with associated movement of the tympanic membrane, and the salpingopharyngeus and superior constrictor muscles. Less frequently the orbicularis occuli, laryngeal musculature, and diaphragm are involved. Such contractions usually range from 60-200 Hz and thus may be confused with a vascular pulse. Patients are classically young, being in their first three decades of life; older patients within their fourth through eight decades have been reported.[4,5] They often had other associated significant neurologic problems. The vibrations responsible for the audible sounds appear to be produced by movement of the Eustachian tube orifice. The audible click in some patients is synchronous with the relaxation phase of the myoclonus, the closure at the tube orifice, and an increase in the intratubal manometric pressure.[6]

The etiology of palatal myoclonus has been ascribed to brainstem infarctions, trauma, multiple sclerosis, syphilis, malaria, and neuroses. Specific lesions have been described in the olivary tracts, reticular formation, dentate nucleus, posterior longitudinal bundle, and central tegmental fasciculi.[4,7] Unlike many involuntary movements, palatal myoclonus usually doesn't disappear with natural or barbiturate-induced sleep, coma, hemiplegia, phonation, or caloric stimulation.[8,9] It may disappear with deep inspiration. It may also temporarily disappear on opening the mouth widely, thereby making the diagnosis difficult for those unfamiliar with this entity. Muscle relaxants, decongestants, tranquilizers, psychotherapy, cervical traction, and hypnosis have all been employed with varying therapeutic response. Section of the levator veli palatini muscle and eliciting contraction of this muscle by blowing cold air on the cornea have successfully eradicated the click. Corneal reflexes have been previously shown to stimulate atonic contraction of the tensor tympani.

Increased Loudness of Normal Sounds. One of the most important causes of objective tinnitus that the otolaryngologist should become more familiar with is the venous hum. This entity is continually rediscovered and discussed extensively in the otolaryngology literature under the name of cephalic murmur or essential objective tinnitus (the *essential* implying no cause should be found).[10-14] Hentzer reported 13 out of 24 patients with vascular objective tinnitus were of this type.[14]

It has remained for others to better document and determine the probable etiology of the venous hum.[15-16] Venous hum occurs normally and can be heard over the fontanelle of infants, in the necks of many children, and in some adults. It may be more pronounced in states of increased cardiac output such as thyrotoxicosis, anemia, and pregnancy. In one case, a venous hum in the neck was the clue to an A-V fistula in the posterior fossa with its own separate bruit.[15] Although technically a continuous murmur, it is usually reinforced by arterial flow and appears to the observer and patient as a pulsatile sound synchronous with systole.[17] Venous hum of the neck is characteristically intensified by deep breathing and reduced by the valsalva maneuver. Turning the head toward the opposite side increases the hum. Two factors may be responsible for this. Ipsilateral contraction of the sternomastoid muscle opens the effective bore of the internal jugular vein, increasing return on that side. Furthermore, it has been shown that the hum may be due to the turbulent flow in the internal jugular vein as it bends around the transverse process of the atlas. This angulation is markedly increased as the head is held to the contralateral side.[16] The sound is decreased by turning the head to the ipsilateral side (reducing agulation and venous return) or by pressure on the neck too light to occlude the carotid artery but occluding the internal jugular vein.

Venous tinnitus may be differentiated from arterial bruits by its dependence on head position and sensitivity to light pressure. A normal cerebral arteriogram is essential to the definitive diagnosis in order to rule out other isolated or coexistent vascular anomalies. Another im-

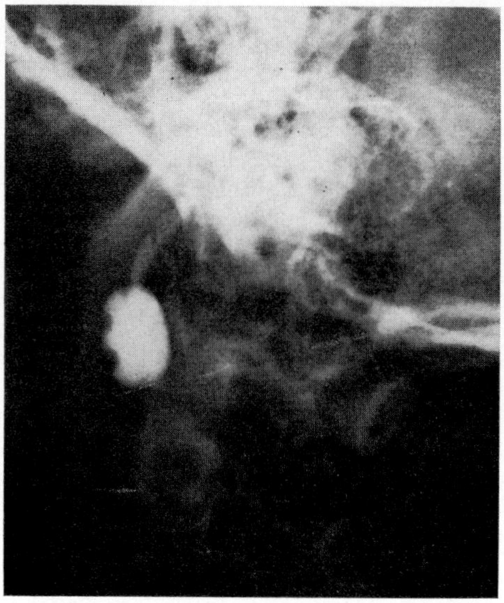

Fig. 1. X-ray of retrograde internal jugular venogram with Fogerty catheter balloon inflated with opaque material. The catheter balloon can be inflated at different levels to determine the optimal level for ligation. In this patient the venous hum was controlled best when the balloon was inflated at the level of the second cervical vertebra.

portant negative study is venous O_2 saturation (which may be done at the time of a retrograde venogram) which may be normal or show a preponderance of cerebral venous drainage to the ipsilateral side. A new test of value used to predict the optimum level of obstruction to eradicate the tinnitus is shown in Figure 1. A Fogerty catheter with a balloon is used to perform the retrograde venogram. The balloon is inflated at different levels in the internal jugular vein in order to detect the optimal level for ligation.

While venous hums have been reported to spontaneously regress, none of the patients currently being followed in our series have experienced this phenomena. In patients with severe tinnitus, particularly when it is so loud that it keeps the companion awake, (as in one of the cases to be presented) the simple ligation of the jugular vein appears warranted. The dramatic decrease or cessation of the tinnitus and bruit following ligation is usually permanent although it has been reported to reappear in some patients.[14] The use of a prosthetic device which provides a constant light pressure on the jugular vein was reported in one case by Cary.[18] With or without therapy, the prognosis is better for this group of patients than that of the arterial group.

CASE REPORTS

The common intracranial arterial abnormalities which are responsible for objective tinnitus, while often diagnosed by the otolaryngologist, are usually within the surgical province of the neurosurgeon, so they will not be presented here. The following are informative and illustrative examples of some of the types of problem cases with extracranial objective tinnitus recently managed successfully and unsuccessfully as reported.

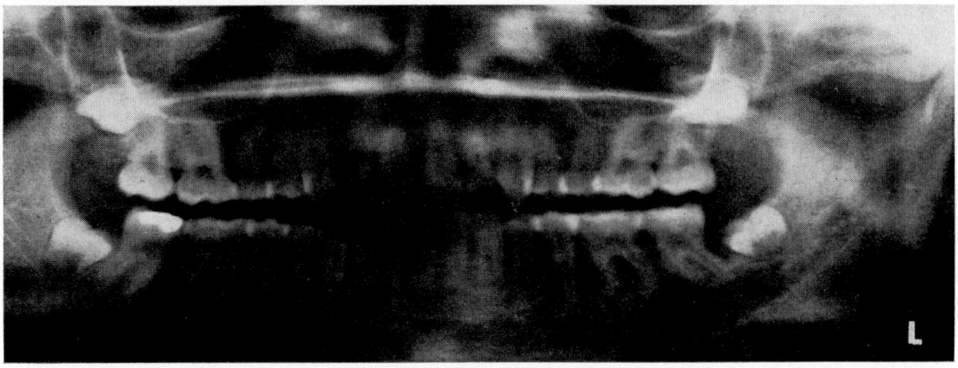

Fig. 2. Panorex x-ray of patient with objective tinnitus caused by a large arteriovenous abnormality eroding the mandible on the left side.

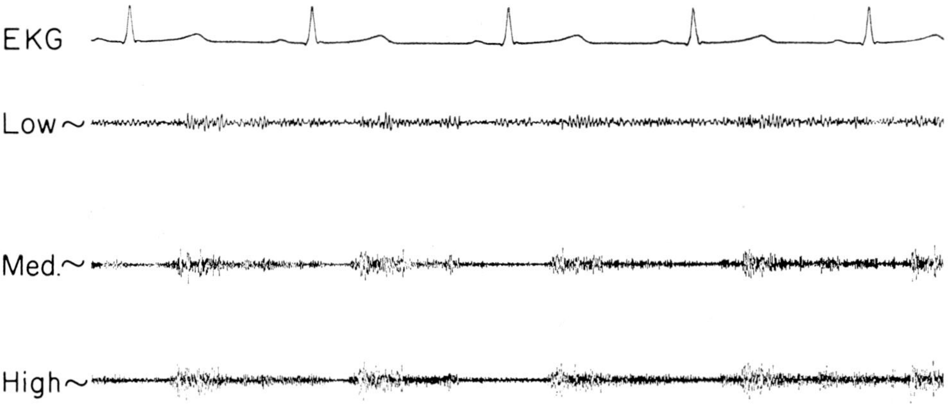

Fig. 3. Photograph of phonocardiograph of bruit emanating from A-V malformations in mandible of Case No. 1. Recording taken in front of left ear shows continuous bruit and the various low, medium, and high frequency components.

Case 1. A 16-year-old Caucasian female had been in good health all her life until approximately one year ago when she noted pain in the first molar tooth on the left and pulsatile tinnitus initially lasting for just a few seconds following vigorous exercise. She also noted bleeding of the peridontal tissue on this side of the mouth.

General physical examination was within normal limits. She had dilated vessels on the left anterior floor of the mouth. No pulsatile lesions were palpable. Auscultation revealed a loud continuous machinery-type bruit heard over the mastoid tip, angle of the mandible, and submental area. Examination of the ears was within normal limits. A panorex x-ray of the mandible showed extensive erosion of the mandibular canal on the left side (Fig. 2). This bruit was recorded by phonocardiography for illustrative purposes (Fig. 3).

Bilateral external and left internal carotid arteriography showed a left mandibular lesion consistent with an A-V malformation with blood supply predominantly from the left facial artery and internal maxillary and minimal supply from the right facial artery. Following arteriography, the patient underwent embolization of both external facial arteries with Gelfoam.®* The left internal maxillary artery had an unfavorable origin and could not be embolized. The patient tolerated this procedure well and had immediate cessation of pulsatile tinnitus. The facial and mastoid bruit could no longer be heard. She did well for several weeks but there was a gradual return of the tinnitus and bruit. She had repeated arteriograms with three additional embolizations with Gelfoam,® followed by plastic spherules during the ensuing seven months after increase in the size of the malformation and bone destruction was noted. In view of the initial success in eradication of the tinnitus and bruit, it was elected to obliterate the vessels permanently with ferromagnetic Silastic®** embolization. This material is held in place by a powerful electromagnet until vulcanization occurs. This procedure was complicated by some of the material entering the tissues of the cheek with resulting mottling of the skin. The patient had several teeth extracted, and her bruit persists. Additional obliterative procedures are contemplated prior to surgical resection, if it becomes necessary.

Case 2. A 34-year-old, mildly obese, Caucasian female presented with a six-week history of pulsatile tinnitus in the left ear and a three-week history of an enlarging neck mass below and around the left ear. The patient related she had had sustained neck trauma during her most recent delivery (by forceps) but had previously noted only transient pain and a few prominent blood vessels on her left neck. She was five months pregnant at the onset of the tinnitus and had had six previous pregnancies, two full term without similar symptoms. There was no history compatible with heart failure or a coagulopathy.

Physical examination revealed a 5 x 7 cm soft mass lesion overlying the left mastoid and upper sternocleidomastoid muscle. There was a diffuse telangiectasia in the skin overlying the mass (Fig. 4). A thrill could be palpated and a loud systolic bruit could be auscultated over the mass and the left ear, which was diminished by pressure over the carotid. The tympanic membranes were clear and freely movable bilaterally and the remainder of the patient's examination was unremarkable. Her blood pressure was 106/78; pulse, 80 and regular; the hematocrit, 32%. After consultation

* The Upjohn Co., Kalamazoo, Mich.
** Dow-Corning Chem. Co., Medical Products Div., Midland, Mich.

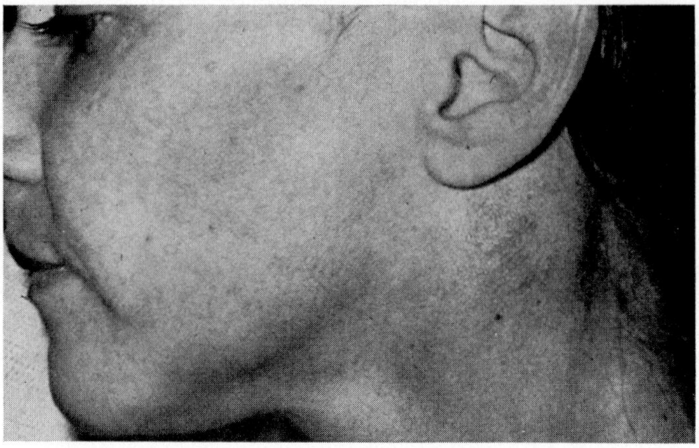

Fig. 4. Photograph of patient with large 5 x 7 cm compressible vascular mass of neck.

with the cardiologist and obstetrician, a left carotid arteriogram was performed. On selective catheterization of the external carotid, a diffuse, large vascular blush was seen along the left aspect of the neck (Fig. 5). The venous phase-emptying channels and vertebral and internal carotid arteries were normal. Skull and cervical spine x-rays were normal. Open biopsy revealed a capillary hemangioma.

By the eighth month of gestation, the mass was 5 x 10 cm, a grade II/VI systolic ejection murmur had appeared at the carotid base, and the tinnitus was more severe. Four months postpartum, the mass was 4 x 5 cm, the telangiectasia had faded considerably, and the tinnitus was gone. The patient was last seen two and one-half years postpartum and with the continued decrease in the size of the mass, she declined elective removal.

Case 3. A 32-year-old female entered with a chief complaint that the ringing in her right ear kept her husband awake at night. The ringing had been present for 18 months and followed a blow to the right mastoid area by a baseball. After the accident the patient had a severe episode of vomiting at which time she stated that she heard a loud pop behind her right ear. The patient dated the onset of her tinnitus to both of these episodes. The patient described her noise as a loud, constant ringing noise which she could eliminate by rotating her head fully to the right or by direct

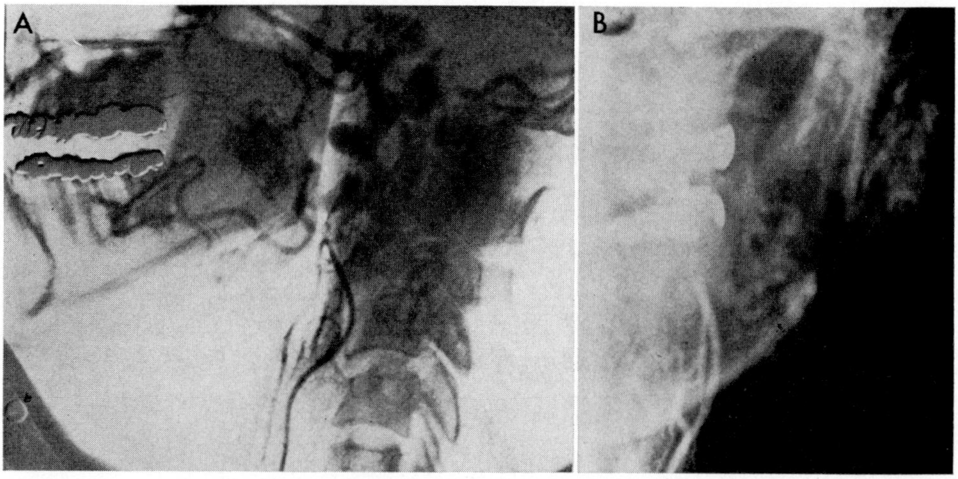

Fig. 5. Left lateral (A) and anterior posterior (B) arteriograms showing the vascular blush of the capillary hemangioma of patient (Case No. 2). Subtraction technique used in (A).

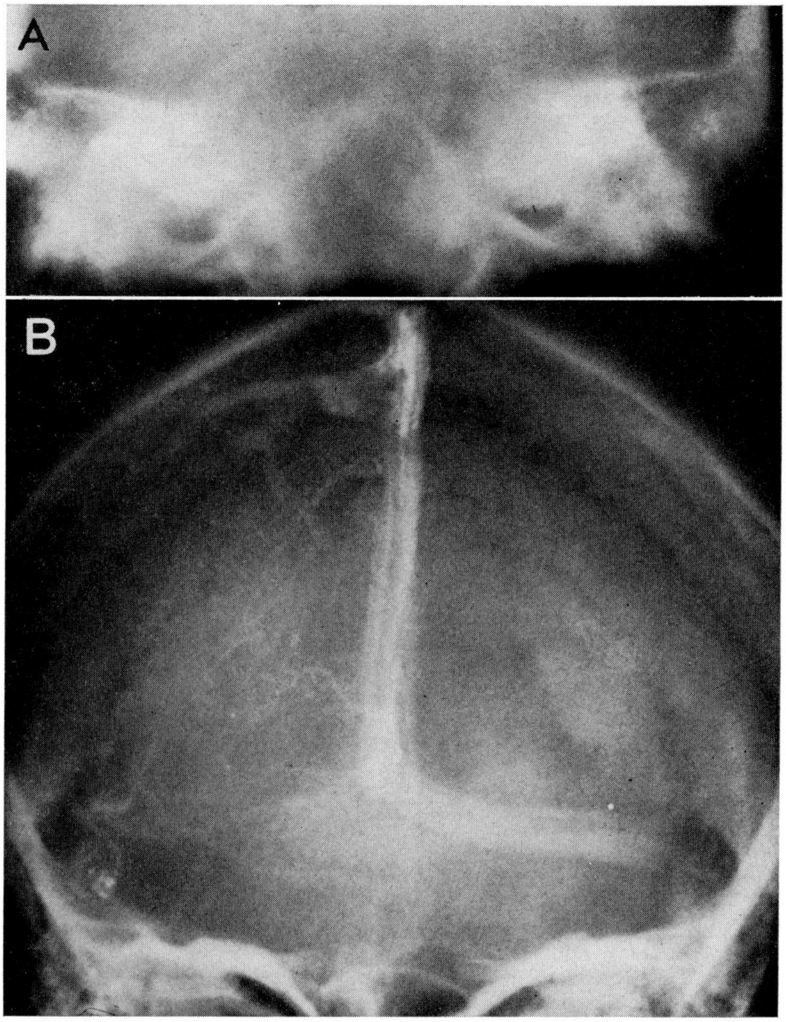

Fig. 6. Laminogram showing enlarged right jugular bulb (A) and retrograde venogram (B) showing dominant right venous drainage system (Case No. 4).

pressure behind the right ear.

Physical examination showed the ears to be normal. There was a high-pitched, pulsating bruit, loudest over the upper one-third of the sternocleidomastoid muscle and the mastoid tip. It could be stopped by mild compression over the sternocleidomastoid muscle. It was exacerbated by turning the head to the opposite side and was diminished by turning the head to the ipsilateral side. Bilateral external carotid, right internal carotid, and right internal maxillary arteriograms showed no abnormalities. A right jugular venogram was performed and was within normal limits. The A-V O_2 difference was within normal limits.

The patient was taken to the operating room, where under general anesthesia a microphone was placed in the right external ear canal and the left neck surgically explored. Selective occlusion of the external carotid, internal jugular vein, and right facial vein were performed independently. Each vessel appeared to decrease the bruit slightly. It was totally eradicated by ligation of the jugular vein. Postoperatively the objective component was no longer audible on auscultation. The patient continued, however, to have a minor subjective component. Two and one-half years after ligation she was doing well without complaints.

Case 4. A 40-year-old obese, Negro female was invovled in an automobile accident two years before her presentation, sustaining a fracture of her right arm and a ruptured spleen and liver. She did not receive any head trauma, and her postoperative course was complicated by pneumonia. Seven months thereafter, she noted the gradual onset of pulsatile tinnitus in her right ear. It was present first only at night. Later it became louder, and she learned that turning her head to the right stopped the noise. She began sleeping on her right side. The tinnitus was not affected by lying down. The patient denied ear infections, vertigo, or hypacusis. She had never been pregnant. The symptoms had gradually increased to the time of her presentation.

Physical examination was entirely normal except for a faint pulsatile sound present over the right mastoid and anterior neck. The tympanic membrane was normal and noted not to pulsate. The sound was eliminated by gentle pressure on the anterior neck or mastoid by turning the head to the right. It was increased when the head was turned to the left. An audiogram was essentially normal, and 75 dB of white noise was necessary to mask out the subjective tinnitus. Mastoid tomograms were normal. Arteriograms were normal and retrograde venogram revealed a dominant right drainage system (Fig. 6). There was concern of possible side effects of ligating the only major vessel of venous return. The patient declined ligation and has continued to live with her symptoms over the past year. The tinnitus and bruit have persisted at essentially the same level.

Case 5. This 35-year-old obese, Negro female underwent a left partial nephrectomy in November 1970 following which she noted blurring of vision, and left-sided constant tinnitus. The tinnitus increased and decreased in pitch and intensity during the day, unrelated to any activity. Generally, when the patient was emotionally upset, the noise increased in intensity. She also had had left frontal headaches intermittently, lasting for up to twelve hours.

An evaluation at another medical center showed bilateral papillaedema which was thought secondary to pseudotumor cerebri. A retrograde right brachial cerebral angiogram was interpreted as normal. The patient was advised to lose weight and was treated with oral glycerol without success. She was followed as an outpatient where evaluation showed inconsistent pure tone audiogram responses. She was thought to have essentially normal hearing on the right and a mild sensorineural loss on the left of cochlear origin. Her past history was unremarkable.

Physical examination showed a Negro female in no distress. Examination of the eyes showed slight blurring of the optic discs bilaterally with normal vasculature. On examination of the ears the tympanic membranes were normal, the Weber was midline, and the Rinne was positive bilaterally. Examination of the head and neck by auscultation revealed a continuous bruit of variable pitch and intensity heard best over the left mastoid tip. The bruit disappeared with light compression over the left upper sternocleidomastoid muscle. Rotating the head to the right side would increase the intensity of the bruit, while turning to the left would decrease the tinnitus. When compression over the left sternocleidomastoid caused objective loss of the bruit, subjectively the patient could still hear the tinnitus, although it had markedly decreased in intensity. From day to day the pitch and intensity varied, and on one occasion, the bruit could not be heard except when the patient was taken to a quiet room. The remainder of the physical examination was normal.

The pure tone audiogram showed symmetrical, mild neurosensory hearing loss. Impedance audiometry was within normal limits. The aural reflex was present bilaterally to broad band noise at 69 and 73 dB sound pressure levels. On arteriography there was no opacification of the right jugular vein. The contrast material was noted to drain from the paracervical venous plexus. A prominent right inferior petrossal sinus was noted. There was no opacification of the right sigmoid sinus. Mastoid tomograms were within normal limits; jugular foramina tomograms showed the left foramina to be larger than the right, but otherwise, unremarkable. An electrocardiogram (EKG) showed possible left ventricular hypertrophy. The left internal carotid PO_2 was 70.5. The left jugular vein PO_2 was 34.4.

Following the above procedure, a Fogerty catheter was introduced into the internal jugular vein to the level of the sigmoid sinus; the balloon was inflated and caused the patient's tinnitus to disappear at the level of the first cervical vertebrae. It is therefore considered that this patient will be a surgical candidate whenever she elects to have surgery.

DISCUSSION

Tinnitus is a bothersome and disturbing symptom for the patient and a perplexing problem for the physician. Patients have been known to become so upset by this symptom that they have committed suicide. Appropriate evaluation of patients with objective tinnitus is imperative since many of the lesions responsible for the symptoms are amenable to surgical correction. The diagnosis and surgical correction of many intra- and extracranial arteriovenous malformations is now possible with risks that are less than the potential complications of the untreated lesion (high output failure, hemorrhage, *etc.*). Careful historical data, physical examination with auscultation and x-rays are important; however, the definitive diagnosis rests upon good selective arteriograms and retrograde venograms.

When the communicating vessels between the arterial system and the venous system are capillaries, there is evidence to suggest that there is some hormone dependence or response. The successful use of steroids to treat hemangiomas in other areas and the decrease in the size of the mass following termination of pregnancy (Case No. 4) supports this concept.

The delineation of venous hum as a nosological entity, formerly called cephalic murmur or essential objective tinnitus, is important for it is an easily treatable lesion. The symptoms and signs are classical with increase in the tinnitus on turning the head to the opposite side and decrease of the tinnitus on turning the head to the same side or on performing a valsalva maneuver. Light pressure over the jugular eradicates the auscultable bruit.

The use of a Fogerty catheter with a balloon during performance of the retrograde venogram and the obstruction of the internal jugular at different levels appears to be a worthwhile diagnostic test. Since the tinnitus or bruit is believed to be caused by eddy currents, this test may indicate the optimal level for ligation of the jugular. Thus far, we have treated these patients with simple ligation of the jugular vein which can be performed under local anesthesia. They have all been informed that if this is unsucessful or if the symptoms return, a clipping of the lateral sinuses through a mastoid approach may be worthwhile.

In only one patient was the balloon test suggestive that obstruction in the sigmoid or lateral sinus would be more effective, and this patient refused surgery. In the patient shown in Figure 2, however, the tinnitus stopped only with occlusion at the body of C_2 and below. While the tinnitus has been reported to subside spontaneously, it has not done so in her case or in several others who been followed up to two years.

The immediate and dramatic improvement experienced in patients following ligation of the internal jugular vein commends its use in patients with venous hum.

Request for reprints should be sent to Paul H. Ward, M.D., Professor of Surgery, University of Calif. School of Medicine, The Center for the Health Sciences, Los Angeles, California 90024.

REFERENCES

1. Arenberg IK, McCreary HS: Objective tinnitus aurium and dural arteriovenous malformations of the posterior fossa. Ann Otol Rhinol Laryngol 80:111-120, 1972

2. Eagle WW: Elongated styloid process. Archives Otol 67:172-176, 1958

3. Cordier G, Garnier H, Durupt L, *el al*: Les allongements anormaux de l'apophyse styloide temprale avec retentissement carotidien. La Presse Medicinale 21 Jun 70 n° 30 p 1547

4. Herrmann C, Crandall PH, Fang HC: Palatal myoclonus — A new approach to the understanding of its production. Neurology 7: 37-51, 1957

5. Bjork H: Objective tinnitus due to clonus of the soft palate. Acta Otolaryngol [Suppl] (Stockh) 116:39-45, 1954

6. Pulec JL, Simonton KM: Palatal myoclonus — A report of two cases. Laryngoscope 71:668-671, 1961

7. Heller MF: Vitratory tinnitus and palatal myoclonus. Acta Otolaryngol (Stockh) 55: 292-298, 1962

8. MacKinnon DM: Objective tinnitus due to palatal myoclonus. J Laryngol Otol 82: 369-374, 1968

9. Quarry JG: Unilateral objective tinnitus a case and a cure. Arch Otolaryngol 96:252-253, 1972

10. Hamburger PL: Head murmurs. Am J Med Sci 181:756-762, 1931

11. Inglauer S: Objective tinnitus aurium. Four cases. Arch Otolaryngol 18:145-151, 1933

12. Bredlau EA: Objective tinnitus aurium. Arch Otolaryngol 28:193-198, 1938

13. Engstrom H, Graf W: On objective tinnitus and its recording. Acta Otolaryngol [Suppl] (Stockh) 95:127-184, 1950

14. Hentzer E: Objective tinnitus of the vascular type. Acta Otolaryngol (Stockh) 66: 273-281, 1968

15. Hardison JE: Cervical venous hum: A clue to the diagnosis of intercranial arteriovenous malformations. New Engl J Med 278: 587-590, 1968

16. Cutforth R, Wiseman J, Sutherland RD: The genesis of the cervical venous hum. Am Heart J 80:488-492, 1970

17. Graf T, Moller T, Mannheimer E: The continuous murmur. Acta Med Scan [Suppl] 196:167-191, 1962

18. Cary FH: Symptomatic venous hum. New Engl J Med 264:869-870, 1961

THIRD W. FRANKLIN KEIM MEMORIAL SEMINAR

The New Jersey Medical School and the United Hospitals Medical Center (Newark Eye and Ear Infirmary) will hold the Third W. Franklin Keim Memorial Seminar on Pathology and Treatment of Head and Neck Tumors October 2-4, 1975.

For further information, contact: Dr. Ki H. Han, United Hospitals Medical Center, 15 S. 9th Street, Newark, New Jersey 07107. Tel.: (201) 484-8000, Ext. 273 or 268.

GOULD FOUNDATION AWARD

The Gould Foundation announces that the recipient of the 1974 Gould Award is Dr. Masafumi Suzuki, Research Associate in the Section of Otolaryngology at Yale University School of Medicine. Dr. Suzuki is being honored for his basic contributions to laryngeal neurophysiology.

Ann Otol 84: 1975

EUSTACHIAN TUBE LYMPHATICS

JACK L. PULEC, M.D.

LOS ANGELES, CALIFORNIA

TOMOKAZU KAMIO, M.D.

TOKYO, JAPAN

MALCOLM D. GRAHAM, M.D.

LOS ANGELES, CALIFORNIA

SUMMARY — Serous otitis media is the most common cause of hearing impairment. The role of lymphatic obstruction in the pathogenesis of serous otitis media is significant. A method for removal of the human Eustachian tube specimen and two techniques for identification of Eustachian tube lymphatic capillaries are described. One involves the antemortem intratympanic installation of Berlin blue. The other utilizes electron microscopy. Lymphatic capillaries cannot be reliably differentiated from blood capillaries with the light microscope. With electron microscopy, lymphatic capillaries can be differentiated from blood capillaries by differences in the basement membrane. The lymphatic capillary has gaps in the basement membrane with large nuclei in the wall. A blood capillary has a continuous basement membrane and sometimes red blood cells can be identified in the lumen. Using these methods, Eustachian tube lymphatic capillaries in the human are described for the first time in this report.

Serous otitis media is the most common cause of hearing impairment, especially in children.[1,2] Despite the prominent role played by the lymphatics of the Eustachian tube in the pathogenesis of serous otitis media, they have not previously been demonstrated in the human. The gross and light microscopic anatomy of the human Eustachian tube has been well described.[3-10] Arnould[11] and Rouviére[12] described the lymphatics of the Eustachian tube which were presumed but not proved to be present. Robison[13-14] described how malignant tumors and infections of the nasopharynx, tonsil, and paranasal sinuses might cause middle ear effusion. He explained that their lymphatic drainage pathways converged on the lateral retropharyngeal nodes and that inflammation would cause blockage at this level, causing the lymphatics around the Eustachian tube isthmus to swell. Porta[15] and Ferriari and Zini[16] demonstrated the nasopharyngeal lymphatics around the Eustachian tube orifice in animals and man by utilizing injections of neoprene and latex. Lymphatic vessels in the middle ear and Eustachian tube of the guinea pig have recently been described by Haye[17] and Lim[9] using electron microscopy. The purpose of this paper is to describe two methods for the study of Eustachian tube lymphatic capillaries and to report for the first time their identification in the human.

METHODS AND MATERIALS

Temporal Bone Study. In order to study normal histology and the anatomic relationship of the Eustachian tube to surrounding structures and to establish a technique for the expedient removal of the Eustachian tube specimen along with the middle ear and a portion of the nasopharynx surrounding the tube orifice, 107 specimens were removed from fresh cadavers during necropsy.* With the skull cap and brain removed, incisions were

* The bones were removed and studied in the laboratories of the Los Angeles County Coroner, Dr. Thomas Noguchi.

From the Otologic Medical Group, Inc. and the Ear Research Institute, Los Angeles, California.

Presented at the meeting of the American Otological Society, Inc., Atlanta, Georgia, April 11-12, 1975.

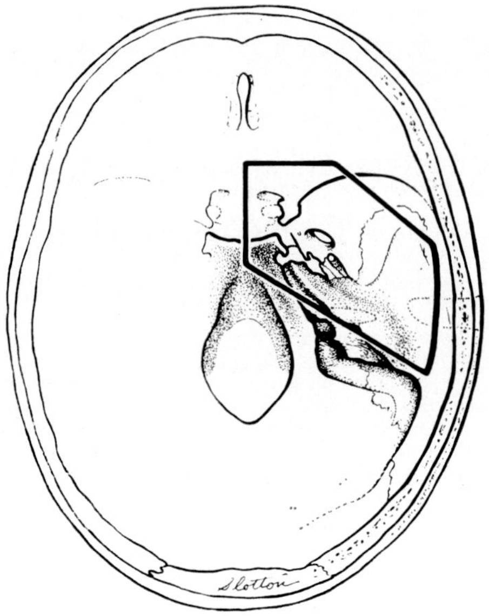

Fig. 1. Bone incisions for removal of Eustachian tube specimen with the temporal bone at necropsy.

developed (Fig. 1) which would provide a satisfactory specimen. We found it important that the anterior bony incision be at least 5 cm anterior to the anterior edge of the external auditory canal (EAC), which places it just anterior to the middle fossa. This cut, with a bone saw, is through the frontal fossa and through the posterior part of the orbit. A midline cut is made and extended back to the foramen magnum. A posterior cut through the posterior fossa in most cases extended through the skull, so that when the zygoma

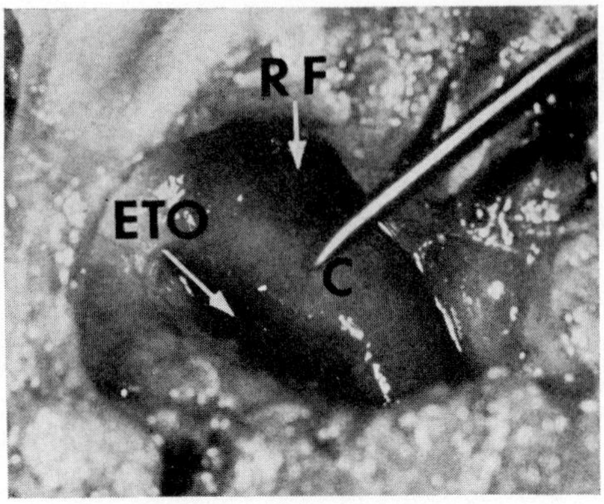

Fig. 3. Eustachian tube orifice (ETO) viewed from the nasopharynx. Rosenmueller's fossa (RF). Cartilage (C).

was transected the specimen included the entire mastoid. Ages at the time of death ranged from 7 weeks to 69 years. All bones were grossly normal and there was no history of otologic disease.

A variety of staining techniques were tried on the cadaver specimens without success, including the application of .5% hydrogen peroxide solution to the middle ear mucosa, the application of Berlin blue and India ink. Injection of the carotid arteries with Berlin blue was unsuccessful. Twenty-seven bones were dissected with the operating microscope in a search for the lymphatics as well as a study of anatomic relationships (Figs. 2A, B and 3). A method for removal of the mucous membrane from the entire length of the Eustachian tube was perfected in order to obtain specimens for light and electron transmission and scanning microscopy.

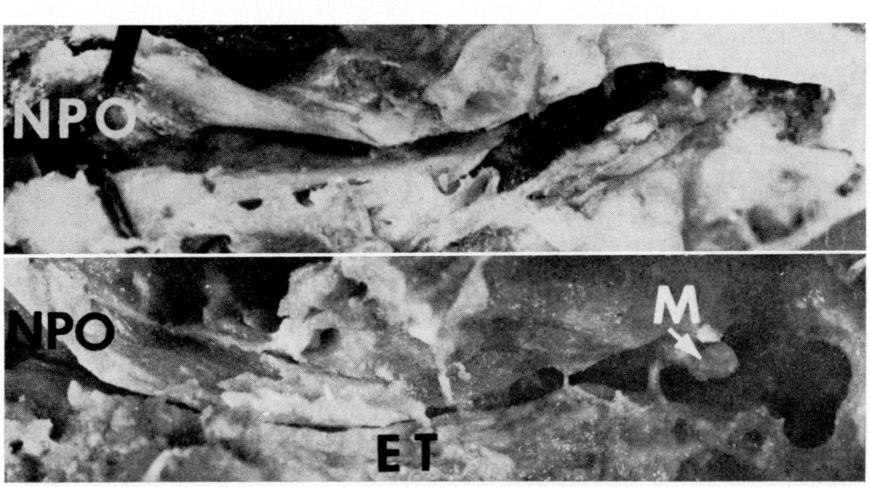

Fig. 2A and B. Gross specimen with Eustachian tube (ET) opened from above oriented to show the nasopharyngeal orifice (NPO) and malleus (M).

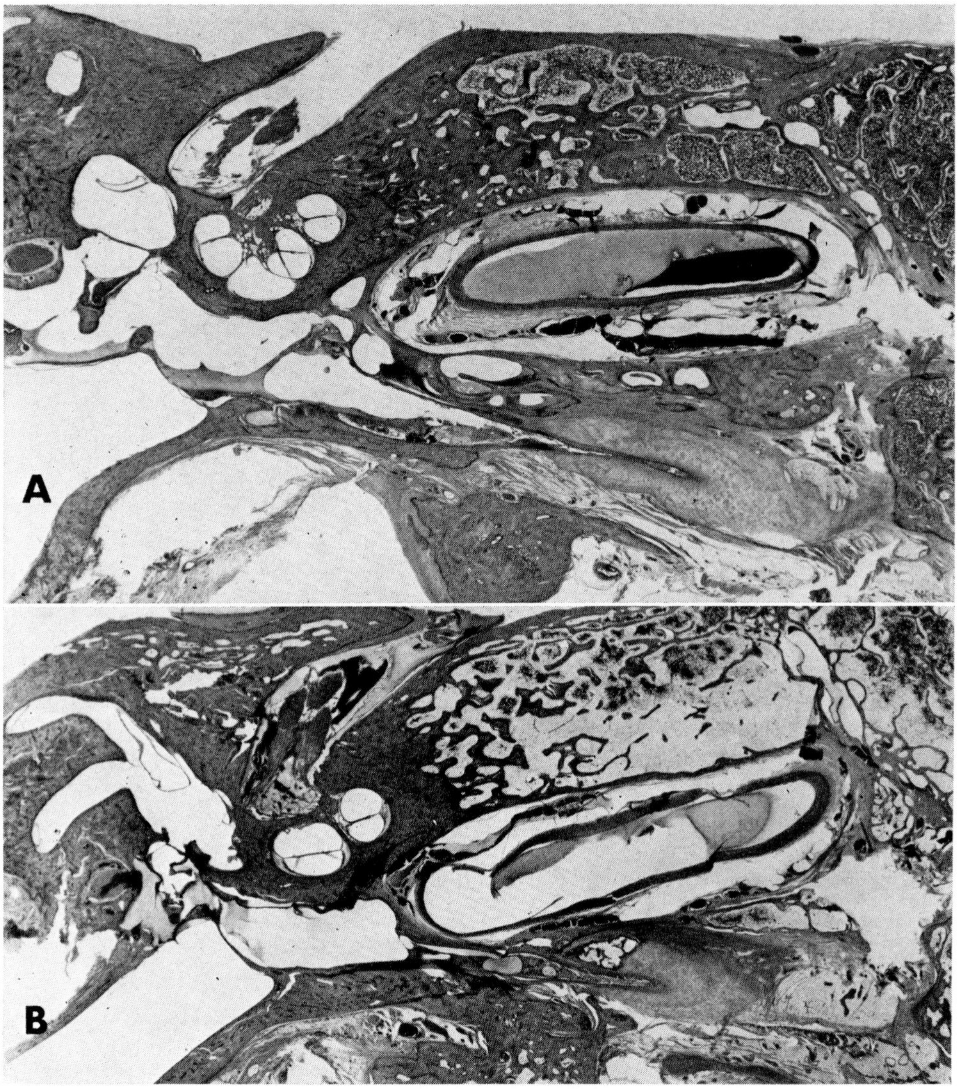

Fig. 4. Temporal bone specimen sectioned horizontally and longitudinally through (A) the protympanum and (B) the bony portion of the Eustachian tube. (H. and E. stain)

Three bones were placed in 10% formalin, decalcified, sectioned, and stained with H. and E. Sections were made horizontally and longitudinally through two Eustachian tube specimens (Figs. 4A, B, C. and D), and transverse to the long axis of the Eustachian tube in a third specimen (Figs. 5A and B).

Fifty-seven bones were dissected in search of the lymphatics using various dyes and stains. Twenty bones were placed in 2% buffered gluteraldehyde for future electron microscopic study.

Staining of Lymphatics and Electron Microscopic Study. A 60-year-old woman had been on a respirator for one full month after the removal of a large left acoustic neuroma. She had been completely unresponsive, had bilaterally dilated fixed pupils, and blood pressure which could not be kept at a normal level since the day of surgery. Her pulse became progressively weaker. Electroencephalogram (EEG) showed no activity. The family of the patient requested that no further unusual steps to prolong life be taken. Since

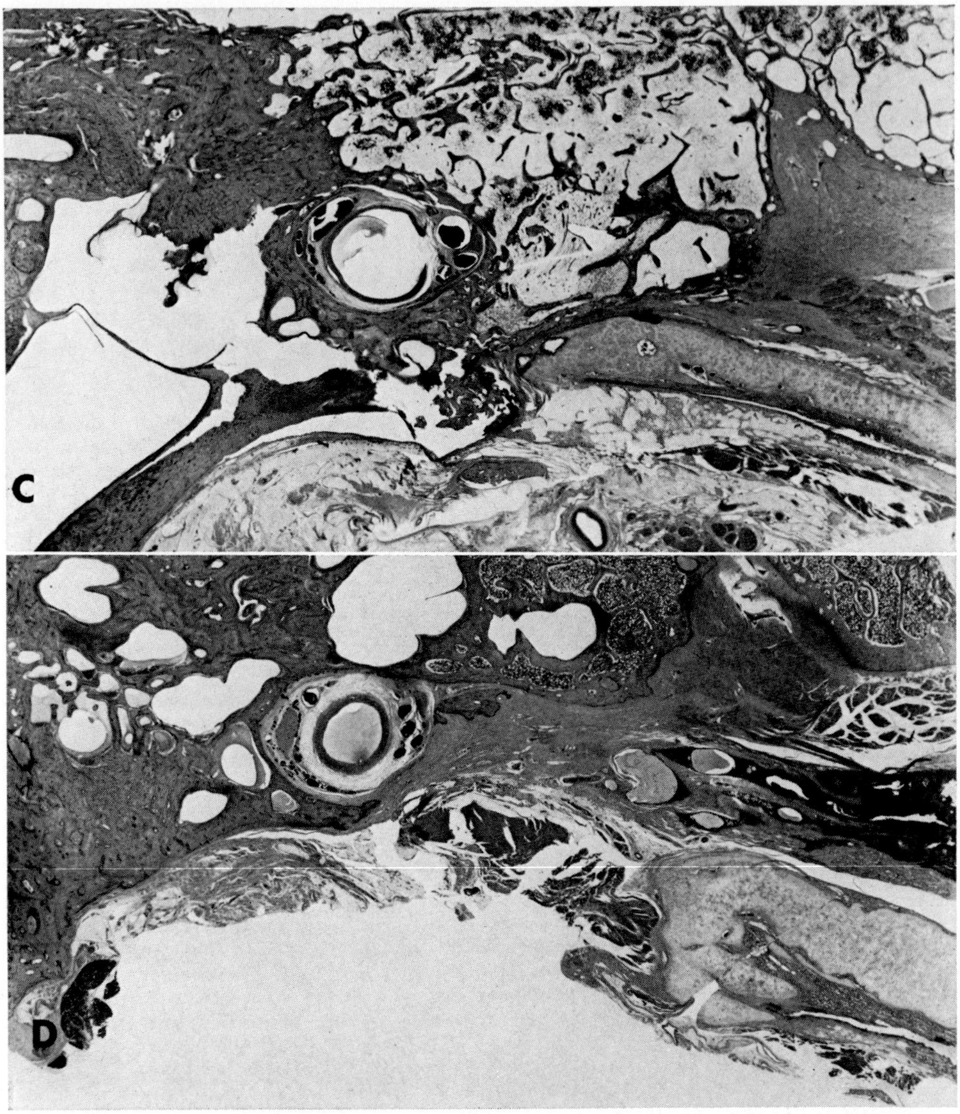

Fig. 4. Temporal bone specimen sectioned horizontally and longitudinally through (C) the fibrocartilaginous portion of the Eustachian tube and (D) the nasopharyngeal opening of the Eustachian tube. (H. and E. stain)

permission was granted for necropsy and examination of the ears, 2 ml of 2% Berlin blue in water was injected through the right tympanic membrane eight hours before death. The Eustachian tube specimen was removed at postmortem examination three hours after death, eleven hours after injection. Ten minutes' time was taken to remove the specimen from the cadaver and within another ten minutes the mucous membrane was dissected from the specimen. The membrane specimen was transected longitudinally. One half was placed in 10% formalin for the preparation of H. and E. stained slides and the other half was immediately placed in 2% buffered gluteraldehyde. It was then transferred to a 1% phosphate buffered osmium tetroxide solution for one hour, dehydrated in graded alcohol, and embedded in Epon.®* Thick and thin sections were prepared with an ultratome** using

* Shell Chemical Co., N. Y., N. Y.

** LKB Instruments, Inc., Rockville, Md.

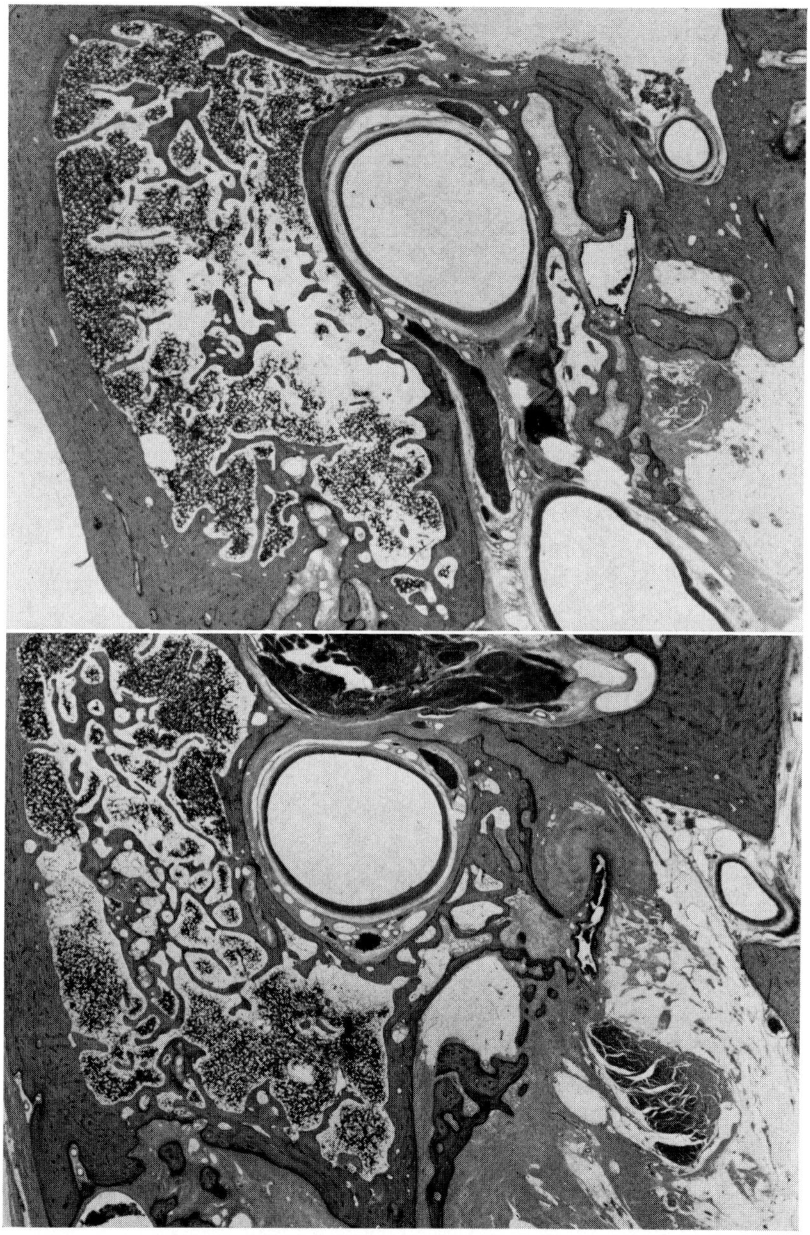

Fig. 5. Temporal bone specimen sectioned transversely through (A) the tubotympanum and carotid artery and (B) the nasopharyngeal orifice of the Eustachian tube and carotid artery. (H. and E. stain)

glass knives, transferred to carbon-coated Formvar membranes, stained with alcohol uranyl acetate and lead citrate, and studied under the transmission electron microscope.

RESULTS

Examination by light microscopy of the mucous membrane of the patient, injected with Berlin blue eight hours before death, revealed only one channel in the submucosa which was stained with the dye (Fig. 6). The specimen is from the nasopharyngeal end of the

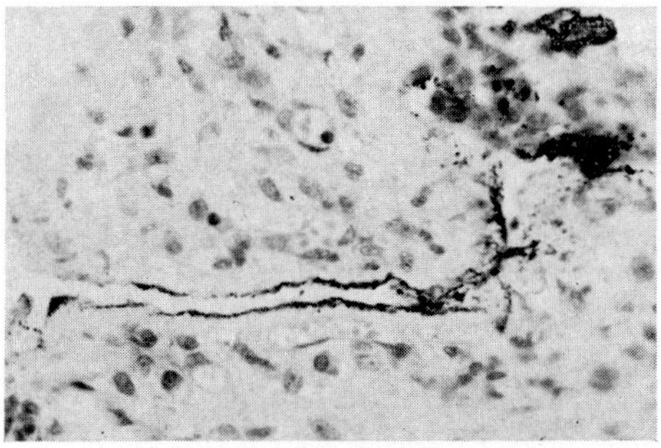

Fig. 6. Lymphatic channel in the submucosa of the nasopharyngeal end of the Eustachian tube stained by antemortem tympanic injection of Berlin blue.

tube and presumably shows a lymphatic vessel.

Specimens studied under the transmission electron microscope revealed the presence of blood capillaries (Fig. 7), as well as lymphatic capillaries (Figs. 8 and 9 A and B). Blood and lymphatic capillaries can be clearly differentiated, not only when red blood cells are seen in the blood capillary but specifically by differences in the basement membrane. Lymphatic capillaries are lined by large, flattened endothelial cells which sometimes have simple end-to-end junctions or overlap, or may have a series of interdigitations with various types of attachment devices between which intercellular gaps may occur. The endothelial cell lining is occasionally interrupted. By contrast, the basement membrane of the blood capillary is continuous and can be traced around the circumference without a gap.

DISCUSSION

Our interest in the lymphatics of the Eustachian tube was stimulated by the serendipitous observation that serous otitis media was regularly the result when Teflon®* paste was injected posterior to the Eustachian tube cartilage in dogs.[18] While doing an experiment to perfect the treatment for abnormally patent Eustachian tubes, it was found that injection of Teflon® paste anterior to the nasopharyngeal orifice in dogs would increase closure of the tube and greatly increase the resistance to the passage of air, but did not result in serous otitis media. Injection of 0.5 ml or more of paste immediately posterior to the nasopharyngeal Eustachian tube cartilage in dogs routinely produced

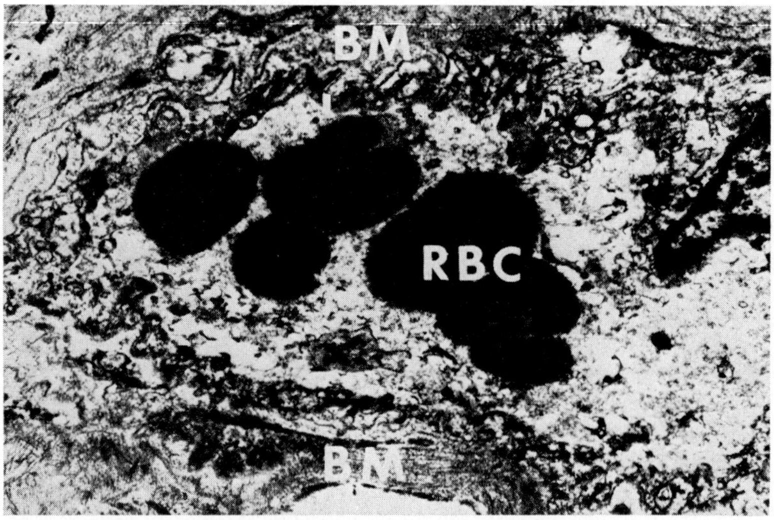

Fig. 7. Electron photomicrograph showing a blood capillary in the human Eustachian tube. The basement membrane (BM) is continuous without interruption. Red blood cells (RBC) are within the lumen. (X6600)

*E. I. DuPont de Nemours and Co., Wilmington, Del.

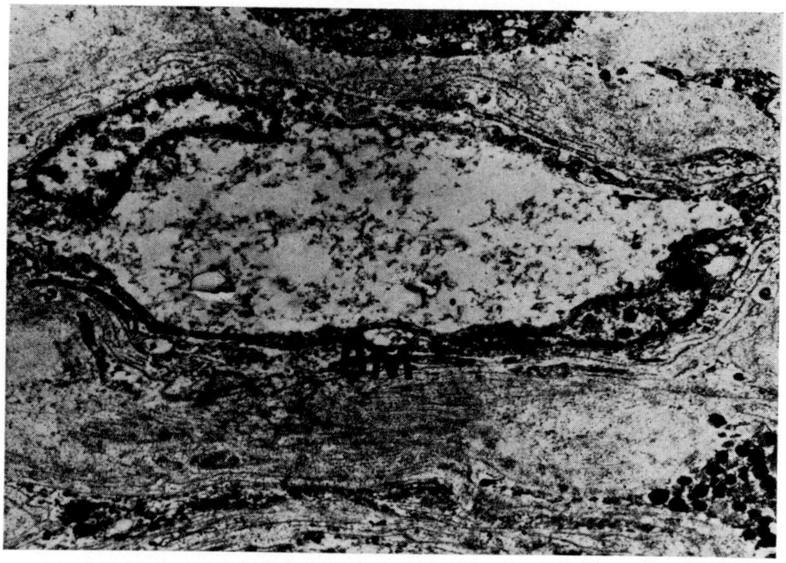

Fig. 8. Electron photomicrograph showing a lymphatic capillary in the human Eustachian tube. Note the large nuclei and gaps in the basement membrane (BM). (X6600)

serous otitis media without increasing the patency or resistance of the Eustachian tube. This observation was further defined and confirmed in a subsequent study.[19] This finding supported the view of Robison[13-14] that one pathogenesis of serous otitis media is lymphatic obstruction in the nasopharynx, specifically involving the lymphatics inferior and posterior to the nasopharyngeal Eustachian tube orifice. The common association, clinically, of serous otitis media with maxillary sinusitis, nasopharyngeal carcinoma, or after heavy radiation to that area would seem to support this thesis.

It would seem likely that serous otitis media associated with infected or inflamed tonsils or adenoid tissue would be the result of a similar mechanism of lymphatic obstruction, rather than the mechanism often casually explained that these tissues physically obstruct the tube orifice.

The possibility that serous otitis media can occur without tubal obstruction and without the production of any vacuum is proved by the observation of the occasional patient who has both serous otitis media and an abnormally patent Eustachian tube on the same side. When the otologist sees a definite fluid level with a conductive hearing loss and at the same time observes the tympanic membrane to move freely in and out with respiration, he usually finds that the patient complains primarily of autophony and fullness in the ear, characteristic of an abnormally patent Eustachian tube. The serous fluid disappears without treatment but the autophony and pressure usually remain.[20]

Obstruction of Eustachian tubal lymphatics may be instrumental as a mechanism of production of serous otitis media from several etiologies, such as inflammation from infected tonsils and adenoids or sinusitis, and from nasopharyngeal tumor, radiation, or allergy.[21] It would seem that knowledge of the normal anatomy of Eustachian tube lymphatics, as well as physiology and the nature of pathologic changes, should be known before routine understanding and effective therapy could be available for serous otitis media.

Despite descriptions in the literature[3,12] based on artists' conceptions of these structures, a good description of

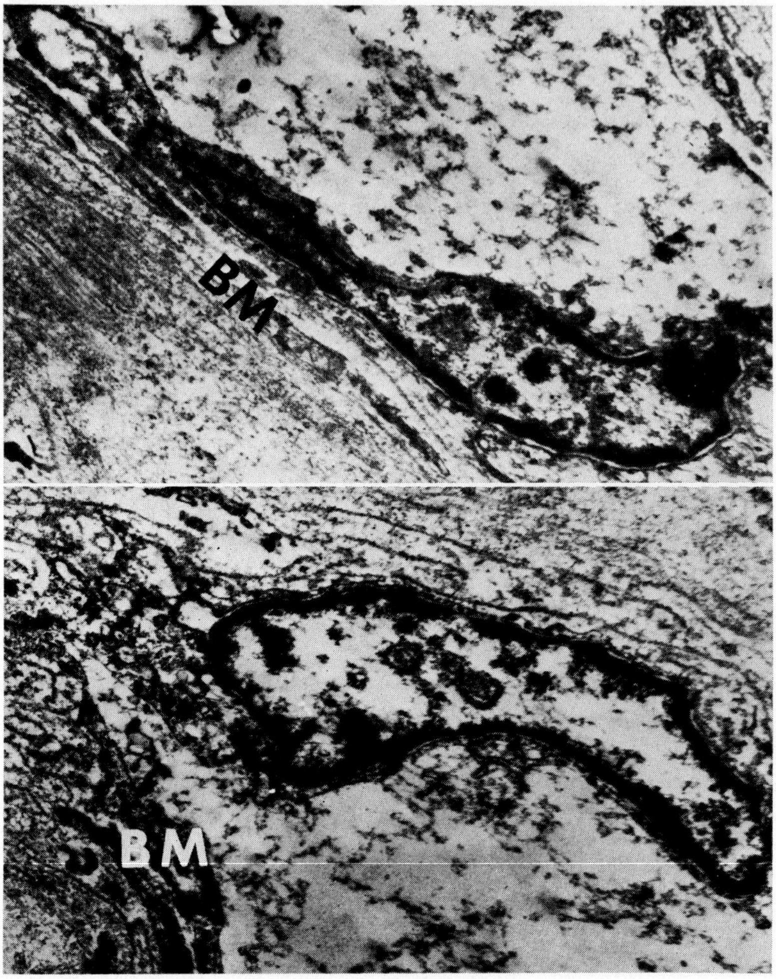

Fig. 9A and B. Electron photomicrograph enlarged view of nucleus within the wall of Eustachian tube lymphatic capillary shown in Figure 8. (X13,800)

the lymphatic drainage of the middle ear mucosa is not yet available. The apparent reason for the lack of this knowledge is quickly evident to one who attempts to study the lymphatics of the Eustachian tube. Most temporal bone specimens are either cores or portions of the bone with part of the Eustachian tube cut away. The deep-seated position within the skull, as well as the need to open widely into the nasopharynx and great vessels, require special techniques. Most human temporal bones cannot have antemortem injection as is possible with experimental animals. If one is to study the lymphatics of the Eustachian tube by injection techniques, timing of the injection as well as having minimal delay before fixation after death is important. In the living, lymphatics clear dye very quickly so that if sometimes death occurs even several minutes after a dye has been instilled, it may already be carried away into the lymphatic system and no longer be visible. If the patient swallows often before death, dye placed in the tympanum will be lost through the Eustachian tube. Large particles such as carbon in India ink do not seem to be absorbed by the middle ear mucous membrane, and it is not possible to place a needle under the membrane to inject this material. The problem of reducing the time lag between injection, death, and acquisition was significantly improved by the development of a cooperative research effort with the County Coroner and in one case by paying careful attention to the timing of these procedures in a patient who was expected to succumb in the hospital. Since opportunities of this sort cannot be planned, the investigator must be thoroughly prepared and able to quickly remove and process the specimen. Care must be taken with the type of dye used. It cannot be toxic if injected in the living, and if it produces discoloration of the skin, it cannot be injected intra-arterially unless the cadaver is to be cremated.

Lymphatic capillaries cannot be reliably differentiated from blood capillaries with a light microscope.[22] The difficulties associated with staining methods are avoided with the electron microscope. Data exists concerning the ultrastructural differentiation of blood and lymphatic capillaries in other organs of the body.[22-24] Haye[17] and Lim[9] demonstrated lymphatic capillaries in the middle ears and Eustachian tubes of guinea pigs using horseradish-peroxidase and transmission electron microscopy. It remained for us in this study to obtain and fix material which would be reasonably free of artifact. We were successful in one case. We feel that these techniques will be useful to study by serial section the course and distribution of lymphatics within the Eustachian tube. Tissue from the same specimen will be studied by the scanning electron microscope in the future.

Request for reprints should be sent to Jack L. Pulec, M.D., Otologic Medical Group, Inc., 2122 West Third St., Los Angeles, California 90057.

ACKNOWLEDGMENTS—The authors are greatly indebted to Dr. Thomas Noguchi, Chief Medical Examiner-Coroner, County of Los Angeles, for his invaluable assistance in the acquisition of anatomic material and for the use of his laboratory; and to Messrs Lawrence E. Irwin and Robert O. Greer for their technical assistance in the Otologic Electron Microscopic Laboratories of the Ear Research Institute; and to Dr. F. H. Linthicum, Jr. for his assistance in the Eccles' Temporal Bone Laboratory of the Ear Research Institute.

REFERENCES

1. Hoople GD: Otitis media with effusion: A challenge to otolaryngology. Trans Am Acad Ophthalmol Otolaryngol 54:531-539, 1950

2. Harrison K, Watson TK: Long-term follow-up of chronic exudate otitis media (glue ears). Proc R Soc Med 62:456-460, 1969

3. Worms G, Colouma VV: Considerations sur la trompe fibro-cartilagineuse et la region pharyngo-tubaire. Societe d'Anthropoligie de Paris. V8, S.8, 1936

4. Kelemen G: The pharyngeal orifice of the Eustachian tube in the aged. Eye Ear Nose Throat Mon 34:809-812, 1955

5. Graves GO, Edwards LF: Eustachian tube. Arch Otolaryngol 39:359-397, 1944

6. Proctor B: Embryology and anatomy of the Eustachian tube. Arch Otolaryngol 86:51-62, 1967

7. Proctor B: Anatomy of the Eustachian tube. Arch Otolaryngol 97:2-8, 1973

8. Schuknecht HF, Kerr AG: Pathology of the Eustachian tube. Arch Otolaryngol 86:45-50, 1967

9. Lim DJ: Functional morphology of the lining membrane of the middle ear and Eustachian tube: An overview. Ann Otol Rhinol Laryngol (Suppl 11) 83:5-26, 1974

10. Tos M: Development of mucous glands in the human Eustachian tube. Acta Otolaryngol (Stockh) 70:340-350, 1970

11. Arnould N: Contribution a l'etude des lymphatiques de l'appareil auditif. Arch Int Laryngol Otologie-Rhinologie 6:696-720, 1927

12. Rouvière H: *Anatomy of the Human Lymphatic System.* MJ Tobias (trans). Ann Arbor, Mich., Edwards Bros Inc. 1938

13. Robison JM: Subacute catarrhal otitis media and mastoiditis with effusion: A symptom and a clinical entity. Southern Med J 35:815-824, 1942

14. Robison JM: Lymphangitis of the mucosa of the paranasal sinuses. Tex Med 40:193-198, 1944

15. Porta CF: Personal communication

16. Ferrari C, Zini C: La vascolarizzazione linfatica del tessuto linfoide bucco-faringeo

(Dell'anello di Waldeyer). *Collana di Monografie de "L'ateneo Parmense."* Parma, No. 4, 1959

17. Haye R: The lymphatic capillaries of the middle ear mucosa in the guinea pig: Ultrastructure and permeability. Z Zellforsch Mikrosk Anat 145:785-189, 1973

18. Brookler KH, Pulec JL: Auditory tube patency after injection of the Teflon paste: An investigation in dogs. Arch Otolaryngol 90:60-64, 1969

19. Reiner CE, Pulec JL: Experimental production of serous otitis media. Ann Otol Rhinol Laryngol 78:880-887, 1969

20. Pulec JL, Hahn Jr FW: The abnormally patulous Eustachian tube. Otolaryngol Clin North Am 3:131-140, 1970

21. Pulec JL, Horwitz MJ: *Diseases of the Eustachian Tube. Otolaryngology.* Philadelphia, W. B. Saunders Co, 1973, vol 2, pp 75-92

22. Lauweryns JM: The blood and lymphatic microcirculation of the lung. Pathol Annu 6:365-415, 1971

23. Leak LV, Burke JF: Fine structure of the lymphatic capillary and the adjoining connective tissue area. Am J Anat 118:785, 1966

24. Lauweryns JM, Boussauw L: The ultrastructure of pulmonary lymphatic capillaries of newborn rabbits and of human infants. Lymphology 2:108, 1969

AMERICAN BOARD OF OTOLARYNGOLOGY

The American Board of Otolaryngology will hold its next certifying examination November 15-21, 1975, at the Palmer House, Chicago, Illinois. The deadline for applying for the 1975 examination is May 1, 1975.

SECOND BRITISH CONFERENCE ON AUDIOLOGY

The Second Conference of the British Society of Audiology will be held at the University of Southampton July 16-18, 1975, in the newly established Medical School. The scientific program will consist of a number of invited papers given by eminent speakers from the United Kingdom and abroad. For further information write: Mrs. O. G. Hyde, Secretary of the 2nd BSA Conference, The Institute of Sound and Vibration Research, The University, Southampton S09 5NH.

Ann Otol 84: 1975

THE COCHLEAR IMPLANT: CURRENT STATUS

ABSTRACT*

WILLIAM F. HOUSE, M.D.

LOS ANGELES, CALIFORNIA

This is the first report in a series of long-term studies on cochlear implants from the vantage point of various specialists. Fifteen patients have been implanted and specifics of each case are presented in case histories. The surgical technique is described and the engineering involved in the development of an electronic prosthesis is detailed. Engineering studies indicate that it is probably feasible to develop a multiple electrode system which can supersede the present single wire appliance. Since there has been considerable controversy about the long-term toxic effects of implanted wires, findings are presented which challenge such pessimism. In one instance, studies under electron microscopy indicate that there is no change either in the insulation material or the electrode wire. Further support comes from another study which indicates that over time there is no evidence of electrolysis. Thirteen patients were given intensive rehabilitation and the results were encouraging because speechreading improved, a wide variety of environmental sounds were understood, and the quality of life seemed improved. Psychologcial studies, which primarily are concerned with describing the problems and methods involved in studying patients with implants, nevertheless have accumulated sufficient data to support the previous view that cochlear implants make a significant difference to the recipient's life. To date, the evidence supports the view that cochlear implants are an important contribution in restoring sound and in improving the quality of life in selected individuals who have sustained a profound hearing loss.

Presented at the meeting of the American Otological Society, Inc., Atlanta, Georgia, April 11-12, 1975.

* The complete manuscript will be published as a supplement and will accompany a future issue of the *Annals of Otology, Rhinology & Laryngology.*

Ann Otol 84: 1975

PRESENT STATUS AND FUTURE DEVELOPMENT OF THE COCHLEAR PROSTHESIS

ROBIN P. MICHELSON, M.D.

MICHAEL M. MERZENICH, PH.D. ROBERT A. SCHINDLER, M.D.

DAVID N. SCHINDLER, M.D.

SAN FRANCISCO, CALIFORNIA

SUMMARY – Presently devised single channel devices generate relatively primitive sensation of hearing. They provide some enhancement of communication skills for the totally deaf. Definite psychological advantages for the totally deaf have been observed. Pitch discrimination is by the mechanism of "periodicity pitch." No "place" pitch encoding is possible. The recognition of complex sounds is not possible. Multiple segments of auditory nerve must be stimulated in a manner which will simulate the complex patterns of neural activity necessary for speech discrimination. Electrodes can be optimized and the pathophysiological consequences of electrical stimulation can be determined in experimental animals. The perceptual consequences of electrical stimulation, however, can best be determined in man himself. How much we will have to rely on known and future methods of aural rehabilitation will depend upon how well perceptual speech patterns can be generated by electrical stimulation of the auditory nerve.

Speech discrimination by ear alone has not been possible with the aid of any cochlear prosthetic device so far devised. The limited sensation of hearing afforded with these devices has, however, been of definite benefit in totally deaf patients. Enhancement of communication skills with lip reading, as well as the awareness of environmental sounds, has resulted. In this manner, the distressing isolation of total deafness has been at least partially overcome.

The synchronous stimulation of a single large segment of auditory nerve, afforded by these single channel devices, produces limited auditory sensation by the mechanism of "periodicity pitch." No "place pitch" encoding is possible with a single channel device. Pitch discrimination is limited to the range of 60-600 Hz although tonal sensation is present when stimulus frequencies are as high as 10 kHz. Thus, it has not been possible to generate neural firing patterns with sufficient information content (and complexity) for the recognition of speech or complex sounds.

The Present Status of Cochlear Prostheses. The question of auditory nerve survival after cochlear implantation has been a major interest to our group. Histopathological studies in animals by Schindler and Merzenich,[1] as well as physiological studies by Merzenich, *et al*, have shown that auditory nerve survives scala tympani implantation almost intact, even though massive hair cell destruction occurs. These studies extend to three and one-half years in animals (Fig. 1). Injury of the basal membrane or fracture of the modiolus produces severe localized degeneration. Implantation of small electrode arrays into the spiral ganglion also results in some localized neural degeneration.[3] Experience with patients correlates well with these observations since no impair-

From the Coleman Memorial Laboratory, Department of Otolaryngology, University of California at San Francisco, San Francisco, California.

Presented at the meeting of the American Otological Society, Inc., Atlanta, Georgia, April 11-12, 1975.

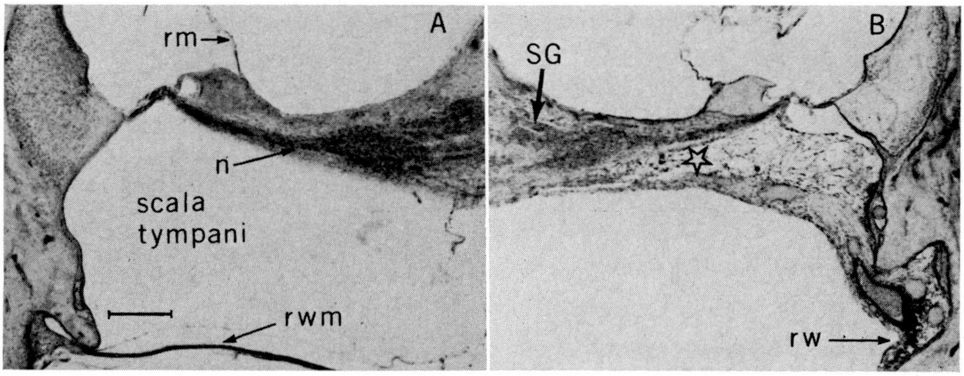

Fig. 1. Midmodiolar section through the basal turn near the round window in a normal cat (A) and an implanted cat (B). rm — Reissner's membrane; n — Radial fibers of the spiral ganglion cells; rwm — Round window membrane; rw — Round window area; SG — Spiral ganglion; star — Connective tissue reaction to the electrode. Note differences in the appearance of the stria vascularis in the normal and implanted cats. The bar at the lower left is 200μ in length.

ment of performance has been noted during a five-year observation period.

Threshold responses of single colliculus units to electrical sine wave stimulation of the auditory nerve in animals correlated well with patient thresholds (Fig. 2).

The sensation of loudness increased in ordered relation to stimulus strength. The upper limit of loudness was taken as a "too loud" response from the patient. No painful or vertiginous sensation ever resulted indicating that the stimulus was limited to the cochlea and was not spreading to the labyrinth or middle ear. The dynamic range of loudness sensation generated by electrical stimulation of the auditory nerve determined in this manner was only 15 dB.

Studies by Merzenich, *et al*[2] have shown phase locked neural responses to electrical sine wave stimulation of the auditory nerve. This "phase locking" breaks up when stimulus frequencies are above 600-700 Hz. This observation correlates well with pitch scaling experiments on implanted patients who show poor pitch discrimination above 700 Hz. Tonal sensation is still present, however, to at least 10 kHz. Paradoxically, these patients are able to detect a tonal quality difference between sine

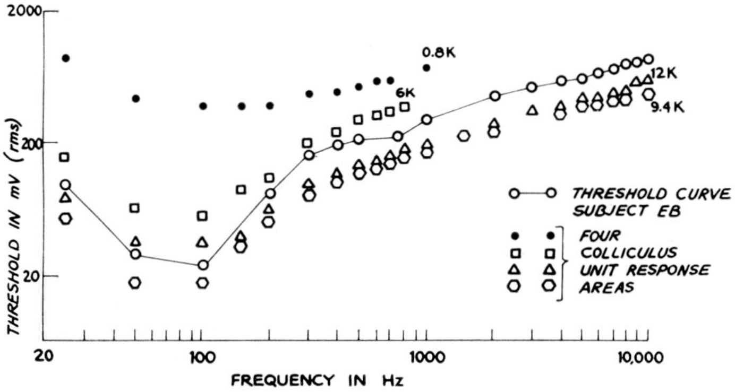

Fig. 2. Threshold responses to electrical stimulation of the acoustic nerve in man (open circles). Response of four colliculus neurons in animals driven by electrical stimulation are also shown.

and square wave electrical stimulation even at high frequencies.

Physiological studies by Merzenich, *et al*[2] also revealed that neural responses to electrical sine wave stimulation occurs over a broad frequency range in contrast to the narrow frequency range to sound stimulation.

Our early prosthetic devices were only capable of synchronously stimulating a broad segment of auditory nerve. The stimulus form was the electrical analog of the acoustic input modified in two ways. First, the frequency response of the system was modified so that patient response thresholds were flat. Second, an automatic gain control was incorporated, which effectively increased patient dynamic range to approximately 50 dB. When these modifications were made, subjects were able to distinguish voices, which had a more "natural" quality. In fact, they were often able to distinguish one voice from another. Unaided speech discrimination, however, was not possible.

A radio frequency carrier was first used to transmit information and power across the intact skin to the internal device. Electromagnetic interference with this system did not present a problem. Failure of some of the internal electronic components, however, was a problem. The broad frequency response range (100 Hz-20 kHz) was a distinct advantage. Later simple electromagnetic coupling proved to be the most reliable, although frequency response was limited to 300 Hz-4 kHz.

Patient acceptance of these devices, in our small series, has been surprisingly good in spite of the mechanical failures necessitating replacement of the implant.

Future Devices and Research Objectives. It is now apparent that if recognizable speech patterns are to be generated with electrical stimulation of the acoustic nerve, multichannel differential stimulation almost certainly will be required. Thus, a means of "place" as well as "periodicity" encoding must be

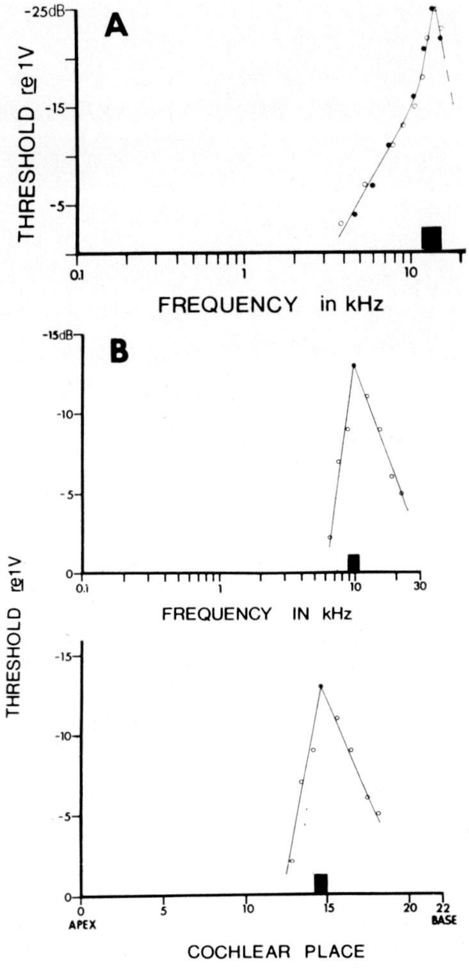

Fig. 3. Colliculus neuron response curves to electrical stimulation of a single segment of basal membrane (electrode contact diameter .003 inch).

provided. Work in our laboratory, principally by Merzenich, *et al*[4], has shown that it is feasible to electrically excite small segments of auditory nerve through the scala tympani. Attenuation between electrically excited segments of basal membrane is approximately 25 dB per octave, presumptive evidence that good isolation can be obtained between channels in a multichannel scala tympani electrode array (Fig. 3). These observations were made with an electrode of .003 inch in diameter. It is conceivable that even better isolation can be obtained with different electrode configurations.

Using bipolar electrodes preliminary observations indicate that performance is degraded if the distance between bipolar elements is less than 200 μ. Exact contact with basal membrane is also critical. Placement against bony modiolus is ineffective. With properly placed electrodes, performance improves with time up to about six weeks, as evidenced by a decrease in threshold stimulus. Histologic studies indicate that the formation of connective tissues around the implant isolates electrode contacts from the surrounding conductive cochlear fluids.

The total number of channels (electrodes) that are feasible will probably be determined by the size of the electrical field that is needed to produce the desired graded neural response in any given segment of basal membrane.

The length of basal membrane that needs to be differentially electrically excited, theoretically, for speech discrimination is 20 mm at the basal end of approximately one and one-quarter turns of the basal coil.

Our group has developed an eight channel array with the mechanical characteristics which allow the device to be inserted safely through the round window for a distance of 23 mm in the human scala tympani. In addition, new molding techniques have provided a more accurate fit to the contours of the scala tympani.

The University of California group at San Francisco have cooperated with the Stanford team led by Simmons.[5] Simmons reports, "The Stanford group (White, Glattke, Simmons) is developing a four-channel stimulating system for placement directly in the auditory nerve. This system will eventually be tried in a small group of human volunteers but only after extensive testing in animals. There are many unique features of this system which are not now available elsewhere, and the most important of these is that the implanted electronics include a computer switch register that is externally programmable by digital instructions to each electrode separately. This will allow considerable flexibility in the translation of sounds into electrical impulses. If the four-channel system proves successful, it will be an easy matter to add additional electrode channels in multiples of four."

"We estimate that we are perhaps 6 to 18 months away from a clinical trial. The implantable electronics have been developed and are now undergoing final preproduction trouble shooting. There is, however, no way to speed up the animal test stage, principally because testing for insulation failures is an important and frustrating bottleneck." Evaluation of both methods will be a joint effort of both groups in the near future.

Future research objectives will include a determination of the safe limits of electrical stimulation of the auditory nerve over a suitable time course, as well as any external environmental hazards to which the implanted patient might be vulnerable.

Past experience has shown that the stabilized implanted electrode is the most reliable part of the cochlear implant system. The implanted electronics appear to be the most failure prone. The NIH workshop on Cochlear Implants held in San Francisco on October 23-24, 1974, concluded that a reliable implanted connector would be desirable. This would allow the replacement of the electronics module with a greatly simplified surgical procedure.

The last but not the least important objective is to determine the most effective mode of stimulation. More exact information on the tissue electrode interface, as well as more exact details of nerve excitation under these conditions, are needed. Three broad methods of encoding information for meaningful excitation of the auditory nerve array within the cochlea seem to warrant investigation.

1. Vocoder Processing: A series of single formant frequencies are extracted

from the incoming speech signal and delivered as a stimulus to the appropriate "frequency place" on the basal membrane.

2. Programmed pulsatile stimulation: Pulses of various repetition rates and amplitude would be delivered to the appropriate "frequency place." Vocoder format could be used on speech filtered into appropriate bands and encoded into pulses.

3. Multiple filters: Speech signals would be divided into predetermined frequency bands and delivered as an analog signal to the corresponding "frequency place."

As indicated above, a versatile programmable pulse-generating device is nearing completion at Stanford. It will deliver symmetrical-graded electrical charges to the auditory nerve via the Simmons modiolar electrode or the scala tympani electrode.

Our group has under design consideration of an implantable device consisting of eight active filters. The frequency elements of the auditory input signal would be delivered as analog stimuli to appropriate locations on the basal membrane.

These devices all have inherent limitations in terms of flexibility. It would be highly desirable to control all variables from outside the subject. With this idea in mind, preliminary engineering studies indicate that a device might be constructed within the required size constraints that would have the following characteristics: 1) independent control of each channel, 2) sufficient channel band-width to allow the delivery of a wide variety of stimulus wave forms including specified pulses, and 3) backward telemetry would be provided to allow monitoring of the actual stimulus and electrode performance *in situ.*

With such a device the perceptual consequences of the various stimulus parameters could be compared in a single individual.

Request for reprints should be sent to Robin P. Michelson, M.D., Coleman Memorial Laboratory, HSE-863, University of California at San Francisco, San Francisco, Calif. 94143.

REFERENCES

1. Schindler R, Merzenich M: Chronic intracochlear electrode implantation: Cochlear pathology and acoustic nerve survival. Ann Otol Rhinol Laryngol 83:202-215, 1974

2. Merzenich M, Michelson RP, Schindler RA, *et al*: Neural encoding of sound sensation evoked by electrical stimulation of the auditory nerve. Ann Otol Rhinol Laryngol 82:486-503, 1973

3. Simmons FB: Cochlear implants. Arch Otolaryngol 89:61-69, 1969

4. Merzenich M, Schindler DN, White MW: Feasibility of multichannel scala tympani stimulation (Symposium on cochlear implants). Laryngoscope 84:1887-1893, 1974

5. Simmons FB: Personal communication

COCHLEAR POTENTIALS AND OXYGEN ASSOCIATED WITH HYPOXIA

MERLE LAWRENCE, PH.D.

ALFRED L. NUTTALL, PH.D. PAUL A. BURGIO, A.B.

ANN ARBOR, MICHIGAN

SUMMARY — In the guinea pig, during general hypoxia produced by shutoff of respiratory air, oxygen-sensitive microelectrodes detect a decrease in oxygen concentration in the fluids of the tunnel of Corti before detecting a decrease in scala media oxygen concentration. The present experiments were designed to measure the cochlear microphonic (CM) potential generated by the organ of Corti when vibrated by a microprobe on the basilar membrane along with the oxygen decline in both tunnel and scala media to see upon which source of oxygen CM is dependent. Because oxygen concentration in both areas can decrease considerably before CM is affected, the recovery following a brief period of hypoxia is a more accurate measure. Because CM starts a recovery before scala media oxygen, the positive endolymphatic potential (EP) was also measured to determine its role in the generation of CM. Our interpretation of the course of events is that CM is partially dependent upon oxygen supplied to the extracellular spaces of the organ of Corti by the spiral vessels and upon EP that, itself, is dependent upon several factors. The data indicate that EP plays a more complex role than that of providing a current flow for modulation by a resistance varying with vibration.

As techniques for the study of the capillaries of the inner ear improve it becomes more apparent that inner ear disorders and the accompanying sensorineural hearing loss are brought about by vascular pathology and changes in the microhomeostatic conditions.[1,2] Capillary involvement has been clearly demonstrated in man and animals, and the observed changes have been found to be associated with aging, toxins, and noise.

The histopathological changes observed in the capillaries have been reported as swollen endothelial cells which occlude blood flow and degenerated capillaries forming intravascular strands and avascular channels.[3] Such pathology would indicate that a deficit in inner ear function results either from the direct effect of local anoxia or from ionic or metabolic imbalance resulting from secondary changes in secretory tissues.

Many experiments have been carried out, starting in 1941,[4] demonstrating the effects of general hypoxia upon the cochlear potentials which have come to be recognized as accurate measures of inner ear function providing these potentials are interpreted correctly.

Békésy[5] showed that the cochlear microphonic (CM) and the DC resting potential of the perilymph (recorded behind the round window), while quite resistant to low-oxygen content of respiratory air, do decrease with anoxia. Later,[6] in an attempt to determine the source of CM and the magnitude of the positive resting potential of the endolymph (EP), he recorded almost par-

---

From the Kresge Hearing Research Institute, University of Michigan Medical School, Ann Arbor, Michigan.

This research was supported by funds from the John A. Hartford Foundation and PHS grants NS-05785 and NS-11731.

Presented at the meeting of the American Otologic Society, Inc., Atlanta, Georgia, April 11-12, 1975.

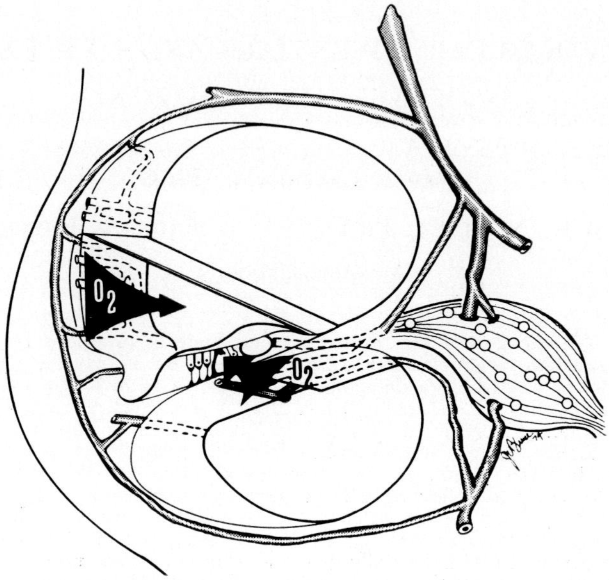

Fig. 1. Sources of oxygen for the organ of Corti with the spiral vessels the most likely.[10] Experiments reported here were designed to determine relationship between CM and O_2 in these fluid spaces.

allel decline in these potentials with anoxia.

There are many other experiments showing the effects of anoxia on cochlear potentials that cannot be reviewed here, but there are a few pertinent to the present study.

Misrahy, *et al*[7] were the first to measure oxygen within the endolymph and to determine the amount of change with anoxia. They concluded that the organ of Corti receives its oxygen from the stria vascularis. In 1961 Rice and Shinabarger[8] sought to correlate the drop in EP and CM with each other and with anoxia. They found the correlation so poor that no direct relation between CM and EP was indicated.

Similarly, other studies have determined the relation between general hypoxia and the decline of the cochlear potentials, but in order to understand the effects of the observed histopathological changes upon the organ of Corti function, it becomes important to know which of the various capillary areas is responsible for the observed decline in electrical potential.

Histopathological changes have been observed in the spiral capillaries and in the capillaries of the stria vascularis, and the evidence indicates that these two areas serve different functions.[9] During general hypoxia the oxygen tension in the tunnel fluid supplied by the spiral vessels falls before the oxygen tension in the scala media endolymph.[10]

Our specific question in the design of the present experiments was whether, with hypoxia, CM generated by the organ of Corti responds to changes in the rapidly changing tunnel oxygen or to the more delayed change in endolymph oxygen. The two sources of oxygen are illustrated in Figure 1 which shows a relatively longer path for diffusion from the stria vascularis to the hair cells than from the spiral vessels to the hair cells.

As can be seen from the results the answer is complex, but the determinations do give a better understanding of inner ear function.

METHODS AND MATERIALS

In order to measure electrical events within the confines of the scala media, especially those affected by the microcirculation, it is essential that the capillaries remain uninjured. To accomplish this we made use of direct microscopic visualization making possible the insertion of an electrode into the tunnel without injury to the spiral capillaries and the insertion of other electrodes into the scala media through the avascular *pars pectinata* of the basilar membrane.

The surgical approach and method of observing the organ of Corti for electrode placement have been described in previous publications.[10-12] Because AC, DC, and oxygen current were to be measured, both platinum and glass-micropipette electrodes were used.

The method of recording oxygen current in both the scala media and tunnel of Corti were the same as described previously except that in certain experiments we recorded both oxygen current and CM through the same platinum electrode. In general this can be accomplished by recording oxygen current with a DC current meter (since oxygen concentration and its changes are essentially DC events and the meter circuit filters out the higher frequencies). An AC amplifier for the CM potentials was connected in parallel to the current meter.

More specifically, a glass-insulated, etched-platinum-iridium microelectrode* with less than 5 μm exposed above a less than 1 μm tip served as an oxygen-reduction cathode while the reduction current was measured by an oxygen-current meter.** This device is basically a very sensitive DC current meter ($< 10^{-10}$ AMPS) and also supplies -0.6 volt bias required for the oxygen cathode. CM potentials picked up by the platinum microelectrode were recorded across a voltage-divider network formed by the resistance of the electrode (~ 10 megohm) and a 5 megohm series resistor. A preamplifier*** was used to separate and amplify the CM.

The positive endolymphatic potential (EP) and also CM were recorded by a glass-micropipette electrode with a tip diameter of 1 μm. These potentials were amplified by an electrometer amplifier,**** the output of which was divided; one branch going to a wave analyzer that does not respond to the DC, and the other branch going directly to the chart recorder.

The chart recorder recorded four events: CM, EP, oxygen current (O_2), and an electrocardiogram (EKG) from electrodes on the chest wall of the animal. This latter was recorded so that any effect on the cardiovascular activity of the animal resulting from the surgical manipulation, anesthesia, or the hypoxia could be monitored.

A microvibrator provided a stimulus either directly to the basilar membrane, or to the head of the stapes. This vibrator consisted of a glass rod with a tip diameter of about 100 μm attached to a precision-tooled steel rod, in ball bearing ways, glued to a rubber diaphragm driven through an air-filled tube by an electromagnetic driver mounted outside the electrically-shielded soundproofed room. For these experiments it seemed to make no difference in the results where the vibrator was placed, so no distinction between placement has been made.

The guinea pigs used were products of our own colony, weighed between 350 and 400 gm, and were anesthetized with diallylbarbituric acid and urethane. Through a tracheostomy, mechanical respiration was provided with rate and air volume adjusted to maintain the animal in good physiological condition. During an experiment which lasted three to four hours, the animals were kept warm by a heating pad.

The respirator used compressed air, and to produce the hypoxia the source was turned off and the tube at the trachea clamped. This procedure is designated as "air off" in the illustrations. The tube to the trachea was unclamped and the air turned on to reestablish the normal condition indicated as "air on."

During the course of these experiments, 224 separate runs with various electrode placement in 39 guinea pigs were made.

RESULTS

The Recorded Data. During an experiment, the data were recorded on the moving chart of a graphic recorder. For tabulation and statistical treatment the instant of decline or increase of each potential following "air off" or "air on" was taken directly from the chart. For visual display of the results and to facilitate the comparison of the exact moment of decline and recovery, the responses were plotted as departures from 100% which represents the pre-hypoxic stabilized output from each electrode. In each of three series of experiments a separate combination of electrodes was used so that different sets of measures could be compared.

Series 1: In this series two platinum microelectrodes were used, one through the zona arcuata, with the tip in the tunnel of Corti, and another passing

---

* No. 30-10-3, Frederick Haer & Co., Ann Arbor, Mich.
** Model 1200, Transidyne General Corp., Ann Arbor, Mich.
*** Model P16, Grass Instrument Co., Quincy, Mass.
**** Model A-35, Medistor Div., Simlog Instruments, Overlake Park, Redmon, Washington.

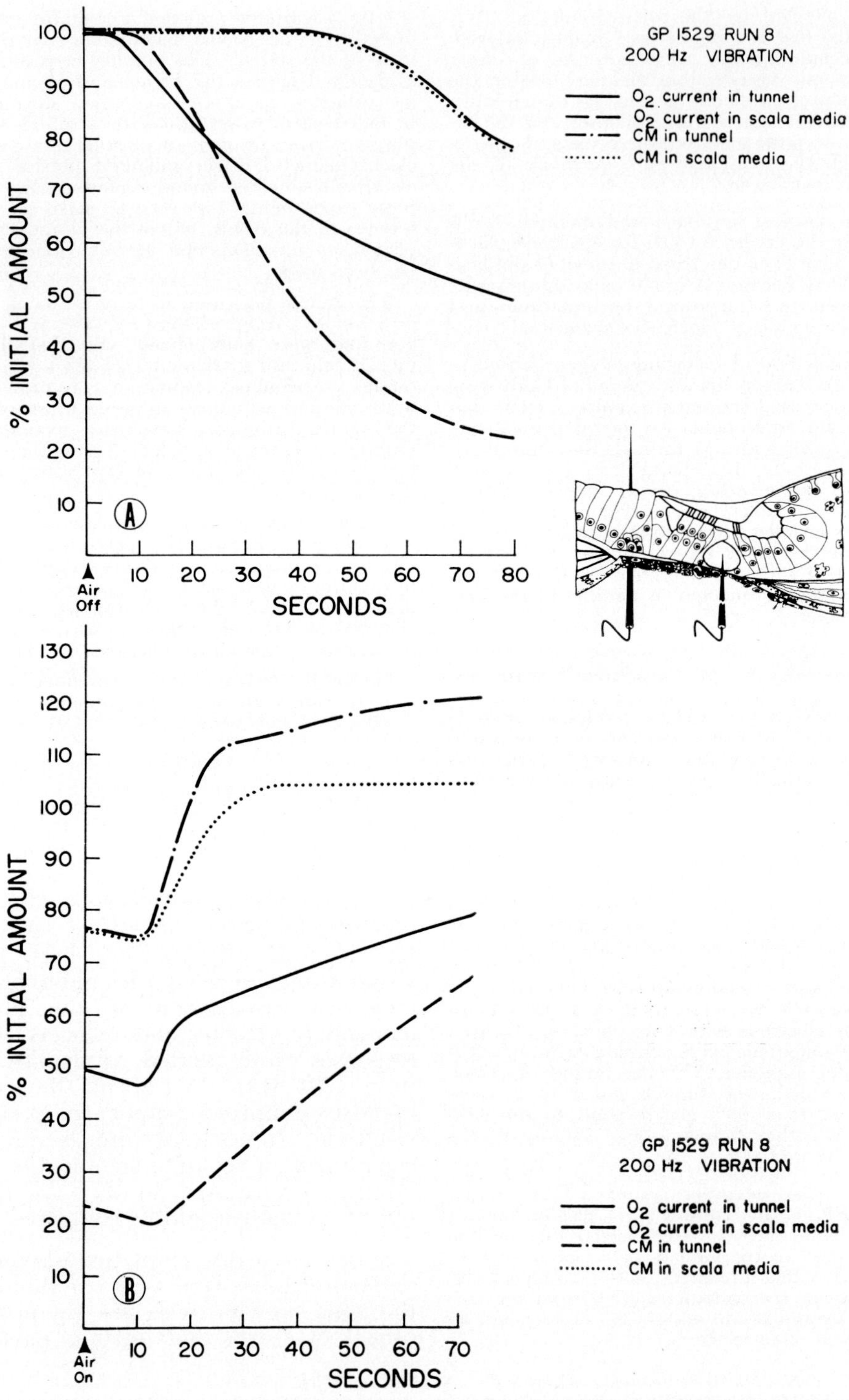

Fig. 2. Decline (A) and recovery (B) of indicated measures determined by platinum electrodes in tunnel of Corti and in endolymph of scala media.

through the zona pectinata and Claudius cells, with the tip in the scala media next to the stria vascularis. From each electrode, changes in oxygen tension and changes in CM to 200 Hz vibrations were recorded simultaneously during induced hypoxia.

Figure 2A portrays graphically the typical decline in responses following "air off." The vibrator amplitude was adjusted to give a CM level between 10 and 30 μV. Differences between initial magnitudes of response from the electrodes, placed in the different areas, were removed by means of the scaling done for graphical presentation. Initial CM magnitudes are not important for the measurement of the delays. This is also true for the oxygen-current data. For reasons stated in our earlier publication,[10] and because each of the two electrodes has a different sensitivity, the data presented are not absolute oxygen-tension measurements.

The important measure is the moment of beginning decline in each of the tracings after respiratory air to the animal is shut off. The amount of decline is immaterial except that an effort was made to return air to the animal before any general changes in the cardiovascular condition, as reflected in the EKG of the animal, were produced.

In this typical run, following shut off of respiratory air, the first recording to decline is that measuring the oxygen content of the tunnel fluid followed by that of the oxygen content of the endolymph. Several seconds later CM starts to decline simultaneously in both recording sites. It would appear that CM generation is maintained for several seconds, in this case about 37 seconds, after the oxygen in the fluid compartments starts to decrease. There apparently is an overabundance of oxygen under normal conditions which must be depleted before CM is affected. Once this storehouse disappears, the relative times of beginning recovery follow a different sequence.

Figure 2B portrays, in a typical animal, the recordings of oxygen current and CM recovery in the two fluid compartments following return of respiratory air. It appears that all recordings start recovery at the same time, but close measurement shows this is not the case. As reported earlier,[10] oxygen concentration in the tunnel fluid begins recovery first. Here we see that this is followed by CM in both the tunnel and scala media. The last measure to start a recovery is that of oxygen concentration in the scala media.

Our interest is in the relationship among the exact points of beginning decline and beginning recovery. In order to present a more exact determination of these responses in the many animals used, the times were recorded and submitted to statistical analysis. The cumulative results are presented in later tables.

Series 2: Because CM starts a simultaneous decline in the two fluid compartments sometime after the oxygen begins to decline, the question was asked whether or not some other factor might not be involved in the maintenance of CM. A prominent theory[13] of the generation of CM is that it is a modulation of the current flow resulting from the presence of the positive EP and negative intracellular potential of the hair cells. If such a condition is operating, one would expect CM and EP to decline and recover together.

In this second series of experiments, in addition to the records of oxygen changes in the tunnel fluid, CM and EP were recorded simultaneously in the endolymph of the scala media by a nonpolarizable glass micropipette electrode.

Figure 3A shows the recordings in a typical animal of these potentials following the shut off of respiratory air. Again the first to decline is the tunnel oxygen. For some reason there was a slight rise in the tunnel oxygen, but the early decline is obvious. The second response to decline is EP and finally, shortly thereafter, the scala media CM starts to decline.

After the respiratory air is turned on,

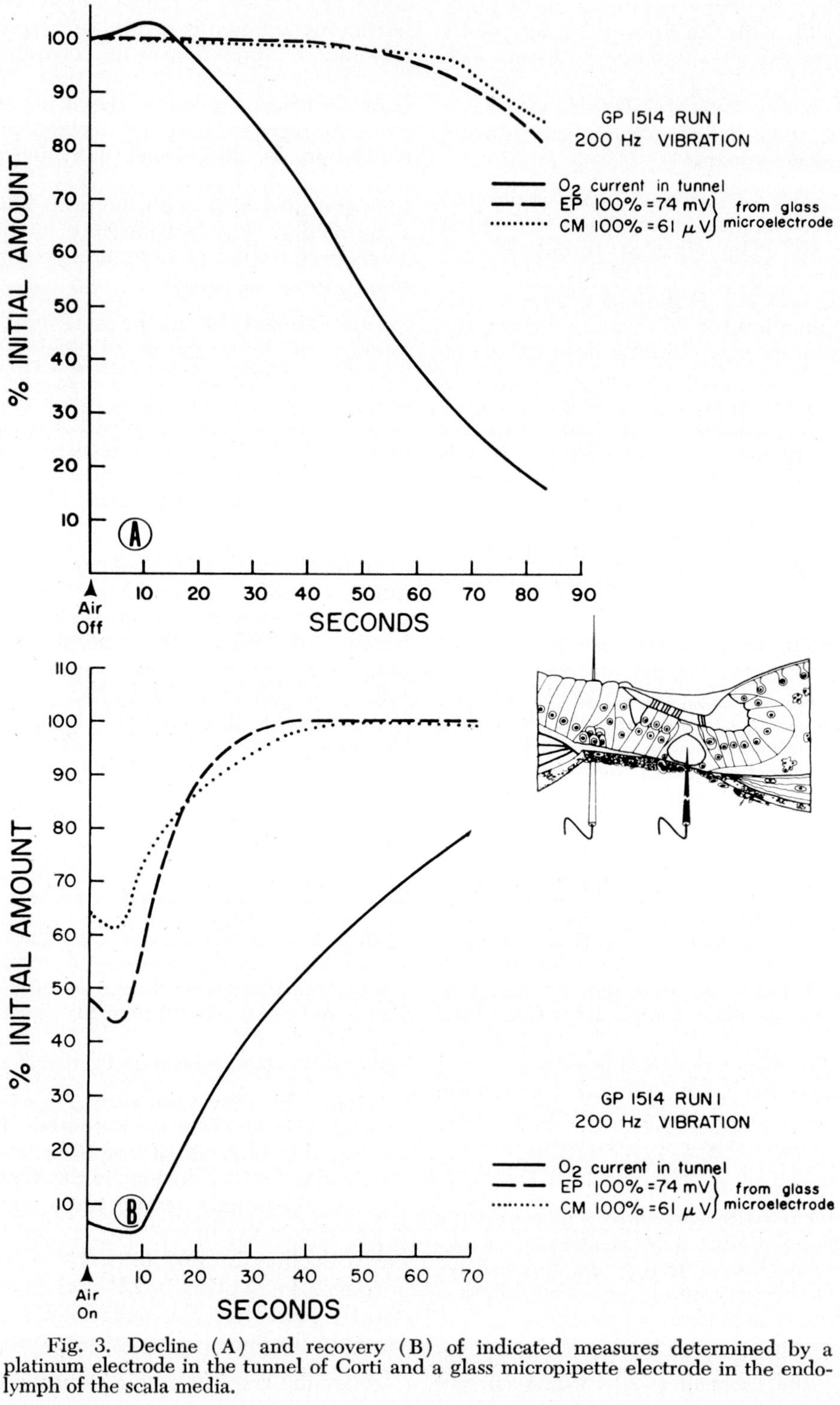

Fig. 3. Decline (A) and recovery (B) of indicated measures determined by a platinum electrode in the tunnel of Corti and a glass micropipette electrode in the endolymph of the scala media.

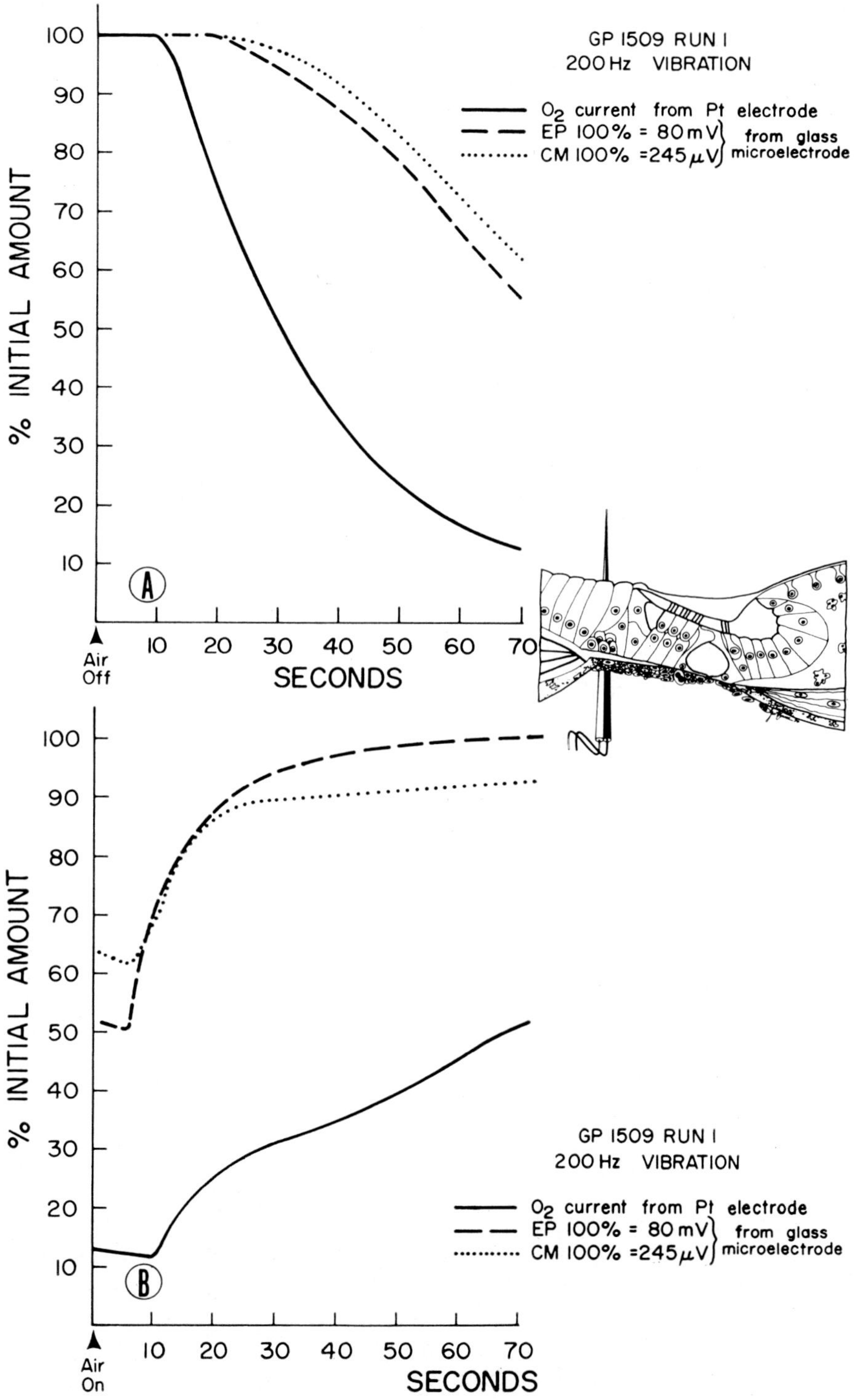

Fig. 4. Decline (A) and recovery (B) of indicated measures determined by a platinum and glass micropipette combined into a double electrode placed in the endolymph of the scala media.

TABLE I

DELAY TIMES FOR RESPIRATORY AIR TURNED OFF OR ON TO DECLINE OR INCREASE IN FLUID OXYGEN. SIMULTANEOUS RECORDINGS

	(a) Air off to O_2 Decline		*(b)* Air on to O_2 Increase	
	Tunnel	*Scala Media*	*Tunnel*	*Scala Media*
N	52	52	11*	11*
μ	12.1 Sec	14.4 Sec	8.1 Sec	9.9 Sec
σ	3.6 Sec	4.8 Sec	1.4 Sec	1.9 Sec
	P<.0005		P<.0005	

* Data from animals with minimal heart-rate change.

all potentials appear to recover at the same instant as shown in Figure 3B. In this particular animal the return of tunnel oxygen was slightly delayed, but as is shown in the later tables, the differences in these recovery measures are not significant. The data from each of the similar runs in all experimental animals are also summarized in the tables.

Series 3: To complete the measurements so as to have similar ones from each fluid compartment, a dual electrode, consisting of a nonpolarizable glass micropipette electrode and a platinum electrode fitted together under a microscope and glued so that the tips were no more than a few microns apart, was inserted into the scala media endolymph.

Figure 4A shows the recordings from a typical animal of the decline of oxygen concentration, EP, and CM from a dual scala media electrode. The first to decline is the oxygen, followed some seconds later by EP and CM. After the respiratory air is turned on (Fig. 4B), EP and CM start to return within a very few seconds followed shortly by the endolymph oxygen. Under these recording conditions the difference between the CM - EP start of recovery and the oxygen concentration start of recovery is quite significant as will be clarified in the tables to follow.

Analysis of Data. Although each animal gave distinct results, consistency was difficult to determine from the graphs, so in order to determine the sequence of events, similar measures for all animals were grouped and analyzed statistically.

This analysis is presented in the following tables, each of which, it will be noted, has a different sample size. The reason for this is that for any statistical comparison only data from paired electrodes in the same animal were considered.

Also it will be noted that the sample sizes for the "on delay" are small. This is because, during the period of hypoxia, the hearts of some animals showed marked changes in beat rate and strength of contraction, delaying recovery of responses until the recorded EKG returned more or less to normal. Therefore, for the analysis, only data from those animals with minimal EKG changes were used.

The total sample size for any data comparison was, of course, much larger, and similar statistical treatment of these figures did not alter the qualitative results as presented in the tables. The reason the smaller sample size has been used is that the data reflect better controlled experimental conditions.

Our earlier publication[10] on the availability of oxygen in the tunnel fluid, as compared with that in the endolymph during hypoxia was, in most instances, made with each electrode placement in a different animal. In the present experiments, the electrodes were paired in each animal as shown in the inset picture of Figure 2. The data in Table I

TABLE II

DELAY TIMES FOR RESPIRATORY AIR TURNED OFF TO DECLINE IN FLUID OXYGEN, COCHLEAR MICROPHONIC (CM) AND ENDOLYMPHATIC POTENTIAL (EP). SIMULTANEOUS RECORDINGS FOR EACH GROUP

	(a)		*(b)*		*(c)*		*(d)*	
	O_2 (Tunnel)	*CM*	*O_2 (Tunnel)*	*EP*	*O_2 (SM)*	*CM*	*O_2 (SM)*	*EP*
N	62	62	31	31	79	79	45	45
μ (Sec)	11.7	37.9	10.9	29	16.6	38.5	14.0	31.4
σ (Sec)	4.0	16.4	3.7	12.9	8.5	19.1	4.1	19.9
	$P<.001$		$P<.001$		$P<.001$		$P<.001$	
	$r=.31$		$r=.23$		$r=.30$		$r=.26$	

SM - scala media

display the delay times, in seconds, for (a) respiratory air turned off to first noticeable oxygen-current decrease and (b) respiratory air turned on to oxygen-current increase. All measurements were paired from two simultaneously-placed oxygen sensitive microelectrodes. "P" is the probability that the mean delay in the tunnel (μ_1) and the mean delay in the scala media (μ_2) are the same, tested against the alternative that $\mu_2 > \mu_1$ (one-tailed Student's t test).

As can be seen in the table, these results are highly significant and confirm the observation in our earlier report[10] that tunnel oxygen starts to decrease before that of the scala media oxygen.

Our first question, as described in the introduction, was whether the decline in CM resulting from the onset of hypoxia correlated with the oxygen decline in the tunnel or with the oxygen decline in the scala media. By combining data from paired recordings as shown in Figures 2-4, delay times for simultaneous recordings could be made.

Table II shows the delay times, in seconds, from shut off of respiratory air to first noticeable decline in oxygen tension in tunnel fluid or scala media endolymph, EP and CM. For comparison of the differences between sample means, the data are grouped. (a) Delays, air off to decrease in tunnel-fluid oxygen tension and air off to decline in CM. (b) Delays, air off to decrease in tunnel-fluid oxygen and air off to decrease in EP. (c) Delays, air off to decrease in scala media oxygen and air off to decrease in CM. (d) Delays, air off to decrease in scala media oxygen and air off to decrease in EP. "P" in this table is the probability that the paired mean delays are the same tested against the alternative that they are not the same (two-tailed Student's t test).

It makes no difference whether the recording is made in the tunnel or in the scala media, the decline in CM shows the same delay after the respiratory air is turned off, and this beginning decline in CM is much later than the beginning decline of oxygen in either tunnel or scala media. Consequently, these data do not tell us which source of oxygen CM is dependent upon.

The table shows that EP starts a decline later than does scala media oxygen, but still ten or more seconds before CM. All the differences between means in this table again are highly significant.

The data for each comparison were also tested for correlation (r = Pearson product-moment correlation coefficient). That is, the measures were tested to see if, in a single pair of measures, early decline in one was followed by an early decline in the other. As can be seen, the means, although their differences would occur by chance

TABLE III

DELAY TIMES FOR RESPIRATORY AIR TURNED ON TO INCREASE IN FLUID OXYGEN, COCHLEAR MICROPHONIC (CM) AND ENDOLYMPHATIC POTENTIAL (EP)

	(a)		*(b)*		*(c)*		*(d)*	
	O_2 *(Tunnel)*	*CM*	O_2 *(Tunnel)*	*EP*	O_2 *(SM)*	*CM*	O_2 *(SM)*	*EP*
N*	19	19	13	13	12	12	7	7
μ (Sec)	8.4	9.2	8.2	8.1	10.2	8.5	10.3	8.6
σ (Sec)	1.5	2.0	1.5	1.5	1.8	2.7	1.0	1.5
	$P < .1$		$P > .1$		$P < .02$		$P < .01$	
	$r = .48$		$r = -.05$		$r = .64$		$r = .67$	

SM - scala media
* Data from animals with minimal heart-rate change

less than once in a thousand, are not very highly correlated, indicating that the two paired-measures are not very dependent on each other.

Because both EP and CM start a decline sometime after oxygen tension in either tunnel or scala media, it would seem that, under normal conditions, there is a storehouse of oxygen which has to be depleted before the discernible changes in the electrical measures are observed. Following the exhaustion of this storehouse, the delay in the return of the various measures after the respiratory air is turned on may be the more realistic determinant of the sequence of events.

Table III shows the delay times in seconds from return of respiratory air to beginning oxygen-tension increase in tunnel fluid or scala media endolymph, and beginning return of EP and CM. All measurements are paired and, again, the data are grouped for comparison of sample means. (a) Delays, air on to increase in tunnel-fluid oxygen tension and air on to beginning recovery in CM. (b) Delays, air on to increase in tunnel-fluid oxygen tension and air on to beginning recovery of EP. (c) Delays, air on to increase in scala media oxygen tension and air on to beginning increase in CM. (d) Delays, air on to increase in scala media oxygen tension and air on to beginning increase in EP. "P" is as defined in Table II.

The first response to start a recovery is the tunnel-fluid oxygen followed immediately, or at the same time by EP and CM. The last measure to begin a recovery is the scala media endolymph oxygen. However, the most significant differences are those between CM and endolymph oxygen, and between EP and endolymph oxygen. There seems to be no relationship at all between tunnel-fluid oxygen and EP. It is interesting to note, however, that the small significance between delays in beginning recovery of tunnel-fluid oxygen and CM would indicate that they start returning at the same time, and this return between the paired measures is somewhat correlated. That is, when tunnel-fluid oxygen shows a relatively early recovery, so does CM. On the other hand, there is no correlation whatsoever between tunnel-fluid oxygen and EP, and their similarity of recovery times are not related to each other ($r = -.05$).

The curious revelation is that scala media oxygen returns last, significantly after both CM and EP. The differences are also fairly well correlated, that is, if CM or EP take a relatively longer time to begin recovery, so does scala media oxygen.

An essential question remains concerning the direct relationship between the beginning decline or recovery of

TABLE IV

DELAY TIMES FOR RESPIRATORY AIR TURNED OFF (a) OR ON (b) TO CHANGE IN ENDOLYMPHATIC POTENTIAL (EP) AND COCHLEAR MICROPHONIC (CM)

	(a)		*(b)*	
	EP	*CM*	*EP*	*CM*
N	44	44	14*	14*
M (Sec)	28.9	33.4	7.9	8.3
σ (Sec)	19.2	22.5	1.3	1.4
	P<.001		P<.1	
	r=.94		r=.85	

* Data from animals with minimal heart-rate change.

CM and EP when simultaneous data are recorded from a single nonpolarizable glass micropipette electrode as shown in Figure 4.

Table IV shows the delay times, in seconds, for (a) respiratory air turned off to beginning decline in EP and CM and (b) respiratory air turned on to beginning return of EP and CM. The sample number for return of respiratory air data is small because all animals that showed changes in the recorded EKG resulting from the hypoxia were eliminated. "P" is the same as described for Table II.

The data of Table IV, with air turned off, clearly show that EP declines significantly ahead of CM and that these declines are highly correlated.

On the return of respiratory air, both EP and CM start recovery at about the same time. Again, EP starts a bit sooner, but the return difference is not as significant as the beginning decline measure. However, the beginning recovery measures are again highly correlated; EP and CM, for any simultaneous recording, return together.

The data from the above tables are summarized in Figure 5. The beginning declines in the various measures are clearly separated following shut off of respiratory air and all the differences are statistically significant. Oxygen in the tunnel starts first, followed by the oxygen in the scala media endolymph. Considerably later, as though an excess of oxygen were being used up, EP starts to decline followed later by CM.

Recovery shows a different picture. Essentially tunnel-fluid oxygen, EP, and CM all start recovery together. The last measure in these experiments to show evidence of return is the oxygen in scala media endolymph.

DISCUSSION

Our experiment was designed to find out if CM decreased with the early decrease in tunnel oxygen or later with scala media oxygen. The results show that CM starts a decline much later than beginning decline of oxygen in either fluid compartment, and actually does not start decreasing until after EP has started to decrease.

There apparently is a storehouse of oxygen in excess of that required to support the generation and maintenance of

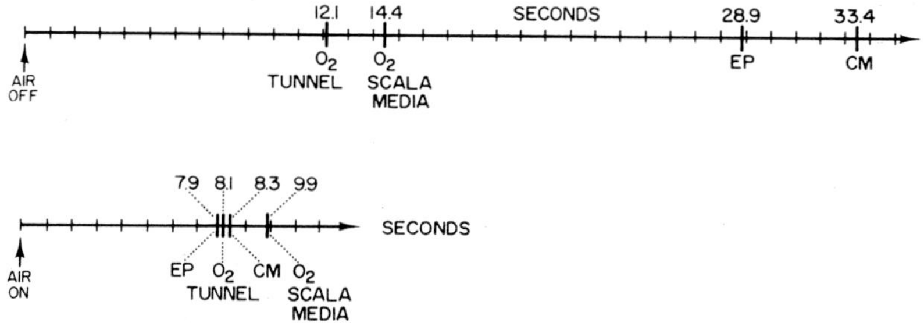

Fig. 5. The time lapse for beginning decline in the indicated measures following shut off of respiratory air and for beginning recovery of the same measures following return of respiratory air.

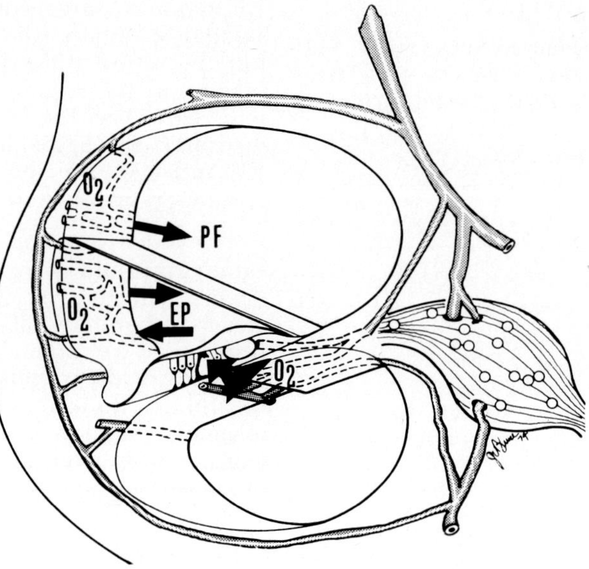

Fig. 6. Oxygen sources and function as indicated by the experiments reported here. The suprastrial capillaries provide oxygen and plasma filtrate (PF) as constituents of perilymph. The positive endolymphatic potential (EP) is brought about by ion transport from perilymph across Reissner's membrane and by special features of the stria vascularis that require oxygen for this function. The generation of CM depends upon tunnel oxygen and EP polarization, but the relationship is not exact.

EP and CM. Since CM is the last to start a decline, one cannot determine to which source of oxygen CM is more responsive, nor does this measure reveal how CM is related to EP. EP and CM could be responding differently to different sources of oxygen, but the correlation figures shown in Table IV indicate a clear relationship between EP and CM.

The high correlation coefficient indicates that the relationship can be represented by a straight line, *i.e.*, large delays in EP correspond to large delays in CM, and also that the experimental variation among animals is greater than the variability within an animal.

Obviously, there is a definite relationship between EP and CM, but the theory suggesting that CM is produced by a variable resistance directly modulating a current flow produced by the relatively high positive voltage of EP is difficult to reconcile since EP and CM do not change together. Such a theory would require a nonlinear element to account for the stability of CM until EP falls to a certain level.

Unexpectedly, the responses during recovery from hypoxia show a different sequence of events. Tunnel-fluid oxygen, EP and CM return together, whereas an electrode in the scala media detects a recovery in EP before there is a change in scala media oxygen. The biophysical mechanism for the generation of EP is obscure, and this difference in beginning recovery times reflects its complexity. Apparently there are other factors contributing to the generation of EP, and one of these factors, more than likely, involves the diffusion of ions from the perilymph across Reissner's membrane.

The suprastrial capillary[14] network lies in the region of spiral ligament just "above" Reissner's membrane. These capillaries are close to the surface and are arranged in a way to allow the formation of a plasma filtrate. These capillaries also would be subject to hypoxia, but oxygen tension in perilymph was not measured in these experiments.

Our interpretation of the course of events is presented in Figure 6. CM is at least partially dependent upon two factors: oxygen supplied to the extracellular spaces of the organ of Corti by the spiral vessels, and EP that itself is dependent upon several factors. Those factors determining EP include the diffusion of ions across Reissner's membrane, the availability of which is controlled by the suprastrial capillaries, and the buildup of the appropriate ion concentrations within the endolymph controlled by the special properties of the stria vascularis which requires oxygen for this function. The oxygen released by the capillaries of the stria vascularis is utilized by the stria vascularis itself[15,16] and is not released for the supply of the organ of Corti.

In the experiments reported here EP, as measured by a microelectrode in the endolymph, is a measure independent of the oxygen content of the endolymph. The oxygen that is measured within the endolymph is that which diffuses from the stria vascularis or through Reissner's membrane from the suprastrial capillaries.

EP itself is directly related to the generation of CM as is also the extracellular-space oxygen of the organ of Corti. However, it appears from the data reported here that the role of EP is more complex than that of providing a current flow for modulation by a variable resistance. The effect of a high-positive polarization without current flow enhancing the transduction process at the extremely low energy levels of threshold hearing is more likely the essential reason for its existence.

In answer to the question posed in the introduction, both capillary areas, the spiral capillaries and those of the stria vascularis are important to the adequate function of the organ of Corti: the spiral capillaries directly and the strial capillaries indirectly. Apparently, the suprastrial capillaries also play an important role.

Request for reprints should be sent to Merle Lawrence, Ph.D., The Kresge Hearing Research Institute, University of Michigan Medical School, Ann Arbor, Michigan.

REFERENCES

1. Hawkins JE Jr: Comparative otopathology: aging, noise and ototoxic drugs. Adv Otorhinolaryngol 20:125-141, 1973

2. Johnsson LG: Vascular pathology in the human inner ear. Adv Otorhinolaryngol 20: 197-220, 1973

3. Johnsson LG, Hawkins JE: Strial atrophy in clinical and experimental deafness. Laryngoscope 82:1105-1125, 1972

4. Wever EG, Bray CW, Lawrence M: The nature of cochlear activity after death. Ann Otol Rhinol Laryngol 50:317-329, 1941

5. Békésy GV: D-C potentials and energy balance of the cochlear partition. J Acoust Soc Am 23:576-582, 1951

6. Békésy GV: Gross localization of the place of origin of the cochlear microphonic. J Acoust Soc Am 24:399-409, 1952

7. Misrahy GA, Hildreth KM, Shinabarger EW, *et al*: Endolymphatic oxygen tension in the cochlea of the guinea pig. J Acoust Soc Am 30:247-250, 1958

8. Rice EA, Shinabarger EW: Studies on the endolymphatic DC potential of the guinea pig's cochlea. J Acoust Soc Am 33:922-925, 1961

9. Lawrence M: Inner ear physiology, in Paparella MM, Shumrich DA (eds): *Otolaryngology*. Philadelphia, W.B. Saunders, vol 1

10. Lawrence M, Nuttall AL: Oxygen availability in tunnel of corti measured by microelectrodes. J Acoust Soc Am 52:566-573, 1972

11. Lawrence M, Nuttall AL, Clapper MP: Electrical potentials and fluid boundaries within the organ of Corti. J Acoust Soc Am 55: 122-138, 1974

12. Lawrence M: Direct visualization of living organ of corti and studies of its extracellular fluids. Laryngoscope 84:1767-1776, 1974

13. Davis H: Biophysics and physiology of the inner ear. Physiol Rev 37:1-49, 1957

14. Hawkins JE Jr, Johnsson LG, Preston RE: Cochlear microvasculature in normal and

damaged ears. Laryngoscope 82:1091-1104, 1972

15. Thalmann I, Matschinsky FM, Thalmann R: Quantitative study of selected enzymes involved in energy metabolism of the cochlear duct. Ann Otol Rhinol Laryngol 79:12-29, 1970

16. Chou JTY, Rodgers K: Respiration of tissues lining the mammalian membranous labyrinth. J Laryngol Otol 76:341-351, 1962

NOTICE

The American Otological Society, Inc., notes with regret that its archives are not complete. The Council desires to remedy this insofar as possible and has directed the Editor-Librarian to seek replacement for volumes depleted from the library.

Accordingly, anyone in possession of any of the following volumes is earnestly requested to notify the Editor-Librarian. If recompense is desired, any fair price will be honored.

Vol. III, 1882-1887

Vol. XV, 1919-1921 (In some cases, these years may be in separate volumes)

Vol. XVIII, 1928

Vol. XXXIV, 1944

Vol. XLVI, 1958

Brian F. McCabe, M.D., Editor-Librarian, American Otological Society, Inc., University Hospitals, Iowa City, Iowa, 52242.

MODERN TRENDS IN OTOLOGIC SURGERY

A course including seminars, discussions, and surgical demonstrations will be presented Oct. 28 - Nov. 1, 1975, by the Department of Surgery, Section of Otolaryngology, Notre-Dame Hospital, Montreal, Quebec. Guest lecturers will include Professor Ugo Fisch, Juan Marquet, M.D., Brian McCabe, M.D., and George Shambaugh, Jr., M.D.

For further information write: Robert A. Bertrand, M.D., Vestibular Laboratory, Notre-Dame Hospital, 1560 Sherbrooke St. East, Montreal, Quebec, Canada, H2L 4 MI.

Ann Otol 84: 1975

CONSERVATIVE MANAGEMENT OF MÉNIÈRE'S DISEASE: FURSTENBERG REGIMEN REVISITED

ROGER BOLES, M.D.
SAN FRANCISCO, CALIFORNIA
DALE H. RICE, M.D. ROGER HYBELS, M. D.
WALTER P. WORK, M. D.
ANN ARBOR, MICHIGAN

SUMMARY — This study reviews twenty years' experience at the University of Michigan with 500 consecutive patients suffering from symptoms of Ménière's disease. An especially strong tradition of medical therapy for Ménière's disease has prevailed at the University of Michigan because of the influence of Albert C. Furstenberg, who developed and promoted the Furstenberg regimen of a low-sodium diet and diuretics. It has been our distinct clinical impression over the years that the Furstenberg regimen has been quite satisfactory in relieving the most disturbing symptoms of Ménière's disease in the vast majority of cases and often in patients who have failed other treatment programs. This study quantifies, as much as possible, our extensive experience with this disease and confirms for us the efficacy of this treatment. Relatively few operative procedures have had to be performed for conservative treatment failures in our hands. The success of this conservative management program has been largely dependent upon the strict adherence by the patient to a professionally prescribed, low-sodium diet. Occasional patients with chronic symptoms which are refractory to medical management continue to be a problem, particularly since it is in this group of patients that bilateral involvement tends to ultimately occur.

Ever since 1861, when Prosper Ménière described the clinical picture of vertigo, hearing loss, and tinnitus as a manifestation of an inner ear disorder, his name has been associated with this specific and distressing combination of symptoms.[1] Ménière, in his treatise, was hopeful that in future years microscopic examination of temporal bones afflicted with these symptoms would ultimately reveal the exact etiology of this disorder and end the "blind empiricism" with which it had been treated so unsuccessfully. In the 114 years since Ménière's original essay, we have essentially failed to meet his charge to find a specific etiology and a rational and scientific treatment for his syndrome, despite extensive attempts by many clinicians and scientists. One such study was carried out at the University of Michigan by Furstenberg, *et al* in the 1930's and was presented before the American Otological Society in Atlantic City in 1934.[2] This study was, in great measure, an expansion of similar work done previously by Dederding which related variations in the body, dietary fluids, and electrolytes to remissions and exacerbations of the symptoms of Ménière's syndrome.[3] From their studies, Furstenberg and his group concluded that the tissues involved in Ménière's disease either have an increased avidity for sodium ions or an unusual sensitivity to them. From this conclusion they tried, with rather clear and dramatic success, a treatment program designed to reduce body sodium by restricting it in the diet and by enhancing its elimination through the kidney with the use of the diuretic, ammonium chloride. This ini-

---

From the Department of Otorhinolaryngology, University of Michigan, Ann Arbor, Michigan.

Presented at the meeting of the American Otological Society, Atlanta, Georgia, April 11-12, 1975.

tial success in 14 patients was confirmed by subsequent trials with this treatment program in 150 patients as reported in 1941.[4] This treatment program of a low-sodium diet and diuretic gained widespread recognition and approval from practitioners both inside and outside of the specialty of otolaryngology, and generally became known as the Furstenberg regimen[5,6] (Fig. 1, Table I).

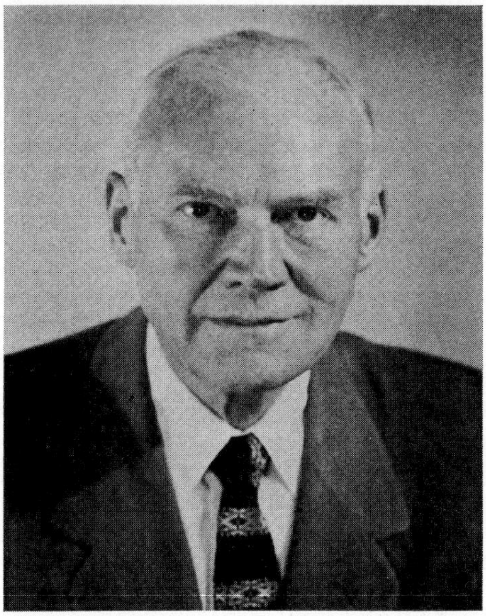

Fig. 1. Albert C. Furstenberg, M.D.; Dean, School of Medicine (1935-1960); Chairman, Department of Otolaryngology (1932-1957); University of Michigan.

Whereas the surgical treatment for Ménière's disease had been partial section of the VIII nerve, after the initiation of the sodium-elimination program, only six of the 150 patients reported by Furstenberg, *et al* in 1941[4] had had to have this surgical procedure because of their failure to respond satisfactorily to medical treatment.

Because of these initial and continued apparent successes, many patients with Ménière's disease and other forms of dizziness have been attracted to the University of Michigan over the ensuing years. Seldom has there been any expression of doubt as to the efficacy of the Furstenberg regimen at this institution, presumably because of considerable patient and physician satisfaction with it. The recent, great attentions given to other methods of treatment, both surgical and medical, and particularly the advocacy of operative procedures of considerable magnitude, suggested that others were not experiencing the same satisfaction that we were with the sodium-restriction program or that perhaps we were not realistically appraising our own results with it. It was largely with this motivation that we reviewed our experience at the University of Michigan with over 500 consecutive cases of Ménière's disease during the past twenty years.

TABLE I

FURSTENBERG REGIMEN

1. 800-1,000 mg sodium diet
2. Avoidance of preparations high in sodium, *e.g.* sodium bicarbonate, sodium salicylates, etc.
3. Diuretic

In order to be included in this study, all patients had to have the classic triad of symptoms and additionally had to have audiometric evidence of sensorineural hearing loss. During the span of time of this study, a number of helpful new audiometric tests were developed and employed as they became available. The same was true for vestibular testing. Whenever there was a serious question as to the accuracy of the diagnosis, the patients were referred to specialists in neurology and internal medicine for their evaluations and opinions.

Once the diagnosis of Ménière's disease was established, our basic treatment program was to start the patient on a low-salt diet and a diuretic. The majority of patients had mild and easily controlled symptoms and required only one or two visits to our clinic before we were willing to return them to their family physicians for long-term maintenance care. This paper will deal with the 125 patients who were followed for longer periods of time, usually because of the severity of their disease.

TABLE II

AGE OF ONSET OF MÉNIÈRE'S DISEASE

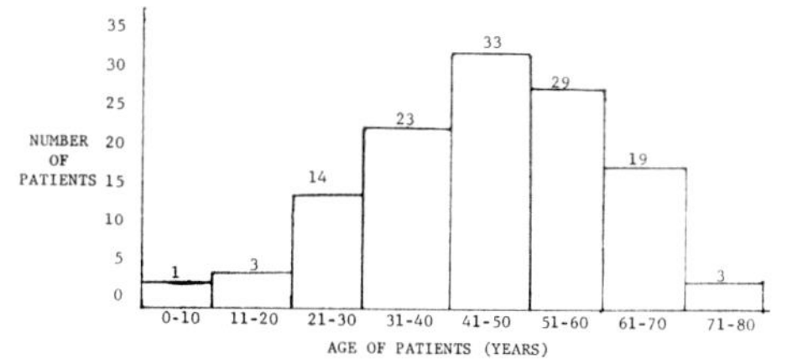

Of this group of 125 longer-term patients, 71 were males and 54 were females. Their ages ranged from 10 to 73 years with the average age being 45.5 years at the time of their first visit (Table II).

The patients in this study group were divided into three classes according to the severity of their disease. If the patient had one or more incapacitating spells a month with nausea or vomiting, he was classified as severe. If a patient had such severe episodes only once or twice every three months, he was classified as moderate. Symptoms less severe than these were considered mild. By these criteria, 103 patients were classified as severe, 18 as moderate, and three as mild. Two could not be accurately classified. Twenty-four patients had bilateral disease.

Almost all patients were treated initially with a low-salt diet which was worked out on an individual basis for each patient by a qualified dietician. These low-salt diets generally allowed the patients 800-1,000 mg Na/day. An occasional patient with mild or moderate symptoms was placed on a no-added-salt diet, which meant adding no salt to one's food either in the cooking process or at the table. In addition, each patient received a diuretic and a variety of other medications. Early in this experience, ammonium chloride was the diuretic used in doses suggested by Furstenberg, specifically 9 g/day. As the thiazides became available, they were used with greater frequency and essentially replaced ammonium chloride. Flushing doses of nicotinic acid were given to many patients. Numerous other preparations were used sporadically, including meclizine hydrochloride, diazepam, and chlorpromazine. The mainstay of treatment, however, was the low-salt diet and the diuretic. If the symptoms continued despite the diet prescribed, the sodium content was reduced further, occasionally to a minimum of 500 mg/day. As symptoms seemed to improve and disappear for two or three months, the treatment program was gradually tapered and titrated against any recurrence of symptoms. This usually consisted of first reducing and finally eliminating the diuretic, followed gradually by a liberalization of the low-salt diet.

The response of the patient to treatment was determined by the degree of relief from vertiginous episodes. If, after the initiation of treatment, the patient had no further spells, the response was considered excellent. If the attacks decreased in severity and occurred no more frequently than one in three months, the response was considered good. If the spells were decreased in severity and occurred no oftener than one per month, the response was considered fair. If more than one attack occurred per month, the response was considered poor. By these criteria, 63 of the 103 patients regarded as severe had excellent responses. Twenty-six of the 103 had good responses. Three had fair responses and eleven had poor responses. Of the 18 patients with moderate symptoms, eight had excellent responses, nine had good responses, and one had a poor response. The three patients followed in the mild group all had excellent responses. (Table III).

TABLE III

RESPONSE TO MEDICAL THERAPY IN MÉNIÈRE'S DISEASE

Severity of Disease	*Quality of Response* Excellent	*Good*	*Fair*	*Poor*	*Totals*
Severe	63	26	3	11	103
Moderate	8	9	0	1	18
Mild	3	0	0	0	3

TABLE IV

CHANGE IN HEARING OVER TIME IN MÉNIÈRE'S DISEASE

Duration of Disease	*Audiogram Results*		
Yrs.	*Air Conduction (Av. at ½, 1 & 2 kHz)*	*Air Conduction (4 kHz)*	*Discrimination %*
5-10	60dB	67dB	55%
11-15	50dB	60dB	55%
16-20	55dB	65dB	54%
>20	50dB	60dB	35%

Furstenberg, *et al* had noted in their early work with the low-salt diet program that not only were patients promptly relieved by this treatment, but also that the return of symptoms was often immediately precipitated by the use of salt.[2] In our current review, 17 of the 125 patients volunteered this same information; namely, improvement of symptoms when avoiding salt and exacerbation upon resumption of salt. All of the patients with good or excellent responses were relatively faithful to their diet.

All but one of the 12 patients who had poor responses to this medical therapy had symptoms classed as severe. Ten of these patients had unilateral disease. All but one patient ultimately had a destructive labyrinthectomy with complete relief of further vertigo. The single surgical patient with bilateral disease had one ear which was much more severely affected than the other and had a destructive labyrinthectomy on the more severely affected ear with good relief from further dizzy spells. Nine of the 11 operative procedures were done via both mastoid and middle ear approaches with opening of each semicircular canal as well as the oval window. Two were performed through the ear canal alone with communication of round and oval windows only. The labyrinthectomy was performed only when the patients' symptoms were uncontrolled by the most intensive medical therapy and only when the involved ear had no further useful hearing. Seven of these 11 patients had poor responses to medical management from the outset and had a destructive labyrinthectomy relatively early in the course of their disease. Four of the 11 surgical patients had a long history of disease which had responded well initially to medical management but which ultimately became reactivated with persistence and worsening of symptoms despite conservative treatment.

The relationship of hearing in the affected ear to the duration of the disease is shown in Table IV. It appears that the hearing loss in the affected ear usually stabilizes within five years of the onset of the disease but that the discrimination score may deteriorate even after many years. Nine patients in this group of 125 had a history of the disease for longer than 20 years. Six of these nine patients eventually developed bilateral disease.

DISCUSSION

Since the etiology and pathophysiology of Ménière's disease remain obscure, treatment of all varieties must still, therefore, be considered empirical. We have generally operated under the principle that under such uncertain circumstances, the most conservative treatment program which will give acceptable relief from symptoms is probably best justified in most instances.

As was stated early by Furstenberg, the success of medical therapy for Ménière's disease will be greatly dependent upon the strictness with which it is prescribed by the physician and dietician and also with which it is followed by the patient himself. We believe much of our continued success with this program is premised on our careful adherence to these principles of close therapeutic control.

Although we have tried a number of auxiliary medications to supplement our basic treatment program through the years, we must emphasize that we have depended most heavily upon dietary sodium restriction as the primary treatment, with the use of diuretics in the more troublesome cases. Patients who will need an operative procedure usually have a poor response to medical management from the outset. The distressing feature of eventual bilateral involvement, in many patients who have long-standing symptoms and who respond poorly to medical management, begs for a better solution to these particular patients' problem than a destructive operation.

CONCLUSIONS

The vast majority of patients with Ménière's disease can be managed adequately with a strict low-salt diet supplemented when necessary with the use of diuretics.

Destructive labyrinthectomy should seldom be necessary but continues to be a satisfactory solution to the problem of unilateral Ménière's disease which is refractory to medical management.

Bilateral Ménière's disease is uncommon, and when it does occur, it is usually in patients with long-standing symptoms which have generally responded poorly to medical treatment.

The pathological processes of Ménière's disease require greater clarification in order to develop more truly rational treatment programs.

Request for reprints should be sent to Roger Boles, M.D., School of Medicine, Department of Otolaryngology, Room 495 U, University of California, San Francisco, California 94143.

REFERENCES

1. Ménière P: Memoire sur de lesions de l'oreille interne donant lieu a des symptoms de congestion cerebrale. Gazette Medicale de Paris 16:597, 1861

2. Furstenberg AC, Lashmet FH, Lathrop F: Ménière's symptom complex: medical treatment. Ann Otol Rhinol Laryngol 43:1035-1046, 1934

3. Dederding D: Our Ménière treatment (principles and results). Acta Otolaryngol (Stockh) 16:404-415, 1931

4. Furstenberg AC, Richardson G, Lathrop F: Ménière's disease; addenda to medical therapy. Arch Otolaryngol 34:1083-1092, 1941

5. Brown MR: Medical treatment (Furstenberg method) of Ménière's syndrome. JAMA 108:1158-1160, 1937

6. Bartels EC: Diagnosis and treatment of Ménière's disease. Med Clin North Am 22: 695-700, 1938

OTOLARYNGOLOGIC ASSEMBLY

The annual Otolaryngologic Assembly of 1975 will be held November 8-14, 1975, in the Eye and Ear Infirmary of the University of Illinois Hospital. The Department of Otolaryngology of the Abraham Lincoln School of Medicine, University of Illinois at the Medical Center offers a condensed basic and clinical program for practicing otolaryngologists under the direction of Emanuel M. Skolnik, M.D., with Burton J. Soboroff, M.D. as co-chairman. Inquiries may be sent to: Otolaryngology, P.O. Box 6998, Chicago, Illinois 60680.

RADIOLOGY CONFERENCE

A Conference on Radiology in Otolaryngology and Ophthalmology will be held on November 28 and 29, 1975, under the guidance of Galdino E. Valvassori, M.D. For further information write to: G. E. Valvassori, M.D., Radiology Department, Abraham Lincoln School of Medicine, P.O. Box 6998, Chicago, Illinois 60680.

Ann Otol 84: 1975

GRAFTING MATERIALS AND METHODS IN RECONSTRUCTIVE EAR SURGERY

RODNEY PERKINS, M.D.

PALO ALTO, CALIFORNIA

SUMMARY – The evolution of tympanic membrane grafting over the past 20 years has been based on biologic tissues of mesodermal origin which contain a collagen matrix. The dominant theme of this evolution has been the modification of these collagen membranes by physical and chemical agents to achieve a more ideal graft. The graft material and the operation should be suited to specific problems. Current operative techniques and graft materials are discussed. It is believed that there will be continued modification and manipulation of collagen in the future to achieve a more ideal graft for tympanic membrane restoration.

Over the past 25 years there has been a progressive improvement in the ability to surgically close perforations of the tympanic membrane. Various materials have been used in combination with a wide variety of surgical procedures in an effort to arrive at a restoration of both structure and function of this unusual and important membrane.

The earlier pioneers employed skin grafts in attempts to restore the integrity of the membrane. Although these epidermal grafts were successful in many cases, they have largely been abandoned and replaced by mesodermal grafts of diverse origins. Today, we see many types of materials of mesodermal origin employed in reconstruction of the tympanic membrane. They are placed in different positions using a plethora of techniques but have generally been accepted by almost all otologists as the material of choice.

It has been found useful in discussing this subject and in organizing my thoughts to think of these mesodermal tissues as material, rather than this tissue or that tissue, treated in this manner or that manner. These are, in fact, all biomaterials. For example, a piece of dried, dehydrated autogenous temporalis fascia is widely used in otologic surgery. This is said to be a "tissue graft." Yes, it is from a tissue source, but it is no longer living tissue. The original nature of the tissue has been dramatically changed by the drying process. It has been devitalized, dehydrated, and slightly denatured by the drying process. It is more appropriate to think of this fascia now as a piece of nonviable biomaterial of autogenous mesodermal origin. By doing so we can better understand the function it serves and develop a basis for understanding the nature of some of the homograft materials now being employed and provide a framework from which we can develop more ideal materials in the future.

THE BASIS OF TYMPANIC MEMBRANE GRAFTING

In some of the earlier literature on tympanic membrane grafts one sees expressed the terms "high metabolic rate" graft and "low metabolic rate" graft. The former is usually applied to autogenous skin grafts and the latter to materials of mesodermal origin. The higher perforation rate of the autogenous skin grafts is said to be due to its "higher metabolic rate," whereas the mesodermal grafts were thought to perforate less due to a "lower metabolic rate." Presumably this meant that the mesodermal grafts required less vascular and nutritive support and therefore in a compromised situation, had a

Presented at the meeting of the American Otological Society, Inc., Atlanta, Georgia, April 11-12, 1975.

higher chance of survival. This line of reasoning does not explain the higher survival of the mesodermal grafts. While it is true that the viable autogenous ectodermal grafts need neovascularization to survive, it is not true for the mesodermal material. The difference in success lies in the fact that these are two different methods of membrane restoration rather than factors related to the "metabolic rate" of the tissues employed. The autogenous skin graft becomes the graft membrane *per se* if successfully neovascularized before skin death. The mesodermal material only serves as a superstructure or scaffolding for growth of epithelium from the adjacent ear canal wall and therefore is only part of the new membrane. Its function is that of superstructure or guide plane for the new epithelium. This superstructure may remain briefly and be replaced by host fibrocytic infiltration and new collagen deposition as with autogenous fascia or may be turned over more slowly, as is thought to occur in aldehyde crosslinked homograft tympanic membranes.

One of the important facts which emerge from this understanding is: superstructure graft materials need not be viable to perform their function in tympanic membrane closure. This should be quite obvious when one considers dried autogenous fascia grafts. These grafts have been dehydrated and frequently heated at supraphysiologic temperatures and still perform quite well as a graft superstructure material.

The Common Denominator. All the superstructure grafts that I have heard about are of mesodermal origin. Autogenous fascia, autogenous perichondrium, autogenous vein, homograft tympanic membrane, homograft dura, homograft fascia, homograft pericardium, homograft omentum, heterograft serosa, heterograft tympanic membrane, and probably others have been used in tympanic membrane restoration. All of these are used in a nonviable state. Why is it that all of these are of mesodermal origin? Why is it that all of these work a certain percentage of the time? What do these tissues have as a common denominator that makes them useful as a superstructure graft? All of these tissues contain a collagen matrix that is the structural layer necessary to perform a graft superstructure function, *i.e.*, support migration of host epithelium.

Modified Collagen Membranes: The Evolutionary Theme. Collagen matrix grafts were introduced to tympanic membrane surgery in the 1950's in the form of autogenous vein and fascia. These were employed essentially as viable and unmodified. Initially, they were employed as a medial surface graft and later were used as a lateral surface graft. However, in both grafting positions the function remains that of a superstructure for epithelial migration.

During the late 1950's and early 1960's we see the beginning of what I believe to be the dominant theme of tympanic membrane grafting evolution: the progressive modification of collagen matrices to achieve a more ideal graft material. These modifications become more apparent with a review of the past 20 years.

Shortly after the introduction of autogenous vein and autogenous temporalis fascia, surgeons began drying or dehydrating the fascia prior to use. I suspect that this was an accident in the beginning as are many things in scientific evolution. One can easily imagine the fascia, drying out on the back table while the operation progressed. However, such a graft was placed, and it worked. Most of us now routinely dry the fascia either by air drying at room temperature or accelerate the process by placing a lighted bulb near the fascia. We do this to facilitate fashioning it to size and to simplify our ability to manipulate it into the desired position before rehydration occurs and the tissue becomes less manageable. However, from an evolutionary point of view, the air drying introduced a modification into the tissue: it devitalized it and dehydrated it. When the lighted bulb adds heat to the tissue, it further alters it by slightly denaturing the protein. What we are in effect doing in

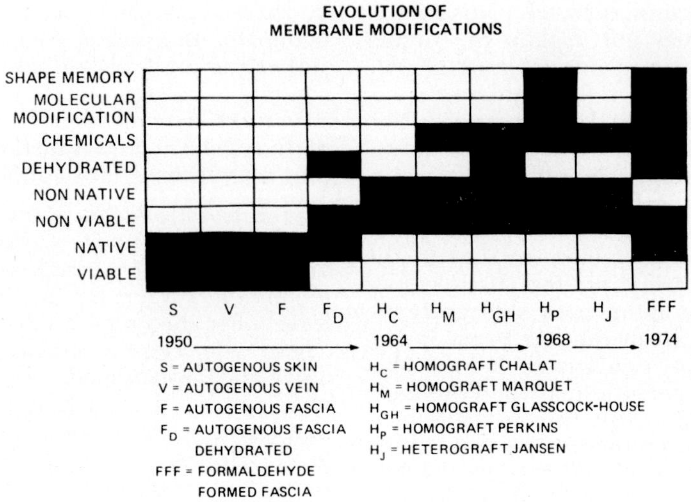

Fig. 1. Chart illustrates progressive modification of grafting materials.

this sequence is trading the viability of the material for the technical advantages that the dehydration affords. We are employing two modifying agents, evaporation and heat, to give us this new nonviable denatured collagen matrix.

We can follow this evolution in more detail by examining further developments in tympanic membrane grafting materials (Fig. 1). During the 1950's, the tissues employed were native and viable. As we have discussed above, the dehydrated fascia (F_D) signalled a change.

In the early 1960's, the report of Chalat on his attempt to use fresh homograft tympanic membrane as a graft material was another significant departure (Fig. 1, [H_c]).[1] The variation here is not so much the modification of a collagen matrix but a change in the source material of this matrix. He did not introduce chemicals into his homograft holding solution, but the collagen matrix did have a different architectural structure than fascia or vein. In that sense, the collagen matrix was modified, but this was accomplished by source selection rather than by chemical or physical modifiers.

Jean Marquet introduced an additional factor by using a chemical agent, Cialit,®* as a sterilizing agent in the solution for storage of homograft tympanic membrane.[2] The Cialit® prevents bacterial growth and, thus, counters the potential effect that proteolytic enzymes from such growth might have on the protein structure of the collagen and its interstitial substance.

In 1968, Glasscock and House reported using two other agents, freezing in combination with isopropyl alcohol (Fig. 1, [H_{GH}]).[3] In this instance, both a physical modification (freezing) and a chemical one, *i.e.*, dehydration by the alcohol, have been employed.

In 1969, our initial experience with homograft tympanic membrane modified with formaldehyde was reported (Fig. 1, [H_P]).[4] The formaldehyde not only serves as an excellent sterilizing agent for both bacteria and for many viruses, but also effects a more specific change in the collagen matrix. The aldehyde interacts chemically with the collagen molecule to give three advantageous modifying effects. It increases tensile strength, and evidence indicates that it reduces the antigenicity.[5,6] In addition, the crosslinking creates a memory in the matrix for its configura-

* Asid Institut, BMBH, Munchen, Lohhof, Germany.

tion at the time of crosslinking. Here, then, from our evolutionary view, we have added a specific chemical alteration of the collagen molecules and created a membrane which retains the desired shape.

In 1973, another departure was introduced by Claus Jansen (Fig. 1, [H_J]).[7] It is a source modification similar to that of Chalat. Jansen used heterograft tympanic membrane of bovine origin in successful closure of perforations. This further supports the migratory plane theory and again emphasizes that the membrane need not be viable, need not be autogenous, nor even homologous. However, it still is a collagen matrix.

The last item in the evolutionary table is the formaldehyde formed autogenous fascia graft (Fig. 1, [FFF]).[8] This modified membrane evolved from seeing the advantages that the conical shape of formaldehyde crosslinked homografts afforded in hearing improvement and reduced blunting and lateral displacement. The graft material and surgical method are described in more detail later in this paper. The graft represents a biomaterial of autogenous fascia modified by dehydration, heat, and chemicals (aldehyde crosslinking) which retains the conical shape of the tympanic membrane during implantation.

Through these years, most of these changes have been made empirically by surgeons in an attempt to improve their results. Each small variation is not noticed as clearly as we can note it with retrospective vision. However, the trend is clear, logical, and will continue to unfold more dramatically in the next few years.

SURGICAL METHODS FOR USE WITH COLLAGEN MEMBRANE GRAFTS

The collagen membrane material is only one facet of the successful restoration of tympanic membrane function. Without a well-designed operative procedure and technique by the surgeon, the type graft employed is a moot point.

Collagen membranes are usually used with techniques that either place the membrane medial to the remnant tympanic membrane or lateral to the de-epithelized remnant. Problems are associated with both of these techniques when used in total tympanic membrane perforations.

Medial surface collagen membrane grafts have been used longer than lateral surface grafts. They are the method of choice in perforations that are clearly posterior to the malleus. Autogenous fascia placed on the medial surface of a posterior perforation has almost assured perforation closure with little chance of complication. However, in total tympanic membrane perforations or in perforations in which there is a substantial portion of the perforation anterior to the malleus, this grafting technique runs into problems and has a higher perforation rate than is acceptable in cases where ossicular anatomy and function are normal. At least a 5% perforation rate is likely.[9]

In these cases, the failures are usually anterior-inferior. This is due to the poor apposition of the graft to the medial surface of the inferior annular rim or to incomplete removal of the epithelium that has migrated over the edge onto the medial surface. This same incomplete removal can also result in residual epithelium in the middle ear.

Lateral surface grafts in similar large or substantially anterior perforations have an exceptionally high rate of closure which in good hands is virtually 100% However, this benefit is too frequently dulled by significant blunting and lateral displacement in the healed membrane and its consequences to hearing improvement. Another less frequent complication of lateral surface autogenous fascia grafts is the late appearance of an expanding epithelial cyst hidden in the blunted anterior sulcus.

Total and Anterior Perforations with Intact Malleus

In an effort to combat the complications of both medial surface and lateral surface grafts and to find a grafting method that could be used with any collagen membrane graft, the following technique has evolved. It can be used in all total tympanic membrane perforations and works well with non-processed autogenous fascia, formaldehyde formed autogenous fascia, homograft tympanic membrane with ossicles en bloc or any other collagen membrane graft materials. It will be described here utilizing a formaldehyde formed autogenous temporalis fascia graft in a total tympanic membrane perforation with no ossicular disease. In my opinion, this biomaterial is the one of choice in this clinical condition.

Preparation of the Formaldehyde-Formed Autogenous Temporalis Fascia. The procedure is done under local anesthesia, if no cholesteatoma is present, in adults. The fascia is obtained from the lateral surface of the temporalis muscle through a separate incision. A separate incision is suggested because the fascia found at the upper extent of a post-auricular incision or an extended post-auricular incision is frequently thicker and more irregular due to its attachment to the skull at the temporal line.

A piece of fascia about 2 cm in diameter is removed and spread on a cutting block. Any attached muscular tissue is removed. The fascia is placed between the layers of a cotton gauze sponge and squeezed between the fingers. This removes any attached blood clot or serum on the graft surface.

At this point a metal male mold,* shaped like the medial external auditory canal and tympanic membrane, is employed (Fig. 2A). The fascia is pulled onto the mold in such a manner that about 3-4 mm of fascia is present on the anterior canal wall portion of the mold. The tympanic membrane portion is completely covered and 5-10 mm of fascia extend onto the posterior superior canal wall portion of the mold (Fig. 2B). Care is taken to eliminate any excess tissue in the anterior sulcus area of the mold. Any bunching or folding of the tissue in that area is worked away toward the posterior superior canal wall area. Redundant tissue is more tolerable in this latter area, whereas it might tend to cause blunting if present in excess in the anterior sulcus zone.

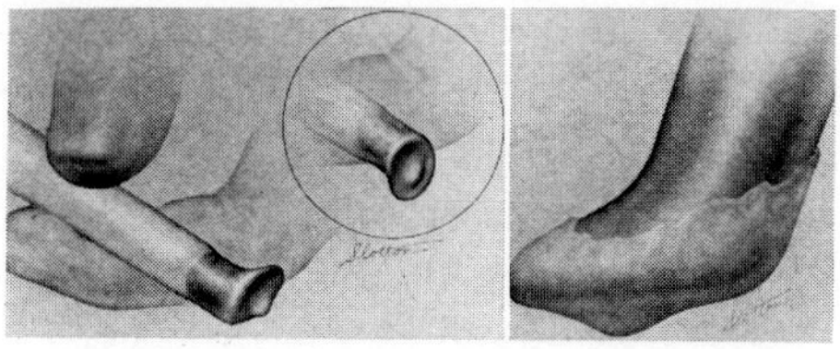

Fig. 2. A) The metal male mold shaped like the medial external auditory canal and tympanic membrane. B) The patient's fascia is draped on the mold, air dried, and fixed with buffered formaldehyde.

The metal mold and fascia are then air dried using a small electric dryer. The dryer is placed about eight to ten inches from the mold. Adequate drying has occurred when the tissue is tested with a blunt probe and all softness is gone, generally taking about five to ten minutes.

The dried fascia and mold are then placed in a solution bath of buffered formaldehyde, 4% pH 5.6, for about six minutes. If a little more stiffness is desired, this can be effected by increasing the time in this solution.

The fascia and mold are then placed in two successive rinsing baths of physiologic irrigating solution for five minutes each. The now formed fascia is then removed from the mold and placed in a third rinsing bath for five minutes. Any rough edges are trimmed at this time and the shaped graft is ready for implantation.

Surgical Implantation Technique. Through the transmeatal approach, an extended posterior vascular strip flap is created (Fig. 3). This flap is retrograde elevated several millimeters using a back-angled elevator.**

A postauricular incision is made and dissection is carried anterio-medially to the posterior lateral bony rim of the external canal. The previously delineated

---

* Hear America Corporation, Sunnyvale, California
** Storz Instrument Co., St. Louis, Mo.

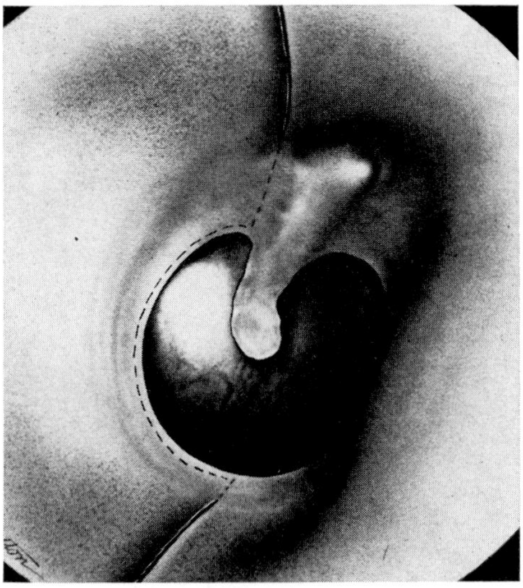

Fig. 3. Canal incisions are made to create a posterior skin flap. The connecting incision (dotted line) is made as near to the posterior rim of the perforation as possible.

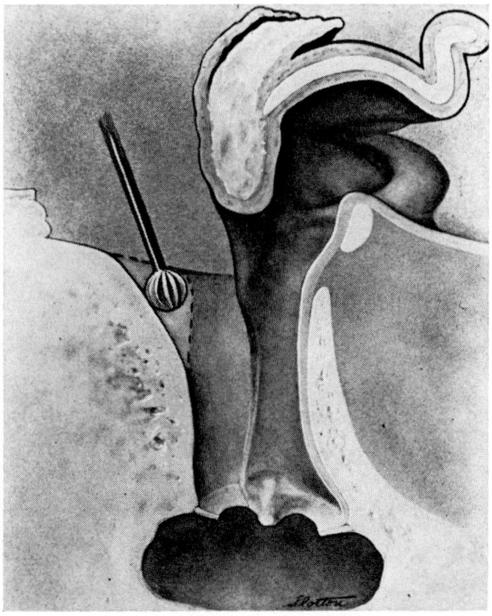

Fig. 4. A small amount of bone removal at the posterior superior rim of the bony external canal facilitates the view of the anterior sulcus.

posterior vascular strip is elevated and retained under the protective blade of a special tympanoplasty retractor.*

In order to clearly view the anterior canal sulcus, it may be necessary to remove a small amount of the rim of the posterior superior bony canal near the spine of Henle (Fig. 4).

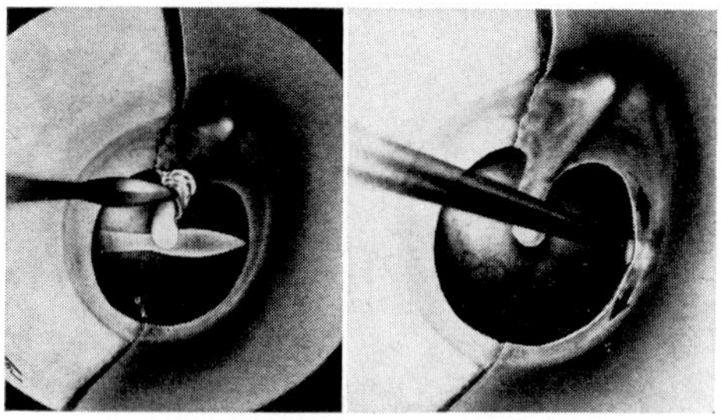

Fig. 5. A) A double-edged sickle knife is used to make an incision in the anterior rim of the perforation and an incision along the posterior periostium of the malleus. B) Using an angled canal elevator the outer squamous epithelium is separated from the middle fibrous layer of the tympanic membrane.

The anterior edge of the tympanic membrane perforation is incised and an incision is made in the posterior periosteum of the malleus (Fig. 5A). The epithelium on the malleus is carefully dissected off in continuity with elevation of the epithelium of the pars flaccida area. The outer squamous epithelium is separated from the middle fibrous layer of the tympanic membrane (Fig. 5B). This dissection is carried forth until the entire remnant tympanic membrane is elevated to the canal wall.

The anterior-superior flap, thus created, is retrograde elevated about 5 mm with the back-angled elevator (Fig. 6). *The remnant tympanic membrane and annulus are then removed.* The formed fascia is then introduced into the canal and placed into anatomical position. Care is taken to be sure the graft is on the bone of the anterior sulcus and on the manubrium of the malleus.

Using a sharpened wood applicator saturated with methylene blue dye, the midpoint of the malleus is marked on

----

* Storz Instrument Co., St. Louis, Mo.

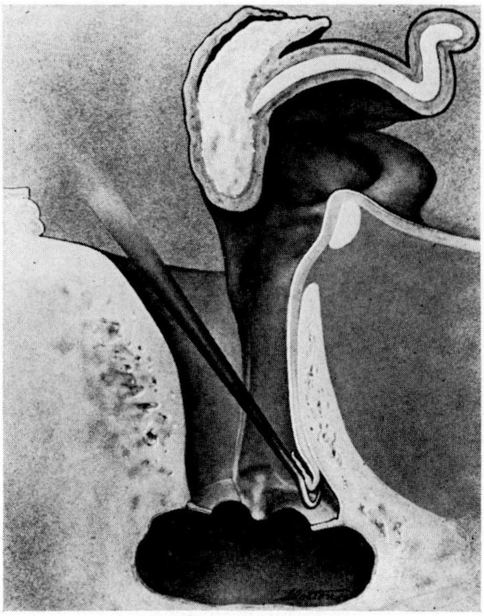

Fig. 6. Using a back-angled canal elevator, the anterior superior skin flap is retrograde elevated.

the lateral surface of the fascia graft. The formed fascia is withdrawn and placed on the cutting block. Using a number 11 scalpel blade, a small incision is made at the dye mark.

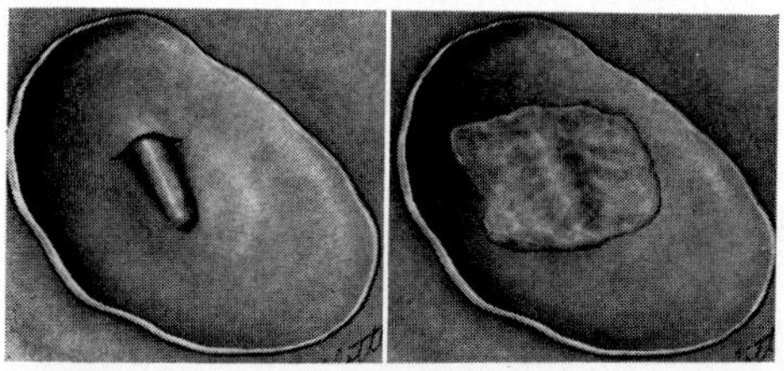

Fig. 7. A) The inferior one-half of the malleus manubrium projects through the slit and lies to the fascia graft. B) A small piece of nonprocessed fascia is placed over the exposed manubrium.

The graft is reintroduced into the canal. The slit is maneuvered over the malleus tip and the graft placed back in its previous position (Fig. 7A). A small piece of dehydrated, but nonformaldehyde treated fascia is then placed over the exposed manubrium (Fig. 7B). The malleolar slit arrangement helps to prevent lateral displacement, both in the early postoperative period due to middle ear bleeding, and in the later period when displacement of the malleus might occur due to graft tightening.

The previously elevated anterior superior canal skin is rolled back over the sulcus flange of the formed fascia. A small slit is made in the canal skin flap to prevent a webbing effect (Fig. 8). The anterior sulcus area is then packed with chloramphenicol soaked gelatin (Gelfoam®)* pledgets. The postauricular wound is closed with interrupted 3-0 subcuticular Dexon suture.

Through the transmeatal view the posterior vascular strip canal skin flap is replaced in its normal position such that it overlies the posterior canal portion of formed fascia graft (Fig. 8). The remainder of the canal is packed with chloramphenicol soaked gelatin (Gelfoam®) pledgets. An expanding plastic

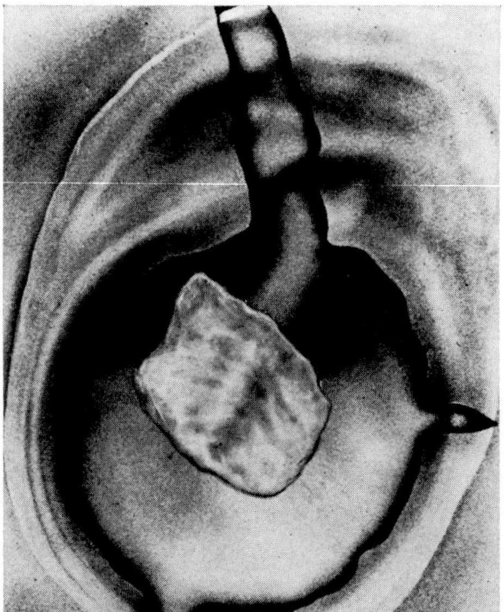

Fig. 8. The anterior and posterior canal skin flaps are placed over the flange of the homograft. A small slit is made in the anterior flap to prevent a webbing effect.

* The Upjohn Co., Kalamazoo, Mich.

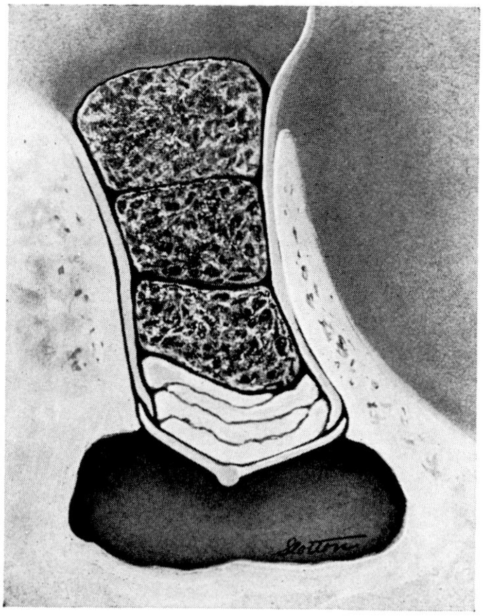

Fig. 9. The medial canal is packed with antibiotic soaked Gelfoam® pledgets and plastic sponge packing is placed in the lateral canal.

sponge pack is introduced into the lateral external meatus with a special applicator (Fig. 9). The plastic packing is removed in the office one week later using the stereo operating microscope. Antibiotic ear drops are used two weeks after the operation to remove the more medially placed gelatin sponge packing.

Results with this chemically modified collagen have been excellent. The perforation rate has been 1% in over 60 cases. It has been particularly effective in reducing blunting and lateral displacement. In the first 41 cases with normal ossicular chains, 71% had closure of the air-bone gap to 1-15 dB.[8]

Large Membrane Perforations with Malleus-Incus Disease

In cases which have pars tensa perforation and significant malleus disease, currently a similar operative technique is used to that just described with the formaldehyde formed fascia. However, in these cases, a formaldehyde crosslinked tympanic membrane with malleus-incus en bloc is employed. The formaldehyde processing is particularly important in en bloc homografts since the incudomalleolar joint is unstable unless strengthened by crosslinking with aldehydes. The homograft incus is placed on the stapes if possible and sometimes connected to the stapes with

CLINICAL CONDITION	OPERATIVE TECHNIQUE	GRAFT MATERIAL: SOURCE	GRAFT MATERIAL: MODIFICATION
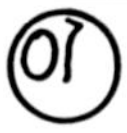 • POSTERIOR PERFORATION	• PERFORATION EDGE REMOVAL • TYMPANOMEATAL FLAP • MEDIAL SURFACE GRAFT	AUTOGENOUS TEMPORALIS FASCIA	• NON VIABLE • DEHYDRATED

CLINICAL CONDITION	OPERATIVE TECHNIQUE	GRAFT MATERIAL: SOURCE	GRAFT MATERIAL: MODIFICATION
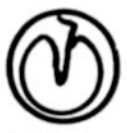 • TOTAL OR ANTERIOR PERFORATION • OSSICLES INTACT	• ANTERIOR CANAL FLAP • REMNANT ANNULUS REMOVAL • SLIT IN GRAFT FOR MANUBRIUM	AUTOGENOUS TEMPORALIS FASCIA	• DEHYDRATED • MOLDED TO ANATOMICAL SHAPE • FORMALDEHYDE CROSSLINKED

CLINICAL CONDITION	OPERATIVE TECHNIQUE	GRAFT MATERIAL: SOURCE	GRAFT MATERIAL: MODIFICATION
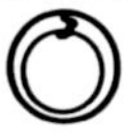 • PARS TENSA PERFORATION • MALLEUS-INCUS DISEASE • WITH OR WITHOUT CHOLESTEATOMA	• ANTERIOR CANAL FLAP • REMNANT ANNULUS REMOVAL • INTACT CANAL WALL TECHNIQUE IF CHOLESTEATOMA	HOMOGRAFT TYMPANIC MEMBRANE WITH MALLEUS-INCUS EN BLOC	• FORMALDEHYDE CROSSLINKED

Fig. 10. Current techniques and biomaterials of choice in tympanic membrane reconstruction.

a wire prosthesis. Continuity with the stapes may be effected with a homograft incus prosthesis (HIP) at a second stage.[10]

The perforation rate in these formaldehyde-processed homografts has been 11%. These are employed in cases that are difficult ossicular reconstructive problems. The 11% perforation risk is worth the marked advantage of having the attached malleus-incus to work with in these difficult ossicular chain problems. Should a perforation occur, they are usually not large and can be repaired at a second stage.

At the present time, the homograft tympanic membrane with ossicles en bloc is the method of choice in such conditions.[10] They have also been used in tympanomastoid reconstructions of ears that have had previous radical surgery. A graphic summary of the indications, technique, and graft material that I currently employ is seen in Figure 10.

CONCLUSIONS

The evolution of tympanic membrane grafting has been the province of the last 20 to 30 years and has followed a rather empirical course. Although numerous graft materials are used, they all have as a common denominator the collagen matrix which forms a superstructure for migration of host epithelium.

During this period, modification of the collagen membrane grafts has evolved. This modification now runs the spectrum from simply drying and devitalizing autogenous fascia to aldehyde crosslinking homologous collagen in tympanic membranes. As in other types of evolution the reason is to gain advantage; in this case: advantage technically, advantage in reducing complications, and, therefore, advantage in restoration of function.

The concept of modification of collagen membranes is not currently embraced by all otologists and valid differences of opinion exist.

The various collagen membrane grafts employed today have different characteristics and each has advantages when they are employed in specific situations. A philosophy that dogmatically employs a singular surgical technique and a singular collagenous material to all cases seems to ignore this evolution and the present state of the art.

Over the next few years, we shall see more sophisticated modifications and manipulations of collagen that will continue the trend toward the utlimate evaluation of a biosynthetic tympanic membrane prosthesis.

Request for reprints should be sent to Rodney Perkins, M.D., 1801 Page Mill Road, Palo Alto, California 94304.

REFERENCES

1. Chalat NI: Tympanic membrane transplant. Harper Hosp Bull 22:27-34, 1964

2. Marquet J: Reconstructive micro-surgery of the eardrum by means of a tympanic membrane homograft. Acta Otolaryngol (Stockh) 62:459-464, 1966

3. Glasscock ME III, House WF: Homograft reconstruction of the middle ear: A preliminary report. Laryngoscope 78:1219-1225, 1968

4. Perkins R: Human homograft otologic tissue transplantation: buffered formaldehyde preparation. Trans Am Acad Ophthalmol Otolaryngol 74:278-282, 1970

5. Furthmayr H, Timpl R: Structural requirements of antigenic determinants in the aminoterminal region of the rat collagen oc 2 chain. Biochem Biophys Res Commun 47: 944-950, 1972

6. Brunner H, Dichtl M, Steffen C: Immunogenitat und Spezifitat von chromstabilisiertem Kalbskollagen. Z Immunitaetsforsch 142:460-470, 1971

7. Jansen C: Heterologous tympanoplasty. Trans Am Acad Ophthalmol Otolaryngol 77: 111-116, 1973

8. Perkins R: Formaldehyde formed autogenous fascia graft tympanoplasty. Presented at the Academy of Ophthalmology and Otolaryngology, Dallas, Texas, Oct. 9, 1974. To be published.

9. Hough JV: Tympanoplasty. Trans Am Acad Ophthalmol Otolaryngol. CETV-OTO, OTO-3, Vol. 1

10. Perkins R: Otologic homograft indications, techniques, and anatomic and functional results. Trans Am Acad Ophthalmol and Otolaryngol 80: 41-46, 1975

Ann Otol 84: 1975

OTOLOGY AND INDUSTRIAL HEARING CONSERVATION

JOSEPH SATALOFF, M.D.

PHILADELPHIA, PENNSYLVANIA

SUMMARY – The Occupational Safety and Health Act is establishing limits for industrial noise exposure The Act may also require physicians to evaluate audiograms and examine almost two million employees annually. Otolaryngologists must take special training and become certified to provide American industry with expertise in industrial hearing conservation.

The Federal Government showed its serious concern for hearing loss by including noise exposure regulations in the Occupational Safety and Health Act (OSHA) of 1971. This law specified 90 dBA as the maximum noise level to which any employee should be exposed for eight hours daily over a period of years. The Department of Labor held inspections to insure industry's compliance with these regulations, but the regulations were too vague. In 1973 the Secretary of Labor instituted a new and appealing approach to writing standards by appointing a fifteen-man committee representing labor, management, government, and science to develop a noise proposal within nine months. The author was a scientific representative on this committee and believes it functioned extraordinarily well and produced an excellent and practical noise standard.

Certain features contained in the proposed noise standard are notable: 1) Certification of occupational hearing conservationists was recognized and defined; 2) No worker should be exposed to noise in excess of the limits shown in Table I; 3) Noise exposures exceeding 90 dBA as specified in Table I should be controlled by feasible engineering methods or administrative controls. If these controls were not immediately feasible, personal hearing protection equipment should be used; 4) All plants should have noise measurements at least annually; 5) Hearing conservation programs should be under the surveillance of a licensed physician; 6) Employees who either use ear protectors or are time exposed to over 85 dBA, Table I,

TABLE I

SOUND LEVEL/DURATION LIMITS TO WHICH INDUSTRIAL WORKERS MAY BE EXPOSED*

Sound Level (dBA)	*Time Permitted (hrs.-mins.)*	*Sound Level (dBA)*	*Time Permitted (hrs.-mins.)*
85	16- 0	101	1-44
86	13-56	102	1-31
87	12- 8	103	1-19
88	10-34	104	1- 9
89	9-11	105	1- 0
90	8- 0	106	0-52
91	6-58	107	0-46
92	6- 4	108	0-40
93	5-17	109	0-34
94	4-36	110	0-30
95	4- 0	111	0-26
96	3.29	112	0-23
97	3. 2	113	0-20
98	2-50	114	0-17
99	2-15	115	0-15
100	2- 0		

* As suggested in the proposed noise standard by the Department of Labor's Committee to propose a noise standard for the Occupational Safety and Health Act.

Presented at the meeting of the American Otological Society, Inc., Atlanta, Georgia, April 11-12, 1975.

should be part of a hearing conservation program that includes annual audiograms. Rules for calibrating all equipment and record keeping were included, and the technique for audiometry was detailed; 7) If the hearing thresholds for any employee showed a change averaging over 10 dB at 2, 3, and 4 kHz in either ear, the employee should be tested within a prescribed period and if the hearing change persisted, the employee should be referred for medical evaluation; and 8) Employees should be notified of their noise exposure and audiometric levels.

Even though all federal standards are based chiefly on the best available scientific information, other influential factors come into play, such as economics, practicability, and even vested interests. It is only natural, therefore, that the proposed noise standard was not accepted unanimously, and certain aspects of the proposal are being challenged. Most notable is that the 90 dBA level should be lowered to 85 dBA or even lower and that the requirement for medical surveillance and referral for medical evaluation should be deleted. The latter issue is of special interest to otologists since the challenge is based on the premise that too few otolaryngologists and other physicians are available with training and experience in industrial hearing conservation and occupational deafness to supply American industry with needed services. It has been estimated that about two million employees might require hearing evaluations annually on the basis of the OSHA medical surveillance requirement, proposed by a representative of Labor and passed unanimously by the Committee. The Committee felt that hearing loss was a medical responsibility and that a trained physician should have the chief responsibility for interpreting audiograms, making a diagnosis, and recommending treatment for patients with hearing problems.

Whether or not OSHA includes medical surveillance in its forthcoming noise regulation, it is essential that otolaryngologists acquire training and expertise to serve industry meaningfully and to help millions of employees with hearing difficulty. More and more, otologists are assuming essential roles in the development of effective hearing conservation programs and are called on to advise management and government in the many important aspects of such programs. The highly specialized problems attending occupational hearing loss and hearing conservation have focused attention upon the need for otologists to acquire training and experience in this field. First, we must become certified hearing conservationists and teachers by taking at least the 20-hour course required by the Council for Accreditation in Hearing Conservation. More desirable, however, is to acquire practical experience by taking more extensive training courses such as the one-week course provided each August for the past 22 years at Colby College in Waterville, Maine. Other courses are available and recommended, but their success depends on the industrial experience of their faculties. The best training courses include lectures on noise measurement, instrument calibration, industrial hearing testing, record keeping, ear protection, motivational programs, noise control, differential diagnosis of hearing loss, workmen's compensation for hearing loss, legislation, and labor relations and management problems.

American otology must also institute training programs in hearing conservation for all our residents, and competence in this field should be required by the American Board of Otolaryngology. We must also make certification courses readily available to practitioners throughout the country.

Otologists have special and unique responsibilities to industrial hearing conservation programs. The otologist must sometimes even coordinate the program and provide a broad understanding that transcends hearing testing or noise measurement.

A proper hearing conservation program requires team work of safety engineers, hygienists, audiologists, hearing conservation technicians, industrial physicians, nurses, and a trained otologist. Among the otologist's singular functions are to interpret hearing tests, to diagnose, and to determine treatment and dispensation. He must also provide medicolegal advice and testify in compensation and legislative proceedings.

Above all, our responsibility is to prevent deafness in all employees and to detect, diagnose, and recommend treatment for all causes of hearing loss. Only with such a broad concept can the objective of our Congress be achieved: to maintain the health of industrial employees.

I am convinced that American otology will meet this challenge so that we may supply the needs of our country and pass on to our successors a specialty broad in horizon, imaginative, and of greater service to our people.

Request for reprints should be sent to Joseph Sataloff, M.D., 1721 Pine Street, Philadelphia, Pa. 19103.

SOFT TISSUE SURGERY

A workshop on basic plastic surgical techniques in soft tissue surgery will be held September 26-28, 1975, at the University of Texas Health Science Center, Dallas, immediately following the annual meeting of the American Academy of Ophthalmology and Otolaryngology sponsored by the University of Texas Otolaryngology Training Programs in conjunction with the American Academy of Facial Plastic and Reconstructive Surgery. The faculty consists of members from various specialties with special guest, John T. Dickinson, M.D., Pittsburgh, Pennsylvania.

For information contact: Jack P. Gunter, M.D., Program Coordinator, Division of Otolaryngology, Suite 314, 8210 Walnut Hill Lane, Dallas, Texas 75231.

MIDDLE EAR MICROSURGERY AND FLUCTUANT HEARING LOSS

The Shambaugh Fifth International Workshop on Middle Ear Microsurgery and Fluctuant Hearing Loss will be held at Northwestern University Medical School, Thorne Hall, March 1-6, 1976. Co-chairmen are George E. Shambaugh, Jr., M.D. and John J. Shea, M.D.

For further information write: American Hearing Research Foundation, Suite 2105, 55 East Washington Street, Chicago, Illinois 60602.

Ann Otol 84: 1975

COMPLICATIONS IN ACOUSTIC NEUROMA SURGERY

MICHAEL E. GLASSCOCK III, M.D.

JAMES W. HAYS, M.D. JAMES P. MURPHY, M.D.

NASHVILLE, TENNESSEE

SUMMARY – The findings in a series of 80 cerebellopontine angle tumors are presented. Complications and results are covered in detail. A new method of controlling postoperative cerebrospinal fluid (CSF) leak is presented. Care of the eye in postoperative facial paralysis is emphasized, and a new type of moisture chamber is introduced.

Acoustic tumors remain a challenge to the otologist both in diagnosis and surgical removal. While the overall morbidity and mortality have been lowered, these tumors are still difficult and dangerous to remove. The complications that occur can be debilitating and, in some instances, fatal. It is important to recognize the more common ones, to know why they occur, and how to prevent them. The purpose of this paper is to review findings in a series of 80 cases and to discuss in detail the results in relation to complications.

DIAGNOSIS AND SURGICAL REMOVAL OF ACOUSTIC TUMORS

When this type of surgery was first attempted, the operative death rate was approximately 80 to 90%.[1] Cushing[2] was able to lower this rate to about 20% by advocating subtotal removals. There were several reasons for this high mortality rate, such as poor operating room conditions, poor general anesthesia, and lack of blood replacement. The chief cause of difficulty, however, was the large size of the tumor at the time of surgery. Most patients were not suspected of having a tumor until they were moribund. This can be attributed only to lack of diagnostic ability. One of Cushing's greatest contributions was his recognition of the natural history of these tumors.[2] He was the first to realize that tinnitus and hearing loss were among the first symptoms of a patient with an acoustic neuroma.

Dandy[3] was able to obtain total removals with an acceptable mortality rate because of better diagnostic tools and improved operating room conditions. The tumors that Dandy removed were, by and large, smaller and detected earlier than those with which Cushing had been left to deal.

Years later, House[4] was able to lower the morbidity and mortality dramatically because of earlier detection. He was able to take advantage of a wide variety of new and sophisticated audiometric and radiological advancements. Dealing largely with much smaller tumors and improved surgical techniques (translabyrinthine and microsurgical), he was able to lower the overall mortality rate to 10%.

While it would be ideal to find these tumors when they are limited to the internal auditory canal (IAC), this is not always possible. Many times the tumors simply do not produce enough symptoms to alert even the most suspicious physician. Until some type of screening test is developed, it would appear that we must continue to deal with medium and large tumors for some years to come.

Presented at the meeting of the American Otological Society, Atlanta, Georgia, April 11-12, 1975.

The key to early detection is a physician with a high index of suspicion who is willing to perform a thorough neurotologic evaluation on all patients with unilateral tinnitus, unilateral sensorineural hearing loss, or any form of spatial disorientation. This evaluation should include: a head and neck examination; screening neurological, audiometric, and vestibular studies; and x-rays of the temporal bone. Should the results of these tests be suspicious, then a posterior fossa contrast study should be performed. The Pantopaque®* examination is highly accurate and will usually indicate the size of the tumor.

There are several operative procedures that are employed at the present time. A certain amount of controversy still remains concerning the best method for the surgical removal of these tumors. At the present time they are being removed through the classical suboccipital route with and without microsurgical technique. House[4] and his disciples[5] continue to advocate the middle fossa approach for small tumors (limited to the IAC), the translabyrinthine for medium, and the transsigmoid or combined procedure for large tumors.

The final test for any procedure or surgeon is the overall morbidity, mortality, and recurrence rate over a period of years. It is only with this experience that the best methods of diagnosis and management can be determined. Certainly, at this point in time, the results of House stand as a yardstick by which others may judge their progress.

To continue our advancement in this type of surgery, it is important for all surgeons to periodically review their cases and make formal reports as to their results and complications. This must be done in a standardized method for the information to be meaningful.

CASE SUMMARIES

In this review of a series of 80 cerebellopontine angle tumors,** there are 79 patients represented. One individual had bilateral acoustic neuromas. Two other patients had neurofibromatosis, but only one tumor has been removed at this time. There were 30 males and 49 females, with 15 large, 62 medium, and 3 small tumors. Seventy-four were acoustic neuromas, four were meningiomas, one was an hemangioma, and one was a ganglioneurolipoma. There were three combined translabyrinthine-suboccipital, one transsigmoid, and three middle fossa procedures performed. The remaining 73 tumors were removed through the translabyrinthine approach.

A tumor confined to the IAC (usually 0.5 to 0.7 cm) is considered small, while one extending out into the cerebellopontine angle is thought of as medium or large. For classification purposes, a tumor is considered large if there are V nerve findings or evidence of increased intracranial pressure. Tumor size in centimeters has been recorded, based on preoperative Pantopaque® studies and observation at the time of removal. Several tumors of 3 to 4 cm have been listed as medium in size because there were no V nerve findings or evidence of increased intracranial pressure. Conversely, some 2.5 cm tumors are listed as large because they did produce V nerve symptoms.

Facial nerve function has been recorded as percentage of loss. Those patients having completely normal function are reported as 0% loss, and those with no function as 100% loss. Any sign of synkinesis is represented as a 10% loss. A 25 to 50% loss signifies some facial weakness although the patient may be able to close the eye, and the face looks normal at rest.

RESULTS

As this paper is concerned primarily with complications of acoustic neuroma surgery, the results of this series will be reviewed in detail. The aim of this study is to better understand how to

* C. G. Armour Medical Corp., Baltimore, Md.

** Detailed tabulation of all 80 cases prepared according to guidelines established by W. F. House, M.D.[4] are available on request to senior author.

prevent complications and how to manage them when they do arise. Experience with these 80 cases has led the authors to change certain aspects of their surgical technique. In addition, it has become necessary to develop new methods of dealing with the sequelae of some of these complications.

FATALITIES

Operative deaths will occur in cases of all tumor sizes from time to time. The surgeon's duty is to obtain a total removal with as little damage to the brain stem and its blood supply as possible. While fatalities are usually associated with injury to the anterior cerebellar artery, they can also occur from cerebral edema, meningitis, or a host of other causes in the immediate postoperative period. In this particular series, there have been no fatalities.

The posterior fossa is a treacherous area of the intracranial cavity for tumor removal. The main reason for this is that the brain stem represents the most primitive portion of the brain and is concerned with the most vital functions of respiration and heart rate. Medium and large tumors usually contact the stem and must be carefully dissected away from it during the removal. At this point in the procedure, the respiratory rate may drop. Even in smaller tumors, the anterior-inferior cerebellar artery may be adherent to the tumor, making its removal extremely difficult. Atkinson has shown that most operative fatalities are associated with injury to this artery.[6] Even if this vessel is not severed in tumor removal, it can still go into spasm and occlude. It is extremely important to avoid contact with this vessel if at all possible. One of the great advantages of the translabyrinthine approach is that the tumor capsule is between the surgeon and this artery throughout the greater part of the procedure. This is in direct contrast to the situation one encounters in the suboccipital approach, where one often finds himself operating past the anterior-inferior cerebellar artery in order to remove tumor.

In order to prevent operative fatalities, microsurgical technique is imperative. Careful dissection of the tumor capsule and bipolar cauterization of all the small blood vessels entering the tumor prevent operative and postoperative hemorrhage.

Bleeding must be kept under control at all times, and there should be no indiscriminate manipulation of the capsule. It must be remembered that these are brain tumors and that the tumor frequently has its blood supply in common with the brain stem. While most fatalities are associated with large tumors, it is certainly possible to injure the anterior-inferior cerebellar artery in removing a medium-sized tumor. In fact, if one were removing a small tumor through the middle fossa, it would still be possible to injure the artery as it frequently loops into the internal auditory canal.

TOTAL VERSUS SUBTOTAL REMOVAL

All tumor removals in this series have been total. We would not hesitate, however, to leave a small piece of capsule attached to the brain stem in order to get the patient off the operating table alive.

Should the tumor recur, House[4] has shown that secondary removal through the translabyrinthine route is less hazardous than through the suboccipital. There is some question as to whether small pieces of capsule survive and cause tumor regrowth.

For standardization when reporting results, it would seem best to simply refer to the removal as being either total or subtotal. The tumor is either totally removed or it is not, and stating whether there was a radical subtotal or partial subtotal is merely confusing and serves no real purpose. In discussing results, a subtotal removal should be considered a complication.

CEREBROSPINAL FLUID LEAK

Cerebrospinal fluid (CSF) leak has been the most frustrating and consistent complication in this series of patients (11%). In the first few cases, temporalis muscle was used in the middle ear and mastoid cavity to prevent a leak. The muscle was sutured into position by using 3-0 silk in the dura. In many women the muscle was very small, and it was difficult to obtain enough bulk to seal the dural defect. Many individuals developed seromas at the donor site due to weeping of the muscle where bleeders had been cauterized, which led the authors to the use of adipose tissue obtained from the abdominal wall. This latter procedure seemed to work well in that the temporalis muscle was left in place and could be used to obtain a water-tight closure of the subcutaneous tissue and did away with the seromas and fluid accumulations under the postauricular skin. Occasionally a patient would develop a postoperative leak, and it would be traced to the middle ear. The adipose tissue did not lend itself to packing in the middle ear. At this point, sternocleidomastoid muscle was obtained for the middle ear, and adipose tissue was used in the mastoid cavity. Leaks still persisted from time to time, leading to the present method of management.

Routine Surgical Technique. Temporalis fascia is taken and put aside to be used later in the closure. After the simple mastoidectomy has been performed, the facial recess is opened, and the incudostapedial joint is separated. The incus is removed and placed in the homograft bank. The head of the malleus is amputated and placed deep into the Eustachian tube. Muscle is cut into small pledgets and inserted into the Eustachian tube behind the head of the malleus. The entire middle ear is then filled with muscle. Special care is taken not to dislodge the stapes from the oval window as this has been a common site for CSF leakage into the middle ear.

Since this method of packing the middle ear and mastoid has been employed, there has been only one leak down the Eustachian tube. There have been nine such CSF leaks requiring a formal closure. This accounts for an overall incidence of 11% for the entire series. Five patients have developed postauricular leaks through the wound that healed spontaneously.

There have been three patients in this series who have had persistent CSF leaks that simply could not be controlled with the usual methods. All had at least one attempt at closure of the leak using all of the methods just described. Finally, in desperation, a totally different approach was conceived to solve the problem.

CASE REPORT

A 42-year-old male underwent the removal of a 4 cm acoustic neuroma in July 1973. The tumor was totally removed and the facial nerve was preserved. He had an uneventful postoperative recovery and was discharged from the hospital one week after surgery. He continued to do well for approximately three weeks. While bending over one day, he noticed a clear drainage from the left nostril. He was readmitted to the hospital, and the wound was explored. The stapes was found to be subluxated, and CSF was flowing freely from the oval window. After the ossicle was removed, the vestibule and Eustachian tube were packed with muscle. Again he had an uneventful postoperative period and did well. Three weeks later he developed another leak. This time it was decided to let the leak remain for awhile to see if it would close on its own. After one month the wound was again examined. CSF was again flowing freely from the oval window. More muscle was placed into the vestibule area, middle ear, and mastoid cavity. The postauricular skin did not look good after so much surgery. Nylon sutures were used to close the wound. The patient did well and went back to work. Almost three weeks later, he started spiking a temperature elevation of 39.4C and he was disoriented. A spinal tap confirmed the diagnosis of bacterial meningitis. With the proper antiobiotic coverage his infection came under control, and his ear was again explored. The leak was still coming through the oval window. Again the ear was filled with muscle. He had an uneventful recovery and went back to work. There was no obvious CSF leak, but he did complain of a salty

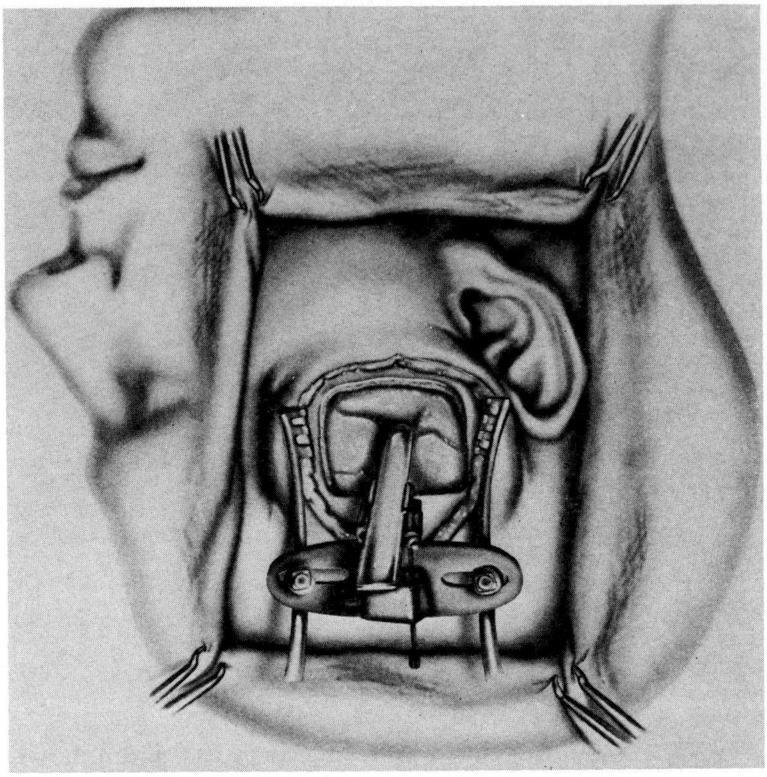

Fig. 1. A routine middle fossa exposure of the temporal bone is accomplished using a House-Urban middle fossa retractor. The surgeon is seated at the head of the table with the patient lying supine with his head turned to one side.

taste. About two months after the episode of meningitis, he suddenly developed ataxia and could not sit or stand in an upright position. An x-ray skull series revealed air in the ventricles and there was evidence of hydrocephalus. There was definitely a leak, and he was producing excessive amounts of CSF. A ventricular-peritoneal shunt was performed and the hydrocephalus came under control. The CSF leak continued. It was obvious that something drastic needed to be done to control his fistula. A middle fossa Eustachian tube closure was performed, and finally we were able to stop the leak. Once it was controlled, he did well. The last surgery was over a year ago. He has had no further signs of a fistula, and he is back to his regular activities.

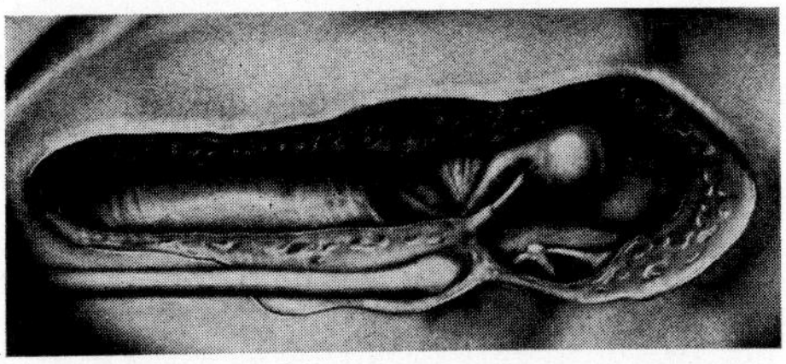

Fig. 2. The tensor tympani muscle is followed to the Eustachian tube, and the superior aspect of the osseous tube is removed down to the isthmus.

MIDDLE FOSSA EUSTACHIAN TUBE CLOSURE

A routine middle fossa exposure (Fig. 1) of the Eustachian tube is accomplished. Once the geniculate ganglion is identified, the bone lying lateral to the ganglion (tegmen tympani) is removed, exposing the middle ear from above. The tensor tympani muscle is followed to the Eustachian tube, and the superior aspect of the osseous tube is removed down to the isthmus (Fig. 2). Next the tensor tympani muscle is

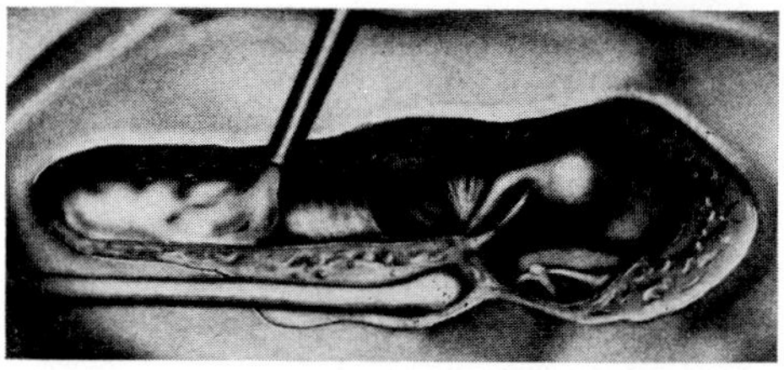

Fig. 3. The orthopedic glue is placed into the Eustachian tube and anterior portion of the middle ear.

stripped from the semicanal, and a small wedge of cortical bone is fashioned so that it fits snugly into the isthmus of the tube. All of the mucosa from the medial wall of the middle ear has usually been removed at the first surgery. Should there be any remaining, it is removed at this time. The scrub nurse now mixes a portion of orthopedic bone glue* and places it in a disposable syringe with a 15 gauge blunt needle. The glue is placed into the Eustachian tube and anterior portion of the middle ear (Fig. 3). Care must be taken to keep the operating field dry so that the glue will become adherent. The chemical reaction that occurs while the glue is solidifying creates an excessive amount of heat. It is important to keep the glue away from the facial nerve during the period of hardening. The carotid artery is in almost direct contact with the glue, but the rapid flow of a large amount of blood quickly dissipates the heat.

The field is kept dry until the glue has solidified and attached itself to the bone of the middle ear and Eustachian tube. The middle fossa retractor is removed, and the temporal lobe is allowed to expand. The wound is closed in layers, and a bulky dressing is applied. The patient is observed in the recovery room overnight where routine craniotomy checks are performed.

PRESERVATION OF THE FACIAL NERVE

We have been able to preserve the facial nerve anatomically in 68 of the 80 cases in this series, representing a success rate of 85%. Two of these nerves, however, failed to regain any function at one year after surgery dropping the percentage to 82.5% for preservation with function. Fifty-one tumors were removed with no loss of function.

For years the sacrifice of the facial nerve was routine in the removal of these tumors. The lesion was lethal, and without microsurgical techniques there was little chance of saving the nerve. House[4] and his development of the translabyrinthine route to the cerebellopontine angle made preservation of the VII nerve a very real and practical goal. While advocates of the microsurgical suboccipital approach are able to preserve the facial nerve, there is no constant bony landmark for its identification, and no one has reported as high an incidence of preservation as has House.[4]

While it is usually easier to preserve the nerve in patients with smaller tumors, size alone is not the most important factor. Often the nerve will dissect from a large tumor quite easily while it is sometimes very adherent to a medium-sized one. In removing the tumor, it is important to take the tumor away from the nerve and not to push or pull too vigorously on the nerve itself. In dealing with the larger tumors, it is important to reduce the size of the tumor until it is about 1 cm in diameter. It is important to have it free of all attachments and completely mobile before the facial nerve is identified at the lateral extent of the IAC at Bill's bar. In this manner, as the tumor is being dissected free from the nerve, it is possible to rotate the tumor and deflect it inferiorly, usually allowing the surgeon to trace the nerve along the side of the tumor, making the line of cleavage much easier to determine.

Occasionally the VII nerve is simply too adherent to the capsule to obtain a separation of the tumor from the nerve. In such a case, regardless of the size of the tumor, the nerve must be sacrificed in order to obtain a total removal. When this occurs, the surgeon

* Simplex®, Howmedica Inc., Rutherford, N.J.

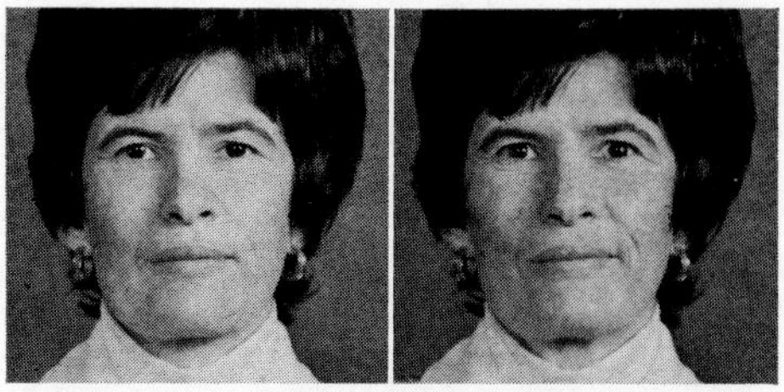

Fig. 4. Note that this patient, who had her facial hypoglossal anastomosis approximately five months before this picture was made, has good tone to her face at rest.

Fig. 5. Voluntary control of the face is relatively good with minimal facial movement. The patient has extremely good control of her eye.

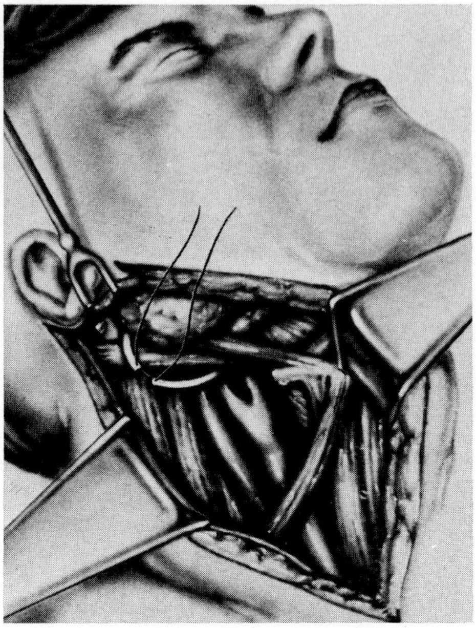

Fig. 6. Microscopic anastomosis should be carried out with four to six well-placed sutures in the sheath of each nerve.

must make the decision to attempt a graft of the facial nerve or to perform some type of anastomosis. Of the 12 nerves that were lost at surgery, seven have been repaired by means of a facial hypoglossal anastomosis. These individuals are considered to have 50% function of their faces.

Nerve Grafts. We have not been able to graft any of the patients in whom the nerve has been severed. Dott[7] reports grafting from the brain stem, but we have seldom been able to find a proximal stump. In attempting a graft, one is committing the patient to a one-year wait to see if there is to be a take. Under most circumstances we have favored a facial hypoglossal anastomosis.

Facial-Hypoglossal Anastomosis. While the facial nerve can be anastomosed with the phrenic or spinal accessory nerves, we have preferred the hypoglossal due to its close proximity to the nucleus of the VII nerve in the brain stem. The loss of function of the involved side of the tongue causes the individuals virtually no difficulty with eating or speech. We feel that it is important to perform this anastomosis early while the facial muscles still have good tone. In the seven cases that have undergone anastomosis, the results have been very gratifying. Figure 4 shows an anastomosis approximately five months postsurgery. At rest, her face appears perfectly normal. When she smiles (Fig. 5), there obviously is a weakness in her face, but this will improve with time. It is important to obtain a good microscopic anastomosis of the two nerves. We use at least four and preferably six to eight sutures in the sheath to obtain good union (Fig. 6).

Care of the Eye. Care of the eye following injury to the facial nerve is extremely important. One of the most valuable methods was suggested to us by a patient. This individual was having difficulty with his eye at night. He obtained some clear plastic food wrap and cut a small square to fit over the eye. He taped this into place with a commercial hair set tape (Fig. 7). This created a moisture chamber for the eye and also kept foreign objects, such as the bed sheets out of the eye. The hair set tape is nonirritating to the skin and peels off easily without pain. We have used this method in a wide variety of cases of facial paralysis now with great success. Patients prefer this method to direct closure of the eye with cellophane or adhesive tape.

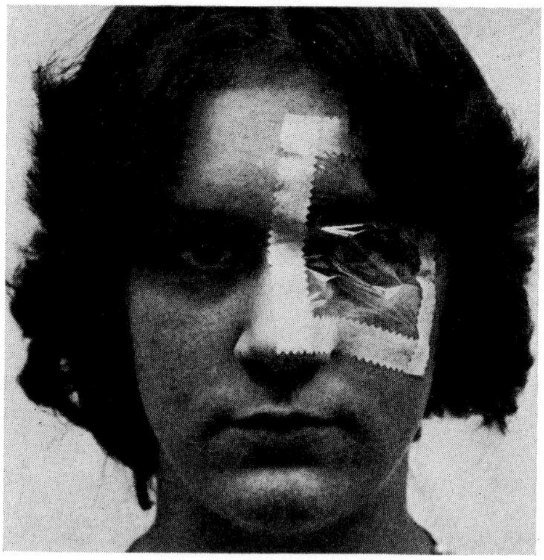

Fig. 7. This square of plastic, when placed over the eye and held in place with the hair set tape, forms a moisture chamber that affords excellent protection. It has the advantage of allowing the patient to keep his eye open and see through the covering.

When there has been permanent injury to the facial nerve and the recovery period may be several months, a tarsorrhaphy is considered. Whether or not one is done depends upon the difficulty the patient experiences with his eye. We have found with the plastic moisture chamber at night and artificial tears during the day, tarsorrhaphies are not needed as often as they were.

MENINGITIS

The most serious complication in this series of patients has been bacterial meningitis (ten cases). This represents an overall incidence of 12.5%. Interestingly, the severe cases have all occurred several weeks after surgery and have been dirctly related to a postoperative CSF leak. There has been only one immediate onset, and it was associated with a postauricular leak that occurred about three days after surgery. There has been no common organism and none that was resistant to antibiotics.

There have been three individuals who developed a low grade chemical meningitis as a reaction to blood in the spinal fluid representing an incidence of 3.5%. These patients experienced some temperature elevation in the range of 37.8-38.3C, headache, and a stiff neck. Spinal fluid taps performed on these individuals revealed a normal sugar level and a cell count of 100 or less. They grew no organisms on culture, and all recovered without antibiotic coverage within three to ten days.

It has been our policy not to use prophylactic antibiotic coverage during the postoperative period. A true bacterial meningitis requires large amounts of potent antibiotics to bring the infection under control. The only way to predict the correct antibiotic is with culture and sensitivity studies. Should the patient be on too small a dosage of a marginally effective prophylactic drug, it will be impossible in many instances to grow a positive culture, making it extremely difficult to treat the infection successfully.

The patient with a bacterial meningitis is easily recognized. His temperature will frequently spike to 38.9-39.4C. He will be confused and disoriented and will very frequently complain of a stiff neck and severe headache. A lumbar spinal puncture must be performed immediately. If the cell count is elevated and the sugar level is low, a true bacterial meningitis should be suspected. It is a good idea to obtain a gram stain as a stat procedure as well. Broad spectrum antibiotics in high doses and in combination should be instituted intravenously until the culture and sensitivity studies are available. Our drugs of choice are penicillin, chloramphenicol, and methicillin. Should the patient be allergic to penicillin, cephalexin monohydrate is substituted. Once the organism is isolated and the sensitivity known, the patient is left on the specific antibiotic, and the others are discontinued.

It has been our feeling that if the postoperative leaks could be kept to a minimum, the number of bacterial meningitis cases could be lowered as well. The length of the operative procedure, when prolonged, is probably another factor in this problem. When a wound is open for several hours, the possibility of contamination is greater.

POSTOPERATIVE INTRACRANIAL HEMORRHAGE

There were no postoperative hemorrhages occurring in this series. The first 24 hours after surgery are the most critical ones in regard to immediate postoperative hemorrhage. The recovery room in our hospital is adjacent to the operating suite. A set of instruments is kept sterile and ready to use at a moment's notice, and a tracheotomy tray is available at all times. A mechanical respirator is kept in reserve in the recovery room.

Routine craniotomy checks are performed every five minutes until the patient is stable and then every 30 minutes for the first 12 hours. Should evidence of increased intracranial pressure occur, the surgeons are notified immediately, and the patient is returned to surgery on an emergency basis to remove a clot from the cerebellopontine angle.

Careful attention to technique and to control of bleeding during surgery will eliminate the problem of postoperative hemorrhage in most cases. The bipolar cautery has been of tremendous value in controlling hemorrhage at the time of surgery. Extreme care must be taken with each blood vessel that enters the tumor capsule. There will be postoperative bleeds, however, regardless of how dry the field is at the end of the procedure. The important fact that must be kept in mind is that the surgeon must be prepared to act decisively and quickly to remove the clot and stop the bleeding. One of the great advantages of the translabyrinthine approach is that this can be done with dispatch in the recovery room if necessary.

POSTOPERATIVE EDEMA

We have had to take only one patient out of 80 back to surgery in the immediate postoperative period. This patient did not respond the morning after surgery. Upon reexposing the operative site, the cerebellum was obviously infarcted and very edematous. His had been a large acoustic tumor, and a self-retaining retractor had been placed on the cerebellum for several hours. The infarcted tissue was removed. The patient recovered and has done well with the exception of some mild ataxia.

Retraction of the cerebellum is the most common cause of postoperative edema. If it is necessary to retract the cerebellum exclusively for exposure, it is better to remove the lateral third of the hemisphere. Another of the advantages of the translabyrinthine approach is that in most cases no retraction of the cerebellum is required for an adequate view of the cerebellopontine angle. It is not necessary to remove the lateral third to gain access with this approach.

One patient had edema of the temporal lobe due to retraction during a prolonged middle fossa procedure. Part of the temporal lobe was removed at the initial surgery, and she did have a postoperative edema. She was placed on dexamethasone MSD for this and made an uneventful recovery.

We have tended to use urea, mannitol, and dexamethasone MSD sparingly due to the rebound phenomenon and bleeding that can sometimes occur with these agents.

MEDICAL PROBLEMS

One patient developed severe pneumonia postoperatively due to a contaminated endotracheal tube. Two other patients had pneumonia, but the cause was not determined. One older patient developed a pleural effusion due to congestive heart failure and melena due to a stress ulcer. Another patient became confused and lethargic about six days after surgery and was found to be suffering from hyponatremia. She responded immediately to intravenous 3% normal saline. Two patients have required tracheotomies because they developed aspiration difficulties due to loss of the X nerve at surgery.

There have been two frank wound infections (2.5% incidence), and these cleared with antibiotic coverage.

We have developed a therapeutic team as well as a diagnostic one for dealing with these patients. An internist sees all of these individuals and follows them with us carefully after surgery.

CONCLUSIONS

These cerebellopontine tumors are treacherous to remove, and operative deaths are going to occur from time to time. While aggressive in tumor removal, we are nonetheless very meticulous and careful in surgical technique. Every attempt is made to control bleeding as the dissection is carried out and the brain stem is handled with great care. The patient is allowed to breathe on his own while the capsule is being removed from the stem. Should the respirations cease, the dissection is stopped until spontaneous respirations occur. This is very tedious and may require several hours of determined effort. Large blood vessels that do not enter the capsule are gently packed away from the tumor with cottonoids, thereby lessening the chance of inadvertent injury.

We have been very fortunate in having superb anesthesia for our patients. Almost without exception, all of them have been responsive and awake at the end of the procedure. The fact that we have only had to take one patient back to surgery in the immediate postoperative period speaks well for anesthesia and the control of hemorrhage and cerebral edema at the time of surgery.

The aggressiveness with which total removals have been sought may account for our lack of facial nerve preservation. While the facial nerve was anatomically preserved in 85% of the cases, it remained functional only 82.5% of the time, a 10% drop since our last report[5] and of great concern to us. We would like to have a better record with facial nerve preservation. While the nerve was simply impossible to save in most cases, there were a few in which it was lost due to technical error. This type of loss can be corrected, and, hopefully, as the series grows, we will be able to improve this aspect.

Eleven (13.7%) of our patients have had serviceable preoperative hearing in the involved ear. Hearing in the opposite ear in all of these individuals (except the bilateral cases) has been good, and we have attempted to save the hearing in the involved ear only three times. All of these were done as middle fossa procedures, and only once were we able to save the hearing. In one case the tumor was too large, and in the other it was adherent to the cochlear nerve.

While interested in preservation of hearing, we are more concerned with total removals, preservation of the facial nerve, and a low mortality rate. At the present time, we feel these goals can best be accomplished through the translabyrinthine approach. We will continue to attempt to preserve the hearing when the tumor is confined to the IAC. In bilateral tumors when there is some hearing present, an attempt will be made to save the labyrinth by means of a combined middle fossa-transsigmoid procedure. We do not feel the suboccipital approach, *per se,* affords good landmarks for the preservation of the facial nerve or furnishes a good route to the cerebellopontine angle and brain stem.

The most bothersome and dangerous complication in this series has been CSF leak with subsequent bacterial meningitis. With improvement in the initial closure, this seems to be coming under control and if it can be kept to a minimum, we feel that the problem of meningitis will also subside.

The best method of lowering morbidity and mortality is to detect these tumors early in their development. Fewer complications occur, and the best results are obtained with small and medium-sized tumors.

Request for reprints should be sent to Michael E. Glasscock, III, M.D., 300 25th Avenue, North, Nashville, Tennessee 37203.

REFERENCES

1. Krause F: Zur Freilegung der hinteren Felsenbeinflache und des Kleinhirns. Beitr Klin Chir 37:728-764, 1903

2. Cushing H: *Tumors of the Nervus Acusticus and the Syndrome of the Cerebello-pontine Angle*, ed 2. New York, Hafner Publishing Co, 1963

3. Dandy WE: Operation for total removal of cerebellopontine (acoustic) tumors. Surg Gynecol Obstet 41:129-148, 1925

4. House WF, ed: Monograph II: acoustic neuroma, Arch Otolaryngol 88:575-715, 1968

5. Glasscock ME, Hays JW: The translabyrinthine removal of acoustic and other cerebellopontine angle tumors. Ann Otol Rhinol Laryngol 82:415-427, 1973

6. Atkinson WJ: The anterior inferior cerebellar artery. J Neurol Neurosurg Psychiatry 12:137-151, 1949

7. Dott NM: Facial nerve reconstruction by graft by-passing the petrous bone. Arch Otolaryngol 78:426-428, 1963

AMERICAN OTOLOGIC SOCIETY GUIDELINES FOR GRANTS

Our objective is clearly the problem of otosclerosis: its diagnosis and management, the possible causes and underlying conditions (such as the hereditary background), and an understanding of the disorder that may lead eventually to its prevention and cure.

Our present lack of understanding of the disorder and the absence, as far as known, of any similar condition in animals below man, makes research in this field particularly difficult. A direct attack on the disease is hardly feasible; therefore, it seems to be sound strategy to try circuitous approaches, such as the investigation of bone development, growth, and repair under various conditions, and the study of other diseases that show suggestive correspondence to this one. It is possible that directions of investigation that may seem initially somewhat remote from otosclerosis itself may provide insights that will eventually lead to success in reaching our goal. Therefore, our policy is to aid and encourage research in the immediate field of otosclerosis and also in adjoining fields if, in our considered opinion, there is a substantial promise that the results obtained will be of assistance in the ways just indicated and may lead to the attainment of our objective.

The Board of Trustees wishes to announce that funds are still available for suitable grants. Application forms may be obtained from the office of the Secretary of the Research Fund Trustees of the American Otologic Society. Write to Maurice Schiff, M. D., Secretary, 7255 Girard Ave., La Jolla, Calif. 92037.

RHINOPLASTY COURSE

The annual basic Rhinoplasty Course of the University of California, Davis, will be held October 26-31, 1975. For further information write: Leslie Bernstein, M.D., D.D.S., Department of Otorhinolaryngology, University of California School of Medicine, Davis, California 95616.

Ann Otol 84: 1975

ELECTRONYSTAGMOGRAPHY: A REVIEW OF 17 YEARS EXPERIENCE

WALLACE RUBIN, M.D.

METAIRIE, LOUISIANA

SUMMARY – The clinical concepts of electronystagmography (ENG) and vestibular testing are simple. They are not mysterious, complicated, nor time consuming. Every patient afflicted with dizziness deserves such a recording as part of the vestibular workup. No one would consider the evaluation of a patient with a hearing loss complete without an audiogram, and in 1975 no patient with a complaint of dysequilibrium has been properly or sufficiently evaluated without an ENG recording of balance function.

The physician must be the captain of the vestibular diagnostic team based on his interest, knowledge, and capability. It is not the electronystagmograph (ENG) instrument used nor the routine battery of vestibular tests with numerical evaluations that provide diagnostic answers. It is the intelligent application and use of the indicated vestibular tests that are practically correlated and clinically evaluated that will give the knowledgeable physician significant information. This can best be accomplished when ENG testing is done in physical proximity to the responsible physician and when the tests used are intelligently ordered and evaluated. Under such circumstances ENG is always helpful and timesaving because the recordings can then assist in answering these clinical questions: 1) Is the vestibular mechanism normal or abnormal? 2) Is the vestibular pathology peripheral or central? and 3) Is the peripheral disease right or left sided?

The data on the recording additionally may be helpful in providing central nervous system (CNS) localizing information based on the ocular tracking tests.

All balance function tests performed (whether with or without electronystagmography) must fall within one of four categories. They must be tests either for: 1) spontaneous nystagmus, 2) positional or positioning nystagmus, 3) induced nystagmus, or 4) nystagmus as a result of tracking moving visual targets.

Spontaneous nystagmus tests are those performed prior to exposing the patient to any stimuli. In these tests the patient may either be seated, lie on an examining table, or stand. Positional or positioning tests are those where the patient has only his head or his head and body moved into certain positions. Tests for induced nystagmus are performed by either rotating the patient as in any of the many rotational tests, irrigating the ear canals with water above and/or below body temperature, or tests wherein a galvanic stimulus is used to induce the nystagmus.

The spontaneous, positional, and induced tests are all related specifically to vestibular function. Any ocular tracking tests such as the gaze test, the optokinetic tests, the pendulum or sawtooth tracking test, or any other ocular tracking tests are tests of ocular function and the results may or may not relate to vestibular abnormalities.

Nystagmus always accompanies ver-

Presented at the meeting of the American Otological Society, Inc., Atlanta, Georgia, April 11-12, 1975.

tigo. It is the one consistent useful objective sign we have available to confirm vestibular abnormalities. Nystagmus which occurs in vestibular disease is best elicited and sometimes only visible when ocular fixation is suppressed or abolished. The only method that allows the physician always to detect the presence of nystagmus is observation of the patient when the patient's eyes are open in a darkened room or when the eyes are closed in a lighted room. There is no better way to accomplish this visualization than with an ENG recorder. Any other method of nystagmus detection (i.e., naked eye or Frenzel's lenses) will miss the majority of nystagmus and will, in addition, not permit accurate evaluation of its characteristics.

ENG rapidly supplies useful differential clinical information when the technique is intelligently combined with a bithermal caloric test and when these responses are interpreted and correlated with the total diagnostic workup. This premise is based on the fact that nystagmus is an algebraically summative phenomenon. When spontaneous nystagmus is present, the ability of an induced thermic nystagmus to inhibit or suppress it and then turn it in the proper physiologic direction is always a better measure of vestibular integrity than the thermic stimulus which would facilitate the spontaneous nystagmus in the same direction. It is this principle that allows for eyeball interpretation of ENG caloric responses and makes it possible to shorten the testing procedure.

Interpreting the caloric responses on an ENG when there is a spontaneous nystagmus present requires primarily a comparison of only two responses. The fundamental question is whether the response to the two stimulations which beat opposite to the spontaneous nystagmus are symmetrical. When the peripheral labyrinth functions in a normal fashion, the spontaneous nystagmus must be slowed, stopped, reversed, and then sustained in the opposite direction. If, for example, there is a right beating spontaneous nystagmus, the two stimulations which should beat left must be compared (R30° and L44°). If there is a left beating spontaneous nystagmus, we must compare L30° and R44°. The results possible with caloric stimulation in the presence of a spontaneous nystagmus are: 1) There will be no change at all of the spontaneous nystagmus with either opposing stimulation; 2) There will be a similar, equal, or symmetrical change with both stimulations; 3) Only one stimulus will slow, stop, or reverse the spontaneous nystagmus or sustain the nystagmus in the opposite direction; and 4) One stimulus will more effectively slow, stop, or reverse the spontaneous nystagmus or will sustain the nystagmus in the opposite direction.

Items 1) and 2) above can occur only with intact peripheral function, while items 3) and 4) indicate pathology of the peripheral labyrinth. The labyrinth least capable of slowing, stopping, or reversing the spontaneous nystagmus or sustaining the induced nystagmus in the opposite direction must be the diseased labyrinth.

When such a testing routine is used and when these concepts are applied, no numbers or formulas are necessary to interpret the ENG. It is also unnecessary to get involved in the problem of adding and/or subtracting the spontaneous nystagmus or to get involved in the directional preponderance controversy. The vestibular end organ algebraically summates the already present and stimulated nystagmic activity and makes these problems moot.

If the caloric responses are recorded from the time of instillation of the irrigating tip and the response is recorded till its completion, then an eyeball comparison of the responses can be made easily and accurately. The correlation of these responses with the spontaneous and positional nystagmus, gaze, and optokinetic (OPK) tests makes it possible to decide normal or abnormal, peripheral or central, right or left peripheral, and possibly to determine CNS localization. This decision can be done easily, quickly, without numbers, without formulas, with less errors, and without the likelihood of overreading an ENG.

Some persons maintain that the "old" method of calorization with ice water and naked eye evaluations of the induced nystagmus is just as accurate as evaluation with ENG. The fallacies of this kind of thinking are: 1) Spontaneous and/or positional nystagmus would have been missed the majority of the time (more than 95%) with naked eye observations. (This is due to ocular fixation suppression of nystagmus); 2) Nystagmus beats to the diseased ear about 35% of the time; therefore, 65% of the time a warm stimulus would give better information than a cool stimulus; 3) With either cold or warm stimulations and depending on the direction of the missed spontaneous nystagmus, the induced nystagmus would have been in a direction that might make the two stimulations look equal if two cool or two warm stimulations are used, and the naked eye is used for evaluation of nystagmus; and 4) In a small but significant number of cases, the observer would report a perverted nystagmus on thermic stimulation because the spontaneous nystagmus was never seen in the first place and the stimulation provoked or facilitated only the spontaneous nystagmus.

Even though ENG is an indispensible part of the vestibular testing procedure, the machine itself does not and cannot make a diagnosis. However, anyone can quickly learn to accurately read a recording. All ENG apparatuses have the same three basic components: 1) electrode pickup, 2) amplification capability, and 3) readout capability. A single channel unit is all that is necessary for the physician's office. Multichannel sophisticated instruments and equipment are useful in research situations but tend to add technical problems and might clutter the clinician's mind with clinically useless data.

There are persons who criticize ENG because they say that there is no standardization and that spurious spikes and pen movements interfere with readings. The fundamentals of recordings and procedure have been agreed upon and documented by the ENG Study Club as long ago as 1968. The differences of opinion regarding technique are nuances of difference that in no way can or should cloud the issue. Experienced neurotologists have no difficulty reading each other's ENG's. Problems arise only in the hands of those persons who are inexperienced and who overread recordings. These reading difficulties do not occur because of extraneous voltages which occur because of large muscle movements such as blinks, swallows, coughing, or body movements. They occur because of lack of understanding by technically untrained individuals. The interpretation of an ENG cannot be the function of the technician. Vestibular tests recorded by ENG must be supervised by a knowledgeable physician who will make the clinical interpretations and decisions.

CONCLUSIONS

The presence of spontaneous and/or positional nystagmus confirms abnormalities of the vestibular mechanism. The responses to the bithermal stimulation separate the peripheral from the central abnormalities and determine sidedness in peripheral problems. The ocular fixation and tracking tests may help in localizing the central abnormalities. Other special tests (not vestibular nor ENG) tell us about etiologic mechanisms.

The clinical concepts of ENG and vestibular testing are simple. They are not mysterious, complicated, nor time consuming. Every patient afflicted with dizziness deserves such a recording as part of the vestibular workup. No one would consider the evaluation of a patient with a hearing loss complete without an audiogram, and in 1975 no patient with a complaint of dysequilibrium has been properly or sufficiently evaluated without an ENG recording of balance function.

Request for reprints should be sent to Wallace Rubin, M.D., 3333 Kingman St., Metairie, Louisiana 70002.

Ann Otol 84: 1975

SENSORINEURAL HEARING LOSS DUE TO COCHLEAR OTOSPONGIOSIS: THEORETICAL CONSIDERATIONS OF ETIOLOGY

FRED H. LINTHICUM, JR., M.D.

LOS ANGELES, CALIFORNIA

ROBERTO FILIPO, M.D.

ROME, ITALY

SIDNEY BRODY, P.E.

LOS ANGELES, CALIFORNIA

SUMMARY – Several theories have been advanced to explain the sensorineural hearing loss that occurs in patients with otospongiosis: toxic substances produced by the otospongiotic focus; vascular shunts between the inner ear vessels and the otospongiotic focus; and atrophy of the organ of Corti and stria vascularis due to unknown causes. Presented here is yet another theory: impingement upon the cochlear walls by the otospongiotic focus, causing a narrowing of the lumen of the cochlea and distortion of the basilar membrane.

There seems to be little question that cochlear otospongiosis can cause sensorineural hearing impairment. But what is the mechanism?

In this paper we will review the various theories and present the results of a study of 100 pairs of temporal bones from the Ear Research Institute collection. Narrowing of the lumen of the cochlea and distortion of the basilar membrane by the otospongiotic focus is another possible cause of sensorineural hearing impairment.

The patients were divided into three groups based upon their ages at the time of the first audiogram: 20 to 29, 30 to 39, 40 to 49. To prevent contamination of our results due to the loss from presbycusis, this loss as determined by Glorig and Davis[1] was substracted from the total sensorineural hearing loss of the patients.

Figure 1 is a chart showing the degree of sensorineural loss after 25 years of repeated examinations and shows a breakdown of the various age groups. It will be noted that in the younger age groups the sensorineural loss is almost twice that one would expect from presbycusis. In the older groups, the loss associated with otospongiosis is equal to that expected in presbycusis for the high frequencies but much greater for the low frequencies. It will be further noted that the low frequencies as well as the high are affected by otospongiosis in distinction to the usually isolated high frequency loss due to presbycusis.

The mechanism by which the otospongiosis produces sensorineural hearing loss, however, is as still uncertain. Probably there is more than one etiology in many cases.

Siebenmann suggested there might be toxic substances, liberated by the otospongiotic focus into the inner ear fluids, that impaired the function of the cochlea.[2] More recently, using electron microscopy, Bretlau, *et al*[3] and Chev-

From the Otologic Medical Group, Inc. and the Ear Research Institute, Los Angeles, California.

Presented at the meeting of the American Otological Society, Inc., Atlanta, Georgia, April 11-12, 1975.

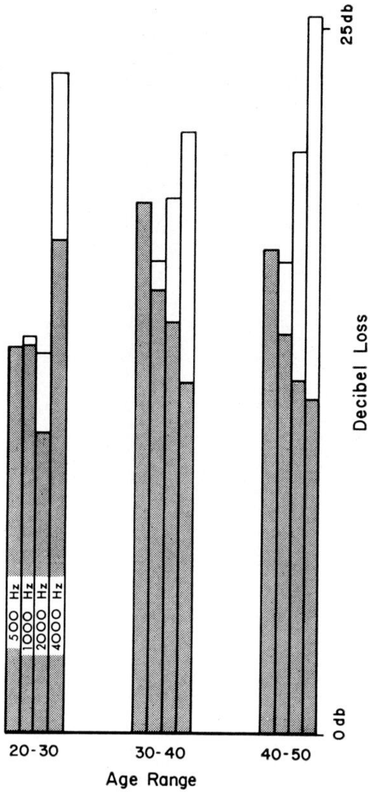

Fig. 1 The graph illustrates the progressive sensorineural hearing loss in 220 patients examined repeatedly over a 25-year period. The total length of each bar indicates the sensorineural hearing loss in the various age groups. The light portion of each bar indicates the expected loss from presbycusis as determined by Glorig and Davis.[1] The patients were divided into age groups to indicate when they had their first audiogram. It will be noted that in the younger age groups the sensorineural loss is almost twice that one would expect from presbycusis. In the older age groups, the loss associated with otospongiosis is equal to that expected in presbycusis for high frequencies but much greater for the low frequencies. It is also obvious that the low frequencies, as well as the high frequencies, are affected by otospongiosis in distinction to the usually isolated high frequency loss seen in cases of presbycusis.

ance, *et al*[4] have demonstrated lysosomes at the margins of the advancing otospongiotic focus. They suspected that these lysosomes might produce a toxic substance that caused absorption of the normal bone and, if liberated into the inner ear fluids, could produce a sensorineural loss. Recently they have demonstrated an increase in enzymes in the perilymph in patients with far-advanced otospongiosis who underwent stapes surgery.

Ruedi described venous shunts between the otospongiotic focus and vessels of the cochlea.[5] He suspects that these might produce venous congestion, interfering with the normal metabolism of the cochlea, thus producing a hearing loss.

Atrophy and hyalinization of the spiral ligament have been found to be associated with the sensorineural hearing loss that occurs in patients with otospongiosis. The mechanism that produces the atrophy and hyalinization is as yet not established.[6]

It is possible that the encroachment of the otospongiotic focus on the cochlear capsule can distort it and the basilar membrane, inhibiting the traveling wave throughout the rest of the cochlea.

METHODS AND MATERIALS

One hundred pairs of temporal bones of patients, with clinical antemortem evidence of otospongiosis, were evaluated. There were complete records on all of these patients which included physical examination and audiometric data including air, bone, and speech. In many patients there were other hearing tests performed, such as Békésy, tone decay, and SISI. Many of these patients had had vestibular tests and X-ray evaluation, either by routine x-ray techniques or polytomography.

The temporal bones were decalcified, embedded in celloidin, and sectioned in 20-micron thicknesses. Every tenth section was mounted and stained with H and E. Occasionally, additional sections were prepared and stained with Gomeri, Mallory, and Bodian stains. We looked for the following: 1) absence (partial or complete) of hair cells, neurons, and ganglion cells; 2) atrophy and hyalinization of the spiral ligament; 3) evidence of vascular shunts between the cochlea and otospongiotic focus; and 4) width of the basilar membrane adjacent to the otospongiotic focus.

RESULTS

Organ of Corti. In some patients numerous hair cells were found to be

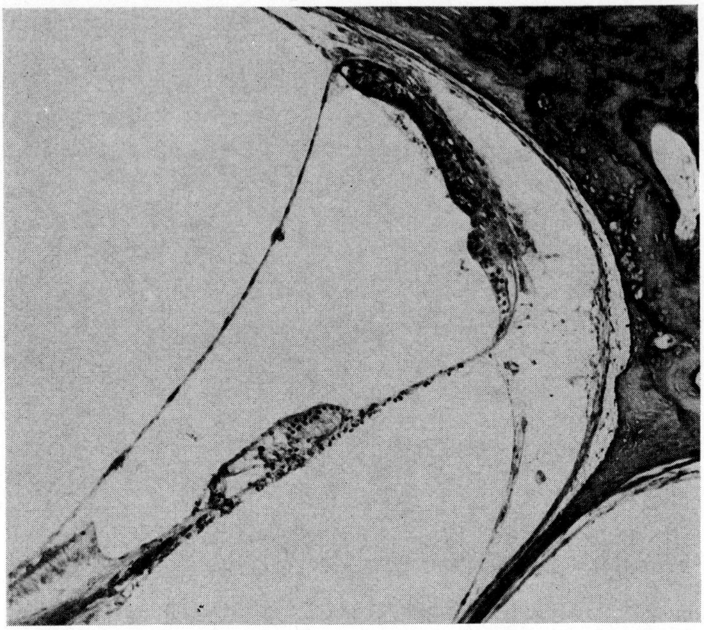

Fig. 2. Otospongiosis involving the endosteum adjacent to the spiral ligament in a patient with an average 50 dB loss in the speech frequencies by bone conduction tests. There is no evidence of an abnormality of the organ of Corti, stria, or spiral ligament with light microscopy. (H. and E., X100)

lacking, particularly the outer cells. This deficiency was most often associated with hyalinization of the spiral ligament. However, there were some patients with clinical evidence of sensorineural hearing loss who demonstrated, by light microscopy, a normally appearing organ of Corti (Fig. 2).

A correlation of the degree of abnormality of the organ of Corti and the sensorineural hearing level could not be made as the sole explanation of the hearing loss.

Spiral Ligament. We have demonstrated a relationship of otospongiosis involving the endosteum adjacent to the spiral ligament.[7] About half of the patients in the Institute collection showing an antemortem bone conduction threshold of 50 dB or more also exhibited hyalinization of varying amounts. This hyalinization always appeared in the peripheral portion of the spiral ligament adjacent to the otospongiotic focus involving the endosteum (Fig. 3). In the turns of the cochlea without otospongiosis, there was no hyalinization (Fig. 4). The cause of this degenerative change in the spiral ligament remains obscure, but it may well be due to the toxic influences of the enzymes secreted by the lysosomes as suggested by Bretlau, *et al* and Chevance, *et al*[3,4] or some abnormal metabolism in the ligament, possibly from hypoxia due to the vascular shunts described by Ruedi.[5]

Vascular Shunts. Ruedi[5] described venous shunts between the venules of the inner ear and the otospongiotic focus adjacent to it (Fig. 5). He postulated that these shunts could produce venous congestion and hence influence the metabolism of the cochlea. This could result in hypoxia and degenerative changes in the spiral ligament such as the hyalinization described in the preceding paragraphs.

Hypoxia due to shunting of blood may also produce new bone formation in the cochlea (Fig. 6) which could also act as an aneurysm, shunting blood

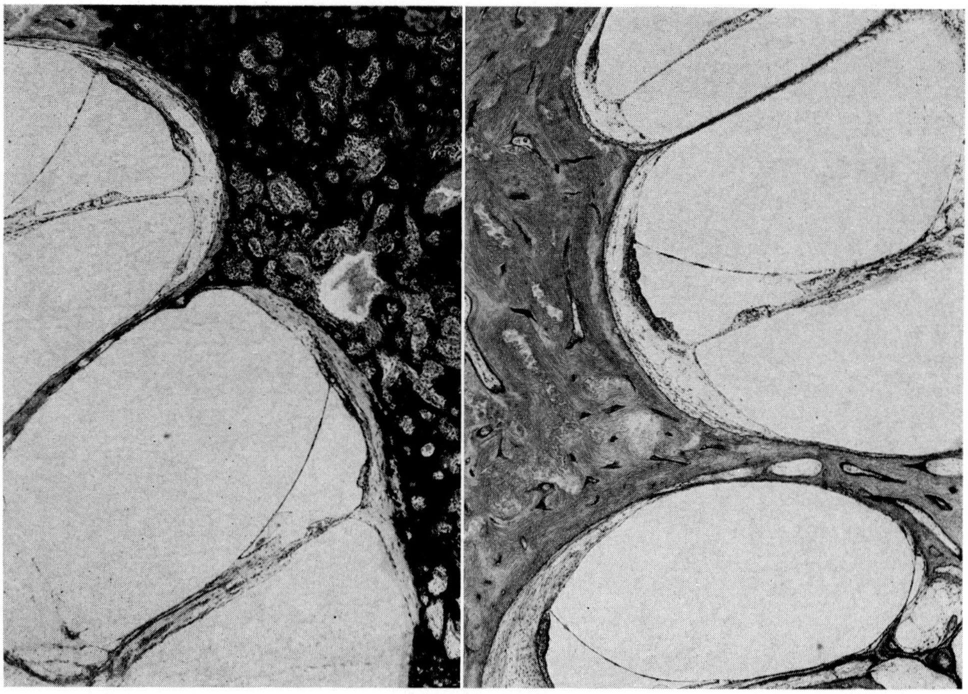

Fig. 3. Active otosclerotic focus adjacent to spiral ligament. Evident is hyalinization and calcification of the spiral ligament, distortion of the cochlear wall, and atrophy of the stria vascularis. (X50)

Fig. 4. Anterior portion of the cochlea of the same patient shown in Figure 3. The stria and spiral ligament appear normal. There is no distortion of the cochlear wall. (X50)

away from the spiral ligament and into the expanding growing otospongiotic lesion. The resulting hypoxia may interfere with the nutrition of the cochlea, much as a hemangioma or aneurysm will impair the growth of a limb or other structure. This might also result in a buildup of metabolites in the cochlear fluids.

Perhaps the stria vascularis, an integral part of the spiral ligament, has a selective absorptive function, rather than secretory and absorptive as some have suggested. Should this be the case, interference of the circulation could result in a buildup of metabolites in the inner ear fluids. Possibly the stria acts like a kidney tubule in being able to selectively absorb certain ions and molecules while rejecting others as the tubule does. This might indicate that the arteries beneath the organ of Corti are analogous to the glomerulus in the kidney and the stria to the kidney tubule. If this were the case, an interference of the circulation to the stria due to vascular shunts could decrease its efficiency. This interference would result in a buildup of carbon dioxide and other products of metabolism and interfere with the normal function of the hair cells in those cases in which there was found, by light microscopy, to be no abnormality.

Toxic Influences. Bretlau, *et al*[3] and Chevance, *et al*[4] have demonstrated lysosomes at the advancing edge of the otospongiotic focus. This explains why bone seems to be absorbed and replaced by the otospongiotic lesion without the evidence of osteoclasts at the advancing edge of the lesion. (Therefore, the multinucleated "osteoclasts" are possibly merely foreign body giant cells absorbing debris rather than cells capable of actually destroying bone.) They

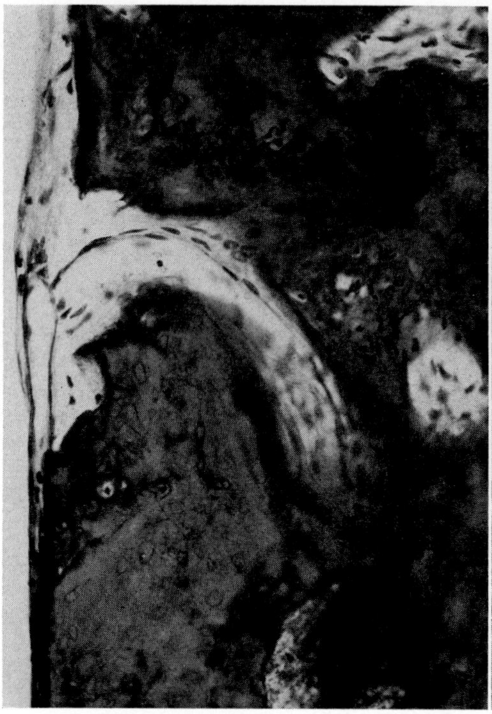

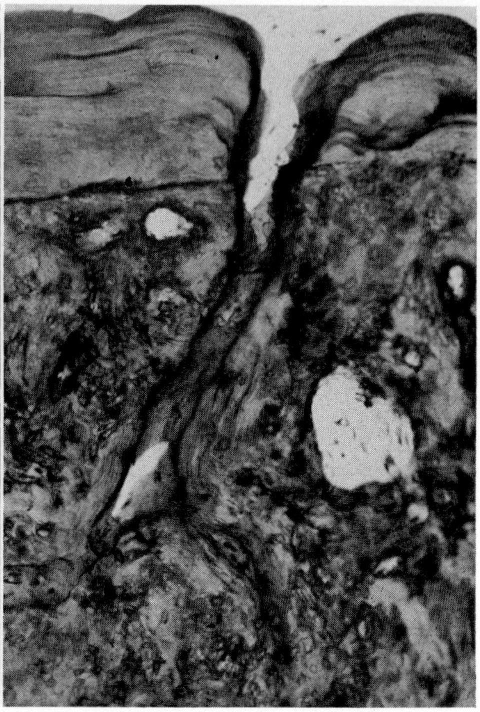

Fig. 5. Vascular shunt between the scala tympani and active otospongiotic focus, similar to those described by Ruedi.[5] Such shunts could alter the metabolism of the inner ear fluids and hence the organ of Corti. (X430)

Fig. 6. Another vascular shunt between the scala tympani and otospongiotic focus. There is lamellar bone present within the scala tympani. Such new bone formation is usually due to hypoxia of an organ. (X430)

postulated that the enzymes secreted by the lysosomes, when liberated into the inner ear fluids, could produce a toxic effect upon the metabolism of the hair cells. In analyzing the perilymph in patients undergoing stapedectomy with mixed hearing losses, they found increased amounts of these enzymes present. This could explain the poor sensorineural function in patients whose temporal bones showed no evidence of damage to the hair cells.

Cochlear Distortion. The propagation of the traveling wave along the basilar membrane was analyzed by Békésy.[8] Later, Tonndorf[9] demonstrated that increased tension on the basilar membrane, as occurs with endolymphatic hydrops, could account for the phenomenon of diplacusis in patients with this condition. However, neither individual, to our knowledge, analyzed what might happen should the basilar membrane insertions be relaxed.

Analysis of the width of the basilar membrane in the posterior basal turn of twelve cochleas with otospongiosis involving the endosteum indicated a median width of .78 mm. The median width of the basilar membrane in sixteen cochleas without otospongiosis was .85 mm, a statistically significant difference.*

This difference suggested the possibility of the cochlear focus encroaching upon the spiral ligament and narrowing the width of the basilar membrane and

* The difference of .07 mm between the two groups yielded a value of 3.80, which is significant beyond the .01 level, 2.77 required with 27 degrees of freedom.[10]

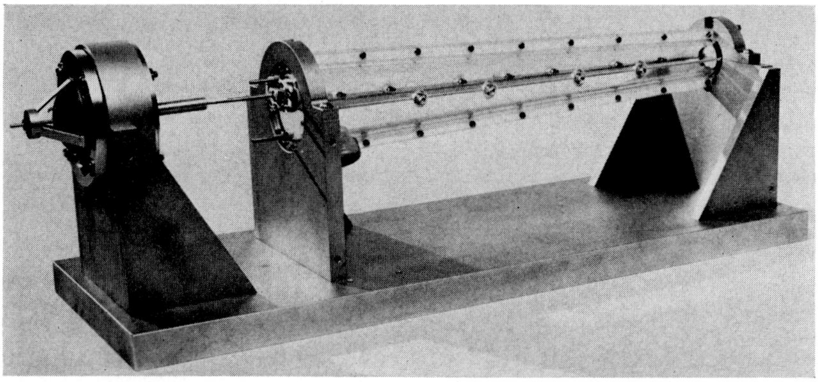

Fig 7. Cochlear model so constructed that the simulated basilar membrane is relaxable throughout the length of the model. It was found that relaxation of the membrane at the basal turn affected the amplitude of the traveling wave. The model is scale 1 cm to 1 mm.

the diameter of the cochlea. This distortion could possibly alter the amplitude of the traveling wave.

A model of the cochlea was constructed in such a manner that the basilar membrane could be narrowed in the simulated basal turn of the cochlea (Fig. 7). It was found that the amplitude of the traveling wave was decreased with the exception of the area where the membrane had been narrowed (Fig. 8). In this area the amplitude increased. This increase was felt to allow energy to be transmitted directly from the scala vestibuli to the scala tympani via the cochlear duct and basilar membrane, thus decreasing the amplitude of the traveling wave along the remainder of the basilar membrane.

These findings suggest that part of the sensorineural hearing loss in patients with cochlear otospongiosis could be due to basilar membrane distortion. Alteration of the diameter of the various turns of the cochlea may also be a factor.

DISCUSSION

Analysis of 36 pairs of temporal bones with otospongiosis involving the endosteum of the cochlea and an antemortem sensorineural hearing loss fails to reveal any single abnormality of the organ of Corti, spiral ligament, configuration of

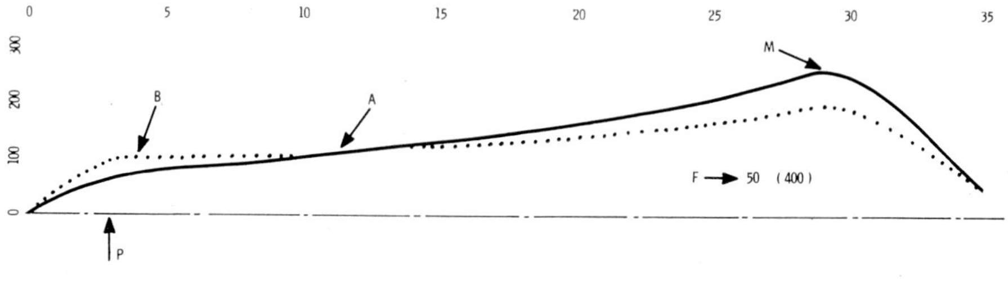

Fig. 8. Traveling waveform in the cochlea model before (solid line) and after (dotted line) relaxation of the basilar membrane in the simulated basal turn. The frequency for this wave pattern was 50 Hz. Note an increase in the amplitude of the wave in the relaxed area "B", indicating an escape of energy from the scala vestibuli to the scala tympani. The amplitude of the rest of the traveling wave is decreased. The numbers on the ordinate represent the distance in centimeters from the round window. The numbers on the abscissa represent the excursion of the basilar membrane in microns. "M" is maximum excursion of wave corresponding at scale to 400 Hz. "A" indicates little difference at high frequencies.

the cochlea, or vascular supply to account for the sensorineural hearing loss present in all cases. Comparison of the hearing level of these patients with nonotospongiosis patients indicates that the sensorineural hearing loss was far greater than one would anticipate in the general population of the same age group. Patients were excluded who had other known causes of hearing loss such as ototoxic drugs, acoustic trauma, and viral infections. It was found that in all but three cases the ear with the greater involvement of the endosteum by the otospongiotic lesion had the greatest sensorineural hearing loss. There is no question in my mind that otospongiosis produces a sensorineural hearing loss. The mechanism by which this occurs is probably multiple: 1) derangement of the vascular supply to the spiral ligament and hence the stria vascularis due to shunting of the blood into the otospongiotic focus; 2) toxic influences due to enzymes secreted by lysosomes at the advancing edge of the otosclerotic focus; and 3) distortion of the cochlear capsule and relaxation of the basilar membrane.

The importance of the roles of these various abnormalities in the production of the sensorineural hearing loss has yet to be determined. The work by Shambaugh[11] indicating that sodium fluoride will change the actively metabolic otospongiotic lesion into the inactive otosclerotic focus and hence prevent the progression of the sensorineural hearing loss is of utmost importance, even though we are as yet not certain of the role played by these various abnormalities in the cochlea as concerns the sensorineural hearing loss.

Valvassori[12] has demonstrated by polytomography that the sodium fluoride treatment does alter the type of otospongiotic focus. More recently we demonstrated the same, using strontium-85 and analyzing the radioactivity in the foot-plates of patients with mixed hearing losses.[13]

Microscopic examination of these foot-plates revealed that half underwent a change from an otospongiotic lesion to an otosclerotic lesion. The other half exhibited an otosclerotic lesion prior to and after administration of sodium fluoride. In spite of the apparent similarity of the type of lesion, the radioactivity was decreased as measured by strontium-85 in all but one patient.

There are, in the temporal bone collection of the Institute, three pairs of temporal bones with cochlear otospongiosis in both ears but stapedial fixation in only one. All three have an equal sensorineural hearing loss in both ears. We believe that the sensorineural loss in all three of these patients was due to the cochlear otospongiosis and that bilateral cochlear otosclerosis without stapedial fixation can occur, based upon the findings of Valvassori and ourselves utilizing the polytomography technique.[12,14] Regardless of the cause of the sensorineural hearing loss in patients with otospongiosis, it appears that sodium fluoride will convert the otospongiotic phase to the otosclerotic phase and prevent the progression of the sensorineural component of the hearing loss. This treatment has been described by Shambaugh[11] and substantiated by polytomography by Valvassori[12] and later, using strontium-85, by us.[13] If the mechanism of the production of the sensorineural hearing loss could be determined, it might be feasible to reverse the sensorineural hearing loss in these patients.

CONCLUSIONS

There is little doubt that otospongiosis involving the cochlear capsule can produce a sensorineural hearing loss. Light microscopic examination of the organ of Corti fails to reveal any abnormality of the hair cells to account for this loss in the majority of the cases.

Several theories have been proposed and passed to account for this hearing loss: toxic substances produced by the otospongiotic focus; vascular shunts between the inner ear vessels and the otospongiotic focus; and atrophy of the organ of Corti and stria vascularis due to unknown causes. In this paper we present yet another possibility: impingement upon the cochlear walls by the otospongiotic focus, causing a narrowing of the lumen of the cochlea and distortion of the basilar membrane. In all probability, more than one of these factors is responsible for the hearing loss in each case.

Analysis of the clinical records of 100 patients with otospongiosis indicates that the degree of sensorineural hearing loss is greater than one would expect from presbycusis. We present microscopic examples of the various factors responsible for the sensorineural hearing loss. A mechanical model of the cochlea demonstrates that if the basilar membrane in the basal turn of the cochlea is loosened or narrowed that the propagation of the traveling wave through the rest of the cochlea becomes decreased, except in the area of relaxation where it is increased. The loosened area corresponds to that area of the basilar membrane that responds to frequencies higher than those tested by routine audiometry.

Sodium fluoride and calcium treatment has been shown to decrease the rapidity of the sensorineural hearing loss due to cochlear otospongiosis. It is hoped that further understanding of the causes of the sensorineural hearing loss will lead to prevention or possibly correction of the hearing loss.

Request for reprints should be sent to Fred H. Linthicum, Jr., M.D., Otologic Medical Group, Inc., 2122 West Third St., Los Angeles, California 90057.

REFERENCES

1. Glorig A, Davis H: Age, noise, and hearing loss. Ann Otol Rhinol Laryngol 70: 556, 1961

2. Siebenmann F: Multiple Spongiosierung der Labyrinthkapsel als Sectionsbefund bei einem Fall von progressiver Schwerhorigkeit. Z Ohrenheilk 34:356-374, 1899

3. Bretlau P, Causse J, Jorgensen MB, *et al*: Histiocytic activity in the otosclerotic bone. Arch Klin Exp Ohren Nasen Kehlkopfheilkd 198:301-316, 1971

4. Chevance LG, Bretlau P, Jorgensen MB, *et al*: Otosclerosis: An electron microscopic and cytochemical study. Acta Otolaryngol [Suppl] (Stockh) 272:1-27, 1970

5. Ruedi L: Histopathologic confirmation of labyrinthine otosclerosis. Laryngoscope 75: 1582-1609, 1965

6. Holleman IL Jr, Harrill JA: Cochlear otosclerosis: Report of a case, with postmortem histologic findings. Laryngoscope 77:493-507, 1967

7. Linthicum FH Jr: Correlation of sensorineural hearing impairment and otosclerosis. Ann Otol Rhinol Laryngol 75:512, 1966

8. Békésy G: *Experiments in Hearing.* New York, McGraw-Hill, 1960, pp 485-534

9. Tonndorf J: Shearing motion in scala media of cochlear models. J Acoust Soc Am 32:238-244, 1960

10. Guilford JP: *Fundamental Statistics in Psychology and Education.* Ed. 4, New York, McGraw-Hill Book Co., 1965

11. Shambaugh GE Jr: Sodium fluoride for inactivation of the otosclerotic lesion. Arch Otolaryngol 89:381-382, 1969

12. Valvassori GE: Otosclerosis: A new challenge to roentgenology. Am J. Roentgenol Radium Ther Nucl Med 94:566-575

13. Linthicum FH Jr, House HP, Althaus SR: The effect of sodium fluoride on otosclerotic activity as determined by strontium^{85}. Ann Otol Rhinol Laryngol 82:609, 1973

14 Britton BH Jr, Linthicum FH Jr: Otosclerosis. Histologic confirmation of radiologic findings. Ann Otol Rhinol Laryngol 79:1, 1970

Ann Otol 84: 1975

RECONSTRUCTION OF THE OPEN MASTOIDECTOMY EAR: A SIX YEAR PROGRESS REPORT

MANSFIELD F. W. SMITH, M.D.

SAN JOSE, CALIFORNIA

SUMMARY – This report deals with 61 mastoid cavities which were revised or reconstructed using homograft techniques over a six-year period. Discussed are the variety of homograft procurement techniques and surgical homograft techniques which have been abandoned and included in a review of 16 consecutive mastoid revisions performed from 1973-1974 utilizing a standard surgical technique.

From 1968 to 1972 a series of mastoid revisions and reconstructions was performed utilizing standard otologic techniques but encompassing a variety of individual techniques incorporating autograft and homograft material. Based on this four-year experience, more standardized techniques of homograft reconstruction evolved, and during 1973 and 1974, these techniques were utilized in all mastoid revisions and reconstructions.

The substance of this report deals with the problems of homograft mastoid reconstructions and with the various surgical techniques which have been unsatisfactory. In addition, it is a review of 21 cases of mastoid reconstruction utilizing a standard surgical technique.

The otologic tissue discussed in this paper was processed and stored in tissue culture medium with Hank's salts with added antibiotic antimycotic mixture.[1]

Obtaining meaningful data on indications, surgical management, and functional results of surgical revision of these problem mastoid cavities is difficult because of varying methods of homograft preparation, changing surgical concepts, and revising prior operated patients. However, it is significant to indicate the combinations of autograft and homograft mastoid surgical reconstruction procedures that have not been satisfactory and why.

During the 1968 to 1972 period certain mastoid revision procedures with otologic homografts were not successful in our hands for a number of reasons. The first and most important reason for poor results was Eustachian tube dysfunction. Occasionally, there was a loss of continuity of the air column between the middle ear and the mastoid cavity. Failure of aeration resulted in loss or displacement of ossicular tissue, the tympanic membrane, and the reconstructed posterior osseous canal.

The second reason, also a major problem, lay in reconstructing the posterior canal and establishing the critical anatomical relationship between the lateral epitympanic plate, ossicles, and mesial wall of the posterior epitympanic space. Often, short-term anatomical appearance of the reconstructed posterior canal and tympanic membrane was good. However, in three to four years, it was not unusual for a posterior superior retraction pocket in the tympanic membrane to occur with resultant

From the Department of Surgery, Division of Otolaryngology, Stanford University and Santa Clara Valley Medical Center, California.

Presented at the meeting of the American Otological Society, Inc., Atlanta, Georgia, April 11-12, 1975.

potential for cholesteatoma behind the reconstructed canal.

These experiences with Eustachian tube dysfunction and posterior superior retraction pockets engendered the following questions: Why convert an open small mastoid cavity into a closed cavity with at least a significant chance of Eustachian tube failure (in our series approximately 25%) with resultant homograft absorption and displacement? The critical question is that if the mastoid reconstruction procedure is going to fail, then what?

We considered it better to revise the mastoid cavity, line it with autograft connective tissue, and reconstruct the tympanic membrane, malleus, and stapes as a myringostapediopexy (Type III, modified radical mastoid) with healthy residual structures plus autografts and homografts when indicated. In this situation Eustachian tube dysfunction does not create an additional problem, and the scutum anatomical dilemma is obviated. Therefore, we have abandoned certain types of homograft processing and have discontinued certain autograft-homograft mastoid revision techniques.

Otologic homografts were prepared and stored in 70% ethanol from 1968 to 1972.* We were not satisfied with alcohol otologic homograft preparation for the following reasons: the healing of soft tissues over posterior osseous canal alcohol prepared homografts was often protracted. Further, the alcohol prepared ossicles behaved as sequestered dead bone, and for a period of between two and four years we noted bone absorption, particularly of homograft stapes. Such agents as alcohol, organic mercurial (ciliate), formalin, and gluteraldehyde all fix the osseous and fibrous otologic tissue. In addition, there are chemical changes in the tissue as well as gross anatomical alterations, such as stiffness of the fibrous tissue, particularly with formalin and gluteraldehyde. Such fixed chemically altered homograft tissue may take on the properties of alloplastic tissue with the potential of ultimate extrusion.

The autograft-homograft techniques that have been discontinued are the following:

Composite Homografts Consisting of the Three Ossicles. In addition to retraction pockets, absorption, and displacement with Eustachian tube dysfunction, the functional results with composite ossicular chain reconstruction have been poor, which has been a result of displacement and fixation of the ossicles.

Autograft Cortical Mastoid Bone Reconstruction of the Posterior Canal. This method is no longer utilized because of the difficulty of establishing the scutum in an appropriate anatomical relationship with a resultant retraction pocket posteriorly and superiorly.

Fibrous Tympanic Membrane Homograft. We have found fascia to be superior to a fibrous tympanic membrane homograft in routine tympanoplastic procedures. However, we occasionally use a fibrous tympanic membrane homograft with attached periosteal cuff after a fascia graft failure, particularly when there has been lateralization. We almost always overlay the fibrous tympanic membrane with fascia. We have not experienced delamination of the fascia from the fibrous tympanic membrane in the tissue culture prepared homograft tissue. The resultant tympanic membrane has been thin and mobile.

SURGICAL TECHNIQUES

The open mastoid cavity is revised by either reconstruction of the posterior canal and conversion to a closed cavity

* All of the homograft otologic tissue discussed in this report was procured, processed, and stored by the Ear Transplant Unit of the Northern California Transplant Bank. The Northern California Transplant Bank is included in the organization of the Institute for Medical Research of the Santa Clara Valley Medical Center which is a nonprofit research organization for the Staff of the Santa Clara Valley Medical Center. The Santa Clara Valley Medical Center is one of the teaching hospitals affiliated with Stanford University.

or revised and relined with a Mosher-Palva flap; thus, the cavity becomes in concept an enlarged external auditory canal (EAC).

Reconstruction of the posterior osseous canal is now carried out only when there is an extremely large mastoid cavity with a high facial ridge. The canal is also reconstructed when there are minor defects in the posterior osseous canal, such as an extensive atticotomy, where approximately 50% of the canal remains. These canal defects are reconstructed with a homograft posterior osseous canal, often with the attached fibrous tympanic membrane and long process of malleus and generous periosteal cuff when total tympanic membrane and malleus long-process replacement is necessary. The advantage of this type of graft is that the relationship of the scutum to the fibrous tympanic membrane are anatomically correct by virtue of the orthotopic homograft. Also, the curvilinear shape of the homograft posterior canal is suitable.

In concept, revision of the open small cavity to a large EAC embodies the following principles: 1) removal of residual disease, 2) exteriorization of all areas of the mastoid and middle ear including an adequate meatoplasty, 3) lining of the cavity, and 4) entrapment of mucous membrane in the middle ear by reconstruction of the tympanic membrane.

All active disease is controlled preoperatively if possible. No open mastoidectomy ears with cholesteatoma of the mastoid were lined with a muscle periosteal flap.

In the following paragraphs, a revision of an open radical mastoidectomy ear without a stapes arch and with a mobile footplate is described. A post-auricular incision with a superior hockey stick extension is made through the superficial fascia with elevation of a post-auricular muscle periosteal flap based on the pinna anteriorly as described by Mosher[2] and Palva.[3] The periosteal epithelial membrane is then dissected from the mastoid cavity over the facial ridge and medial aspect of the middle ear to the anterior osseous canal wall at the level of the fibrous annulus. The mastoid cavity is appropriately revised, all residual disease is removed, the facial ridge lowered, and, if there is a large mastoid tip, the osseous tip structure is removed to allow superior displacement of the digastric muscle to reduce the inferior portion of the mastoid cavity.

The recipient mobile foot-plate is denuded of all soft tissues. This is done in an anterior to posterior orientation with a fine sharp needle. The soft tissue is deflected from the foot-plate towards the VII nerve superiorly and onto the promontory inferiorly. In most instances, an envelope of soft tissue is developed inferior and superior to the oval window. The donor stapes foot-plate is placed adjacent to the recipient foot-plate without any interposition of soft tissue. The previously elevated soft tissues are then placed back over the foot-plate of the donor. A 4x4 mm .005 inch medical grade Silastic®* sheeting is cut on the diagonal to 0.1 mm of a corner. Each side of the halved square of silicone sheeting is placed on the promontory and the other on the facial nerve area. The intent in using the Silastic® is to prevent fibrous adhesions and ultimate displacement or fixation of the stapes. Gelfoam®** pledgets are then placed on the silicone sheeting to stabilize the stapes.

Reconstruction of the malleus is accomplished by inserting a homograft fibrous tympanic membrane with attached generous periosteal cuff of the donor EAC and also the attached long process of the incus. All epithelium has been removed from this graft. The head of the malleus has been removed because it is unnecessary in the shallow middle ear cavity of the open radical

* Dow-Corning Chem. Co., Medical Products Div., Midland, Mich.
** The Upjohn Co., Kalamazoo, Mich.

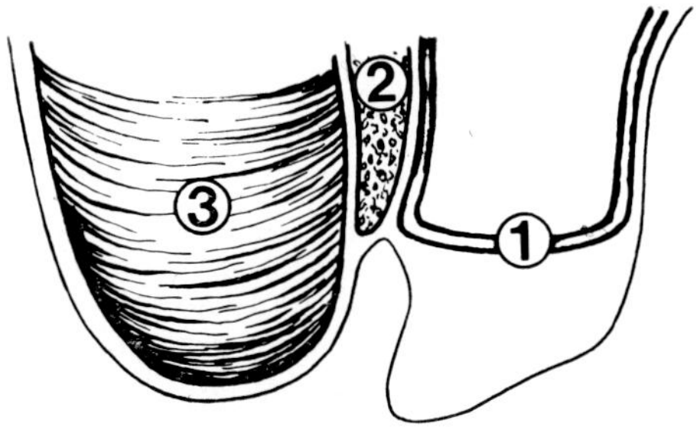

Fig. 1. Diagrammatic representation of middle ear and mastoid demonstrating the use of two pedicled soft tissue flaps and homograft bone. 1) Pedicled epithelial periosteal flap. 2) Homograft bone. 3) Pedicled muscle periosteal flap.

mastoidectomy ear. Any residual fibrous tympanic membrane and fibrous annulus are removed from the recipient preventing the problem of retained epithelial tissue in the fibrous annulus, particularly in the anterior sulcus. If there is residual osseous tympanic sulcus, the homograft annulus is then positioned into this sulcus. The periosteal cuff is incised from lateral to medial to the annulus at approximately the six o'clock position in order to drape the periosteal cuff onto the anterior osseous canal. The fibrous vascular strip area is placed superiorly onto the area of the horizontal semicircular canal. Temporalis fascia is placed onto the lateral aspect of the fibrous tympanic membrane and incised from inferior to superior in the area that would be adjacent to the long process of the malleus. In this manner the fascia adapts to the normal conical shape of the homograft reconstructed drum. The fascia is carried posteriorly into the mastoid cavity, and the previously prepared periosteal muscle flap is placed into the mastoid cavity defect and onto the lateral aspect of the fascia and homograft fibrous posterior extension. Because of the shallow middle ear space, the homograft fibrous tympanic membrane is now draped over the homograft reconstructed stapes arch, thus forming a myringostapediopexy. If any of the residual epithelial periosteal membrane that was elevated from the mastoid cavity is healthy, it can be placed against the anterior limit of the periosteal muscle flap that is now in filling the mastoid defect (Fig. 1). This periosteal epithelial membrane that has been dissected from the mastoid cavity is based on the medial aspect of the pinna but anterior to the base of the muscle periosteal flap. Often this residual periosteal epithelium is healthy and allows for quick epithelialization of the Mosher-Palva flap on its anterior limit. These pedicled flaps do not obliterate the mastoid cavity in the long term, but they do afford excellent lining of the mastoid cavity and often substantially reduce the size of the cavity. The external auditory meatus is revised through an end aural incision as described by Stacke.[4] The area of the reconstructed tympanic membrane is then packed with Gelfoam® soaked in 10% Chloromycetin®* out to the level of the meatus. The post-auricular incision is repaired, and a mastoid pressure dressing is applied for at least one week.

RESULTS

From 1968 to 1974, 61 patients with open mastoid cavities have been revised. Part of these patients came from the author's private practice and the other part were supervised staff patients of the Stanford Otolaryngology Service at the Santa Clara Valley Medical Center. From January 1968 to June 1972, 40 open mastoid cavities were revised. However, because of varying methods of homograft preparation, changing surgical concepts, and revisions of prior patients. no meaningful data were obtained. However, the autograft homograft procedures for open mastoid cavity revision that have not been successful have been indicated.

From 1973 to 1974, 21 patients with open radical mastoid cavities were reconstructed. Five of the 21 patients were lost to follow-up, so 16 consecutive patients were observed. Preoperatively, eight of the 16 patients had re-

* Parke, Davis & Co., Detroit, Mich.

current drainage. All 16 were interested in having improved hearing. The primary interest of four of the 16 was having a "waterproof ear," enabling them to participate in water sports. In all 16 patients active infection was controlled preoperatively by conservative care. Eustachian tube patency or function or both was assessed clinically without unusual apparatus, and only one of the 16 patients had a proven preoperative air-containing middle ear space, in this situation a cavum minor.

At the time of surgery three patients were noted to have active cholesteatoma. The status of the stapes in the 16 patients at the time of surgery is as follows: 1) stapes arch present in five patients, 2) stapes arch absent in 11, 3) stapes foot-plate mobile in 15, and 4) stapes foot-plate fixed in one (One of the five patients with an intact arch).

Postoperative results were as follows: 1) the anatomic appearance of the cavity was dry, clean, and shallow, in 16 of 16 patients; 2) the tympanic membrane was satisfactory in 12 of 16; unsatisfactory in four because of retraction and hypomobility in three and perforation in one; 3) the malleus position was satisfactory in 15; unsatisfactory in one; and 4) the middle ear was air-containing in 12 of 16; fluid in one; atelectatic in three.

The following describes the functional results. Two of the 16 patients were converted to normal hearing. One had a mild sensorineural loss of greater than 20 dB. All patients preoperatively had normal speech discrimination, which remained normal postoperatively. The maximum gain in hearing was a speech reception threshold (SRT) of 38 dB from a preoperative SRT of 74 and a postoperative SRT of 36. The average gain in the SRT was 17 dB.

DISCUSSION

The advantages of converting the open radical mastoid ear to a modified radical mastoidectomy with homograft and autograft material and lining of the disease free mastoid cavity with a Mosher-Palva flap are: 1) involves a one stage procedure, 2) does not require alloplastic material, 3) embodies well-defined ear surgical techniques with proven long-term anatomical and functional results, and 4) if there is failure of middle ear aeration, the procedure does not create any additional problems for the patient, such as absorption of a reconstructed posterior osseous canal or retraction of epithelium into a recreated closed mastoid cavity.

SUMMARY

Revision and reconstruction experience with 61 problem radical mastoid cavities over a six-year period is the basis of this report. Reconstruction of the posterior osseous canal with homograft osseous canal is carried out both in patients with very large mastoid cavities that have partially intact posterior canals, and also in patients with relatively minor defects in the posterior osseous canal regardless of the size of the mastoid cavity.

Included are the details of surgery and the anatomical and functional results of converting open radical mastoid cavities to a modified radical mastoid cavity using homograft and autograft material and lining of the mastoid cavity with an anterior pinna based periosteal muscle flap.

The tympanic membrane and malleus is reconstructed with homograft material consisting of the fibrous tympanic membrane, attached long process of the malleus and attached periosteal cuff of the EAC. The fibrous tympanic membrane contacts the stapes capitulum with a resultant myringostapediopexy. Forty-five patients with reconstructed open mastoid cavities, operated prior to 1973, were summarized by indicating the operative procedure used and the reason for its discontinuation.

Results of 16 consecutive revised radical mastoid cavities done in 1973 and 1974 were satisfactory. All 16 patients developed dry, clean, shallow cavities. Twelve of the 16 patients developed an air-containing middle ear space. However, four of the 16 (25%) did not have satisfactory Eustachian tube function, three developed atelectatic middle ears, and one, a serous otitis media. The average gain in the SRT of the 16 revised mastoid cavities was 17 dB.

Request for reprints should be sent to Mansfield F. W. Smith, M.D., 751 South Bascom Ave., San Jose, Calif. 95128.

REFERENCES

1. Smith MFW, Downie D: Otologic homograft indications, techniques and results. Trans Am Acad Ophthalmol Otolaryngol 80: 47-51, 1975

2. Mosher HP: A method of filling the excavated mastoid with a flap from the back of the auricle. Laryngoscope 21:1158-1168, 1911

3. Palva T: Surgery of chronic ear without cavity: results in 130 cases with musculoperiosteal flap and fasciotympanoplasty. Arch Otolaryngol 77:570-580, 1963

4. Stacke L: Stackes Operationsmethode. Arch Ohrenheilk 35:145, 1893

X-RAY OF THE MONTH

GUEST EDITORS

JAMES RHEA, M.D.

ALFRED L. WEBER, M.D.

BOSTON, MASSACHUSETTS

PATIENT

The patient is a 38-year-old male with congenital malformation of the right ear, who underwent reconstructive procedures of the auricle between 1944 and 1949. In September 1974 he noted a "fullness" deep in the right ear which failed to respond to antibiotic therapy. The above radiographic studies were obtained in January 1975 prior to surgery.

RADIOGRAPHS

Towne's view (Fig. 1) demonstrates a large, well-defined cavity (arrows) in the region of the right mastoid antrum. Tomographic sections (Figs. 2 and 3) reveal absence of the external auditory canal with a moderately thick bony atresia plate, hypoplasia of the right tympanic cavity, malformation of the ossicles, and destruction of the tegmen (arrow).

DIAGNOSIS

Surgical exploration was carried out and revealed an abscess cavity in the right mastoid with erosion of the tegmen.

DISCUSSION

Gill[1] reported that mastoid infection was present in 46 of 83 cases of surgically treated congenital atresia. The severity of infection ranged from indolent granulations to pus under pressure with bone destruction. In only two of the 46 cases were there clinical signs of infection. Not only was the presence of infection difficult to detect clinically, but postoperative results were less satisfactory in those cases having severe infections.

Tomography is of value in determining the extent of deformity in congenital malformation of the ear and in detecting the presence of infection when there is either bone destruction or increased density in normally lucent areas.

REFERENCE

1. Gill NW: Congenital atresia of the ear. J Laryngol Otol 83:551-587, 1969

From the Departments of Radiology, Massachusetts General Hospital and Massachusetts Eye and Ear Infirmary, Boston, Massachusetts.

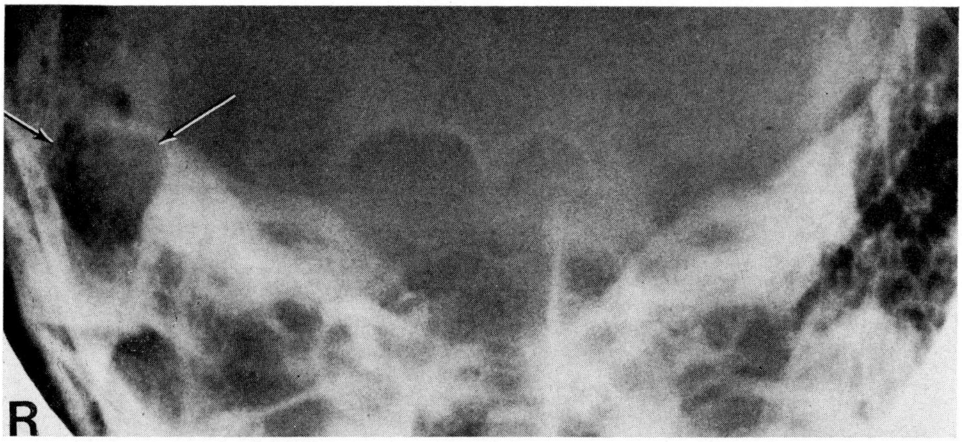

Fig. 1. Conventional Towne's view showing the large radiolucent defect (arrows) in the right mastoid area.

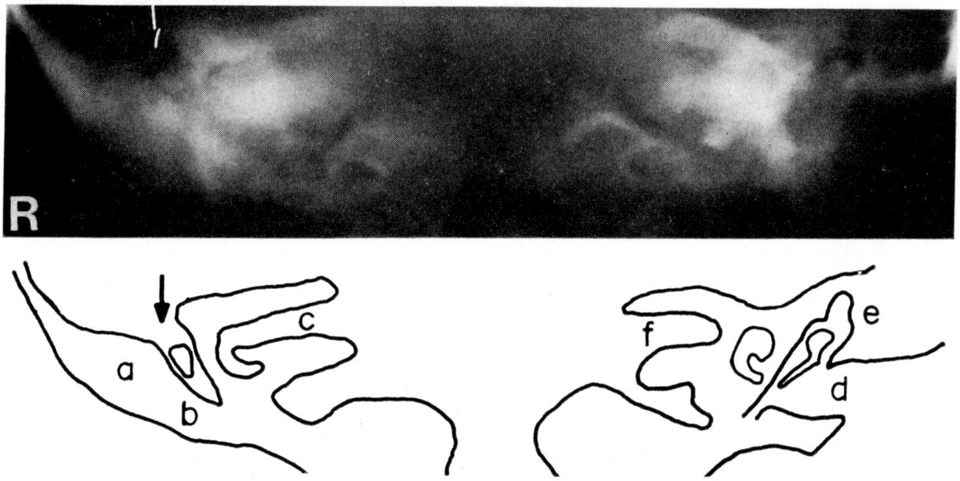

Fig. 2. Frontal tomogram and explanatory outline drawing through both temporal bones. The arrow points to the area of destruction in the tegmen on the right (R). Note the thick bony atresia plate (a), the hypoplastic tympanic cavity with a malformed ossicular mass (b), and a normal internal auditory canal (c) on the right side. Compare to the normal left middle ear and external auditory canal (d), epitympanum with a normal malleus (e), and normal internal auditory canal (f).

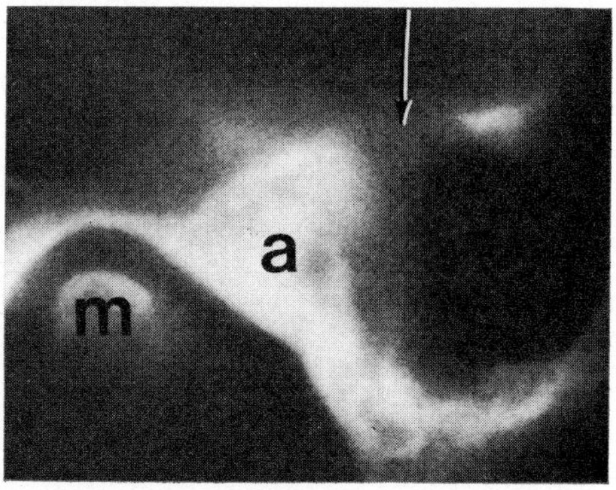

Fig. 3. Lateral tomogram of the right ear demonstrating the area of destruction in the tegmen plate (arrow). Note the dense bony atresia plate (a) and the proximity of the mandibular condyle (m).

COMMUNICATIONS

CONFERENCE ON ANIMAL MODELS OF AGING IN THE AUDITORY SYSTEM

David E. Crowley, Ph.D.
St. Louis, Missouri

SUMMARY — A conference was held to consider conceptual issues, methodological problems and preliminary findings related to auditory research with aging animals. Current concepts from various areas of experimental gerontology were discussed in relation to research on the aging auditory system and to the problem of human presbycusis.

On November 4, 1974, a small group, consisting of auditory researchers, experimental gerontologists, and veterinary specialists, met informally at Washington University in St. Louis to discuss research in which the auditory systems of aging experimental animals are studied to gain insights into the fundamental processes of human presbycusis.

H. T. Blumenthal, M.D., of Washington University, began the meeting by reminding participants of the fundamental relationship between disease and the aging process. He stated a view, generally held among gerontologists, that the gradual elimination of various diseases as major contributors to human mortality results in progressively more rectangular survivorship curves, as a greater proportion in each successive generation lives past middle age. Accordingly, as each disease is brought under control, it ceases to be part of the aging process, and the population survival statistics begin to reflect the basic cellular processes which ultimately limit lifespan. He then presented some of the concepts emerging from current research on aging at the cellular level, including the hypothesis that errors in transcription of genetic information from DNA to messenger RNA result in the production of deleterious protein which may lead to cell death, to cellular mutation, or to autoimmune reactions. He described some recent findings suggesting that the accumulation of mutant cells in certain organs could account for some of the major diseases of the aged, such as cancer, diabetes, and cardiovascular disease. Finally, he presented Hayflick's finding[1] that the number of doubling generations observed in cultures of normal fibroblasts is roughly proportional to the remaining lifespan of the human being or animal from which the cells were obtained, a finding which is consistent with the concept of a genetically-programmed cellular aging process.

J. Botwinick, Ph.D., also of Washington University, reviewed some of the experimental design problems complicating research on aging animals and emphasized the need for adequate control groups and for the careful application of statistical methods. He also pointed out that difficulties in interpreting differences between old and young animals as age effects can be overcome in part through the use of special research designs introduced by Schaie,[2] among others, in which differences due to time of birth and time of measurement are controlled.

Several auditory investigators then presented research designs and preliminary data from their animal experiments. M. L. Feldman, Ph.D., of Boston University, reported a variety of ultrastructural changes in the cochlear nucleus of aging male Sprague-Dawley rats, including alterations in mitochondria, loss of synaptic endings, and gliosis. His data from the rat's auditory cortex show that synaptic spine counts decrease monotonically with age.[3] J. M. Harrison, Ph.D., of Boston University, has developed behavioral methods, which he reported, for measuring absolute auditory thresholds and sound localization to be used on aging rats prior to morphological study by Feldman. His preliminary data do not reveal profound age differences in auditory thresholds. D. E. Crowley, Ph.D., of Washington University, presented a research design for studying age-related inner ear changes in male Wistar rats raised under conditions favoring the preservation of hearing and general health. His design employs the Schaie strategy[2] and provides for quantification of ambient noise levels to avoid noise-induced cochlear damage. J. W. Coleman, B.Sc., of the University of London, submitted a written description of his studies of age-related hair cell degeneration in guinea pigs. Considerable loss of outer hair cells can be detected as early as three months of age, according to his preliminary findings. In discussing Coleman's paper, V. Dayal, M.D., of the University of Toronto, reported that his study of the aging guinea pig's cochlea shows hair cell loss to begin in the apical turn.

D. C. Gibson, D.V.M., of the National Institute of Child Health and Human Development in Bethesda, Maryland, discussed various ways in which aging research has been seriously hampered in the past by difficulties in obtaining disease-free aged rodents with known biological characteristics.[4] He then described a contract program, established to overcome this problem, in which aging inbred rats and mice are maintained in special barrier facilities at Charles River Breeding Laboratories, Inc. for use by investigators conducting pilot studies or whose own aging colonies are decimated by epizootics or other disasters.

S. McQueen, D.V.M., of Washington Uni-

From the Department of Otolaryngology, Washington University School of Medicine, St. Louis, Missouri 63110.

The conference was supported in part by the Department of Otolaryngology.

versity, presented a detailed description of murine chronic respiratory disease (CRD), the most troublesome epizootic of laboratory rats and mice. She discussed the acute and chronic stages of CRD which can involve the entire lower and upper respiratory system, including the middle ear, but which are difficult to detect in the intact animal. Since the responsible organism *Mycoplasma pulmonis*[5] is apparently resistant to most conveniently administered antibiotics, she suggested that the avoidance of CRD requires a careful choice of animal suppliers and good methods of animal care.

In discussions throughout the meeting, a number of technical problems relevant to auditory research with aging animals were covered, including morphological methods, experimental design, and noise specifications in the maintenance and shipment of animals. A consideration of whether to use male or female animals ended with a general concensus that males are preferable at this early stage of research in the field, due to estrous-induced variability in females.

Several topics of more general interest were also covered during the various discussions. The question of genetic contributions to the variability observed in many data from aged human beings and animals was raised at several points and was discussed with respect to human longevity, to early auditory degeneration in certain inbred mice, and to the possibility of breeding animals for performance on certain auditory tasks.

H. Davis, M.D., of the Central Institute for the Deaf, St. Louis, stressed the importance of obtaining information on the interaction of age and noise exposure, due to the practical problem of separating these effects in humans seeking compensation for occupational hearing loss. However, the applicability of age changes observed in the auditory system of short-lived rodents to human presbycusis was questioned by Harrison. In reply, Gibson suggested the viewpoint, proposed by Heston,[4] that animal models, in general, are very useful in pointing the way to important variables in human disease, but should not be expected to replicate a human disorder exactly.

The meeting ended with a general discussion which focused on aspects of age-related changes in the central nervous system (CNS) and their role in audition. Blumenthal pointed out that the loss of neurons with advancing age now appears to be restricted to certain cortical loci and may not occur in the brain stem. Moreover, he added, current data suggest that vascular changes do not play a primary role in the loss of neurons with advancing age, for instance, or in some other age-related changes in the CNS, as was held in the past. Finally, he recommended that studies be made of amyloid deposits in the aging auditory nervous system, since amyloid is found elsewhere in the aging nervous system, and may represent a failure of the immune system to protect the CNS.

REFERENCES

1. Weiss AK: The Hayflick hypothesis. Gerontologist 14:492-493, 1974

2. Schaie KW: Age changes and age differences. Gerontologist 7:128-132, 1967

3. Feldman ML: Degenerative changes in aging dendrites. Gerontologist 14:36 (No. 5, pt. 2), 1974

4. Gibson DC (ed): *Development of the Rodent as a Model System of Aging.* Bethesda, NICHD, 1972. DHEW Publ. No. (NIH), pp 72-121

5. Cassell GH, Lindsey JR, Overcash RG, *et al*: Murine mycoplasma respiratory disease. Ann NY Acad Sci, 225:395-412, 1973

BOOK REVIEWS

Psychiatric Assessment by Speech and Hearing Behavior

By *Clyde L. Rousey, Ph.D. (editor).* Hard cover, indexed and referenced, not illustrated, 376 pp. Charles C Thomas, 301-327 East Lawrence Avenue, Springfield, Illinois 62703. 1974. Price $18.75

The editor is sharing "a set of premises relating the sounds used in our spoken language to various aspects of personality functioning." Rejecting the generally accepted "motoric speech development notion" as outdated, he proposes that productions of certain consonants reflect oral, anal, and phallic periods of psychosexual developments. He notes that some of the ideas presented in this book which have been previously published have met with skepticism and resistence, but he and his colleagues are willing to "let these ideas and efforts stand the test of time and scrutiny by others." Unfortunately, the premises of this book (approx. 60 pages) are such that they will not be a clear challenge to any clinician or investigator proficient in the psychiatric assessment of a child or adult. The danger is that the book may be picked up and its premises accepted by someone interested yet uninformed concerning speech, hearing, and/or psychiatry.

Since the ample reference listings contain no more than five published research-oriented studies of speech and hearing characteristics of psychiatric patients, the reader must accept or reject the premises presented primarily in relation to the case histories (approx. 250 pages) or reports of in-house studies (approx. 40 pages).

Examples of inferences follow:

"The substitution of w for r occurs in underachieving persons." One is fascinated also to read that the same substitution "reflects conflict over anal aspects of psychosexual development and dependence on obsessional styles of thinking." Still later one is told that "The misarticulation of the vowel r reflects lack of impulse control and minimal neurological dysfunction." One is almost relieved to read that w for r substitution "suggests at least average and probably above average intelligence when there are no sound omissions and the patient is able to demonstrate normal speech discrimination on the W-22 and Rush-Hughes recordings." These inferences do not, however, prepare the reader for the case study which involves the statement, ". . . based on the w for r substitutions, we would expect the child to have continued toilet training difficulties."

Some sections which attempt to differentiate psychiatric from neurological dysfunction could lead some readers to assume that diseases of unknown origin have a psychological explanation. These sections are spotty; for example, unusually weak intensity of speech is mentioned as representing inhibition of aggression, but the possibility of a dysarthria is not raised.

One cannot help but agree with the authors that psychiatrists, alone, can miss important speech and hearing problems. The impression left is that, in addition to Speech and Hearing specialists, specialists in ENT and Neurology frequently are needed.

LINDA SWISHER, PH.D.

Diagnosis and Treatment of Dento-Facial Abnormalities

By *Viken Sassouni, D.D.S.* and *George C. Sotereanos, D.M.D.* Hard cover, indexed by author and subject. Charles C Thomas Publishing Co., 301-327 East Lawrence Avenue, Springfield, Illinois 62703. Price $29.75

This book is written on the philosophy that the treatment of patients with dental-facial anomalies demands a team approach, in which the various skills of several specialties may be brought to bear as one unified management concept. Dental-facial abnormalities resulting from either congenital or acquired developmental defects, or from trauma, need considerable attention from various specialties, such as plastic surgery, otolaryngology, pediatrics, orthodontics, prosthodontics, oral surgery, and social services. In order that such a diversified group of specialists can work together so that their patient may receive good care, it is necessary that these specialists have a background of knowledge in each other's particular area.

In this text, the authors provide information about photography and radiographic techniques used by the various specialties, as well as about several surgical procedures that they have used over the last ten years in care of their patients. The techniques which they have used are outlined step-by-step, so that each specialist should be able to gain an understanding of how the patient was treated from diagnosis to complete rehabilitation. In this way, their patients have not been limited by the ability of any one specialty area. Through cooperation and teamwork the individual specialty areas have been able to extend what they can do towards the ultimate goal of patient rehabilitation. It may have also been beneficial for the authors to have included a glossary of specialized terms from the various specialty areas.

This book should be especially interesting to those residents and students who are just becoming interested and involved in the treatment of dental-facial abnormalities.

WILLIAM E. LAVELLE, D.D.S.

Detection of Hearing Loss and Ear Disease in Children

By *Kenneth S. Gerwin, M.D.*, and *Aram Glorig, M.D.* Hard cover, 190 pp, not referenced, indexed, nor illustrated. Charles C Thomas Publishing Co., 301-327 East Lawrence Avenue, Springfield, Illinois. Price $12.50

A strong and well-documented argument in favor of improved screening procedures for ear pathologies in children is presented. Serious weaknesses inherent in most school hearing screening programs are pointed out, and recommendations are made for their improvement. Important among these weaknesses are the following: a) the unwarranted assumption that absence of hearing loss implies "normality" or absence of ear pathology; and, b) insufficiently low screening levels (related to unfavorable testing-room noise).

Among the authors' suggestions for improvement are the inclusion of measurements of middle ear impedance, the use of an effective medical questionnaire, and better control of background noise so that screening levels can be lowered 10 to 15 dB.

These important points are perhaps obscured by an unnecessarily detailed description of the Callier Study. This study compared the effectiveness of a word-screening test (VASC) and, although it is an important report, a summary could have been sufficient. In the opinion of this reviewer, if this book were half as long, it would be twice as good.

DONALD P. PASCOE, PH.D.

Otolaryngology Case Studies

By *C. T. Yarington, Jr., M.D.* Paperback, 173 pp, illustrated, indexed and referenced. Medical Examination Publishing Co., Inc., 65-36 Fresh Meadow Lane, Flushing, New York. Price $10

Those who enjoy the case study approach as a didactic technique will find a particularly useful and informative compilation in this recent publication. Edited by C. T. Yarington, Jr., with contributions from 12 others, this book contains 60 case studies which cover the spectrum of disorders frequently encountered in clinical otolaryngology.

The general format includes presentation of a brief history, physical examination, laboratory data, and, where indicated, illustrations and visual aids. Relevant multiple-choice questions on diagnosis and management of the clinical problem are included. The answers to these questions are accompanied by lengthy discussion and pertinent references.

The cases are well selected and range from such common entities as tonsillitis and serous otitis to rare but important disorders as malignant myopathic hyperthermia and nasal septal melanoma. The inclusion of 417 references, including numerous review articles, is one of the highlights of the book.

Considering the fact that there are few unequivocal, indisputable, clinical statements possible in otolaryngology, the editor and his contributors are to be commended for a thoughtful, conservative, and useful presentation. It has obvious appeal to residents and practicing otolaryngologists. Hopefully, it will also come to the attention of pediatricians, internists, family practitioners, and others who encounter the problems discussed.

FRANK E. LUCENTE, M.D.

Handbook of Sensory Physiology. Vol. 6/1. Vestibular System

By *H. H. Kornhuber (ed).* Hard cover, referenced, indexed (by subject and author), 198 black and white illustrations, 680 pp. Springer-Verlag New York Inc., 175 Fifth Avenue, New York, New York 10010. Price $102.10

This is the basic sciences volume of a two-volume set on the complete vestibular system and its interactions with other sensory and motor systems. It is as impressive a collection of basic data on one central theme as I have encountered in any handbook. There are in excess of 2,440 bibliographical entries in the fourteen chapters, beginning with a well-written review on invertebrate motion detection systems, and ending with an indepth review on central nervous system influences on mammalian body tonus and rapid eye movement sleep.

The editor has chosen internationally recognized authorities in each field and the chapters progress in a classical fashion from comparative morphology, through endorgan anatomy, biochemistry, innervation, to physiology. Central nervous system anatomy and physiology are similarly reviewed in the second one-half of this volume. It is definitely not the type of handbook one would choose for casual browsing, but it is a book which will undoubtedly be the first reference source for many years for the serious student of the vestibular system.

A work of this magnitude cannot be produced overnight and was undoubtedly several years in preparation. Some contributors met their deadlines and others may have been tardy, resulting in an unevenness in the most recent bibliographical entries among chapters. Some were completed as early as 1968, and some were updated through 1973. However, this is more of a minor annoyance compared to the overall value of this handbook. If the second volume on the psychophysics and clinical aspects of the vestibular system is as complete and scholarly, the clinician will have at hand a truly complete source book for attempting to make some sense out of a very complex subject.

F. BLAIR SIMMONS, M.D.

A Short Textbook. Ear, Nose and Throat (Second Edition)

By *R. Pracy, F.R.C.S., J. Siegler, F.R.C.S.,* and *P. M. Stell, F.R.C.S.* Paperback, indexed, 156 pp, black and white line drawings, appendixed. J. B. Lippincott Co., Medical Books Division, East Washington Square, Philadelphia, Pa. 19105. Price $7

A Short Textbook: Ear, Nose and Throat, in contradistinction to more elaborate works on the subject, is just what it purports to be. In a 156-page paperback addition, the authors have collected the basic essentials of everyday otolaryngology and present them in a concise text nicely bolstered with self-explanatory line drawings.

Of particular note are the succinct chapters dealing with vertigo, stridor in childhood, and tracheostomy, all subjects which the medical student may be expected to confront, and with the aid of this book, in a quite organized fashion.

My only criticisms are limited to therapeutic philosophy. For example, serous otitis medial "will usually mean an antrum wash-out . . . . " Sinus irrigation is again relied upon for the initial treatment of sinusitis, with complete omission of nasal or systemic decongestants. The chapter on laryngeal cancer fails even to mention conservation surgery, a probably unforgiveable omission in the light of twenty years of partial laryngectomy. The second indication (p. 28) for closing a tympanic membrane perforation: "to help the patient to join one of the armed services," should be taken *cum grano salis!*

These few shortcomings are easily overcome with concurrent clinical experience, and I heartily recommend this inexpensive book to the medical student and general practitioner.

NICHOLAS L. SCHENCK, M.D.

Sensations and Measurements — Papers in Honor of S. S. Stevens

By *H. R. Moskowitz, B. Scharf,* and *J. C. Stevens* (eds.). Hard Cover, 469 pp. D. Reidel Publishing Co., Dordrecht, Holland: Boston, U.S.A., 1974.

This book was planned as a *Festschrift* for the occasion of S. S. Stevens' (1906-1973) anticipated retirement as Director of the Psychophysical Laboratory at Harvard University in 1974. It turned out to become a memorial volume for him since Dr. Stevens died, unexpectedly, on January 18, 1973, while attending the annual winter conference on Brain Research at Vail, Colorado, and doing some skiing on the side.

"Smitty" Stevens, whose name is probably not too familiar to most Otolaryngologists, was a man who put psychophysics on the map. (It had been founded a century earlier by G. T. Fechner in Germany.) Psychophysics is a discipline that deals with the measurement of sensations in response to well-defined stimuli; hence, psycho - physics, and also the title of this volume: *Sensation and Measurement.* Smitty fought a life-long war to convince people that sensations can be measured with almost the same precision as physical entities; voltages, for example. They can even be measured, as Smitty once emphasized, when the experimenter is unable to verbalize what he wants his subject to measure; as long as he can demonstrate to him two or three samples that markedly differ with respect to the parameter he wants assessed. That all this is the very basis of audiometry should be plain to the reader.

Despite his own claims to the contrary, Smitty was a first-class teacher, perhaps not for undergraduates in the classroom, but definitely for postdoctorates in the laboratory. The majority of the forty contributors to this volume were such students of Smitty's; the older ones worked in the old Psychoacoustic Laboratory in the basement of Memorial Hall at Harvard, and the younger ones in the new Psychophysical Laboratory at James Hall.

A few more of the contributors were lifelong friends and collaborators of Smitty's at Harvard, such as, Békésy and Davis, although Békésy must have "learned" some psychophysics from Stevens which he was able to apply with great benefit to his later studies on the skin, taste, *etc.* Even though all of the contributors became eminent "psychophysicists" in their own right, the guiding spirit of the book, and its unifying principle, is Smitty's.

The contributions are somewhat arbitrarily classed into four parts. Part I: Psychophysics, Measurement, Sensory Physiology (17); Part II: Hearing and Speech (15); Part III: Vision, Taste, and Warmth (8); and Part IV: Smitty's own brief *Notes for a Life Story* which he had put together in 1970. This is a fitting conclusion of the book; it is full of the things that never find their way into scientific papers: the joys and disappointments of a scholar and researcher.

It would be presumptuous to single out any of the forty contributions. They were written by some of the foremost people in the field. They are not easy reading, but highly rewarding for those who make the effort.

JUERGEN TONNDORF, M.D.

Traite de Radiodiagnostic

By *Secretaire General: H. Fischgold; Secretaire Adjoint: D. Doyon.* Hard cover. 453 pp, indexed, referenced, black and white illustrations. Masson & Cie, Editeurs, 120, Boulevard Saint-Germain, Paris, France, 1974

This book is a unique reference of radiology. It has features of both an atlas and a textbook. It is extremely well illustrated with a generous display of anatomical and radiological material for comparison. Where appropriate, very illustrative line drawings are included. The greater bulk of the volume is dedicated to the radiology of the ear. The first part of this section is a lavishly illustrated review of the anatomy and sectional anatomy. This part is followed by a section on radiographic technique with short text and abundant illustrations and a correlative section on polytomography and thin sectional anatomy in an atlas form. A brief discussion of the physiology, pathophysiology, and clinical signs is interposed to form a smooth transition to the section on the radiologic features of different disease conditions which is well classified and very well illustrated.

Angiography is lightly touched in conjunction with chemodectomas of glomus and the carotid body, as well as in a brief section on vertebrobasilar insufficiency that followed in a natural sequence after Ménière's disease. The section on the nasal cavity and paranasal sinuses and temporomandibular joints is less detailed but quite adequate. Nasopharyngeal lesions are not discussed.

The book is a good reference for both the otoradiologist and the clinician. The difficulty that one might expect from the fact that the book is written in French is greatly ameliorated by the abundant provision of clear illustrations of high quality and the relatively short texts.

MOKHTAR H. GADO, M.D.

RESEARCH FORUM

Sponsored by

COMMITTEE FOR RESEARCH IN OTOLARYNGOLOGY, AAOO
ASSOCIATION FOR RESEARCH IN OTOLARYNGOLOGY

September 20-21, 1975, Dallas, Texas

Program Chairmen: Owen Black, M.D., University of Pittsburgh
William Melnick, Ph.D., Ohio State University

SEPTEMBER 20

HEAD AND NECK - GENERAL

Techniques for Demonstrating the Existence of Tumor Specific Antigens in Carcinomas of the Head and Neck. Deyan Popovic, M.D., George Sisson, M.D., and Byron Anderson, Ph.D., Northwestern University Medical School.

Serum Immunoglobulin A (IgA) Levels in Cancer of the Head and Neck. Arnold E. Katz, M.D., Tai-June Yoo, M.D., Ph.D., Lee A. Harker, M.D., University of Iowa.

Collagenase Activity in Tumors of the Head and Neck. Cheng-chun Huang, Ph.D. and Maxwell Abramson, M.D., University of Iowa.

Epithelization of Dermal Grafts in Dogs. G. C. Swanson, M.D., T. E. White, M.D., R. E. Swain, M.D. and T. F. Miller, M.D., Naval Regional Medical Center, Oakland.

Experimental Results of Autogenous Cancellous Bone Chips Transplanted into the Infected Canine Frontal Sinus Cavity. Robert L. Eason, D.V.M., Allan L. Abramson, M.D., William H. Pryor, Jr., D.V.M., Naval Medical Field Research Laboratory, Camp Lejeune.

Anatomy of the Eustachian Tube in Normal and Cleft Palate Human Fetuses. Wilma M. Dickson, Ph.D., David R. Dickson, Ph.D., Steward Rood, Ph.D., University of Pittsburgh and Mercy Hospital.

HEAD AND NECK - LARYNX AND TRACHEA

Survival and Growth of Syngeneic and Allogenic Fetal Larynx and Trachea. Marcelo Obando, M.D., Augustin Peale, M.D., Narasimha Rao, M.D., Kam Chang, M.D., Charles Norris, M.D., F.A.C.S. and Frederick A. Reichle, M.D., F.A.C.S., Temple University Health Sciences Center.

Perichondrial Flap Reconstruction of the Larynx. William K. Zollinger, M.D., William A. Alonso, M.D. and Joseph H. Ogura, M.D., Washington University School of Medicine.

Hyoid Arch Transposition. Norman S. Druck, M.D., William A. Alonso, M.D., Joseph H. Ogura, M.D., Washington University School of Medicine.

VESTIBULAR PHYSIOLOGY

Reciprocal Synapses in the Crista Ampullaris: A Possible Mechanism for Hair Cell Interaction. R. F. Dunn, Ph.D., UCLA School of Medicine.

Response Properties of Spontaneously Inactive First-Order Afferents Innervating the Isolated Guitarfish Semicircular Canal. Dennis P. O'Leary, Ph.D. and Conrad Wall, III, Ph.D., University of Pittsburgh School of Medicine.

Neurophysiological Correlates of Nystagmus. D. Reingold, V. Honrubia, M.D. and P. H. Ward, M.D., UCLA School of Medicine.

The Characteristics of Eye Movements Induced by Semicircular Canal Stimulation with Angular Accelerations in Normal and Labyrinthectomized Cats. David E. Owens, M.D., Herman Jenkins, M.D. and Vicente Honrubia, M.D., UCLA School of Medicine.

Brain Stem and Vestibular Neuron Behavior During Eye Movements Evoked by Cerebellar Stimulation. Joseph Kimm, Ph.D., Barbara Cogdell, Ph.D., and Michael Hassul, Ph.D., University of Washington.

VESTIBULAR FUNCTION - CLINICAL APPLICATIONS

Evaluation of Air Caloric Response in a Chronic Monkey Preparation. Daniel Kozie, M.D., and Joseph Kimm, Ph.D., University of Washington.

A Method for Adjusting the Stimulus Intensity of the Air Caloric Test. Preliminary Report. Leonard R. Proctor, M.D., Rollin C. Dix, Ph.D., and Werner Metz, University of Chicago.

A Rapid OKN Test: Comparison with Standard Testing. Andrew W. Sills, Ph.D., UCLA School of Medicine.

The Impulsive Vestibular Test in Man. Horst R. Konrad, M.D., UCLA School of Medicine.

ENG Findings in Dyslexic Children. Charles W. Stockwell, Ph.D., Earl S. Sherard, M.D., and Jean V. Schuler, M.A., Ohio State University College of Medicine and Children's Hospital.

AUDITORY SYSTEM - ANATOMY AND PATHOLOGY

In Vitro Study of Fate Mapping of the Mouse Otocyst. Chung W. Li, Ph.D., Thomas R. Van de Water, M.S., and Robert J. Ruben, M.D., Albert Einstein College of Medicine of Yeshiva University, Bronx.

Spiral Migration Hypothesis of the Cochlear Duct Formation. Joel M. A. Shugar, M.D.C.M., Mt. Sinai School of Medicine.

Outer Hair Cell Loss and Alterations in Glycogen in the Inner Ear Following Treatment with Tobramycin Sulfate. D. Postma, J. Pecorak, J. Prazma, M.D.,

S. Logue, University of North Carolina School of Medicine.

Ototoxicity and the Olivocochlear Bundle. Mary Jane Capps, Ph.D. and Arndt J. Duvall, III, M.D., University of Minnesota College of Medicine.

Basal Turn Cochlear Lesions Following Exposure to Low Frequency Noise. Marvin P. Fried, M.D., Stanley E. Dudek, M.D., and Barbara Bohne, Ph.D., Washington University School of Medicine.

An Examination of an Electro-chemical Mechanism for Noise-Induced Hair Cell Loss, i.e., Noise with Aminooxyacetic Acid (AOAA). Richard P. Bobbin, Ph.D., Mary S. Guth, and Arthur B. Mines, M.A., Louisiana State University Medical Center, Kresge Hearing Research Laboratory of the South.

Effect of Impulse Level on the Interaction between Impulse and Continuous Noise. William J. Hunt, M.D., Roger P. Hamernik, Ph.D., and Donald Henderson, Ph.D., State University of New York, Upstate Medical Center and Department of Mechanical and Aerospace Engineering, Syracuse University.

Toxicity of Ethacrynic Acid in Different Blood pO_2. J. Prazma, M.D., N. D. Fischer, M.D., J .B. Pecorak, T. Logan, University of North Carolina School of Medicine.

The Blocking Effect of Pressure on the Visceral Motor (Salivary Flow) and the Somatic Muscle (Facial Muscle) Functions of the Facial Nerve. Charles W. Parkins, M.D., and David Rodriguez, M.D., State University of New York, Upstate Medical Center.

The Microfissure between the Round Window Niche and the Posterior Ampulla. Yasumasa Okano, M.D., University of Pittsburgh School of Medicine, Eye and Ear Hospital.

An Inflammatory Agent in Middle Ear Effusion. L. Pickford, M.D. and R. T. Jackson, Ph.D., Emory University School of Medciine.

ANNUAL BUSINESS MEETING ASSOCIATION FOR RESEARCH IN OTOLARYNGOLOGY (ARO)

SEPTEMBER 21

NASAL RESEARCH

Treatment of Epistaxis with Porcine Stripped Packing. Barbara B. Heywood, M.D., Richard B. Davis, M.D., and Anthony J. Yonkers, M.D., University of Nebraska Medical Center.

Intranasal Trigeminal Detection of Chemical Vapors by Humans. Richard L. Doty, Ph.D., and Bruce Jafek, M.D., Monell Chemical Senses Center, University of Pennsylvania.

AUDITORY PHYSIOLOGY

Role of Inner and Outer Hair Cells in Neural Excitation. David Strelioff, Ph.D., Steven Sitko, and Vicente Honrubia, UCLA School of Medicine.

Source and Maintenance of the Endocochlear Potential. Steven Sitko, David Strelioff, Ph.D., and Vicente Honrubia, M.D., UCLA School of Medicine.

The Effect of Hyperosmotic Agents on Perilymph Osmolarity. S. K. Juhn, M.D. and S. Prado, M.D., University of Minnesota Medical School.

Effects of Low and High Frequency Noise Bands in Producing a Physiological Correlate of Loudness Recruitment in Mice. Gregory R. Bock and James C. Saunders, Ph.D., University of Pennsylvania, School of Medicine.

Audiological Implications of Transmission Losses Caused by Experimental Tympanic Membrane Perforations in Cats. Barbara Kruger, M.A. and Juergen Tonndorf, M.D., City University of New York and Columbia University.

Tone Burst Electrocochleography in Humans. Daniel F. Mouney, M.D., John K. Cullen, Jr., Ph.D., Maria Gondra, B.A. and Charles I. Berlin Ph.D., Kresge Hearing Research Laboratory, Louisiana State University School of Medicine.

AUDITORY BEHAVIOR

Pure Tone Masking in the Parakeet *(Melopsittacus Undulatus).* James C. Saunders, Ph.D. and Page V. Else, University of Pennsylvania School of Medicine.

Effects of Sensorineural Loss on Hearing Speech in Noise. R. C. Bilger, Ph.D., M. S. Stiegel, Ph.D. and N. Stenson, Bioacoustics Laboratory, Eye and Ear Hospital, Pittsburgh.

Extraction of Speech Messages by Central Auditory Pathways. Charles I. Berlin, Ph.D., John K. Cullen, Jr., Ph.D., Daniel F. Mouney, M.D., and Harriet L. Berlin, B.A., Kresge Hearing Research Laboratory, Louisiana State University School of Medicine.

Dynamic Properties of Acoustic Reflex Adaptation. Harold J. Kaplan, M.D., Samuel Gilman, M.S., and Donald D. Dirks, Ph.D., UCLA Medical School.

Auditory Manifestation of Alport's Disease Syndrome. William F. Rintelmann, Ph.D. and Ellen K. Leroi, M.A., Michigan State University.

EUSTACHIAN TUBE FUNCTION

Osmolarity Effects in the Eustachian Tube. W. Parker, M.D., L. Pickford, M.D., and R. T. Jackson, Ph.D., Emory University School of Medicine.

A New Selectively Permeable Membrane for Tympanic Ventilation Tubes. John B. Castelli, M.D., Joseph P. Murray, M.D. and Hugh O. deFries, M.D., National Naval Medical Center.

Ann Otol 84: 1975

PHYSIOLOGY AND PATHOPHYSIOLOGY OF THE LOWER ESOPHAGEAL SPHINCTER

CAPT. DONALD O. CASTELL, MC USN

BETHESDA, MARYLAND

SUMMARY – The physiologic factors controlling lower esophageal sphincter (LES) function are interrelated in a complex fashion and include the autonomic nerve supply, gastrointestinal hormones, and specific characteristics of the circular smooth muscle at the esophagogastric junction. It might be expected that a defect in any of these three controlling mechanisms would result in a clinically recognizable symptom complex. Abnormalities with either high or low LES pressure have been shown to relate to these specific aspects. Studies of the effects of various foods and other agents which decrease or increase LES pressure are of therapeutic interest in relating to patients with reflux symptoms. Decreases in LES pressure occurring after fat ingestion may explain a mechanism for many cases of fatty food intolerance. Pressure decreases after chocolate ingestion, after smoking, and after alcohol all have strong therapeutic implications in patients with chronic heartburn. Gastric alkalinization will increase pressure for up to one hour in patients with basal sphincter hypotension and reflux symptoms. Recent studies with drugs that work through the cholinergic mechanism have important therapeutic considerations. Anticholinergic agents produce definite decreases in LES pressure and are to be avoided in treatment of patients with reflux symptoms. On the other hand cholinergic drugs such as bethanechol have been shown to increase LES pressure in normal subjects and in patients with chronic sphincter incompetence. Recently, a double-blind therapeutic trial with bethanechol in patients with chronic heartburn has indicated that this drug, when given on a regular basis, is an effective adjunct to therapy in these patients.

Although a specific muscular structure defining the sphincteric mechanism at the esophagogastric junction has never been identified anatomically in man, there is no question that such a sphincter exists functionally. This lower esophageal sphincter (LES) is readily identified both manometrically and radiographically. The past few years have seen a remarkable information explosion relative to physiology and pathophysiology of this smooth muscle structure. This new information has resulted in major changes in our understanding of esophageal disease and its therapy. It is now clear that the LES performs two major functions in digestive physiology: 1) relaxation from its usually tonic state during swallowing to allow free passage of ingested material from esophagus to stomach, and 2) maintenance of an effective high pressure zone preventing the reflux of acid gastric material from the stomach to the esophagus. It might be anticipated that a defect in either one of these normal functions of the LES would be manifest in a clinically recognizable disorder.

PHYSIOLOGIC CONTROLS OF LES FUNCTION

Through refinements in manometric techniques and the use of animal models, the factors of importance in normal control of the function of the LES have been clarified. Three major components have been identified to be crucial in regulation of sphincter function: the nervous supply to the sphincter muscle; gastrointestinal hormones, particularly gastrin; and the intrinsic

---

From the Clinical Investigation Center and Gastroenterology Division, Internal Medicine Service, U.S. Naval Hospital, Philadelphia, Pennsylvania 19145.

This work was supported by Bureau of Medicine and Surgery Clinical Investigation Program #5-05-530R.

Presented at the meeting of the American Broncho-Esophagological Association, Atlanta, Georgia, April 7-8, 1975.

sphincteric smooth muscle itself.

Studies using either *in vitro* smooth muscle preparations or *in vivo* animal experiments in the cat or opossum have revealed that the circular smooth muscle at the esophagogastric junction is indeed unique in its ability to respond to pharmacologic and hormonal stimulation.[1,2] Thus, although a definite anatomic sphincter has not been identified at the distal end of the esophagus, chemical identification of a unique muscle segment has been shown.

The full details of the neural control of LES function remain to be elucidated. One clear observation from numerous studies is that vagotomy, whether intraabdominal or cervical, does not result in a change in resting LES pressure.[3,4] This observation at least suggests that the parasympathetic nervous system has little effect in maintenance of the resting tone of the LES. However, pharmacologic doses of cholinergic or anticholinergic compounds markedly raise or lower LES pressure respectively.[5,6] Further studies with cervical vagotomy in the opossum have revealed that stimulation of the distal end of the transected vagus produces LES relaxation.[4] This observation indicates that LES inhibitory tracts are contained within the vagus nerve. Additional studies in man and cats have revealed supersensitivity to both a cholinomimetic agent and to pentagastrin after truncal vagotomy at the esophagogastric junction, possibly due to release from these inhibitory pathways.[7] Studies in the opossum have revealed that the sympathetic nervous system may account for a portion of the resting tone of the LES, and that the alphaadrenergic portion of this system exerts a major effect.[8] Finally, recent observations in animal models suggest that nonadrenergic inhibitory fibers (the so-called purinergic nervous system) may be responsible for the normal relaxation of the LES during swallowing.[9]

In 1970 the effect of pentagastrin on this sphincteric mechanism was first shown.[10] Following the injection of pentagastrin, marked increases in lower esophageal sphincter pressure occurred in normal subjects. Other studies indicated that not only did exogenous pentagastrin affect this sphincter, but the stimulation of the release of endogenous gastrin from the gastric antrum, would also increase pressure in this area.[11] Numerous studies have been performed on the effect of gastrointestinal hormones on the LES. It is now clear that pharmacologic doses of gastrin will increase LES pressure, but to date this is the only hormone that has been shown to result in increases in sphincter pressure.

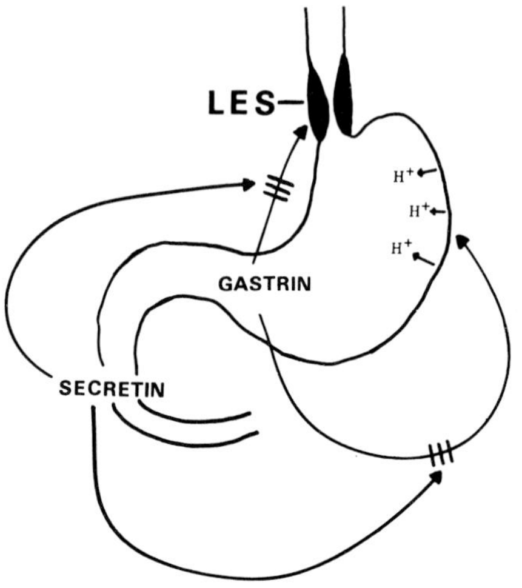

Fig. 1. Schematic representation of the interaction of gastrin and secretin on the lower esophageal sphincter (LES) and gastric acid (H^+) production.

Subsequent studies have demonstrated that besides gastrin other gastrointestinal hormones, particularly secretin, may affect this sphincter.[12] These interrelationships are shown schematically in Figure 1. The effect of secretin in blocking the gastrin stimulatory effect on the sphincter is illustrated. This is not surprising, since secretin is a known inhibitor of gastric acid stimulation by gastrin. The hormones cholecystokinin and glucagon have also been studied, and both result in decreases in sphincter pressure, with the mechanism apparently due to competitive inhibition of gastrin stimulation.[13,14]

TABLE I

CLINICAL DISORDERS OF LES FUNCTION

Disorder	LES Pressure (mmHg)	Proposed Defect
Normal	15-20	–
Achalasia	40-60	Neural
Scleroderma	<10	Neural (Smooth Muscle)
Zollinger-Ellison Syndrome	25-30	Excess Endogenous Gastrin
Pernicious Anemia	8-10	Smooth Muscle
Gastroesophageal Reflux	<10	Deficient Endogenous Gastrin (Smooth Muscle)

Changes in LES pressure occurring with gastric alkalinization and acidification were initially proposed as evidence for the role of endogenous gastrin in the physiologic control of LES pressure. However, recent studies measuring LES pressure and serum gastrin concentrations simultaneously, have raised numerous questions about the specificity of this relationship.[15] It now appears that although gastric alkalinization increases LES pressure, the mechanism of this effect is probably not through increases in circulating endogenous gastrin.[16] Recent studies have shown that continuous intravenous infusions of the synthetic heptadecapeptide of human gastrin I at rates producing serum gastrin levels similar to those occurring after a meal result in significant increases in LES pressure.[17] In addition, the simultaneous increases in LES pressure and serum gastrin following a protein-rich meal give support to a physiologic role for gastrin in regulation of sphincter pressure, but the exact details of this mechanism, and its interaction with other GI hormones and nerves, remain to be clarified.

DYSFUNCTION OF THE LES

Clinical disorders of LES function are listed in Table I. As stated above, a defect in either of the two primary physiologic functions of the LES can be expected to result in clinical symptoms. Abnormality of the normal relaxation of the sphincter with swallowing will result in dysphagia, and failure of the sphincter to maintain a competent anti-reflux barrier produces the symptom of heartburn.

Achalasia. Dysphagia is a prominent symptom in achalasia. Manometrically this disease is characterized by an absence of peristalsis in the body of the esophagus, a hypertensive LES, and an incomplete relaxation of the LES with swallowing. The high sphincter pressure producing the cardiospasm of this entity has been recently postulated to be due to a supersensitivity to endogenous gastrin, secondary to the denervation of the sphincteric area which occurs in this disease.[18]

Scleroderma. This connective tissue disease often affects the gastrointestinal tract. Manometric findings include weak-to-absent peristalsis in the distal two thirds (smooth muscle portion) of the esophagus and a low-to-absent LES pressure. Although dysphagia occurs occasionally in scleroderma patients, the defective anti-reflux barrier usually results in more prominent heartburn symptoms. Recent studies have suggested that the mechanism for this defect may be primarily neural in nature, although possible associated atrophy of the gastrointestinal smooth muscle has also been described.[19]

Zollinger-Ellison syndrome is characterized by extremely high levels of circulating endogenous gastrin, and has recently been shown to be associated with increased resting LES pressure.[20] This observation supports the importance of endogenous gastrin in the control of resting LES pressure. It should be noted, however, that dysphagia does not occur in these patients, since the relaxation of the LES during swallowing is not impaired.

Pernicious anemia (PA) patients are also characterized by extremely high levels of serum gastrin. This finding led to early speculations that the LES pressure might also be elevated in the PA patients. However, resting LES pressures were found to be low in these patients when compared to an appropriate control group; and in addition the LES of PA patients showed a defective response to pharmacologic and hormonal stimulation.[21] It has been proposed that the defect in the LES in PA is primarily one of smooth muscle atrophy. In spite of the hypotensive LES, heartburn is not a common symptom in PA, primarily because of the achlorhydria also present in these patients. However, a recent report has described heartburn secondary to bile reflux across both an incompetent pyloric and lower esophageal sphincter in a patient with PA.[22]

Gastroesophageal Reflux. The classical manometrical finding in patients with chronic heartburn is a hypotensive LES. Pressures are generally found to be less than 10 mm Hg above intragastric pressure. Although circumstantial data has suggested that a major defect in these patients might be a deficient release of endogenous gastrin,[23] recent studies comparing simultaneous LES pressure measurement and serum gastrin concentrations have failed to confirm this hypothesis.[15] Fasting serum gastrin values were found to be somewhat lower in patients with chronic reflux than in control subjects, but the differences were not significant. These slight differences were out of proportion to the marked differences in LES pressures found between the control and reflux patients. Furthermore, intravenous doses of pentagastrin which produce serum levels far exceeding those occurring under physiologic conditions failed to result in absolute LES pressure levels in reflux patients similar to those in the control subjects. Following the stimulation of a protein meal reflux patients appeared to have a somewhat deficient release of endogenous gastrin. At present, it would appear that although a deficient production of endogenous gastrin may partially account for the hypotensive sphincter of reflux patients, the basic defect is probably a compound one which includes abnormal sphincteric smooth muscle.

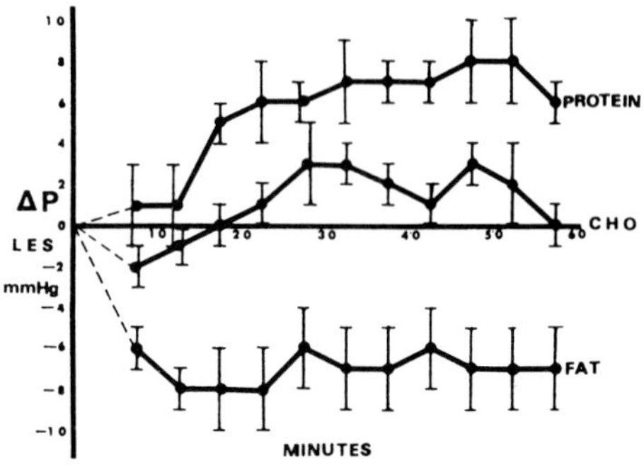

Fig. 2. Lower esophageal sphincter (LES) pressure changes (ΔP) for ten normal subjects after meals of protein, carbohydrate (CHO), or fat. Dots indicate mean values and vertical lines ± SEM.

EFFECT OF FOODS AND OTHER AGENTS

Patients with symptomatic gastroesophageal reflux commonly complain of their heartburn after ingestion of foods of many kinds. Since gastrointestinal hormones are know to be released in response to the ingestion of foods, it would seem reasonable to study the relative effects of food on LES pressure. Gastrin stimulates this sphincter; therefore, it had been postulated that a protein meal would most likely increase sphincter pressure, since protein has been known for years to be a stimulator of endogenous gastrin release. But what about the effects of other common foods? This question has been recently attacked vigorously in studies of the effects of relatively pure foods on LES pressure.[24] These studies were performed on a group of normal volunteers after an overnight fast. Each subject then ingested on successive days each of three test meals of protein, carbohydrate, or fat. Each consisted of 150 calories in a total volume of 150 ml of water. Following the ingestion of each meal, these subjects were studied for an additional 60-minute period.

Figure 2 shows the results of these studies. After ingestion of the protein meal, significant increases in sphincter pressure occurred in all subjects studied. The pressure began to rise within the first 10 to 15 minutes, and reached

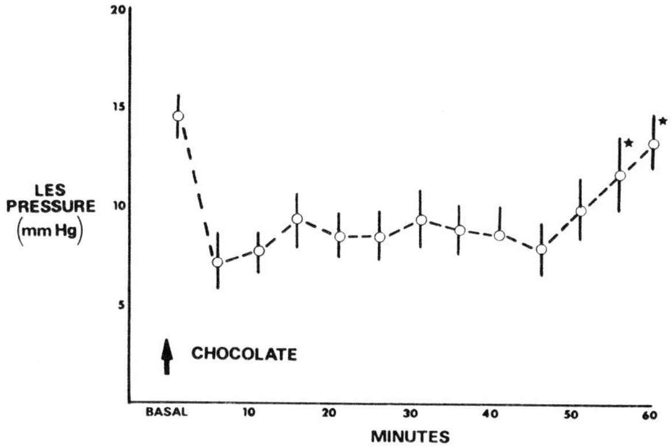

Fig. 3. Lower esophageal sphincter (LES) pressure for ten normal subjects basally and after ingestion (arrow) of chococlate. Open dots indicate mean values and vertical lines ± SEM. Stars note values not significantly lower than basal value.

a mean peak pressure change of 8 mm Hg at 45 minutes. This response was predictable from previous observations of gastrin and its effect on sphincter pressure. After ingestion of the glucose solution, slight increases in sphincter pressure were noted. Significant increases in pressure occurred only at 30 and 45 minutes and were but 3 mm Hg. After ingestion of fat, all subjects had marked decreases in LES pressure. Pressure fell rapidly and remained decreased for the full 60 minutes of testing. The average peak fall in pressure was 8 mm Hg.

The striking inhibitory effect of fat on the LES offers an attractive explanation for some forms of fatty food intolerance. That is, the patient with the incompetent or borderline-competent sphincter pressure might note ready reflux of acid gastric contents into the esophagus following the ingestion of a fatty meal.

An additional clinical observation which has been studied in our laboratory is the effect of chocolate on LES pressure. As with fat, rapid and sustained decreases in LES pressure are seen in normal subjects after the ingestion of chocolate syrup[25] (Fig. 3). Although originally the mechanism was felt to be due to the high fat content of chocolate, it now seems more likely that this effect may result from the methylxanthine (caffeine and theobromine) content of chocolate. In addition, the dramatic effect of cigarette smoking in decreasing LES pressure and promoting ready reflux of gastric content has been demonstrated[26] (Fig. 4). Table II summarizes the many chemical and hormonal agents that have been shown to produce decreases in LES pressure. Many of these compounds have obvious clinical implications in that the patient suffering from chronic reflux may well be properly advised to avoid the use of such agents.

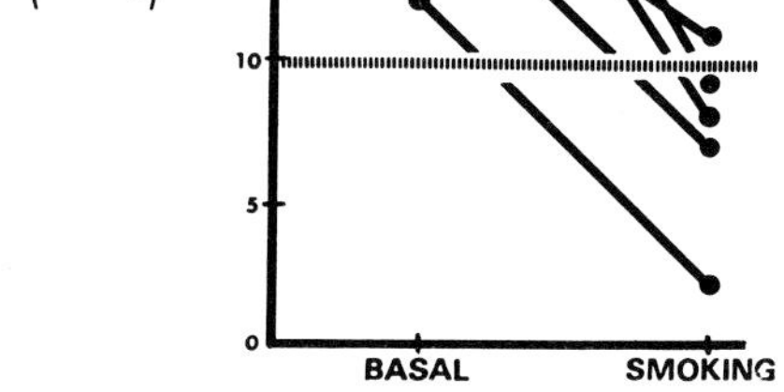

Fig. 4. Lower esophageal sphincter (LES) pressure for six normal subjects basally and during cigarette smoking. Broken line indicates usual separation of competent and incompetent sphincter (10 mm Hg).

TABLE II

AGENTS PRODUCING DECREASED LES PRESSURE

Secretin	Theophylline
Cholecystokinin	Caffeine
Glucagon	Gastric acidification
Prostaglandins E_1, E_2, A_2	Fat meal
Beta adrenergic agonist (isoproterenol)	Chocolate
Alpha adrenergic antagonist (phentolamine)	Smoking
Anticholinergic (atropine)	Ethanol

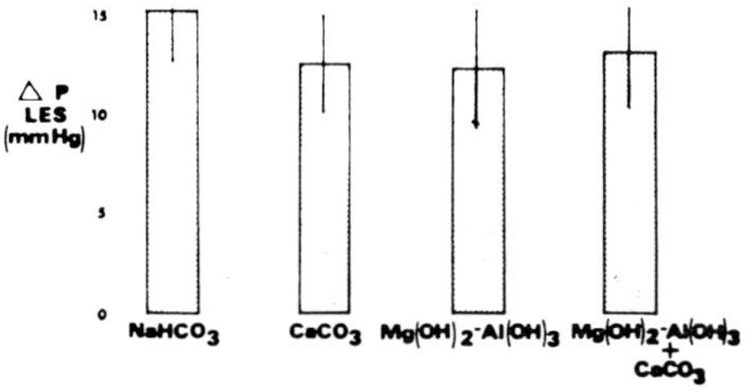

Fig. 5. Lower esophageal sphincter (LES) pressure changes (ΔP) for ten normal subjects after gastric alkalinization of four common alkalies in usual therapeutic doses. Bars indicate mean maximal increases and vertical lines $\pm$ SEM.

Of even greater clinical importance from a therapeutic point of view may be those agents producing increased LES pressure, as summarized in Table III. Gastric alkalinization has been repeatedly demonstrated to cause increased LES pressure, with pressure increases occurring after a variety of alkalizing agents[16] (Fig. 5). These studies have led to the conclusion that the use of antacids in the treatment of heartburn has a dual effect, not only neutralizing the acidic gastric contents, but also increasing the sphincteric antireflux barrier.

TABLE III

AGENTS PRODUCING INCREASED LES PRESSURE

Gastrin/Pentagastrin
Prostaglandin $F_{2}\alpha$
Alpha adrenergic agonist (norepinephrine; phenylephrine)
Cholinergic (bethanechol; methacholine)
Anticholinesterase (edrophonium)
Betazole
Gastric alkalinization
Metoclopramide
Protein meal

The ability of cholinergic agents to raise LES pressure is well documented. Not only has bethanechol been shown to increase LES pressure after subcutaneous administration in both normal subjects and patients with sphincter incompetence,[5] but a 25 mg oral dose of this drug will produce significant increases in LES pressure in chronic reflux patients for up to two hours.[27] These observations raised the possibility of a therapeutic role for oral bethanechol in patients with chronic reflux. Recently, a controlled clinical trial with bethanechol, 25 mg four times a day, has revealed that this agent will effectively decrease reflux symptoms and antacid use in patients with chronic heartburn.[28] This study has led to a strong recommendation that bethanechol be given a definite place in medical therapy of gastroesophageal reflux.

Based on the clinical studies presented above, the treatment of heartburn would still seem to include the avoidance of specific aggravating foods such as fat, chocolate, smoking, and alcohol. In addition, the interaction of gastric alkalinization and bethanechol as agents to increase LES pressure would seem to have important therapeutic implications.

Our studies of the physiology and pathophysiology of the lower esophageal sphincter have broadened our horizons concerning the action of this antireflux mechanism. Experimental support for many of our clinical "truths" has been obtained and studies now in progress offer promise of new therapeutic vistas for the heartburn sufferer.

Request for reprints should be sent to Donald O. Castell, M.D., Chairman, Department of Internal Medicine, National Naval Medical Center, Bethesda, MD 20014.

ACKNOWLEDGMENT—The assistance of Mrs. Linda Yeck in preparation of this manuscript is appreciated.

REFERENCES

1. Christensen J: Pharmacologic identification of the lower esophageal sphincter. J Clin Invest 49:681-691, 1970

2. Lipshutz W, Cohen S: Physiological determinants of lower esophageal sphincter function. Gastroenterology 61:16-24, 1971

3. Mazur JM, Skinner DB, Jones EL, *et al*: Effect of transabdominal vagotomy on the human gastroesophageal high-pressure zone. Surgery 73:818-822, 1973

4. Rattan S, Goyal RK: Vagal control of the lower esophageal sphincter. Clin Res 22: 366A, 1974

5. Roling GT, Farrell RL, Castell DO: Cholinergic response of the lower esophageal sphincter. Am J Physiol 222:967-972, 1972

6. Lind JF, Crispin JS, McIver DK: The effect of atropine on the gastroesophageal sphincter. Can J Physiol Pharmacol 46:233-238, 1968

7. Higgs RH, Castell DO: Increased sensitivity of the lower esophageal sphincter after truncal vagotomy. Clin Res 23:16A, 1975

8. DiMarino AJ, Cohen S: The adrenergic control of lower esophageal sphincter function. J Clin Invest 52:2264-2271, 1973

9. Goyal RK, Rattan S: Mechanism of the lower esophageal sphincter relaxation. J Clin Invest 52:337-341, 1973

10. Castell DO, Harris LD: Hormonal control of gastroesophageal-sphincter strength. N Engl J Med 282:886-889, 1970

11. Giles GR, Mason MC, Humphries C, *et al*: Action of gastrin on the lower oesophageal sphincter in man. Gut 10:730-735, 1969

12. Cohen S, Lipshutz W: Hormonal regulation of human lower esophagel sphincter strength: Interaction of gastrin and secretin. J Clin Invest 50:449-454, 1971

13. Resin H, Stern DH, Sturdevant RA, *et al*: Effect of octapeptide of cholecystokinin on lower esophageal sphincter pressure in man. Gastroenterology 62:797, 1972

14. Jennewein HM, Waldeck F, Siewert R, *et al*: The interaction of glucagon and pentagastrin on the lower oesophageal sphincter in man and dog. Gut 14:861-864, 1973

15. Farrell RL, Castell DO, McGuigan JE: Measurements and comparisons of lower esophageal sphincter pressures and serum gastrin levels in patients with gastroesophageal reflux. Gastroenterology 67:415-422, 1974

16. Higgs RH, Smyth RD, Castell DO: Gastric alkalinization: Effect on lower esophageal sphincter pressure and serum gastrin. N Engl J Med 291:486-490, 1974

17. Freeland GR, Higgs RH, Castell DO, *et al*: Lower esophageal sphincter and gastric acid responses to intravenous infusions of synthetic human gastrin heptadecapeptide I. Gastroenterology 68:700, 1975

18. Cohen S, Lipshutz W, Hughes W: Role of gastrin supersensitivity in the pathogenesis of lower esophageal sphincter hypertension in achalasia. J Clin Invest 50:1241-1247, 1971

19. Cohen S, Fisher R, Lipshutz W, *et al*: The pathogenesis of esophageal dysfunction in scleroderma and Raynaud's disease. J Clin Invest 51: 2663-2668, 1972

20. Isenberg J, Csendes A, Walsh JH: Resting and pentagastrin-stimulated gastroesophageal sphincter pressure in patients with Zollinger-Ellison Syndrome. Gastroenterology 61:655-658, 1971

21. Farrell RL, Nebel OT, McGuire AT, *et al*: The abnormal lower oesophageal sphincter in pernicious anaemia. Gut 14:767-772, 1973

22. Orlando RC, Bozymski EM: Heartburn in pernicious anemia. N Engl J Med 289:522-523, 1973

23. Lipshutz WH, Gaskins RD, Lukash WM, *et al*: Pathogenesis of lower-esophageal-sphincter incompetence. N Engl J Med 289: 182-184, 1973

24. Nebel OT, Castell DO: Lower esophageal sphincter pressure changes after food ingestion. Gastroenterology 63:778-783, 1972

25. Babka JC, Castell DO: On the genesis of heartburn. The effects of specific foods on the lower esophageal sphincter. Am J Dig Dis 18:391-397, 1973

26. Dennish GW, Castell DO: Inhibitory effect of smoking on the lower esophageal sphincter. N Engl J Med 284:1136-1137, 1971

27. Farrell RL, Roling GT, Castell DO: Stimulation of the incompetent lower esophageal sphincter. A possible advance in therapy of heartburn. Am J Dig Dis 18:646-650, 1973

28. Farrell RL, Roling GT, Castell DO: Cholinergic therapy of chronic heartburn. A controlled trial. Ann Intern Med 80:573-576, 1974

Ann Otol 84: 1975

SURGICAL MANAGEMENT OF SEVERE LYE BURNS OF THE ESOPHAGUS BY COLON INTERPOSITION

WALLACE P. BERKOWITZ, M.D.

CHARLES L. ROPER, M.D. DONALD G. SESSIONS, M.D.

GERSHON J. SPECTOR, M.D. JOSEPH H. OGURA, M.D.

ST. LOUIS, MISSOURI

SUMMARY – Thirty-seven patients with severe esophageal and hypopharyngeal burns from lye ingestion are reviewed. Preliminary surgical procedures consisting of gastrostomy, esophagostomy, esophagectomy, and tracheotomy were often performed prior to definitive esophageal bypass with colon interposition. The technical aspects of the two-team approach to colon interposition are described with particular emphasis placed on the cervical anastomosis. Common postoperative complications included aspiration, delayed tracheal decannulation, and restenosis in the anastomotic area. Functional restoration of deglutition and phonation was successful in most cases. Attention is focused on management of early and late complications. Results of colon transposition are discussed with references made to other surgical procedures. Functional evaluation of patients followed over a long period is described.

The techniques used in reconstruction of the lye-damaged upper alimentary tract are numerous.[1-4] While no specific approach to hypopharyngeal and cervical esophageal stenosis appears to have a decided advantage, colon interposition has been a satisfactory method.[5]

This study analyzes the management of patients with severe hypopharyngeal and cervical esophageal lye-induced strictures. The initial, definitive, and revisional surgery that was required, along with early and late postoperative complications are reviewed. The technique of Ogura for hypopharyngeal and cervical esophageal anastomosis with colon transposition is described.[2] Long term assessment of deglutition and phonation is presented.

CLINICAL MATERIAL

All patients who underwent colon interposition for severe esophageal and hypopharyngeal stricture from lye ingestion at Washington University Medical Center from 1959 to 1972 were included in the study. Analysis was made of the initial treatment, definitive surgical management, and the early and late results of this management. Patients who were longer than two years post-colon interposition and not under therapy were felt to be eligible for long-term assessment of deglutition and phonatory function. Deglutition was considered good if the patient led a normal life without special consideration, tolerated a regular diet, and maintained weight and nutrition. Deglutition was adequate if swallowing function interfered with normal living. Barium x-ray studies confirmed the subjective impression in all cases. Phonation was considered good if the patient had a normal sounding voice, fair if voice was hoarse, and poor if voice was breathy.

From the Departments of Otolaryngology and Surgery, Division of Thoracic Surgery, Washington University School of Medicine, St. Louis, Missouri.

Supported in part by NIH Training Grant 5T01 NSO 519015 from NINDS.

Presented at the meeting of the American Broncho-Esophagological Association, Atlanta, Georgia, April 7-8, 1975.

PRINCIPLES AND TECHNIQUE OF COLON INTERPOSITION

Principles. Anatomical restoration of the upper alimentary tract may be a one or more stage procedure. Possible mediastinal contamination from an infection complicating a tracheotomy is the prime consideration for a staged procedure. Tracheotomy is necessary when pharyngeal reconstruction is required. Unless it is needed for the initial management of the patient, tracheotomy and pharyngeal repair is best delayed until the second stage.

Extensive supraglottic resection may be performed without impairing deglutition or phonatory function significantly. Accommodation of the swallowing mechanism occurs early in the postoperative period.

Technique. The first team opens the abdomen through a midline incision and mobilizes the right and transverse colon. The middle colic artery is isolated and along with the colon segment is passed posterior to the stomach and delivered through the gastro-hepatic omentum. A median sternotomy allows anterior mediastinal placement of the colon segment. The transverse colon is divided and an end-to-end ileo-transverse colostomy is performed. The proximal free end of the transverse colon is then anastomosed high on the anterior aspect of the fundus of the stomach. A pyloroplasty completes the abdominal part of the procedure unless a gastrostomy has not been performed earlier.

A second team works simultaneously to prepare the cervical area for cecal anastomosis. Either an end-to-end high cervical esophago-cecal or an end-to-side pharyngo-cecal anastomosis is performed depending upon the extent and location of pharyngeal scarring. This scarring is determined by prior endoscopic evaluation. The skin is incised along the anterior border of the sternocleidomastoid muscle from the suprasternal notch to the angle of the mandible. The dissection is carried down to the esophagus carefully avoiding the recurrent laryngeal nerve. The esophagus is mobilized and transected. The distal end is closed by interrupted 3-0 silk sutures, and the proximal end is anastomosed to the cecum in two layers. The sternal head of the clavicle and part of the manubrium are often removed to provide room for the colon.

To prepare for the pharyngeal anastomosis, the skin incision is made on the side opposite the most severe scarring. The skin and subcutaneous tissues are elevated over the larynx, and dissection is carried toward the posterolateral border of the thyroid cartilage. The sternohyoid, thyrohyoid and omohyoid muscles are divided transversely at the superior border of the thyroid cartilage, and the medial constrictor muscles are divided along the thyroid cartilage edge. The perichondrium is elevated inferiorly and the cartilage is incised obliquely from the thyroid notch to a point just superior to the inferior cornu.

The internal perichondrium and the hypopharyngeal area are exposed after the cartilage is resected. The pyriform sinus is identified. The hypopharynx is opened vertically, and the arytenoid eminence is identified. The incision is extended superiorly to the level of the epiglottis. The cecum is opened along one tenia for approximately 3 cm for an end-to-side anastomosis with the hypopharynx. The esophagus distal to the anastomosis is closed. Drains are placed into the neck and upper mediastinum prior to wound closure.

If a pharyngeal repair is required, it is performed two weeks after colon interposition. A paramedian tracheotomy using local anesthesia is followed by administration of general anesthesia. A transverse incision is made at the level of the hyoid bone. The suprahyoid muscles are partially separated and the hyoid bone is split in the midline. The pharynx is entered at the vallecula. The midline incision may be extended down to the thyroid notch for additional exposure. All epiglottic and glossoepiglottic folds are cut on

TABLE I

COLON INTERPOSITION FOR ESOPHAGEAL AND HYPOPHARYNGEAL STRICTURE (N = 37)

	No. Occurrences	*% Occurrences*
Colon interposition (staged)	16	43%
Colon interposition (unstaged)	21	57%
(a) End-to-end anastomosis (cecum to esophagus)	12	33%
(b) End-to-side anastomosis (cecum to hypopharynx)	9	24%

each side taking great care to avoid accidental incision into the colon. The arytenoid cartilage should not be traumatized since vocal cord fixation may result. Dissection may be carried into the endolarynx to below the false cords and into the ventricles. The epiglottis together with the remaining scarred supraglottic tissues are excised, taking care to preserve the pyriform mucosa, and a cuff of mucosa at the cecal-pharyngeal anastomosis. Split thickness skin grafts are used to cover the raw supraglottic area. A Negus stent is used to secure the skin graft in position. The distal end of the stent is placed into the colon stoma. The neck wound is then closed after the hyoid bone is reapproximated.

The stent is removed in two to three weeks. Deglutition is attempted after the pharynx is healed and the laryngeal airway has been reestablished. If the tracheotomy tube is patent, a cork stopper must be used to allow the expired air column to assist clearing the larynx. The tracheotomy tube is removed when aspiration is no longer a significant problem.

RESULTS

Thirty-seven patients with severe lye burns of the esophagus and hypopharynx underwent colon interposition between 1959 and 1972. There were 26 males and 11 females. Age at the time of ingestion varied. The peak incidence occurred with adults over 18 (14). Children and young adults (23) were subdivided into infants less than one year (4), children one to ten years (13), and young adults 10 to 18 years (6). Initial evaluation in all patients included a barium swallow roentgenographic contrast study and endoscopy. Initial management with corticosteroids, antibiotics, and endoscopic dilatation did not prevent eventual esophageal stricture in these patients.[6,7]

Gastrostomy and esophagostomy were performed to maintain nutrition in 29 and 7 patients, respectively. Esophagectomy was required subsequent to esophageal perforation and mediastinal infection in seven patients.[8] Laryngeal edema with airway obstruction necessitated tracheotomy in six cases.

The severity of the stricture determined whether reconstruction of the upper airway and alimentary tract was performed in one or two stages. Table I illustrates the definitive surgical management of these patients. In the 16 patients requiring two-stage reconstruction, the colon interposition was done initially with repair of the hypopharyngeal stenosis done secondarily. All of these patients had significant hypopharyngeal stenosis, as well as esophageal stricture. A single-stage procedure was possible in 21 patients who had esophageal stricture with minimal hypopharyngeal involvement.

An end-to-end (cecum to esophagus) anastomosis was performed in 12 cases while an end-to-side (cecum to hypopharynx) anastomosis was accomplished in nine patients. Stenosis was distal to

TABLE II

EARLY POSTOPERATIVE COMPLICATIONS AND SURGICAL MANAGEMENT (N = 37)

Complication	*No. Occurrences*	*% Occurrences*	*Surgical Management*
Airway: significant aspiration	9	24%	
prolonged tracheal cannulation	5	13%	
tracheal stenosis	2	5%	
Alimentary: cervical restenosis	7	19%	4 anastomotic dilatation
cervical anastomotic leak	2	5%	3 anastomotic revision
colon necrosis	2	5%	2 abdominal exploration
General: wound infection	5	13%	5 incision and drainage
operative mortality	1	2%	

the cricopharyngeus muscle in the former and involved the muscle in the latter nine cases.

Table II indicates the incidence and treatment of early postoperative complications. Aspiration of food and saliva was noted in nine patients. Late spontaneous improvement in symptoms occurred in all but two. Extensive cervical scar resection and slow development of a swallowing technique were factors observed in patients with significant aspiration. Tracheal stenosis was noted in two patients.

Early stenosis of the cervical colon anastomosis occurred in seven patients. Endoscopic dilatation was successful in four while revision of the anastomosis was required in three patients with severe lumen narrowing. Two patients had a small dehiscence at the pharyngeal anastomosis stricture. Both cases underwent surgical revision and are included with those cases requiring early revision of the cervical anastomosis. Abdominal exploration for intestinal obstruction was performed on two occasions. Necrosis of the transposed colon segment was observed in both cases. One patient died during surgery. In the second case, necrotic colon was excised and the stomach anastomosis was closed. The patient later underwent

TABLE III

LATE-OCCURRING COMPLICATIONS AND SURGICAL PROCEDURES PERFORMED

Late Complications	*No. Occurrences*	*% Occurrences*
Airway: persistent aspiration	3	8%
supraglottic stenosis	3	8%
persistent tracheal stenosis	2	5%
Alimentary: cervical anastomotic restenosis	5	13%
Surgical Procedures	*No. Occurrences*	
Airway: resection of tracheal stenosis	2	
resection of recurrent pharyngeal stenosis	3	
Alimentary: cervical anastomotic dilatation	5	
cervical anastomotic revision	3	
resection of esophageal diverticulum	1	
left colon interposition	1	

TABLE IV

LONG-TERM RESULTS OF THERAPY (N = 37)

Evaluation Completed (27)		*Evaluation Not Completed (10)*	
Deglutition Function		Surgery less than 2 yrs	4
Good	25	Therapy continuing	3
Adequate	2	Therapy terminated	2
Phonation Function		Operative death	1
Good	21		
Fair	4		
Poor	2		

successful left colon bypass. Five patients with superficial wound abscesses were treated by incision and drainage procedures with healing occurring secondarily.

Table III summarizes the incidence of late-occurring complications and the surgical procedures performed during this period. Five patients continued to require tracheal cannulation for pulmonary toilet as a result of aspiration. Tracheal stenosis recurred after excision and end-to-end anastomosis. Restenosis of the colon anastomosis occurred with five patients and initially all were dilated successfully. Eventually three underwent surgical revision because repeated dilatation gave only transient relief of dysphagia. Three patients developed stenosis within the supraglottic area during the late postoperative period. Surgical revision was initially successful in all, but repeated scar formation occurred in two necessitating a second revision and skin graft.

Symptoms of dysphagia in one patient were related to a diverticulum at the colon-esophageal anastomosis. Surgical resection of the pouch relieved his symptoms.

Throughout the postoperative period, recurrent scarring was the predominant factor in most complications seen. There were no complications related to gastric acid reflux into the transposed colon segment.[4] Anastomosis of the colon to the fundus of the stomach seemed to be significant in this regard. In some reports, esophageal bypass involving transposition of a gastric tube or segment of jejunum was complicated by frequent distal stenosis with occasional necrosis resulting from acid reflux. Split thickness skin grafting for hypopharyngeal restoration has a high incidence of restenosis.[5,9] Graft failure occurs more frequently when skin is secured about a stent rather than sutured directly to the denuded pharynx before positioning of the stent to maintain lumen size. Even slight movements of a stent may prevent or disrupt skin adherence.

Table IV summarizes the long term results of therapy. Twenty-seven of the 37 patients had completed therapy. There was one operative death. In four patients colon interposition was performed within the past two years. Two patients terminated therapy prematurely. Three patients were undergoing further management for restenosis. Deglutition was considered good in 25 patients (Fig. 1) and adequate in two patients. One of these two experienced intermittent symptoms of dysphagia with no evidence of stricture noted on barium-swallow roentgen examination. The second patient had good objective evidence of colon patency but continued to depend on gastrostomy feeding as he had done during repeated revisions for an anastomosis stricture.

Phonatory function was good in 21 patients, fair in four, and poor in two. The four patients with a fair voice had required surgical revision for supraglottic and hypopharyngeal restenosis. The two patients with poor phonation had tracheal stenosis and a permanent tracheostomy.

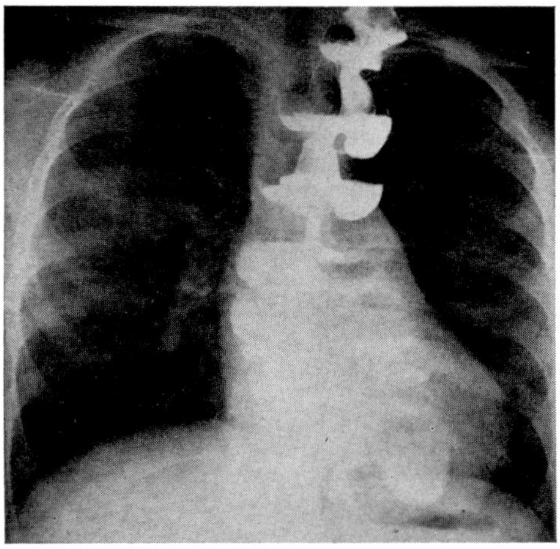

Fig. 1. Good deglutition following colon interposition.

DISCUSSION

Proper treatment of esophageal lye burns requires knowledge of the extent of damage.[6,7] Esophagoscopy and barium-swallow x-rays should be performed as soon as possible. Extensive burns may be noted on the lips and within the oral cavity. Indirect mirror examination of the oro- and hypopharynx, along with direct endoscopic assessment, dictate the course of therapy to be implemented. With severe burns of the esophagus and hypopharynx, corticosteroids and early endoscopic dilatation are of no value and may be detrimental when esophageal perforation is imminent. Tracheotomy and other immediate life-support measures are often required in these patients before endoscopic evaluation can be performed.

Tertiary burn of the hypopharynx and cricopharyngeal area is seen in cases that eventually require esophageal bypass and is the main factor for considering early therapy. The average time lapse from ingestion to definitive surgery was four months in this series. Esophagoscopy must be terminated at the first sign of a third degree burn to avoid esophageal perforation. Once the severity of the burn has been verified, appropriate therapy can be started. Laryngeal and supraglottic edema requiring immediate tracheotomy also suggest extensive hypopharyngeal burns.

Repeated dilatation of esophageal stricture by bougienage has been a successful method restoring deglutition when the pharynx and proximal cervical esophagus is uninvolved with signficant scarring. An extensive review of esophageal dilatation has recently been published.[10] Relatively little has been published on long-term follow-up and retrospective analysis of patients with hypopharyngeal and proximal cervical esophageal strictures. Techniques of hypopharyngeal reconstruction with free skin grafts,[9] skin flaps from neck and chest,[11] laryngotracheal autografts,[12] and modified Z-plasty procedures[13,14] have been described as successfully restoring anatomical integrity necessary for deglutition in selected cases.

The technique of pharyngeal reconstruction and esophageal replacement described by Ogura *et al*[2] was employed in the cases reviewed. Successful restoration of deglutition by objective roentgenographic appraisal occurred in all patients. Barium swallow x-ray studies confirmed the subjective appraisal of deglutition. On subjective appraisal, two patients felt their swallowing efforts were labored, and their general activities were not entirely normal. Phonatory function was likewise subjectively assessed. Good results were achieved in over three-fourths of the patients. Long-term success using the technique described appears to be excellent.

Wound dehiscence, poor skin graft take, residual unexcised scar, a narrow lumen, and foreign body irritation were some of the factors in stricture formation. On the other hand, successful long-term management seemed to rely on meticulous attention to technique for anatomical restoration. The relatively low complication rate with colon interposition accounts for its wide acceptance.

Aspiration occurred in all patients requiring hypopharyngeal and supraglottic reconstruction. Once swallowing was successful, aspiration subsided. Prolonged aspiration occurred in those patients finding swallowing difficult to relearn. Most cases resolved spontaneously once a technique of swallowing was mastered. Hospitalization in these instances was prolonged by a few days. In a few patients, pulmonary therapy was required for retained secretions. Tracheal decannulation was delayed as a result.

Neck and chest flaps[5,11,15] have been used for hypopharyngeal repair. A three-stage procedure for complete reconstruction is often required, but the incidence of restricture is low.

The stomach and jejunum have been acceptable alternatives to colon interposition in patients with minimal hypopharyngeal involvement.[3,4] The incidence of jejunum necrosis following vascular compromise is high. The jejunal segment is often limited by its length and blood supply to esophageal replacement.

SUMMARY

Management of severe cervical esophageal and hypopharyngeal lye-induced strictures has been reviewed in this study. The indications, technique, and complications resulting from colon interposition as the procedure used to reestablish upper alimentary tract continuity are presented and analyzed. Postoperative complications and management are separated into early and late manifestations. Long-term results of deglutition and phonatory function are emphasized. Return to full function and original life style is the goal for every patient. Colon interposition with cervical esophageal and hypopharyngeal reconstruction seems to be a successful approach to attain this goal.

Request for reprints should be sent to Wallace P. Berkowitz, M.D., Dept. of Otolaryngology, Wash. Univ. School of Medicine, 517 S. Euclid, St. Louis, Mo. 63110.

REFERENCES

1. Wookey H: The surgical treatment of carcinoma of the hypopharynx and the oesophagus. Br J Surg 36:249, 1947-48

2. Ogura JH, Roper CL, Burford TH: Functional restoration of the food passages in extensive stenosing caustic burns of the pharynx and esophagus. Laryngoscope 71: 885-902, 1961

3. Rienhoff WF: Intrathoracic esophagojejunostomy for lesions of the upper third of the esophagus. South Med J 39:928, 1945

4. Heimlich HJ: Esophagoplasty with reversed gastric tube. Review of fifty-three cases. Am J Surg 123:80-92, 1972

5. Leonard JR, Holt GD: Reconstruction of the hypopharynx and cervical esophagus. Otolaryngol Clin North Am 5:(3)435-446, 1972

6. Middlekamp JN, Cone AJ, Ogura JH, *et al*: Endoscopic diagnosis and steroid and antibiotic therapy of acute lye burns of the esophagus. Laryngoscope 71:1354-1362, 1961

7. Viscomi GJ, Beekhuis GJ, Whitten CF: An evaluation of early esophagoscopy and corticosteroid therapy in the management of corrosive injury of the esophagus. J Pediatr 59:356-360, 1961

8. Ritter FN, Gago O, Kirsh MM, *et al*: The rationale of emergency esophagogastectomy in the treatment of liquid caustic burns of the esophagus and stomach. Ann Otol Rhinol Laryngol 80:513-520, 1971

9. Rabuzzi DD, Camp HL: Repair of hypopharyngeal stenosis. Arch Otolaryngol 97:256-258, 1973

10. Tucker JA, Turtz ML, Silberman HD, *et al*: Retrograde esophageal dilatation 1924-1974 – a historical review. Ann Otol Rhinol Laryngol 83:1-35 (Suppl. 16), 1974

11. Bakamjian VY: A two-stage method for pharyngoesophageal reconstruction with a primary pectoral skin flap. Plast Reconstr Surg 36:173, 1965

12. Som ML: Laryngoesophagectomy. Arch Otolaryngol 63:474, 1956

13. Gross CW, Harris AS: Relief of stricture in the cervical esophagus by Z-plasty technique. Laryngoscope 81:658-662, 1971

14. Bernstein L: Z-plasty in head and neck surgery. Arch Otolaryngol 89:574-584, 1969

15. Edgerton MT: One-stage reconstruction of the cervical esophagus or trachea. Surgery 31:239, 1952

Ann Otol 84: 1975

EARLY LUNG CANCER DETECTION AND LOCALIZATION

DAVID R. SANDERSON, M.D.

ROBERT S. FONTANA, M.D.

ROCHESTER, MINNESOTA

SUMMARY – The Mayo Lung Project was established to develop and evaluate a screening program for early lung cancer in high-risk subjects. Men who are more than 45 years of age and who smoke one package of cigarettes or more daily are screened by the use of thoracic roentgenograms, three-day pooled sputum cytology, and lung health questionnaires at four-month intervals. These data are compared with data from similar subjects screened only on entry into the project. During the past three years, 34 patients who had no roentgenographic evidence of lung cancer were identified and examined because of carcinoma cells in sputum. Of these 34 patients, 27 have had bronchoscopic localization of their tumors and definitive treatment, and 3 had upper respiratory tract neoplasms and also have been treated. Of the remaining four, one patient died suddenly after myocardial infarction and three patients have not had localization or treatment because of other severe complicating medical problems. Localization of roentgenographically occult lung cancer is reliable by the use of bronchofiberoscopy and meticulous, thorough sampling from the tracheobronchial tree. A search must be made for upper airway cancers in the same high-risk population, and the possibility of second primary bronchogenic tumors also must be considered. Although follow-up is short, 22 of the 27 treated lung cancer patients were found with stage I disease. The outlook for 19 of these 27 is encouraging an average of 16 months after surgical resection.

Bronchogenic carcinoma continues to increase as a major public health problem. The American Cancer Society estimates that 91,000 new cases will be diagnosed in 1975 and that there will be 81,000 deaths.*[1] Some observers have expressed doubt whether curable lung cancer can be detected effectively by any means.[2] However, data from the American Joint Committee for Cancer Staging and End Results Reporting (AJC) show definite differences in long-term survival, depending on the histologic classification of the lesion and its stage when treatment is accomplished.[3]

The National Cancer Institute has established a Cooperative Early Lung Cancer Group to develop and evaluate a program for screening high-risk subjects.[4] Multidisciplinary groups at Johns Hopkins Hospital, Memorial Sloan-Kettering Cancer Center, and Mayo Clinic were assigned the task of determining whether screening will make it possible to lower the mortality rate due to bronchogenic carcinoma from that in a matched population not screened regularly.

The Mayo Lung Project (MLP) was established to screen men who are more than 45 years of age and who smoke one package of cigarettes or more daily (or who have done so within the previous year) from a population that presents for routine health examinations.[5,6] Persons are excluded who already have respiratory cancer, who

----

* Incidence estimates are based on rates from the National Cancer Institute's Third National Cancer Survey.

From the Mayo Clinic and Mayo Foundation, Rochester, Minnesota.

This investigation was supported in part by Research Grant CB-53886 from the National Institutes of Health, Public Health Service.

Presented at the meeting of the American Broncho-Esophagological Association, Atlanta, Georgia, April 7-8, 1975.

have other serious illnesses that make five-year survival unlikely, or who have a respiratory reserve so severely diminished that surgical resection of at least one lobe of the lung is impossible. With these criteria for exclusion, the population is randomized into two groups. One group is followed regularly at four-month intervals, at which time a three-day pooled sputum cytology examination, 14- by 17-inch thoracic roentgenogram, and lung health questionnaire are completed. Every effort is made by mail or telephone to ensure completion of each screening procedure. The other group is advised, at the initial enrollment, of the desirability of getting regular annual sputum tests and chest roentgenograms, but the person must initiate such action. All persons in either group are to be followed for at least five years. Any patient in whom carcinoma of the lung develops will be treated as promptly as possible, depending on type of tumor, its localization, and other medical considerations. All patients treated for lung cancer will continue to receive frequent follow-up indefinitely.

When the thoracic roentgenogram demonstrates a persistent new lesion compared with the previous normal film, the likelihood of malignancy is high and early resection probably will follow. However, when the roentgenogram of the chest is normal but sputum cytology examination indicates suspicion or conclusive evidence of malignancy, the task of localizing the source of the exfoliated cancer cells presents a major challenge.

A specific protocol for investigating patients with this problem has been evolved by the Cooperative Early Lung Cancer Group (CELC Group).[4] Earlier reports from Johns Hopkins[7] and Mayo Clinic[8] have outlined the procedures to be followed.

PRE-ENDOSCOPY EXAMINATION

After a patient with positive sputum cytology and normal routine chest roentgenography is identified, a series of prebronchoscopy tests is completed. A complete physical examination, routine laborary studies (including hemogram, blood chemistry profile, and urinalysis), and electrocardiography are carried out. Roentgenographic studies include stereoscopic paired posteroanterior views at 140 kvp and lateral chest roentgenograms, whole lung tomograms, and a 14- by 17-inch posteroanterior projection made at 350 kvp. Pulmonary function is assessed by standard spirometry to measure VC, FEV_1, MBC, and MMF* (before and after nebulized isoproterenol is given). If doubt exists regarding respiratory reserve, arterial blood gas measurements are also obtained. Special attention is given to examination of the larynx and oropharynx in search of lesions of the upper respiratory tract. The patient is asked to discontinue smoking for one to two weeks before the examination. Oral bronchodilators and antibiotics may be given in an effort to improve the underlying chronic bronchitis. The patient is then hospitalized and bronchoscoped while under general anesthesia, as described by Perry and Sanderson.[9] Care is taken to ensure the maintainence of optimal levels for arterial blood gases during and after the prolonged examination of the tracheobronchial tree.

PROTOCOL FOR BRONCHOSCOPIC EXAMINATION

The methods employed are modified after the description of Marsh and colleagues[7] and subsequently standardized by the CELC Group.[4]

After induction of anesthesia, an open rigid ventilating bronchoscope with inflatable cuff placed distally is inserted. One hundred percent oxygen is insufflated, and the bronchoscope is positioned in the left main bronchus. Lavage is repeated on the left side two or three times before the cuff is deflated. After another one- to two-minute interval with the patient breathing 100%

---

* VC — Vital capacity. FEV — Forced expiratory volume. MBC — Maximum breathing capacity. MMF — Maximal midflow.

oxygen, the bronchoscope is positioned in the right main bronchus just proximal to the right upper lobe orifice and the cuff is reinflated. The right side is again lavaged two or three times, and washings are submitted separately for examination. The cuff is deflated, and ventilation is resumed before withdrawal of the open bronchoscope. A cuffer endotracheal tube of 9 or 10 mm internal diameter is inserted in order to complete the procedure. A specially fitted T-adapter permits access with the bronchofiberscope while controlled ventilation and general anesthesia are maintained. Both sides of the tracheobronchial tree are inspected completely, and the entire accessible bronchial mucosa area is recorded on video-tape using color television. Any locally suspicious areas are also documented with still photography using a 35 mm half-frame camera.

Brush, curette, and forcep biopsy specimens are obtained when an obvious bronchogenic carcinoma is seen. However, if no grossly abnormal lesion is seen, samples are taken from all accessible segmental and subsegmental branches, and each sample is labeled and submitted separately for examination. Generally, all brush and curette samples are taken before the multiple biopsy collections are begun because the latter is more likely to cause bleeding, which may obscure subtle mucosal changes. After bronchoscopic sampling has been completed, the patient is allowed to waken and is transferred to the postoperative recovery room for further observation. Arterial blood gases are monitored during and after the procedure to ensure adequate, safe oxygenation and alveolar ventilation.

RESULTS

Since Jan. 1, 1972, 34 patients with no roentgenographic evidence for cancer localization have been evaluated by the MLP because of sputum cytology positive for carcinoma cells. Fifteen of these patients were included in an earlier report on roentgenographically occult lung cancer, and the others have been seen since that time.

These 34 patients represent three categories of presentation. Ten had sputum positive on initial screening of an ambulatory outpatient population of male smokers more than 45 years of age ("prevalence"). Five had sputum that became positive after initial negative screening ("incidence"). The remaining 19 were referred to the Mayo Lung Project for localization because of known positive sputum cytology after initial negative findings elsewhere.

All patients were men whose ages averaged 61 years and ranged from 46 to 79 years. All patients had initial reports that were frankly positive for malignant squamous cells or squamous metaplasia with marked atypia on cytologic examination. Those with the latter interpretation had subsequent confirmation of malignant cells on repeat sampling. The initial specimen in each patient was a pooled three-day collection of spontaneous deep-cough sputum fixed in 50% alcohol and 2% Carbowax®* according to the technique of Saccomanno *et al.*[10]

Untreated Patients. Of the 34 patients, 4 have not been treated for their cancer. A 73-year-old man had endoscopic lateralization to the left side of the bronchial tree but, because of other medical problems, has not had further localization or treatment. Roentgenographically, the chest remained negative 12 months after discovery of carcinoma cells. A 67-year-old man had endoscopic lateralization to the right side of the bronchial tree, and further bronchoscopic examination was planned. He died after an acute myocardial infarction, and a small squamous cell carcinoma was found in the right lung at postmortem examination. A 52-year-old man with severe chronic obstructive lung disease and cor pulmonale was too ill to tolerate any treatment, even if localization had been accomplished. Twenty-four months after the initial sputum diagnosis, the patient

* Doak Pharmacal Co., Inc., Westbury, L.I., New York.

TABLE I

BRONCHOSCOPIC LOCALIZATION OF PRIMARY LUNG CANCER IN PATIENTS WITH INITIAL POSITIVE SPUTUM CYTOLOGY AND NEGATIVE CHEST ROENTGENOGRAM

Procedure	*Total No. Patients*	*Lesion Localized*	*No Lesion Detected*
Initial bronchoscopy	27	13	14
Initial random biopsy	14	3	11
Second bronchoscopy required	11	3	8
Third bronchoscopy required	8	4	4
Fourth bronchoscopy required	4	2	2
Fifth bronchoscopy required	2	2	0

developed roentgenographic evidence of lung tumor. He is still alive but doing poorly with palliative therapy. The fourth patient was 79 years old when positive sputum cytology was discovered. He also had severe disabling chronic obstructive lung disease, with emphysema and generalized cardiovascular disease precluding any definitive treatment. Thirty months later, he is still alive with no roentgenographic evidence of localization of his cancer. In all four of these patients, results of upper airway examination have been negative.

Patients With Upper Respiratory Tract Cancers. Three patients had upper respiratory tract cancers that have been treated. Two of these had positive cytology on initial sputum screening. A 59-year-old man had a tiny tumor at the base of the tongue, which has been treated with radiation therapy. A 69-year-old man had cautery excision of the right vocal cord, after suspension and biopsy. A 58-year-old man presented with positive sputum after initial negative screening and also underwent cautery excision of an early lesion on the right vocal cord. All three patients had bronchoscopic examination, with no visible or pathologic evidence for malignancy below the glottis. Each has had follow-up sputum cytology reported as negative since treatment for the upper respiratory tract cancer.

Patients With Primary Lung Cancer. The remaining 27 patients have been treated for primary bronchogenic squamous cell carcinoma. These patients were asymptomatic at the time of diagnosis except for mild-to-moderate sputum production, which they invariably ascribed to "smoker's cough." One man developed mild hemoptysis during the week before bronchoscopic examination, but none of the remaining 26 patients had expectorated blood.

In spite of negative findings on chest roentgenograms, nearly half (13 patients) of this group had grossly visible, albeit often small, endobronchial tumors on initial examination. Biopsy or brush cytology samples confirmed the localization of tumor and permitted definitive therapy. In the other 14 patients, the initial bronchoscopic inspection failed to disclose specific localization. In these patients, multiple samples from all accessible portions of the tracheobronchial tree provided the definitive localizing information, although repeated bronchoscopy was necessary in 11 of the 14 patients (Table I).

For all 27 patients, the time interval from initial sputum cytology to localization ranged from one week to 24 months. Excluding two patients with known positive cytology who were referred to us for localization, the mean time required from diagnosis until treatment was 2.6 months. With greater experience, the interval from diagnosis to treatment has been shortened to two months during the last 1½ years.

The most fruitful sampling technique in this series has been spur biopsy; that is, microbiopsy of the bronchial mucosa at a bronchial bifurcation. Of the 14 patients with no grossly visible lesion at initial examination, 11 had the lesion localized by spur biopsy, 3 by brush cytology, and none by curettage. When only brush cytology was positive, we required confirmation at a separate examination before we planned surgical resection.

Of these 27 patients, 24 underwent surgery and 3 received primary radiation. Of the three given radiation, two had tumors on the main carina and distal trachea as well as other medical problems that made resection and reconstruction unduly hazardous. The third patient developed a new primary tumor eight years after pneumonectomy for a previous lung cancer. Of those who underwent operation, 6 had pneumonectomy, 2 had bilobectomy (including 1 with left upper lobectomy and right lower lobectomy for synchronous primary tumors), and 16 had lobectomy (including 1 with left upper lobectomy that completed pneumonectomy in which the initial resection had been done nine years before).

According to the AJC classification, 5 patients had stage III disease and 22 had stage I disease.

There were no operative deaths in this group of patients. As of Mar. 1, 1975, five of the 27 patients have died. One patient who had left pneumonectomy for stage III disease developed metastasis and died 20 months after operation. Four other patients have died, but they had no evidence of recurrent bronchogenic carcinoma. Three of these died of cardiovascular disease, whereas the fourth patient had a separate laryngeal cancer involving the upper esophagus and died of aspiration pneumonitis.

The mean duration of follow-up through Mar. 1, 1975, among the 22 survivors was 16 months. Two of these patients have developed what may be separate new primary tumors; one has received radiation and the other is awaiting treatment. One of the patients who had radiation therapy to the carina and distal trachea remains well, with negative sputum after 14 months. The other patients continue to be free of recurrent disease at intervals from 4 to 34 months after treatment.

DISCUSSION

Although the number of patients with treated lung cancer is small and the duration of follow-up is relatively short, several preliminary impressions are justified.

First has been the excellent record of patient acceptance and cooperation in a screening program. More than 90% of patients initially enrolled have continued under close surveillance.[6] Screening has produced results in diagnosing lung cancer in a presymptomatic phase when treatment is more likely to be effective. Localization of roentgenographically occult lung cancers can be done reliably, although the procedure is time-consuming and often must be repeated.

The discovery of three patients with upper respiratory cancer by sputum cytology examination illustrates the usefulness of screening and emphasizes that patients at risk for lung cancer also share sharply increased risks for laryngeal and other upper respiratory tract tumors.

The discovery of multiple primary lung lesions is not new,[11,12] but the occurrence of such lesions is unusually high for this series of patients. In total, the 27 patients with primary lung cancer have had 34 apparently separate primary lung lesions. Two patients had synchronous but remotely situated tumors; and five had metachronous tumors, but the location, appearance, and time interval suggested new primary tumors rather than metastatic lesions. If this trend continues or increases, the therapeutic value of surgical resection could be diminished, although such a trend underscores the importance of conservative resection in order to preserve useful lung function.

Finally, survival among this population with occult lung cancer at time of treatment appears to be better than survival after treatment when the lesion is at a more advanced overt stage. One could argue that this method only identifies a presymptomatic interval and does not actually prolong life, but data accumulated in this and the companion studies of the Cooperative Early Lung Cancer Group should ultimately furnish this answer.

Request for reprints should be sent to Dr. D. R. Sanderson, Mayo Clinic, Rochester, MN 55901

REFERENCES

1. American Cancer Society: *'75 Cancer Facts and Figures.* New York, 1974

2. Boucot KR, Weiss W: Is curable lung cancer detected by semiannual screeing? JAMA 224:1361-1365, 1973

3. American Joint Committee for Cancer Staging and End Results Reporting: *Clinical Staging System for Carcinoma of the Lung.* Chicago, September 1973

4. National Cancer Institute, Cooperative Early Lung Cancer Group: *Manual of Procedures,* Jan. 1, 1975

5. Fontana RS, Sanderson DR, Miller WE, *et al*: The Mayo Lung Project: preliminary report of "early cancer detection" phase. Cancer 30:1373-1382, 1972

6. Fontana RS, Sanderson DR, Woolner LB, *et al*: The Mayo Lung Project for early detection and localization of bronchogenic carcinoma: a status report. Chest 67:511-521, 1975

7. Marsh BR, Frost JK, Erozan YS, *et al*: Flexible fiberoptic bronchoscopy: its place in the search for lung cancer. Ann Otol Rhinol Laryngol 82:757-764, 1973

8. Sanderson DR, Fontana RS, Wollner LB, *et al*: Bronchoscopic localization of radiographically occult lung cancer. Chest 65:608-612, 1974

9. Perry LB, Sanderson DR: Anesthesia for prolonged bronchoscopy. Ann Thorac Surg 19:248-253, 1975

10. Saccomanno G, Saunders RP, Ellis H, *et al*: Concentration of carcinoma or atypical cells in sputum. Acta Cytol (Baltimore) 7: 305-310, 1963

11. Merrick DK, Carr DT, Payne WS, *et al*: Multiple primary cancer of the lung. Geriatrics 27:71-79, 1972

12. Martini N, Beattie EJ Jr, Cliffton EE, *et al*: Radiologically occult lung cancer: report of 26 cases. Surg Clin North Am 54: 811-823, 1974

ERRATA

In the article "Benign Granular Cell Tumors of the Larynx: A Review of 36 Cases with Clinicopathologic Data," by John Campagno, M.D., *et al,* which appeared in the Annals of Otology, Rhinology and Laryngology 84:308-314, a correction should be made on page 308 in line 8 of the Summary as follows: " . . . often simulating squamous cell carcinoma."

The article entitled "Hypersomnia Caused by Upper Airway Obstructions" by Drs. Simmons and Hill (83:670-674, 1974) contains an error in the Summary. The word "cured" was inappropriately applied to the patient whose sleep problems were helped, not cured, by a submucous resection. We would also like to acknowledge the collaboration of Drs. William C. Dement and Christian Guilleminault of the Stanford Sleep Laboratory.

Ann Otol 84: 1975

DELAYED CLEARANCE OF TANTALUM BY RADIOLOGICALLY OCCULT CANCER

FREDERICK P. STITIK, M.D.

DONALD F. PROCTOR, M.D.

BALTIMORE, MARYLAND

SUMMARY — The best current treatment of bronchogenic carcinoma is prompt surgical excision of early lesions before mediastinal and extrathoracic spread occurs. Bronchoscopy, in a patient with a positive cytology and a negative chest radiograph, is a long, time-consuming procedure. Tantalum bronchography done prior to the bronchoscopy will significantly reduce the time necessary for bronchoscopy. Tantalum is cleared solely by mucociliary action. Early bronchogenic carcinoma, when sufficiently large enough, will destroy the ciliated epithelium, thus impairing mucociliary clearance and altering mucus secretion. Tantalum bronchography has localized these early x-ray negative lesions, both by minimal mucosal irregularity and by delayed clearance. In the past three years we have localized the radiologically occult malignancy in four out of five patients.

Bronchogenic carcinoma is the most common cause of death from malignancy in males in the United States. In 1975 an estimated 80,000 people will die of this disease.* Although there have been recent advances in the immunotherapy and the chemotherapy of bronchogenic carcinoma, at the present time surgical excision remains the treatment of choice. If survival rates are to be reduced in this disease, the best current hope lies in the earliest possible localization and resection of the malignancy before mediastinal or extrathoracic spread occurs.

Early bronchogenic carcinomas usually shed malignant cells into the sputum years before they become radiologically apparent.[1] Prompt and accurate localization of these early malignancies for the surgeon is mandatory. Fiberoptic bronchoscopy in a patient with a positive cytology and a negative chest radiograph is a long and tedious procedure. Meticulous search of all lobes, segments, and subsegments with repeated washings and brushings requires two or three hours. Even if one is fortunate enough to locate a lesion early in the search, it is desirable to examine for a second cancer. Our experience has indicated that tantalum bronchography may uncover very small areas in which malignant change has disrupted mucociliary clearance. Prior evaluation by tantalum bronchography and serial clearance films may significantly reduce the time needed for bronchoscopic localization. This paper reviews our experience with bronchography performed with the experimental contrast agent tantalum in patients with bronchogenic carcinoma and a normal chest radiograph.

METHODS AND MATERIALS

Three patients with a positive cytology and a normal chest radiograph were detected by cytologic screening as part of an NIH-NCI

* Levin ML: Personal communication.

From the Department of Radiology and Department of Laryngology and Otology, The Johns Hopkins Hospital, Baltimore, Maryland.

This work was supported by NCI Contract: N01-CB-92172.

Presented at the meeting of the American Broncho-Esophagological Association, Atlanta, Georgia, April 7-8, 1975.

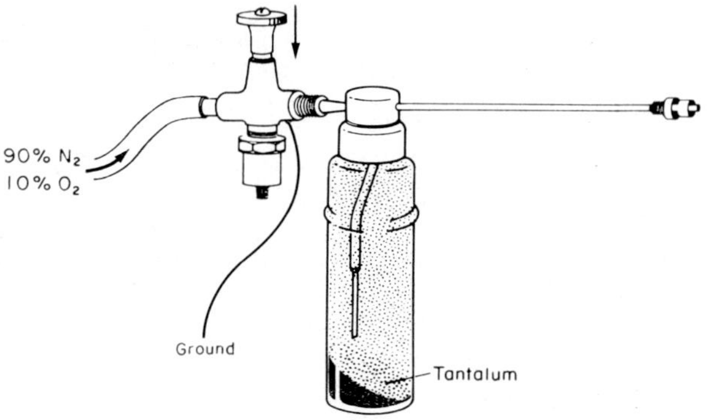

Fig. 1. Tantalum generator. The valve is a one way valve allowing insufflation of the tantalum and insufflating gas only when the plunger is depressed as shown by the arrow.

contract to detect early lung cancer.[2] The other two patients were referred to the Johns Hopkins Hospital for tantalum bronchography because of intermittent wheezing.

The five patients' PA and lateral chest radiographs were reviewed prior to the procedure. The patient was questioned regarding allergies to local anesthetic agents as well as to contraindications to atropine. Atropine was injected intravenously in 0.2 to 0.3 mg increments until the peripheral pulse reach 120/min or a total of 2 mg of atropine had been administered. The usual dose ranged from 1.4 to 1.7 mg of atropine given over three to five minutes. Topical anesthesia with 4% Xylocaine®* was applied to the pharynx, larynx, and trachea. One percent Xylocaine® was subsequently administered through a catheter into the segmental bronchi.

The tantalum powder used was the commercially available, dry 5 μ powder.** The tantalum was generated from a modified powder blower (Fig. 1)*** The generator was connected to a Selector Catheter System.**** The catheter most frequently used was the 13 French - 65 cm catheter. Under careful fluoroscopic control, tantalum was insufflated selectively into lobes or segments of the lung. A complete bilateral bronchogram could usually be performed by repositioning the catheter six or seven times. The insufflating gas was a 90% nitrogen - 10% oxygen mixture. Short bursts of five to ten seconds were necessary to completely coat the desired lobe or segment. Insufflating pressures ranged from 10 pounds per square inch (psi) to 20 psi. Throughout the entire procedure the generator and the patient were electrically grounded.

During the bronchogram, spot films were obtained where necessary. After a complete bronchogram, PA, lateral, and both oblique

TABLE I

PATIENTS WITH RADIOLOGICALLY OCCULT BRONCHOGENIC CANCER

Case	*Patient*	*Age*	*Sex*	*Site*	*Morphologic Abnormality*	*Delayed Clearance*
1	W.K.	57	M	LUL	−	+
2	R.P.	26	M	Bronchus intermedius	+	+
3	M.H.	57	F	Apical-posterior segment, LUL	+	+
4	L.V.	30	M	Left main stem bronchus	+	Not done
5	W.J.	47	M	LUL	−	−

* Astra Pharmaceutical Products, Inc., Worcester, Mass.
** Fansteel Corporation, Baltimore, Md.
*** No. 175, The DeVilbiss Company, Somerset, Pa.
**** Medi-Tech Division, Cooper Scientific Corporation, Watertown, Mass.

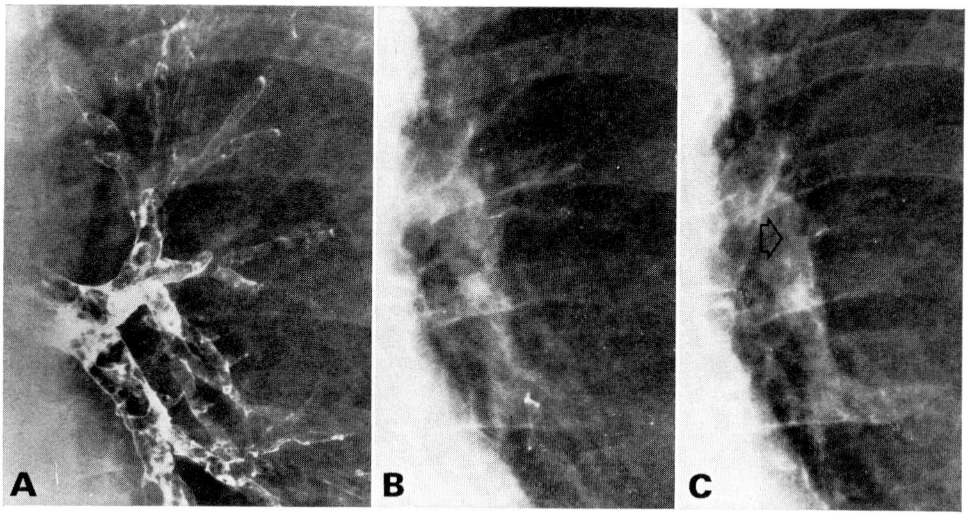

Fig. 2. Case 1. W.K. A) AP tantalum bronchogram of the left lung. No definite morphologic abnormality is demonstrated. There is moderate mucus and diffuse irregular mucosal irregularity suggestive of bronchitis. B) 24-hour clearance radiograph. Small linear collection of tantalum in the left upper lobe. Minimal tantalum coated mucus in the left lower lobe. C) 48-hour clearance radiograph. Linear delayed clearance by a bronchogenic carcinoma in the left upper lobe (arrow). There is no residual tantalum in the left lower lobe.

radiographs were obtained. A cine examination of all regions of the tracheobronchial tree in deep inspiration and deep expiration was also obtained. PA and lateral chest radiographs were obtained at 24, 48, 72, and 96 hours after the bronchogram. Areas of delayed clearance were identified by comparison to adjacent airways of similar caliber.

RESULTS

From 1972 through 1974 we have studied five patients with bronchogenic carcinoma and normal chest radiographs. Three patients had squamous carcinoma, one had oat cell carcinoma, and one had a bronchial carcinoid. In four of these, the area of occult malignancy was localized by tantalum bronchography. Localization of the malignancy was either by morphologic abnormalities in the airways or by delayed clearance by the bronchogenic carcinoma. Two patients showed both morphologic abnormalities and delayed clearance (Table I). The delayed clearance was most obvious on the 48-hour clearance films. In this small group of patients, cine examination of the airways was not helpful in localization. We anticipate that in more invasive lesions there will be focal alteration in bronchial dynamics.

CASE REPORTS

Two representative cases are described below. Case 3 (M.H.) has been described in detail previously.[3]

Case 1. (No morphologic abnormality, delayed clearance). The patient (W.K.) is a 57-year-old white male. Two years earlier the patient had a right lower lobe resection for bronchogenic carcinoma. The patient returned with a positive sputum cytology. PA and lateral chest radiograph and full chest tomography showed only signs of the previous resection. On the right side, tantalum bronchography demonstrated only the previous surgical procedure. On the left side, no definite morphologic abnormality was seen on the initial bronchogram (Fig. 2A). The 24-hour film showed minimally retained tantalum in the left upper lobe bronchus and the left posterior basal bronchus (Fig. 2B). The 48-hour clearance films showed a linear area of retained tantalum only in the left upper lobe bronchus (Fig. 2C). Subsequent bronchoscopy and thoracotomy confirmed this as the only site of bronchogenic carcinoma.

Case 2. (Morphologic abnormality and delayed clearance). The patient (R.P.) is a 26-year-old white male that presented with

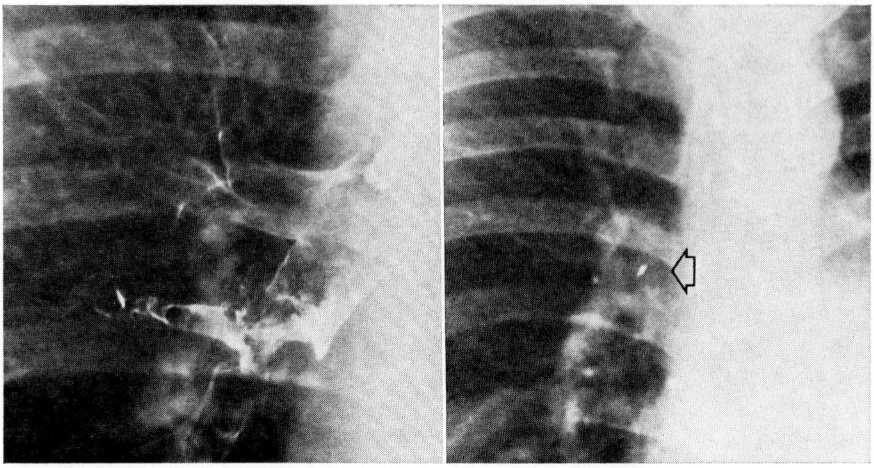

Fig. 3. Case 2. R.P. A) AP bronchogram, right lung. Large mass in the bronchus intermedius. B) Focal delayed clearance on the area of bronchial carcinoid (arrow).

intermittent wheezing of two year's duration. One year earlier a Dionosil®* bronchogram at another hospital had shown minimal irregularity of the bronchus intermedius. Bronchoscopy and biopsy at that time revealed only minimal granulation tissue. Treatment with corticosteroids resulted in no significant improvement. Bilateral tantalum bronchography demonstrated a mass in the bronchus intermedius (Fig. 3A). Forty-eight hour clearance films showed retained tantalum on the mass (Fig. 3B). Subsequent bronchoscopy and thoracotomy confirmed the mass to be a bronchial carcinoid.

DISCUSSION

In 1968, Nadel introduced powdered tantalum as an experimental contrast agent for bronchography.[4] Since 1969, we have been coinvestigators in the study of tantalum bronchography in humans. Our initial hope that a good quality double contrast bronchogram could be performed without significantly altering pulmonary function was realized.[3,5] In localizing radiologically occult tumors we had anticipated that the fine mucosal detail afforded by tantalum would be the major means of detecting these early malignancies. Since tantalum powder is cleared solely by mucociliary action, early bronchogenic carcinomas which interrupt mucociliary flow, should demonstrate delayed clearance.

Many factors can alter mucociliary clearance. These include: 1) impaired ciliary function; 2) altered mucus secretion; 3) obstruction; 4) trauma; 5) local inflammation; and 6) pharmacologic agents.

Impaired Mucociliary Function and Altered Mucus Secretion. In 1973 Gamsu *et al* reported a case of bronchogenic carcinoma demonstrated by tantalum bronchography that showed delayed clearance. He reported " . . . the delay appeared out of proportion to the degree of bronchial narrowing. Tantalum was also retained in the area of the carcinoma."[6] We believe his case and our three demonstrate delayed clearance due to a destroyed ciliated epithelium. Our concept of tracheobronchial mucociliary clearance postulates the following mechanism: 1) Cilia beat in a thin periciliary fluid which reaches just beyond the cilia tips; 2) In the peripheral pulmonary airways, beyond the region where goblet cells normally appear, surface materials are very slowly cleared in this fluid; 3) In bronchi where goblet cells begin, small patches of mucus appear on the surface of this fluid and, as they are swept along, they carry with them surface materials; and 4) As we proceed up the

* Glaxo Laboratories, Ltd., Greenford, Middlesex, England. Distributed by Picker Corp., Cleveland, Ohio.

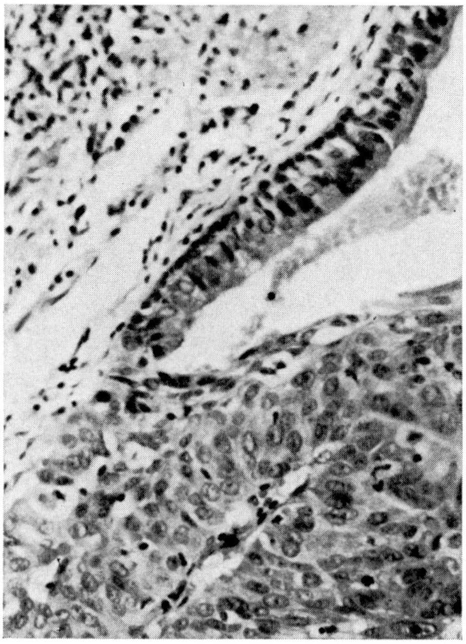

Fig. 4. High power photomicrograph of *in situ* squamous carcinoma with abrupt alteration from normal mucosa.

airway, mucous glands appear and add to the frequency and size of the mucus patches, and the clearance of surface materials becomes more rapid. In the region where most early bronchogenic cancers begin, clearance is by the method mentioned in 3 and 4 above.

Interference with clearance can result from impaired ciliary activity or alterations in airway secretions. Each bronchial spur interferes with clearance as the mucus stream must deviate from its path to circumvent these areas. Small areas of poor clearance may lead to penetration of some materials into underlying cells, and thus may be a factor in lung and laryngeal cancer pathogenesis. But, surface particles at such areas are caught up by mucus flowing nearby and cleared. Only when the size of a dead spot reaches sufficient dimensions, possibly one mm or more, will surface particle retention be significantly prolonged.

In carcinoma *in situ* there is a small sharply defined contiguous area where cilia disappear and airway secretions are probably altered (Fig. 4). When this area becomes large enough, prolonged retention of a surface material such as tantalum will ensue. We failed to localize one bronchogenic carcinoma. At bronchoscopy it was a 2 mm area of squamous carcinoma. This lesion has not been removed, though we expect the total extent of epithelial destruction is very small.

Twelve patients with gravely atypical cells in their sputum have been studied by tantalum bronchography. The initial bronchogram showed varying degrees of bronchitis. Three of these patients had minimal delayed clearance. We feel that these few false positives are acceptable as the areas biopsied at bronchoscopy often showed severe squamous metaplasia. These areas are the most severely damaged by inhaled carcinogens and presumably would be the site of early bronchogenic carcinoma. Cancer was not found at bronchoscopy in any of these 12 patients. None have developed bronchogenic carcinoma in a two to three year follow-up period.

Bronchiectasis which destroys a large contiguous area of epithelium has also been shown to exhibit delayed clearance.[7] The destruction in bronchitis is often spotty, ill-defined, and noncoalescent. Clearance from these areas occasionally can be delayed but is usually grossly normal. These very small areas probably do not effectively alter overall mucociliary clearance. The tantalum is probably removed by neighboring mucus streams.

Obstruction. Obstruction will delay mucociliary clearance. This type of delayed clearance is usually seen as tantalum coated mucus distal to the obstruction. The fine linear area of delayed clearance by early bronchogenic carcinoma is quite dissimilar radiologically. To evaluate further the role of obstruction in delayed clearance by carcinoma, we compared the clearance in a patient with subglottic carcinoma of the trachea, to that of a patient with a similar degree of obstruction due to

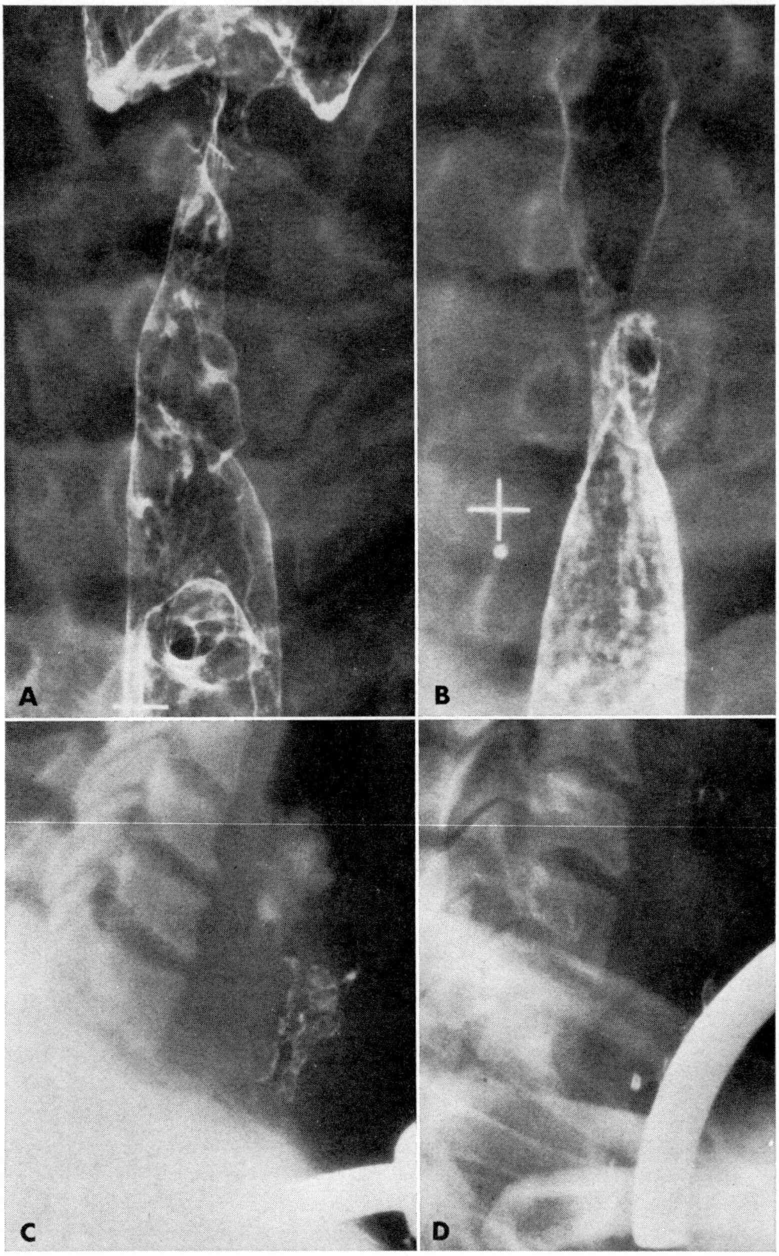

Fig. 5. Comparison of tracheal carcinoma to tracheal stenosis. AP tracheogram: A) Carcinoma. B) Tracheal stenosis. The ring-like area below the narrowing is the tantalum coated tracheostomy tube tract seen enface. Six hour lateral clearance radiograph. C) Tracheal carcinoma has tantalum demarcating the carcinoma from the normal mucosa. D) The subglottic stenosis has minimal tantalum coated mucus distal to the narrowing.

tracheal stenosis secondary to prolonged endotracheal tube intubation (Figs. 5A, B, C and D). The carcinoma of the trachea shows complete clearance by the surrounding normal mucosa. In the patient with subglottic tracheal stenosis there is minimal retained tantalum. This retained tantalum is in the form of tantalum coated mucus distal to the tracheal stenosis.

Trauma. The work of Wood *et al*[8] indicated that the trauma produced by catheter techniques can significantly alter mucociliary clearance of tantalum in dogs. All of our patients were studied without prior localization of the cancer. Trauma from the catheter may have played a role in the delayed clearance in Case 2 where there was a large endobronchial mass. In the other patients the morphologic abnormality, if present, was not detected during insufflation under fluoroscopy. Subsequently, catheter repositioning to insure a complete bilateral bronchogram was performed in all of these patients. The trauma therefore was presumably identical in all regions of the major bronchi.

Local Inflammation. Localized infection, such as pneumonia, has been shown to significantly alter mucociliary clearance.[9] We feel that infection was not a cause of delayed mucociliary clearance in the patients presented in this report. No patient had radiologic or clinical evidence of pneumonia before the procedure or in the subsequent week. The delayed clearance demonstrated with acute infection represents an "alveolarization" of the contrast material rather than a focal linear area of delayed clearance as demonstrated by the destroyed mucociliary epithelium.

Pharmacologic Agents. Pharmacologic agents play a role in slowing the clearance of tantalum from the airways. However, these agents should have a diffuse effect and should not cause the focal delayed clearance as shown in our patients.

SUMMARY

Tantalum bronchography both by its fine mucosal detail and physiologic assessment of mucociliary clearance may play a significant role in localizing radiologically occult bronchogenic carcinomas. Tantalum bronchography does not establish a tissue diagnosis, but it does allow the bronchoscopist confronted with the problem of a positive cytology and a negative chest radiograph, to concentrate his efforts on an area or areas of suspicion. The time of bronchoscopic search for radiologically occult malignancy can be significantly shortened by careful evaluation of the tantalum bronchogram and subsequent clearance films.

Request for reprints should be sent to Frederick P. Stitik, M.D., Department of Radiology, The Johns Hopkins Hospital, 601 North Broadway, Baltimore, Md. 21205

REFERENCES

1. Carbone PP, Frost JK, Feinstein AR, *et al*: Lung cancer: perspectives and prospects. Ann Intern Med 73:1003-1024, 1970

2. Baker RR, Marsh BR, Frost JK, *et al*: The detection and treatment of early lung cancer. Ann Surg 179:813-818, 1974

3. Stitik FP, Swift DL, Proctor DF: Bronchography with the experimental contrast agent tantalum, in Johnston R (ed): *Pulmonary Care.* New York, Grune and Stratton Inc., 1973

4. Nadel JA, Wolfe WG, Graf PD: Powdered tantalum as a medium for bronchography in canine and human beings. Invest Radiol 3:229-238, 1968

5. Nadel JA, Wolfe WG, Graf PD, *et al*: Powdered tantalum: a new contrast medium for roentgenographic examination of human airways. N Engl J Med 283:281-286, 1970

6. Gamsu G, Weintraub RM, Nadel JA: Clearance of tantalum from airways of different caliber in man evaluated by a roentgenographic method. Am Rev Respir Dis 107:219, 1973

7. Gamsu G, Weintraub RM, Nadel JA: Clearance of tantalum from airways of different caliber in man evaluated by a roentgenographic method. Am Rev Respir Dis 107: 214-224, 1973

8. Wood PB, Nagy E, Pearson FG, *et al*: Measurement of mucociliary clearance from the lower respiratory tract of normal dogs. Anaesth Soc J 20:192-206, 1973

9. Friedman PJ, Tisi GM: "Alveolarization" of tantalum powder in experimental bronchography and the clearance of inhaled particles from the lung. Radiology 104:523-535, 1972

Ann Otol 84: 1975

TRANSBRONCHIAL LUNG BIOPSY THROUGH THE FIBEROPTIC BRONCHOSCOPE IN DIFFUSE LUNG DISEASE

LEE R. JOYNER, M.D.

DAVID J. SCHEINHORN, M.D.

WASHINGTON, D.C.

SUMMARY – Transbronchial forceps biopsy (TBB) of the lung through the fiberoptic bronchoscope was performed in 74 patients. A histological diagnosis compatible with the clinical course, and roentgenographic appearance was obtained in 47 (64%) patients. There were six cases with inadequate tissue and ten cases where TBB was both nondiagnostic and of no other benefit in the subsequent management of the patient. This procedure was of particular value in evaluation of acutely ill patients with diffuse parenchymal disease. TBB either gave a specific diagnosis or correctly influenced patient management in 14 (89%) of 16 acutely ill patients with diffuse parenchymal disease. There was no uncontrollable hemorrhage; in one patient (15%) pneumothorax occurred. The safety and diagnostic value of this technique in the diagnosis of diffuse lung disease is proven.

Lung tissue is frequently required for a definitive diagnosis in cases of diffuse lung disease. We have recently reported the adaptation of the transbronchial lung biopsy (TBB) technique of Andersen and Fontana[1] for use with the flexible fiberoptic bronchoscope.[2] It is felt that this technique will become the procedure of choice in the initial evaluation of patients with diffuse lung disease. Open biopsy should be reserved for patients with a nondiagnostic TBB and a clinical situation or course which requires definitive diagnosis. This paper reports the results of 74 TBB in both acute and chronic diffuse lung disease encountered by our pulmonary service in an 18 month period.

METHODS AND MATERIALS

Twenty-six outpatients and 48 inpatients were biopsied. Patients were selected on the basis of a chest roentgenogram showing diffuse parenchymanl involvement without prior tissue diagnosis. In most patients the involvement was bilateral although patients with diffuse involvement of a single side were also included. Patients with limited, segmental disease were not biopsied. One exception was patients who were felt to have sarcoidosis. Some of these patients had bilateral hilar adenopathy without visible parenchymal disease on chest x-ray. Biopsies were not performed in patients felt to have significant pulmonary hypertension, a clinical bleeding diathesis, or a sufficiently unstable ventilatory condition such that pneumothorax would result in unmanagable decompensation. The procedure for transbronchial biopsy has been described elsewhere.[2]

Patient preparation included no food for at least five hours prior to biopsy, coagulation studies, and supplemental oxygen at the time of biopsy if the resting PO_2 was less than 60 torr. At least three biopsies were done on each patient to insure adequate alveolar tissue. Extra samples were obtained in special cases when additional diagnostic procedures were desirable, *i.e.,* lung tissue was cultured for AFB and fungi with special stains in cases of suspected diffuse granulomatous disease or opportunistic infection and lung tissue was studied with electron microscopy and immunofluorescence in cases of suspected dust or autoimmune disease.

Chest x-rays were obtained immediately after biopsy and were repeated 24 hours later to check for pneumothorax. Outpatients were allowed to go home after the postbiopsy x-ray was reviewed and returned to normal activities

From the Pulmonary Disease Service, Walter Reed Army Medical Center, Washington, D.C.

Presented at the meeting of the American Broncho-Esophagological Association, Atlanta, Georgia, April 7-8, 1975.

TABLE I

RESULTS OF TRANSBRONCHIAL BIOPSY OF THE LUNG IN 74 PATIENTS

Diagnosis Confirmed by TBB	*Acutely Ill**	*Chronically Ill*	*Total No.*
Usual interstitial pneumonia	2	12	14
Sarcoidosis	2	11	13
Pneumocystis carinii pneumonia	4	1	5
Radiation pneumonitis	1	2	3
Lymphangitic carcinoma (Histology Shown in Fig. 1)	0	2	2
Goodpasture's syndrome	0	2	2
Histoplasmosis	2	0	2
Aspiration pneumonia	1	0	1
Idiopathic pulmonary hemosiderosis	0	1	1
Lymphosarcoma	1	0	1
Pigeon breeder's lung	0	1	1
Acute diffuse alveolar damage	1	0	1
Lipoid pneumonia	0	1	1
Clinical Diagnosis at Time of Biopsy in Patients with Negative TBB			
R/O *Pneumocystis carinii* pneumonia**	8	0	8
Sarcoidosis	0	11	11
Hodgkin's disease	0	1	1
Alveolar cell carcinoma+	1	0	1+
Metastatic carcinoma	0	1	1
Lymphocarcinoma	1	0	1
TOTAL	24	46	70++

* Symptomatic for less than two weeks.

** None subsequently were proven to have pneumocystic by other techniques and none were treated empirically for pneumocystis. Four had rise in titer for cytomegalovirus and three were receiving drugs capable of causing interstitial disease.

\+ Proven with open biopsy.

++ Four with inadequate tissue for biopsy making total number biopsied 74.

if no pneumothorax was present at 24 hours. All histopathologic specimens were reviewed by the authors, the Pathology Department at Walter Reed Army Medical Center, and in some cases, the Lung Branch of the Armed Forces Institute of Pathology.

RESULTS

A histopathological diagnosis compatible with the clinical course and roentgenographic appearance was obtained in 47 of 74 patients (64%). Even with our multiple specimen technique, there were six cases with inadequate alveolar tissue for evaluation. A diagnostic accuracy of 70% was obtained when these cases were excluded (47 of 68 biopsies with adequate tissue). In spite of what was considered to be adequate tissue, there were ten cases in which TBB was both nondiagnostic and of no other benefit in the subsequent management of the patient. The results are summarized in Table I.

COMPLICATIONS

As reported earlier, transbronchial lung biopsy through the fiberoptic bronchoscope has a very low attendant morbidity.[2] Andersen, *et al*[3] in over 500 cases of transbronchial lung biopsy through the rigid bronchoscope reported 11% incidence of pneumothorax with less than 1% incidence of significant bleeding. The biopsy forceps employed with the fiberoptic scope is smaller and not serrated. Levin, *et al*[4] reported no

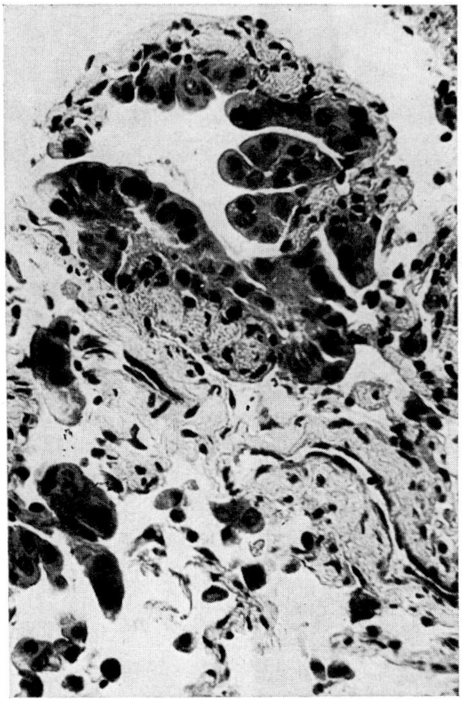

Fig. 1. Metastatic Adenocarcinoma. Adenocarcinoma cells seen lining alveolar walls and lying free in alveolar spaces. Chest film showed diffuse picture of mixed alveolar/interstitial infiltrates. (Metastatic breast carcinoma) 400X.

significant complications in 33 patients using the flexible fiberoptic bronchoscope, and we have had a single pneumothorax with 74 biopsies. It has become our policy to avoid even mild sedation in our patients to insure maximal cooperation at the time of biopsy.

We also have had no cases of uncontrollable hemorrhage. The "routine biopsy" results in a small amount of blood visible immediately in the subsegmental orifice from which the biopsy was taken. This blood can usually be cleared with suction prior to the next biopsy. On four occasions, there was immediate, explosive hemorrhage of greater than 100 ml, requiring that the procedure be terminated. Two of four specimens obtained at the time of hemoptysis showed a more sizable vessel than routinely encountered. The third patient had a platelet count of less than 20,000 with platelet transfusion prior to biopsy. In the fourth case, there was no explanation for the increased bleeding. No special measures were employed, and in each case the hemoptysis terminated spontaneously without harm to the patient.

Three patients had platelet counts less than 20,000 at the time of biopsy but were felt to have acceptable coagulation properties if transfused with fresh platelets prior to biopsy by our hematology service. In each case, there existed life-threatening acute diffuse lung disease with a high suspicion of opportunistic infection. In addition, two biopsies were performed with patients on volume ventilators at the time of biopsy without complications.

DISCUSSION

The efficacy of transbronchial lung biopsy through the fiberoptic bronchoscope now seems well established. Levin, *et al*[4] showed a high correlation (73%) between results of TBB and open lung biopsy in 15 cases subjected to both procedures. Although the specimens obtained are small, many cases of diffuse lung disease are sufficiently diffuse for even small samples to be diagnostic. In addition, the ability to take multiple specimens compensates significantly for the small size of individual biopsies.

Pneumocystis Carinii Pneumonia. Acute diffuse lung disease was encountered in 16 patients with a compromised immune status. These were either patients with malignancy reeiving chemotherapy or renal transplant recipients. In each, the difficult differential of opportunistic infection, drug induced lung disease, and diffuse lung malignancy existed. In five patients, a diagnosis of *Pneumocystis carinii* was established by TBB with 100% recovery on pentamidine therapy (Fig. 2). There were no "false negatives" and no empiric treatment for pneumocystis was given when TBB was negative. It was our policy to biopsy all patients suspected of having pneumocystis as soon as this diagnosis was

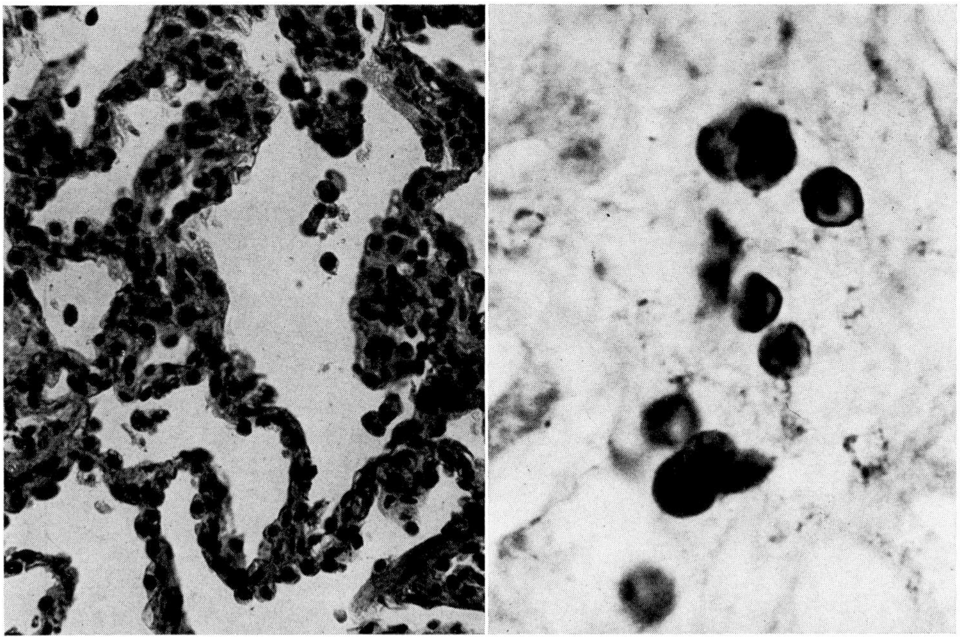

Fig. 2. A) *Pneumocystis Carinii* Pneumonia. Lung tissue showing diffuse increase in cellularity, *i.e.,* interstital pneumonitis with thickening of alveolar septa. 110X. B) *Pneumocystis Carinii* Pneumonia. Gomors methenamine silver stain of the same specimen showing *Pneumocystis Carinii* organism. 400X.

deemed remotely possible. Our experience was similar to others[5] in that pneumocystis was correctly diagnosed before absolute changes in chest x-ray had occurred in two patients. A third patient represented a more chronic course of pneumocystis in a renal transplant recipient with low grade fever, dry cough, and slowly progressive chest x-ray changes over a one-month period.

Of the remaining 11 patients, a diagnosis was subsequently established in eight. Four showed an acute interstitial pneumonitis on biopsy with rise in titer for cytomegalovirus. All four recovered without specific therapy. Two patients were felt to have diffuse parenchymal involvement with lymphosarcoma. In one, the lung biopsy showed lymphocytes diffusely throughout the interstitium of the lung with invasion of the bronchial mucosa also obtained with transbronchial biopsy. In the second, there was also an increase in interstitial lymphocytes but not to the extent suggesting diffuse lympho-sarcomatous involvement of lung. The interstitial picture resolved with blenomycin therapy. A classic picture of acute diffuse alveolar damage (Fig. 3) was encountered in a young patient with Hodgkin's disease following Gram negative sepsis and shock. This was felt to represent the early pathological change of shock lung. The subsequent course was that of an adult respiratory distress syndrome ending in death. No other explanation for the diffuse lung problem was found at autopsy.

In four patients, TBB showed essentially normal lung. Three of the four either resolved their x-ray abnormality or failed to progress during the period of follow-up. These patients were felt to represent either viral pneumonia or drug-induced lung disease. In the two patients in this group with residual change on x-ray, drugs capable of causing interstitial fibrosis were discontinued. One of these two patients underwent open lung biopsy which also showed a nonspecific interstitial re-

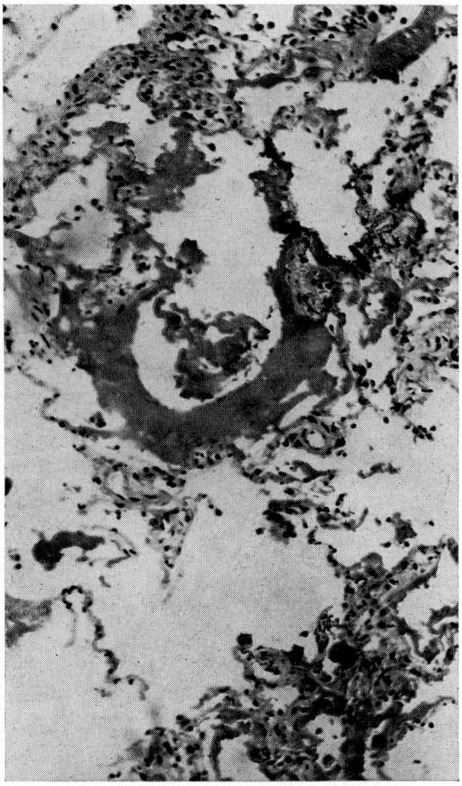

Fig. 3. Shock Lung. Fragments of lung showing diffuse thickening of alveolar walls with hyalin membrane formation. (Shock lung with diffuse alveolar damage — etiology gram negative sepsis.) 110X.

action. The fourth patient was a 29-year-old renal transplant recipient with progressive alveolar infiltrates. Subsequent open biopsy showed alveolar cell carcinoma, apparently reflecting the increased propensity for malignancy with immunosuppressive therapy.

In this very difficult diagnostic group, TBB either gave a specific diagnosis or correctly influenced patient management in 14 of the 16 patients. Of specific note is the exclusion of pneumocystis from the four patients with cytomegalovirus infection since these two infections frequently coexist.[6] In two patients TBB was misleading. Both patients had a subsequent clinical course inconsistent with the biopsy picture leading to empiric therapy with blenomycin in probable lymphosarcoma of the lung and to open lung biopsy in the case of the alveolar cell carcinoma.

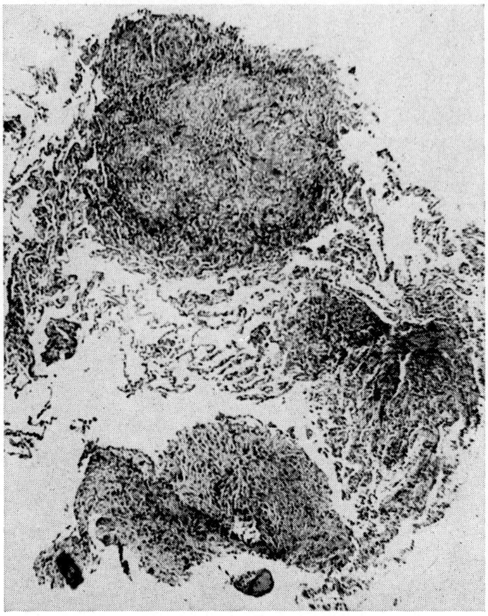

Fig. 4. Sarcoidosis. Noncaseating granulomas within lung showing considerable crush artifact. 110X.

Sarcoidosis. Sarcoidosis was the clinical diagnosis in 24 patients. There were two biopsies with inadequate tissue and 13 positive biopsies (Fig. 4) for a diagnostic accuracy of 60%. The most common x-ray pattern in patients with positive biopsies was bilateral hilar adenopathy (BHA) without parenchymal disease visible radiographically (8/13). Four of the five remaining patients with positive biopsies had stage II disease (BHA + interstitial disease) with one positive biopsy in a patient presenting with stage III disease (interstitial disease only. These data again demonstrate that sarcoidosis has a high incidence of lung parenchymal involvement in the presence of clear chest x-rays and that the granulomatosis is sufficiently diffuse to allow diagnosis with a small biopsy. These data probably do not truly indicate that patients with BHA only on chest x-ray (stage I) are more likely to have a positive TBB. It just happened that most of our patients (15/24) presented with stage I involvement. We recommend TBB before liver biopsy and mediastinoscopy in suspected cases of sarcoidosis. The diagnostic yield of 60% is somewhat less than liver biopsy but should be more specific, and when a positive biopsy is obtained, it avoids the risk of general anesthesia and suprasternal scar resulting from mediastinoscopy.

Goodpasture's Syndrome and Idiopathic Pulmonary Hemosiderosis. We report two patients with Goodpasture's syndrome and one patient with idiopathic pulmonary hemosiderosis (IPH). All presented very similar clinical histories with recurrent hemoptysis and fleeting bilateral alveolar densities on chest x-ray over a two- to three-year period. The patient with IPH showed no evidence of renal involvement and both patients with Goodpasture's had received previous renal biopsies showing characteristic linear immunofluorescence. H. and E. stain of the specimens obtained showed essentially normal lung in all three patients except for hemosiderin-laden macrophages in the alveolar spaces, particularly abundant in the patient with IPH. Immunofluorescent linear deposits on the alveolar basement membrane with anti-complement and anti-immunoglobulin G stains were easily demonstrated in two of the three cases.

Lipoid Pneumonia. Transbronchial biopsy was performed in a 72-year-old male with chronic alveolar infiltrates in both lower lobes near the cardiac silhouette. The histology showed the alveolar spaces to be filled with large macrophages. The macrophages contained numerous intracytoplasmic vacuoles with positive staining for lipid. The patient related a long history of mineral oil ingestion, and barium swallow showed free reflux of the barium meal high into the esophagus. We feel that diffuse alveolar filling diseases are particularly amenable to diagnosis with TBB.

SUMMARY

Transbronchial lung biopsy through the fiberoptic bronchoscope is easily accomplished, has low morbidity, and is of value as a diagnostic aid in a great variety of diffuse lung diseases. We feel that it was of greatest benefit in our management of patients with acute diffuse disease. In this group, clinicians in the past have been reluctant to obtain lung tissue because of the morbidity of the procedures available. TBB was highly effective in diagnosing *Pneumocystis carinii* pneumonia (100% in our patients), and we feel it is the procedure of choice for this infection in the adult. In sarcoidosis it is an attractive, initial procedure with advantages over liver biopsy and mediastinoscopy. In the past several years, thoracic surgery assisted our medical service with 10-15 open biopsies each year. During the 18 months of this study, open biopsy was necessary on two occasions.

Request for reprints should be sent to Lee R. Joyner, M.D., Maj. MC, 435-60-2900, Chief, Pulmonary Disease Service, Tripler General Hospital, Honolulu, Hawaii.

REFERENCES

1. Andersen HA, Fontana RS: Transbronchoscopic lung biopsy in diffuse pulmonary disease. Chest 48:187-192, 1965

2. Joyner LR, Scheinhorn DJ: Chest. To be published

3. Andersen HA, Miller WE, Bernat PE: Lung biopsy: Transbronchoscopic, percutaneous, open. Surg Clin North Am 53:785-793, 1973

4. Levin DC, Wicks AB, Ellis JH: Transbronchial lung biopsy via the fiberoptic bronchoscope. Am Rev Resp Dis 110:4-12, 1974

5. Friedman BA, *et al*: Roentgenographically atypical *Pneumocystis carinii* pneumonia. Am Rev Resp Dis 111:89-96, 1975

6. Goodell B, Jacobs JB, Powell RD, *et al*: *Pneumocystis carinii*: The spectrum of diffuse interstitial pneumonia in patients with neoplastic disease. Ann Intern Med 72:337-340, 1970

Ann Otol 84: 1975

CLINICAL EXPERIENCE WITH PLEUROSCOPY UTILIZING THE BRONCHOFIBERSCOPE

GERALD R. KERBY, M.D.

GEORGE PIERCE, M.D. WILLIAM E. RUTH, M.D.

KANSAS CITY, KANSAS

SUMMARY – The gas sterilized bronchofiberscope has been utilized as a pleuroscope for visual exploration of the pleural space and forceps biopsy of abnormal lesions in 16 patients with undiagnosed pleural disease. The instrument was inserted through a small (1-2 cm) incision. Aspiration of pleural fluid and instillation or aspiration of air to produce a controlled pneumothorax are easily accomplished through the instrument's suction channel. In eight patients with undiagnosed pleural effusion, biopsy of visualized nodules established the diagnosis of carcinoma. Three patients with bronchogenic carcinoma and pleural effusion had no pleural metastases at pleuroscopy which was confirmed in two patients who had thoracotomy and lung resection. Parenchymal subpleural nodules of metastatic carcinoma were confirmed by pleuroscopic biopsy in one patient. Biopsy via the pleuroscope was unsuccessful in two patients, one with pleural fibrosis, probably related to asbestosis, and one with mesothelioma. Both required open surgical biopsy of the pleura. There has been minimal patient discomfort and no serious complications.

Thoracoscopy was originally introduced by Jacobeus for lysis of pleural adhesions during pneumothorax therapy for pulmonary tuberculosis.[1] The diagnostic use of pleuroscopy was described by Branco,[2] and subsequently several reports confirmed the high diagnostic yield of the procedure in patients with pleural effusion.[3-7]

Despite these reports, pleuroscopy has not been generally included in the approach to the patient with pleural disease. The reasons are unclear but may relate to lack of widespread availability of instruments and also that their caliber and rigid nature limited the range of observation.

The flexible fiberoptic bronchoscope has recently acquired widespread popularity and use in the diagnosis of bronchopulmonary disease. Its size and flexibility have significantly increased the diagnostic yield from bronchofibroscopy as compared to examination by rigid bronchoscopy. The size and flexibility of the instrument are also advantageous in exploration of the pleural space. The widespread availability of these instruments may reawaken interest in pleuroscopy. In addition to our early experience,[8] others have reported on the bronchofiberscope in exploration of the pleural space.[9,10] The present report relates our experience with the technique in sixteen patients.

METHODS AND MATERIALS

Patients were selected because of undiagnosed pleural disease after the usual studies on pleural fluid and/or needle biopsy with the Abrams needle.* One patient was examined because of postoperative bronchopleural fistula following an upper lobe lobec-

* Abrams Instrument Corp., Lansing, Michigan.

From the Division of Pulmonary Disease, Departments of Medicine and Surgery, University of Kansas School of Medicine, Kansas City, Kansas.

Supported by NIH Grants 5 K07 HL 70073 and 3 T01 HL05991.

Presented at the meeting of the American Broncho-Esophagological Association, Atlanta, Georgia, April 7-8, 1975.

tomy for carcinoma of the lung to determine whether or not the resection line was free of tumor. Another patient developed a peripheral pleural based lesion after nephrectomy for renal cell carcinoma. One patient with cervical carcinoma had pleural thickening without fluid. Thirteen patients had undiagnosed pleural effusion.

A bronchofiberscope* was used for the procedure after gas sterilization. Fifteen of the procedures were carried out in the operating room, 12 with local anesthesia, and 3 with general anesthesia. In one patient, who had a thoracostomy tube for a bronchopleural fistula, pleuroscopy was performed through the chest tube in the intensive care unit with no anesthesia.

The patients were placed either in a sitting position or in a lateral thoracotomy position. The site of insertion was usually along the posterior axillary line. After skin preparation and draping, the site was infiltrated with local anesthetic. A 1 to 2 cm incision was made in the skin and a purse-string suture of No. "0" silk placed around it. With sharp dissection the incision was extended through the intercostal muscles. By blunt dissection the pleural space was entered. The sterilized bronchofiberscope was then inserted into the pleural space with the purse-string ligature maintaining an airtight seal. Pleural fluid was removed through the suction channel of the bronchoscope for appropriate studies and to clear the pleural space. Air was introduced as needed through the suction channel to produce a small controlled pneumothorax for better visualization. The pleural space was then systematically explored visually with the bronchofiberscope. Since landmarks are few, the examination was somewhat random, but it was usually possible to visualize the entire costal surface of pleura and portions of the mediastinal and diaphragmatic pleural space. If a lesion was encountered, the biopsy forceps was inserted through the suction channel and a sample of the lesion was obtained for histopathological study and appropriate cultures. Several biopsies were usually taken. Still photographs were obtained to provide a permanent record of the lesions seen. Following examination, air was evacuated by suction through the bronchoscope; the bronchoscope was withdrawn, and the purse-string suture tied. A postpleuroscopy chest roentgenogram was obtained to determine the presence or absence of residual pneumothorax. Vital signs were monitored at frequent intervals for the next 24 hours.

RESULTS AND DISCUSSIONS

The results of pleuroscopy in 16 patients are summarized in Table I. The procedure provided a tissue diagnosis of malignancy in eight patients who were undiagnosed by pleural fluid cytology and/or needle biopsy. In these patients, the malignant implants visualized were scattered randomly over the pleural surface; therefore, it is not surprising that few exfoliated cells were present in the effusion and that random needle biopsy was unproductive. Pleuroscopy is probably of greatest value in these patients as it conclusively provides a diagnosis and avoids full scale thoracotomy which would otherwise be required.

As illustrated by the second group of patients, normal findings at pleuroscopy may also provide useful information in clinical management. In patients with pleural effusion who have radiographic or bronchoscopic findings of bronchogenic carcinoma, the question usually arises as to whether the effusion is due to malignant pleural implants or is inflammatory because of pneumonia distal to the tumor. Normal pleuroscopy permitted an attempt at curative surgical resection in two patients.

In two other patients with apparently benign pleural effusion, normal findings at pleuroscopy supported the decision for follow-up without therapy in one patient and with antituberculous therapy in another.

Pleuroscopic biopsy was unsuccessful in two patients who subsequently required open surgical biopsy to obtain adequate tissue for pathologic study. Both had thick pleural plaques, one from fibrosis and the other due to mesothelioma where the small biopsy forceps was technically unable to obtain an adequate specimen.

The complications have been relatively minimal. Pain after the procedure is likely related to removal of pleural fluid so that the visceral and parietal pleura oppose. The single residual pneumothorax was small and resolved without aspiration. The cause of fever is unclear. No subsequent infection has been encountered.

Our experience to date suggests that

* Model No. BF-5B-2, Olympus Corp. of America, New Hyde Park, N.Y.

TABLE I

RESULTS OF PLEUROSCOPY IN 16 PATIENTS

Pt	*Sex*	*Age*	*Problem*	*Pleural Fluid Cytology*	*Needle Pleural Biopsy*	*Pleuroscopy Visual*	*Pleuroscopy Biopsy*	*Complications*	*Subsequent Findings*
				A. Diagnosis Achieved by Pleuroscopy Biopsy					
FD	F	59	L. pleural effusion	Atypical cells nondiagnostic	Neg. X2	Nodules	Anaplastic carcinoma		
ED	F	54	L. pleural effusion	Neg.	Not done	Nodules	Anaplastic carcinoma	Fever small pneumo- thorax	
MV	F	49	R. pleural effusion	Atypical cells nondiagnostic	Neg. X2	Nodules	Adenocarcinoma or mesothelioma	Transitory pain & hypotension	
GH	M	62	R. pleural effusion	Carcinoma post procedure	Not done	Nodules	Poorly differentiated carcinoma		
MT	F	38	R. pleural effusion	Atypical nondiagnostic	Neg.	Occas. nodule	Adenocarcinoma signet-ring type		
GS	F	33	L. pleural effusion	Neg.	Not done	Nodules	Poorly differentiated carcinoma	Pain	
EB	F	60	L. pleural mass carcinoma cervix	No fluid	Not done	Pleural mass	Squamous cell carcinoma		
VE	M	55	L. lung mass prior renal carcinoma	No fluid	Not done	Nodules	Small cell carcinoma		

B. Negative Pleuroscopy - Subsequently Confirmed									
JF	M	63	R. pleural effusion & lung mass	Not done	Neg.	Neg.	Not done	Fever	R.U. lobectomy bronchogenic carcinoma no pleural involvement
HH	M	55	R. pleural effusion bronchogenic carcinoma	Neg.	Neg.	Neg.	Not done		Rt. pneumonectomy no pleural involvement
DH	M	41	R. pleural effusion ? chest trauma	Neg.	Neg.	Fibrinous adhesions	Chronic pleuritis		Effusion resolved no recurrence
AC	M	51	R. pleural effusion active pulm. TBC carcinoma pancreas	Neg.	Giant cell no granuloma	Adhesions inflam-mation	Chronic inflammation		Effusion resolving on TBC R_x
HS	M	65	Broncho-pleural fistula bronchogenic carcinoma			Neg.	Neg.		Patient died
C. Pleuroscopy Incorrect or Unconfirmed									
RT	M	62	Bilat. pleural effusion	Neg.	Neg.	Pleural plaques	Unsuccessful		Open biopsy pleural fibrosis ? asbestosis
FK	M	66	R. pleural effusion	Neg.	Reactive mesothelium	Large nodules	Reactive mesothelium		Open lung & pleural biopsy - mesothelioma
LR	M	71	R. pleural effusion	Not done	Neg.	Neg.	Not done		Findings not confirmed. Sub-sequent metastatic carcinoma to brain & liver

pleuroscopy is a useful adjunct in the diagnosis of pleural disease. The bronchofiberscope is generally available and provides an adequate instrument. The procedure is simple and the complications to date have been minimal.

Request for reprints should be sent to Gerald R. Kerby, M.D., Division of Pulmonary Disease, Department of Medicine, University of Kansas School of Medicine, Kansas City, Kansas 66103.

REFERENCES

1. Jacobeus HC: The cauterization of adhesions in artificial pneumothorax treatment of pulmonary tuberculosis under thorascopic control. Proc R Soc Med 16:45-62, 1923

2. Branco JMC: Thoracoscopy as a method of exploration in penetrating injuries of the thorax. Dis Chest 12:330-335, 1946

3. Bloomberg AE: Thoracoscopy in the diagnosis of pleural effusions. NY State J Med 70:1974-1977, 1970

4. Bergquist S, Nordenstrom H: Thoracoscopy and pleural biopsy in the diagnosis of pleurisy. Scand J Respir Dis 47:69-74, 1966

5. Hatch HB, DeCamp PT: Diagnostic thoracoscopy. Surg Clin North Am 46:1405-1410, 1966

6. Lloyd MS: Thoracoscopy and biopsy in the diagnosis of pleurisy with effusion. Q Bull Seaview Hosp 14:128-133, 1953

7. Fleishman SF, Lichter AI, Buchanan G, *et al*: Investigation of idiopathic pleural effusions by thoracoscopy. Thorax 11:324-327, 1956

8. Gwin E, Boggan M, Pierce G, *et al*: Pleuroscopy and pleural biopsy with the bronchofiberscope. Am Rev Respir Dis 109: 690, 1974

9. Senno A, Moallem S, Quijano ER, *et al*: Thoracoscopy with the fiberoptic bronchoscope: a simple method in diagnosing pleuropulmonary diseases. J Thorac Cardiovasc Surg 67:606-611, 1974

10. Ben Issac FE, Simmons DH: Fiberoptic pleuroscopy. Chest 64:388-389, 1973

EAR SURGERY COURSE

The J. Brown Farrior Ear Surgery Course will not be conducted in 1976. The next course will be held March 13-16, 1977.

PLASTIC SURGERY RESEARCH AWARDS

The American Academy of Facial Plastic and Reconstructive Surgery, Inc., invites entries in its annual competition for original research in head and neck plastic surgery.

The Ira J. Tresley Research Award consists of a $500 prize and is open to any physician who has been Board certified for three years or longer.

Residents and Fellows in otolaryngology are invited to compete for the annual Benjamin Shuster Memorial Awards offered for outstanding research papers. Papers can cover any clinical or research study in the field of plastic and reconstructive surgery of the head or neck. Only original, non-published papers will be considered. $250 is awarded for first prize and $100 for second prize.

Notification of intent to enter the competition must be sent to the Academy by November 30, 1975. All papers must be received by January 31, 1976, for final judging. Notice and paper should be sent to: G. Jan Beekhuis, M.D., 573 Fisher Bldg., Detroit, Michigan 48202.

Ann Otol 84: 1975

TREATMENT OF PAPILLOMATOSIS OF THE LARYNX WITH TRANSFER FACTOR

CEDRIC A. QUICK, M.D.   HANS W. BEHRENS, M.D.

MINNEAPOLIS, MINNESOTA

MARGO BRINTON-DARNELL, PH.D.   ROBERT A. GOOD, M.D.

MINNEAPOLIS, MINNESOTA   NEW YORK, NEW YORK

SUMMARY — Transfer factor was used in two patients with laryngeal papillomatosis in an attempt to influence the thymus dependent small lymphocytes to become immunologically effective in their attempt to control the lesions. Following transfer factor, therapy laboratory tests showed altered reactivity of the lymphocyte stimulation tests for delayed hypersensitivity, and the results of the *in vitro* lymphocyte cytotoxic assay suggested that transfer factor improved the ability of lymphocytes to kill the tumor cells. Clinically, a change in the skin responses to the tests of delayed hypersensitivity was observed, and a change in the endoscopic appearance of the lesions occurred. Histologically, the specimens showed a marked influx of immune cells when transfer factor was being administered. Finally there was a significant clinical improvement in the disease state.

The most common neoplasm of the larynx in children is the papilloma. Although classified histologically as a benign neoplasm, this tumor has proved to be quite resistant to current methods of surgical therapy. Untreated or uncontrolled, this tumor can spread throughout the larynx, the trachea, and the lower respiratory tract, leading to partial or complete airway obstruction. The patients, predominantly children, become respiratory cripples and require many hospital admissions for treatment of this condition.

Because of the lack of success in eradicating the tumor from the respiratory tract (and reflecting the frustrations of the physicians treating this disease), juvenile papillomatosis continues to be the subject of much clinical investigation. Antibiotics, hormones, electrocoagulation, ultrasound, cryotherapy, radiation, surgical excision, carbon dioxide laser beams, and autogenous vaccines have all been used with varying degrees of success. These methods have failed to consistently eradicate this neoplasm in all patients. At the present time, the usual method of controlling this disease is by some form of physical removal of the lesions.

A new immunological approach designed to arrest the growth and prevent the spread of papillomas was undertaken. This paper presents an initial report of the effect of transfer factor therapy in two cases of papillomatosis of the larynx.

ETIOLOGY

Laryngeal papillomas are thought to be produced by a tumorogenic double-stranded DNA containing virus belonging to the papova virus group. Although a virus has been isolated from several animal wart tissues and from human

From the Departments of Otolaryngology and Microbiology, The University of Minnesota, and from the Sloan-Kettering Institute, New York, New York.

Aided by Grants CA-08748 from the Immunobiology and American Cancer Society and Grants from the Minnesota Medical Foundation.

Presented at the meeting of the American Broncho-Esophagological Association, Atlanta, Georgia, April 7-8, 1975.

cutaneous papillomas,[1-3] virus isolation has not been reported from any human laryngeal papilloma. In spite of the failure to isolate a virus from laryngeal papilloma, clinical and histological similarities of these lesions to other papillomas provides circumstantial evidence that a papilloma virus of the papova virus group may be the causative agent.

Papova viruses can either cause a productive infection or transform cells into tumor cells. The genetic properties of the host cell are thought to determine which type of infection occurs. A productive infection results in death of the host cell and the release of progeny virus. In transformed cells viral DNA is probably replicated with the cell DNA and passed to both daughter cells at cell division.[4] These transformed cells produce no progeny virus, but because they are transformed, they multiply faster than normal cells. In the case of the papillomas it is likely that cells that allow transformation and cells which can support virus production are present in one lesion. Noyes has demonstrated that only the keratinized superficial cells of the Shope papilloma yield infectious virus.[5] It is possible that in certain environmental conditions, such as the process of cell death or physiologic stress, transformed cells may be changed to allow whole virus production to commence. This could explain why virus particles are only found histologically in the dead keratin layers of cutaneous papillomas. Since laryngeal papillomas do not have a well-defined keratin layer, this may be the reason that whole virus particles are rarely found in sections of surgical tissue.[6]

IMMUNOLOGICAL BACKGROUND

Lewis Thomas first postulated that in the survival of multicellular organisms, cell-mediated immunity had to be evolved if mutant cells or neoplastic cells were to be recognized as foreign cells.[7] This function has been called immunologic surveillance and further development of this theory by Burnett and others has led to a revival of interest in the immunological approach to treatment of neoplastic diseases.[8] The early attempts to demonstrate the involvement of cellular immunity in human neoplasms have been equivocal, one of the reasons being the difficulty in distinguishing and isolating the unique antigens on the tumor cell surface. However, the principle of surveillance is sound, and if these unique antigens were available, they could theoretically be used for immunization to enhance the host's ability to immunologically destroy the tumor cells.

The discovery by Landsteiner and Chase that delayed hypersensitivity could be transferred by cells from sensitized guinea pigs to nonsensitized guinea pigs has been explored extensively.[9] It is now known that a select group of cells called "thymus-dependent small lymphocytes" is responsible for these functions.[10]

Lawrence described the specific transfer of cutaneous hypersensitivity to tuberculin in man. A soluble extract of human leukocytes,[11] termed "transfer factor," was used. Such soluble, dialyzable extracts, containing active molecules of low molecular weight, have been shown to be as effective as whole leukocytes in transferring delayed cutaneous sensitivity and have the advantage of being nontoxic.

Transfer factor is not an immunoglobulin, and several studies have shown that it is not itself immunogenic since it does not induce formation of specific antibodies even when given in large amounts.[12]

The moiety within these extracts which is capable of transferring cellular immunity has not been identified, but it has been shown to resist inactivation by DNAase, RNAase, and trypsin. Thus, a molecule which does not appear to be an antibody, a DNA, or a single-stranded RNA has been found to possess the capacity for changing lymphocytes *in vivo* from the nonsensitized state to the sensitized state, thus, converting recipients from nonreactors to reactors.

Transfer factor has been used clinically in the therapy of immunodeficiency diseases, such as the Wiskott-Aldrich syndrome, mucocutaneous candidiasis, coccidiomycosis, and of malignancies, such as osteogenic sarcoma and malignant melanoma.[13,14]

It is an elementary principle that any new method of therapy should be evaluated experimentally. For this reason an *in vitro* assay model was developed using the techniques of tissue culture and a modification of the lymphocyte cytotoxicity assay.[15,16] The results of these laboratory experiments seemed to confirm that transfer factor could increase the cytotoxic effect of lymphocytes.[17] It was considered justifiable, therefore, to continue with the clinical experiments.

The immunological treatment of laryngeal papillomas with transfer factor was started at this institution in May 1973. Transfer factor was used in an attempt to influence the thymus-dependent small lymphocytes to become immunologically effective in their attempt to control the transformed cells of the laryngeal papilloma.

METHODS AND MATERIALS

Two patients were selected for transfer factor therapy. C.N. is a four-year-old child whose diagnosis of papillomatosis of the larynx was made at the age of one year. Since the initial diagnosis, the patient has been admitted to the hospital 38 times, and surgery has been necessary on 37 occasions. Papilloma recurrence, manifested by increased hoarseness and stridor, required surgical removal at four to five week intervals. D.S. is a 13-year-old female who developed the disease at the age of ten years. In this patient, the severity of the disease was not quite as marked, and laryngoscopy with removal of papillomas was necessary to relieve airway obstruction at intervals of approximately eight weeks.

In addition to the routine clinical evaluation, these children underwent full immunological screening tests. These tests consisted of quantitive immunoglobulins, total lymphocyte count with a percentage of small lymphocytes, PHA, NBT, liver function battery, full hemolytic complement studies, and skin tests to PPD, SK/SD, mumps, and trichophyton. In addition to the delayed hypersensitivity skin tests, *in vitro* lymphocyte challenge was performed using the same antigens.

Initially, transfer factor was made from the white cells contained in approximately 500 ml of whole blood obtained from the younger child's mother, who was chosen as a donor because she had a history of being successfully treated for lesions of condyloma acuminata which were present during pregnancy and delivery of the affected child. Subsequently, a more suitable donor was obtained. A 19-year-old female, with a ten-year history of the disease prior to a gradual remission of the lesions at puberty, was chosen. Transfer factor was subsequently prepared from lymphocytes obtained by continuous separation leukophoresis.* The lymphocytes were isolated by density gradient centrifugation using ficoll/Hypaque®.** Further preparation of the dialyzed transfer factor was performed by the method described by Levin and his coworkers.[18] Each dose consisted of the extract from 10^9 lymphocytes divided into 2-3 subcutaneous injections. Doses were given at weekly intervals and each patient received more than one series of doses. To date the first patient (C.N.) has received a total of 16 doses of transfer factor and the second patient (D.S.) a total of nine doses. The skin tests for delayed hypersensitivity and the *in vitro* lymphocyte challenge were repeated before and after administration of transfer factor.

RESULTS

Initial immunological screening showed normal humoral and cellular immune competence in each patient. The results of all other laboratory tests were also within normal limits. Skin testing with specific antigen showed that the mother of C.N. reacted to SK/SD, while the patient C.N. did not. *In vitro* lymphocyte stimulation demonstrated that while in both mother and child a normal positive response to PHA occurred, the mother's cells also responded to SK/SD, while those of the patient did not. Following therapy with transfer factor prepared from the mother, the child showed conversion of skin reactivity to a positive SK/SD response, as well as a positive *in vitro* lymphocyte response.[19] The second patient's (D.S.) skin tests showed positive reactivity to SK/SD, mumps, and trichophyton and a negative response to PPD. Following administration of transfer factor from the second donor,

---

* American Instrument Co., Silver Springs, Maryland.
** Winthrop Laboratories, New York, N.Y.

a conversion to a positive PPD skin test and positive *in vitro* lymphocyte stimulation by PPD was noted. Skin tests and *in vitro* lymphocytic stimulation tests were not repeated on the first patient (C.N.) when transfer factor from the second donor was given.

No side effects were noticed in the two patients following the administration of transfer factor. There was an occasional rise in temperature of one-half to one degree, but this subsided spontaneously without medication, and was felt to be of no significance. The initial treatment of patient C.N. was curtailed after three doses because the child developed rapid increase of respiratory difficulty, subsequently found to be due to the combined effect of papilloma regrowth and an upper respiratory tract infection and possibly not due to transfer factor. Subsequently, with the use of transfer factor from the second donor, a significant response in the clinical state of both children was observed. Whereas the laryngeal papillomas in patient C.N. previously had to be removed surgically at four-to-five-week intervals to maintain an adequate airway, the frequency of surgical excision was now reduced to eight-week intervals and never on an emergency basis. This elective surgery was performed for documentation of the course of the disease and because it was presumed that reduction of the tumor mass would make transfer factor therapy more effective. Similarly, the second patient also required less-frequent surgery.

Direct observation of the papillomas in the larynx at surgery, several weeks after transfer factor therapy, showed a significant change in the appearance of the papillomas. Prior to transfer factor therapy, all of the lesion appeared to have a rough surface and were of a pale pink color. They frequently had stalks and considerable resistance was encountered when removing them with laryngeal-cupped forceps. Following transfer factor therapy, the majority of the lesions were observed to have a glistening surface and were a dark pink color and much flatter. These tumor masses were very friable, bled easily, and were considerably less resistant to mechanical removal. However, other small papillomas which were of the original consistency were also present and seemed to be new lesions.

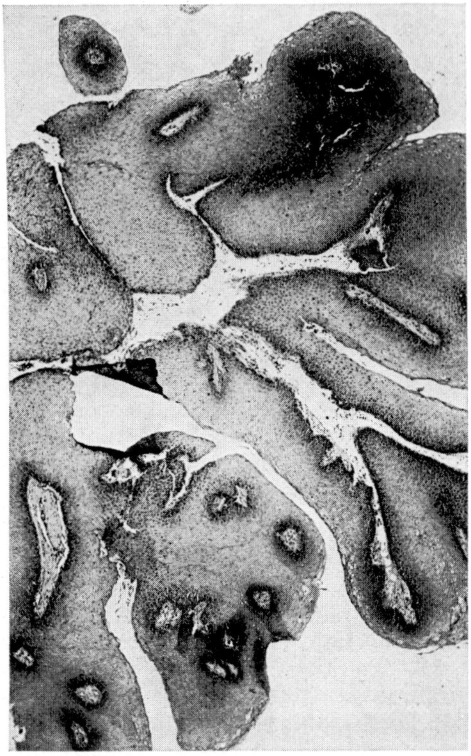

Fig. 1. Normal histologic appearance of laryngeal papilloma showing deep foldings of squamous epithelium and a sparse cellular stroma. (Approx. X100)

Histological examination of specimens often showed marked differences before and after transfer factor treatment. Prior to treatment, the laryngeal papillomas consisted of deep epithelial folds with sparse cellular content in the stroma (Fig. 1). After transfer factor therapy, a marked increase in the number of lymphocytes and plasma cells was present in the stroma of the papilloma (Figs. 2A and B), which was consistently seen in the majority of specimens. In some specimens of patient D.S., areas of necrotic degeneration, in addition to the increased cellu-

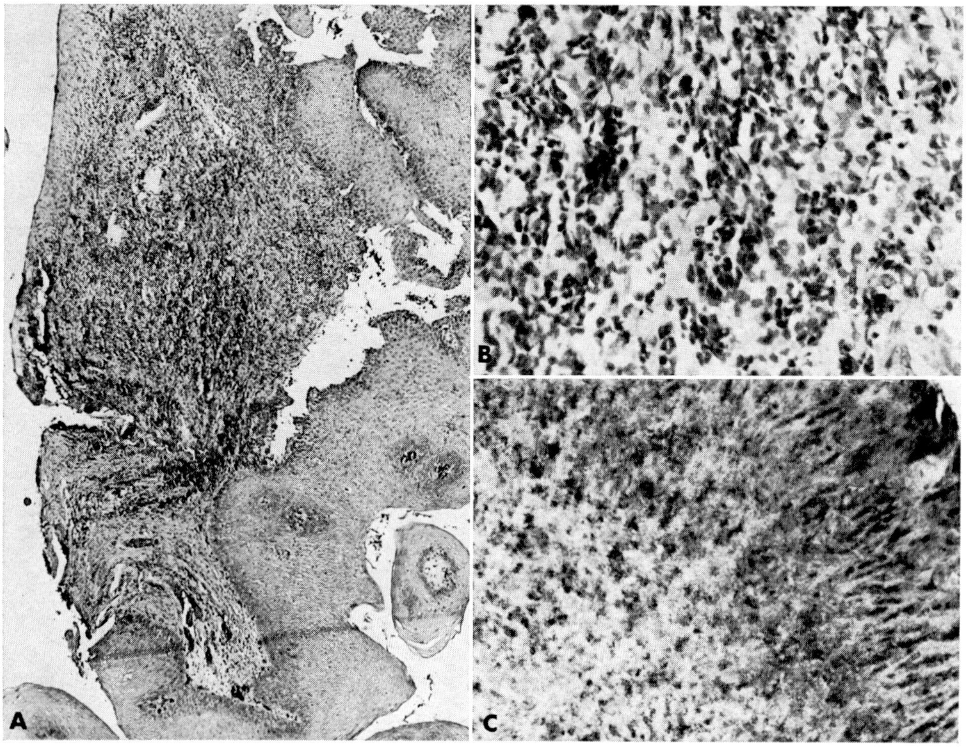

Fig. 2. A) Histologic appearance of laryngeal papilloma after transfer factor therapy showing marked increase of plasma cells and lymphocytes in the stroma. (Approx. X100). B) High power magnification of papilloma stalk showing marked increase of round cell infiltrates. (Approx. X400). C) Histologic appearance of necrotic papilloma after transfer factor therapy. (Approx. X400)

lar infiltration, was noted (Fig. 2C). The histological changes noted above were observed only when patients were receiving transfer factor. During a four-month interval when transfer factor was not given, the original pattern of sparse cellular infiltrates in the stroma was again seen. The influx of lymphocytes and plasma cells recurred after restarting transfer factor therapy.

DISCUSSION

Thirteen patients, ten females and three males, with laryngeal papillomatosis are presently being treated at this center. The average age of onset is 2½ years, and the oldest patient is 62 years. These patients are treated by surgical excision of the papillomas. Microsurgical techniques and cryosurgical removal of the papillomas are the mainstays of treatment. Tracheostomy is avoided, if at all possible, because it is felt that it leads to seeding of the papillomas at the site of the tracheostomy and subsequently further down the tracheobronchial tree.

The histological pattern, in over 120 pretreatment specimens of laryngeal papillomas reviewed for this paper, was remarkably consistent. In approximately two-thirds of the specimens, the stroma consisted of sparse connective tissue with no round-cell infiltrates. Minimal infiltrates of lymphocytes and plasma cells in the stroma were observed in the remaining one-third of the specimens. These infiltrates were seen more frequently in older patients or in younger patients whose disease had been present for several years.

In comparison, papilloma specimens from the two patients treated with transfer factor showed a marked increase in the number of cells in the stroma. These cells were almost entirely lymphocytes and plasma cells. Since the small lymphocyte is the agent of cellular immunity, it is not unreasonable to assume that this marked increase of lymphocyte infiltration represents a change in the cellular immunity of the host.

Tagami *et al*, in their histological study of cutaneous warts, postulated that the change in cellular immunity of the host was responsible for the massive lymphocyte infiltration and subsequent spontaneous regression of the warts.[20] However, Matthews and Shirodaria found little evidence of cellular infiltrates in regressing warts and declared that cellular immunity apparently plays a minor role in regression.[21] In addition to the significant change in the histological apearance of the tumors of our patients, transfer factor was responsible for an alteration in the response to the tests for delayed hypersensitivity. Collectively, this represents strong evidence that a change in the cellular immunity of the host has been invoked. Despite this change, however, new papillomas were seen to emerge during transfer factor therapy.

Evidence from cutaneous warts suggests that each papilloma represents a clone of descendents from a single transformed cell.[4] If the etiological agent of laryngeal papilloma is similar to that of cutaneous papillomas, then each new laryngeal lesion results from the multiplication of either previously transformed dormant cell or a newly infected cell. Furthermore, if a specialized environment is necessary to initiate virus replication, then the physiological stress created by transfer factor might stimulate virus production. This would conceivably lead to increased infection of neighboring cells because transfer factor does not provide the humoral immunity presumed to be necessary for virus neutralization. The appearance of new papillomas during transfer factor therapy therefore, would not be unexpected.

The synergistic action of humoral immunity to prevent reinfection and cellular immunity to suppress the tumor cells may be necessary to completely eradicate the papilloma from the larynx. Transfer factor seems to provide one of these modalities, but until much more experimental and clinical work has been performed, this form of therapy must remain under the strict control of investigative use. These encouraging clinical observations, however, urge that further studies of the influence of transfer factor be attempted in patients with laryngeal and other forms of papilloma. Studies particularly indicated should determine whether the transfer factor used must be specific or whether it can be nonspecific; studies must be carried out in a blindfold fashion to establish beyond any question the usefulness of this approach to this neoplastic disease.

Request for reprints should be sent to Cedric A. Quick, M.D., Department of Otolaryngology, University of Minnesota, Hospital Box 406, 412 Union St. S.E., Minneapolis, Minnesota 55455.

REFERENCES

1. Straus MJ, Shaw EW, Bunting H, *et al*: Crystalline virus-like particles from skin papillomas characterized by intra-nuclear inclusion bodies. Proc Soc Exp Biol Med 72:46-50, 1949

2. Williams MG, Howatson AF, Almeida JD: Morphological characterization of the virus of the human common wart. Nature 189: 895-897, 1961

3. Almeida JD, Howatson AF, Williams MG: Electron microscope study of human warts; sites of virus production and nature of the inclusion bodies. J Invest Dermatol 38: 337-345, 1962

4. Murray RF, Hobbs J, Payne B: Possible clonal origin of common warts (verruca vulgaris). Nature 232:51-52, 1971

5. Noyes WF: Studies on the shope rabbit papilloma virus. II. The location of infective

virus in papillomas of the cottontail rabbit. J Exp Med 109:423-427, 1959

6. Boyle WF, Riggs JL, Oshero LS, *et al*: Electron microscope identification of papova virus in laryngeal papilloma. Laryngoscope 83:1102-1107, 1973

7. Thomas, quoted by Lawrence HS: *Immunobiology*. Good RA, Fisher DW (eds), Connecticut, Sinauer Associates Inc. 1972, p 112

8. Burnett Sir FM: *Self and Cellular Immunology, Book 1*. New York, Cambridge University Press, 1969

9. Landsteiner K, Chase MW: *The Specificity of Serological* Reaction. Cambridge, Mass., Harvard University Press, 1945

10. Lawrence JL: *Immunobiology*, ed 4. Connecticut, Sinauer Associates Inc, 1972, p 104

11. Lawrence HS: The transfer in humans of delayed skin sensitivity to streptococcal M substance and to tuberculin with disrupted leukocytes. J Clin Invest 34:219-230, 1955

12. Lawrence HS, Valentine FT: Transfer factor in delayed hypersensitivity. Ann N Y Acad Sci 169:269, 1970

13. Lynn E, Spitler AS, Levin DP, *et al*: The Wiskott-Aldrich syndrome: The results of transfer factor therapy. J Clin Invest 51: 3216-3224, 1972

14. Fudenberg HH, Levin AS, Spitler LE, *et al*: The therapeutic uses of transfer factor. Hosp Pract 9:95-104, 1974

15. Hellstrom IL, Hellstrom KE, Sjogren HO, *et al*: Demonstration of cell-mediated immunity to human neoplasms of various histological types. Int J Cancer 7:1-16, 1971

16. Jagarlamoody SM, Aust JC, Tew RH, *et al*: *In vitro* detection of cytotoxic cellular immunity against tumor-specific antigens by radioisotopic technique. Proc Nat Acad Sci 68:1346-1350, 1971

17. Quick CA, Behrens HW: An in-vitro model for assay of cellular immunity of laryngeal papilloma. In preparation.

18. Levin AS, Spitler LE, Stites DP, *et al*: Wiskott-Aldrich syndrome, a genetically determined cellular immunologic deficiency. Clinical and laboratory responses to therapy with transfer factor. Proc Nat Acad Sci 67: 2821-2828, 1970

19. DuPont B, Ballow M, Hansen JA, *et al*: Effect of transfer factor therapy on mixed lymphocyte culture reactivity. Proc Nat Acad Sci 71:867-871, 1974

20. Tagami H, Ogino A, Takigawa M, *et al*: Regression of plane warts following spontaneous inflammation. Br J Dermatol 90:147-154, 1974

21. Matthews RS, Shirodaria PV: Study of regression warts by immunofluoresence. Lancet 1:689-691, 1973

CURRENT CONCEPTS OF TEMPORAL BONE PATHOLOGY

The A.F.I.P., A.A.O.O. and the National Temporal Bone Banks Center are sponsoring a symposium on Current Concepts of Temporal Bone Pathology in Washington, D.C., December 1-3, 1975. The faculty will include Drs. H. F. Schuknecht, O. Black, G. Nager, E. Myers and V. J. Hyams. The scope of this symposium will include histological correlations of clinical entities as well as anatomic-pathologic entities. Registration fee is $25.00. For registration forms contact The Director, A.F.I.P., Washington, D.C., 20305.

Ann Otol 84: 1975

CARCINOMA AND JUVENILE PAPILLOMATOSIS

Paul R. Zehnder, Jr., M.D.

George D. Lyons, M.D.

New Orleans, Louisiana

SUMMARY – A 41-year-old male presented with a fungating squamous cell carcinoma growing through the skin around his tracheostomy site. His history revealed a long-term laryngeal growth treated only by tracheostomy in 1955. He had been followed intermittently since age 25 and in 1968 a biopsy diagnosis of juvenile papillomatosis was made. This case is outlined until his death and the literature is reviewed concerning malignant changes in papillomatosis with and without radiation treatment. Malignant degeneration is reported in 3-14% of squamous papillomas. Critical histologic evaluation of such lesions is required to establish the diagnosis. When the criteria of maligancy are strictly adhered to, malignant change is considered exceedingly rare.

Laryngeal papilloma is the most common benign neoplasm of the larynx. Nevertheless, to this day it remains an enigma with regard to etiology, pathogenesis, therapy and prognosis. Numerous papers have proposed theories of its evolution and invoked various modes of therapy which invariably have fallen short of expectation. The papilloma has been declared a completely benign neoplastic entity and yet subsequently been incriminated in malignant degeneration by other authors.

This presentation is deliberately limited in its scope. A single case is presented where spontaneous malignant degeneration of benign laryngeal papillomatosis appears to have occurred. This patient may represent the only one or one of few in which malignant change has occurred without previous radiation therapy. Such change is considered much more rare than suggested in previous reports. In fact, of 141 patients, both children and adults, admitted to Charity Hospital over a 20 year period, this patient is the only one known to have malignant change, or an incidence of 0.7%.

CASE REPORT

A 37-year-old black male first presented to Charity Hospital of New Orleans in 1968 for a gunshot wound of the chest. During the course of his hospital stay, otolaryngological consultation was sought when a tracheostomy tube was noted in place upon admission.

Direct laryngoscopy revealed a diffuse, irregular mass of warty tissue filling the glottis. There was normal range of motion of the cords. Biopsies taken (Figs. 1 and 2) were compatible with multiple benign squamous papillomas.

The patient had been treated at another hospital in 1960 for growths in his larynx which had been present all his life, and a tracheostomy was performed in 1955 at age 24. He visited the Otolaryngology Clinic of that hospital again four years later where indirect laryngoscopy revealed large obstructive papillomas. He failed to return for his scheduled admission and was lost to follow-up.

His final admission was in 1971 at age 41. His symptoms were difficulty in swallowing and a cervical ulcer of six weeks duration. Examination revealed a chronically wasted man with a massive ulcerating tumor of the anterior neck surrounding the tracheostomy tube (Fig. 3). Biopsies of the tumor show moderately well-differentiated squamous cell carcinoma (Figs. 4A and B). Over the next three months, he received lymphocyte immunotherapy and cobalt 60 irradiation to the neck and larynx. He developed a tracheo-

----

From the Department of Otorhinolaryngology and Biocommunications, Louisiana State University School of Medicine, New Orleans, Louisiana.

Presented at the meeting of the American Broncho-Esophagological Association, Atlanta, Georgia, April 7-8, 1975.

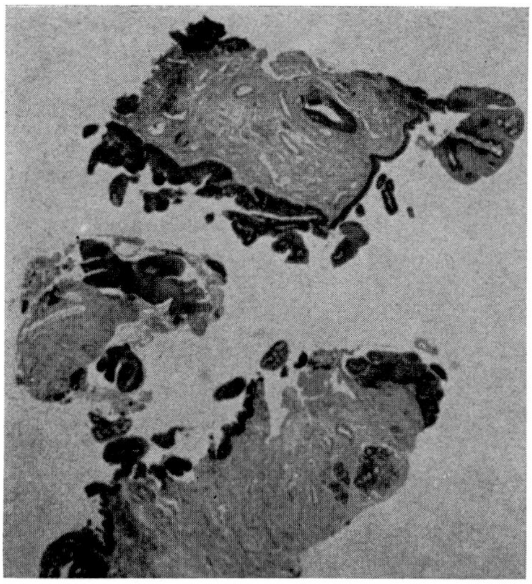

Fig. 1. Under low power, multiple papillomatous projections of squamous epithelium are seen to arise from the mucosal surface.

esophageal fistula, but the tumor regressed remarkably in size (Fig. 5). He was permitted to return home prior to a scheduled laryngectomy but failed to return. The tumor registry reveals his death a year later of unknown causes.

DIAGNOSIS

Juvenile laryngeal papillomatosis is a clinical diagnostic term which has been applied for years to the condition of multiple laryngeal papillomas thought to occur primarily in children. Holinger[1] and others have subsequently pointed out that the incidence of squamous papillomas is actually as great or greater in adults. Nevertheless, perhaps because of the protracted clinical course and repeated recurrences in children, the term juvenile papillomas has persisted. There is no histologic difference between true laryngeal papillomas as found in adult patients and the "juvenile papillomas" of children.

A number of excellent papers[2-4] have outlined the various laryngeal lesions presenting as papillary projections from the vocal folds. These include squamous papilloma, hyperkeratotic papilloma (or papillary keratoses), and verrucous carcinoma.

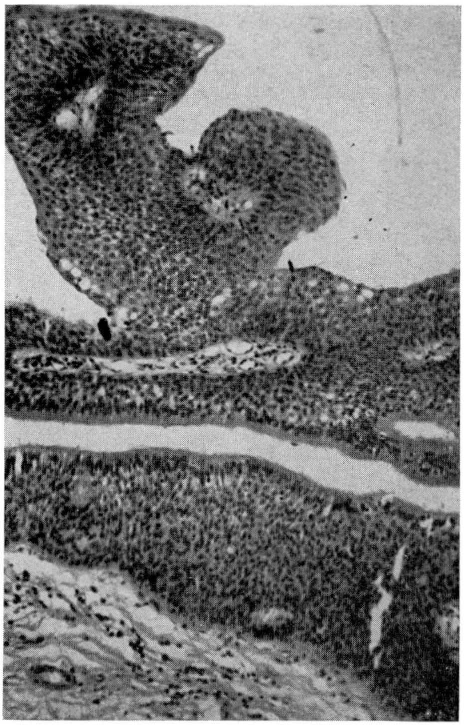

Fig. 2. Under higher power, the tissue consists of respiratory epithelium and connective tissue. The papillary projections have small cores of connective tissue containing moderately dilated blood vessels. There is no hyperkeratosis of the squamous epithelium and no significant variation in size and shape of individual nuclei. There is no dyskeratosis.

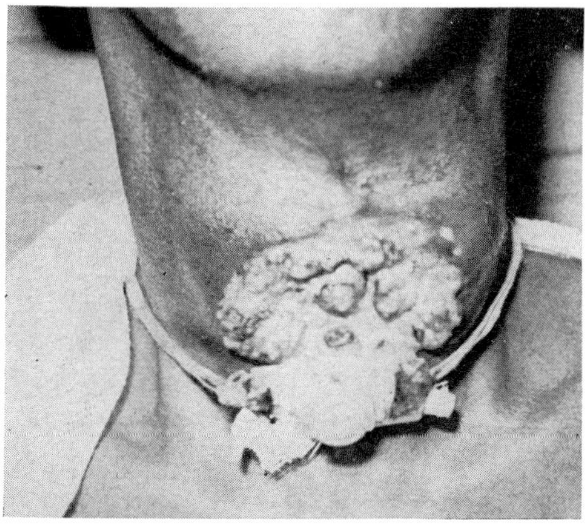

Fig. 3. Massive ulcerating tumor of the anterior neck surrounding the tracheostomy tube.

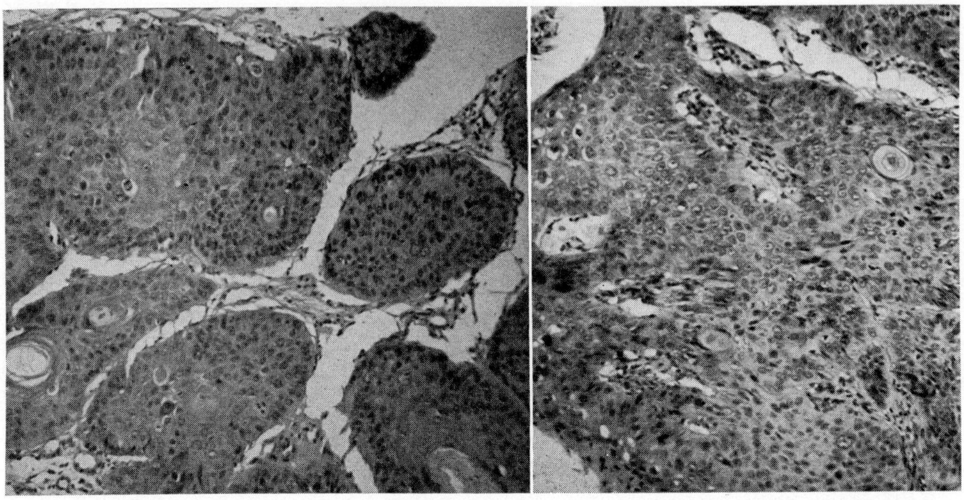

Fig. 4. A) Fragments of squamous epithelium in which there is evidence of hyperkeratosis with fairly marked acanthosis and extensive atypical dyskeratosis. B) Marked variation in size and shape of individual nuclei and many nuclei have frankly malignant cytologic features. Mitoses are numerous. In some areas, the lesion is fairly well-differentiated with formation of epithelial pearls. There is superficial connective tissue invasion.

Squamous papilloma is an exophytic proliferation of squamous epithelium and stroma. It is characterized grossly as a glistening, elevated nodule that varies in coloration from pink to red. Microscopically, it consists of a connective tissue stalk covered with epithelium which is generally relatively thick and well differentiated, with varying degrees of keratosis and parakeratosis.[4] The so-called juvenile papilloma is also such a lesion.

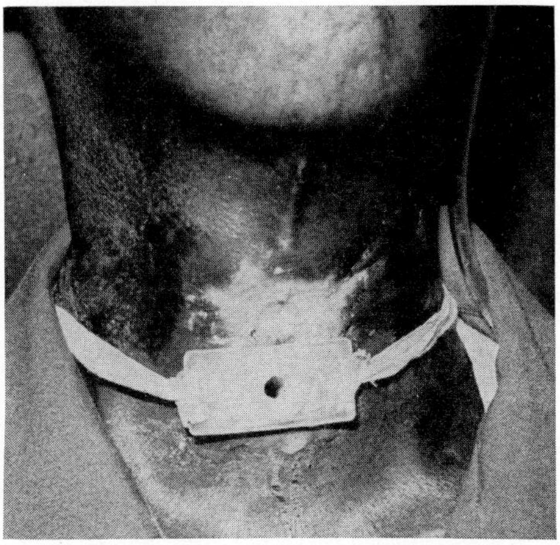

Fig. 5. Evidence of marked regression in size of tumor.

Hyperkeratotic papilloma is a distinctly different lesion. Clinically and histologically it resembles the senile keratosis of the skin, with varying degrees of dyskeratosis and possible intraepithelial pearl formation.[4] There is no question that this keratosis is a potentially malignant lesion.

Verrucous carcinoma can likewise present as a papillary growth. Although difficult to diagnose histologically, the gross appearance makes the clinical differentiation from the other papillomas easy.

The estimates of malignant transformation in all types of laryngeal papillomas range from 3-14%. It has also been stated that there is a higher potential for this change to occur in the adult form of papilloma. We feel, as do other authors[2-3] that the failure to adhere to strict histologic criteria between papilloma and keratotic lesions has resulted in the discrepancy of statistics concerning the malignant potentiality of the squamous papilloma.

LITERATURE REVIEW

The literature was reviewed in regard to reported cases of malignant transformation of papillomas of the larynx.[5-15] A similar review was performed by Fechner[15] in an excellent case presentation of invasive papillomatosis without malignancy. Our findings concur with his that the majority of reported cases can be characterized as: 1) involving the tracheobronchial tree; 2) having received x-ray or radium treatment; or 3) failure of illustration or description of pathological material to allow meaningful independent interpretation.

Only two cases were found in the literature that truly resemble ours, *i.e.*, a long history of laryngeal papillomas with subsequent development of carcinoma without irradiation.[3,17] Yet 16 cases have been reported that developed malignant change after radiation therapy.[5,6,10,11,13]

The cancerogenic possibility of radiation has become known in the past two decades. The number of patients who have developed malignancies after such treatment for nonneoplastic conditions have been documented.[12] Accordingly, radiation therapy is no longer advocated and is contraindicated in the treatment of benign laryngeal papillomas.

CONCLUSION

When this case first came to our attention we felt it represented a most unusual clinical picture. Initially, in reviewing the literature, it appeared that there were a number of similar cases. However, after critical review of these reports, we have come again to our original presumption: spontaneous malignant degeneration of benign squamous papilloma of the larynx is extremely rare. Our case also supports the view that malignancy is more common in tracheobronchial tree involvement.

We, therefore, feel that a figure of 3% is exaggerated. Furthermore, the so-called "adult" papilloma (if, in fact, histologically confirmed as benign squamous papilloma) does not represent a potentially malignant lesion of any proportion. The extreme rarity of malignancy in papilloma is an important concept for the clinician.

Request for reprints should be sent to Paul R. Zehnder, Jr., M.D., 225 Bendel Road, Lafayette, La. 70501.

REFERENCES

1. Holinger PH, Johnston KC, Conner GH, *et al*: Studies of papilloma of the larynx. Ann Otol Rhinol Laryngol 71:443-447, 1962

2. Holinger PH, Schild JA, Maurizi DG: Laryngeal papilloma: review of etiology and therapy. Laryngoscope 78:1462-1474, 1968

3. Friedberg SA, Stagman R, Hass GM: Papillary lesions of the larynx in adults: a pathologic study. Ann Otol Rhinol Laryngol 80:683-692, 1971

4. Ash JE, Beck MR, Wilkes JD: Tumors of the upper respiratory tract and ear in Atlas of Tumor Pathology, sec. 4. Armed Forces Institute of Pathology, Wash DC, 1964

5. LeJeune FE: The story of Warren Bell. Ann Otol Rhinol Laryngol 50:905-908, 1941

6. McCart H: Tracheal and bronchial papillomatous implants showing malignant changes. Ann Otol Rhinol Laryngol 63:498-499, 1954

7. Ogilvie OE: Multiple papillomas of trachea with malignant degeneration. Arch Otolaryngol 58:10-18, 1953

8. Bjork H, Teir H: Benign and malignant papilloma of the larynx in adults. Acta Otolaryngol (Stockh) 47:95-104, 1957

9. Galloway TC, Soper GR, Elsen J: carcinoma of the larynx after irradiation for papilloma. Arch Otolaryngol 72:289-294, 1960

10. Walsh TE, Beamer PR: Epidermoid carcinoma of the larynx occurring in 2 children with papilloma of the larynx. Laryngoscope 60:1110-1124, 1960

11. Putney FJ: Borderline malignant lesions of the larynx. Arch Otolaryngol 61:381-385, 1955

12. Vlodyka J: The cancerogenic effect of x-ray on the larynx. Arch Otolaryngol 76:372-276, 1962

13. Al-Saleem T, Peal AR, Norris CM: Multiple papillomatosis of the lower respiratory tract: a clinical and pathologic study of eleven cases. Cancer 22:1173-1184, 1968

14. Altmann F, Basek M, Stout AP: Papillomas of the larynx with intraepithelial anaplastic changes. Arch Otolaryngol 62:478-485, 1955

15. Fechner RE, Goepfert H, Alford BR, *et al*: Invasive laryngeal papillomatosis. Arch Otolaryngol 99:147-151, 1974

16. Ballenger JJ: *Diseases of the Nose, Throat and Ear,* ed 11. Philadelphia, Lea and Febiger, 1969

17. Toso G: Epithelial papillomas – benign or malignant? Interesting findings in laryngeal papilloma. Laryngoscope 81:1524-1531, 1971

SOCIETY FOR EAR, NOSE AND THROAT ADVANCES IN CHILDREN

The third annual meeting of the Society for Ear, Nose and Throat Advances in Children (SENTAC) will be held at the Hospital del Niño IMAN (Institucion Mexicana de Asistencia a la Niñez) in Mexico City November 5-9, 1975. Papers of 10 to 20 minutes' duration are invited; abstracts should be submitted by September 15 either to Ernesto Deutsch, M.D., Servicio de Otorrinolaringologia, Hospital del Niño IMAN, Insurgentes Sur 3700-C, Mexico 22, D.F., or to Sanford E. Gerber, Ph.D., Department of Speech, University of California, Santa Barbara, CA 93106. For information concerning travel and accommodations write to Dr. Deutsch.

COSMETIC SURGERY OF THE NOSE AND FACE

The First Panamerican Course of Cosmetic Surgery of the Nose and Face, sponsored by the Panamerican Association of Otolaryngology will be held February 12-17, 1976 at the Intercontinental Hotel, Medellin, Colombia, South America. For further information write: Dr. Jaime Florez, 4220 Central Ave., St. Petersburg, Florida 33711.

Ann Otol 84: 1975

EXTRALUMINAL FOREIGN BODIES (COINS) IN THE FOOD AND AIR PASSAGES

King F. Yee, M.D.

Joyce A. Schild, M.D. Paul H. Holinger, M.D.

Chicago, Illinois

SUMMARY – Four children with foreign bodies found outside the lumen of the upper food and air passages are presented. The diagnostic difficulty of such extraluminal foreign bodies and the importance of accurate localization by endoscopy and radiologic examination prior to external surgical removal are discussed.

Foreign bodies in the food and air passages occur commonly in children, and removal is generally accomplished by peroral endoscopy.[1] Foreign bodies that reach the stomach will usually pass spontaneously, although uncommonly sharp, pointed objects are known to perforate the alimentary tract.[2-5] More rarely, foreign bodies in the mediastinum have been reported which resulted from external penetrating injuries.[6]

This report presents four cases in which swallowed foreign bodies were found outside the lumen of the upper food and air passages. It illustrates the diagnostic difficulty of such extraluminal foreign bodies and the importance of accurate localization by endoscopy and radiologic examination prior to external surgical removal.

CASE REPORTS

Case 1. D.K., a four-year-old caucasian female, swallowed a penny while eating a banana one year previously. Following the accident, she refused food for several days. Thereafter, she ate poorly, but no medical advice was obtained. Three weeks prior to admission she developed a cold, and a chest x-ray revealed a coin in the esophagus.

On physical examination, there were rhonchi bilaterally throughout the chest with equal expansion. The rest of the examination was normal. A chest x-ray confirmed the coin at the level of the aortic arch with some impingement of the trachea. When the esophagoscopy was performed, extensive granulation tissue was found on the posterior wall of the esophagus 15 cm from the incisor teeth. The foreign body was not seen, nor could it be palpated. Esophagoscopic examination under cine- fluoroscopy showed the coin lying entirely outside the posterior wall of the esophagus. Three days later right thoracotomy was performed, and the coin was removed.

Case 2. B.J., a two-year-old female, was found to have a coin in the esophagus when a chest x-ray was taken because of high fever and symptoms of upper respiratory tract infection. The parents could not recall any incident that might have indicated when the child had swallowed the coin. On esophagoscopy, in a local hospital, removal was not successful, and the child was referred to Children's Memorial Hospital for treatment.

She was admitted with a temperature of 39.4 C with moderate inspiratory stridor and bilateral rhonchi. In the chest x-ray, the coin appeared to be lodged in the upper esophagus with impingement on the trachea (Fig. 1). Because of the previous unsuccessful esophagoscopy, the possibility of the coin being outside the lumen of the esophagus was entertained, and an esophagram revealed that the coin was lying outside the anterior wall of the esophagus with a sinus tract leading to it.

From the Department of Otolaryngology, Abraham Lincoln School of Medicine, University of Illinois Eye and Ear Infirmary, University of Illinois at the Medical Center, Chicago and The Children's Memorial Hospital, Chicago.

Presented at the meeting of the American Broncho-Esophagological Association in Atlanta, Georgia, April 7-8, 1975.

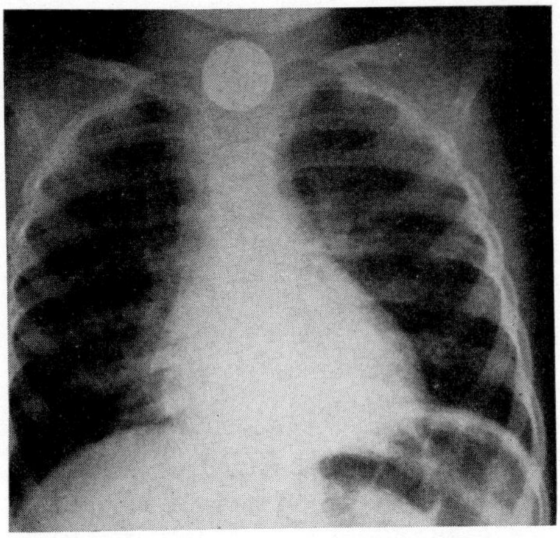

Fig. 1. Case 2. Coin lodged in the esophagus at the level of the cricopharyngeus on conventional chest x-ray.

Marked thickening of the party wall between the trachea and esophagus was also apparent (Fig. 2).

On esophagoscopy, at 10 cm distance from the upper incisor teeth, granulation tissue could be seen, but no foreign body was found. Because of the level at which the granulation tissue was found, a low cervical esophagostomy approach was performed. The coin was found at the level suspected and was removed.

Case 3. K.K., an eight-year-old Negro male, had a tracheoesophageal fistula (TEF) repaired in infancy. He was well until three weeks prior to admission when he was treated for tracheobronchitis for two weeks without improvement. A chest x-ray showed a coin apparently in the right main bronchus with atelectasis of the lung distal to the coin. He was admitted to a local hospital where bronchoscopy was performed on two occasions. The coin could be seen in the right main bronchus but could not be extracted, and he was transferred to Children's Memorial Hospital for further treatment.

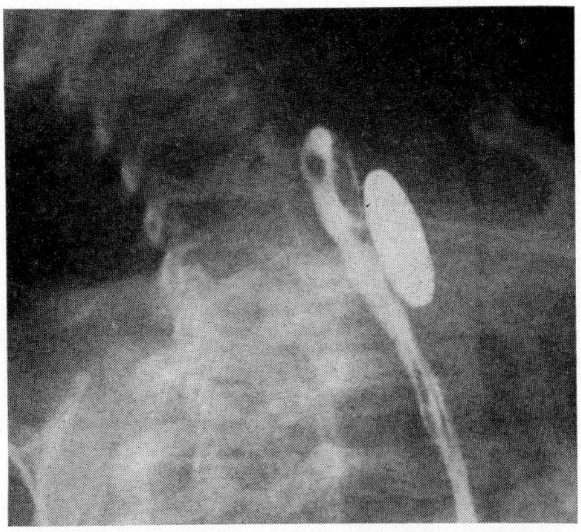

Fig. 2. Case 2. In contrast to Figure 1, the esophogram shows the coin lying outside the cervical esophagus with a sinus tract. A marked compression of the upper trachea is evident.

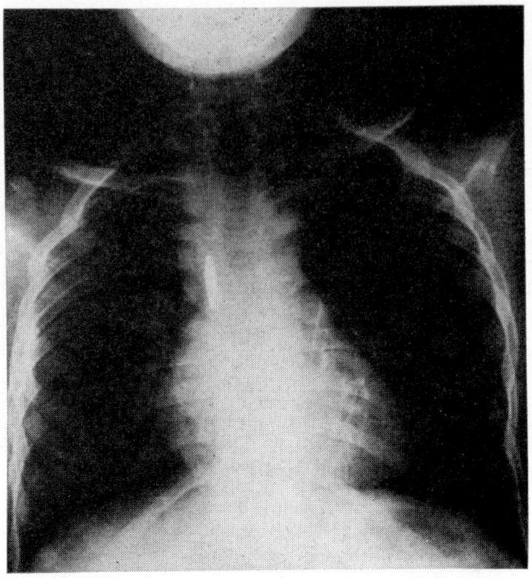

Fig. 3. Case 3. Chest x-ray showing the inferior half of the coin in the lumen of the right bronchus with the superior portion projecting outside the tracheobronchial tree.

On admission, careful questioning failed to document a definite time when the coin had been swallowed. The history and size of the coin were not compatible with aspiration. On examination, the child was in no respiratory distress, in spite of markedly decreased breath sounds over the right chest, with dullness of percussion. Chest x-ray again demonstrated that the coin obstructed the right main bronchus (Fig. 3), but only one-half of the coin was in the lumen of the bronchus with the superior portion seeming to project into the trachea. Because of the unusual position of the foreign body and the history of TEF repair, cine-fluoroscopy was done. It showed that one-half of the coin was in the lumen of the right main bronchus, and the superior half was outside the lumen. A fistulous connection between the esophagus and the bronchus around the coin could be demonstrated (Fig. 4).

Bronchoscopy and esophagoscopy were done to identify further the location of the coin. During bronchoscopy, a small diverticulum at the site of the previous TEF repair was noted on the posterior wall of the trachea, 1 cm above the carina. The edge and a part of the coin were seen at the origin of the right main bronchus covered by a large

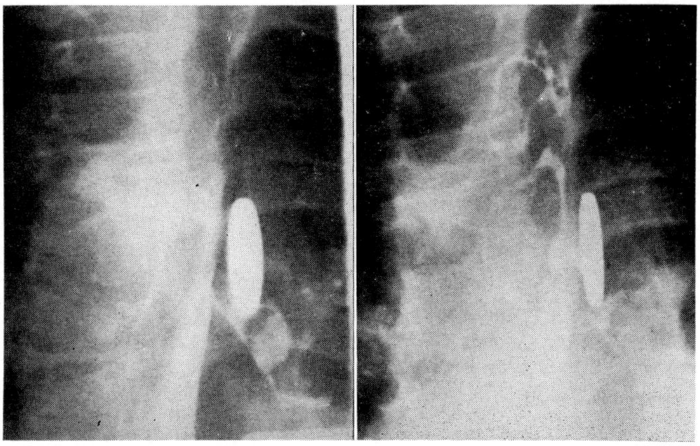

Fig. 4. Case 3. Cine-fluoroscopy delineates the inferior half of the coin in the lumen of the right bronchus. B) The superior half is lying between the bronchus and the esophagus with a fistulous connection communicating through the coin.

amount of granulation tissue. No attempt to remove the coin was made as the coin was much too large for manipulation in the bronchus or trachea. Esophagoscopy revealed a diverticulum on the right anteriolateral wall of the esophagus at 18 cm distance from the upper incisor teeth, corresponding to the level of the carina. No foreign body was found, and no fistulous connection between the esophagus and trachea or bronchus could be determined at endoscopy.

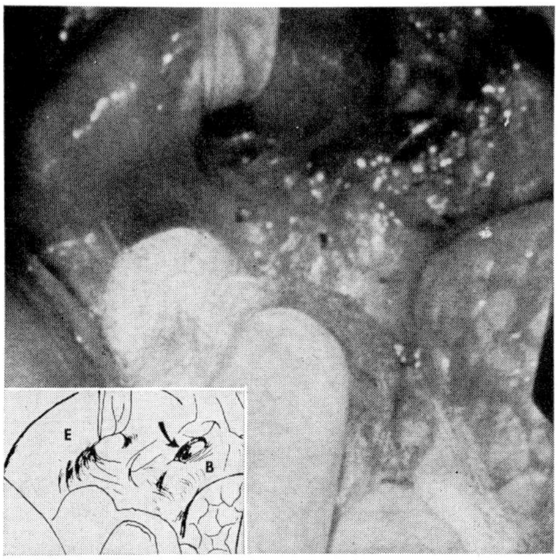

Fig. 5. Case 3. After isolation in the mediastinum, the exposed portion of the coin (arrow) is found outside the esophagus (E) and the hidden portion is in the right bronchus (B). After removal of the coin, the bronchoesophageal fistula can be demonstrated. Insert: line drawing for key to photograph.

Five days later, thoracotomy was performed. A moderate inflammatory reaction was found in the mediastinum making dissection quite difficult. Aided by the information from endoscopy and fluoroscopy, the surgeon was able to isolate the coin lying between the esophagus and the right bronchus (Fig. 5). As had been noted endoscopically, part of the coin was in the lumen of the bronchus. After removal of the coin, a definite fistula was found between the esophageal diverticulum and the right bronchus and the fistula was closed. Three days after surgery, a gastrografin study of the esophagus revealed the fistula had reopened. However, within four weeks of conservative management, aided by a feeding gastrostomy, the fistula closed spontaneously.

Case 4. K.D., a two-year-old caucasian male, was thought to have bronchitis because of croupy respiration and wheezing. He had been treated for eight months by his family physician without improvement. A chest x-ray showed a coin in the proximal esophagus although the parents cannot recall any incident that might indicate when the child had swallowed the coin. On esophagoscopy, at a local hospital, the coin could be palpated in the anterior wall of the esophagus, but it could not be seen. He was then referred to Children's Memorial Hospital for treatment.

On admission, physical examination revealed moderate inspiratory stridor with wheezing bilaterally. Croupy cough was also noted. Two days later, under general anesthesia, an esophagram with gastrografin was done prior to esophagoscopy under fluoroscopy. The coin was noted in the upper chest and was seen to be outside the esophagus. The inferior portion of the coin apparently communicated with the esophagus. Multiple spot films demonstrated the coin between the esophagus and

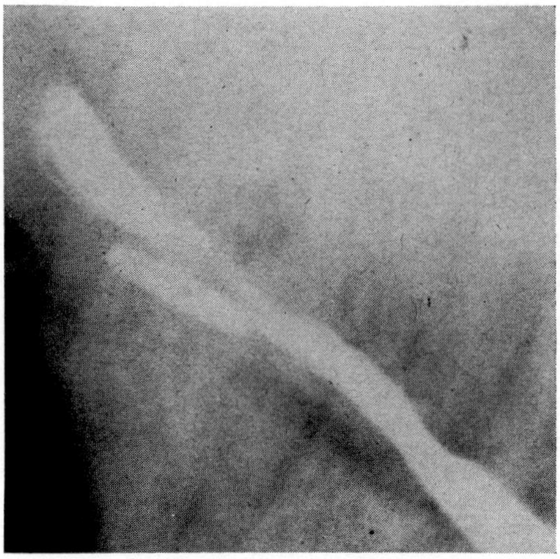

Fig. 6. Case 4. Esophogram shows the coin lying between the esophagus and trachea with moderate tracheal compression. The inferior portion of the coin communicates with the esophagus.

the trachea with moderate tracheal compression (Fig. 6).

On esophagoscopy, the coin and some granulation tissue could be seen in the anterior wall 2 cm below the cricopharyngeus. The coin, however, was embedded in such a manner that it could not be grasped. Consequently, extraction was not possible.

Four days later the coin was removed through a left cervical esophagostomy approach. Recovery was uneventful with complete resolution of the stridor, croupy cough, and wheezing.

DISCUSSION

With extraluminal foreign bodies present in the upper food and air passages, respiratory symptoms are a result of tracheobronchial compression, as seen in the four cases presented in this report. Depending on the level of the pathology, these symptoms can result in respiratory embarrassment. They can be potentially fatal if left unchecked as the tracheal compression may occur at a level below that for routine tracheostomy.

Sharp objects penetrating the alimentary tract can be easily understood. However, with blunt foreign bodies, such as coins, pressure from the object itself, foreign body tissue reaction, and time must interact to allow erosion of the wall of food and air passages. In young children, all of these factors are especially favorable. In our Case 3, the coin must have created the esophageal diverticulum at the site of the previous TEF repair and eroded through the wall and into the right main bronchus. The diverticulum found on the posterior wall of the trachea was above the coin. It was the residual of the superior part of the lower esophageal segment at its original point of attachment to the trachea.

Current radiologic techniques often provide invaluable assistance to the endoscopist. Accurate localization of the foreign body must be obtained by proper radiologic studies. Incomplete studies may lead to errors in diagnosis, and the endoscopist may find himself attempting frustrating, ineffective procedures.

Flat objects in the esophagus most often lie in the coronal plane on the anteroposterior plain film. On the lateral soft tissue film of the neck, they lie parallel to the vertebral column. Any deviation from this axis should arouse suspicion that the foreign body is in an unusual location and possibly is not in the lumen of the esophagus. Additionally, the small caliber of the airway of the child could never admit a coin. Significant tracheal compression, especially when combined with a deviation of the axis of the foreign body from the usual, should forewarn the endoscopist that the foreign body is in an abnormal location. Supplementary contrast material studies such as esophagram, bronchogram, and/or cine-fluoroscopy are warranted to define the relation of the foreign body to the surrounding tissue. However, contrast materials should be used with caution and only after plain films have been found to be inadequate.

Endoscopy is important in localizing the foreign body even when extraction is not possible. The level of the foreign body or its telltale sign of granulation tissue can be located accurately at endoscopy. Biplane fluoroscopic techniques with television monitoring add a third dimension of perspective to the endoscopic view if employed during the procedure.

Detailed information obtained from endoscopy and radiologic studies will facilitate external surgical removal. In difficult cases peroral endoscopy can be performed concomitantly with exploratory surgery. This endoscopy will help in localizing the foreign body by enabling the surgeon to palpate the tip of the endoscopic instrument adjacent to the foreign body.

While extraluminal foreign bodies are infrequently encountered, the possibility of such unusual migration should be recognized in the management of foreign bodies.

SUMMARY

Coins swallowed by four children were undetected for up to one year when respiratory symptoms led to chest x-rays that revealed their presence. Fluoroscopic and endoscopic studies demonstrated them to be outside the lumina of the esophagus; and, in one case, it had eroded into the bronchus. Removal necessitated surgical exploration of the mediastinum where each coin was found.

Request for reprints should be sent to King F. Yee, M.D., Dept. of Otolaryngology, Abraham Lincoln School of Medicine, Univ. of Ill. Eye and Ear Infirmary, Chicago, Ill. 60612.

ACKNOWLEDGMENT—Dr. John Raffensberger removed the coins in Cases 1 and 2 and Dr. Joseph Sherman operated in Cases 3 and 4.

REFERENCES

1. Holinger PH: Foreign bodies in the air and food passages. 17th Wherry Memorial Lecture. Trans Am Acad Ophthalmol Otolaryngol 66:193-210, 1962

2. Abel RM, Fischer JE, Hendren WH: Penetration of the alimentary tract by a foreign body with migration to the liver. Arch Surg 102:227-228, 1971

3. Persky L, Frank ED: Foreign body perforations of the gastrointestinal tract: a report of six cases. New Engl J Med 246:223-224, 1952

4. Kobak NW: Transit of foreign bodies from the intestinal tract through the abdominal wall: report of an instance of passage of toothbrushes. Surgery 55:574-575, 1964

5. Gupta KR, Kakar PK, Saharia PS: Impacted foreign body of retropharyngeal space. J Laryngol Otol 86:519-521, 1972

6. Matsaniotis N, Karpouzas J, Katsaras H: Foreign body in mediastinum. Int Surg 55: 293-296, 1971

CERVICAL LYMPH NODE METASTASIS

An International Symposium on Cervical Lymph Node Metastasis will be held in Milan, Italy November 24-28, 1975, sponsored by Gruppo Italiano Oncologia Cervico-cefalica della Società Italiana di Cancerologia; Institut "Gustave-Roussy", Villejuif, France; Clinica Otorinolaringologica dell'Università di Milano; Instituto Nazionale per lo Studio e la Cura dei Tumori, Milano.

For information write: Miss Lucia Manfredi, Ufficio Attività Didattiche, Instituto Nazionale per lo Studio e la Cura dei Tumori, Via G. Venezian, 1, 20133, Milan, Italy.

Ann Otol 84: 1975

THE PROBLEM OF THE OPEN SAFETY PIN

BERNARD R. MARSH, M.D.

BALTIMORE, MARYLAND

SUMMARY – The open safety pin lodged in the stomach or esophagus presents a challenge to surgical judgment and technical skill. Most foreign bodies causing trouble lodge in the esophagus. Once in the stomach, uneventful passage can be expected in 80 to 90% of cases. Active intervention is reserved for those where intestinal performation is likely or where there is failure to progress. We have used the fiberesophagoscope to remove three open safety pins from the stomachs of two patients whose symptoms and threat of perforation required intervention. The microbiopsy forceps was used successfully to retrieve the open pins, but a newly developed grasping forceps for use with the fiberesophagoscope now provides a more secure hold on such foreign bodies. Rigid instruments retain their value for selected cases, but the flexible equipment now provides an important advance in the management of the open safety pin in the stomach.

The open safety pin lodged in the stomach or esophagus presents the endoscopist a challenge both to his surgical judgment and technical skill.

The majority of ingested foreign bodies causing trouble lodge in the esophagus. Once a foreign body has entered the stomach, uneventful passage through the intestinal tract can be expected in 80 to 90% of cases.[1,2] Eldridge reported his experience of 36 years at St. Elizabeth's Hospital in Washington, D. C., where many patients swallowed open safety pins, and in only one such case did laparotomy become necessary.[3]

In a series of 660 patients under age 16 with foreign body ingestion, only 43 of 412 patients not subjected to esophagoscopy required operative intervention. In a series of 35 patients who had ingested pins and needles, only three required operative removal, while the rest were managed with radiological observation in the hospital.[4]

The technical difficulty in retrieval of open safety pins from the stomach and the experience that they frequently pass uneventfully has led to the practice of watchful waiting in the hospital. Active intervention is reserved for patients who are symptomatic, when perforation seems likely, and when the foreign body fails to progress.

Chevalier Jackson recorded that "Any foreign body that has reached the stomach through the esophagus can be brought back the same way." But he added, "The indications for doing so are not present in all cases."[5] Various methods for such removal have been described including the use of the rigid gastroscope, special forceps or magnets, and more recently the fiberoptic gastroscope.[4,6]

In two patients we have recently been consulted regarding the removal of open safety pins from the stomach. It is the purpose of this report to describe our use of the fiberesophagoscope in the management of these cases where foreign body removal seemed indicated.

CASE REPORTS

Case 1. A 47-year-old Negro female was admitted complaining of chest and

---

From the Department of Laryngology and Otology, The Johns Hopkins University School of Medicine, Baltimore, Maryland.

Presented at the meeting of the American Broncho-Esophagological Association, Atlanta, Georgia, April 7-8, 1975.

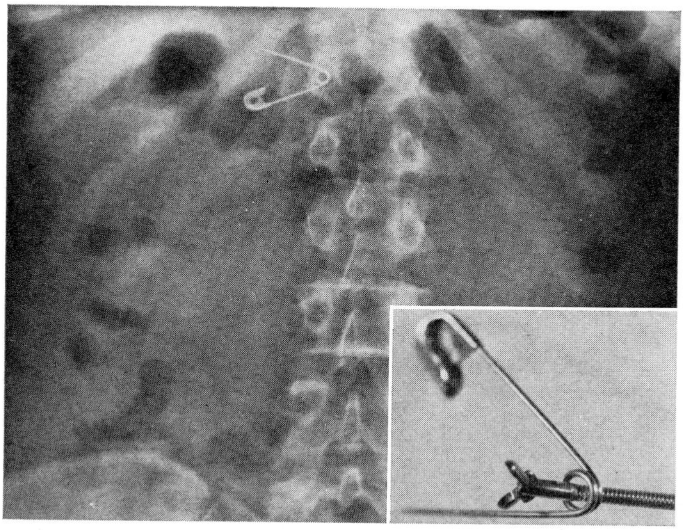

Fig. 1. Case 1, open safety pin lodged in pylorus. Insert: microbiopsy forceps prepared for pin removal.

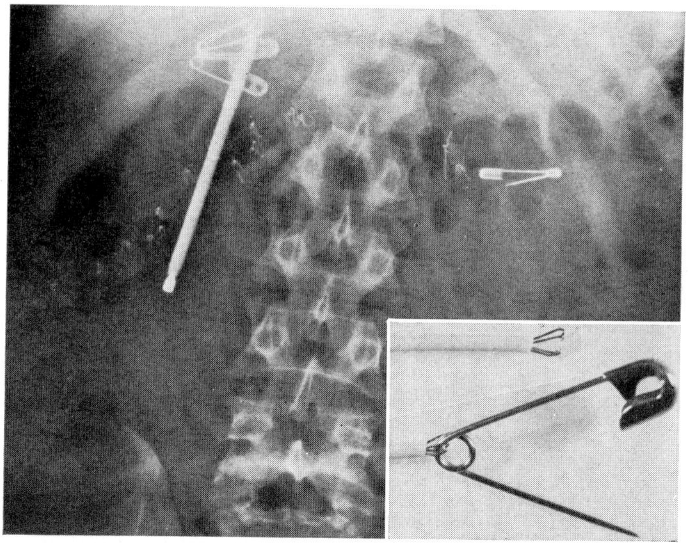

Fig. 2. Case 2, multiple foreign bodies in abdomen. Insert: open safety pin, grasping forceps.

back pain. Earlier in the day she had swallowed an open safety pin which x-rays demonstrated as being just below the cricopharyngeus. Others attempted its removal by endogastric version, but the pin became dislodged and lost in the stomach. After 24 hours the patient complained of epigastric pain, and x-rays revealed the pin keeper lodged in the pylorus with the point forward making further progress both unlikely and hazardous (Fig. 1). Endoscopic removal was advised. The patient was positioned on the fluoroscopy table and the fiberesophagoscope* was passed to the pylorus. A microbiopsy forceps was

* Olympus Corp. of Amer., New Hyde Park, N. Y.

inserted through the spring of the safety pin and the forceps jaws opened to extract the foreign body, point trailing, into the lower esophagus (Fig. 1, insert). At this point the microforceps proved too weak for further removal. An open tube esophagoscope was then introduced under fluoroscopic control so as not to override the pin (now point down) and the spring grasped with a rotation forceps for removal through the esophagoscope. The patient made an uneventful recovery.

Case 2. A 25-year-old Caucasian male was referred from a State mental institution complaining of sharp abdominal pain radiating to the back. He had a history of five laparotomies, three related to foreign body ingestion in the past. X-rays revealed a cluster of four open safety pins lodged at the pylorus, a thermometer in the duodenum and an additional pin in the colon (Fig. 2).

We felt that the four pins represented a significant hazard and, based on our previous success, recommended endoscopic removal. At fibergastroscopy we were able to disengage the first two pins and removed them without use of the open tube esophagoscope. On our return for the remaining two pins, we were chagrined to discover that a peristaltic wave had stolen them from our view and cast them out of reach.

The following day the patient was pain free and over the next three days demonstrated continued progress of the remaining pins. During his fourth postop day he disappeared from the hospital without benefit of medical approval.

A recently developed grasping forceps* now allows a much better grip on the safety pin than provided by the microbiopsy forceps making accidental dislodgment less likely (Fig. 2, insert).

SUMMARY

The advent of flexible instruments has given us yet another valuable tool in the management of gastric foreign bodies. This technique is associated with minimal morbidity, is technically simpler, and probably safer in most hands than the open tube approach to gastric foreign bodies. Yet, as we have experienced in Case 1, the open tube instrument retains its value in selected circumstances. It is unwise to attempt the management of such cases without a full complement of foreign body instruments and the requisite skill to use them when indicated.

While gastric foreign bodies frequently pass harmlessly through the gastrointestinal tract, circumstances may dictate removal when there is a failure to progress or a threat of perforation. Perhaps these newer techniques warrant a re-examination of our criteria for gastric foreign body removal when there exists even a remote risk of intestinal perforation.

---

* Medi-Tech, Watertown, Mass.

Request for reprints should be sent to B. R. Marsh, M.D., U.S. Public Health Service Hospital, 3100 Wyman Park Drive, Baltimore, Maryland 21211.

REFERENCES

1. Maleki M, Evans WE: Foreign body perforation of the intestinal tract. Arch Surg 101:475-477, 1970

2. Spitz L: Management of ingested foreign bodies in childhood. Br Med J 4:469-472, 1971

3. Eldridge WW Jr: Foreign bodies in the gastrointestinal tract. JAMA 178:665-667, 1961

4. Swarbrick ET, Lancaster-Smith MJ, Areling W, *et al*: Removal of darning needle with fibreoptic gastroscope. Br Med J 3:470, 1972

5. Jackson C: Foreign bodies in the air and food passages, in Maloney W (ed): *Otolaryngology,* Hagerstown, Harper & Row Pub, 1972, vol. 5, chap 1, p. 92

6. Fiser B: Magnetic tube for removal of ferrous foreign bodies from the stomach and duodenum in children. Lancet 1:76, 1972

Ann Otol 84: 1975

UNEXPECTED RADIOGRAPHIC FINDINGS RELATED TO FOREIGN BODIES

Wilfred T. Morioka, M.D. Robert H. Maisel, M.D.
Thomas W. Smith, M.D. Robert W. Cantrell, M.D.
San Diego, California

SUMMARY – In two asymptomatic patients, routine preoperative radiographs revealed three pennies in the esophagus in one patient and a spring from a toy in another patient. In contrast, two symptomatic patients, one with a flip-top cap from a beer can in the esophagus and the other with a piece of photographic film in the larynx, had negative findings on their radiographs. Salient points of the cases are that diagnois can be delayed by inadequate history, misinterpretation of signs and symptoms, and unexpected radiographic findings. Special attention should be focused on the flip-top cap ingestion case. Sixty-five percent of 677 people polled have placed flip-top caps into full cans. Fifty-two people almost swallowed a flip-top cap. Otolaryngologists should be alerted about the radiolucency of this metallic foreign body, and the general population should be discouraged from this dangerous practice.

Radiographs taken of patients who have swallowed or aspirated foreign bodies may not reveal them,[1-3] and routine x-rays may show unsuspected foreign bodies. Two patients with unsuspected foreign bodies, three coins in the esophagus of one and a spring in the right bronchus intermedius of the other, had these foreign bodies discovered on routine preoperative chest x-rays. Two symptomatic cases suspected of having foreign bodies had negative findings on x-ray. Endoscopy performed due to clinical symptoms located a flip-top cap of a can in the esophagus of one patient and a piece of photographic film in the larynx of another patient. These cases are presented to alert otolaryngologists to unexpected radiographic findings in cases involving foreign bodies.

CASE REPORTS

Case 1. A three-year-old male was admitted to the ophthalmology service with esotropia. Preoperative chest x-ray revealed a right middle lobe infiltrate and three coins in the midthoracic esophagus (Fig. 1). There was no history of pulmonary or gastrointestinal problems. After the x-rays, the parents stated that the child had been a poor eater for two years with occasional minor episodes of dysphagia, but no previous pulmonary problems were mentioned. He had been evaluated two years previously for gastrointestinal problems, which were attributed to emotional problems.

Esophagoscopy was performed, and three pennies were found. The coins were removed without complications. Mild mucosal erythema was evident, but no other abnormalities were noted. Bronchoscopy revealed small amounts of purulent material in both main stem bronchi. No anatomical deformity in the airway was seen.

Case 2. A six-year-old boy was ad-

From the Department of Otolaryngology, Naval Regional Medical Center, San Diego, California.

The opinions or assertions contained herein are those of the authors and are not to be construed as official or as reflecting the view of the Department of the Navy.

Presented at the meeting of the American Broncho-Esophagological Association, Atlanta, Georgia, April 7-8, 1975.

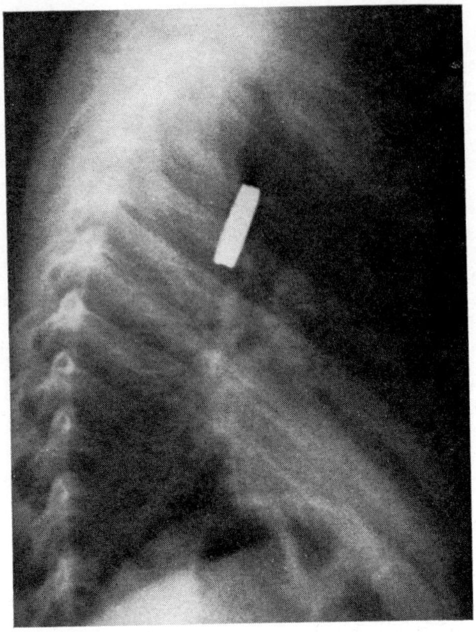

Fig. 1. (Case 1) Preoperative chest x-ray revealing three coins in the esophagus.

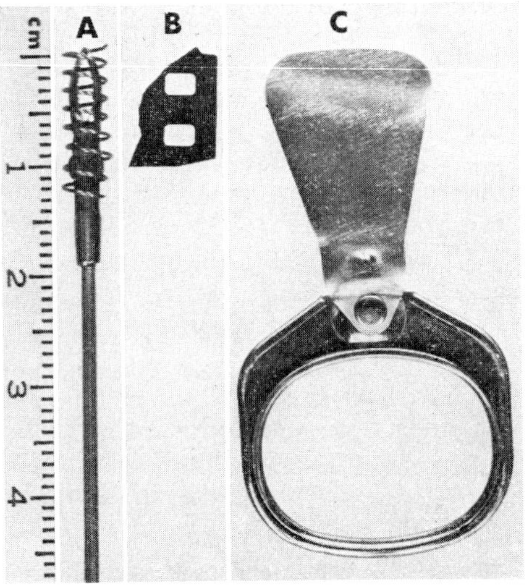

Fig. 2. A) (Case 2) Coiled spring removed with grasping forceps during bronchoscopy. B) (Case 3) Piece of photographic film which was found wedged between the vocal cords. C) (Case 4) Flip-top cap removed by esophagoscopy.

mitted to the otolaryngology service for myringotomies and insertion of ventilating tubes. Preoperative chest x-ray showed a coiled spring in the right bronchus intermedius. The parents reported a bout of severe coughing which subsided after a few minutes two months previously. A mild, intermittent nonproductive cough persisted. During bronchoscopy a 1½ cm coiled spring was removed. The spring was imbedded in the mucosa. Removal was accomplished by inserting the grasping forceps into the lumen of the spring, opening the forceps, and withdrawing the spring into the bronchoscope (Fig. 2A).

Case 3. An eleven-month-old female was admitted to the pediatric service with a diagnosis of laryngotracheobronchitis. Three days prior to admission, she developed an expiratory wheeze. On the day of admission the patient had a fever of 39.5 C, a barking cough, tachypnea, and inspiratory and expiratory stridor. The epiglottis appeared normal. The diagnosis was laryngotracheobronchitis with a differential including foreign body, subglottic stenosis, and laryngeal polyp. The child was treated initially with a mist tent with nebulized racemic epinephrine and epinephrine subcutaneous. After the first day the child was afebrile, and the cough was diminished. Stridor persisted during agitation, and the cry was weak. Soft tissue x-ray of the neck revealed no foreign body. Chest x-ray showed a suggestion of subglottic swelling. Four days after admission, diagnostic laryngoscopy was performed to determine the cause of the persistent stridor. A small piece of photographic film was found wedged between the vocal cords (Fig. 2B). After removal of the film the child became asymptomatic.

Case 4. A 31-year-old male was admitted after accidentally swallowing the flip-top cap from a beer can. He placed the flip-top cap into the full can of beer to prevent littering. As he was drinking the beer, he felt the cap enter his mouth but was unable to avoid swallowing it.

X-rays of the neck, chest, and abdomen were negative for this metallic foreign body. He complained of a mild ache in the retrosternal area. The patient was admitted for observation. The next morning the retrosternal ache increased. Esophagoscopy was performed and the flip-top cap (Fig. 2C) was located and removed from its location 34 cm from the upper incisor teeth. A mucosal abrasion was noted at 30 cm, but his postoperative course was uneventful.

DISCUSSION

Most cases of foreign body ingestion or aspiration are readily diagnosed and treated. In some cases, there are factors that can confuse and delay diagnosis.[2,4,5]

In Cases 1 and 2, the unusual foreign bodies discovered on preoperative chest x-rays were unexpected. The patients were thought to be asymptomatic, and there was a significant delay in the diagnosis. The delay related to: 1) the young age of the children; 2) the parents not observing the ingestion or aspiration; 3) parents observing the incident but assuming that coughing had expelled the foreign body; and 4) symptoms being disregarded or misdiagnosed.

In Case 1 the parents did not observe the child actually ingesting the coins. His subsequent symptoms of "poor feeding" and occasional dysphagia were noticed, but they were attributed to "emotional problems." This case points out three factors that delay diagnosis: 1) young children cannot communicate adequately their symptoms or difficulties; 2) parents do not always know what their children have ingested; and 3) the symptoms can be disregarded or attributed to other causes by parents and physicians.

The second patient was observed during his aspiration incident, but his mother thought he had coughed up the foreign body. His subsequent symptoms of intermittent mild cough were disregarded. Without the radiographs, the foreign body most likely would have remained for a long period with probable damage to the bronchus.[6]

Patient No. 3 was admitted with a diagnosis of laryngotracheobronchitis. During hospitalization foreign body was repeatedly mentioned in the differential diagnosis. Due to negative x-ray findings and improvement of the patient, diagnosis was delayed. Four days after admission, laryngoscopy and removal of the segment of photographic film stopped the stridor. With the increase of radiolucent material[3,4,7] that can be ingested or aspirated, pediatricians, radiologists, and otolaryngologists must be suspicious of negative radiographs and think of foreign bodies in children with esophageal or respiratory symptoms.

Patient No. 4 ingested a flip-top cap from a beer can. Cervical, chest, and abdomen x-rays were negative for a metallic foreign body. As shown in this patient, thin metallic objects can be radiolucent. Eight hours after admission due to persistent symptoms, esophagoscopy was performed with removal of the flip-top cap. Repeat chest x-ray with the flip-top cap taped to the chest wall did not show the foreign body.

A survey was conducted to determine the incidence of placing flip-top caps into a full can. Four hundred and forty-one (65%) of 677 people polled stated that they have placed flip-top caps into a full can. Two hundred eighty people still continue the practice. Of the 161 who have stopped, 130 stated that they had read or heard about the danger in magazines, newspapers, or on the radio. Of the 441 people who did place caps into full cans, 52 or 12% said they almost swallowed a flip-top cap.

SUMMARY

Preoperative radiographs in asymptomatic patients revealed three pennies in the esophagus in one patient and a spring from a toy in the bronchus of another patient. Two symptomatic patients, one with a flip-top beer can cap in the esophagus and another with a piece of photographic film in her larynx, had negative findings on their radiographs. Diagnosis and treatment may be delayed due to: 1) young children cannot give an adequate history; 2) parents may be unaware of the ingestion of aspiration; 3) parents may believe that the foreign body was expelled during coughing; 4) the signs and symptoms are misinterpreted; and 5) radiolucent foreign bodies. The ingestion of a flip-top cap from a can deserves special attention. The practice of placing flip-top caps into full cans is common and we feel this practice should be discouraged.

Request for reprints should be sent to Wilfred T. Morioka, M.D., Department of Otolaryngology, Naval Regional Medical Center, San Diego, California 92134.

REFERENCES

1. Kim IG, Brummitt WM, Humphry A, *et al*: Foreign body in the airway: a review of 202 cases. Laryngoscope 83:347-354, 1973

2. Brooks JW: Foreign bodies in the air and food passages. Ann Surg 175:720-732, 1972

3. Winship WS, Le Roux PD, Le Roux BT: Retention of radiotranslucent foreign bodies in the oesophagus as a cause of stridor. S Afr Med J 48:831-832, 1974

4. Smith PC, Swischuk LE, Fagan CJ: An elusive and often unsuspected cause of stridor or pneumonia (the esophageal foreign body). Am J Roentgenol Radium Ther Nucl Med 122:80-89, 1974

5. Steichen FM, Fellini A, Einhorn AH: Acute foreign body laryngo-tracheal obstruction: a cause for sudden and unexpected death in children. Pediatrics 48:281-285, 1971

6. Jackson C: Observations on the pathology of foreign bodies in the air and food passages. Otolaryngol Clin North Am 1:3-35, 1968

7. Pyman C: Radiolucent foreign bodies. Aust Paediatr J 8:166, 1972

NOTICE

The American Otological Society, Inc., notes with regret that its archives are not complete. The Council desires to remedy this insofar as possible and has directed the Editor-Librarian to seek replacement for volumes depleted from the library.

Accordingly, anyone in possession of any of the following volumes is earnestly requested to notify the Editor-Librarian. If recompense is desired, any fair price will be honored.

Vol. III, 1882-1887

Vol. XV, 1919-1921 (In some cases, these years may be in separate volumes)

Vol. XVIII, 1928

Vol. XXXIV, 1944

Vol. XLVI, 1958

Brian F. McCabe, M.D., Editor-Librarian, American Otological Society, Inc., University Hospitals, Iowa City, Iowa, 52242.

Ann Otol 84: 1975

SPECIAL NEW LOW RESISTANCE TO FLOW TUBE AND ENDOTRACHEAL TUBE ADAPTER FOR USE DURING FIBEROPTIC BRONCHOSCOPY

EDWARD CARDEN, FRCP(C)

PHULCHAND P. RAJ, M.D.

LOS ANGELES, CALIFORNIA

SUMMARY — This paper describes endotracheal tubes and adapters which are designed specially for fiberoptic bronchoscopy; the tubes are designed in such a way that they are wide at the upper part but are narrow and thin walled in the part of the tube which goes through and below the cords. By designing tubes in this manner, the resistance to flow of gas through the tube when the fiberoptic bronchoscope is in place is very much reduced and the safety of the whole precedure is enhanced. A special adapter for use under these circumstances is also described which utilizes a commercially available swivel tracheostomy adapter with a special silicone diaphragm fitted onto the top to enable the fiberoptic bronchoscope to be placed through the diaphragm and keep a sealed system. A plug is available for the hole in the diaphragm when the fiberoptic bronchoscope is not being used. Clinical and laboratory data show that these pieces of equipment perform the function for which they were designed.

Fiberoptic bronchoscopy is a relatively new art which has gained much prominence over the last two or three years. With the advent of the fiberoptic bronchoscope, peripheral regions of the lungs can be viewed and previously undiagnosable conditions seen, biopsied, and diagnosed. There are, however, problems in the use of the fiberoptic bronchoscope when it is utilized during general anesthesia or during local anesthesia if an endotracheal tube is used as a sheath down which to slide the bronchoscope. The two problems which are the most prominent are the fact that, firstly, with the fiberoptic bronchoscope inside an endotracheal tube, the resistance to flow of gas through the tube rises very significantly and may be high enough to impair the respirations of the patient being bronchoscoped;[1] secondly, when the patient is being ventilated with positive pressure ventilation during the bronchoscopy, an adapter through which to slide the fiberoptic bronchoscope is needed which will seal the bronchoscope and not allow anesthetic gases to leak out into the atmosphere. The purpose of this paper is to describe a new endotracheal tube for use during fiberoptic bronchoscopy and a special adapter to go with the tube to simplify the management of patients under general anesthesia.

TUBE DESIGN

Adult endotracheal tubes (Fig. 1) were made in the same design as the Cole tube[2] used in infant anesthesia in that the upper section of the tube was made with a large diameter but the section of the tube which goes through the cords was of a smaller diameter. Tubes were manufactured from silicone elastomer, the narrow section of the tube being specially thin-walled with the external diameter equivalent to that of a normal 8.0, 8.5 or 9.0 silicone endotracheal tube but being 8.75, 9.25 and 9.5 mm in internal diameter respectively. In the narrow section of the tube a Murphy eye was present, as was a

Presented at the meeting of the American Broncho-Esophagological Association, Atlanta, Georgia, April 7-8, 1975.

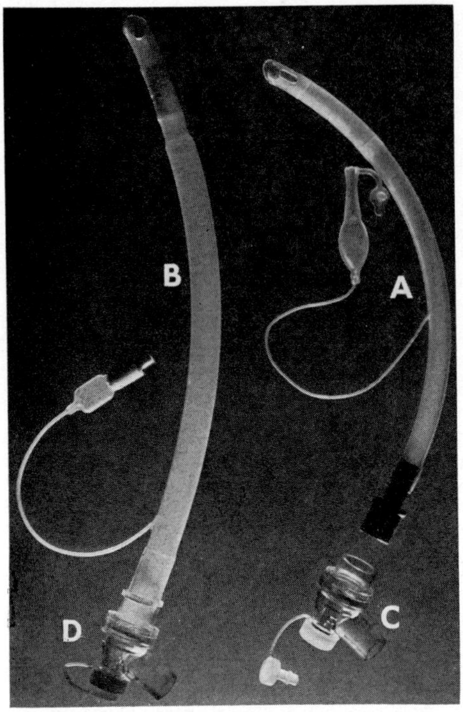

Fig. 1. A) Standard 8.0 mm endotracheal tube. B) Special endotracheal tube. C) Special adaptor (plug out). D) Special adaptor connected to tube (plug in place).

short cuff only approximately one inch long as opposed to the normal 1½ to 2 inches long. The upper parts of the tubes were manufactured with tubing of 11 mm internal diameter and into the top of these tubes an endotracheal tube adapter was fitted with a conventional 15 mm male taper for connection to anesthesia apparatus. At the point where the wide section of the tube and the narrow section of the tube meet, the internal parts of the tube were streamlined to minimize turbulence. The outside parts of the tube were also smoothed, so that when resting against the cords, trauma would not occur.

SPECIAL ADAPTER DESIGN

A commercially available, swivel, tracheostomy adapter* was obtained

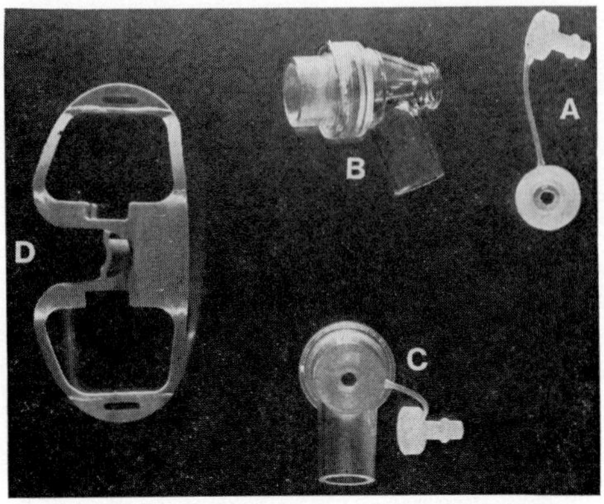

Fig. 2. A) Diaphragm with attached plug. B) Swivel tracheostomy adaptor. C) A and B assembled, end on view. D) Portex endotracheal tube anchoring device.

and a special silicone elastomer diaphragm made to slip over the end of it (Fig. 2). The diaphragm has a hole in the center of it which is approximately 3 mm in diameter but which will stretch to accommodate anything from a 3 to a 6.5 mm rod placed through it. A special plug was also made to fit into this hole in the diaphragm. The plug was attached to the cap by a 1" length of 16 gauge Silastic®** tubing. The intention was that general anesthesia would be maintained with the plug in place, and when fiberoptic bronchoscopy is going to be carried out the plug is removed and the bronchoscope inserted. The connection to the endotracheal tube is of a conventional 15 mm female type and the connection to the anesthesia machine is of the conventional 15 mm male type.

EXPERIMENTAL DATA

Tubes from the same manufacturer of 8, 8.5 and 9 mm internal diameter were obtained, and the resistance to flow through these tubes compared to the new tubes of equivalent external diameter in the distal portion with the fiberoptic bronchoscope inside them. In order to do this a flow rate of 20, 30 and 40 1./min was used through the endo-

* Harris Lake, Inc.
** Dow Corning Corp., Midland, Mich.

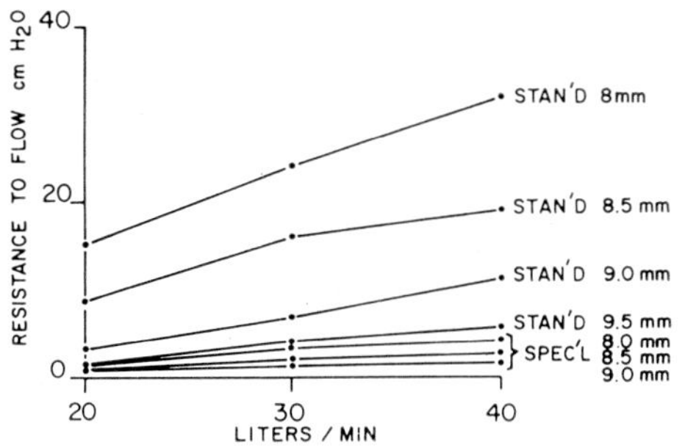

Fig. 3. Resistance to flow through standard and special endotracheal tubes with fiberoptic bronchoscope in place.

tracheal tube. Utilizing the special adapter described above, a 5.7 mm external diameter fiberoptic bronchoscope was placed inside these endotracheal tubes and the resistance to flow of gas through these tubes measured on a manometer. These results can be seen in Figure 3.

CLINICAL STUDIES

Patients who were to have fiberoptic bronchoscopy under general anesthesia were anesthetized utilizing a conventional anesthetic technique with Pentothal,®* Anectine;®** this was followed by intubation with the special tube, inflation of the cuff, and ventilation with nitrous oxide/oxygen mixtures using a Monaghan volume-cycled ventilator.*** The tube was anchored in the mouth with tape or a Portex tube anchoring device (Fig. 2) and arterial blood gas samples were obtained in heparinized syringes and analyzed for oxygen, CO_2 and pH prior to the insertion of the fiberoptic bronchoscope and ten minutes after beginning the fiberoptic bronchoscopy. No increases in arterial pCO_2 levels were found in the 15 cases studied all using the smallest diameter tube.

The following clinical questions and observations were made. 1) Was the tube as easy to insert through the cords as a normal endotracheal tube? 2) Was there any tendency for the tube to come out with the upward and downward movement of the bronchoscope? 3) Did the patient suffer any trauma to the vocal cords with the wide section of the tube resting upon them? 4) Did anesthetic gases leak from around the diaphragm whilst the fiberoptic bronchoscope was being used? 5) Would the bronchoscope slide in and out through the diaphragm and tube without undue friction? 6) Could the anesthesia equipment be easily hooked up to this apparatus?

RESULTS

The results of the laboratory studies (Fig. 3) confirm that the resistance to flow through these tubes is significantly less than an equivalent sized endotracheal tube. As noted earlier, rises of pCO_2 did not occur during bronchoscopy. Further clinical observations: 1) The tubes were found to be easy to insert. 2) The tendency to come back out through the cords was minimal despite the use of a shorter than normal cuff length. 3) Careful viewing of the vocal cords following the endoscopy showed no evidence of trauma to the vocal cords from the shoulder of the tube resting upon them. 4) Provided the bronchoscope was lubricated with a water soluble gel, there was little tendency for gas to leak from around the diaphragm during the bronchoscopy procedure unless excessively high ventilation pressures were needed (*i.e.*, over 40 cm H_2O). 5) Provided that lubrication of the bronchoscope was carried out, there was very little friction noticed by the operator either from the inside of the tube or the diaphragm. 6) The tube was very simple to hook up to the standard anesthetic equipment and its use was made even easier by the fact that the adapter would swivel around its base.

DISCUSSION

The principle used in the design of the tube is that embodied in the Cole tube used in infants. The resistance to

* Abbott Laboratories, North Chicago, Ill.
** Burroughs Wellcome Co., Research Triangle Park, NC
*** Monaghan, Div. Sandoz-Wander, Inc., Littleton, CO

flow down the upper part of the tube is negligible. The high resistance to flow occurs in the narrow section of the tube; and since the narrow section of the tube is approximately one fourth of the total length of the tube, the total resistance to flow through this endotracheal tube would be expected to be approximately one fourth the resistance to flow through a tube of equivalent internal diameter, but of normal configuration (*i.e.*, the same diameter throughout the whole length).

In order to enhance the effectiveness of the tube, the terminal section was made with special thinwall tubing, thereby increasing the effective internal diameter and hence reducing the resistance to flow even more.

To eliminate the possibility of the cuff overriding the end of the tube, the cuff has been made shorter and slightly stiffer than the normal silicone elastomer cuff. Its wall pressure in the trachea is still very much less than conventional smooth cuffed endotracheal tubes, but its sealing is just as adequate.

In carrying out the procedure of fiberoptic bronchoscopy, really critical resistance to flows occur when the difference between the external diameter of the fiberoptic bronchoscope and the internal diameter of the tube in which it is placed becomes less than 3½ mm.[1] and very small changes in this difference can make large changes in resistance to flow. Should the resistance to flow become too high, then we would expect to be able to blow a gas into the patient's lungs utilizing a ventilator. However, the patient may not have time to exhale, which may lead initially to an increase in arterial CO_2 levels, an increase in mean intrathoracic pressure with a fall off of cardiac output, and possibly to the development of a pneumothorax. It is therefore critical that resistance to flow of gases through these endotracheal tubes be as low as possible to minimize the occurrence of these complications. These tubes accomplish this.

Requests for reprints should be sent to Edward Carden, FRCP(C), VA Wadsworth Hospital Center, Anesthesiology Section, Wilshire and Sawtelle Blvd., Los Angeles CA 90073.

REFERENCES

1. Lindholm CE: Flexible fiberoptic bronchoscopy in the critically ill patient. Ann Otol Rhinol Laryngol 83:786-794, 1974

2. Cole F: A New Endotracheal Tube for Infants. Anesthesiology 6:87-88, 1945

AMERICAN BOARD OF OTOLARYNGOLOGY

The American Board of Otolaryngology will hold its next certifying examination November 15-21, 1975, at the Palmer House, Chicago, Illinois. The deadline for applying for the 1975 examination is May 1, 1975.

Ann Otol 84: 1975

EVALUATION OF MAJOR AIRWAY LESIONS USING THE FLOW-VOLUME LOOP

ROBERT E. HYATT, M.D.

ROCHESTER, MINNESOTA

SUMMARY – The flow-volume (FV) loop is another way of representing spirometric data from combinations of forced expiratory and forced inspiratory vital capacity breaths. The FV loop is of use in identifying, and often localizing, lesions of the larynx and the trachea (down to the carina). Three general patterns have been recognized. When the lesion behaves in a fixed fashion (as might occur with an artificial orifice), maximal expiratory and inspiratory flows are almost equally compromised. This results in a rectangular FV loop, irrespective of whether the lesion is located intrathoracically or extrathoracically. When the lesion behaves in a variable fashion, two distinct patterns are seen, depending on the location of the lesion (intrathoracic or extrathoracic). The variable lesion acts as a fixed lesion during one phase of forced respiration only. The extrathoracic variable lesion results in a predominant reduction in forced inspiratory flow, with little effect on expiratory flow, whereas the intrathoracic variable lesion produces a characteristic reduction in expiratory flow. These patterns reflect the transmural forces existing at the site of the lesion.

There is a relatively simple test that can be useful in detecting and evaluating lesions of the major airways. The major airways involve the larynx as well as the trachea as far down as the carina.

FLOW-VOLUME CURVE

The flow-volume curve is another method of representing data from a spirogram. The spirogram (Fig. 1A) shows a plot of volume versus time for a person breathing quietly. The subject inhales to total lung capacity, does a forced expiration, and immediately follows this with a forced inspiration. A trace of volume versus time enables one to measure the rate of airflow by placing a line tangent to the tracing and measuring the slope of the line. At the three volumes (indicated by the horizontal arrows), flow in liters per second has been calculated at one, two, and three liters of volume (columns in center of figure). These flows are then plotted as a function of volume, producing a flow-volume curve (Fig. 1B). The open circles represent the values measured from the spirogram on the left. Expiratory flow is plotted above zero flow, and inspiratory flow is plotted below zero. If flow was measured at many volumes, the flow-volume curve would appear as the continuous dashed line. A normal flow-volume loop, showing the relationships of maximal expiratory and maximal inspiratory flows to volume, is seen in Figure 1B.

Rather than using a spirogram and laboriously drawing tangents to obtain flow-volume data, one can use many other techniques for obtaining flow and volume signals that can be plotted simultaneously to provide a flow-volume loop (Fig. 2): flow and volume can be measured directly from a waterless spirometer (left); flow and volume can be measured with a pneumotachograph and volume is sensed from a potenti-

From the Mayo Clinic and Mayo Foundation, Rochester, Minnesota.

This investigation was supported in part by Research Grant HL-12229 from the National Institutes of Health, Public Health Service.

Presented at the meeting of the American Broncho-Esophagological Association, Atlanta, Georgia, April 7-8, 1975.

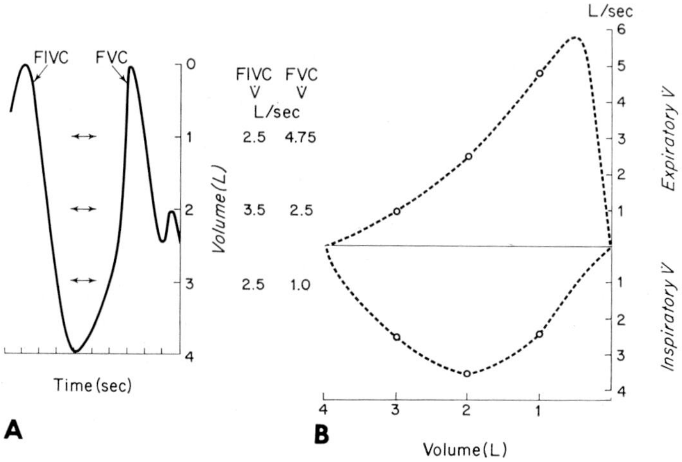

Fig. 1. A) Spirographic tracing of forced expiration (FVC), followed by forced inspiration (FIVC). B) Flow versus volume representation of these maneuvers.

ometer attached to the wheel of the spirometer (middle); and flow can be integrated to obtain the value for volume (right).

There are a number of important mechanical determinants of the normal expiratory limb of the flow-volume curve. Figure 3A shows a model with devices for measuring flow and volume. The trachea and cords are shown, and a model lung is contained in a thorax, which can be ventilated. Note the bronchi; the irregular lines represent the elastic parenchymal support. The lung is in the state of maximal inspiration, with a negative pressure of 30 cm H_2O in the pleural cavity; the airways and alveoli are all at zero or atmospheric pressure.

Figure 3B shows the events during a forced expiration in which volume has changed and pleural pressure is positive at 150 cm H_2O. Alveolar pressure is 160 cm, and there is a point in the airways where the pressure is 140 cm. Because the outside of the airway is essentially exposed to pleural pressure, a pressure difference of 10 cm H_2O exists across the airway; this difference causes airway compression at approximately the sites indicated. This is an example of dynamic compression, and this narrowing or compression determines the maximal expiratory flow at any given lung volume; the downstream (toward the mouth) pressure has decreased to about 15 cm H_2O. Dynamic compression occurs during the lower two-thirds of the vital capacity. The expiratory flow-volume limb of such a maneuver is shown in Figure 3C.

There are also a number of important mechanical determinants of forced in-

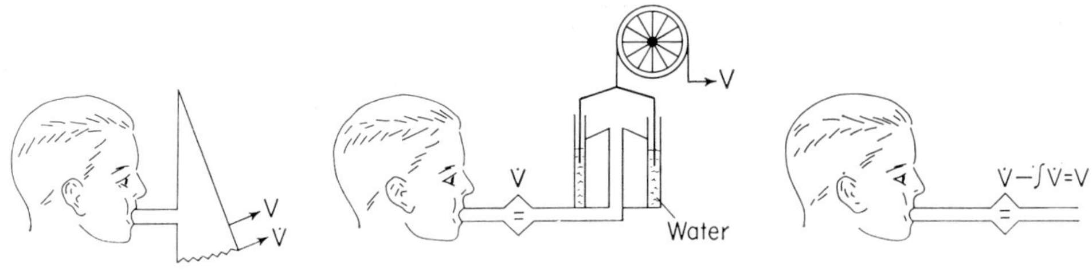

Fig. 2. Three methods of obtaining simultaneous measurements of flow and volume.

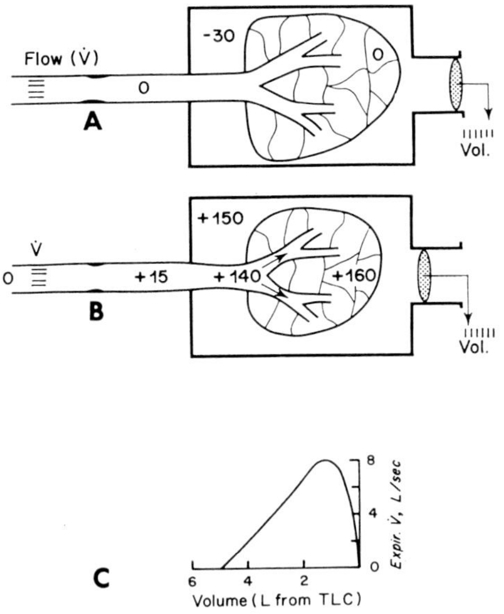

Fig. 3. A and B) Basic mechanical determinants of normal expiratory limb of flow-volume curve. C) Normal expiratory flow-volume curve.

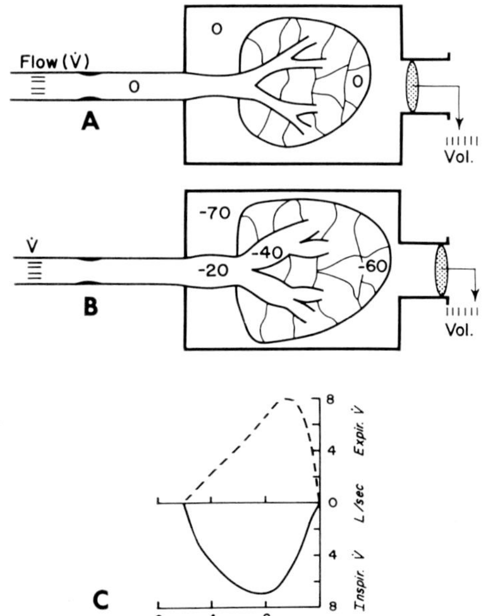

Fig. 4. A and B) Basic mechanical determinants of inspiratory limb of normal flow-volume loop. C) Normal inspiratory curve.

spiratory flow and, hence, of the inspiratory flow-volume limb (Fig. 4). The subject starts at full expiration, or residual volume (Fig. 4A). Pleural pressure is approximately 0 cm H_2O, as are the other pressures. During forced inspiration a point is reached in which the intrapleural pressure is –70 cm H_2O and the pressure is decreasing along the bronchial tree from –20 to –60 cm H_2O (Fig. 4B). The pressure difference in this situation favors dilatation of the airways, because –70 cm H_2O is more negative than –20 cm H_2O. A characteristic normal inspiratory limb of the curve is shown in Figure 4C; the dotted expiratory limb from Figure 3 defines the full flow-volume loop.

Because many major airway lesions are initially misdiagnosed as asthma or chronic obstructive lung disease, it is important to consider both the mechanical events that occur in obstructive disease and the resulting flow-volume loop (Fig. 5). The model in Figure 5A depicts the situation in chronic bronchitis associated with emphysema, but the flow curve in asthma would be similar. The chronic bronchitis and emphysema are represented in the model by the narrowing of the airways, the pile up of mucus, and the loss of some of the parenchymal supports; this leads to a decrease in recoil at maximal inflation, in this instance, to –15 cm H_2O. Figure 5B shows that, with forced expiration, dynamic compression of the airway occurs but that both the dynamic compression and the transbronchial pressure are greater than in the normal situation. The disease of the parenchyma and airways causes the maximal achievable flow during expiration to be considerably reduced (Fig. 5C). Maximal flow decreases gradually as volume decreases, much as is seen in the normal subject. Similarly, maximal inspiratory flow is reduced (also due to the disease process), which is depicted by the dashed inspiratory limb in Figure 5C. The flow-volume loop is similar to a miniature normal loop, but with flows reduced at every lung volume.

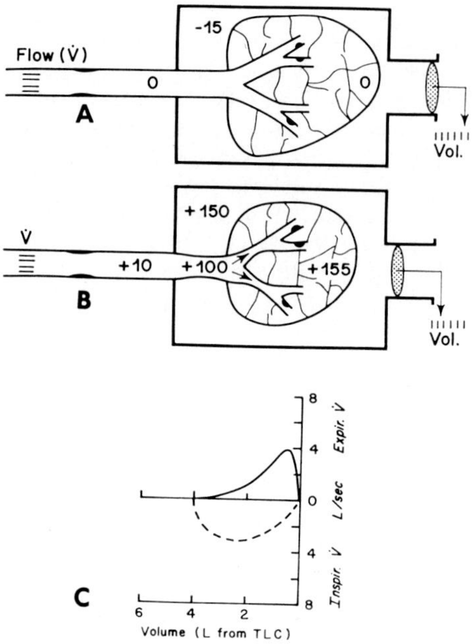

Fig. 5. A and B) Models showing lung during forced expiration in chronic obstructive lung disease. C) Typical expiratory limb in this condition (solid line), along with a typical inspiratory limb (dashed line).

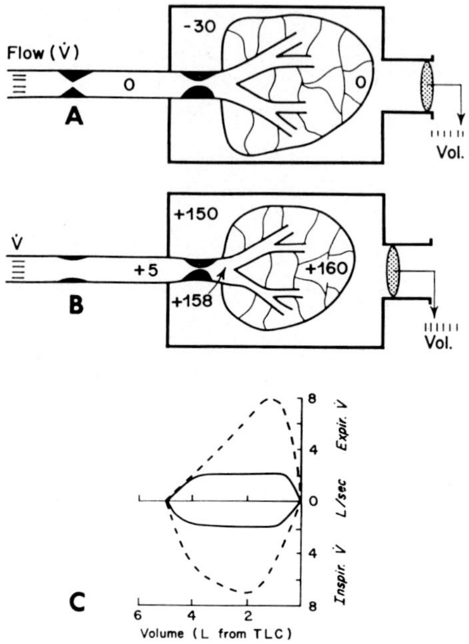

Fig. 6. A and B) Basic mechanical determinants of flow-volume loop in fixed major airway disease. C) Flow-volume loop for fixed lesion of major airway.

FLOW-VOLUME CURVE AND MAJOR AIRWAY LESIONS

The flow-volume loop can be of aid in the detection and understanding of certain major airway lesions. These lesions can be functionally classified as fixed or variable, and each can be further classified as to location — extrathoracic or intrathoracic. The important features are whether the lesion has a fixed size or changes size during both inspiration and expiration or whether the lesion changes size during inspiration or expiration; that is, does the lesion act as a fixed lesion only during one phase of forced respiration. If the lesion is a variable one, whether it is extrathoracic or intrathoracic makes a considerable difference. If the lesion is a fixed one, location has no significant effect on the flow-volume loop.

Fixed Lesions. The fixed lesion behaves like an orifice. In Figure 6A, two types of fixed lesions are illustrated. One involves the cords, and the other is an intrathoracic tumor. In this situation, the airways, parenchyma, and lung recoil are all normal. Figure 6B illustrates the behavior of the intrathoracic tumor; the same results would be obtained from a fixed extrathoracic lesion, such as bilateral cord paralysis. In this situation, there is a significant pressure decrease across the lesion, namely a decrease from 158 to 5 cm H_2O. There is no dynamic compression of the intraparenchymal airways because their pressure is greater than that existing in the pleural cavity (158 versus 150 cm H_2O). Dynamic compression occurs only at low lung volumes when the orifice-like effect of the tumor no longer determines flow. The loops (Fig. 6C) show the typical expiratory limb associated with this lesion, as well as a dashed normal expiratory limb. These loops meet only near residual volume, which indicates that normal dynamic

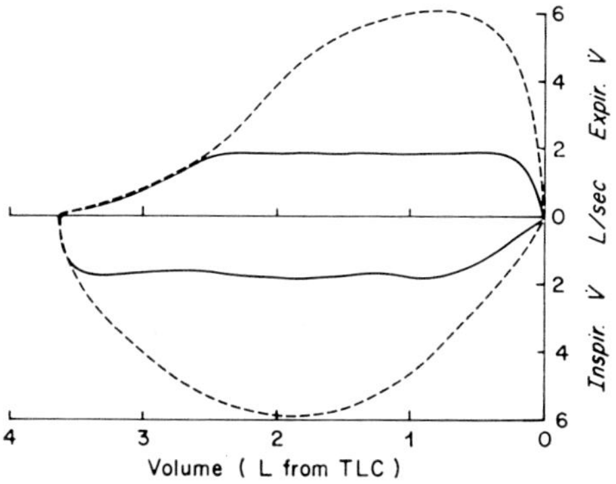

Fig. 7. Solid line depicts loop from patient with fixed lesion, while predicted normal flow-volume loop is represented by dashed line.

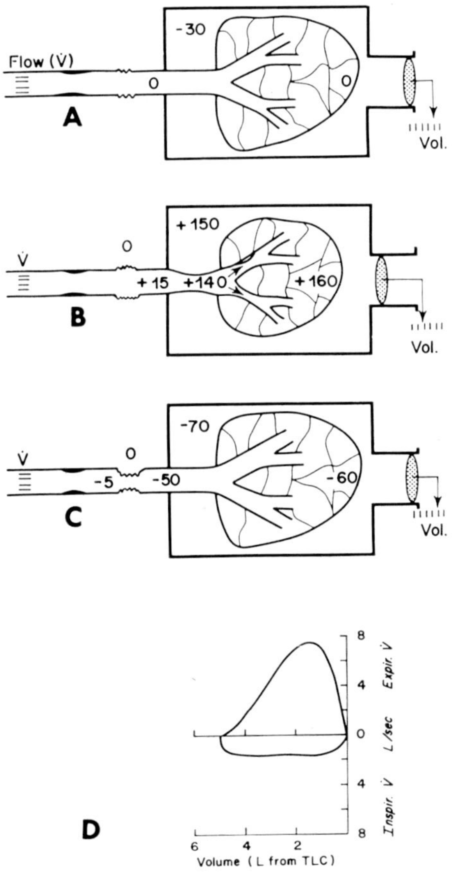

Fig. 8. A, B and C) Basic mechanical determinants of flow-volume loop in variable extrathoracic airway disease. D) Resulting flow-volume loop with its severe reduction in inspiratory flow.

compression is occurring. Because this lesion presumably has the same configuration during inspiration, inspiratory flow is equally reduced. This produces the rectangular flow-volume loop shown by the solid curve (Fig. 6C). Such a loop suggests the presence of a fixed lesion, but does not indicate whether the lesion is located within or without the thorax.

Figure 7 shows a flow-volume loop of a fixed lesion (the solid line); the predicted normal curve is shown by the dashed line. This curve is from a 38-year-old woman who had thyroid surgery four years before admission (in which the surgery produced bilateral cord paralysis). She had noted the onset of difficulty in breathing 1½ years before admission. Routine pulmonary function tests showed only a decrease in the maximal breathing capacity. The patient also had inspiratory stridor. Examination revealed fixation of the cords, with orifice-like behavior. The loop is consistent with what was predicted from the model, showing essentially equal reduction in maximal expiratory and inspiratory flow. For example, at midvital capacity, the ratio of expiratory to inspiratory flow is about one (which is nearly normal), but the loop is abnormal.

Variable Lesions

Extrathoracic Location. The usual cause of such a lesion is a paralyzed cord or tracheal damage after prolonged intubation with a cuffed endotracheal tube. This latter situation is illustrated in three panels of Figure 8 by the irregularity of the extrathoracic trachea. The pressure relationships of this lung are normal at full inflation (Fig. 8A), and during forced expiration, normal dynamic compression of the airways occurs (Fig. 8B). The pressure in the trachea tends to hold the lesion open since the pressure is +15 cm H_2O and the pressure around the trachea is 0 or atmospheric. A relatively normal expiratory limb of the curve is obtained (Fig. 8D). But during forced inspiration (Fig. 8C), the lesion makes its presence

	Estimated normal	Observed
Vital capacity (L)	4.7	6.0
MVV (L/min)	115	45
MMF (L/sec)	〉2.0	3.3

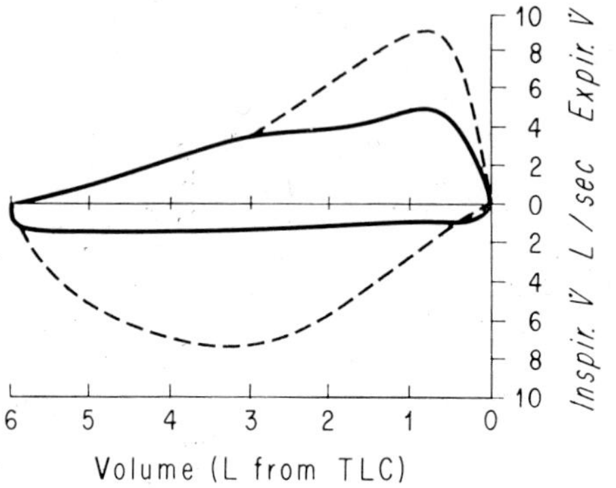

Fig. 9. Solid line represents flow-volume loop in variable extrathoracic disease while dashed lines indicate expected normal loop for this patient. (With permission from Miller RD, Hyatt RE: Obstructing lesions of the larynx and trachea: clinical and physiologic characteristics. Mayo Clin Proc 44:145-161, 1969.)

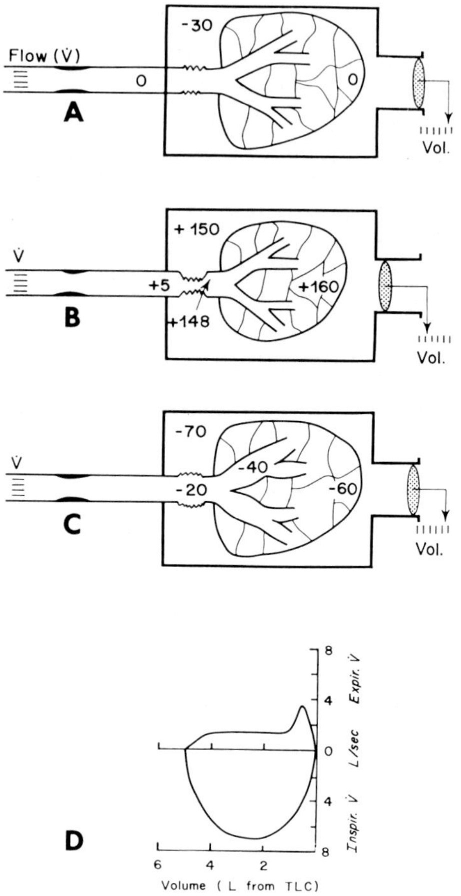

Fig. 10. A, B and C) Important mechanical determinants of flow-volume loop in variable intrathoracic disease. D) Typical flow-volume loop in this disease. Note severe reduction in expiratory flow.

known. The subatmospheric intratracheal pressure collapses the lesion, which quickly acts like an orifice with a large pressure decrease across it, that is, from –5 to –50 cm H_2O. This compressed fixed segment restricts inspiratory flow substantially, as is shown by the inspiratory limb in Figure 8D. The ratio of expiratory to inspiratory flow at midvital capacity is abnormally high, being about four to one.

Figure 9 shows a flow-volume curve from a patient with a variable extrathoracic lesion. The patient was a 53-year-old man who had poliomyelitis in 1946 and in recent years has experienced considerable tension and fatigue. In addition, he had cough and dyspnea. At examination, he was depressed, and initially he was thought not to have organic disease. Routine pulmonary function studies revealed a normal vital capacity and a normal maximal midexpiratory flow but a significant reduction of the maximal breathing capacity. These findings indicated a possible lesion of the major airway. These studies were followed up by obtaining the flow-volume loop shown by the solid lines. There is some reduction in peak expiratory flow, but the most striking reduction occurs on the forced inspiratory limb. Later examination revealed inspiratory stridor, a fixed right vocal cord, and a left cord that moved only about 4 mm; the dashed line is the normal predicted loop for this patient.

Intrathoracic Location. Typically, such lesions are due to invasive tumors that weaken the bronchial wall (Fig. 10). The lungs and pressures are nor-

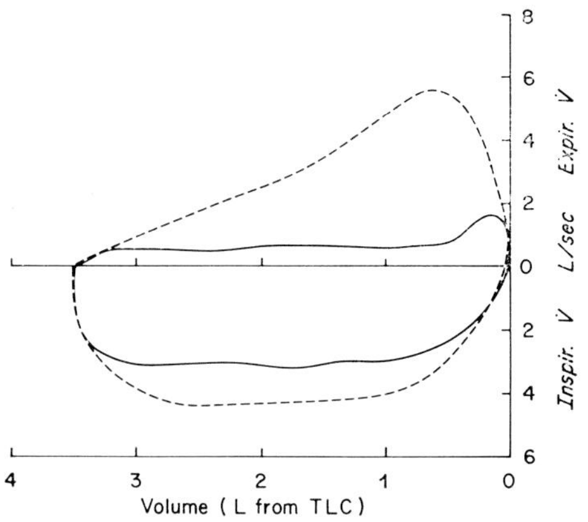

Fig. 11. Solid lines depict flow-volume loop obtained from 68-year-old man with variable intrathoracic lesion. Dashed lines represent predicted normal loop for this patient.

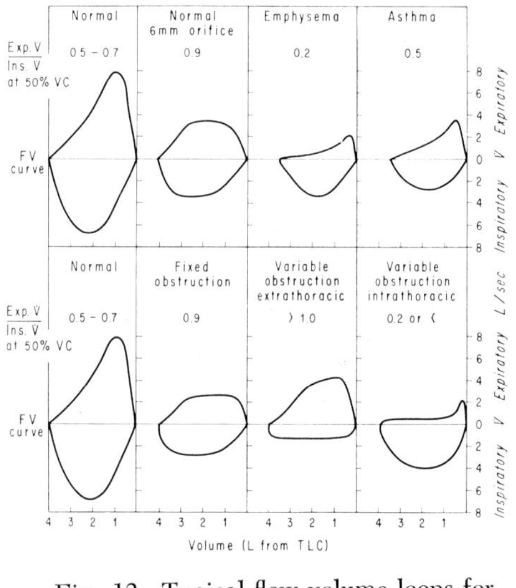

Fig. 12. Typical flow-volume loops for normal person, normal person breathing through an orifice, and patients with obstructive lung disease and various types of major airway lesions. Ratio of expiratory to inspiratory flow at midvital capacity for each loop is shown.

mal, but with forced expiration, the lesion becomes apparent. The lesion collapses quickly and acts like a fixed orifice. The pressure decreases significantly across the lesion from about 148 to 5 cm H_2O (Fig. 10B). The flow is greatly reduced on the expiratory limb (Fig. 10D). There is no dynamic compression of the airways because the major pressure decrease is occurring across the lesion. The spike of expiratory flow (Fig. 10D) presumably occurred while the lesion was undergoing collapse. During inspiration (Fig. 10C) the pressure across the tracheal wall tends to hold the lesion open and inspiratory flow is affected little, as reflected in the relatively normal inspiratory limb of the flow-volume curve (Fig 10D).

The typical loop for a variable intrathoracic lesion is shown in Figure 11. The solid flow-volume loop was obtained from a 68-year-old man who, six weeks before admission, had developed cough, phlegm and wheezing, all of which had onset after a cold. The patient had smoked but had stopped about one year before admission; he had no prior symptoms of chronic bronchitis. Initially, the patient was seen by an allergist, who referred him to a chest physician, who in turn ordered pulmonary function tests, which showed an obstructive pattern. In addition, special lung mechanics studies were requested; these included the flow-volume loop.

The studies revealed no evidence of emphysema but did demonstrate a very abnormal expiratory limb of the flow-volume loop. The flow spiked initially during expiration and then, essentially, flattened during expiration. In contrast, inspiratory flow was affected little. This expiratory pattern differs from that in typical obstructive lung disease (Fig. 5). The ratio of expiratory to inspiratory flow at the midvital capacity is about 0.2, similar to that in obstructive lung disease, but the flow-volume loop has a distinctive and unusual contour of the expiratory limb.

SUMMARY

Figure 12 shows a series of flow-volume loops and the ratios of expiratory to inspiratory flow at midvital capacity in normal and disease states. The variations in flow-volume loops can be helpful in diagnosing and analyzing lesions of the major airway. The flow-volume loop test is easy to perform, being a combination of a maximally forced expiratory vital capacity breath, followed by a maximally forced inspiratory vital capacity breath. Visualizing these maneuvers in terms of flow and volume can permit a much better recognition of the presence of a major airway lesion than can examination of the spirogram.

Request for reprints should be sent to Dr. R. E. Hyatt, Mayo Clinic, Rochester, MN 55901.

MODERN TRENDS IN OTOLOGIC SURGERY

A course including seminars, discussions, and surgical demonstrations will be presented Oct. 28 - Nov. 1, 1975, by the Department of Surgery, Section of Otolaryngology, Notre-Dame Hospital, Montreal, Quebec. Guest lecturers will include Professor Ugo Fisch, Juan Marquet, M.D., Brian McCabe, M.D., and George Shambaugh, Jr., M.D.

For further information write: Robert A. Bertrand, M.D., Vestibular Laboratory, Notre-Dame Hospital, 1560 Sherbrooke St. East, Montreal, Quebec, Canada, H2L 4 MI.

OTOLARYNGOLOGIC ASSEMBLY

The annual Otolaryngologic Assembly of 1975 will be held November 8-14, 1975, in the Eye and Ear Infirmary of the University of Illinois Hospital. The Department of Otolaryngology of the Abraham Lincoln School of Medicine, University of Illinois at the Medical Center offers a condensed basic and clinical program for practicing otolaryngologists under the direction of Emanuel M. Skolnik, M.D., with Burton J. Soboroff, M.D. as co-chairman. Inquiries may be sent to: Otolaryngology, P.O. Box 6998, Chicago, Illinois 60680.

Ann Otol 84: 1975

HYOID AUTOGRAFT REPAIR OF CHRONIC SUBGLOTTIC STENOSIS

DOUGLAS A. FINNEGAN, M.D.

MATTHEW L. WONG, M.D. HASKINS K. KASHIMA, M.D.

BALTIMORE, MARYLAND

SUMMARY — A previously unreported surgical technique has been evaluated for the correction of chronic subglottic (cricoid) stenosis. The principle of skeletal support as the primary means of repair was examined. Severe stenoses were created in sixteen adult, mongrel dogs. One to three months later a hyoid bone autograft on a sternohyoid muscle pedicle was employed for repair. The dogs were sacrificed at regular intervals from two weeks to six months. The majority of the animals maintained a widely patent lumen after repair. Vocal cord mobility remained normal in every case. The results are illustrated by photographs and histologic sections. This study convincingly demonstrates a successful surgical technique for correcting a most difficult laryngeal lesion.

Chronic subglottic stenosis of various etiologies has been a most difficult problem to correct. Several recent cases of infant and adult chronic subglottic (cricoid) stenosis at our affiliated hospitals have reiterated the difficulty of managing such lesions. The basic problem involved is the reestablishment of a permanent airway without compromise of vocal cord function. Primary resection of the stenosis with direct tracheothyroid anastamosis has been successfully accomplished.[1-6] Careful review of case reports, however, generally reveals that the great majority had bilateral adductor vocal cord palsies preoperatively. An arytenoidpexy was usually part of the procedure. Voice quality generally seemed to be poor in these patients postoperatively, and the chance of new or further recurrent laryngeal nerve injuries was great.

Other clinical and experimental reports have described less radical surgical repairs of this lesion. Bennett[7] reported the partially successful repair of chronic cricoid stenosis using an autogenous free hyoid bone graft in one patient. Alonso, *et al*[8] reported one patient repaired with an interposed free autogenous hyoid graft. No final conclusion could be made, however, as the intraluminal stent was still in place at the time of publication.

Lapidot, *et al*[9] reported an experimental study on piglets using a thyroid alar chondroperichondrial "trap door" flap to immediately repair a cricoid defect created by resecting part of the anterior arch. This surgery seemingly did not adversely affect normal growth in this area, and the airway apparently was maintained. However, there was no mention of vocal cord function, and the number of experimental animals was too small to draw firm conclusions.

Delahunty, *et al*[10] and Alonso, *et al*[11] reported an experimental study on anterior cricoid arch homotransplantation in four dogs. Six months follow-up showed some resorption of the transplants, and at one year the homografts had been completely replaced by fibrous tissue. Vocal cord function had

Presented at the meeting of The American Broncho-Esophagological Association, Atlanta, Georgia, April 7-8, 1975.

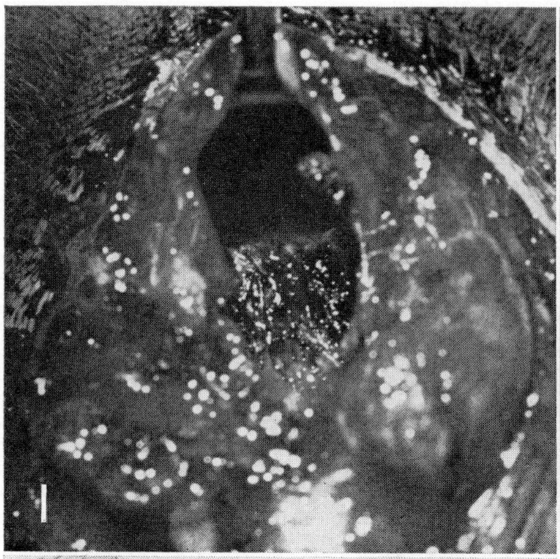

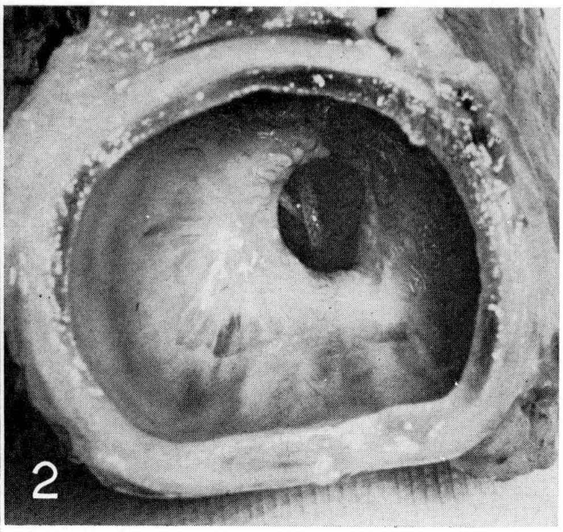

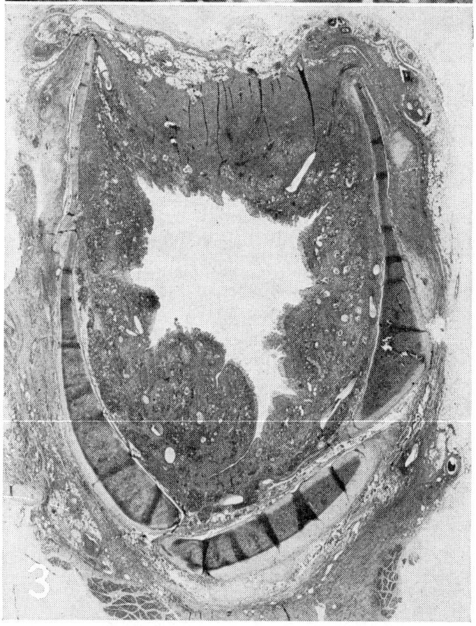

Fig. 1. The anterior 40-50% of the cricoid arch has been resected and mucosal/submucosal tissues electrocoagulated.

Fig. 2. Resultant severe chronic subglottic stenosis.

Fig. 3. Subglottic stenosis with absent anterior cricoid cartilage and cicatricial intraluminal scarring.

been preserved. It is quite obvious today that the problem of tissue rejection has not been solved. Additionally, the availability of appropriate donors remains a most difficult problem.

Fearon[12] reported an experimental study on monkeys using a thyrochondral flap similar to Lapidot's. He enlarged the lumen by interposing the flap between two cut ends of the anterior cricoid arch. In most of his models, the repair was immediate with no stenosis created. Apparently, the lumens remained widely patent but no length of follow-up was given.

Alonso, *et al*[13] reported the autotransplantation of free hyoid grafts in four dogs immediately after resecting the anterior cricoid arch. Again, however, no stenosis had been created before repair.

Our study was initiated to test the efficacy of skeletal support as the primary means of permanently correcting severe chronic cricoid stenosis, while at the same time maintaining vocal cord function.

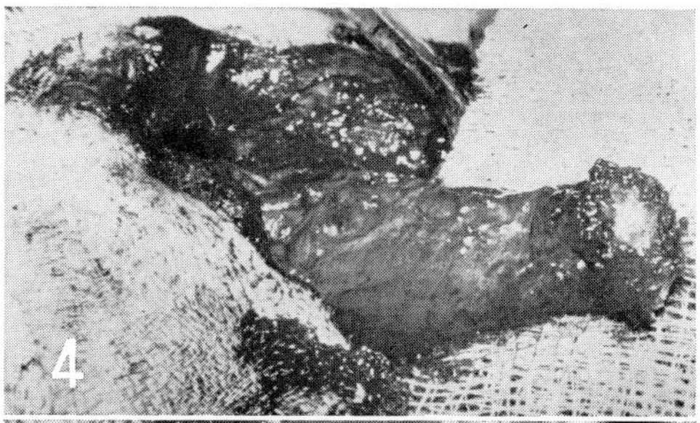

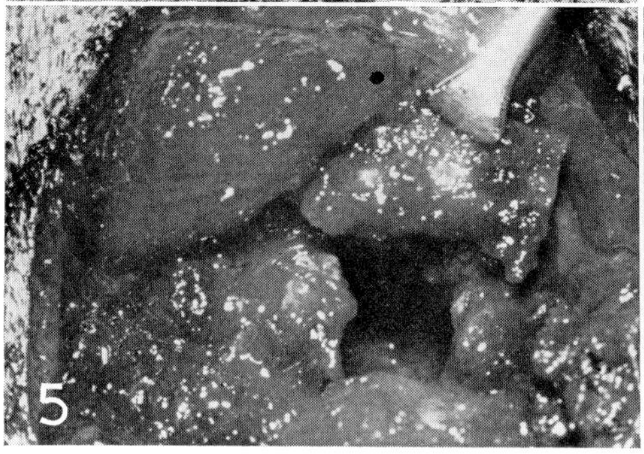

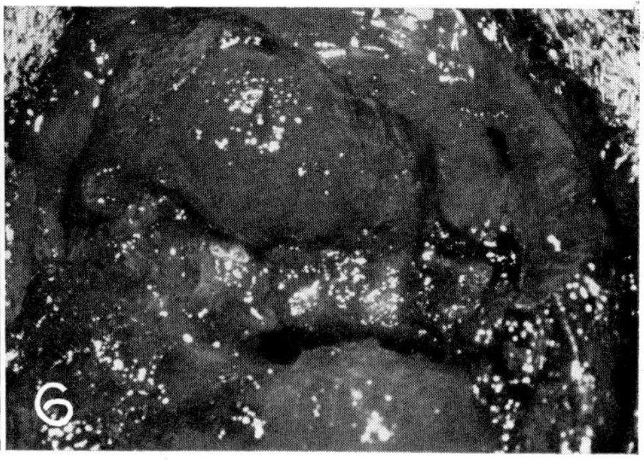

Fig. 4. Hyoid bone-sternohyoid muscle pedicle graft.

Fig. 5. Cricoid stenosis incised, opened, and cartilage ends dissected.

Fig. 6. Graft interposed anteriorly.

METHODS AND MATERIALS

Thirty-five adult mongrel dogs weighing between 11 and 30 kgs. were used. Of these, 19 died after the initial surgical procedure of creation of subglottic stenosis. The remaining 16 were used for the repair. Nembutol®* (22 mgs/kgs), intravenously, and 1% Xylocaine®** with 1:100,000 Epinephrine®***, locally, were used for anesthesia. Intravenous Ringer's lactate was given intraoperatively and in the immediate postoperative period. Intramuscular penicillin (300,000 μ) and streptomycin (400 mgs) were administered postoperatively for seven days.

First, a severe cricoid stenosis was created. Through a vertical midline incision the larynx, cricoid, and trachea were exposed. A permanent tracheostomy was performed excising an anterior window including tracheal rings 7 through 10. The trachea was then sutured to the skin. The origins of the anterior cricoarytenoid muscles were sharply detached, and the anterior 40-50% of the cricoid arch was resected. The posterior cricoid arch was then incised sharply in the midline. Next, the subglottic mucosal and submucosal tissues were electrocoagulated to effect maximum scarring (Fig. 1). Lastly, the remaining cricoid ring was crushed and sutured together with 0 Chromic catgut. Examples of resultant stenoses are well shown in Figures 2 and 3.

Between one and three months later the stenoses were repaired. The middle third of the hyoid bone was resected (including periosteum) with one sternohyoid muscle attached (Fig. 4). The cricoid stenosis was incised and opened anteriorly. The ends of the remaining cricoid cartilage were dissected free of scar tissue and the hyoid muscle pedicle graft interposed (Figs. 5 and 6). Finally, the autograft was sutured into place with two 28 gauge stainless steel wires. The wound was then closed in layers including the tracheostomy. No intraluminal stenting or steroids postoperatively were used.

Two animals each were sacrificed at the following intervals: 2 weeks, 1, 2, 3, 4, 5 and 6 months. Two animals will be sacrificed at one year. The larynges were removed for serial sectioning and photomicrographs. Luminal measurements were made of the original cricoid areas, after creation of the stenoses, immediately after repair, and upon sacrificing.

RESULTS

The resultant lumens after stenosis ranged from 6% to 50% of the original cricoid areas. 12 dogs (86%) had at least 67% stenosis. The mean percent remaining lumen after stenosis was 23%. The repaired subglottic areas ranged from 54% to 148% of the original lumens.

---

* Abbott Laboratories, N. Chicago, Ill.
** Astra Pharmaceutical Products, Inc., Worcester, Mass.
*** SMP Division, Cooper Laboratories, San German, P.R.

TABLE I

SUBGLOTTIC AREAS AFTER CREATION OF STENOSIS AND AFTER REPAIR

Dog No.	Original Area (mm²)	Stenosis Area (mm²)	% Lumen After Stenosis	Repair Area (mm²)	% Lumen After Repair
6	452	60	13	246	54
73	201	50	25	132	66
22	314	104	33	260	83
28	380	78	21	525	138
77	414	60	14	462	112
66	283	70	25	420	148
74	380	190	50	314	83
27	283	50	18	306	108
69	282	28	10	190	67
12	314	20	6	201	64
55	314	52	17	247	79
23	314	70	22	288	92
53	456	228	50	396	87
76	369	60	16	330	89
Mean:	340 mm²	80 mm²	23%	308 mm²	91%

The mean percent restoration of the original lumen was 91% with four dogs overcorrected (Table I).

Nine of fourteen animals (64%) maintained the initial repair. Five (36%) demonstrated later reduction of cricoid area (Table II). There was no correlation between the severity of the original stenosis and the incidence of later reduction (Table III). Moreover, there was no correlation between loss of cricoid area and length of follow-up (Table IV).

TABLE II

% REDUCTION OF SUBGLOTTIC AREAS AFTER REPAIR

Dog. No.	Immediate Repair Area (mm²)	Follow-Up Repair Area (mm²)	% Reduction of Repair
6	246	246	0
73	132	132	0
22	260	260	0
53	396	396	0
76	330	330	0
74	314	314	0
12	201	201	0
66	420	394	6
77	462	420	9
55	247	192	22
28	525	375	29
69	190	120	37
23	288	180	38
27	306	160	48

TABLE III

ORIGINAL % STENOSIS AS COMPARED TO % REDUCTION OF REPAIR

Dog No.	% Luminal Stenosis	% Reduction of Repair
6	87	0
73	75	0
22	67	0
53	50	0
76	84	0
74	50	0
12	94	0
66	75	6
77	86	9
	Mean 74%	
55	83	22
28	79	29
69	90	37
23	78	38
27	82	48
	Mean 82%	

TABLE IV

LENGTH OF FOLLOW-UP
AS COMPARED TO
% REDUCTION OF REPAIR

Dog No.	*Length of Follow-Up*	*% Reduction of Repair*
6	2 wks.	0
73	2 wks.	0
22	1 mo.	0
77	2 mos.	9
66	2 mos.	6
74	3 mos.	0
12	4 mos.	0
53	6 mos.	0
76	6 mos.	0
28	1 mo.	29
27	3 mos.	48
69	4 mos.	37
55	5 mos.	22
23	5 mos.	38

The successful restoration of the subglottic airway is clearly demonstrated in Figures 7, 8, and 9. Cross sectional photomicrographs of three and six months repairs are shown in Figures 10 and 11, which illustrate the intact hyoid muscle pedicle autograft. The lining epithelium is normal ciliated pseudostratified columnar (Fig. 12).

Vocal cord mobility was examined prior to sacrificing. In every animal mobility was normal.

DISCUSSION

The use of hyoid bone grafts for correction of glottic stenosis is not new. Looper,[14] Woodward,[15] and Ogura and Biller[16] have used this technique with success. Only Bennett[7] and Alonso, *et al*[8] have attempted subglottic stenosis repair with hyoid bone. These repairs have utilized free autografts. Conley[17] has reported the successful use of bone-muscle pedicle grafts in mandibular and facial reconstruction. In an attempt to insure a more reliable blood supply, we selected a muscle pedicled hyoid autograft. This selection also provided us with a rigid graft which could be interposed to correct a stenotic subglottis. We reasoned that skeletal support could be provided without intraluminal stenting, thus reducing postoperative morbidity and avoiding further procedures. Likewise, recurrent laryngeal nerve damage could hopefully be avoided.

The data presented confirm our impressions about the appropriateness of an autogenous hyoid bone muscle pedicle graft. Approximately two-thirds of our repairs showed no significant resorption. In the dogs with resorption, all had a resultant restenosis less than 50%. No consistent reason could be determined for the restenosis. Gross examination of the larynges upon sacrificing revealed all the muscle pedicles to be viable. All 14 animals were able to breathe easily throughout the follow-up period. Recurrent laryngeal nerve function was not disturbed.

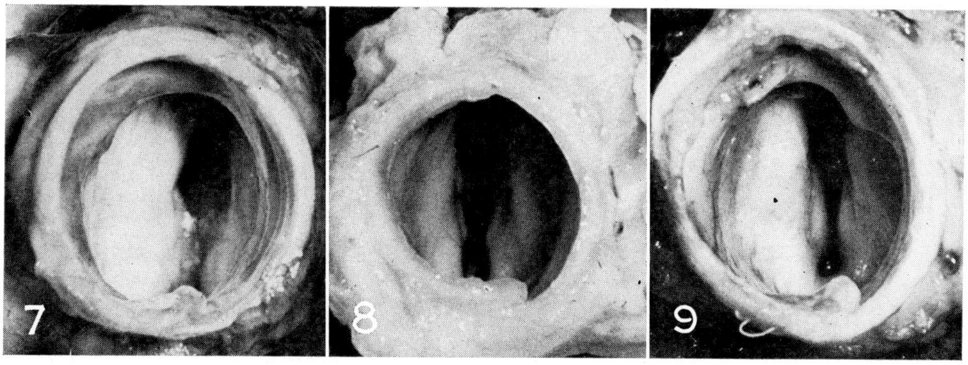

Fig. 7. Dog. No. 22. One month after repair.
Fig. 8. Dog. No. 74. Three months after repair.
Fig. 9. Dog. No. 76. Six months after repair.

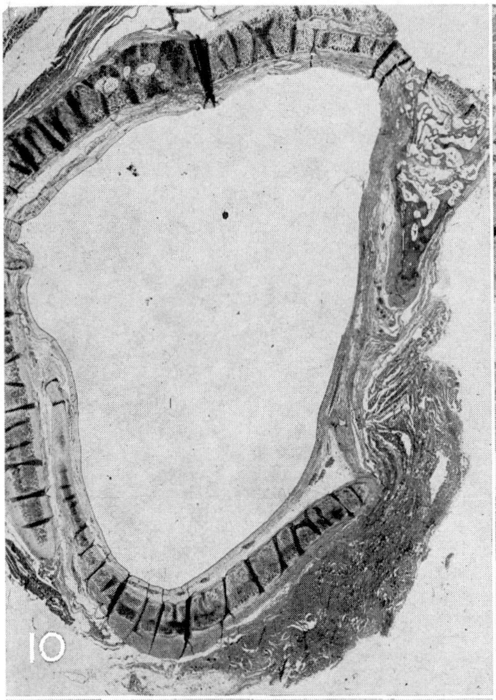

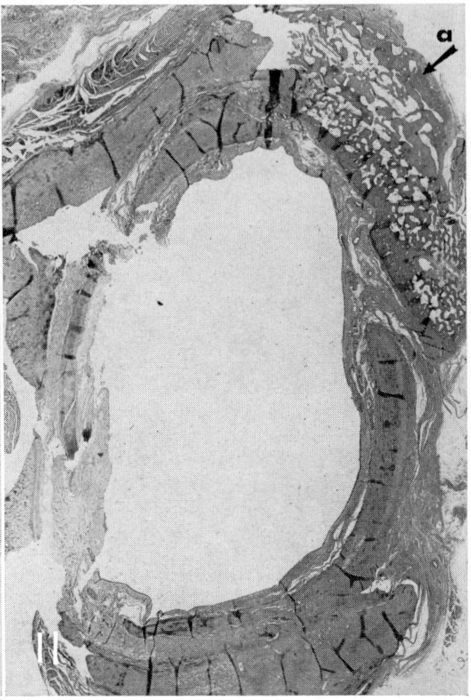

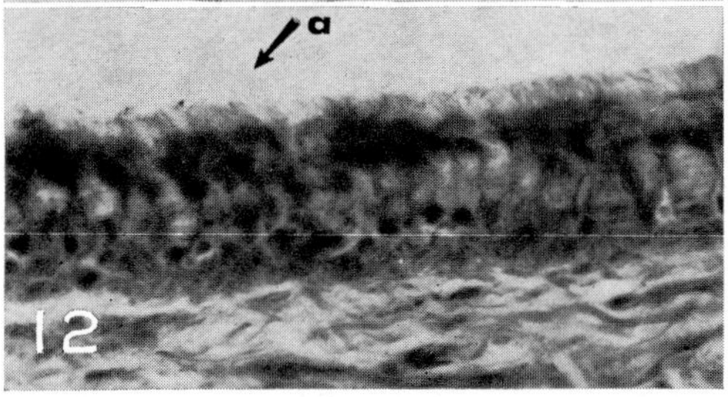

Fig. 10. Dog. No. 74. Note the widely patent lumen and intact hyoid bone.

Fig. 11. Dog. No. 76. a - Interposed hyoid bone with intact mucosa.

Fig. 12. Dog. No. 76. a - Normal respiratory mucosa.

CONCLUSIONS

From the previous study the following conclusions can be drawn.

Skeletal support with a hyoid bone muscle pedicle autograft is an effective means of correcting chronic subglottic (cricoid) stenosis.

The problem of restenosis is not severe and appears to be a sporadic occurrence unrelated to severity of stenosis or length of time following repair.

Normal vocal cord mobility is maintained.

Intraluminal stenting is not necessarily required.

This experimental operation seems applicable for adults with this lesion.

A parallel study has been initiated with puppies to ascertain the feasibility of such surgery on the infant larynx.

ACKNOWLEDGMENT—The authors would like to express their gratitude to Mr. Richard Evans and Mr. Joseph Claggett for their excellent technical assistance and to Mr. Donald Meyers for his preparation of the histologic sections.

Request for reprints should be sent to Douglas A. Finnegan, M.D., Department of Otolaryngology, The Johns Hopkins Hospital, Baltimore, Md. 21205.

REFERENCES

1. Conley JJ: Reconstruction of the subglottic air space. Ann Otol Rhinol Laryngol 62:477- 495, 1953

2. Shaw RR, Paulson DL, Kee JL: Traumatic tracheal rupture. J Thorac Cardiovasc Surg 42:281-297, 1961

3. Rush BF Jr: Repair of the injured larynx following destruction of the cricoid cartilage. Surg Gynec Obst 112:507-510, 1961

4. Ogura JH, Roper CL: Surgical correction of traumatic stenosis of larynx and pharynx. Laryngoscope 72:468-480, 1962

5. Morrow RC, Muldowny TJ: One-stage correction of subglottic stenosis. The Eye, Ear, Nose and Thorat Monthly 49:119-124, 1970

6. Gerwat J, Bryce DP: The management of subglottic laryngeal stenosis by resection and direct anastomosis. Laryngoscope 84:940-957, 1974

7. Bennett T: Laryngeal strictures. South Med Jour 53:1101-1104, 1960

8. Alonso WA, Pratt LL, Zollinger W.K., *et al*: Complications of laryngotracheal disruption. Laryngoscope 84:1276-1290, 1974

9. Lapidot A, Sodogar R, Ratanaproshtporn S, *et al*: Experimental repair of subglottic stenosis in piglets. Arch Otolaryngol 88:529-535, 1968

10. Delahunty J, Alonso WA, Bordley JE: Cricoid arch transplantation. Laryngoscope 80:137-144, 1970

11. Alonso WA, Bridger GP, Youngblood J, *et al*: Cricoid arch transplantation. Long term follow-up. Laryngoscope 81:1968-1970, 1971

12. Fearon B, Cotton R: Surgical corrections of subglottic stenosis of the larynx. Ann Otol Rhinol Laryngol 81:508-513, 1972

13. Alonso WA, Druck NS, Griffiths CM, *et al*:Cricoid arch replacement in dogs. Arch Otolaryngol 101:42-45, 1975

14. Looper EA: Use of the hyoid bone as a graft in laryngeal stenosis. Arch Otolaryngol 28:106-111, 1938

15. Woodward FD: The surgical correction of cicatricial stenosis of the larynx. Ann Otol Rhinol Laryngol 59:488, 1950

16. Ogura JH, Biller HF: Reconstruction of the larynx following blunt trauma. Ann Otol Rhinol Laryngol 80:492-506, 1971

17. Conley JJ: Regional bone - muscle - skin pedicle flaps in surgery of the head and neck. Trans Amer Acad Ophthalmol Otolaryngol 76:963-967, 1972

RADIOLOGY CONFERENCE

A Conference on Radiology in Otolaryngology and Ophthalmology will be held on November 28 and 29, 1975, under the guidance of Galdino E. Valvassori, M.D. For further information write to: G. E. Valvassori, M.D., Radiology Department, Abraham Lincoln School of Medicine, P.O. Box 6998, Chicago, Illinois 60680.

Ann Otol 84: 1975

FOREIGN BODY REMOVAL:
A NEW ROLE FOR THE FIBEROPTIC BRONCHOSCOPE

DONALD C. ZAVALA, M.D.

MITCHELL L. RHODES, M.D.

IOWA CITY, IOWA

SUMMARY – Artificial and animal lung models initially were used to investigate the removal of foreign bodies from the tracheobronchial tree with the flexible fiberoptic bronchoscope. Different extraction instruments (claw, basket, forceps, and balloon catheter) were passed separately through the channel of the bronchofiberscope, and tested for usefulness prior to human application. The Fogarty balloon catheter served as a valuable aid in dislodging impacted objects so that the operator could then grasp them with the claw, basket or forceps. The wire claw recovered many of the metallic and organic objects, the wire basket was successful in retrieving only the bulky objects and the forceps (ACMI) was effective in capturing all of the metallic foreign bodies. These techniques, developed in our laboratory, are now being used to augment rigid bronchoscopy in the removal of foreign bodies from adults and older children. At the present time fiberoptic foreign body removal is not recommended for pediatric cases because of the small diameter of the trachea and glottis in infants and young children.

Aspiration of foreign bodies remains a significant clinical problem. The majority of objects in the tracheobronchial tree can be removed by rigid bronchoscopy with an extraction forceps or special instruments.[1-8] However, if conventional methods fail, then early thoracotomy and transpleural bronchotomy must be performed to prevent increased complications and mortality.[9]

Because the flexible fiberoptic bronchoscope can visualize areas of the tracheobronchial tree inaccessible to the rigid instrument, we investigated its application in the removal of foreign bodies from the airway. Improvement in fiberoptic scope designs, better bronchoscopic techniques, and the recent development of new extraction instruments inserted through the channel of the scope made this a promising area of investigation. Prior to use on humans, we employed artificial and animal (dog) lung models.[10]

METHODS AND MATERIALS

In the experimental studies, the methods and materials used were as follows:

1. An Olympus fiberoptic bronchoscope*, an 8.5 mm endotracheal tube, and a tracheal tube adapter** with oxygen inlet (Fig. 1).

2. A steel wire basket,*** wire claw,*** biopsy forceps, and a variety of metallic and organic foreign bodies (Fig 2). The wire basket was mounted in a 1.6 mm teflon tube and passed down the channel of the bronchofiberscope (BFS) with the basket retracted inside the tube. Under endoscopic control the tip of the tube was advanced just beyond the foreign body. At this point the basket was opened

---

* Model BF-5B2, Olympus Corp. of America, New Hyde Park, N.Y.

** Med-Econ Plastics, Upland, Calif.

*** Medi-Tech Corp., Watertown, Mass.

From the Department of Medicine, University of Iowa College of Medicine, Iowa City, Iowa.

This work was supported in part by a grant from the American Lung Association of Iowa.

Presented at the meeting of the American Broncho-Esophagological Association, Atlanta, Georgia, April 7-8, 1975.

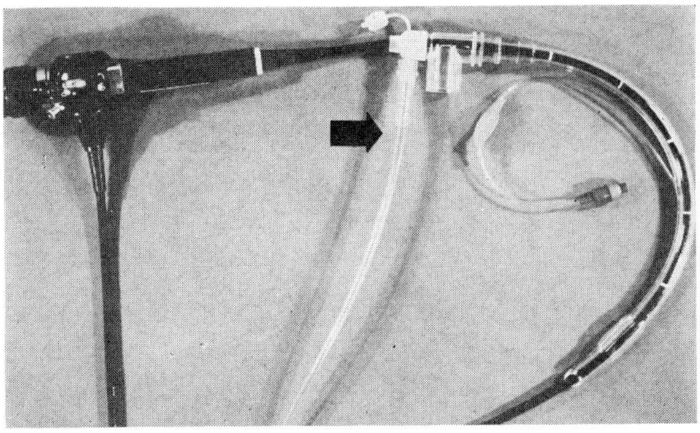

Fig. 1. Set-up for foreign body extraction: an Olympus BF-5B2 fiberoptic bronchoscope inserted through an 8.5 mm endotracheal tube. Arrow indicates the oxygen line running to the tracheal tube adapter.

and pulled back so that the object became enveloped by the separated wires, then entrapped when the basket was closed, as shown in Figure 3A. Upon visible evidence of a successful capture, the entire bronchoscope was withdrawn. The steel wire claw operated in a fashion similar to the basket; however, the foreign body was captured by the direct approach as demonstrated in Figure 3B. Two biopsy forceps, Olympus and ACMI models,* were used as extraction tools (Fig. 3C).

3. Fogarty** and Swan-Ganz** catheters, size 7F (Fig. 3D). Both balloon catheters were utilized to dislodge impacted objects in swollen bronchi so that the operator could reach them with the claw, basket or forceps. The catheter was passed alongside or piggy-backed to the shaft of the BFS. The tip of the catheter was positioned beyond the foreign body. Then the balloon was inflated and drawn back, thus freeing the object for retrieval by one of the extraction instruments.

4. An artificial lung model* (Fig. 4). To gain expertise, the foreign bodies were dropped into and removed from a flexible plastic reduplication of the tracheobronchial tree.***

5. Four mongrel dogs. Each animal upon several different occasions, was anesthetized by neuroleptanalgesia using Innovar®**** plus atropine. When asleep, the dog was secured on a tilt able and intubated. Each foreign body was maneuvered with the BFS into a segmental or subsegmental bronchus of the

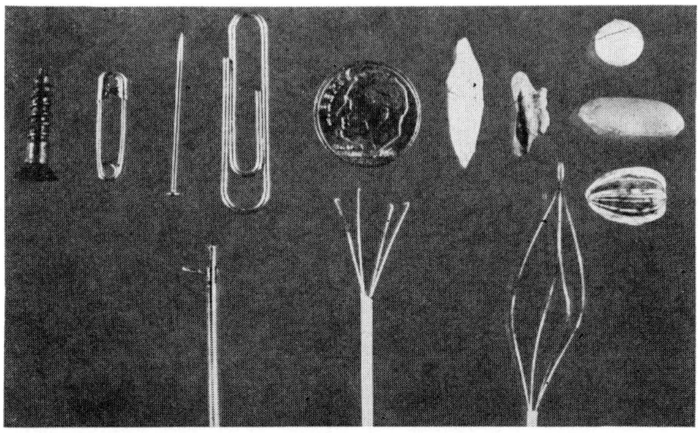

Fig. 2. Foreign bodies from left to right: screw, safety pin, straight pin, paper clip, dime, incisor tooth, chicken vertebra, bean, peanut, and sunflower seed. Extraction tools, located below: forceps, steel wire claw and basket.

----

* American Cystoscope Makers, Inc., Pelham Manor, N.Y.

** Edwards Laboratories, Div. Amer. Hosp. Supply Corp., Santa Ana, Calif.

*** This model was conceived in our laboratory and is now being manufactured by the Medi-Tech Corporation.

**** 1.0 ml = 0.4 mg of fentanyl (analgesic) + 20 mg of droperidol (tranquilizer). McNeil Laboratories, Inc., Fort Washington, PA

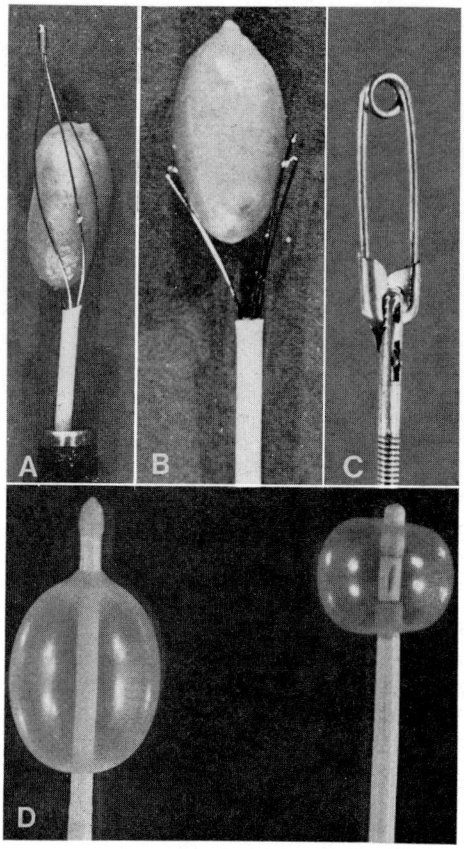

Fig. 3. A) Capture of a peanut with the wire basket. B) Capture of a peanut with the wire claw. C) Capture of a safety pin with the ACMI forceps. D) Two balloon catheters used to dislodge impacted objects, Fogarty on the left and Swan-Ganz on the right.

lower lobe before recovery was attempted. A dime and a peanut, because of their large diameters, had to be inserted and removed without the endotracheal tube. Two persons were required for the recovery maneuver, one to operate the bronchoscope and the other to assist in handling the extraction instruments. Capture of the foreign body was carried out with the head of the dog elevated so that the object, if inadvertently dropped during recovery, would not become lost in the subglottic area.

In the human studies, the instruments and techniques were the same as those used experimentally in the animal laboratory.

RESULTS

Of the different extraction tools employed experimentally in this study, no

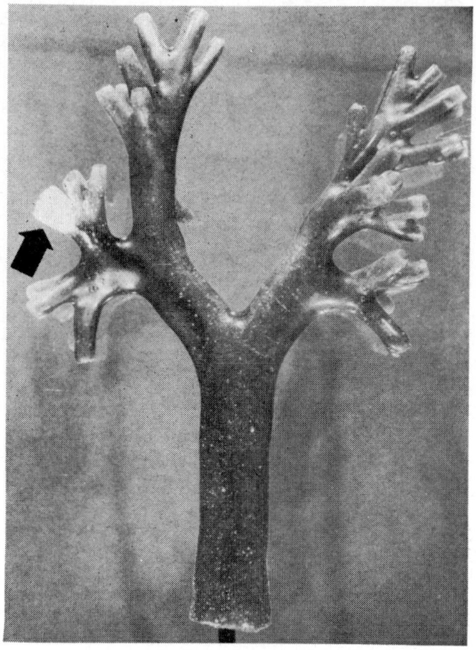

Fig. 4. Plastic model of the human tracheobronchial tree. Arrow points to lighted bronchus (LB^4) where the tip of the fiberscope is located.

single one was successful in removing all of the foreign bodies. The Olympus forceps with its small jaws was satisfactory only for removal of the straight pin, whereas the ACMI forceps with its long jaws was capable of removing any of the metallic objects. The organic objects such as the peanut, broke into pieces at application of the forceps, making complete removal impossible. The basket worked well in recovering all of the bulky, organic objects (peanut, bean, chicken vertebra) but failed to retain the thin items (safety or straight pin, paper clip, screw). The claw recovered most metallic and organic objects except for the straight pin which was too slender and the bean and sunflower seed which were too smooth to grasp. The single instance of recovery failure was when the screw become firmly impacted in a segmental bronchus of the dog's lung with the tip pointing distally, a situation which probably would have required a bronchotomy if it had occurred in a human.

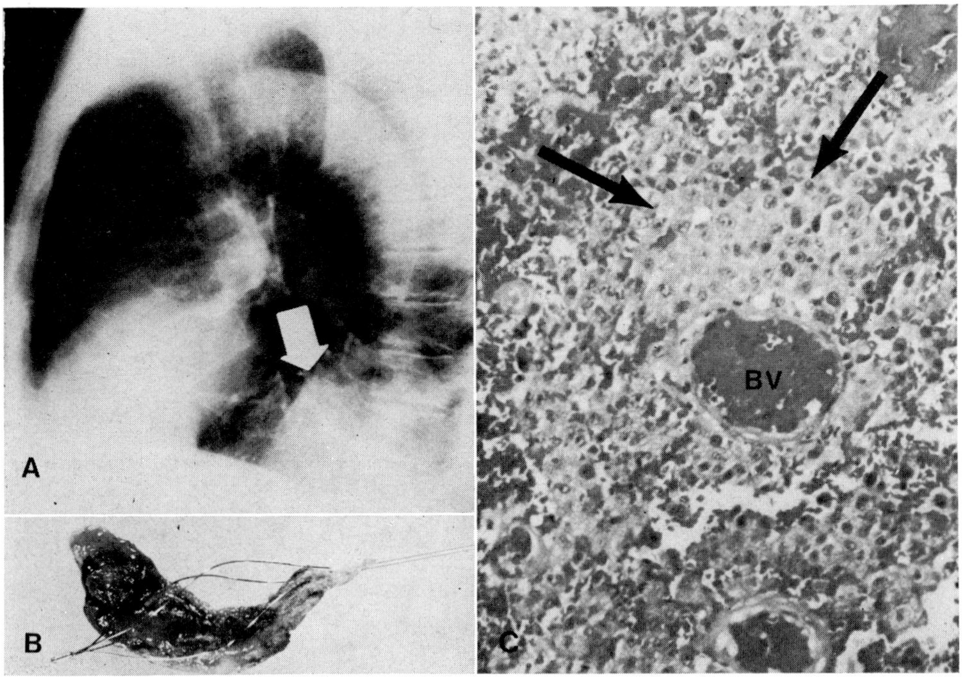

Fig. 5. Case 1. A) Lateral chest x-ray showing atelectasis of the posterobasal segment (B^{10}) of the left lower lobe (note arrow). B) Wire basket is shown grasping a large "piece of meat", removed from the left inferior mainstem bronchus. C) Pathology consisting of large, undifferentiated malignant cells (note arrows) around blood vessels (BV).

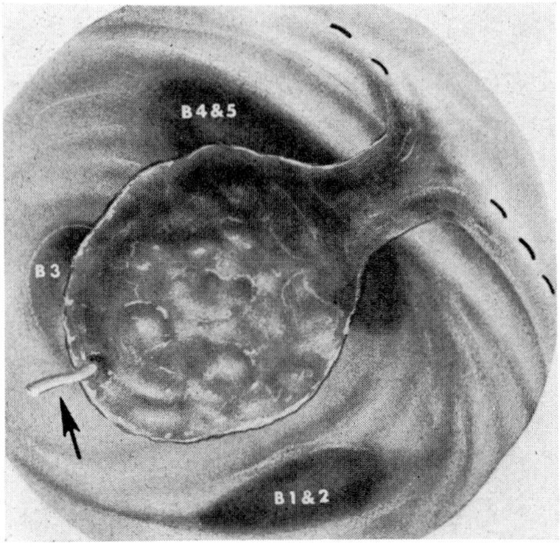

Fig. 6. Case 2. Artist's drawing of the left upper lobe as seen by the endoscopist. Arrow points to the tip of a suture barely projecting from the top of a polypoid mass. B1 & 2: apical-posterior segment (left upper lobe), B3: anterior segment (left upper lobe), B4 & 5: superior and inferior segments (lingula).

To date, our experience using these techniques on humans is limited to the following two patients who presented with a clinical picture resembling a foreign body in the tracheobronchial tree. Their brief case histories illustrate use of the Fogarty balloon catheter, wire basket, and forceps inserted through the channel of the BFS:

CASE 1

The first patient is a 75-year-old, semi-invalid retired farmer who developed a pneumonia of the left lower lobe that did not clear after 5 weeks of antibiotic therapy (Fig. 5A). Prior to his acute illness, the patient's wife had been trying to "fatten him up" by force feeding him with fried chicken. He was edentulous and noted to have great difficulty swallowing. Fiberoptic bronchoscopy revealed a large, elongated "piece of meat" filling the left inferior mainstem bronchus. The mass was removed with the wire basket (Fig. 5B), after first dislodging it with a 7F Fogarty catheter. Bleeding was negligible at the site of its distal attachment near the B-10 bronchial orifice. To our surprise, pathology revealed

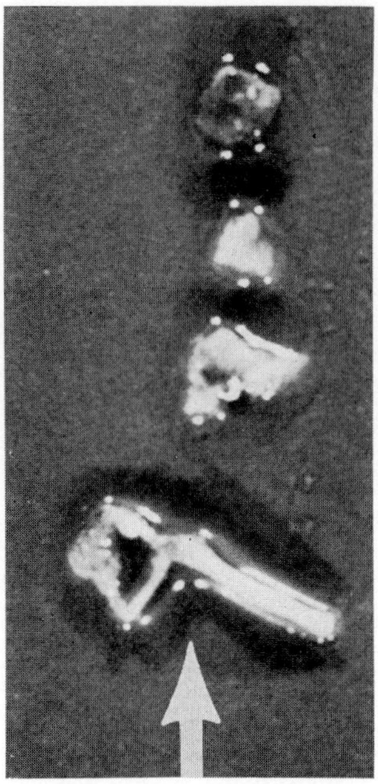

Fig. 7. Case 2. Gross specimen with suture material (arrow) and pieces of the "polyp".

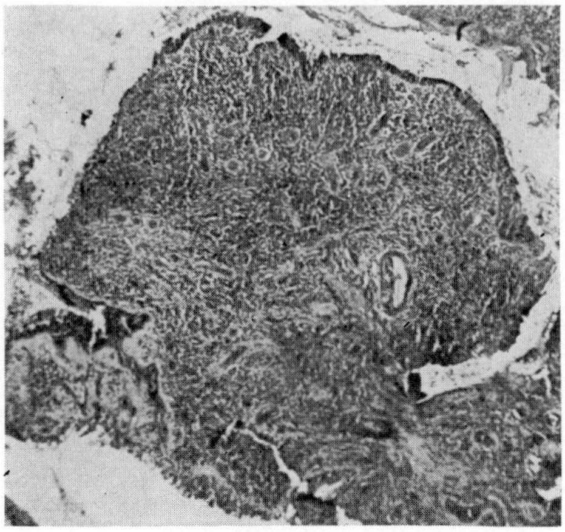

Fig. 8. Case 2. Microscopically, the specimen consisting of dense fibrous and granulation tissue covered with surface epithelium.

an undifferentiated large cell carcinoma (Fig. 5C).

CASE 2

The second patient is a 29-year-old housewife who had had a left lower lobectomy three years previously for a bronchial adenoma (carcinoid). The onset of her symptoms coincided with a visit to the dentist's office one month prior to hospital admission. A piece of her denture was noted to be missing. She related that when lying on her left side something would cut off her breathing. Her symptoms were relieved by changing position and by coughing. Chest x-rays were not remarkable except for evidence of previous surgery. Fiberoptic bronchoscopy revealed a polypoid mass projecting from the suture line of the left lower lobectomy. Each time the patient was turned on her left side the mass was observed to swing laterally, resulting in almost complete occlusion of the left upper lobe bronchus (Fig. 6). The tip of a suture could be seen barely projecting from the top of the tissue mass. A forceps, inserted through the channel of the fiberscope, was used to remove the suture and to resect the granulomatous polyp at its base (Fig. 7). Pathology reported no microscopic evidence of a recurrent carcinoid (Fig. 8).

DISCUSSION

Prior to use on humans, foreign body removal by flexible fiberoptic bronchoscopy was investigated thoroughly in artificial and dog lung models.[10] Different extraction tools (claw, basket, forceps, and balloon catheter) were passed through the channel of the BFS and guided to the foreign body under endoscopic control.

Various standard biopsy forceps are readily available for fiberoptic work, but the ACMI model is more effective in grasping metallic objects because of its larger jaws. The use of a claw or basket as an extraction tool is not new, but the miniturization and enclosure of these devices in a tiny Teflon®* tube is unique. The claw is a good extraction instrument for metallic and organic foreign bodies unless the objects are too slender or slippery. The basket works best on bulky objects.

The Fogarty balloon catheter also has been employed previously by endoscopists, but only with the rigid bronchoscope. This catheter is ideal to dislodge an impacted foreign body prior to its capture by an extraction instrument.[6] Of the two different types of

* E.I. DuPont de Nemours and Co., Wilmington, Delaware.

balloon catheters used in this study, we prefer the Fogarty model because it is less expensive than the Swan-Ganz catheter and also does not bend as easily when inserted past an impacted object. When dealing with an aspirated organic object *e.g.*, peanut, one may anticipate having to use a Fogarty catheter initially because of entrapment of the object by swollen bronchial mucosa. Metallic bodies, however, have been known to lie in the tracheobronchial tree for many months with almost no inflammatory reaction, usually making their removal easier.

The techniques of bronchofiberscopic foreign body removal were utilized on two patients, both of whom were thought to have aspirated foreign objects. The "large piece of meat" recovered from the first patient was a bronchogenic carcinoma, and the missing piece of denture in the second patient was a foreign body granuloma secondary to suture material from previous surgery. Although neither of these patients actually had aspirated foreign bodies, flexible fiberoptic extraction methods were successfully carried out as demonstrated previously in our laboratory.

In 1974, Ikeda reported removing an aspirated fish bone and the tip of a small dental drill by using a forceps inserted through the fiberoptic bronchoscope.[11] Prior rigid bronchoscopy was unsuccessful in both patients. Barrett and colleagues, also in 1974, reported using a flexible fiberscope to remove two foreign body fragments from the right lower lobe with a forceps.[12] Recently in a communication, Harrell* stated that he had removed aspirated foreign bodies from 25 patients, the majority of objects being organic, using the same extraction tools and fiberoptic methods described in this report. In one case, two previous attempts to remove a gold dental crown by the rigid bronchoscope resulted in further impaction of the foreign body.

Prior training in flexible fiberoptic methods of foreign body removal is essential, otherwise harm to the patient may result. Any of the following complications could occur because of faulty or improper techniques: 1) Displacement of the foreign body to an unfavorable position so that recovery would require bronchotomy; 2) Trauma to the bronchial tree resulting in infection, bleeding or perforation; 3) Airway obstruction secondary to losing the foreign body in the subglottic area during recovery. The head of the patient should be kept elevated to prevent this serious, potential complication; 4) Breaking an organic object (*e.g.*, peanut) into pieces by application of the wrong extraction tool (forceps) so that retrieval becomes difficult if not impossible; 5) Attempting to remove aspirated foreign bodies in infants and young children. The rigid (hollow tube) and not the flexible fiberoptic bronchoscope (solid shaft) should be used in pediatric cases because of the small diameter of the trachea and glottis in these young patients; 6) Hypoxemia and possible cardiac arrest because of failure to utilize supplemental oxygen.

----

* J. Harrell, University of California Medical School, San Diego, Calif.

Request for reprints should be sent to Pulmonary Division, Department of Medicine, University of Iowa College of Medicine, Iowa City, Iowa 52242.

REFERENCES

1. Abbott OA: Recommended principles relative to the use of bronchoscopy and tracheotomy in infants and children. Dis Chest 52: 117-123, 1967

2. Camarata SJ, Salyer JM: Management of foreign bodies in air passages and esophagus under general anesthesia. Amer Surg 31:725-738, 1965

3. Jackson C, Jackson CL: *Bronchoesophagology.* Philadelphia, W.B. Saunders Co., 1950, pp 68-109

4. Equen MS: The Alnico Magnet: An aid to bronchoscopy and esophagoscopy. Ann Otol Rhinol Laryngol 54:178-182, 1945

5. Roach GS, Majoros M: Removal of a toy bullet from the lung with a new instrument.

Arch Otolaryngol 82:403-404, 1965

6. Ullyot DG, Norman JC: The Fogarty catheter — An aid to bronchoscopic removal of foreign bodies. Ann Thorc Surg 6:185-186, 1968

7. Armstrong BW, Hart VK: Removal of plastic bullet from tracheo-bronchial tree with a bronchoscopic cautery. Ann Otol Rhinol Laryngol 62:217-219, 1953

8. Schaller R, Goff WF: A new mini-cork-screw for bronchoscopic foreign bodies. Laryngoscope 80:1740-1743, 1970

9. Carter R: Bronchotomy: The safe solution for an impacted foreign body. Ann Thorac Surg 10:93-94, 1970

10. Zavala DC, Rhodes ML: Experimental removal of foreign bodies by fiberoptic bronchoscopy. Am Rev Respir Dis 110:357-360, 1974

11. Ikeda S: *Atlas of Flexible Bronchofiberscopy.* Tokyo, Igaku Shoin Ltd., 1974, p 220

12. Barrett CR Jr, Vecchione JJ, Bell ALL Jr: Flexible fiberoptic bronchoscopy for airway management during acute respiratory failure. Am Rev Respir Dis 109:429-434, 1974

AMERICAN OTOLOGIC SOCIETY GUIDELINES FOR GRANTS

Our objective is clearly the problem of otosclerosis: its diagnosis and management, the possible causes and underlying conditions (such as the hereditary background), and an understanding of the disorder that may lead eventually to its prevention and cure.

Our present lack of understanding of the disorder and the absence, as far as known, of any similar condition in animals below man, makes research in this field particularly difficult. A direct attack on the disease is hardly feasible; therefore, it seems to be sound strategy to try circuitous approaches, such as the investigation of bone development, growth, and repair under various conditions, and the study of other diseases that show suggestive correspondence to this one. It is possible that directions of investigation that may seem initially somewhat remote from otosclerosis itself may provide insights that will eventually lead to success in reaching our goal. Therefore, our policy is to aid and encourage research in the immediate field of otosclerosis and also in adjoining fields if, in our considered opinion, there is a substantial promise that the results obtained will be of assistance in the ways just indicated and may lead to the attainment of our objective.

The Board of Trustees wishes to announce that funds are still available for suitable grants. Application forms may be obtained from the office of the Secretary of the Research Fund Trustees of the American Otologic Society. Write to Maurice Schiff, M. D., Secretary, 7255 Girard Ave., La Jolla, Calif. 92037.

Ann Otol 84: 1975

SWYER-JAMES SYNDROME: A CAUSE OF HYPERLUCENT LUNG

JACOBO GUZOWSKI, M.D.

ARNDT J. DUVALL III, M.D.

MINNEAPOLIS, MINNESOTA

SUMMARY — Swyer-James syndrome consists of an abnormal radiolucency of one lung or lobe, secondary to obliterative bronchiolitis with distal air trapping. The etiology of the bronchiolar inflammatory process is quite diverse. The syndrome will simulate the presence of a foreign body in the bronchial tree, and the patients will usually undergo bronchoscopy with that presumptive diagnosis. Two cases are presented and the pathogenesis, clinical picture, and differential diagnosis are outlined. The separation of this condition from hypoplasia of the pulmonary artery is discussed.

Swyer-James syndrome is a radiological entity, that consists primarily of an abnormal radiolucency of one lung or lobe due to obliterative bronchiolitis with air entrapment. Other causes of this finding, such as an obstruction of a major bronchus by a foreign body, a large emphysematous bulla, compensatory expansion, or congenital lobar emphysema, must be ruled out.[1]

In 1953, Swyer and James first described the syndrome in a six-year-old patient[2] and Macleod detailed nine more cases in 1954.[3] Since then, more than 100 cases have been reported, none of them in the otolaryngologic literature. Alternate nomenclature has been applied, such as Macleod syndrome, unilateral emphysema, unilateral lung transradiancy, and hyperlucent lung.

The syndrome is characterized by a marked difference between the radiolucency of the lungs or lobes in the chest roentgenogram, caused by an increase in the air content and decreased vascular markings in the affected lung or lobe. The corresponding hilum is small, but present. There is a shift of the mediastinum toward the affected side on inspiration and to the opposite side on expiration, indicating air entrapment.[4] Thus, the syndrome can be easily confused with a ball valve foreign body mechanism.

CASE REPORTS

Case 1. This previously healthy six-year-old male was seen initially in December 1972 for pneumonia. The etiologic agent determined from sputum cultures and antibody titer studies was *Mycoplasma pneumoniae.* The patient improved with antibiotic treatment, but required readmission one month later with cough, fever, and lethargy. Chest x-ray revealed hyperexpansion of the left lower lobe, with collapse of the left upper lobe. Bronchoscopy was done twice without positive findings. Upon referral to our institution in October 1973, pulmonary studies showed a severe impairment of his respiratory function with values six standard deviations below normal (Forced Expiratory Volume: .53, Vital Capacity: .94) The chest x-ray still revealed a hyperlucent left lower lobe and collapse of the upper lobe. A shift of the mediastinum to the left on inspiration and to the right on expiration was demonstrated (Fig. 1). Due to these findings another bronchoscopy was suggested to rule out a foreign body in the left main stem bronchus creating a ball valve phenomenon. In view of the clinical history, the endoscopy was not performed and treatment with bronchodilators was initiated. No significant improvement ensued. In January 1974, a bronchogram showed no evidence of

Presented at the meeting of the American Broncho-Esophagological Association, Atlanta, Georgia, April 7-8, 1975.

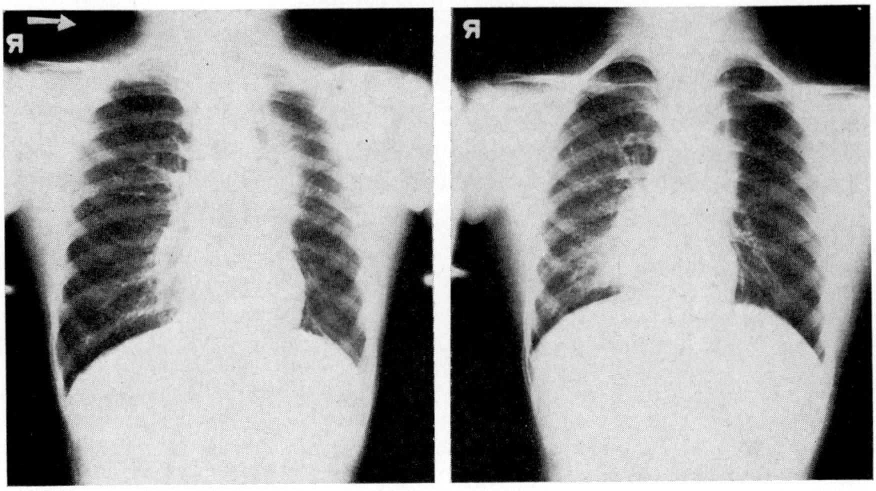

Fig. 1. Case 1. Inspiratory and expiratory chest radiographs demonstrate the hyperlucency of the left lower lobe and the mediastinal shift to the right on expiration.

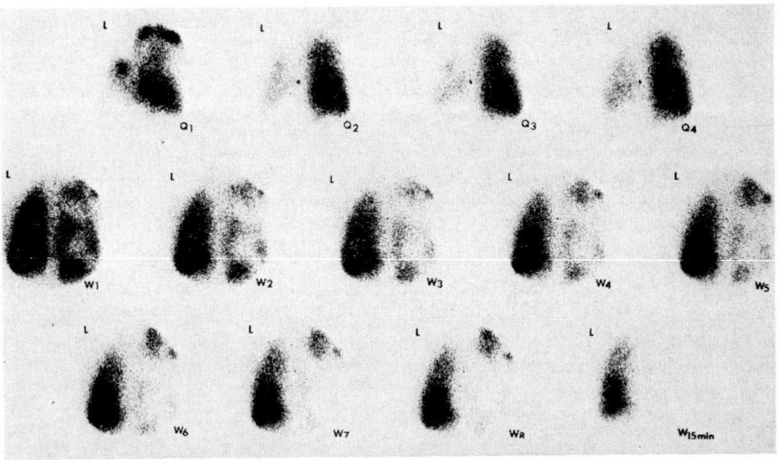

Fig. 2. Case 1. Xenon lung scan. After I.V. injection of the labeled isotope, a very slow uptake in the left lung takes place, indicating decreased perfusion (Q1-4). Once the gas is in the alveoli, it will remain there for a long time (W1-8W15 min), indicating poor ventilation

obstruction in a major bronchus, but there was a marked decrease in the bronchial tapering pattern and several areas of stenosis. These findings, combined with a small hilar shadow and decreased vascular markings reflecting a decreased flow in the left pulmonary artery, suggested Swyer-James syndrome.

A Xenon lung scan demonstrated decreased perfusion with a very delayed washout of the medium from the affected left lung (Fig. 2). An exploratory thoracotomy was subsequently done and the findings of a very emphysematous left lower lobe and collapse of the upper lobe were confirmed. Biopsy specimens demonstrated bronchiolitis and dilated and ruptured alveoli.

Case 2. In January 1974, this 16-month-old female experienced respiratory difficulty without fever or cough. Auscultation revealed a clicking sound in the right chest. Roentgenographically, there were infiltrates in the left lung and evidence of air trapping in the right. A shift of the mediastinum to the left on expiration was found on inspiratory and expiratory films. On January 26, 1974, a bronchoscopy was performed, and a pop corn hull was

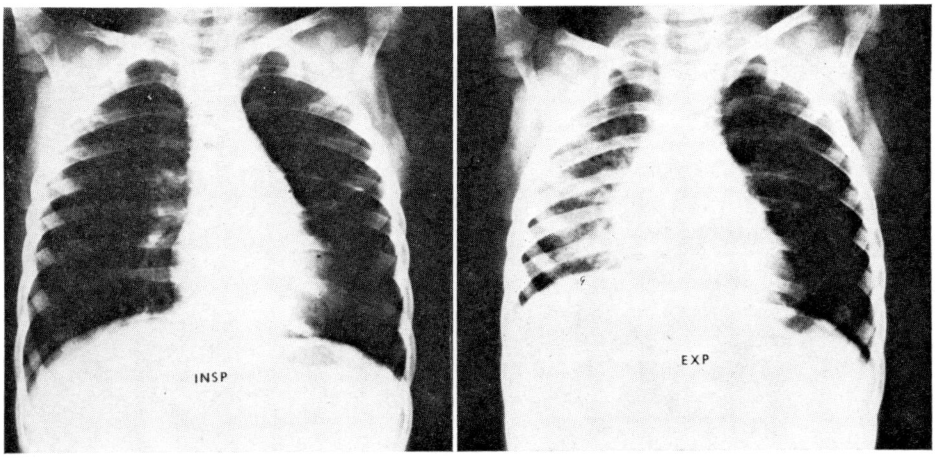

Fig. 3. Case 2. Inspiratory and expiratory films demonstrate a shift of the mediastinum towards the normal lung on expiration. Similar findings would result from a ball valve foreign body in the left main stem bronchus.

removed from the right main stem bronchus. Follow-up chest x-ray revealed a persistent left lower lobe infiltrate, and bronchoscopy was repeated in February 1974. No foreign body could be found this time. The patient was asymptomatic until December 1974 when another respiratory infection developed. A chest x-ray then demonstrated a hyperlucency of the left lower lobe. Physical examination was unremarkable except for short stature and diffuse rhonchi in the left lung. Inspiratory and expiratory films showed a shift of the mediastinum towards the right on expiration (Fig. 3). Contemplating the possibility of a foreign body in the patient's tracheobronchial tree, a bronchoscopy was done with negative results. Bronchography revealed a collapse of the left lower lobe major bronchi on expiration and the presence of distal bronchiectasis (Fig. 4). A lung scan confirmed the clinical impression of poor perfusion and ventilation of the left lung.

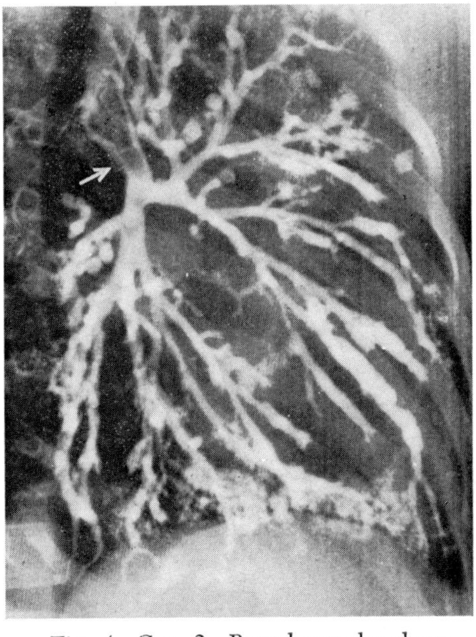

Fig. 4. Case 2. Bronchography shows expiratory collapse of the left lower lobe major bronchi (arrow), as well as distal bronchiectasis.

CLINICAL DESCRIPTION

Most patients with Swyer-James syndrome have been children or young adults. The majority are asymptomatic, and the hyperlucency of a lung or lobe is found on a routine chest radiograph. Some complain of repeated respiratory tract infections and/or dyspnea on exertion. Six cases reported in the literature have presented with hemoptysis.[5]

In over 60% of the cases, history of a severe acute respiratory tract infection during childhood can be recollected.[1] MacPherson *et al*[6] described six patients with a history of adenoviral pneumonia. A number of other etiologies have been reported, including infection with respiratory syncitial virus, measles,[7] radiation, hydrocarbon ingestion, foreign body aspiration,[8] and tuberculosis.[9,10] All of these agents can produce an acute bronchiolitis with obliteration of small airways, up to the eighth order bronchioles.[1] The peripheral parenchyma is then ventilated by collateral air drift through the pores of Kohn, and the bronchiolar obstruction acts as a multiple check valve mechanism with air trapping and overdistention of the affected lung or lobe.[5] One of our patients (Case 2) also demonstrated involvement of major bronchi by the inflammatory process. We suspect that there were foreign bodies in the left lung which were not removed; later these were eliminated or were dissolved. In the interval, the process leading to bronchiolar obstruction was initiated.

Radiologically, patients with Swyer-James syndrome have an increased translucency of one lung or lobe, more marked on expiration. The affected lung or lobe is usually of smaller size, and it has been noted that the earlier the age of the original insult, the smaller the size will be. The left lower lobe is more commonly affected for unknown reasons. On inspiration, the mediastinum can be in the normal position or deviated towards the affected lung, but on expiration, the mediastinum always makes an excursion towards the normal side. Movement of the diaphragm is decreased on the affected side, which can be well demonstrated by fluoroscopy. Rigid bronchoscopy is usually performed with no abnormal findings.

Bronchography will reveal a wide fanning of the branches of the bronchial tree, without significant bronchial displacement, as is found in bullous emphysema. The smaller bronchi are mildly dilated and show a beaded appearance, with buds or smooth pockets projecting from the ends or sides of the bronchi. There is a lack of alveolar filling, which speaks in favor of bronchiolar obstruction as the pathogenesis of the disease.

Xenon lung scans show a decreased perfusion, but more important, there is a delayed washout of the medium, with trapping of the gas in the alveoli due to decreased ventilation.

Physiologically, the problems are poor perfusion and aeration. Studies of pulmonary function will show obstruction to air flow, reduction in vital capacity, and, to a lesser extent, reduction in respiratory flow. Unilateral bronchospirometry may show that the ventilation in the affected side is decreased by as much as 90%.[8]

DIFFERENTIAL DIAGNOSIS

The differential diagnosis will include conditions which cause unilateral emphysema, and these can be divided into three categories:[11] 1) asymmetric chest wall; 2) unilateral obstructive emphysema; and 3) pulmonary undercirculation.

The first condition occurs in congenital absence of the pectoralis muscle, scoliosis, or after surgical procedures such as mastectomy. This group can be ruled out readily by the history and physical examination of the patient, the absence of mediastinal shift on inspiratory and expiratory films, and by the normal appearance of the pulmonary vessels.

The obstructive emphysema due to a foreign body check valve mechanism in one of the major bronchi is best ruled out by bronchoscopy and/or bronchography. The size of the lung is increased in obstructive emphysema. In the Swyer-James syndrome the volume is decreased. This difference, however, cannot be considered an absolute criterion. The possibility of unilateral diffuse or bullous emphysema must be eliminated by bronchography which shows, in this case, arcuate patterns around the bullae and attenuation and elongation of the small bronchi.

Swyer-James syndrome has to be distinguished from unilateral alteration of the pulmonary vasculature, such as obstruction of a large pulmonary artery or its congenital absence or hypoplasia. In the latter conditions, there is an increased lucency due to a decrease in vascularization. There is no mediastinal shift, and in the absence of a pulmonary artery, the hilum is very small or absent. Nevertheless, it is recognized that hypoplasia of the pulmonary artery may be the most difficult differential diagnosis, and only a pulmonary angiogram will establish the underlying pathology.

There has been a controversy as to whether or not the hypoplastic pulmonary circulation found in the Swyer-James syndrome is responsible for poor ventilation or vice versa. Some authors have tried to implicate the pulmonary undercirculation as the pathophysiological mechanism for the Swyer-James syndrome, as opposed to the theory of obliterative bronchiolitis. Reed and Simon[12] and Cumming *et al*[1] have been able to document the presence of normal bronchovascular markings prior to the development of the hyperlucent lung, indicating that the disease is acquired and that the probable sequence of events is first airway obstruction and then decrease in vascularity. The hypofunctioning lung fails to grow and the pulmonary artery remains relatively small. When the insult occurs after growth is completed, the hypoplasia of the pulmonary artery is less evident.[1]

We believe that both situations (Swyer-James syndrome and hypoplasia of the pulmonary artery) are totally separate entities, even though both will result in an increased lucency of the affected lung parenchyma.

Treatment is based on the fact that the process is essentially benign, and a lobectomy or pneumonectomy should be contemplated only in the face of repeated infections, hemoptysis, or severe dyspnea on exertion.[4,5,13] In Case 1, only an exploratory thoracotomy was performed, and no benefit to respiratory function ensued. However, resection of a hyperexpanded, nonfunctioning lobe might allow expansion of the remaining normal lung, with improvement of respiratory function.

Request for reprints should be sent to A. J. Duvall III, M.D., Dept. of Otolaryngology, Univ. of Minn., 2630 University Ave. S.E., Minneapolis, Minn. 55414.

REFERENCES

1. Cumming GR, McPherson RI, Chernick V: Unilateral hyperlucent lung in children. J Pediatr 78:250-260, 1971

2. Swyer P, James GCW: A case of unilateral pulmonary emphysema. Thorax: 8:133-136, 1953

3. Macleod WM: Abnormal transradiancy of one lung. Thorax 9:147-153, 1954

4. Fraser GF, Pare JAP: *Diagnosis of Diseases of the Chest.* Philadelphia, W.B. Saunders, 1970. volume 2, p 1033

5. Eliades S: Place du syndrome de Macleod dans le groupe des hyperclartés poulmonaires unilatérales. Praxis 59:991-1002, 1970

6. McPherson RI, Cumming GR, Chernick V: Unilateral hyperlucent lung: A complication of viral pneumonia. J Canad Ass Radiol 20:225-231, 1969

7. Lepercq G, Poupuiet S, Saad R, *et al*: Aspects évolutifs du poumon hyperclair unilatéral. Ann Pediatr (Paris) 19:21-28, 1972

8. Kogutt MS, Swischuk LE, Goldblum R: Swyer-James syndrome (unilateral hyperlucent lung) in children. Am J Dis Child 125:614-618, 1973

9. Mengoli V, Mastella G, Castellarin T, *et al*: Il polmone iperchiaro nel bambino. Pediatria (Napoli) 78:842-853, 1970

10. Brum J, Perrin-Fayolle M, Kofman J: Hyperclartés poulmonaires unilatérales séquellaires de primo infection tuberculeuse et discussion sur le limits du syndrome de Macleod. J Fr Med Chir Thorac 24:785-796, 1971

11. Margolin HN, Rosenberg LJ, Felson B, *et al*: Idiopathic unilateral hyperlucent lung. Amer J Roentgen 82:63-75, 1959

12. Reed L, Simon G: Unilateral lung transradiancy. Thorax 17:230-239, 1962

13. Hazel B, Perras P, Thubert D, *et al*: Hypertransparence unilaterale du poumon. Syndrome de Swyer-James-Macleod. Union Med Can 99:85-89, 1970

Ann Otol 84: 1975

OBJECTIVE EVALUATION OF VOCAL PATHOLOGY USING VOICE SPECTROGRAPHY

EUGENE RONTAL, M.D.

MICHAEL RONTAL, M.D. MICHAEL I. ROLNICK, PH.D.

SOUTHFIELD, MICHIGAN

SUMMARY – Permanent objective evaluation of vocal changes associated with laryngeal pathology is a goal which has been difficult for the laryngologist and speech pathologist to attain. Most attempts at achieving objective records have focused on direct visual examination of the larynx using techniques such as high speed photography, x-ray studies or histologic sectioning. However, the important subjective qualities of the voice are difficult to translate into objective visual patterns. In order to produce these patterns, certain individual components of the voice (*i.e.*, breathiness, periodicity and formant structure) must be analyzed. Recently, modifications of the sound spectrograph have enabled the clinician to objectively visualize these components. The patterns produced by the spectrograph may be applied to a variety of clinical situations. For example, the technique aids greatly in determining the success or failure of medical and surgical management for vocal cord lesions. Secondly, voice spectrography can readily show improvements or deficiencies in vocal rehabilitation for functional dysphonia. Lastly, this method provides an objective, permanent record of the voice which may be useful from a medicolegal standpoint. Sound spectrographic analysis of vocal pathology is an important diagnostic tool for the clinician. Its future use should be encouraged as a more precise aid in the evaluation of the voice.

Permanent objective evaluation of vocal changes associated with laryngeal pathology is a goal which has been difficult for the laryngologist and speech pathologist to attain. Most attempts at achieving objective records are focused on direct visual examination of the larynx, using techniques such as high speed photography, x-ray studies, or histologic sectioning. However, the subjective qualities of the voice are difficult to translate into objective visual patterns. In order to produce these patterns, the individual components of the voice must be analyzed.

Clinical modifications in voice spectrographic analysis have allowed adequate visualization of these components. Once these patterns are formalized, they can be applied to a variety of clinical situations. Although attempts have been made in the past to use spectrography in the evaluation of certain types of hoarseness, direct clinical application to voice problems has been a recent development. This paper is a presentation of our use of spectrography in a clinical situation for evaluation of vocal rehabilitation, surgical treatment and medical management of a variety of vocal cord disorders.

DESCRIPTION OF VOICE SPECTROGRAPHY

The voice spectrograph is not a new method of voice analysis. Potter *et al*[1] first developed this technique at the Bell Telephone laboratories in the 1940's. Spectrography has been a useful tool in voice research since its first development.[2-6] It differs from a visible speech translator in that an actual graphic analysis of the speech pattern rather than a display in a cathode ray tube is produced. The graphic display is known as a spectrogram.

Presented at the meeting of the American Broncho-Esophagological Association, Atlanta, Georgia, April 7-8, 1975.

Iwata and Von Leden[7] have discussed the use of spectrograms in the study of laryngeal disease. They suggested that different laryngeal diseases might yield different spectrographic characteristics. Cooper[8] reported spectrographic analysis as a tool to describe and compare fundamental frequencies and hoarseness in dysphonic patients before and after vocal rehabilitation. Isskiki *et al*[9] have presented a classification system for hoarseness using spectrograms. Rontal *et al*[4] pointed out the usefulness of spectrographic analysis as a clinical tool in evaluation of the voice following Teflon®* paste injection of paralyzed vocal cords. In spite of these contributions to the literature, few laryngologists or speech pathologists are utilizing this important, objective method of voice analysis.

Sound spectrography, through a series of filters, presents a picture of the intensity, frequency and duration characteristics of the voice. These characteristics are translated into an electrical impulse represented by an electrical stylus which prints out the pattern on a rotating paper graph. Either steady state vowels such as "ah" or "ee" or spoken words and sentences can be evaluated by this technique. Depending on the information desired, a number of different patterns can be elucidated. A trained individual may then "read" the spectrograms produced and view the phonatory, articulatory and resonance qualities of the human voice.

The technique called "voice printing" has confused the clinical application of voice spectrography. The voice print is a form of voice spectrogram used to identify individuals for criminal purposes, based on vocal characteristics of their spoken words. The voice spectrograph, on the other hand, analyzes the specific components of the voice by relating acoustic energy to physiology, so that vocal function can be assessed.

The sound spectrogram best analyzes steady state vowels for the purpose of evaluation of phonatory characteristics. The patient is asked to produce a vowel in front of the input microphone for a period of 2.4 seconds. A recording is made on a special tape loop in the spectrograph. This sample is then repeated many times and analyzed through a series of filters. The analysis can be performed in approximately three minutes. Broad band spectrograms are made for the analysis of phonation and can be kept permanently in a patient's file. A spectrographic analysis of phonatory characteristics is performed at periodic intervals so that changes during treatment can be monitored.

SPECTROGRAPHIC CHARACTERISTICS OF THE NORMAL VOICE

In order to adequately understand voice spectrography, the normal physiology of voice production at the level of the glottis must be understood.[10,11] This physiologic sound production is then related to the graphic display on the spectrogram. Sound is the alternate compression and rarefaction of air molecules. Subglottic air, trapped in the trachea by the closed vocal cords, is compressed by the accessory muscles of respiration. As the pressure beneath the glottis increases, the vocal cords are separated, allowing the escape of the compressed air. When subglottic pressure falls, the vocal cords cannot be held open. They move back passively by their intrinsic tension. The subglottic pressure can then build to produce another wave of compressed air. The result is a train of compressions and rarefactions and the result is sound.

The sound spectrogram will show the various physiologic characteristics of the normal voice. In this range of normality, there are certain definable differences, such as different characteristics between a male and a female voice, the characteristics of trained singers, the whisper voice and vocal fatigue.

In the analysis of the spectrographic characteristics of the normal voice,

* E.I. DuPont de Nemours and Co., Wilmington, Delaware.

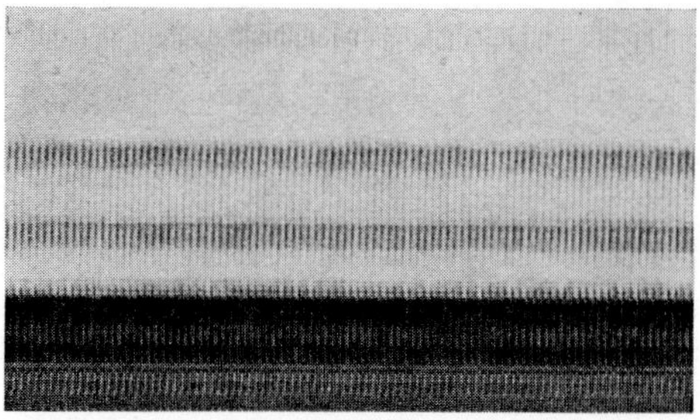

Fig. 1. Spectrogram of a normal male "ah" vowel produced by an individual with no vocal pathology. Regular, periodic vertical striations indicate synchronous vocal cord movements with no irregularity of the vibratory pattern. The horizontal bars going across the pattern are formants and represent frequency regions of energy selectively amplified by the resonating cavities. The top half of the spectrogram is relatively clear, indicating that no excessive breathiness exists.

phonatory samples are made from steady state vowels. Because of interference from articulatory characteristics, spoken words are less apt to give reproducible, analyzable data. The patterns visible on the spectrogram are evaluated in terms of acoustic parameters (Fig. 1).

Periodicity of vocal cord movement is a measure of the regularity of the opening and closing of the vocal cords. It is translated on the spectrogram as the vertical striations seen (Fig. 1). The synchronous, periodic opening and closing of the vocal cords in a normal voice will produce a corresponding regularity in the vertical striations seen. While periodicity is measured by the pattern of individual vertical striations, certain pitch characteristics of the voice can be observed in the closeness of the vertical striations on the spectrogram.

The spectrogram also measures the formants of the normal voice. These formants are the horizontal bars represented as the darker bands on the spectrogram (Fig. 1). These bars or formants relate to the size and shape of the resonating cavities of the vocal tract. Formants will shift position during connected speech and with each sound being produced. On the spectrogram, clear

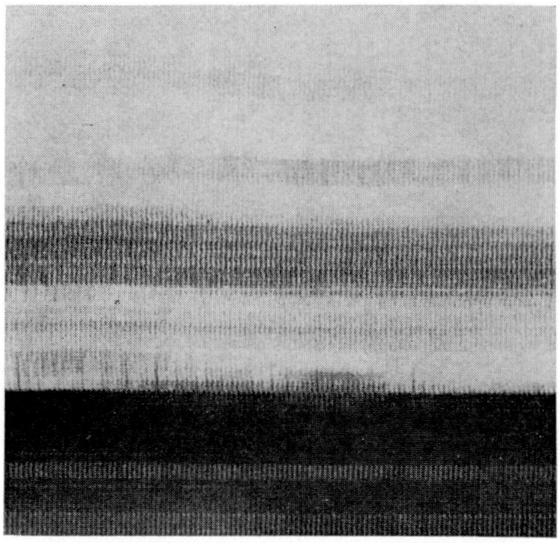

Fig. 2. "Ah" vowel produced by a female speaker. Normal periodicity of vocal cord movement is seen by the regularly spaced vertical lines. These vertical lines differ from the male voice in Figure 1 inasmuch as they are closer together. This is due to the higher pitched voice. The horizontal bars or formants are typical of the female voice. A lack of breathiness in the upper half of the spectrogram indicates good closure of the vocal cords.

and adequate formant structure is dependent upon a good resonating system and a lack of breathiness, as well as normal periodicity of vocal cord movement.

Differences between the male and female voice are demonstrable on the spectrogram (Fig. 2). In the female voice, the fundamental pitch is generally higher. Subsequently, the rapid vibrations of the vocal cords are represented by closer vertical striations. The remainder of the spectrographic characteristics are usually the same. A child's voice closely parallels the female voice in fundamental pitch and resonance characteristics. Until vocal changes associated with pubescence occur, both the male and female child will exhibit a similar spectrographic pattern.

The singing voice differs from the spoken voice. Vocal cord closure is too rapid to distinguish individual striations on the pattern produced (Fig. 3). The extra formant structure present is indicative of a finely tuned vocal mechan-

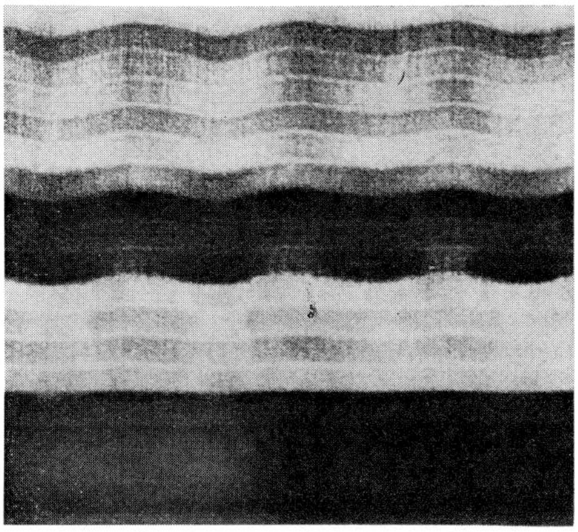

Fig. 3. A trained singer singing an "ah" vowel at a very high pitch. The vertical lines are blurred together although they make up the actual spectrogram. Extra formant structure can be seen at different frequency regions on the spectrogram. The wavy characteristic relates to tremulo so often found in the trained singing voice.

ism. This is one of the distinguishing features of the voice that is trained, or voice involved in the singing act. The regular wavy motion to the formant structure is indicative of the vibrato commonly heard in a singer's voice.

Other variations of the normal voice can produce distinct changes on a spectrogram. A whispered voice with no vocal cord movement shows a distinct pattern (Fig. 4). The excessive energy throughout the pattern is created by air escaping through a constricted, partially open glottis. Frequency is represented in the vertical axis of the spectrogram from 0 to 8,000 Hz. When the whispered or breathy voice is produced, energy is present in the highest frequency regions of the spectrogram. Further, vocal fatigue will also be indicated as a normal variant in a voice spectrogram (Fig. 5). Cords which are able to move in a regular, periodic manner may suddenly go into an aperiodic, low-pitched tone with subsequent return to a normal voice. This can occur in a normal individual's phonatory pattern at some time during the speaking day, when the vocal cords are fatigued or mucus rests upon them.

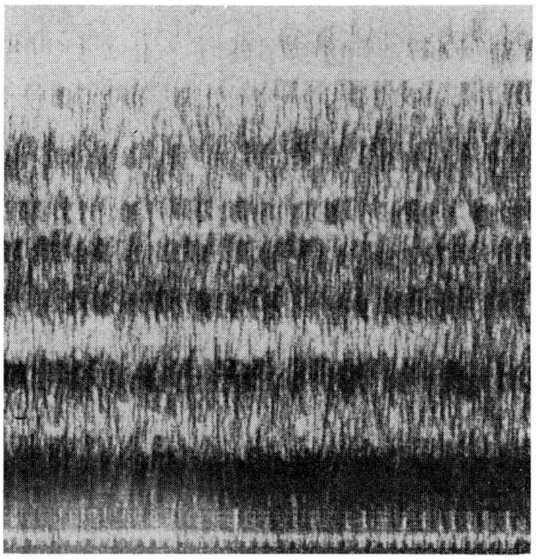

Fig. 4. Whispered vocal quality showing no evidence of vocal cord movement. Only frictional, random noise is present, caused by escape of air through a partially opened glottis. This glottal fricative sound can be produced in isolation, resulting in a whispered voice or with phonation resulting in a breathy vocal quality. The formant structure can be seen occurring due to the fact that the glottal fricative sound is being resonated by the resonating cavities.

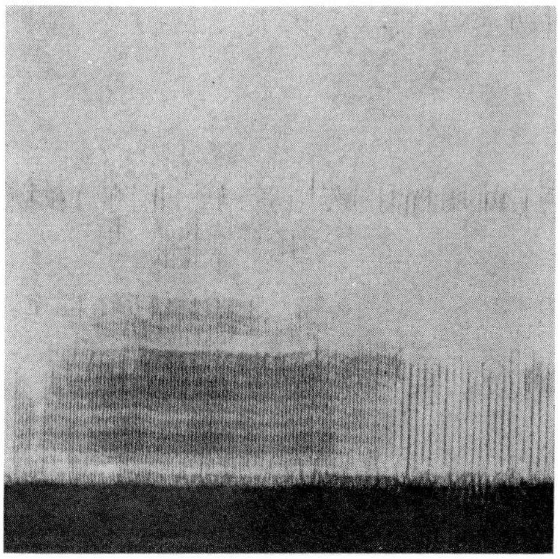

Fig. 5. Example of a normal speaker producing an aperiodic voice due to mucus on the vocal cords. No laryngeal pathology is present. This is a normal occurence that can take place at different times during the speaking day. This type of pattern can also be caused by vocal fatigue. The spectrograph is capable of picking up and portraying these normal variations of the voice.

The sound spectrograph was designed to show a graphic representation of the energy involved in the phonatory act. Consideration of the spectrographic characteristics of the normal voice show what is occurring on a physiologic basis. An extension of this would then allow an observation of the acoustic end result of various dysphonic or pathological problems. in doing so, certain characteristics can be identified as representing specific spectrographic aspects of dysphonia. In order to evaluate the voice adequately, each parameter of the spectrogram must be analyzed: 1) aperiodicity or loss of regular vocal cord closure is observed; 2) breathiness or increase in energy in the high frequency regions of the spectrogram is also evaluated; and 3) a breakdown in the formant or energy resonance of the voice must also be analyzed. Individual abnormalities or combinations of abnormal conditions would create spectrograms characteristic of vocal cord pathology. Correction of vocal cord problems will be reflected by an improvement in the abnormalities of each of these three factors.

USES OF VOICE SPECTROGRAPHY IN THE EVALUATION OF VOCAL REHABILITATION

Both organic and functional disturbances of the vocal cords are frequently amenable to vocal rehabilitation. An objective description of the acoustic end result of the vocal cord pathology is important to the subsequent treatment program. Spectrographic analysis allows both the speech pathologist and the patient to be aware of ongoing improvement in the voice. Vocal cord nodules, vocal paralyses, hyperkinetic dysphonia and dysphonia plica ventricularis are just a few examples of disorders in which the spectrograph was an important tool in the total program of vocal rehabilitation.

The presence of vocal nodules prevents adequate movement of the vocal cords with a subsequent aperiodic breathy voice. Some patients with these nodules will respond well to vocal hygiene and rehabilitation. This is especially true in children. The objective

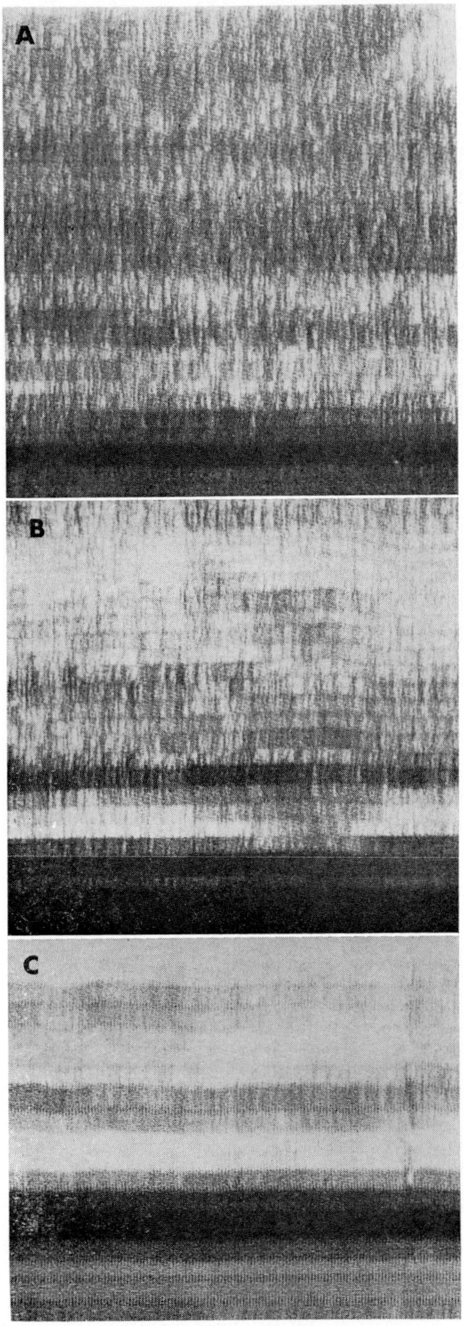

Fig. 6. Three spectrograms A, B and C, in serial order showing improvement in dysphonia related to the resolution of vocal cord nodules. As the nodules reduce in size one can see a lessening of the breathiness, better periodicity of vocal cord movement, and more distinct formant structure.

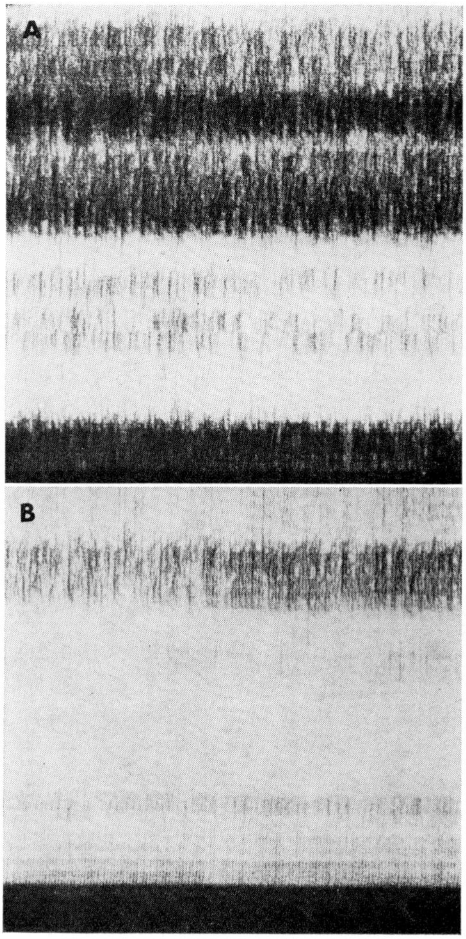

Fig. 7. Improvement in the voice of a patient with unilateral vocal cord paralysis (A). While the post treatment spectrogram (B) is obviously improved with the reduction in high frequency breathiness, and noticeably more adequate periodicity of vocal cord movement, continued problems are still evident. There is a continuation of high frequency breathiness indicating that complete closure of vocal cords is not possible due to remaining problems.

measurement of change in the voice during the process of vocal rehabilitation can be accurately assessed by the voice spectrogram. Therefore, one may be able to see the exact progression of events in correction of the vocal pathology. Serial spectrograms made at different stages in treatment can clearly show a decrease in dysphonic characteristics (Fig. 6).

Vocal cord paralysis shows most of the abnormal spectrographic characteristics of the voice. There is evidence of aperiodicity, breakdown of formant structure and breathiness. Vocal rehabilitation programs related to this condition involve improvement of each of these abnormal components of the voice. The spectrogram allows observation of the change in the voice following treatment. Both vocal rehabilitation and surgical correction of vocal cord paralysis have been used. In the vocal rehabilitation program, the voice spectrogram can evaluate the efficacy of the treatment technique. This type of program generally involves forced adduction exercises. The documentation of the improvement through spectrographic analysis makes a meaningful visual presentation to the referring laryngologist, speech pathologist and the patient (Fig. 7). Lack of resolution of high frequency energy indicative of continued breathiness will aid in the clinical consideration of vocal cord injection.

Vocal rehabilitation is the prime modality of treatment is functional dysphonias. Hyperkinetic dysphonia and dysphonia plica ventricularis are common examples of this type of vocal disorder. In hyperkinetic dysphonia, there is an incoordination of vocal cord movement. This is commonly associated with stressful situations or prolonged vocal strain. With spectrography, the before and after treatment progress of the patient is made visible (Fig. 8). Treatment generally involves hypofunctional voice use with specific attention to decreased vocal strain.

Dysphonia plica ventricularis is another example of a functional neuromuscular vocal disorder which can be treated effectively by vocal rehabilitation. In this situation, the false vocal cords meet in the midline before the true cords. This is clearly demonstrable on indirect laryngoscopy. The dysphonic characteristics of the voice in

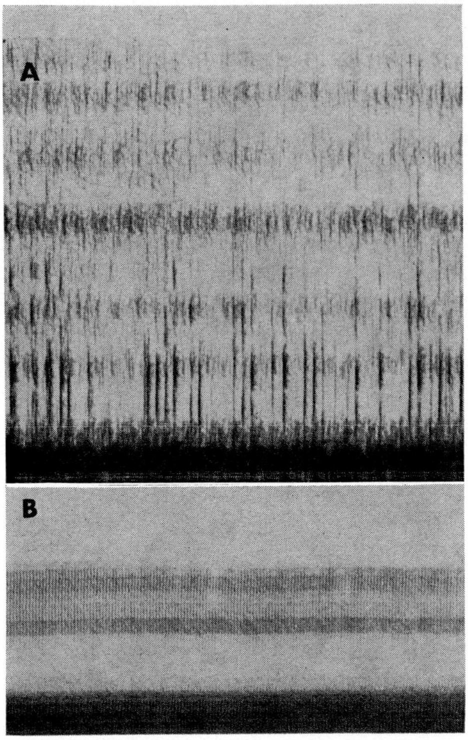

Fig. 8. Dramatic improvement in the voice of a patient with hyperkinetic dysphonia. A severely dysphonic voice with very little evidence of periodic vocal cord movement (A) was vastly improved through the use of a hypofunctional approach to voice production. The post treatment spectrogram (B) shows marked improvement in periodicity. All of the breathiness has cleared due to more adequate vocal fold closure.

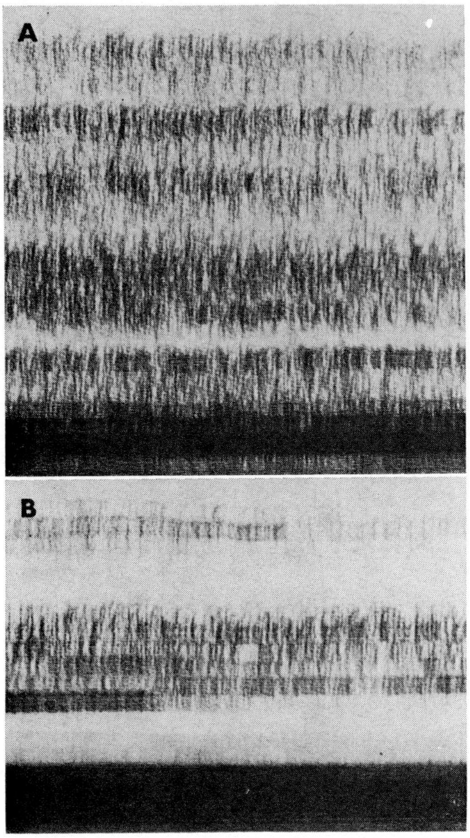

Fig. 9. Patient wtih dysphonia ventricularis (A) exhibits a much improved voice after a hypofunctional approach to treatment. A major acoustic characteristic that has been eliminated in the posttreatment spectrogram (B) is the excessive breathiness found throughout the pretreatment pattern.

dysphonia plica ventricularis are related to an attempt by the false vocal cords to participate in the phonatory act (Fig. 9). There is an extreme amount of breathiness throughout the pattern, represented by high frequency energy. The formant structure is hidden within the breathiness which is caused by the escape of air through an apparently tense and nonactive pair of vocal cords. Vocal rehabilitation involves the use of the hypofunctional approach to voice production. With the emergence of formant structure and the decrease in breathiness as indicated by the posttreatment spectrogram, voice use is encouraged. As can be seen in each of these examples, the voice spectrograph is extremely useful in demonstrating objective changes in voice, related to the vocal rehabilitation program.

EVALUATION OF SURGICAL PROCEDURES OF THE LARYNX

Voice spectrography is useful in evaluation of certain surgical procedures of the larynx. Vocal cord injection, conservative laryngeal operations for carcinoma of the larynx and evaluation of pre- and postoperative vocal cord stripping procedures have all been successfully evaluated by the use of voice spectrograms. The objective evidence

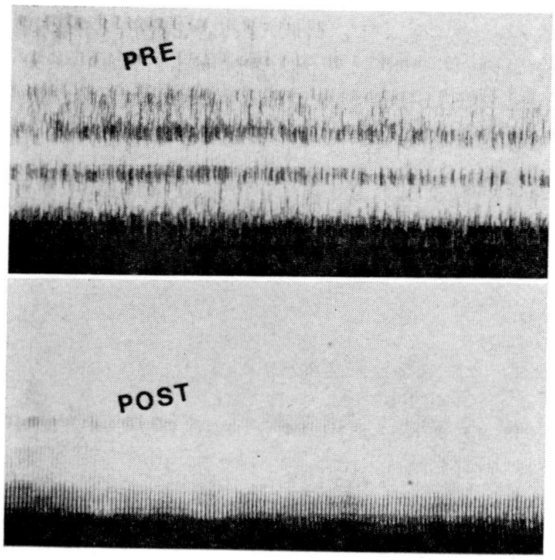

Fig. 10. Pre- and postspectrograms of a patient who underwent Teflon® paste injection for unilateral vocal cord paralysis. The postsurgical spectrogram shows an essentially normal voice with none of the aperiodicity, breathiness or formant breakdown noted in the presurgical example.

indicated by spectrographic analysis is useful both in the management of the patient in the clinical situation, and in the professional evaluation of the voice by both the laryngologist and speech pathologist.

As mentioned previously, vocal cord paralysis can be treated by vocal rehabilitation. However, many of these patients are amenable to vocal cord injection with dramatic results. Widely displaced cords in the intermediate position or vocal cords paralyzed in the paramedian position with breathiness are all subjects for potential vocal cord injection. The voice spectrogram has been advocated in the evaluation of vocal cord injections with Teflon.®[4] This is becoming increasingly useful in the proper evaluation of the pre- and post operative voice (Fig. 10). As mentioned previously, the abnormalities of aperiodicity, breakdown of formant structure and breathiness are all seen in vocal cord paralysis. Their correction by vocal cord injection is dramatic when pre- and postoperative spectrograms are compared. Persistent abnormalities of the spectrogram can give information to the laryngologist and help him decide whether a second injection may be necessary.

Voice spectrography is also useful in evaluation of the voice associated with the various types of glottic reconstruction following vertical hemilaryngectomy. Vertical hemilaryngectomy has been advocated as an excellent means of removal of carcinoma of the true cord with sparing of the voice. Excessive breathiness and hoarseness following this procedure has prompted a variety of laryngoplasties to be advocated as a means of reconstructing tissue opposite to the normally mobile cord in an attempt to achieve glottic closure. Although several techniques have been advocated, there is no uniform opinion as to which is the best. An evaluation of these techniques by spectrography is helpful on an objective basis to decide which technique is most efficacious in the improvement of the voice following this surgical procedure. In a limited series, we have compared the results of sternohyoid muscle grafts to the use of hemilaryngectomy alone without laryngoplasty. The spectrograms when analyzed are compared with the normal voice. The objective evidence produced by the spectrograms would indicate that there is no improvement by laryngoplasty in the long-term follow-up of these individuals. However, it must be emphasized that only large studies with long-term follow-ups can be adequately used to produce a final statement on this problem.

Lastly, vocal cord nodules and polyps are frequent inciting etiologies responsible for many vocal cord strippings. The pre- and postoperative voice attained has not until this time been adequately evaluated. Frequently, hoarseness persists after vocal cord stripping. An objective evaluation of the pre- and postoperative voice is essential for the laryngologist to adequately evaluate his patients. Frequently, the ability to produce a spectrogram and show the patient that though the voice has not returned to normal levels but has been dramatically improved is extremely im-

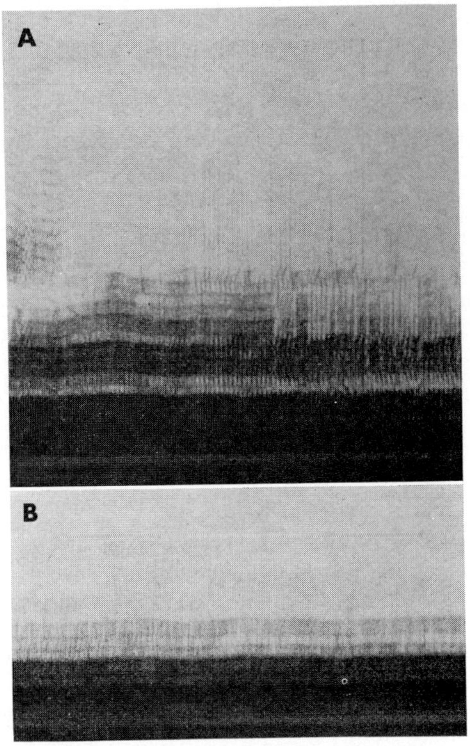

Fig. 11. Pre- and postsurgical example of phonation related to vocal cord stripping for bilateral nodules. The presurgical example (A) shows noticeable evidence of breathings and aperiodicity of vocal cord movement. The postsurgical example (B) reflects an essentially normal voice with no evidence of dysfunction.

portant in the postoperative management of these individuals (Fig. 11). Again, the objective evidence of vocal cord change cannot be overemphasized as an essential component in the adequate evaluation of laryngeal surgical candidates.

EVALUATION OF MEDICAL MANAGEMENT OF VOCAL CORD LESIONS

The voice spectrogram will in the future have significant use in the evaluation of medical treatment for certain illnesses causing laryngeal disorders. Both hypothyroidism and myasthenia gravis have distinct vocal cord changes associated with their respective metabolic disturbances. Improvement in the metabolic condition is frequently associated with marked improvement in the voice. The changes subjectively seen in the treatment program will actually be demonstrable based on objective changes seen in the spectrogram. It is further hoped that in the future the end point in the so-called Tensilon®* test for myasthenia gravis may be indicated more readily by close evaluation of the voice spectrogram. An improvement in periodicity in patients with myasthenia gravis could be an objective indication of improvement with injected Tensilon.® This may help establish the diagnosis of myasthenia gravis. Further studies will be needed for complete evaluation of this technique.

Further, the objective determination of the voice is of vital interest from a medicolegal standpoint. A quality tape recording can be a great asset in assessing the exact nature of the voice. The accompanying spectrogram produced from this tape will give increasing objective evidence of the laryngeal disorders described by the clinician. Just as the audiogram helps in evaluating the pre- and postoperative condition of the ear, so too the spectrogram will help in evaluating the pre- and postoperative condition of the voice. As the legal implications of laryngeal surgery become more and more important, the voice spectrogram will have increased usage.

LIMITATIONS OF VOICE SPECTROGRAPHY

As in any other objective technique, the limitations of voice spectrography should be well understood. The exact quantification of spectrogram measurements is not feasible. It is the visual qualitative change of pattern in the parameters of the voice on the spectrogram rather than the actual measureable degree of change in formant structure, periodicity or breathiness, that is the significant aspect of voice spectrography. The spectrogram as such produces a clinically usable objective evaluation of the voice.

* Roche Laboratories, Nutley, New Jersey

To date, spectrograms cannot differentiate between different types of vocal cord lesions. Vocal cord nodules do not produce acoustic characteristics different from a contact granuloma. Furthermore, dysphonic characteristics, as indicated on a spectrogram, cannot indicate the existence or nonexistence of a malignant lesion. It is important to remember that many types of vocal cord pathologies yield similar resultant acoustic characteristics as seen on the spectrogram.

Spectrograms should not be used in place of indirect laryngoscopy to determine whether or not lesions have been resolved. Spectrograms are not a substitute for direct or indirect observation of the larynx. It should be emphasized that voice evaluation by spectrography should not be used as a substitute for good clinical acumen. Again, the final judgements of vocal conditions should be an evaluation of all the parameters available to the clinician and not on the basis of a single test.

Request for reprints should be sent to Eugene Rontal, M.D., 21700 Northwestern Hwy., Tower 14, Suite 545, Southfield, Mich. 48075.

ACKNOWLEDGMENT—The authors acknowledge the assistance of Mrs. Sydnor Gilbreath for her generous support of these research activities through the Gilbreath Voice Analysis Laboratory, Speech and Language Pathology Department, William Beaumont Hospital, Royal Oak, Michigan. Technical assistance was given by the Audio-Visual Department at William Beaumont Hospital.

REFERENCES

1. Potter R, Kopp G, Green H: *Visible Speech.* New York, D. Van Nostrand Company, Inc., 1947

2. Arnold GE: Vocal rehabilitation of paralytic dysphonia: IX Technique of intracordal injection. Arch Otolaryngol 76:358-368

3. Rolnick MI, Hoops HR: Plosive phoneme duration as a function of palato – pharyngeal adequacy. Cleft Palate J 8:65-76, 1971

4. Rontal E, Rontal M, Rolnick MI: The use of spectrograms in the evaluation of vocal cord injection. Laryngoscope 85:47-56, 1975

5. Yanagihara N: Significance of harmonic changes and noise components in hoarseness. J Speech Hearing Res 10:531-541, 1967

6. Holbrook A, Fairbanks G: Diphthong formants and their movements. J Speech Hearing Res 5:38-58, 1962

7. Iwata S, Von Leden H: Voice prints in laryngeal disease. Arch Otolaryngol 91:346-351, 1970

8. Cooper M: Spectrographic analysis of fundamental frequency and hoarseness before and after vocal rehabilitation. J Speech Hearing Disord 39:286-297, 1974

9. Isshiki N, Yanagihara N, Morimoto M: Approach to the objective diagnosis of hoarseness. Folia Phoniatr (Basel) 18: 183-192, 1964

10. Koyama T, Kawasaki M, Ogura JH: Mechanics of voice production, regulation of vocal intensity. Laryngoscope 79:337-354, 1969

11. Timcke R, Von Leden H, Moore P: Laryngeal vibrations; measurement of the glottic wave. Part I. The normal vibratory cycle. Arch Otolaryngol 68:1-19, 1958

Ann Otol 84: 1975

HYPOGEUSIA, DYSGEUSIA, HYPOSMIA, AND DYSOSMIA FOLLOWING INFLUENZA-LIKE INFECTION

R. I. HENKIN, M.D.

A. L. LARSON, M.D. R. D. POWELL, M.D.

BETHESDA, MARYLAND

SUMMARY — Hypogeusia, with or without dysgeusia, and hyposmia, with or without dysosmia, followed an influenzal-like infection in 87 of 143 consecutive patients who presented at the Taste and Smell Clinic at the NIH with taste and smell abnormalities. Findings in this disease included pale nasal mucous membranes with marked patency of the nasal airway, a positive Rudolph sign, elevated detection and recognition thresholds for several tastants and odorants, disruption of the pore region of the taste bud observed on electron microscopy and infiltration of the upper lamina propria of the nasal mucous membrane with chronic inflammatory cells observed on light microscopy. These findings, taken together, are relatively specific for the diagnosis of this surprisingly common disorder.

We have recently described a syndrome characterized by hypogeusia, with or without dysgeusia, and hyposmia, with or without dysosmia.[1,2] Eighty-seven of 143 consecutive patients studied at the Taste and Smell Clinic at the NIH developed the above symptoms following an influenza-like illness. The purpose of this report is to describe in detail the clinical findings of these 87 patients and to relate these symptoms, where possible, to specific pathophysiological changes. For convenience, we will refer to this clinical entity as postinfluenza-like hypogeusia and hyposmia (PIHH).

Patients. One hundred forty-three consecutive patients with taste and smell symptoms presented at the Taste and Smell Clinic of the National Institutes of Health. Eighty-seven patients who developed these changes following an influenza-like illness served as subjects in this study. Patients ranged in age from 19-83 years (mean, 54 years), were of both sexes, of varied ethnic and racial groups, and residents of various geographical regions in the world.

Clinical History. In each subject the onset of PIHH followed an upper respiratory illness which was clinically of viral origin and usually occurred in the winter or spring months. Patients who developed their respiratory illness in the winter-spring of 1968-69 were said to have had "Hong-Kong flu" by their local physician. The illness began as a severe coryza with fever, chills, malaise, anorexia, arthralgia, and myalgia. Lower respiratory and gastrointestinal symptoms were occasionally present but not prominent. During the period 1968-69 the onset of this respiratory illness was occasionally associated with vertigo, decreased auditory acuity and tinnitus, symptoms previously described.[3] However, during the winter-spring of 1969-70 or 1970-71 these latter symptoms were not prominent in patients who developed upper respiratory illnesses and subsequently PIHH. Although patients often referred to this influenza-like illness as "the worst cold I ever had," most did not visit their family physician. Of those treated by their family physicians medications consisted of antihistamines, antipyretic agents, sympathomimetic agents, and occasionally, antibiotics. The admini-

From the Section on Neuroendocrinology, National Heart and Lung Institute; Pathological Anatomy Branch, National Cancer Institute, National Institutes of Health, Bethesda, Md.

stration of these drugs could not be consistently related to the development of any subsequent taste or smell abnormalities. Indeed, many untreated patients also developed these abnormalities. With or without treatment the acute symptoms of the coryza waned within six days to two weeks as did the vertigo, decreased auditory acuity, and tinnitus.

At the onset of the coryza the patients usually noted an abrupt decrease in taste acuity (hypogeusia) and smell acuity (hyposmia). At first, most patients were not overly concerned about these changes since many had experienced similar hypogeusia and hyposmia with previous influenza-like illnesses.[1,2] However, during the recovery period, they noted that their taste and smell acuity did not return to normal although their auditory symptoms, if present, did. In most patients the hypogeusia and hyposmia persisted without significant improvement or variation. Approximately one-half of the patients also developed symptoms of dysgeusia* and dysosmia*. These symptoms usually began during the recovery period. In about one-half of these latter patients the dysgeusia and dysosmia became increasingly severe with time, whereas in the other half they fluctuated in intensity, usually decreasing and disappearing over the next six months.

Following the influenza-like illness and the development of PIHH, patients began to note dryness of their nasal passages and decreased frequency and quantity of nasal discharge. Neither nasal crusting nor epistaxis was prominent, and nasal stuffiness was uncommon. There was no reported associated decrease in tearing or secretion from other glands. Patients never complained of any associated oral ulcerations, gingivitis, "cold" or "canker" sores. Swelling of the parotid or other salivary glands was never evident, and lymphadenopathy in the head and neck region was not a common feature either during the acute or recovery phase of the influenza.

Following the development of PIHH, over 75% of the patients noted either a decreased frequency or complete absence of further attacks of influenza-like illnesses or coryza. Among those who did experience these diseases, the intensity was greatly attenuated.

Patients were referred to our clinic by physicians who had exhausted all their knowledge of diagnosis or treatment of these distressing symptoms. Patients were referred from local family physicians, neurologists, otorhinolaryngologists, and psychiatrists.[1,2]

Physical Examination of the Head and Neck. Patients were examined three months to ten years following their initial illness.

Nose. The most prominent consistent clinical feature of PIHH was in the nose where the tenacious, clear, occasionally white, mucous blanket normally found was not observed. The nasal mucous membranes were moist but neither shiny nor glistening. The membranes were often pale in color, but not similar to the pale, boggy bluish tinge commonly observed in allergic rhinitis or the reddish tinge seen in infectious rhinitis. Nasal membranes looked similar to those following the topical application of a vasoconstrictor agent, such as Neo-Synephrine.®** A second consistent feature was the patency of the nasal airway. This patency was such that the deeper structures of the nasal cavity were easily seen by anterior rhinoscopy without the use of vasoconstrictor agents. The openings of the glands of the nasal mucous mem-

* Dysgeusia: inappropriate, usually unpleasant, taste sensations. Aspects of dysgeusia include cacogeusia, an obnoxious taste produced by food, phantogeusia, a taste perceived without an appropriate taste stimulus (*e.g.*, a persistent metallic or salty taste in the mouth) and heterogeusia, a consistently inappropriate taste sensation produced by food or drink but not necessarily obnoxious (*e.g.*, all food tastes, sweet or bitter). Dysosmia: inappropriate, usually unpleasant smell sensations. Aspects of dysosmia are similar to those noted above for dysgeusia and include cacosmia, phantosmia, and heterosmia.[4]

** Winthrop Laboratories, N.Y., N.Y.

branes were not prominent. Membranes were not edematous, and there was little vascular congestion or turgor. Purulent secretions, crusting, or bleeding were not commonly observed. Two patients (2/87) had unilateral nasal polyps.

Mouth. There were no distinctive changes observed in the oral cavity. The buccal mucous membranes, tongue, palate, and all other oral structures visualized were within normal limits. Fungiform, circumvallate, and palatal papillae were normal in number and appearance, as were the minor salivary glands of the palate.

Ear. There were no distinctive changes observed in the external auditory canal (EAC) or tympanic membranes. However, three patients had perforations of the tympanic membrane, two unilateral, one bilateral, all apparently secondary to prior chronic otitis media unrelated to the present illness. A fourth patient had previously undergone a successful unilateral myringoplasty for treatment of a perforated tympanic membrane, and a fifth patient had bilateral otosclerosis. Each condition antedated the onset of PIHH.

Neck. No significant adenopathy was present in the neck. Indirect mirror laryngeal examination was within normal limits in all patients.

ROENTGENOGRAPHIC EXAMINATIONS

Paranasal Sinuses. Roentgenographs of the paranasal sinuses including Waters, Caldwell, submento-vertex, and lateral views were obtained in each patient. Roentgenographs were considered to be abnormal in 16 patients (18%). Of these, a rudimentary frontal sinus was the only abnormality present in two. Of the remaining 14, two had evidence of acute sinusitis manifested by air fluid levels, one in the left antrum, and other in the right frontal sinus. Four exhibited thickening of the mucosa of the antrum of mild to moderate degree without evidence of an air-fluid level. One had an antral osteoma and three had mucoceles, one in the left antrum, one in the right antrum, and one, bilaterally. Four exhibited bilaterally small, sclerotic, well-aerated antra. Although there was no antecedent history of chronic sinusitis or treatment of sinus disease, the radiographic interpretation of these changes in these latter four patients was that of chronic maxillary osteitis.

Of the two patients with nasal polyps, one had an air-fluid level in the frontal sinus, and the other had no abnormalities of the paranasal sinuses on roentgenographic examination.

Only three of the 16 patients had local unilateral disease of the sinuses which in time of onset and degree of severity could be related to the PIHH. These patients were included in this study because their local disease was unilateral.

Temporal Bones. Roentgenographs of the temporal bones, including Stenver's, Law and Towne's views, were obtained in each patient. Although normal variation was considerable, ranging from small, contracted mastoid air cells to well-pneumatized, extensive air cell systems, only two patients exhibited unilateral sclerosis which was interpreted to be consistent with chronic otitis media. Each of these patients had perforations of the tympanic membrane on the affected side. One patient exhibited asymmetry of the sphenoidal ridges which was interpreted to be within normal limits. No evidence of a space occupying lesion of the internal auditory canal (IAC) was observed in any patient.

Skull. Roentgenographs of the skull including frontal and lateral views were obtained in each patient. Two patients exhibited calcification of the falx cerebri, while one exhibited hyperostosis frontalis interna. Roentgenographs of all other patients were considered to be within normal limits. No evidence of an olfactory cleft tumor was found in any patient.

Chest. Posterior, anterior, and lateral roentgenographs of the chest were obtained in each patient. No active pulmonary lesion was found in any patient.

Radionuclide Studies. Brain scanning

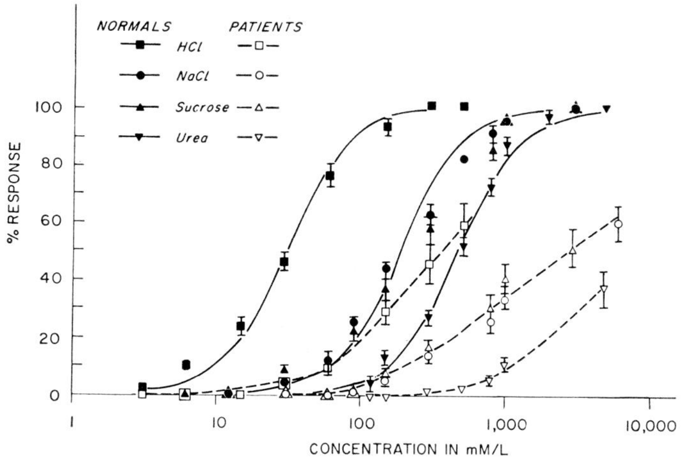

Fig. 1. Mean forced scaling measurements for the taste of HCl, NaCl, sucrose, and urea in 25 normal volunteers and in 65 patients with untreated PIHH. Vertical bars indicate ±1 standard error of the mean (SEM).

following an intravenous injection of technetium-99m was carried out in each patient. While no intrinsic pathology of the brain was observed in any patient, accumulation of technetium-99m in the nasal region was observed on both frontal and lateral views in 40% of the patients. This accumulation was previously observed in 82% of a group of patients with Sjögren's syndrome,[5] has been termed Rudolph sign, and has previously been related to the intensity of inflammation in the nasal mucous membrane.[5]

Other Studies. Electroencephalography (EEG) was carried out in each patient as a screening test for intrinsic abnormalities of the brain; no signs of intrinsic brain abnormalities were observed.

A neurological examination did not reveal abnormalities in any cranial nerve other than related to taste and smell. Evaluation of each patient also included a complete hematological work-up, urinalysis, and examination of liver and renal function; results did not relate the PIHH to any abnormality revealed by these tests.

SENSORY EXAMINATIONS

Taste. Detection and recognition thresholds for representatives of each of four taste qualities (NaCl for salt, sucrose for sweet, HCl for sour, and urea for bitter) were determined in each patient on at least two occasions by a forced-choice, three-stimulus drop technique.[1,2] Median values were determined for the patient group. Forced scaling measurements were also determined during each of these examinations.[1,6] These results were compared with those obtained in normal volunteers and in patients with various acute and chronic diseases who had normal taste acuity.[1,2,6] Median detection and recognition thresholds for the patients with PIHH were elevated above normal levels for salt, sour, and bitter, whereas for sweet, median detection and recognition thresholds were at the upper limit of normal (Table I). Forced scaling patterns for the patients were significantly different from those of the controls for each taste quality tested (Fig. 1).

Smell. Detection and recognition thresholds for representatives of each of three vapors (pyridine, nitrobenzene, and thiophene) were determined in each patient on at least two occasions by a forced-choice, three stimulus, sniff technique.[1,2,7] Median values were determined for the group. These results were compared with those obtained in

TABLE I

MEDIAN AND RANGE OF DETECTION AND RECOGNITION THRESHOLDS FOR FOUR TASTE QUALITIES IN 87 PATIENTS WITH PIHH AND 150 CONTROL SUBJECTS

	Patients		*Controls*	
Taste Quality	*MDT/MRT (mM/liter)*	*Range (mM/liter)*	*MDT/MRT (mM/liter)*	*Range (mM/liter)*
NaCl	90/150	12-*/30-*	12/30	6-60/6-60
Sucrose	60/60	6-*/12-*	12/30	6-60/6-60
HCl	15/90	0.5- > 500/3- > 500	3/6	0.5-6/0.8-6
Urea	500/800	60- > 8000/90- > 8000	120/150	60-150/60-150

MDT - median detection threshold
MRT - median recognition threshold
* - inability to detect or recognize saturated solutions of NaCl or sucrose.

normal volunteers and in patients with various acute and chronic diseases who had normal smell acuity.[1,6-8] Median detection and recognition thresholds for the patients with PIHH were elevated above normal levels for each vapor tested (Table II).

Hearing. Air and bone conduction thresholds were obtained in 79 of the 87 patients on at least one occasion. Each was seated alone in a single walled sound chamber.* Using a clinical audiometer,** pure tone thresholds were obtained by the method of limits using frequencies from 250-8000 Hz and bone conduction using frequencies from 500-4000 Hz. The same audiologist, who had no knowledge of the clinical status of the patients, performed each test.

Twenty-six of 79 patients (31%) had no history of hearing loss and had normal hearing thresholds upon testing; thirty-five (44%) gave a history of hearing loss prior to the onset of their influenza and had abnormalities demonstrated by testing; eighteen (25%) noted the onset of hearing abnormalities at or during the time of the influenza, and

TABLE II

MEDIAN DETECTION AND RECOGNITION THRESHOLDS FOR THREE VAPORS IN 87 PATIENTS WITH PIHH

	Patients		*Normal Subjects*	
Vapor	*MDT/MRT in M/L*	*Range*	*MDT/MRT in M/L*	*Range*
Pyridine	$10^{-1}/1$	10^{-3}-†/10^{-1}-†	$10^{-7}/10^{-3}$	10^{-9}-10^{-5}/10^{-5}-10^{-2}
Nitrobenzene	A/A	10^{-2}-†/10^{-1}-†	$10^{-6}/10^{-3}$	10^{-7}-10^{-5}/10^{-5}-10^{-2}
Thiophene	A/A	10^{-2}-†/10^{-1}-†	$10^{-7}/10^{-3}$	10^{-8}-10^{-5}/10^{-4}-10^{-2}

MDT - median detection threshold
MRT - median recognition threshold
A - ability to detect or recognize an absolute solution
† - inability to detect or recognize an absolute solution

* Model 401-A, Industrial Acoustics Co., Inc., Bronx, N.Y.
** Model MA-11, Maico Hearing Instruments, Minneapolis, Minn.

TABLE III

RESULTS OF AUDIOMETRIC TESTING IN THE 53 PATIENTS WITH PIHH WITH HEARING LOSSES

		Sensorineural Losses				Mixed Losses
	No. of Patients	*Notch at 4K*	*High frequency mild*	*High frequency moderate-severe*	*Peaked Curve*[9]	
Changes in auditory acuity unrelated in time to PIHH	35	26%	46%	11%	0	17%
Changes in auditory acuity related in time to PIHH	18	22%	56%	11%	11	0

hearing losses of various types were observed (Table III).

None of the 18 patients with hearing losses related in time to the influenza gave a history of otitis media at the time of the acute illness. Each developed a sensorineural hearing loss, eight of them, unilateral losses, and ten, bilateral losses. Ten (56%) exhibited a mild high frequency loss (loss of 30 dB or less in the speech range with further losses in the frequencies above 2 kHz), two (11%) a moderate-severe high frequency loss (loss of 30-60 dB in the speech range), four (22%) a "notch" at 4 kHz, and two (11%), a "peaked curve."[9]

MICROSCOPIC EXAMINATIONS

Taste Buds. Taste buds from patients with PIHH were examined by light and electron microscopy[1] and compared with taste buds removed from normal volunteers and from patients with various acute and chronic diseases in whom taste acuity was normal. Taste buds from patients with PIHH showed severe disruption of the pore region of the bud with marked diminution in the number and organization of the neurosecretory granules, absence of the dense, extracellular material, amputation of the finger-like projections from cells which extend into the pore region, and the presence of many large and small vacuoles (Fig. 2).

Nasal Mucous Membranes. Biopsies from the nasal mucous membranes of patients with PIHH were examined by light microscopy and compared with similar tissue taken from normal volunteers undergoing local nasal procedures for cosmetic reasons and from patients with various acute and chronic diseases in whom olfactory acuity was normal.

Biopsies were taken from the nasal septum in the area immediately posterior to the nasal limen. This area was initially infiltrated with 1% Xylocaine®* containing 1:100,000 Epinephrine.®** A 3-4 mm Hayes Martin punch biopsy of the entire thickness of the mucous membrane, to but not including the perichondrium, was removed and placed into B5 medium,*** embedded in paraffin, sectioned, and prepared for examination by light microscopy. Bleeding was usually minimal and, if present, was controlled with the placement of a small cotton pledget in the area of the biopsy.

Representative biopsies from a subject with normal olfactory acuity and from a patient with PIHH and hyposmia are compared in Fig. 3. The biopsy from the patient with PIHH demonstrates thickening of the surface epithelium, with mild cellular atypia, moderate thickening of the basement

----

* Astra Pharmaceutical Products, Inc., Worcester, Mass.
** SMP Division, Cooper Labs, Inc., San German, P.R.
*** B5 medium consists of 6 g mercuric chloride, 1.25 g anhydrous sodium acetate, 90 cc distilled water, and 10 cc concentrated formaldehyde added just before use.

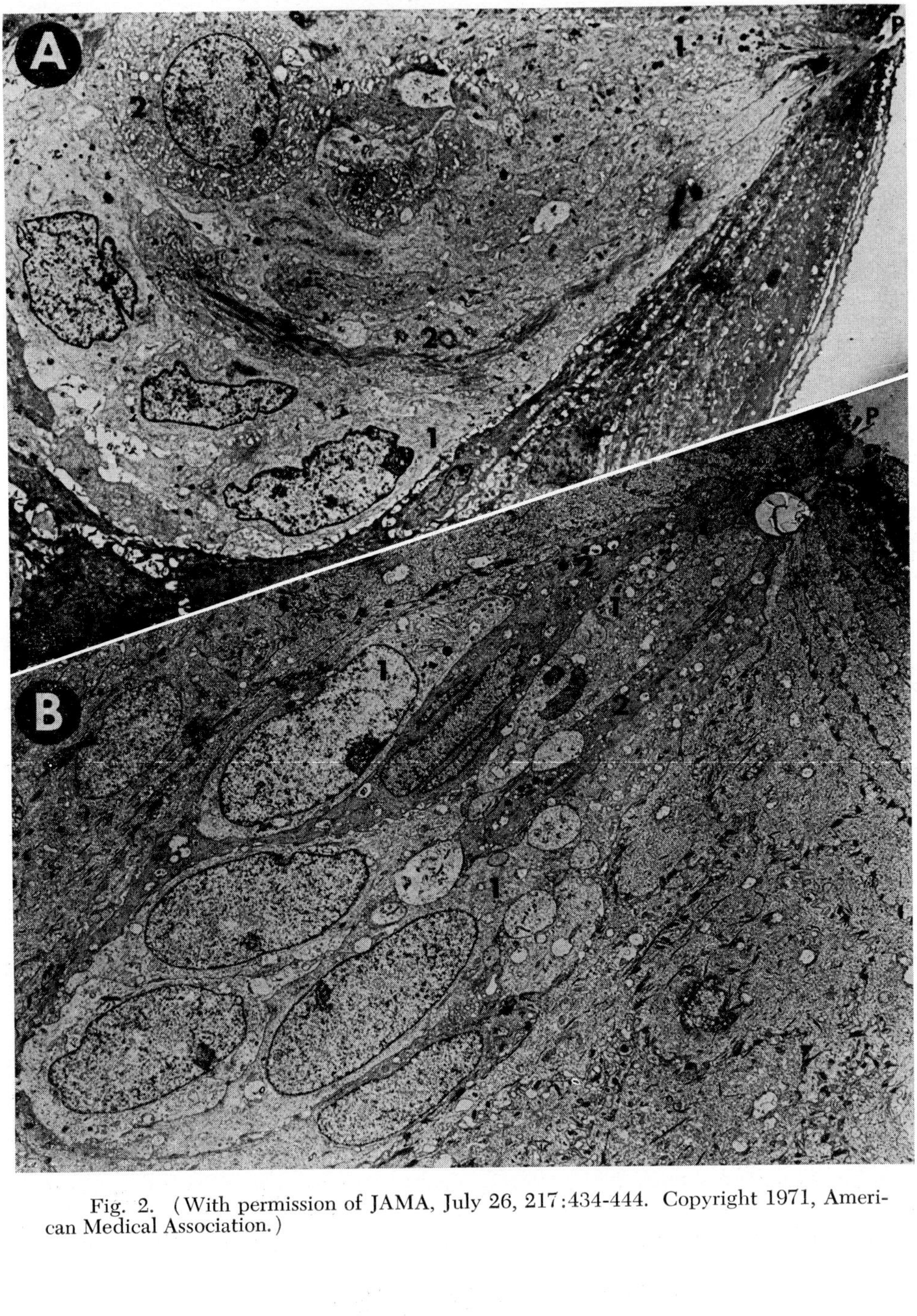

Fig. 2. (With permission of JAMA, July 26, 217:434-444. Copyright 1971, American Medical Association.)

membrane and, most characteristically, infiltration of the upper lamina propria with chronic inflammatory cells. These cells are mainly small lymphocytes, but some plasma cells were also observed. Relatively little, if any, inflammation was present in the submucosal glands. Significant sclerosis and fibrosis of the upper lamina propria was also commonly observed. Both serous and mucous glands were decreased in number, but serous gland were decreased to a much greater degree. Dysplasia of the ducts of some mucous glands was observed.

DISCUSSION

The syndrome of PIHH is a clinical pathological entity characterized by decreased taste and smell acuity following an influenza-like illness. Distortion of taste and/or smell perceptions also occur. These sensory abnormalities are commonly associated with pathological changes in taste buds and in nasal mucous membranes. Dry, pale nasal mucous membranes with decreased turgor and patulousness of the nasal airway are characteristic findings in the nose.

This syndrome can be differentiated from several other pathological processes which affect the nose and which may have hyposmia as one of their symptoms. Since crusting, inspissated mucous, and localized infection were not seen in the nasal mucous membrane of patients with PIHH, ozena and/or atrophic rhinitis can be excluded as etiological factors.

The nasal mucous membrane in PIHH is similar in some ways to that observed in Sjögren's syndrome except that crusting and marked dryness are more common in Sjögren's syndrome. In addition, decreased secretion from lacrimal, oral, cervical, and aural glands is common in Sjögren's syndrome and not in PIHH. Patients with Sjögren's syndrome also exhibit an associated collagen vascular disease, whereas this is an uncommon accompaniment of PIHH. Further, the nasal mucous membrane biopsy in Sjögren's syndrome characteristically features periglandular infiltration with chronic inflammatory cells,[10] whereas in PIHH the infiltration is primarily in the upper lamina propria and includes both acute and chronic inflammatory cells. Sjögren's syndrome is almost unformly observed in women, whereas PIHH occurs in both sexes.

Fig. 2 A) Representative taste bud from a circumvallate papilla of a man with normal taste acuity (X3000). The entire papilla was amputated at its root with a fine iris scissors following infiltration of Xylocaine® just external to the lingual foramen and at the posterior base of the tongue. The specimen was placed immediately into buffered glutaraldehyde and fixed, sectioned, and examined as previously described.[1] The most external area of the bud is the pore (P) which communicates with the oral cavity. Within the pore region there are numerous fine, fingerlike cytoplasmic projections and dense extracellular material. Small dense core or neurosecretory granules are stratified in Type I (1) cells and extend into the pore region. Fingerlike cytoplasmic projections from Type II (2) cells also extend into the pore region. Type II (2) cells commonly contain a characteristic bundle of tonofilaments which may function as a protective, contractile element of the taste bud. This bundle is clearly shown in one of the Type II cells in this micrograph. Type II (2) cells are characteristically vacuolated, as observed. Each of the three major cell types (I, II, III) which comprise the bud extend throughout the length of the bud, but only Type I (1) and II (2) cells are clearly observed in this figure. Similar anatomical structures were observed in papillae excised from five other subjects with normal taste acuity. B) Representative taste bud from a circumvallate papilla of a man with PIHH with both hypogeusia and hyposmia (X3000). The papilla was excised and handled in a manner similar to that used for the subjects with normal taste acuity.[1] The pore (P) which communicates with the oral cavity is clearly observed. The fine, fingerlike cytoplasmic projections are decreased in number and the dense, extracellular material is absent. Occasional large and small vacuoles are present throughout the pore area and also in other areas of the cytoplasm. Fewer dense core granules are observed in Type I (1) cells, and they appear less stratified than in the normal bud. Type II (2) cells are also observed but contain many more and also larger vacuoles than in the normal bud. The normal cellular organization near the pore area is markedly altered. Similar results were observed in several other taste buds found in this same patient and in four patients with PIHH.

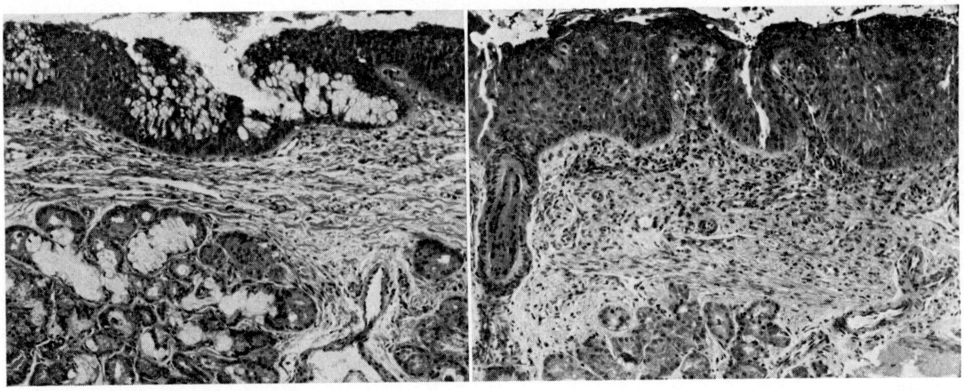

Fig. 3. Biopsies of the nasal mucous membrane from a representative subject with normal olfactory acuity (left) and from a representative patient with PIHH and hyposmia (right) (H. and E. X40). Both biopsies show similar areas of the nasal mucous membrane including the surface epithelium, basement membrane, upper lamina propria and mucous and serous glands. Compared with that from the normal subject, the biopsy from the patient with PIHH shows thickening of the surface epithelium, moderate to marked thickening of the basement membrane, and, most characteristically, infiltration of the upper lamina propria with chronic inflammatory cells.

Since the nasal mucous membranes of patients with PIHH were not pale, boggy, or watery, but were occasionally bluish, and upon biopsy did not exhibit eosinophilia in the upper lamina propria, these patients may be differentiated from those with acute and chronic allergic rhinitis. In both allergic rhinitis and vasomotor rhinitis patients commonly exhibit edematous nasal mucous membranes with marked airway obstruction; this condition was never seen in PIHH. Since the nasal mucous membrane in PIHH was not reddened, injected, purulent, or crusted and upon biopsy did not exhibit a marked infiltration of acute inflammatory cells in the surface epithelium and the number of acute inflammatory cells in the upper lamina propria was slight, these patients may be differentiated from those with acute or chronic infectious rhinitis of various types. Patients with chronic granulomatous processes involving the nasal mucous membrane may be differentiated clinically from patients with PIHH by their crusted inflamed nasal mucous membrane and by biopsy where marked, extensive infiltration with chronic inflammatory cells may occur and occasionally multinucleated giant cells are found, at times to the point of replacement of glandular elements. In Wegener's granulomatosis, vasculitis and multinucleated giant cells usually are observed, and in leishmaniasis the organisms may be observed intracellularly.[11]

Patients with hypogeusia and hyposmia produced by various pathogenetic mechanisms have presented to our clinic. Of the first 143 consecutive patients, 87 (59%) had PIHH. Others developed their symptoms following a variety of disorders, including: scleroderma; porphyria; viral encephalitis; head trauma and/or skull fracture; cerebral vascular accidents; facilitating myesthenic syndrome and other muscle disease; multiple sclerosis; untreated hypothyroidism; primary amyloidosis; congenital hyposmia; postsurgical hypogeusia and hyposmia; X-irradiation of the head and neck; occult malignancy; overt malignancy including leukemia, lymphoma, and carcinoma of the lung, ovary, or stomach and brain tumors of several types (excluding esthesioneuroblastomas); Wegner's granulomatosis and midline granuloma of the face; tertiary syphilis; drug-induced hyposmia and hypogeusia; xerostomia of several causes; several malabsorption syndromes. There may be instances without any prior historical event. The diagnosis of each disease underlying the changes in taste and smell was made by appropriate means. However, biopsy of the nasal mucous membrane was useful in the establishing of some diagnoses. It is clear that in this sense taste and smell abnormalities may be secondary to some underlying metabolic or other disease process or, as in PIHH, may be the result of some direct insult to those organs which directly support or are directly involved in taste and smell function.

Those hearing losses which developed in patients with PIHH with the influenza-like illness were primarily sensorineural in character and were similar to those observed in patients with PIHH whose hearing losses antedated their illness. However, two patients who exhibited a peaked curve[9] developed their hearing loss and PIHH simultaneously.

Two patients with unilateral air fluid levels and two patients with unilateral nasal polyps were included in the study because their disease was localized and unilateral and therefore presumably not responsible for their generalized taste and smell loss.

Many patients, who present to an otorhinolaryngologist complaining of taste loss, in actuality have experienced a smell loss. In this sense patients complain that they have lost their ability to "taste" their food, whereas, in actuality, it is their ability to smell or obtain flavor from food, which is primarily related to olfactory acuity which has been decreased.

The incidence of PIHH has not been clearly established. However, estimates suggest an incidence of 1 in 400 or in the United States, approximately 500,000 patients.[1,2] Since the number of patients who suffer from influenza-like illnesses each year is not definitely established, it is not possible to establish the frequency with which PIHH occurs following an influenzal-like illness.

The diagnosis of PIHH may be made by an appropriate history, observing characteristic changes in the nose, demonstrating abnormalities in taste and smell perception, demonstrating specific changes in nasal mucous membrane upon biopsy, and by demonstrating the presence of Rudolph sign following intravenous injection of technetium 99m. Although taken separately, these findings may be nonspecific; taken together they are relatively specific for this surprisingly common disorder.

Request for reprints should be sent to Robert I. Henkin, M.D., Center for Molecular Nutrition and Sensory Disorders, Georgetown University Medical Center, Washington, D.C. 20007.

REFERENCES

1. Henkin RI, Schechter PJ, Hoye RC, *et al*: Idiopathic hypogeusia with dysgeusia, hyposmia and dysosmia: A new syndrome. J Am Med Assoc 217:434-1971

2. Schechter PJ, Friedewald WT, Bronzert DA, *et al*: Idiopathic hypogeusia: a description of the syndrome and a single blind study with zinc sulfate, in Pfeiffer C (ed): *International Review of Neurobiology*, Suppl 1. New York, Academic Press, 1972, pp 125-140

3. Sataloff J, Vassallo L: Head colds and viral cochleitis. Arch Otolaryngol 87:56-69, 1968

4. Henkin RI: Disorders of taste and smell. J Am Med Assoc 218:19-46, 1971

5. Jones AE, Larson AL, Powell RD, *et al*: Localization of 99^{m} Technetium in the region of the nose in Sjögren's syndrome. Ann Otol Rhinol Laryngol 83:370-378, 1974

6. Henkin RI, Bradley DF: On the mechanism of action of carbohydrate active steroids on tastant detection and recognition, in Sawyer C, Gorski R (eds) *Steroid, Hormones and Brain Function.* Los Angeles University of California, 1971, pp 339-353

7. Marshall JR, Henkin RI: Olfactory acuity, menstrual abnormalities and oocyte status. Ann Intern Med 75:207-211, 1971

8. Henkin RI: The definition of primary and accessory areas of olfaction as the basis for a classification of decreased olfactory acuity, in Hayashi T (ed) *Olfaction and Taste II.* London, Pergamon Press, 1967, pp 235-252

9. Henkin RI, Lifschitz MD, Larson AL: Hearing loss in patients with osteoporosis and

Paget's disease of bone. Am J Med Sci 262: 383-393, 1972

10. Powell RD, Larson AL, Henkin RI: Nasal mucous membrane biopsy in Sjögren's syndrome: A new diagnostic technique. Ann Intern Med 81:25-31, 1974

11. Larson AL, Powell RD, Henkin RI: Unpublished observations

RHINOPLASTY COURSE

The annual basic Rhinoplasty Course of the University of California, Davis, will be held October 26-31, 1975. For further information write: Leslie Bernstein, M.D., D.D.S., Department of Otorhinolaryngology, University of California School of Medicine, Davis, California 95616.

COURSE IN NEUROTOLOGY

The Department of Otolaryngology of the Abraham Lincoln School of Medicine and the University of Illinois Hospital Eye and Ear Infirmary, University of Illinois at the Medical Center, will conduct a continuing education course in Neurotology, March 22-25, 1976.

The four day intensive course will offer a didactic and practical review of clinical neurotology under the direction of Nicholas Torok, M.D. It will be held at the Eye and Ear Infirmary and will include basic vestibular physiology and pathophysiology, commonly used testing methods applied in functional examination of the vestibular organ.

Enrollment is limited to 15. For application forms write: Department of Otolaryngology, 1855 West Taylor Street, Chicago.

Ann Otol 84: 1975

NEW APPROACH TO CALORIC STIMULATION OF THE VESTIBULAR RECEPTOR

LEONARD R. PROCTOR, M.D.

ROLLIN C. DIX, PH.D.

CHICAGO, ILLINOIS

SUMMARY – A new caloric testing method is described. During continuous aural irrigation, fluid is switched between hot and cold values at times computed according to a mathematical model of heat conduction in the labyrinth area. As a result, the induced temperature difference across the lateral semicircular canal describes an approximately sinusoidal time course, reaching peak values of equal magnitude but opposite sign. The magnitude of the caloric stimulus may be selected by choosing appropriate irrigation durations from a graph or table. Application of the test to clinical subjects demonstrated that the heat conduction model and analysis used in timing the sequence of thermal pulses was accurate. The new procedure causes less patient discomfort and requires less time to complete than does the conventional Fitzgerald-Hallpike test.

The caloric test is currently the primary clinical method for testing vestibular function and the procedure described in 1942 by Fitzgerald and Hallpike[1] is the most widely accepted technique for administering the caloric stimulations. As a result of empirical studies among normal subjects and patients with vestibular abnormalities, they recommended a standardized technique consisting of four separate aural irrigations (30C left; 30C right; 44C left; 44C right) using a high flow rate and carefully controlled irrigation temperatures. They intended to produce independent stimulations that were all of equal strength so that small differences in excitability between labyrinths as well as between right-beating versus left-beating nystagmus could be detected and measured. Although most clinicians continue to use, either literally or in principle, the Fitzgerald-Hallpike (F-H) method for administering caloric stimulations, there are significant problems inherent in this technique which could be largely overcome through a new approach to caloric stimulation described below.

One objectionable feature of the F-H method is its duration which makes the procedure fatiguing to patients and time consuming to the person applying the tests. Fitzgerald and Hallpike noted the time taken for a single test was about four minutes and advised an interval between tests of at least five minutes, thus requiring a minimum of 31 minutes to complete the series of tests.

A more subtle problem is presented by the fact that the prolonged and unphysiologic duration of individual stimulations contributes an element of inaccuracy and confusion to the interpretation of test results. In this regard it is important to take into account certain experimental evidence that indicates caloric-induced nystagmus normally ends long before the inciting physical stimulus has subsided. The observation of Fitzgerald and Hallpike[1] that among normal subjects with eyes open nystagmus ends after 1.2 to 2.4 minutes must be compared with temporal bone temperature measurements in living human subjects which have shown that a sig-

From the Department of Surgery (Otolaryngology), Pritzker School of Medicine, University of Chicago and the Department of Mechanics and Mechanical and Aerospace Engineering, Illinois Institute of Technology.

This work was supported in part by USPHS Grants 2-R01 NS-09613-02 and 2-R01 NS-09613-03A1.

nificant thermal disturbance continues far beyond the time nystagmus ends[2,3] and may last for more than ten minutes.[4] In a recent nystagmographic study, Hood[5] demonstrated that a caloric stimulus capable of producing nystagmus will persist for at least 11 minutes.

Hood explained the cessation of nystagmus in the face of a persisting caloric stimulus as an adaptive process of the vestibular neural elements, brought into play during sustained cupular deviations. It is of particular interest that the adaptive process to which Hood referred depends not upon cupular deviation per se but rather upon the length of time such deviation is maintained.[6] Thus, we must consider the probability that a persisting caloric stimulus will interfere with responses to successive F-H method irrigations, both directly by a sustained influence upon the receptor and indirectly through a modification of vestibular responsivity induced by such prolonged action. Furthermore, the magnitude of interaction between successive stimuli will vary with such factors as the amount of water left in the aural canal following each irrigation and the time elapsing between irrigations.

An additional argument against the use of prolonged caloric stimulations is based upon the demonstration that nystagmus intensity measurements taken during the peak of the reaction are much better correlated with vestibular stimulus intensities than is the duration of the induced nystagmus.[7] For this reason, most clinicians have come to depend upon that period when maximum nystagmus intensity is expected for their interpretation of the caloric test. In light of these considerations, there does not appear to be any compelling reason for maintaining caloric stimulation beyond the time when maximum response intensity has been established.

Finally, we must consider the difficulty of assuring that in practice we achieve the goal of producing four stimulations of equal magnitude when using the F-H method of aural irrigations. For example, Dohlman[8] showed that considerable variations in heat transmission will occur if the irrigation stream is directed at different parts of the aural canal. Other potential causes of variations in stimulus magnitude are entrapment of air in the aural canal during irrigation,[9] changes in head position relative to the gravity vector,[10,11] and the quantity of water remaining in the canal following irrigations. Thus, with each irrigation there is a danger that one of the above factors may exert a minor or major influence upon the strength of the stimulus. These considerations assume still more significance when we note that no method is used to monitor the strength of the stimulus which finally acts upon the vestibular receptor. Consequently, we are sometimes uncertain whether an altered nystagmus response represents an abnormality of the vestibular system or an inadvertent departure from precise irrigation technique.

Experiences with temperature recordings in living cats[9] and the availability of mathematical models and data concerning heat transmission in the labyrinth area[8,12,13] led us to try a new approach to caloric labyrinthine stimulation. This report describes a new caloric test method which provides selected peak stimulus values of equal magnitude but opposite sign, with rapid removal of the caloric stimulus at the conclusion of each test. As a result, stimulations are shorter and more physiologic, less time is taken to complete the test procedure and an improved control is achieved over stimulus magnitudes.

THEORETICAL CONSIDERATIONS

Aural irrigation with cold or hot water produces a temperature gradient across the labyrinth attended by changes in endolymph density, making possible the generation of forces acting to displace the endolymph-cupula system and thereby stimulate the vestibular receptor. The lateral semicircular canal is primarily responsible for the nystagmus response[1,8,11] and the temperature difference across this canal is nearly proportional to the physical stimulus acting upon the vestibular receptor, so long as the orientation of the semicircular canal with respect to gravity is controlled.[8,12,13] In our calculations we have ignored the fact that only the component of the temperature vector orthogonal to the gravity vector contributes to endolymph-displacing forces,[10,11] and we have assumed the labyrinth area can be treated as a solid of uniform thermal characteristics.

The time course of the temperature difference across the lateral semicircular canal (ΔT) resulting from a varied irrigation temperature may be calculated from a model assuming unidirectional conduction of heat through a homogeneous solid.[12,13] With this model, standard formulas[14] show that beginning irrigation with water at aural canal temperature plus T_1 degrees produces a temperature gradient after t seconds of

$$(1) \qquad dT/dx = \frac{-T_1}{\sqrt{\pi at}} e^{-x^2/4at}$$

The temperature difference across the canal, ΔT, is simply the gradient dT/dx times the distance across the canal, L. Therefore,

$$(2) \qquad \Delta T = \frac{-LT_1}{\sqrt{\pi at}} e^{-x^2/4at}$$

Where

T_1 = difference between irrigation water temperature and initial aural canal temperature in degrees, centigrade. In our method T_1 has a value of 44C − 37C = 7C.

L = distance across lateral semicircular canal, millimeters.

ΔT = temperature difference across lateral semicircular canal, degrees centigrade.

a = thermal diffusivity of temporal bone surrounding lateral semicircular canal, mm^2/sec.

x = distance between external aural canal and center of lateral semicircular canal, millimeters.

t = time elapsing from onset of irrigation, seconds.

e = natural logarithm base.

In the present study we used values for the above parameters determined by Young[13] for human temporal bones: L = 6 mm, a = .25 mm^2/sec, and x = 10.5 mm. With a, L, x and T_1 constant equation (2) may be simplified to read

$$(3) \qquad \Delta T = \frac{-A}{\sqrt{t}} e^{-B/t}$$

where A and B are constants. This equation predicts that for a continued irrigation the absolute magnitude of the temperature difference (ΔT) increases to a maximum value and then diminishes. For example, continuous irrigation with water at 44C would result in an absolute maximum ΔT value of 1.93C after 220 seconds.

However, we have chosen to interrupt the 44C irrigation by quickly changing the temperature of the irrigation to 30C and equation (3) must be expanded to account for this condition. After irrigating at the initial hot temperature (44C = 37C + T_1) for a duration of t_1 seconds the irrigation water is switched to a cold temperature (30C = 44C − $2T_1$). Thereafter the temperature difference across the lateral semicircular canal may be found by

$$(4) \qquad \Delta T = \frac{-A}{\sqrt{t}} e^{-B/t} + \frac{2A}{\sqrt{t-t_1}} e^{-B/(t-t_1)}$$

Equation (4) indicates that within certain limits the maximum value of ΔT produced by the initial (hot) irrigation can be controlled simply by adjusting the duration of this irrigation (t_1). An extension of equation (4) shows that the maximum value of ΔT produced by the second (cold) irrigation can be controlled by similarly adjusting the duration of the second irrigation.

METHOD

Our goal was to produce contiguous hot and cold caloric stimulations of equal magnitude and thereafter remove the stimulation as quickly as possible. This was to be accomplished by beginning with hot irrigation for t_1 seconds, switching to cold irrigation for t_2 seconds, switching back to hot for t_3 seconds and then stopping the irrigation. As explained above, the maximum value of ΔT produced by the second (cold) irrigation depends upon the duration of this second irrigation (t_2). We denote the peak temperature difference associated with the hot irrigation as $-\Delta T^*$ and the peak temperature difference of the cold irrigation $+\Delta T^*$. If we cause $-\Delta T^*$ and $+\Delta T^*$ to reach equal values, we consider our goal of equal hot and cold stimulations to be satisfied.

The correct values for irrigation durations t_1 and t_2 were determined using a computerized, interval-halving search procedure.[15] The first step was to find the value of t_1 in equation (4) which would result in a selected value of $-\Delta T^*$. The duration of the second (cold) irrigation (t_2) was then found by performing a search for $+\Delta T^*$ using an extension of (4). The duration of the final warm irrigation (t_3) is currently estimated with the intention of returning the labyrinth area to uniform temperature as soon as possible.

RESULTS

We selected an arbitrary stimulus value of $\pm\Delta T^* = .84C$ and, using the computerized search procedure described above, determined that this stimulus magnitude would be produced by irrigation at 44C for 38 seconds, switching to 30C for 58 seconds and then back to 44C. A general indication of the time course of the thermal disturbance in the region of the lateral semicircular canal caused by this irrigation sequence may be found in Figure 1, where temperature as a function of distance in the labyrinth area is plotted at uniform time intervals. Values for the plots in Figure 1 were determined by computer, using equation (1) and a modification and extension of equation (4). In agreement with temporal bone temperature recordings,[2-4,8,12,13] our calculations indicate a latency between thermal events in the aural canal and their effects in the region of the lateral semicircular canal. Thus, a significant temperature difference does not appear until about 15 seconds after beginning the first irrigation. Also, the effect of the initial hot irrigation continues to predominate for some time after switching to a cold irrigation (see 45 and 60 seconds plots in Fig. 1). Note that the temperature difference (ΔT) between the lateral and medial aspects of the lateral semicircular canal grows first negative, then positive, and then quickly falls to very low values.

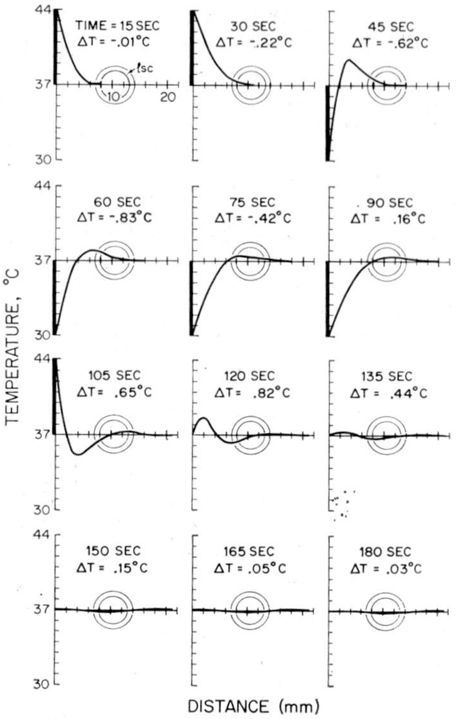

Fig. 1. Predicted temperature changes in the labyrinth area resulting from continuous aural irrigation at 44C for 38 seconds, 30C for 58 seconds, 44C for 20 seconds, and 37C thereafter. Temperature versus distance is plotted at 15 seconds intervals. The temperature difference (ΔT) across the lateral semicircular canal (lsc) as derived from formulas (2) and (4) is indicated above each figure.

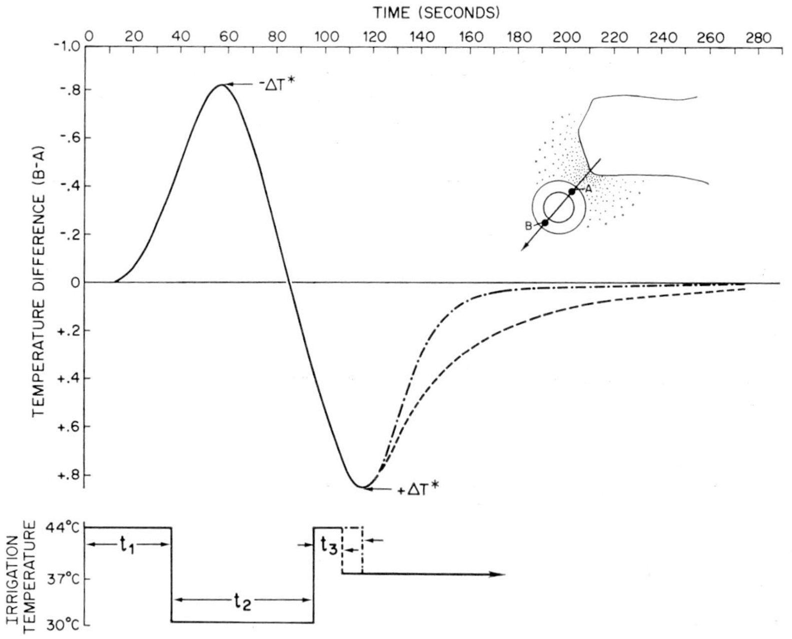

Fig. 2. Time course of predicted temperature difference across the lateral semicircular canal produced by step temperature changes during continuous aural irrigation. $-\Delta T^*$ and $+\Delta T^*$ are peak temperature differences associated with the initial hot phase (t_1) and the succeeding cold phase (t_2) of irrigations, respectively. The terminal course of the temperature difference is predicted for 2 cases, based upon a return of the irrigation temperature to 37C at 108 seconds (- - -) and 117 seconds (- • • -). (See text).

As explained above, the temperature difference across the lateral semicircular canal (ΔT) may be taken as an approximation of the intensity of the caloric stimulation. Consequently, the time course of the caloric stimulus is appropriately represented by a plot of values for ΔT versus time as determined by computer and shown in Figure 2. As can be seen, irrigation at 44C for 38 seconds, switching to 30C for 58 seconds and then back to 44C would produce an approximately sinusoidal ΔT curve with peak values of equal magnitude ($\pm$.84C ΔT^*) occurring at 58 and 117 seconds. The latency between changes in temperature at the aural canal surface and the effect of these thermal events upon the temperature difference (ΔT) across the lateral semicircular canal is once more evident (Figs. 1 & 2). After a latency of about 15 seconds, the value of ΔT increases rapidly as a result of the initial hot irrigation. Despite switching to the cold irrigation temperature at 38 seconds, the effect of the hot irrigation continues until a peak value is reached ($-\Delta T^*$) at 58 seconds. Similarly the cold irrigation ends at 96 seconds ($t_1 + t_2 = 96$ seconds), but $+\Delta T^*$ does not occur until 117 seconds. The final course of ΔT (broken lines, Fig. 2) is estimated as explained below.

The computerized search procedure was used to determine sets of values for t_1 and t_2 which would be required for several arbitrary stimulus magnitudes and the results are shown in Table I. Values for t_3 in Table I are estimated according to clinical experience. The computer-determined time courses of ΔT which would result from the irrigation sequences of Table I form smooth curves as shown in Figure 3. Note that all curves are similar and conform to a sinusoidal pattern.

A very important practical finding was the observation that a nearly linear

TABLE I

IRRIGATION DURATIONS REQUIRED TO PRODUCE VARIOUS STIMULUS MAGNITUDES.*

Desired Stimulus Magnitude	Irrigation durations (seconds) t_1	t_2	t_3 (estimated)
.25	15	27	4
.5	24	41	7
.75	34	54	10
1.0	45	68	14
1.2	56	80	17

* Stimulus magnitudes are expressed as peak temperature differences ($\pm\Delta T^*$) in degrees, centigrade.

relationship exists between switching times and peak stimulus strengths through the major portion of the plotted values (Fig. 4). This indicates that any values of stimulus strength between approximately .25C and 1.75C can be induced by a proper selection of irrigation times from the graph.

After the final hot irrigation is terminated, temperature at the aural canal surface returns slowly toward normal body temperature.[7] However, the specific course of the aural canal surface temperature during this period is unknown; therefore, we are unable to predict with certainty the final course of ΔT (broken lines, Figs. 2 & 3). For purposes of the computer search procedures and the computer determination of data shown in Figures 1, 2 and 3, we arbitrarily assumed the final course of ΔT could be predicted according to a continuation of the irrigation with temperature set at 37C following the final

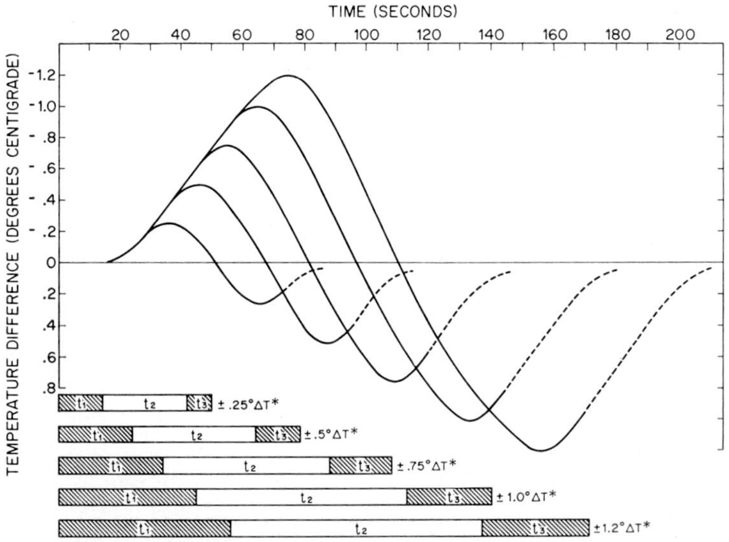

Fig. 3. Computer-determined time courses of stimulus strengths (ΔT) resulting from various irrigation sequences. Broken lines indicate course of ΔT based upon a return of irrigation temperature to 37C following the final hot irrigation. The final irrigation times shown (t_3) are those used for the mathematical model and are not recommended for clinical use (see Fig. 4).

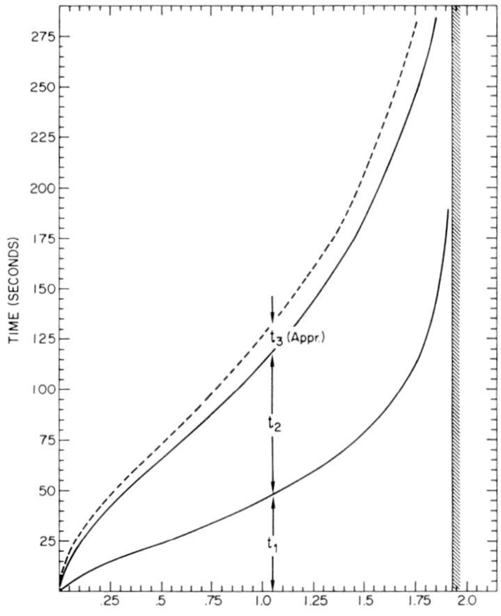

Fig. 4. Duration of irrigations (seconds) required for various stimulus strengths (degrees centigrade, $\pm\Delta T^*$). t_1, duration of initial hot irrigation. t_2, duration of second (cold) irrigation. t_3, duration of final (hot) irrigation.

hot irrigation. With this assumption, we searched for values of t_3 which would be most effective in rapidly returning the magnitude of ΔT to zero value. The result was that appropriate values for t_3 were usually close to $.6t_1$.

Although the relationship $t_3 = .6t_1$ is appropriate according to the mathematical model and presumptions described above, a final irrigation with water at 37C was not applied during our clinical trials. Instead, we simply terminated the irrigation. Consequently, the mathematical model is not representative of the actual test procedure so far as determinations of t_3 are concerned. When the irrigation is terminated without applying a final 37C phase, our clinical experience indicates the value of t_3 should be set at approximately $.3t_1$, and we have therefore recommended this value in Table I and Figure 4.

In a clinical trial of the $\pm.84$C ΔT^* stimulus (described below), we used a value of 12 seconds for t_3. To estimate the course of the physical stimulus resulting from this t_3 duration, we plotted computer-determined values for both $t_3 = 12$ seconds and $t_3 = 20$ seconds. Thus, the true course of ΔT should lie between the broken lines of Figure 2.

CLINICAL TRIALS

We have explained above the derivation of a new sinusoidal bithermal caloric (SBC) test method designed to produce rapid, balanced hot/cold stimulations of the vestibular receptor. Next we would like to describe briefly the results of a preliminary study among human subjects in which we tested the accuracy of our calculations and evaluated the practicality of the new method.

The new SBC test procedure was applied to several normal volunteers and then to patients referred to the clinical vestibular laboratory. Water was directed against the posterosuperior part of the aural canal under visual control from an irrigation handle[16] containing a temperature sensor. Continuous recordings from the sensor enabled us to monitor irrigation temperatures and switching times. A valve connected two water baths with external circulation to the irrigation handle, providing a means for quickly changing the temperature of the irrigation water from 44C to 30C and vice versa. Although this apparatus requires further development, we were able to control irrigation temperature with accuracy sufficient for the present study. Responses were recorded electronystagmographically (ENG) using a dynograph* and commercial silver-silver chloride skin electrodes at the outer canthi. We used 10 mm/sec paper speed, 3 seconds time constant, and "slow" setting for filters. Calibration (10° eye movement = 10 mm pen displacement) was adjusted immediately before the series of caloric stimulations, whch were performed with the patient recumbent and head raised 30° above

* Type R, Beckman Instruments, Inc., Fullerton, Calif.

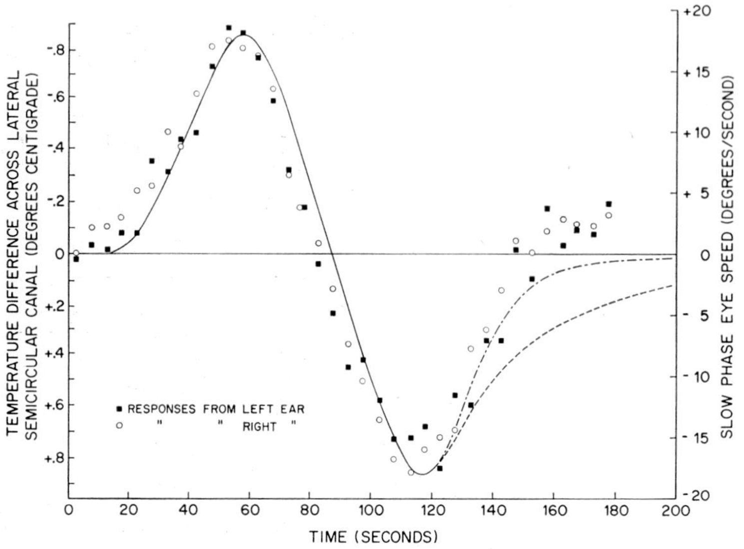

Fig. 5. Average slow phase eye speed for 13 "normal" subjects tested with new caloric stimulation procedure (see Figs. 1 & 2). Note close agreement between predicted stimulus strength (ΔT, solid and broken lines) and the direction and intensity of averaged nystagmus responses.

horizontal. Subjects were instructed to keep their eyes closed, and were "alerted" with arithmetic tasks. Testing was carried out in a dimly-lit room and caloric stimulations were preceded by oculomotor and positional tests.

An initial group of 18 patients was tested with an irrigation sequence which produces a relatively weak stimulation of $\pm.5C\ \Delta T^*$. The responses of most patients were sufficiently intense and clearly formed to provide a full picture of caloric-induced vestibular responsivity. However, we felt it was necessary to rely upon conventional caloric stimulations in those cases where responses to this stimulus were uncertain or absent.

It was our impression that a stronger SBC stimulus would be more suitable for routine clinical use and we, therefore, tested a second group of patients with the stronger stimulus discussed above ($\pm.84C\ \Delta T^*$; Figs. 1 & 2). The appropriate irrigation sequence (44C x 38"; 30C x 58"; 44C x 12") was applied to 32 unselected patients referred for vestibular evaluation. Separate hot irrigations (44C x 30") were also applied to these subjects so that responses to conventional stimulations could be compared with responses to the new SBC test. All responses from this second patient group were analyzed by determining from the ENG recordings the mean slow phase eye speed for each 5 seconds of the responses. Nystagmus beats were assigned positive and negative values when the fast phase of the beat was directed toward the stimulated or opposite ear, respectively.[17] Average slow phase eye speed was calculated for the 20 seconds period during which response to the hot mode stimulus of the new SBC test was strongest (usually 45 to 65 seconds; see Fig. 5) and for the time period when response to the cold mode stimulus was strongest (usually 105 to 125 seconds). Differences in excitability between labyrinths and between right-beating versus left-beating nystagmus were determined in relation to total excitability as recommended by Jongkees and Phillipszoon.[18]

Unilateral hypoexcitability score:

$$\frac{(1+2)-(3+4)}{(1+2+3+4)} \times 100\%$$

TABLE II

MEAN SLOW PHASE EYE SPEED* OF NYSTAGMUS INDUCED BY SINUSOIDAL BITHERMAL** AND CONVENTIONAL HOT CALORIC STIMULATIONS

	Sinusoidal Bithermal Caloric Test		*Conventional Test*
	Hot mode responses	*Cold mode responses*	*Hot responses*
Normal subjects (13)	17.75	18.40	28.20
All subjects (32)	16.95	16.81	22.41

* degrees/second
** ±.84 C ΔT*

Directional preponderance score:

$$\frac{(2+3)-(1+4)}{(1+2+3+4)} \times 100\%$$

Where

1 = Hot mode stimulus, left ear

2 = Cold mode stimulus, left ear

3 = Hot mode stimulus, right ear

4 = Cold mode stimulus, right ear

Since we have not as yet determined normative performance for the SBC test, we arbitrarily applied the same normative values to our data as those reported by Jongkees and Philipszoon[18] for the conventional caloric test. These authors used a 30 seconds irrigation and recorded responses with their subjects' eyes closed. From calculations of maximum slow phase eye speed, they determined that the limits of normal for unilateral hypoexcitability (UH) scores were ±15% and for directional preponderance (DP), ±18%. According to these values thirteen of our patients had normal SBC responses, six had UH alone, three had DP alone, and ten showed combined abnormalities.

The first question to be considered regarding the practicality of the new caloric test method was whether the SBC stimulations achieved sufficient magnitude and acted long enough to test properly the responsivity of the lateral semicircular canal receptor. We found responses to the .84C SBC stimulus were usually less intense than responses to the conventional hot stimulus (Table II). Average slow phase eye speed during maximal 20 seconds periods of all responses to SBC hot mode stimulations was 16.95°/sec, compared with an average value during maximal 20 seconds periods of all responses to conventional hot stimulations of 22.41°/sec. The difference in mean response intensities is partly explained by the fact that the SBC stimulus declines more rapidly after reaching a peak value than does the conventional stimulus. If desired, response intensity of the SBC test could be increased by selecting longer irrigation durations (t_1, t_2, t_3) as shown in Table I and Figure 4. However, in the present study, there were only four instances where the response to conventional hot stimulation was well formed and easily recognized (64 stimulations), while in the same subject the response to SBC hot mode stimulation was not also clearly recognizable. Among most subjects it appeared the SBC stimulus acted long enough that responses were clearly recognized even in cases where nystagmus was feeble, poorly formed, or obscured by the presence of spontaneous nystagmus.

A second question to be considered was what benefits would result from the reduced duration of the new SBC stimulations. As our clinical study progressed, it soon became obvious that practical benefits were indeed to be realized by reducing the discomfort and fatigue of patients subjected to the new test and reducing the time required for its completion. Patients reported less intense vertigo and definitely less discomfort from the SBC test than from the conventional hot stimulations. The complete SBC test procedure usually required about ten minutes, since we allowed a resting period between left and right stimulations. This is a very significant saving in time over the 31 minutes or longer required for the conventional bithermal test procedure.[1]

The accuracy of our calculations can be judged by examining the intensity and direction of nystagmus induced by the new test procedure. Mean slow phase eye speed was calculated for each five-second interval during the responses of all 13 "normal" subjects and plotted as a function of time as shown in Figure 5. The time course of the stimulus strength, ΔT, is superimposed for comparison. Note that the intensity of nystagmus beating toward the irrigated ear rises to a peak value at approximately the predicted time, falls to zero, and then begins to beat in the opposite direction, reaching a second peak intensity also at the predicted time. When nystagmus was well developed, even in subjects with abnormal responses, there was usually a close correspondence between the time of occurrence of peak slow phase eye speed and predicted peak temperature differences ($\pm\Delta T^*$).

Among normals the mean of all hot mode SBC responses was 17.75°/sec compared to mean cold mode responses of 18.40°/sec. This gives strong supportive evidence that our efforts to produce equal peak stimulus magnitudes ($-\Delta T^* = +\Delta T^*$) were successful. However, we have not ruled out the possibility that some unseen order effect may act differentially upon the two responses. For example, a state of vestibular adaptation may influence the intensity of cold mode responses.

As can be seen in Figure 5, the terminal course of nystagmus did not conform to our predictions. Following subsidence of the second (cold mode) nystagmus phase, there usually appeared a third nystagmus phase, beating once more toward the irrigated ear. A third phase nystagmus appeared in 20 of the 32 subjects in this study. In five cases the phenomenon could be attributed to the return of spontaneous nystagmus which had been beating toward the irrigated ear before stimulation was applied. In the remaining 15 cases no clinical explanation was evident. Among most of our subjects nystagmus either ended or reversed direction before about 160 seconds.

The frequent occurrence of third-phase nystagmus could mean the final hot irrigation is too long or improperly terminated, causing a third temperature difference to appear and stimulate the vestibular receptor. On the other hand, the physical stimulus may be essentially ended at about 180 seconds, and nystagmus appearing at this time may be related to the vestibular adaptive process discussed above.[5,6,19,20] It is of interest that a nystagmus reversal comparable to SBC third-phase nystagmus does not normally occur following conventional unilateral stimulations.[6] Rapid termination of the thermal stimulus offers certain practical advantages and the possibility of new approaches to studying vestibular responsivity. However, precise control of stimulus termination must await further studies concerning the time course of temperature within the aural canal and labyrinth following cessation of the irrigation sequence.

DISCUSSION

By removing both hot and cold caloric stimuli soon after they reach maximum intensity, we have reduced the duration of the physical stimulus and eliminated the long waiting periods required when using conventional methods. In this way we have made the stimulations more physiologic, as well as reduced patient discomfort and the time required to complete the tests. The strength of the SBC stimulation can be increased or decreased by adjusting irrigation durations (t_1, t_2, t_3), and in practice it may be useful to employ more than one stimulus strength routinely. We have calculated switching times for a three cycle sinusoidal stimulus pattern which produces progressively larger $\pm\Delta T^*$ values but consider such a procedure less attractive from a practical standpoint than the single cycle pattern described in this report.

Since variations in temporal bone anatomy may cause changes in some of the physical constants of equation (2), we intend to determine what effect such variations might have upon the ΔT curve and upon the nystagmus response. None of our subjects had detectable temporal bone abnormalities, however, and the close correlation between the predicted ΔT curve and nystagmus intensity curves found in most of our subjects indicates that the heat conduction model and analysis used in timing the sequence of thermal pulses was accurate.

By apposing hot and cold irrigations, we improve the possibility that uniformity is maintained within a single (unilateral) test as regards adequacy of irrigations, direction of irrigation stream, and head position. This helps to insure that equal hot/cold stimulus strengths are delivered during single irrigations though, of course, it does not affect the control of variability among successive irrigations.

We believe further investigation will prove this new caloric test method to be not only less time consuming and distressing to patients, but also superior to conventional methods in diagnostic sensitivity and reliability.

Department of Surgery (Otolaryngology), Pritzker School of Medicine, University of Chicago, Illinois 60637.

Request for reprints should be sent to L. R. Proctor, M.D., Associate Professor of Surgery (Otolaryngology), Pritzker School of Medicine, 950 East 59th St., Chicago, Illinois 60637.

REFERENCES

1. Fitzgerald G, Hallpike CS: Studies in human vestibular function: I. Observations on the directional preponderance ("Nystagmusbereitschaft") of caloric nystagmus resulting from cerebral lesions. Brain 65:115-137, 1942

2. Kleinfeldt D, Dahl D: Temperaturmessungen am menschlichen Bogengang nach thermischer Reizung. Acta Otolaryngol (Stockh) 68:411-419, 1969

3. Kleinfeldt D, Dahl D: Die Abhangigkeit des thermischen Nystagmus von Temperaturveranderungen am horizontalen Bogengang. Acta Otolaryngol (Stockh) 70:136-141, 1970

4. Cawthorne T, Cobb WA: Temperature changes in the perilymph space in response to caloric stimulation in man. Acta Otolaryngol (Stockh) 44:580-588, 1954

5. Hood JD: Persistence of response in the caloric test. Aerosp Med 44:444-449, 1973

6. Aschan G, Bergstedt M: The genesis of secondary nystagmus induced by vestibular stimuli. Acta Soc Med Upsaliensis 60:113-122, 1955

7. Henriksson NG: Speed of slow component and duration in caloric nystagmus. Acta Otolaryngol [Suppl] (Stockh):125, 1956

8. Dohlman G: Physikalische und physiologische Studien zur Theorie des kalorischen Nystagmus. Acta Otolaryngol [Suppl] (Stockh):5, 1925

9. Proctor LR: (Unpublished observations)

10. Brünings W: Beitrage zur Theorie, Methodik und Klinik der kalorimetrischen Funktionsprüfung des Bogengangapparates. Z Ohrenheilk 63:20-99, 1911

11. Proctor LR: Testing the vestibular system. Value of the caloric test, in *International Vestibular Symposium.* Naunton RF, Fernandez C (eds), New York, Academic Press, 1974

12. Schmaltz G: The physical phenomena occurring in the semicircular canals during rotatory and thermic stimulation. Proc R Soc Med 25:359-381, 1932

13. Young JH: *Analysis of Vestibular System Responses to Thermal Gradients Induced in the Temporal Bone,* thesis. University of Michigan, Ann Arbor, 1972

14. Carslaw HS, Jaeger JC: *Conduction of Heat in Solids.* Oxford, Oxford University Press, 1959

15. Carnahan B, Luther HA, Wilkes JP: *Applied Numerical Methods.* New York, John Wiley, 1969

16. Proctor LR, Byrnes RG: Irrigation handle with temperature sensor and flow control. Laryngoscope 83:1717-1721, 1973

17. Proctor LR, Carli T, Davis S: Analysis of thermal vestibular responses in the cat. A preliminary report. Ann Otol Rhinol Laryngol 81:114-127, 1972

18. Jongkees LBW, Philipszoon AJ: Electronystagmography. Acta Otolaryngol [Suppl] (Stockh):189, 1964

19. Young LR, Oman CM: Part II: A model for vestibular adaptation to horizontal rotation, in *Fourth Symposium on the Role of the Vestibular Organs in Space Exploration.* Washington, D.C., NASA SP-187, National Aeronautics and Space Administration, 1970, p. 363

20. Malcolm R: Part III: Quantitative study of vestibular adaptation in humans, in *Fourth Symposium on the Role of the Vestibular Organs in Space Exploration.* Washington, D.C., NASA SP-187, National Aeronautics and Space Administration, 1970, p. 369

FACIAL PLASTIC SURGERY: TELEVISION SEMINARS

A continuing education workshop devoted to all aspects of facial plastic surgery (including rhinoplasty) will be held February 1-5, 1976 on Key Biscayne, Miami, Florida.

Sponsored by the American Academy of Facial Plastic and Reconstructive Surgery, Inc. in cooperation with the Department of Otolaryngology, University of Miami, the workshop will include a broad interdisciplinary faculty of national prominence. Course directors are Robert Simons, M.D. and M. Eugene Tardy, Jr., M.D. For applications and reservations write: M. Eugene Tardy, Jr., M.D., 2800 Lake Shore Drive, Chicago, Illinois 60657.

SYMPOSIUM ON CONTROVERSIAL AREAS IN SURGERY OF HEAD AND NECK

The University of California at San Diego School of Medicine announces the Fifth Annual Symposium on Controversial Areas in Surgery of the Head and Neck, February 12-15, 1976 in San Diego, California.

For information write: Alan M. Nahum, M.D., University Hospital, 225 West Dickinson, San Diego, Ca. 92103.

FACIAL NERVE RECONSTRUCTION AND ITS PROGNOSIS

J. Sadé, M.D.

Kfar Saba, Israel

SUMMARY – This study of the functional end results of successful surgical repair of the traumatized facial nerve trunk shows more or less homogenous results, whether the procedure was end-to-end suture or grafting, and independent of the site of the lesion. The expected results are: 1) excellent tonus at rest; 2) the ability to close the affected eye to a useful degree when the other eye is closed; 3) some ability to close the affected eye in association with some mass action of the affected face; 4) in a small proportion of patients, the ability to produce a faint smile, but not to move the corner of the mouth, to smile fully or to whistle; and 5) though all patients seemed to be able to move their faces "en masse," none could move isolated groups of muscles as a healthy person can. Thus, though appreciable results are obtained, important limitations of movements are inevitable. The reason for these uniformly deficient results stems from the fact that in the facial nerve the peripheral axons are not arranged in a separate specific compartmental fashion. Instead, they intermingle and are distributed among the various bundles which constitute together the main nerve trunk; each bundle will therefore represent the whole face and not one specific region of the face. The result of this intermingling is that when axons regrow after traumatic repair, they have scarcely any chance to be redirected to their original regional muscular plate, due to inevitable crossover phenomena during regeneration.

Surgical repair of the traumatically severed facial nerve trunk is often described in general terms as yielding very successful results.[1-8] Theoretical considerations[9] do, however, pose limitations on restoration of full facial movement after such surgery – even if technically perfect, whether the repair is direct end-to-end anastomosis or through grafting.

The aim of the present study is to evaluate as precisely as possible how much and what kind of facial movement can be regained after the continuity of a severed nerve has been restored surgically. Surgical repair of the peripheral branches and twigs which branch off the main trunk of the facial nerve is not discussed.

METHODS AND MATERIALS

Six patients were examined who had facial nerve trunks either anastomosed or grafted within two weeks after surgical accidents. One patient was grafted intratympanically, two anastomosed intratympanically, and three anastomosed near the stylomastoid foramen (after parotid surgery). The patients were surgically treated two to eight years ago (average five years).

The state of the face at rest (tonus), as well as evidence of performance of various facial movements, was estimated. Tests were given for: 1) simultaneous closure of both eyes, and 2) closure of each eye by itself. Lips were checked for the ability: 1) to smile, 2) to whistle, and 3) to move each corner of the mouth by itself. Also, the frequency and amount of associated movements were looked for.

Nerve excitability tests were made on the exposed nerve at the site of surgery in the ear, in patients where the lesion was within the Fallopian canal. This was possible in all three patients where the lesion was intra-aural, as these patients were left with a radical mastoidectomy by the original surgical procedure. In these patients, the nerve was blocked by injecting 10 ml of 2% Procaine®* into the stylomastoid region and the nerve was restimulated.

RESULTS

All six patients had excellent tonus, evaluated as between 90-100% (ave.

* Abbott Laboratories, North Chicago, Ill.

From the Meir Hospital and the Weizmann Institute of Science.

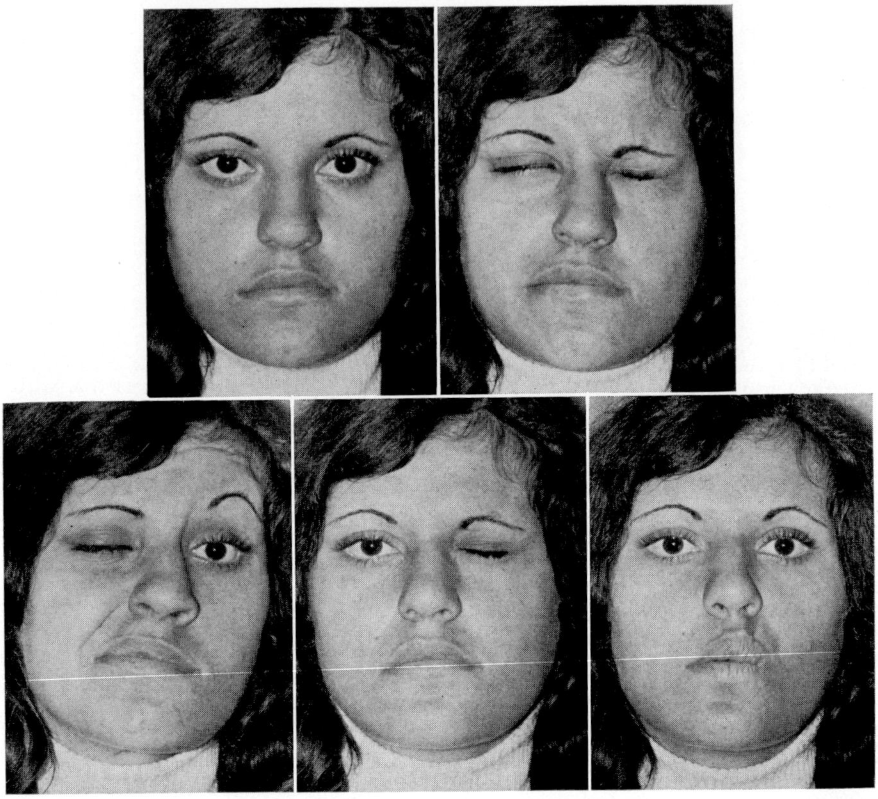

Fig. 1. A) Perfect facial tonus (face at rest) in a patient who had her right facial nerve sutured after it was cut in its intratympatic course. B) Same patient, both eyes closed. Note right eye closed to a lesser degree than the left eye and slight associated movement of the right cheek and upper lip. C) Same patient, closure of right eye by itself. Note accompanying "mass movement" of most of the right side. D) Same patient, closure of left (unaffected) eye, shown for comparison. E) Same patient, showing patient being unable to whistle. Corner of her mouth on right side shows no movements.

95%) (Fig. 1A). Simultaneous closure of both eyes was feasible in all six patients (Fig. 1B), with a score ranging from 80-100% (ave. 90%) of closure of the affected eye in comparison with the unaffected one. Some associated movement of the affected cheek and lip was apparent in three (50%) of the patients. Closure of the affected eye by itself was performed successfully by four patients (Figs. 1C and 1D), with a score of 70-90% (ave. 80%) in comparison with the healthy eye; this action was accompanied in all patients by considerable associated mass movement of the affected part of the face. In three patients (50%) movements of the lips were practically absent while only slight movements were possible in three patients (50%). The slight movement seen in these three latter patients might represent the ability to produce a faint smile, at times reported in the literature. None of the patients were able to move the affected lips when asked to whistle (Fig. 1E). Ability to move the affected corner of the mouth was present to some degree in three (50%) of the patients (20-50% degree of movement compared to the normal side) and was always accompanied by associated movements.

Nerve excitability tests were performed in three patients applying a current of 0.5 milliamps over the exposed nerve at the vicinity of the tensor tympani (above the lesion) in the exposed middle ear cavity. On electrical stimulation, the three patients showed violent contraction of all the facial muscles; most branches, including those to the platysma, contracted violently, the only exception being the frontal region. To block the nerve, Procaine® (2%, 10 ml) was injected into the stylomastoid region in the same three patients. No facial contraction occurred when the nerve was thereafter directly stimulated at the previous spot. Voluntary facial movements weakened very considerably in one patient and facial paralysis occurred in the other two. However, in all three patients, the ability to close the eye was not totally abolished.

DISCUSSION

From a technical point of view, the facial nerve, the dread of otologists at the beginning of the century,[10] became quite exposable surgically in the last decades. Exposure of the nerve in the ear without disturbing the sound-transmitting mechanism, through a posterior tympanotomy,[11-12] and endaurally[12] became practical, and now the intracranial segment has also become accessible.[13,15] Once exposure of the facial nerve became feasible, indications for surgical treatment of facial nerve diseases soon followed.

However, perhaps partly due to difficulties in evaluating therapeutic results on the one hand and enthusiasm for the surgery itself on the other, some controversy has ensued regarding the postoperative results, and the desirability of some of the operations proposed on the facial nerve has been questioned.

Thus, the advisability of surgery in Bell's palsy has been queried on theoretical grounds,[16-18] raising doubts which were later confirmed to some degree by clinical and statistical data.[19-21] Some of the results claimed more recently in hemifacial spasm (another sphere of enthusiastic facial nerve surgery) have also received adverse comment.[9,22] Over-enthusiasm for surgical repair of the injured facial nerve may have resulted in an over-optimistic concept of what can be achieved, though the positive indications for surgical intervention in these patients are usually beyond doubt. Results in such patients have been described as 90% satisfactory,[7,8,23] good,[4,24] excellent,[1,6] most gratifying,[23] and complete or near complete recovery.[5] Restoration of facial function[3] and regaining of emotional expression have been claimed as well.[1,2] Surgical urgency was also advocated.[1,7,24] However, theoretical considerations cast doubt on the degree of postoperative recovery. Indeed, various facial nerve surgeons and neurologists[25-29] have already been cognizant for some time that only partial results could be achieved in the repair of facial nerve injuries and that associated movements were frequently an aftermath.

In spite of the enthusiastic approach to facial nerve repair, data on the procedure are surprisingly sparse and a complete and truly detailed analysis of the surgical results has not been attempted. Reports not presenting photographic evidence usually state that "the procedure was successful."[5,7] Fortunately, other reports supplement such statements with photographs. I have found and examined 54 such photographs presented in publications by six authors.[1,8,24,26-28] In these 54 patients good tonus was almost always achieved; closure of both eyes was reported in 80% of the patients (with a score of about 95% or normal performances and associated movements in 30% of them), while closure of one eye was reported in only 20% of the patients, and it was always accompanied by associated movements. Fifteen percent of the patients were able to move their lips slightly and about 30% produced a faint smile, or trace of a smile.

The similarity of this analysis with the findings in my smaller series suggests that these findings are representative of what can usually be achieved in reparative facial nerve surgery. It would seem that in principle the end results are not dictated by whether a direct anastomosis or a graft is done, or by the type of suture or glue used to approximate the nerve ends, but on factors inherent in the procedure which probably are related to the microanatomy of the facial nerve trunk.

Facial Movements and their Limitation after Facial Nerve Repair. This study shows what we can expect from a practical point of view when facial nerve trunk restoration is successful, and this is also dependent on surgical skill. Excellent tonus can be expected, as well as satisfactory ability to close and protect the affected eye. The eye cannot be closed by itself as efficiently as the nonaffected eye. In order to close the affected eye, the patient usually has to call into play other muscles than those of the eye itself; thus, the affected eye will close either in association with the healthy eye or in association with most of the muscles of the homolateral side (mass movement).

This is true for other motions as well; no single muscle or muscle group movement can act independently, *i.e.*, closure of one eye, movement of one cheek, movement of one lip, or of one corner of the mouth. Essentially, only partial or total mass movements can be performed on the affected side. These missing single movements are, however, required to express various emotions or mimicry by facial movements. The patient in all probability will be unable to express these to any degree of refinement. If he tries, he will either fail or will be able to produce such expressions only as part of a total or subtotal contraction of the homolateral face.

At times no movement, and otherwise only very limited movements, of the corner of the mouth can be performed and these mostly in association with other muscles of the same side. Most patients cannot smile symmetrically. However, those who can move the corners of their mouths to a limited degree may train themselves to produce a faint, semisymmetrical smile. A complete spontaneous smile or symmetrical laughter was never documented and the aim of achieving "restoration of emotional expression"[1,3] can in all probability not be realized. Obviously, these rules should not be viewed in a totally rigid way and in a group of patients some variations might be expected, some doing better, others less, yet in principle all will conform to the above description.

Innervation of the Facial Nerve after its Surgical Restoration. Direct stimulation of the nerve proxymal to the site of repair resulted in mass movement of the whole affected face, demonstrating continuity of active nerve fibers through the anastomosis to most (except possibly frontal) facial muscles. Therefore, spontaneous postoperative limitation of facial movements should not be blamed on an insufficient reinnervation of the face, but on some basic alteration of neural transmission as a result of the trauma and its repair.

Since some voluntary closure of the eye was still possible after Procaine® injection, the claim that the face, and mainly the orbicularis oris, may be innervated to some extent by extra facial nerve(s), seems to be supported,* assuming that the Procaine® injection brought about a total facial paralysis, an effect which is not always easy to obtain.

Facial Nerve Microanatomy. The peripheral branches of the facial nerve are traditionally considered as carrying impulses to definite limited and specific regions of the face. The same definite representation is supposed to be also preserved throughout the length of the main facial trunk as a compartmental (*i.e.*, nerve bundle) arrangement of the various peripheral fields.[29] We have termed this concept the "specific regional representation theory"[9] (Fig. 2). This theory may, however, be viewed

---

* The notion that facial muscles may also be innervated either from the contralateral side or by another nerve such as the trigeminus, has been proposed by several authors.[30-39] This contention is based on observations that patients whose facial nerves were totally sacrificed during mutilative cancer surgery may eventually end with less than total facial paralysis. Kettel[2] argued vehemently against any such notions.

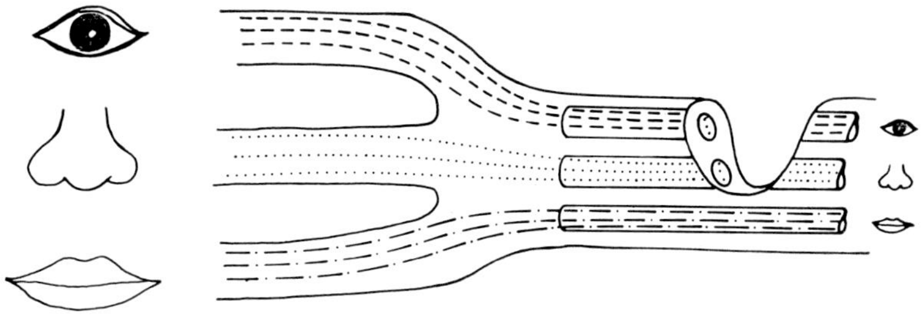

Fig. 2. Diagrammatic representation of facial nerve tracts or bundles as viewed through the "specific regional representation theory," and the obligatory regional paralysis which should follow after Scoville's operation. (Reproduced by permission from: Sadé J: Subtotal Evulsion of the Facial Nerve in Hemifacial Spasm. Acta Otolaryngol (Stockh) 78: 410-417, 1974.)

with some skepticism for the following reasons.

The operations performed for facial spasm by Scoville on the main trunk[33] of the facial nerve consist essentially of dividing and sacrificing an important part of its width together with the compartments, bundles, and fibers which pass through it. This operation should bring about a selective or regional paralysis of those parts innervated by the cut fibers (or by the sacrificed compartments) if the specific regional representation theory truly reflects the intimate anatomy of the facial nerve trunk (Fig. 2). However, such selective paralysis does not happen. Furthermore, as we have noted previously,[9] those operations which aim at alleviating hemifacial spasm by sacrificing several of the peripheral facial nerve branches[34,35] should also lead to specific regional paralysis if each branch represents a definite specific region exclusively. This does not happen either. What indeed seems to be the case is that each peripheral branch "represents" a rather large part of the whole face. When some are cut, the remaining branches (even if only one or two) suffice to carry movements to the entire face, or most of it; this can probably only come about through a very extensive peripheral anastomosing network. At the same time, each small

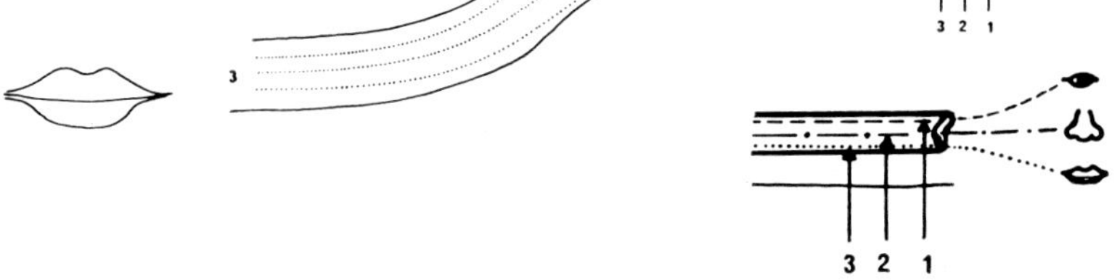

Fig. 3. Diagrammatic representation of the facial nerve tracts of bundles showing crossing over of axons in a way which will allow for facial movements after partial injury of the nerve (including Scoville's and Greenwood's operations). (Reproduced by permission from: Sadé J: Subtotal Evulsion of the Facial Nerve in Hemifacial Spasm. Acta Otolaryngol (Stockh) 78:410-417, 1974.)

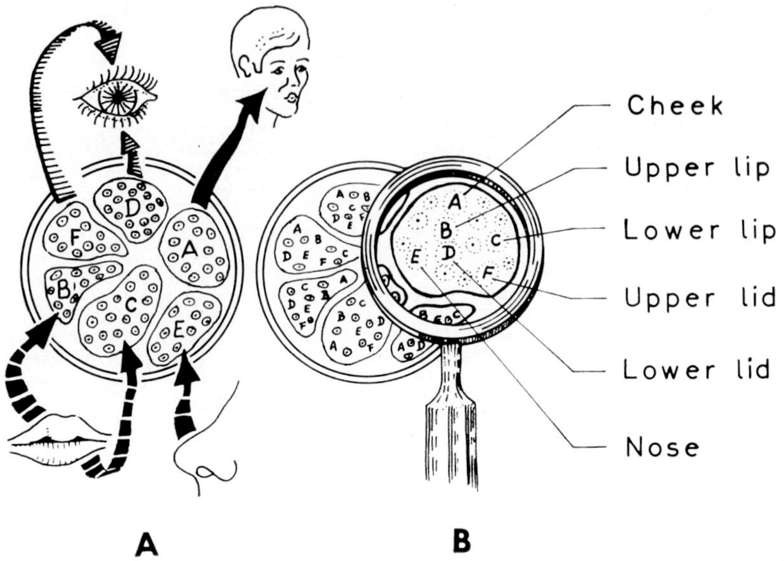

Fig. 4. Schematic drawing of the facial nerve trunk showing: A) Distribution of axons according to the "specific regional representation theory" where each bundle represents axons from a specific region in the face. B) Alternative distribution of axons where each bundle contains axons from each region in the face.

section of the main trunk also has enough axons representing a major part of the face (Fig. 3). This may be the result of an intraneural arrangement of axonal mixing and intermingling, so that the various peripheral regions represented in the main trunk are arranged in several bundles, each bundle representing the whole face or its greater part (Figs. 4, 5). These observations cast doubt on the validity of the specific regional representation theory. The main concept which does emerge from these observations is that in the main trunk a specific axon (let us assume from the eye region) will be near

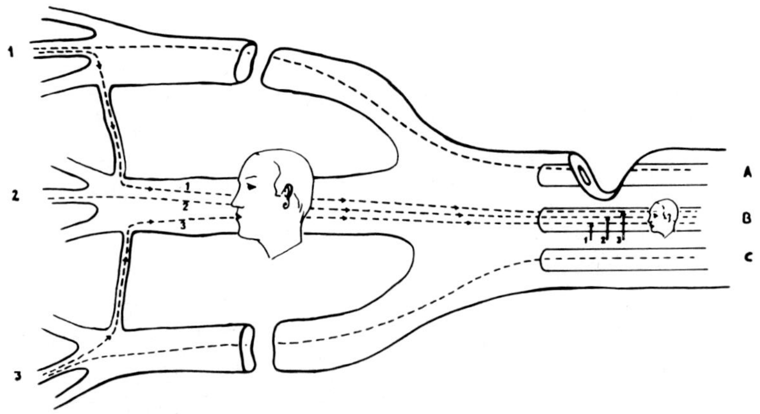

Fig. 5. Schematic drawing of the facial nerve tree showing how a peripheral branch can represent the face as a whole while other peripheral branches are cut, and how a section of the main trunk may represent the face. (Reproduced by permission from: Sadé J: Subtotal Evulsion of the Facial Nerve in Hemifacial Spasm. Acta Otolaryngol (Stockh) 78:410-417, 1974.)

an axon from a different region (let us say the lips). All the axons from the eye will probably not be grouped together and all those from the lip will not be grouped together.

These anatomical conclusions, derived from surgical observations, have also received strong support from the experimental work of Duel and Fowler,[36] as well as of Harris,[37] and from microanatomical dissections of the facial nerve by Cossar and Sunderland[38] and White and Verma.[39] However, this sort of arrangement is not universally accepted, thus May[29] has discussed the concept at length and rejected it.

The Inherent Difficulties of Facial Nerve Repair. When axons regrow in a healing nerve they have a tendency to deviate and even to branch off, shifting from the original axon-plate relationship.[40] If the specific regional representation theory would have been valid, mixed axon reinnervation might possibly be of minor consequence; as much of the crossover would probably occur within the specific bundles, *i.e.*, each specific region would experience mixing within itself, the eye axons with the eye axons, the upper lip axons with the upper lip axons, *etc.* However, if the axons of each specific region (lips, eyes, *etc.*) are not grouped together, but distributed among the various bundles, then the fact that axon-to-axon fitting does not happen is of consequence. What will result is significant mixing of axons from various specific regions ending in the inability of the patient to move specific facial regions selectively; rather, he will be from now on limited to more or less mass movements of his face, or associated movements. These imperfections were indeed noticed in the past by both otologists and neurologists,[41-46*] especially by Conly.[47]

At first, when one observes the limited abilities of a surgically repaired patient, one may think that the surgical repair was not perfect and that the anastomosis itself was only partly successful. However, stimulation of the facial main trunk has shown that all the face (except the frontal muscle) does indeed contract en masse; no selective contraction is obtained no matter where one puts the stimulating electrode. This implies that all the muscles which contracted are axonally connected, though in a mixed way, with the repaired main stem and can be stimulated.

The importance of realizing the limitation of the surgically-repaired facial nerve function cannot be too strongly stressed. Many surgeons have become exasperated (not to mention their disappointed patients) when they achieved the highest results possible but kept striving for even better results. Surgeons have contemplated performing secondary surgery on patients (whose primary repairs may or may not have been made by them) who had already regained practically everything that the best surgery could restore. Moreover, it is conceivable that partial facial restoration after skull fracture and trauma, in conformity with the results described here, may also have the same mechanism of limitation and is often better left untouched.

From the theoretical point of view, we should consider whether a partially injured nerve trunk might serve the patient better if left unrepaired, in those cases where the uninjured part is judged to suffice as far as innervation of the face is concerned. This can best be assessed by electrical stimulation of the remaining part of the nerve. If such stimulation results in good movement of the face, approximation of the injured part can only add misdirected axons and the resulting associated movements.

---

* From Fish's report,[48] one may deduce that the same rules apply to the intracranial facial nerve trunk.

Anastomosis between peripheral branches of the nerve casts doubt on whether suturing such severed branches, while some branches have remained intact, has much surgical or functional value.

Request for reprints should be sent to Prof. J. Sadé, Meir Hospital, Kfar Sada, Israel.

Dr. Sadé is an Established Investigator of the Chief Scientist's Bureau, Ministry of Health, Israel.

REFERENCES

1. Kettel K: *Peripheral Facial Palsy.* Copenhagen, Munsgaad, 1959

2. Kettel K: Surgical repair versus expectant treatment in traumatic facial palsy. Arch Otolaryngol 71:623-627, 1960

3. Campbell JB, Luzio J: Facial nerve repair: New surgical technique. Trans Am Acad Ophthalmol Otolaryngol 68:1069-1074, 1964

4. Martin RC: Late results of facial nerve repair. Ann Otol Rhinol Laryngol 64:861-869, 1955

5. Leventon G, Kraus P, Man A: Treatment in surgical trauma of the facial nerve. Harefuah 68:333-335, 1965

6. Kitamura T, Towaga K, Tsukamoto K *et al*: Extratemporal facial nerve surgery. Arch Otolaryngol 95:269-275, 1972

7. Ballance C, Dule AB: The operative treatment of facial palsy. Arch Otolaryngol 15:1-70, 1932

8. Drake CG: Facial function after intracranial repair of facial nerve. Arch Otolaryngol 95:420-425, 1972

9. Sadé J: Subtotal excision of the facial nerve in hemifacial spasm. Acta Otolaryngol (Stockh) 78:410-417, 1974

10. Cawthorne T: Intratemporal facial palsy. Arch Otolaryngol 90:137-147, 1969

11. Wulstein HL: Die Methode der Decompression des Nervus Facialis von Austritt aus dem Labyrinth bis zu dem Foramen Stylomastoideum ohne Beeintrachtigung des Mittelohres. Arch Klin Exp Ohren Nasen Kehlkopfheilkd 172:582-587, 1958

12. Sadé J, Levy E, Chace J: Surgery and pathology of Bell's palsy. Arch Otolaryngol 82:594-602, 1965

13. House WF: Middle cranial fossa approach to the petrous pyramid: Report of 50 cases. Arch Otolaryngol 78:460-469, 1963

14. Fish N, Esslen E: Total intratemporal exposure of the facial nerve. Arch Otolaryngol 95:335-341, 1972

15. Shiff M: Early response after facial nerve decompression. Arch Otolaryngol 81: 509-517, 1965

16. Taverner D: The prognosis and treatment of spontaneous facial palsy. Proc R Soc Med 52:1077-1080, 1959

17. Sadé J: Pathology of Bell's palsy. Arch Otolaryngol 95:406-414, 1972

18. Miler H: Facial paralysis. Br Med J 3: 815-819, 1967

19. Adour KK, Swanson PJ: Facial paralysis in 403 consecutive patients. Trans Am Acad Ophthalmol Otolaryngol 75:1285-1301, 1971

20. Mechelese K, Goor G, Hinzing EH *et al*: Bell's palsy: Prognostic criteria and evaluation of surgical decompression. Lancet 57-59, 1971

21. McNeill R: Facial nerve decompression. J Laryngol Otol 88:445-456, 1974

22. McCabe BF: Management of hyperfunction of the facial nerve. Ann Otol Rhinol Laryngol 79:252-259, 1970

23. Kettel K: Management of peripheral facial palsies due to trauma. Proc R Soc Med 52:1069-1074, 1959

24. Botman WM, Jongkees LBW: The results of intratemporal treatment of facial palsy. Pract Oto Rhinol Laryngol 17:80-100, 1955

25. Papparella MM, Shumrick DA: *Otolaryngology.* Philadelphia, Saunders Co, 1973 vol 2, pp 274

26. Martin, RC: Surgical repair of the facial nerve. Arch Otolaryngol 23:458-466, 1936

27. Scaramella LF, Tobias E: Facial nerve anastomosis. Laryngoscope 83:1834-1840, 1973

28. Laage-Hellmann, LE: Facial nerve in parotidectomies. Arch Otolaryngol 81:527-533, 1965

29. May M: Anatomy of the facial nerve (spatial orientation) of fibers in the temporal bone). Laryngoscope 83:1311-1329, 1973

30. Miehlke A: Discussion. Arch Otolaryngol 95:345, 1972

31. Baumel JJ: Trigeminal-facial nerve. Communications. Arch Otolaryngol 99:34-44, 1974

32. Martin H, Helsper JT: Supplementary report on spontaneous return of function fol-

lowing surgical section or excision of the seventh cranial nerve in the surgery of parotid tumors. Ann Surg 151:436-541, 1960

33. Scoville WB: Partial section of proximal seventh nerve trunk for facial spasm. Surg Gynecol Obst 101:495-497, 1955

34. Greenwood J: The surgical treatment of hemifacial spasm. J Neurosurg 3:506-510, 1946

35. Fish U, Esslen E: The surgical treatment of facial hyperkinesis. Arch Otolaryngol 95:400-405, 1972

36. Fowler PE: Abnormal movements following injury to the facial nerve. JAMA 113: 1003-1008, 1939

37. Harris WD: Topography of the facial nerve. Arch Otolaryngol 88:264-267, 1968

38. Sunderland S, Lossar FD: The structure of the facial nerve. Anat Rec 116:147-164, 1953

39. White A, Verma PL: Spatial arrangement of facial nerve fibers. J Laryngol Otol 87:957-962, 1973

40. Cajal R: *Degeneration and Regeneration of the Nervous System.* Oxford University Press, New York, 1928

41. Martin RC: Prognosis in traumatic peripheral facial paralysis. Laryngoscope 61: 1004-1009, 1951

42. Martin RC: Recent experiences with operation on the facial nerve. Arch Otolaryngol 32:1071-1075, 1941

43. Lathrop FD: Facial nerve grafting. Trans Am Acad Ophthalmol Otolaryngol 68: 1060-1063, 1964

44. Wartenberg R: Associated movements in oculomotor and facial muscles. Arch Neurol 55:439-488, 1946

45. Ford FR, Woodhall B: Phenomena due to misdirection or regenerating fibers of cranial, spinal and autonomic nerves. Arch Surg 36:480-496, 1938

46. Kettel K: Repair of the facial nerve in traumatic facial palsies. Arch Otolaryngol 66: 634-672, 1957

47. Conly J: Facial nerve grafting. Arch Otolaryngol 73:322-327, 1961

48. Fish H: Facial nerve grafting. Otolaryngol Clinic North Am 7:517-529, 1974

MIDDLE EAR MICROSURGERY AND FLUCTUANT HEARING LOSS

The Shambaugh Fifth International Workshop on Middle Ear Microsurgery and Fluctuant Hearing Loss will be held at Northwestern University Medical School, Thorne Hall, March 1-6, 1976. Co-chairmen are George E. Shambaugh, Jr., M.D. and John J. Shea, M.D.

For further information write: American Hearing Research Foundation, Suite 2105, 55 East Washington Street, Chicago, Illinois 60602.

Ann Otol 84: 1975

GRAND ROUNDS
CLINICAL PATHOLOGICAL CONFERENCE*
MASSACHUSETTS EYE AND EAR INFIRMARY

Chairman: HAROLD F. SCHUKNECHT, M.D.

BOSTON, MASSACHUSETTS

PARTICIPANTS:

TERENCE STEWART, M.D., *Boston, Mass.*
JAMES SHEEHY, M.D., *Los Angeles, Calif.*
AZIZ BELAL, M.D., *Boston, Mass.*
ROGER WEHRS, M.D., *Tulsa, Okla.*
MENDELL ROBINSON, M.D., *Providence, R.I.*
ROBERT FULK, M.D., *Wilmington, N. Car.*
NELSON KIANG, M.D., *Boston, Mass.*
HERBERT SILVERSTEIN, M.D., *Sarasota, Fla.*
MICHAEL GLASSCOCK, M.D., *Nashville, Tenn.*
WILLIAM LAVELLE, M.D., *Boston, Mass.*
ALFRED WEISS, M.D., *Boston, Mass.*
MICHAEL PAPARELLA, M.D., *Minneapolis, Minn.*
WALTER KLESTEDT, M.D., *Fall River, Mass.*
ALFRED WEBER, M.D., *Boston, Mass.*

Dr. Harold F. Schuknecht: Today, we have six interesting cases to present. Four of the patients are here and you will have an opportunity to question them or examine them if you wish.

CASE REPORTS

Case 1

Dr. Terence Stewart: Mr. C. is a 32-year-old male who, in 1961, began to have attacks of spinning vertigo with nausea and vomiting, associated with right-sided hearing loss. However, he had been free of attacks of vertigo from 1965 until two months prior to our first examination in December 1971. During these two months, he experienced ten episodes of vertigo, associated with fluctuating right-sided hearing loss and tinnitus and could not satisfactorily perform his work as a travel agent. There was no relevant family history. Nose and throat examination was negative. An audiogram revealed a mild high tone hearing loss on the right side. He was told to return for re-examination during the next episode of hearing loss. Three weeks later he returned with a right sensorineural hearing loss of 50-60 dB and a speech reception threshold (SRT) of 46 dB. Speech discrimination (phonetically balanced) was 60%, and loudness recruitment was present. The diagnosis was right Ménière's disease. He continued to have attacks during the following four months. He stated that on some occasions, the hearing would improve dramatically at the onset of the vertigo, only to decrease again after three or four days.

He was advised to have an endolymphatic sacotomy, which was performed on May 19, 1972. The first slide (Fig. 1) shows audiometric findings prior to the surgical procedure.

The next slide (Fig. 2) shows his hearing status thirteen months following surgery. In addition to a mild sensorineural loss, there is a mild conductive loss. Examination reveals a normal right tympanic membrane with full mobility of the malleus.

Dr. Schuknecht: Tell me a little bit about these dizzy spells? How big a problem were they?

* Held at the Massachusetts Eye and Ear Infirmary, June 18, 1973.

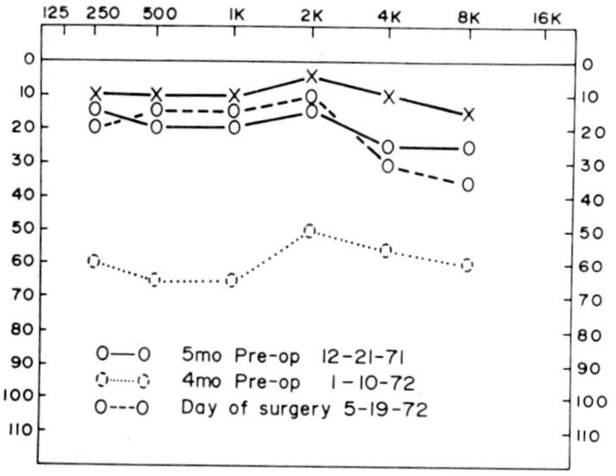

Fig. 1. Case 1, Ménière's disease. Air conduction thresholds prior to surgery. Right ear (O), left ear (X).

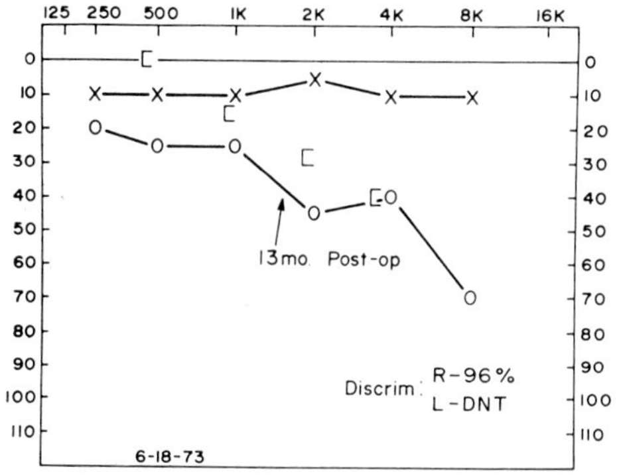

Fig. 2. Case 1, Ménière's disease. Postoperative audiogram.

Mr. C.: The dizziness was a considerable problem. It lasted anywhere from an hour to twenty-four to thirty-six hours.

Dr. Schuknecht: With vomiting?

Mr. C.: Yes, considerable.

Dr. Schuknecht: And your hearing would sometimes improve with an attack?

Mr. C.: Almost immediately after vomiting. It improved and stayed improved.

Dr. Schuknecht: You mean with the first vomiting? Is that when the hearing improved? Or was it after several hours?

Mr. C.: Let us say that by the time I had cleaned myself up is when the ear would clear up.

Dr. Schuknecht: So that is the Lermoyez type of manifestation of this disease, which is rare in my experience. I think it is only a variant of Ménière's and pathologically no different from the usual Ménière's, but it is an interesting clinical manifestation. Mr. C., I often considered advising a labyrinthectomy, but your hearing was too good at times.

Mr. C.: Correct, and as a patient I did not know what to do either. I was faced with either having an operation or just living with it; however, I could not live with it much longer as I had been dizzy at least once a week over a period of four months. The business I am in requires a lot of travelling and I was tied down. I could not leave home.

Dr. Schuknecht: So we decided to do an endolymphatic sacotomy. The procedure was performed by exposing the sac through a mastoid approach, slitting it, and introducing a Silastic®* drain. The drain extends from inside the sac into the mastoid cavity. In this patient, a piece of temporalis fascia was laid over the silastic implant, although this is not always done. The idea is to increase the surface area of the sac rather than to shunt into the subarachnoid space. I have not seen Mr. C. for a while. Would you describe how you have been feeling?

Mr. C.: For the most part, well. I do have my "off" days. I have been trying to keep a record since the humidity and atmospheric pressure has a lot to do with the hearing. On days that are extremely warm, my hearing plugs up terribly.

Dr. Schuknecht: How about the dizzy spells?

Mr. C.: None as severe as I have had. Sometimes I am a bit lightheaded but nothing bad.

Dr. Schuknecht: Would you say that

* Dow-Corning Chem. Co., Medical Products Div., Midland, Mich.

there has been a definite change in the character of the disease since the surgery?

Mr. C.: Yes, quite definitely. The surgery did about 99% more good than harm.

Dr. Schuknecht: We have done only five of these procedures to date. This is not a difficult procedure. All of these patients have had a diminution in the severity of vertigo; however, one lost the hearing totally in the operated ear. In this case, the operation went very smoothly, and he had no postoperative vertigo. The posterior canal was not opened, nor were the oval or round windows exposed. I had hoped that this would be a perfectly safe operation and could even be done in only hearing ears. I cannot take that approach now. The other finding of significance is the conductive hearing loss which developed after surgery. Jim, what did I do wrong?

Dr. James Sheehy: Hal, I do not think you could possibly do anything wrong! (Laughter)

Dr. Schuknecht: Now you know that is not true!

Dr. Sheehy: I am sure that the most likely thing that happened here is that somehow the incus got dislocated.

Dr. Schuknecht: I did not even expose it, I just got a peek at the incus. I have another explanation for it.

Dr. Sheehy: In sac operations, when you end up with a conductive impairment and you have a mobile ear drum, the most likely conclusion is that somehow you have some disarticulation problem.

Dr. Schuknecht: No, I think bone dust was washed into the middle ear through the aditus and settled down around the ossicles, possibly the stapes. You remember, Jim, on many of the stapes operations on previously fenestrated ears how often you will find a mass of bone dust around the crura and the oval window niche? Well, somebody recently has written or talked about the importance of plugging the aditus with a plug of Gelfoam®* during endolymphatic sac procedures.

Dr. Sheehy: Have you done an impedence test? It could give you some interesting information. If it is a fixation problem, the test might be normal but if it showed a very high compliance, it would suggest a loose system.

Postscript: When last interviewed by phone (March 1975), the patient felt well and had experienced no vertigo during the previous year. His hearing was fluctuating but unchanged subjectively.

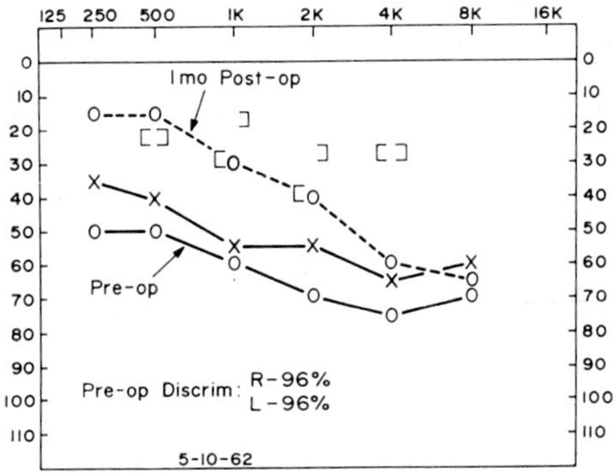

Fig. 3. Case 2, audiometric findings showing improvement of hearing immediately following stapedectomy.

Case 2

Dr. Aziz Belal: Mrs. E., a 50-year-old female, first presented in May 1962, with a long history of progressive hearing loss and having had a fenestration operation in the left ear in 1947. In 1962, Dr. Schuknecht performed a stapedectomy and fat-wire implant on the right ear. The hearing was improved as shown in the slide (Fig. 3). She was not seen again until May 1973 when she presented with a five-day history of hearing loss, a sensation of vibration, and poor understanding of speech in the right ear. Hearing tests now show the left ear essentially unchanged and on the right, a small bone-air gap and

* The Upjohn Co., Kalamazoo, Mich.

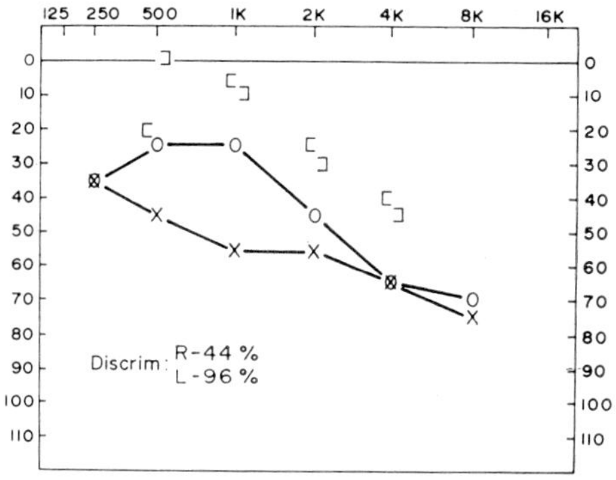

Fig. 4. Case 2, eleven years after right stapedectomy. Sudden discrimination loss in right ear.

a discrimination score of 44% (Fig. 4).

Dr. Schuknecht: We have a lady who had a good result from a right stapedectomy for eleven years and then experienced a hearing loss. Mrs. E., would you please tell us what happened?

Mrs. E.: I woke up one morning with a marked loss in hearing; then, listening to anything mechanical, like the radio, television, or my car, just sounded loose or vibrating. I could hear a vibration in human voices, too. It just got worse.

Dr. Schuknecht: You told me it was a scratchy sensation, like a bad phonograph needle.

Mrs. E.: As if there were parts loose in the television or radio or automobile.

Dr. Schuknecht: Was it an off-and-on situation? Would it come and go in a few seconds, or was it constant?

Mrs. E.: It was constant.

Dr. Schuknecht: Did it involve high frequencies or low frequencies?

Mrs. E.: I think it did involve high frequencies.

Dr. Schuknecht: Was it an irritating sensation?

Mrs. E.: Quite, plus the loss of hearing. I was unable to comprehend at the same time.

Dr. Schuknecht: Let us look at this audiogram once again (Fig. 4), The one showing the situation at the time she was complaining. Although she said that her hearing dropped, you can see that the principal change is a decrease in speech discrimination, tested to be 44%. Mrs. E., did you have any dizziness?

Mrs. E.: No.

Dr. Schuknecht: Dr. Wehrs, what would you do?

Dr. Roger Wehrs: I have seen, of course, a sudden loss in hearing in individuals who have never had ear surgery. It often comes on overnight. However, since she has had an operation, you could explore the ear.

Dr. Schuknecht: You would explore the ear. What would you look for?

Dr. Wehrs: It is possible that she has developed a fistula.

Dr. Schuknecht: You are suggesting that as the most probable cause of her symptoms?

Dr. Wehrs: Yes.

Dr. Mendell Robinson: The other possibility might be a loose prosthesis or a partial incus necrosis. This may not account for the drop in her discrimination. Was the discrimination done with masking in the opposite ear?

Dr. Schuknecht: Yes, oh yes, you have to assume that we use infallible audiometric techniques on all our cases. (laughter)

Dr. Sheehy: Has she been subjected to any pressure change?

Dr. Schuknecht: Mrs. E., have you been flying in an airplane or scuba diving?

Mrs. E.: No.

Dr. Belal: An exploratory tympanotomy was done immediately as an emergency procedure. The prosthesis was found to be loose on the incus. It was tightened.

Dr. Schuknecht: The packing was removed and her hearing tested on the

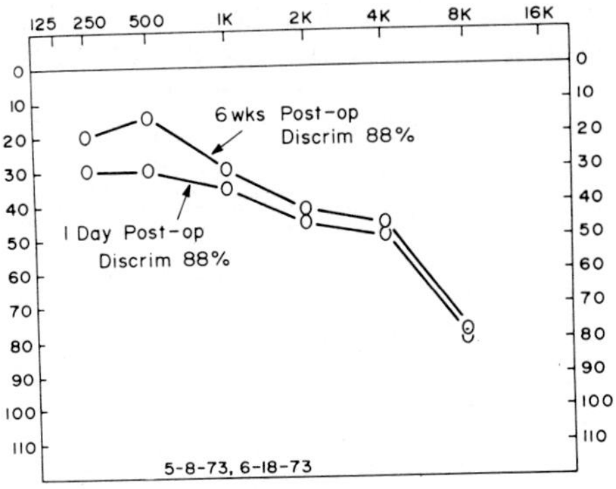

Fig. 5. Case 2, improvement in thresholds and discrimination following wire-tightening procedure.

day following surgery (Fig. 5). The audiogram shows the discrimination up to 88%, but there was still a small bone-air gap. This morning's audiogram (six weeks postoperative) shows speech reception at 28 dB and discrimination again at 88%. Mrs. E., is your hearing back to where it was before this recent incident?

Mrs. E.: Yes.

Dr. Schuknecht: Was it improved immediately after surgery? I do not mean in the operating room but after the packing was removed one day later?

Mrs. E.: Yes, it was.

Dr. Schuknecht: (to the audience) What happened here? Is it true that the discrimination loss was caused by a loose linkage between incus and prosthesis? This is the first time I have seen such strong evidence to favor such a thesis. I turned the flap, put a pinch on that wire, put the flap back, and nothing else. It took about ten minutes, and that is it.

Dr. Sheehy: I think you have to seriously consider that the hearing improvement was coincidental to the surgery. If your thesis is correct, then we should have many similar cases with intact drums and loose linkage. We see many loose linkage situations following stapes operations but rarely an associated discrimination impairment. This may have been coincidental.

Dr. Schuknecht: It is possible, I suppose, that it was coincidental to the hearing improvement. But I believe it is more probable that the surgery in this case corrected a unique kind of acoustic distortion.

Dr. Sheehy: We have had a number of discussions over the past ten years, and I remember some of them with you, concerning whether high tone hearing impairments would result in discrimination impairments. If I remember correctly, it was your feeling at the time that they did. I remember a study performed, not to prove you were incorrect, of course, in which audiograms were made the day after surgery, a week later, *etc.* Almost invariably, the day after surgery there was a mass type of conductive hearing curve where the bone-air gap was closed for the low frequencies, but a severe loss existed for the highs. This probably accounts for the patient's feeling the hollowness in the ear. Invariably at suprathreshold intensities of 20 to 25 dB, they did not show significant impairment of speech discrimination, so I would not think that a loose prosthesis, as such, in the vast majority of cases is going to result in a loss of discrimination.

Dr. Schuknecht: For the majority of cases, I would agree with you. I have seen many loose wires and usually it just causes fluctuating hearing. I think it is one of the most common problems we have. I am perfectly aware of that, but I think we have a different situation here. Do you remember, Mrs. E., that we tested you during the operation? Were you awake enough?

Mrs. E.: No.

Dr. Schuknecht: After I tightened the wire, did you notice any difference in hearing right in the operating room. Can you recall listening to voices. *etc.*?

Dr. Robert Fulk: I was in the operating room and she did get nine out of ten PB list words correct.

Dr. Schuknecht: Well, I suppose that does not mean too much.

Dr. Fulk: No, but she was hearing very well!

Dr. Schuknecht: I think I asked her whether or not this corrected her problem after I tightened the wire and I think she said it sounded better. Would anyone like to discuss acoustic transmission as it might relate to this case?

Dr. Nelson Kiang: Acoustic distortion can obviously affect speech discrimination, and a loose stapedectomy wire can conceivably generate such distortion. The patient's description of her hearing problem as everything sounding "loose or vibrating" is vivid and enlightening. This is, in fact, what happened to the wire prosthesis as verified at surgery. Tightening the prosthesis relieved the problem as it should have. The only wonder is why this problem does not appear more often? It may be that this particular type of looseness is rare. On the other hand, it may also be that otologists are too dogmatic in associating low speech discrimination only with sensorineural lesions. There is every theoretical reason to expect that certain kinds of distortion in the middle ear transmission mechanism could account for some instances of low discrimination ability. I should think that appropriate tests for acoustic distortion products by sensitive microphones or impedance measurements could help to determine whether the ossicular chain is defective in these ways. If it turns out that there are some patients whose low discrimination scores are attributable to middle ear conditions, then present surgical techniques could constitute adequate treatment. Certainly otologists should be aware of these possibilities.

Dr. Herbert Silverstein: I was just wondering if the wire could loosen enough as the sound waves were transmitted so that the wire was actually making noise against the incus.

Dr. Schuknecht: An interesting thought!

Postscript: One year later (June 1974) the patient's hearing was subjectively good, and she had no complaints.

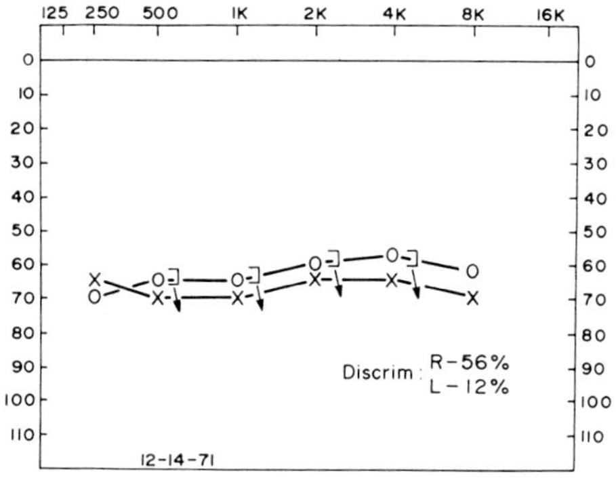

Fig. 6. Case 3, audiometric findings showing a bilateral hearing loss (worse on the left), climaxing a ten-year history of tinnitus and vertiginous attacks.

Case 3

Dr. Robert Fulk: Mr. B. is a computor systems analyst who was first seen in 1971 when he was forty-six years of age. He gave a history, going back to 1958, when he had the onset of tinnitus in the right ear and mild vertiginous episodes, which over the next ten years became progressively worse. During this time, he began also to experience bilateral fluctuating hearing loss. In 1969, the vertigo subsided, and hearing was maintained at a good level. He was receiving no treatment. In 1971, he began having vertiginous attacks about once a week, lasting three to six hours, associated with nausea and vomiting. He was able to work an average of one day per week. An audiogram showed a bilateral hearing loss, worse on the left (Fig. 6). On caloric testing, he demonstrated diminished vestibular response on the right.

Dr. Schuknecht: Mr. B., we just presented the problem as it existed at the time we saw you in 1971, when you were disabled with recurring attacks of dizziness and bilateral hearing loss. We have a few questions before we go on. In 1971, was your hearing fluctuating, or was it pretty much remaining at the low level of hearing?

Mr. B.: Just about the low level.

Dr. Schuknecht: How long was it at this low level of hearing?

Mr. B.: For the last five years it was decreasing, so finally in 1971 it was at its lowest.

Dr. Schuknecht: Did it fluctuate at all?

Mr. B.: Somewhat, but not much.

Dr. Schuknecht: How long were you disabled?

Mr. B.: I attempted to get to work every morning. Several mornings, my coworkers picked me up at my desk and took me in a wheelchair to the medical unit to sleep off these attacks. Finally, it came to the point where something had to be done.

Dr. Schuknecht: What would you gentlemen in the audience do with this man who has severe bilateral Ménière's disease and cannot work as a computer analyst?

Several in Audience: Treat with streptomycin!

Someone in Audience: Did he have an allergic history or workup?

Dr. Fulk: Beginning January 24, 1972, he received intramuscular streptomycin sulfate at a rate of 2 g/day. By the seventh day he was having slight ataxia, and by the fourteenth day the ataxia was moderately severe. Streptomycin was then increased to 3 g/day, and by the twenty-first day he had severe ataxia, and he had lost his caloric response to ice water. Streptomycin was discontinued at this time after a total of 56 g had been given. His period of compensatory recovery lasted approximately two months during which time the ataxia decreased. He has had no vertiginous episodes since this therapy. The immediate posttreatment audiogram showed speech perception thresholds to be essentially the same as before treatment; however, there was slight improvement in discrimination. The next audiogram taken two-and-a-half months after completion of therapy shows hearing to be markedly improved with speech discrimination of 96%.

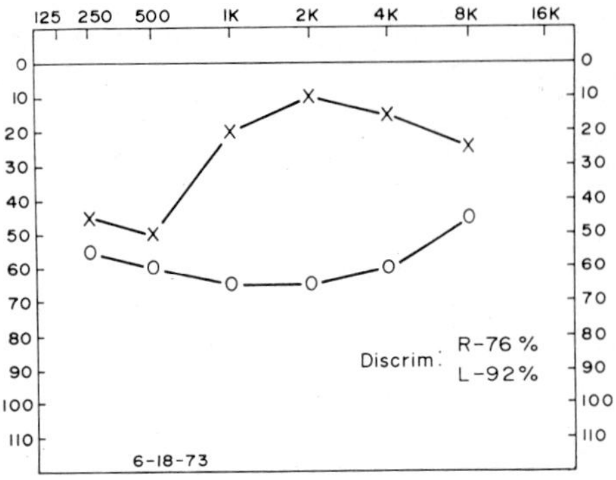

Fig. 7. Case 3, audiometric findings six months following completion of streptomycin therapy.

Dr. Schuknecht: This morning's audiogram, as seen on this slide (Fig. 7), shows a speech reception level (SRL) on the left of fourteen and discrimination of 92%. The opposite side shows some improvement over pretreatment levels. Mr. B., how long was it after the streptomycin treatment before your hearing improved?

Mr. B.: I received the streptomycin in February, and it was April 2 when my hearing came back. It was fantastic; I went into church, and I used the stereo ear phones. I put the ear phones on and turned them to the lowest possible volume I could; and it was too loud, so I took them off and listened to the service on the public address system. It was a miracle!

Dr. Schuknecht: Let us see him walk! (Mr. B. walks back and forth, showing no significant ataxia.)

Dr. Schuknecht: Mr. B., I was worried about you for a while because you were terribly ataxic. You wobbled all over the place. The ataxia was really quite frightening for the first few weeks following treatment. You have made a good recovery. Let us now turn off the lights. He is doing very well, so he must be getting some visual cues.

Improvement in hearing does happen to a small percentage of these streptomycin-treated patients. I remember the first one I treated in 1949, when I was a resident at the University of Chicago. The patient had bilateral Ménière's and the same thing happened to him, except that both ears improved. Of the twenty patients I have personally treated, I have seen this happen in five cases. The hearing in all of these patients has subsequently been maintained at good levels. What could cause this improvement? The only thing I can think of is that streptomycin, in addition to destroying the sensory cells of the vestibular system, may have damaged the endolymph-producing secretory cells of the inner ear. This may have improved the fluid physiology of the inner ear. I have no evidence to prove that.

Similar spectacular improvement of hearing has been observed following surgical procedures for Ménière's disease, such as endolymphatic sacotomy, section of the superior division of the vestibular nerve, and fenestration of the lateral semicircular canal. Could it be possible that all of these procedures, including streptomycin therapy, induce a diffuse reaction in the membranous labyrinth which reduces secretory activity and thus improves the fluid physiology of the inner ear?

What would be alternative therapies for a man with disabling bilateral Ménière's? Do we have anybody here who would do bilateral endolymphatic sacotomies or vestibular nerve sections?

Dr. Michael Glasscock: I was interested in this patient when you first presented him, but I was not aware of the workup. Did he have a full workup with x-ray studies, *etc.*?

Dr. Schuknecht: No, my workup did not include x-ray studies. Why? What are you considering other than Ménière's?

Dr. Glasscock: Well, you must consider bilateral acoustic tumors; what about congenital lues?

Dr. Schuknecht: If an ophthalmologist cannot see evidence of interstitial keratitis, I do not consider congenital lues. He had none of the stigmata of congenital lues. I think congenital lues is an entirely different disease, and I do not worry about that if the corneas are clear.

Dr. Glasscock: I think you certainly could treat bilateral Ménière's disease with bilateral endolymphatic shunt procedures, but in my experience shunts give about 50% long-time cure rate. The other surgical procedure is bilateral nerve section, and that is a pretty good-sized procedure to put a patient through, so I think streptomycin therapy would be far superior to that.

Postscript: At the last examination, two years following treatment, the patient's hearing for pure tones had decreased somewhat in the left ear (Fig. 8).

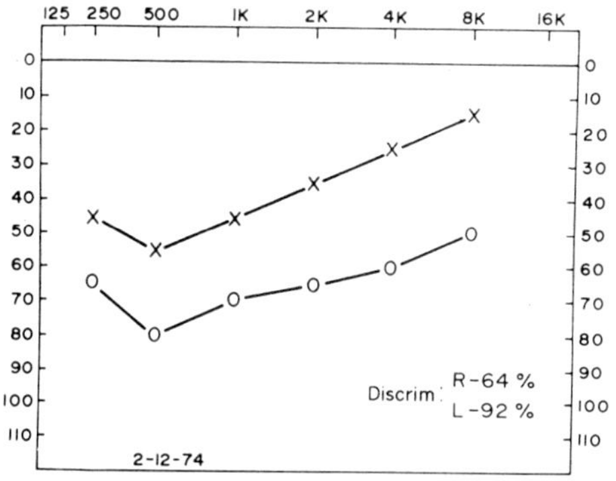

Fig. 8. Case 3, audiometric findings one year following completion of streptomycin therapy.

Case 4

Dr. William Lavelle: Mr. M. is a 35-year-old male who presented in August 1972. When he was in the military service in 1963, he was told he had bilateral high tone hearing loss from noise exposure. Following discharge from the service, he noticed bilateral tinnitus. In 1966, he experienced a severe attack of vertigo with unsteadiness persisting for four weeks. He recalls being nauseated and vomiting on several occasions. Over the next eight years he had two similar episodes, each of which subsided in two to three weeks. During this time, he had no change in his hearing. In April

1972, he had a severe attack of vertigo following which he was very ataxic and could walk only with assistance. Again, he was nauseated and vomited on several occasions. At the same time, he noticed a hearing loss in both ears, more severe on the right. The hearing in the left ear returned to normal in twenty-four hours, but the loss on the right remained. At that time, he was admitted to the Peter Bent Brigham Hospital and had an extensive examination. Except for the loss of hearing in the right ear and severe persisting ataxia, all examinations were normal.

Dr. Schuknecht: Tell us again very briefly what hapened to you. What was the first thing you noticed, hearing loss or dizziness?

Mr. M: Dizziness is the first thing I noticed. It began approximately eight years ago. I was treated at the time with Antivert.®* The dizziness went away after a month, stayed away for a few years, then recurred in a more severe degree, and was treated again with different medicines. Again, it went away, was inactive for a period of time, and then just recently, about a year-and-a-half ago, I had a very severe "attack" if you want to call it that. I could not stand or keep my eyes open, and if I opened my eyes for a few minutes, I would get sick to the point of vomiting. At that time, I went into the Peter Bent Brigham Hospital and was under the care of a neurologist, who did all kinds of tests.

Dr. Schuknecht: When did you lose your hearing in your right ear?

Mr. M.: I lost my hearing while I had the last severe attack, in April 1972. I lost the hearing in both ears for a period of a day and night. The next day, the hearing in my left ear came back but the hearing in my right ear never came back.

Dr. Schuknecht: What were the caloric responses?

Dr. Lavelle: The calorics, using ice water, showed absent response on the right and diminished response on the left, and these results were confirmed with ENG.

Dr. Schuknecht: Here is an audiogram of August 1972 showing normal hearing on the left and a profound loss on the right (Fig. 9). How is his hearing today?

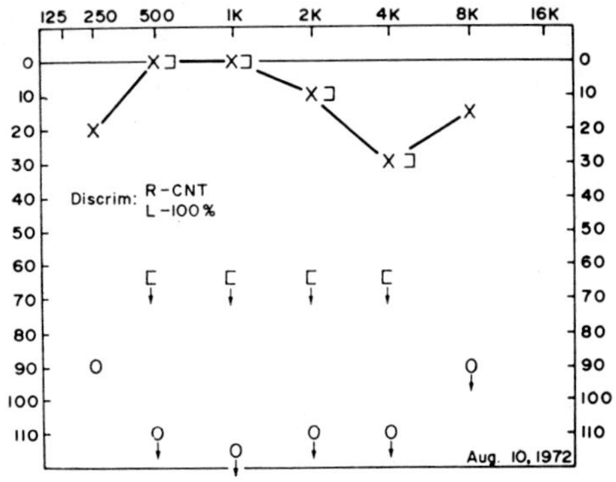

Fig. 9. Case 4, audiogram showing profound loss of hearing in the right ear.

Dr. Lavelle: Today's test is the same.

Dr. Schuknecht: The thing that amazed me, Mr. M., was the way you were walking at that time. We have a movie of you taken at that time, which shows that you can just barely walk without assistance. [Movie shown]. How long had it been that you were so unsteady?

Mr. M.: Since April 1972. The movie was made in August, four months later.

Dr. Schuknecht: You could just barely get around, and you were not getting any better?

Mr. M.: Not until recently. Of course, I had the labyrinthectomy in the meantime.

Dr. Schuknecht: You spilled the beans! I was going to ask the audience what they would do. On December 4, 1972, I performed a transcanal labyrinthectomy on the right ear under local anesthesia. During the several weeks

* Roerig, N.Y., N.Y.

following the operation, I could see no significant change in his symptoms. I imagine most of you would have done a right labyrinthectomy, as I did. Quite frankly, this ataxia seemed to me to be inconsistent with a unilateral loss of vestibular function. This man could barely walk four months after the acute attack. We were afraid to let him walk, unaided, the few steps from the waiting room into our examining room for fear he might fall down. Show us how you can walk today! You're better! I did not realize you had improved so much. I have not seen him for six months. He still has a wide gait and takes a few side steps. Are you feeling better?

Mr. M.: No, I still have headaches and am feeling "rotten," in general.

Dr. Schuknecht: We performed the procedure under local anesthetic to determine if he had any remaining vestibular function in that ear. He became very vertiginous on the operating table. Did you vomit in the operating room?

Mr. M.: No. Afterwards I did.

Dr. Schuknecht: Do you remember whether the room was spinning around?

Mr. M.: Very much so.

Dr. Schuknecht: So, in spite of the absent ice water caloric, we did have a functional vestibular system.

Dr. Silverstein: Did you take any fluid from his ear?

Dr. Lavelle: Fluid was taken. Sodium was 100 mEq and potassium was 17 mEq, which is normal for perilymph and mitigates against Ménière's disease.

Mr. M.: Excuse me a minute. Something I might add is that I have been on Vontrol®* since January.

Dr. Michael Paparella: I am confused! Do you have x-ray and other studies of this gentleman?

Dr. Lavelle: During the neurological workup, he had vertebral arteriography, internal carotid arteriography, posterior fossa myelogram, spinal taps, polytomography of the skull, and brain scan. All the studies were negative.

Dr. Schuknecht: I did not order them; the neurologist did. I think you are right though, Dr. Paparella. Such studies are indicated for unusual cases. When I get into these very difficult problems, I ask for the help of the otoneurologists. I would not do a labyrinthectomy in such a case unless I had their support that this is the right action to take. At the moment, we have not made a diagnosis on this man. I have never seen Ménière's disease behave in this way. I am delighted to see that you are getting better, Mr. M. Are you back to work now?

Mr. M.: No, not yet.

Dr. Schuknecht: Cannot work yet?

Mr. M.: No, I still have good days and bad days, and on the bad days I spend a good part of my time lying down.

Dr. Silverstein: After you did the labyrinthectomy, was there a change in the symptomatology?

Dr. Schuknecht: No, he did not show any improvement whatsover during the several weeks I observed him following surgery.

Member of the Audience: What was the preoperative diagnosis?

Dr. Schuknecht: We did not have one. What we did here was a labyrinthectomy in an ear that exhibited no auditory or vestibular function with the hope that we might help this man. I doubt that the labyrinthectomy did a thing as he had no improvement postoperatively. But now after six months, I can see that he is doing much better.

Question from the Audience: Was a spinal culture done?

Dr. Schuknecht: This was done and it was normal. The neurologist ran him "through the works."

* Smith, Kline & French, Philadelphia, Pa.

Question from the Audience: Did he have any slurred speech?

Dr. Schuknecht: Have you had any slurred speech?

Mr. M.: I would say that it is normal.

Question from the Audience: Is there any neurological evidence of a demyelinating process?

Dr. Schuknecht: No, the neurologist cannot find a thing on him.

Dr. Walter Klestedt: This does not mean that he did not have such a condition. Vestibular, medullar, and cerebellar symptoms can be confusingly alike.

Dr. Schuknecht: There are still these unusual cases where we just cannot make a diagnosis. Anyway, I thought I would like to share this interesting problem with you. Mr. M., thank you very much for coming.

Postscript: When last seen twenty-one months later, the patient was ambulating better but still could not drive an automobile and was not working.

Case 5

Dr. Robert Fulk: Mrs. G. is thirty years old. Her history goes back to 1963 at which time she first noted a hearing loss in the left ear. In 1965, she consulted an otolaryngologist who found a large exostosis filling the left ear canal. He did a surgical exploration and removed the bony exostosis. Behind the exostosis, he saw a soft tissue mass, which on biopsy proved to be salivary tissue. About a year later, the exostosis had apparently recurred, and she reported to another otolaryngologist who explored through a postauricular incision. He identified the mastoid antrum and the ossicles and identified a fibrous track which led down to a normal tympanic membrane. He did a canalplasty and lined the canal with skin grafts; however, within six months stenosis had occurred again. He repeated the operation, again lining the newly created canal with skin. However, the canal stenosed again and in 1970 she was referred to Doctor Schuknecht. Examination revealed a stenosed left auditory canal. Audiometry showed a severe conductive loss in her left ear as shown on the slide (Fig. 10).

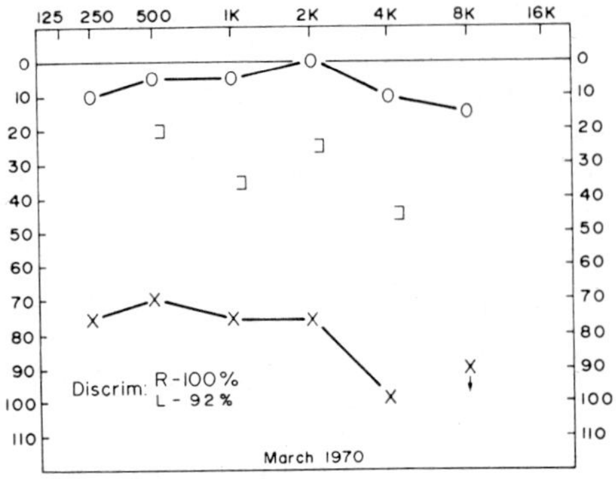

Fig. 10. Case 5, audiometric findings showing a severe conductive loss in left ear.

Dr. Schuknecht: The only thing I did at that time was to inject her left ear canal locally with some Xylocaine,®* then incise the canal area to make certain that she did not have a cholesteatoma of the external auditory canal, deep to the stenotic area. I was able to work around the bony mass down to a fibrous tract and follow it until I thought I was down to the level of the drum and middle ear. I could not see much. There was no evidence of cholesteatoma, so I told her we wished to observe the ear. She came back in a year and presented with a very interesting osseous lesion.

Dr. Alfred Weber: Anteroposterior (AP) and lateral skull studies of the petrous bones show a sclerotic process which involves the mastoid and petrous portion of the left temporal bone (Figs. 11A and B). The bone is homogeneously dense and there are no lytic areas. No mastoid air cells are visible; they have been replaced by the sclerotic process. The squamosal portion of the left temporal bone, the skull table, the remaining structures of the skull, in-

* Astra Pharmaceutical Products, Inc., Worcester, Mass.

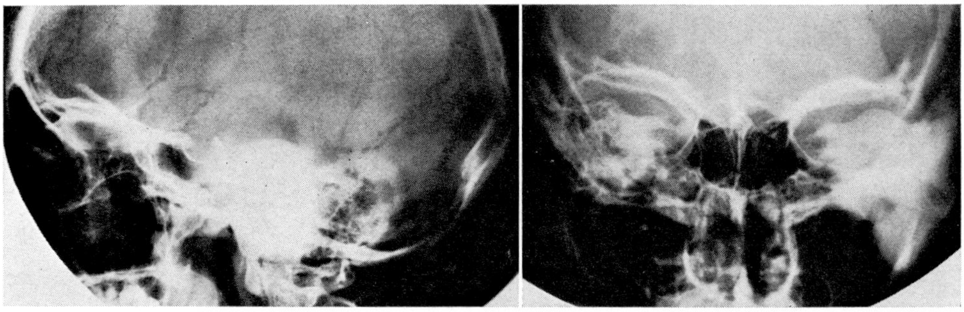

Fig. 11A and B. Case 5, anterioposterior (AP) and lateral views of skull and petrous bones showing a sclerotic process involving the mastoid and petrous portion of the left temporal bone.

cluding the right petrous bone and facial bones, are normal. For detailed assessment, AP polytome cuts were obtained of the left petrous bone (Fig. 12A). These demonstrate almost complete obliteration of the external canal. There is a decrease in size of the left tympanic cavity. The ossicles are not clearly defined. The vestibule, semicircular canals, cochlea, and internal auditory canal appear normal but are surrounded by the sclerotic bone. The left facial canal is poorly defined and partially obliterated by the abnormal bone.

The right petrous bone was studied for comparison, and all visualized anatomic structures, including the ossicles and external canal, are normal (Fig. 12B).

In conclusion, there is a diffuse, homogeneous, sclerotic process involving the petrous and mastoid portion of the left temporal bone. There is no involvement of the squamosal portion. The remaining skull, including facial bones, is normal. The radiologic appearance is consistent with monostotic fibrous dysplasia.

In the differential diagnosis, lesions that should be considered are: osteoma, meningioma, Paget's disease, and systemic diseases that cause sclerosis of bone and involve the skull. Osteoma cannot be excluded but is unlikely to involve the entire petrous bone in a generalized fashion as seen in this case. Osteoma is usually limited to the external canal and occurs commonly in the sinuses and external table. Menin-

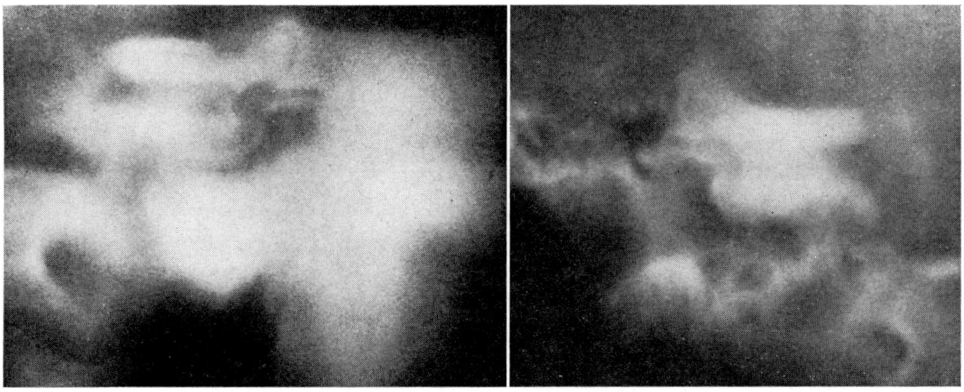

Fig. 12. A) Case 5, AP polytome cut of the left petrous bone demonstrating almost complete obliteration of the external canal. B) Cut of right petrous bone showing normal anatomic structure.

gioma, likewise, does not involve the petrous bone in a homogeneous manner and is usually associated with osteolytic destruction. Paget's disease, not uncommonly, involves the petrous bone but is then usually associated with diffuse involvement of the skull table. In addition, Paget's disease causes expansion and poor definition of the involved bone. In all cases of Paget's disease involving the petrous bone, the individual anatomic structures such as cochlea and internal auditory canal are poorly delineated and are difficult to define on close analysis. The patient has a negative history for other diseases; therefore, systemic sclerotic processes such as osteopetrosis, Engleman's disease, and Pyle's disease are excluded.

There are different types of fibrous dysplasia, such as the monostotic form, as in this case, and the polyostotic form. The monostotic form commonly occurs in the skull, particularly the base, and causes nerve deficits, hearing loss, and impaired vision secondary to involvement of the skull foramina including the optic canal. There usually is progression up to puberty and then the process reveals less active growth. The course, however, is difficult to predict, and in the severe cases marked deformity occurs in the skeleton in the polyostotic variety. The radiographic appearance varies from a diffuse homogeneous sclerotic process to a cystic form of fibrous dysplasia and a mixed form composed of cystic and sclerotic components. The monostotic form never converts into the polystotic form of fibrous dysplasia. In rare instances, malignant degeneration has been reported. A variant of fibrous dysplasia is the ossifying fibroma that often involves facial bones and sinuses and many likewise lead to considerable deformity.

Dr. Schuknecht: So, we have a thirty-year old lady who is beginning to have a little deformity here in the preauricular area. The zygomatic process is bulging out just a little bit and the facial canal is beginning to narrow. What should we do?

Comment from Audience: Give her sodium fluoride.

Dr. Schuknecht: Does anyone here know anything about sodium fluoride?

Dr. Weber: I do not think that anyone would give sodium fluoride for fibrous dysplasia.

Comment from Audience: Sodium fluoride is supposed to harden, mature, and correct bone growth, is this not so?

Dr. Schuknecht: Well, maybe so. The thing that worries me is whether she is going to have a facial palsy. Osteopetrosis (marble bone disease) sometimes causes recurring facial palsy presumably because of narrowing the facial canal. Herman Hammersma of Pretoria, South Africa, made a study of these cases and has operated on several and has described the problem. I should think that fibrous dysplasia would be very similar. Does anyone here want to comment about whether you would take prophylactic surgical action, assuming that it is going to progressively involve the facial canal and nerve?

Dr. Silverstein: I would wait until facial paralysis develops and then if the nerve excitability test indicates degeneration of the facial nerve, treat this with a total decompression of the facial nerve through the combined middle fossa and mastoid approaches.

Dr. Schuknecht: I find it fascinating that the fibrous dysplasia has not invaded the labyrinth. The lesion seems to have replaced the normal bony labyrinth while honoring the integrity of the inner ear spaces.

Member of Audience: I think a biopsy should be done.

Dr. Schuknecht: How would you biopsy this?

Member of Audience: It should be fairly simple to biopsy this lesion from the zygoma or mastoid.

Postscript: One year later, (June 1974) polytomography revealed no obvious progression of the disease; however, the patient had experienced some

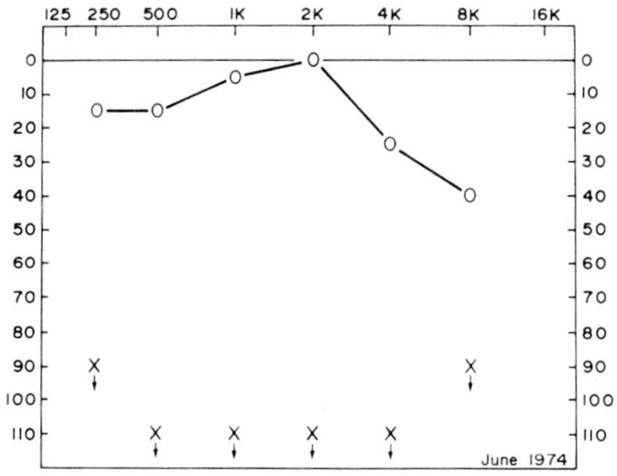

Fig. 13. Case 5, audiogram one year later showing a profound sensorineural hearing loss of the left ear.

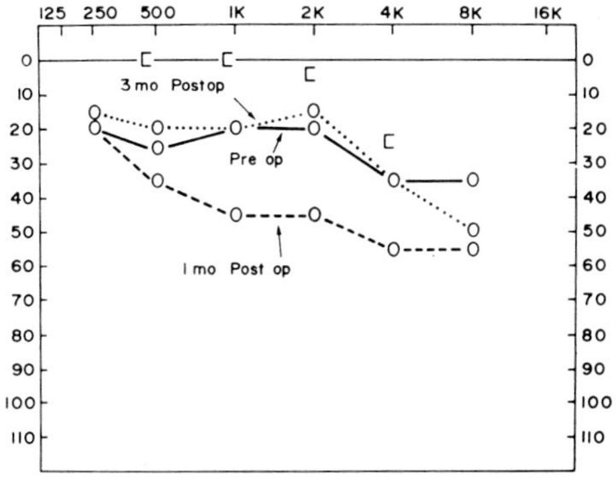

Fig. 14. Case 6, audiometric findings preoperative and one month and three months postoperative.

vertigo and had a profound sensorineural hearing loss (Fig. 13).

Post Postscript: Examination of the ear in June 1975 revealed a recurrence of the attic cholesteatoma. The patient has been scheduled for another atticotomy procedure.

Case 6

Dr. William Lavelle: Mr. C. is fifty-two years old who, in 1966, had a left transcanal type III tympanoplasty. The procedure consisted of enlarging the bony canal and removing a cholesteatoma through an atticoantrostomy opening. Postoperatively, he developed a posterior perforation and drainage from the ear. In 1972, he underwent a left mastoid obliteration procedure and closure of the perforation. Also, during the next six years, a steadily deepening attic retraction pocket was observed in the *right* ear. The audiogram at this time showed the right ear to be the better hearing ear. In April 1973, he underwent a right transcanal attico-antrotomy and canalplasty and a reconstruction of the bony defect with a cartilage graft.

Dr. Schuknecht: So, we have a patient who had two surgical procedures on his left ear with a fair hearing result but now has an attic cholesteatoma in his opposite better hearing ear.

He is a business executive and is quite satisfied with the present hearing level. Actually, his ears are asymptomatic. Now we have to tell him he has to have surgery on his good right ear. The following movie will show you the type of procedure I did here. You can tell me whether or not you agree with this approach. [Movie shown]

This is a transcanal approach to the epitympanum, and you can see that after removing a little scutum, I am trying to get the cholesteatoma sac out of the epitympanum. I could not get it out; therefore, I removed bone of the lateral epitympanic wall. The sac extends beyond the area of vision, so we are creating a larger epitympanic opening. We are hoping to find the deepest extension of this sac before too long, or we are going to have an atticotomy opening too large for a simple atticotomy procedure. The sac is finally visualized in its entirety and can be peeled out. Now the question is what to do with the atticotomy opening? If we simply place a temporalis fascia graft over the defect, it may retract into the epithymanum and create another retraction pocket and cholesteatoma. The head of the malleus, the anterior epitympanic cell, the lateral process of the manubrium, and the incus can be seen. The procedure used in this case is a cartilage graft closure of the epithmpanic defect. Conchal cartilage is removed through an incision on the posterior surface of the auricle, trimmed to accurately fit the defect, and then covered with an overlying fascial graft. The cartilage graft is carefully trimmed to fit the defect and care is taken to avoid contact with the ossicles. Being the better hearing ear, this is a very touchy situation.

The first postoperative audiogram is seen in Figure 14. The patient is wearing a hearing aid temporarily, and, of course, he is worried as am I. Then, one month later his hearing improved suddenly. His ear looks excellent, and his hearing remains good to date.

Question from Audience: Can this procedure be done through an ear speculum?

Dr. Schuknecht: It is better performed through an endaural incision.

Question from Audience: Why did you let this condition develop before your own eyes? Could that attic disease have been arrested before surgery was required?

Dr. Schuknecht: I know of no method to prevent this from happening. Does anyone else use this technique?

Dr. Roger Wehrs: Yes, I do essentially the same thing, but I use a homograft cartilage graft.

Postscript: Two years following the surgical procedure, the patient's ear appears excellent, and the hearing level is stable at a good threshold level.

Request for reprints should be sent to Harold F. Schuknecht, M.D., Department of Otolaryngology, Massachusetts Eye and Ear Infirmary, 243 Charles Street, Boston, Mass. 02114.

X-RAY OF THE MONTH

GUEST EDITORS

GUILLERMO F. CARRERA, M.D.

ALFRED WEBER, M.D.

DEPARTMENT OF RADIOLOGY
MASSACHUSETTS EYE AND EAR INFIRMARY
BOSTON, MASSACHUSETTS

PATIENT

This patient is a 20-year-old male diagnosed as having a squamous cell carcinoma of the right vocal cord and laryngeal ventricle approximately two years before the current examination. He was treated with radiation therapy (7,000 R total dose) and was followed without evidence of recurrence.

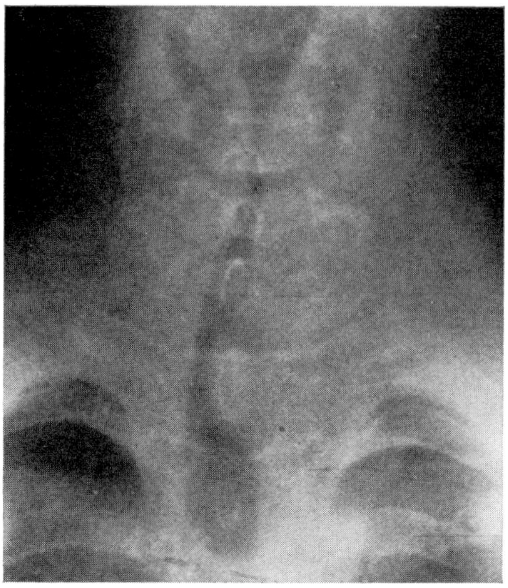

Fig. 1

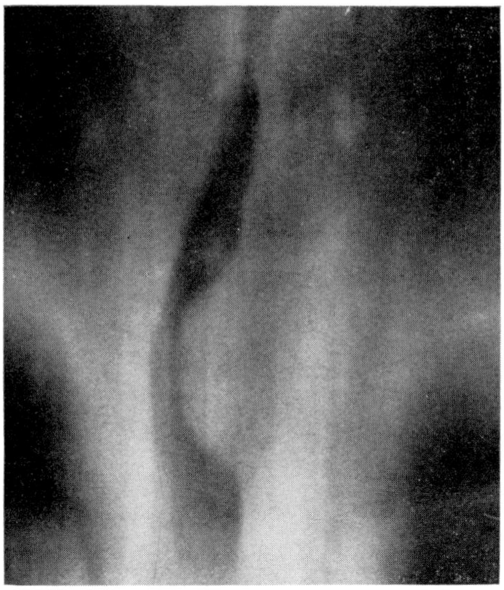

Fig. 2

RADIOGRAPHS

A plain film (Fig. 1) and tomographic study (Fig. 2) of the upper mediastinum and neck reveal a large soft tissue mass projecting into the tracheal lumen from the left wall of the trachea. The mass is irregular, lobulated, and involves a considerable length of the cervical trachea. The remainder of the visualized structures appear normal.

DIAGNOSIS

Evaluation revealed a squamous cell carcinoma of the trachea extending from 1 cm below the vocal cords to 6 cm above the carina, which apparently represents a second primary tumor. It involved the anterior and left wall of the trachea and invaded the left lobe of the thyroid and serosa of the adjacent esophagus. The larynx was free of disease.

Treatment in this case has consisted of total laryngectomy with a four-ring cervical tracheal resection and left hemithyroidectomy. Postoperative radiation to a total dose of 6,000 R to the neck and 4,500 R to the mediastinum was delivered over one year. At the present time, there is evidence of recurrent tumor involving the stoma and adjacent soft tissues.

DISCUSSION

The trachea represents a very unusual site of origin for squamous cell carcinoma. The true incidence of this lesion is difficult to establish but has been estimated to be about 1% or less of bronchogenic carcinoma.[1] This case is very unusual because of the young age of the patient, as well as the coincidence of extensive laryngeal carcinoma as an independent primary tumor. Carcinoma of the larynx has also been reported as a very rare lesion in young patients.[2] The explanation for simultaneous occurrence of multiple malignant tumors of the respiratory tract is not known. Direct spread, true metastasis, and coincident occurrence of separate diseases have all been proposed.[3] The role of common causative factors in the development of simultaneous primary tract tumors is still speculative.

REFERENCES

1. Ranke EJ, Presley SS, Holinger PH: Tracheogenic carcinoma. JAMA 182:519-522, 1962

2. Donnely JP: Extensive carcinoma of the larynx in a girl aged 19 at diagnosis. J Laryngol Otol 86:853, 1972

3. Sakula A: Multiple primary carcinomas of the respiratory tract. Br J Dis Chest 68: 128-135, 1974

BOOK REVIEWS

Handbook of Sensory Physiology, Volume VI/2: Vestibular System. Part 2: Psychophysics, Applied Aspects and General Interpretations

By *H. H. Kornhuber* (ed). Hard cover, 680 pages, 198 figures, indexed. Springer-Verlag, Berlin-Heidelberg-New York, 1974

This is the second of two volumes on the Vestibular System. Like the first, it is a scholarly work, amply annotated and indexed with a comprehensive bibliography. The authors are acknowledged authorities in vestibular psychology, human physiology and neurology, and cybernetic theory, which is what this book is all about. The first one-third is devoted to perceptual phenomena, sensation thresholds, after-images of motion, body position judgements, visual influences and their interaction in normal man. The next three hundred pages (eleven chapters) are orientated more towards an understanding of the pathophysiology of the vestibular system. The clinician will more likely be interested in the chapters on nystagmus in otoneurology, arousal and habituation, vestibulo-spinal reflexes, motion sickness and pathological vestibular sensations than in the occasionally lengthy discussions of human responses to angular and linear acceleration or animal studies of single neurons. The final section contains two conceptualized models of how all this might fit together as a system concept of vestibular function, and more broadly yet, how the vestibular system fits within the body's total motor behavior.

Though well written, this volume is definitely not bedside reading or a clinical handbook for the differential diagnosis of disequilibrium. While the facts about disrupted spatial disorientation are there, surprisingly little attention is devoted to clinical syndromes *per se*. The reader has to dig a little in several places to put it together. I had perhaps naively expected this second volume to magically provide me with instant complete understanding of the damaged vestibular system. It did not, but an impressive number of the pieces of the puzzle are there for the reader who wants to try. It is an excellent source book for serious students of the vestibular system and for clinical neurologists and otoneurologists.

F. Blair Simmons, M.D.

An Introduction to the Laboratory Study of the Ear

By *David M. Lipscomb, Ph.D.* Hardcover, 282 pp, referenced, illustrated, indexed. Charles C Thomas, Springfield, Ill., 1974. Price $19.75

This ten-chapter volume covers all procedures and techniques necessary to conduct experimental anatomical studies on the inner ear. Basic information such as solution preparation and record keeping are included in addition to actual preparative techniques for morphological studies of cochlear tissue and observation and recording of findings.

The intent of this book, as described by the author, is to provide a basic grounding in fundamental techniques for the serious student of the ear and to serve as a useful reference for those currently engaged in auditory research. Unfortunately, the book falls short of its intended goals.

It appears that much of this book was written on the basis of casual observation of procedures rather than actual experience, which has resulted in some inaccuracies or confusing descriptions of the theoretical bases of techniques and also the actual methodology.

In some cases, the terminology used to refer to certain structures or cells or parts of cells is erroneous or demonstrates a lack of understanding of the pertinent literature. For example, the following phrases are used in the text: *hollow* modiolus; *cilia* on sensory cells; cytoplasm is cell inner *tissue;* OHC apparently has *4 points* of attachment to the reticular membrane.

In addition, to be a good basic text, illustrations should be clearly and completely labelled. Many of the book's figures are not labelled at all. Structures must be identified from the verbal descriptions given in the text. A few judiciously placed arrows, along with identification of important landmarks, would have improved the instructiveness of the illustrations. Unlabelled structures which are clear to the experienced investigator may not be seen at all by the novice.

Another point of particular importance to a teaching text is an accurate and representative list of references. In this volume, several authors cited in different chapters are not included in the list of references. In some cases, the original work is cited in a footnote, but in other cases only a name and page number are given so that it would be extremely difficult to locate the original work.

In view of the shortcomings just mentioned, it is impossible to give this book a good recommendation as either a teaching text or a reference book.

BARBARA A. BOHNE, PH.D.

Pathology and Surgery of the Salivary Glands

By *Jose Yoel, M.D.* Hard cover, indexed, referenced, illustrated. Charles C Thomas Publishing Co., 301-327 East Lawrence Avenue, Springfield, Illinois. Price $132.50

This is a most comprehensive manuscript pertaining to salivary gland disorders. In fact, it is so comprehensive that it stands alone in publications regarding this subject.

The text is divided into five sections: General, Parotid Glands, Submaxillary Glands, Sublingual Glands, and Accessory or Minor Salivary Glands.

Special pathology is considered. At the end of each section, surgery and complications are discussed. Surgery is clearly shown in atlas form. Ductal disorders are depicted for the parotid and submaxillary glands. It is enlightening to have disorders of the sublingual glands put forth so succinctly and understandable. One of the outstanding features of this textbook is its illustrations which are numerous, clear, and apropos.

This is a reference source which should be in the libraries of all persons interested in the disorders of the salivary glands.

WALTER P. WORK, M.D.

Physiologie des Gehörs, Akustische Informationsverarbeitung, Einführung für Ärzte, Biologen, Psychologen und Nachrichtentechniker

(Auditory Physiology, the Processing of Acoustic Information, An Introduction for Physicians, Biologists, Psychologists, and Communication Engineers)

By *W. D. Keidel* (Editor). Paperbound, 409 pp, indexed, referenced, illustrated. Georg Thieme, Stuttgart, West Germany. Price DM 24.00 ($9.50)

This pocket book is written and published in a time-honored German tradition. Books of this kind are printed on inexpensive paper and are low priced to keep them within the reach of the average reader. Yet, they are written by well-recognized authorities in their respective fields.

Chapters and sections of the present book were written by members of the staff of the First Physiological Institute, University of Erlangen: W. D. Keidel, E. David, P. Finkenzeller, S. Kallert, K.-H. Plattig, G. Rinsdorf, and M. Spreng; some emphasis quite naturally is on their own work.

The content ranges from a description of the input signal to a discussion of cortical processing. Much space is devoted to neural coding and decoding, something in which the Erlangen Institute has an interest of long standing. Otologists should be particularly interested in the discussion of objective auditory responses, ranging from electrocochleography to evoked cortical responses. The varied background of the contributors (physiology, biology, bioengineering) assures that each subject area is discussed from a number of different aspects, usually culminating in a section employing the tools of engineering network analysis. It is probably for this reason that the book addresses itself to "Physicians, Biologists, Psychologists, and Communication Engineers." I am not at all sure that every one of these readers will be able to obtain a maximum of information from every chapter of the book. Physicians and engineers do not look at a given problem in the same manner nor do they speak the same language. Should we, therefore, come to the conclusion that the book has failed its stated purpose? I think not. Books like this one *should* be read by persons with varying backgrounds, and although a physician will not derive the same information from a chapter on network analysis as an engineer does, the book provides an incentive to learn something about the tools and approaches that the other person uses, so that they can discuss problems together in a fruitful manner. The opposite is also true. Too often, engineers think only in terms of the equivalent network and largely disregard the actual anatomical structure. This is a brave attempt to bridge the gap.

J. TONNDORF, M.D.

ABSTRACTS OF CURRENT ARTICLES

Congenital Aneurysm of the Extracranial Carotid Arteries

Hammon JW, Silver D, Young WG: Ann Surg 176:777, 1972

The authors discuss extracranial aneurysms of the carotid artery and present two of their patients. These particular instances are believed due to a developmental cleft in the media of the vessel. The high mortality of expectant observation is stressed. These lesions should be considered in the differential diagnosis of neck masses. Treatment is best accomplished by resection of the aneurysm and restoration of vascular continuity.

STAGMAN

Basal Cell Adenoma of Minor Salivary Gland Origin

Christ TF, Crocker D: Cancer 30:214, 1972

A review of a series of 55 tumors of minor salivary gland origin revealed three instances of basal cell adenoma. All three arose in the upper lip and were mobile, suggesting mucocele. Surgical excision is curative. The importance of recognition of this entity histologically is to allow differentiation of the canalicular type of basal cell adenoma from the much more aggressive adenoid cystic carcinoma. Histologic features of this lesion are presented and contrasted with those of adenoid cystic carcinoma.

STAGMAN

Fiberoptic Bronchoscopy

Schoenbaum SW, Pinsker KL, Rakoff SJ, et al: Radiology 109:571, Dec., 1973

The authors describe the combination of endoscopy, biopsy, culture and bronchography into a single procedure by the use of the fiberoptic bronchoscope.

Two tables, six radiographs, 12 references are presented.

PAYNE

Benign Osteoblastoma of the Mandible

Brady CL, Browne RM: Cancer 30:329, 1972

The authors report two instances of benign osteoblastoma of the mandible. Histologic features are identical to the much more commonly occurring osteoblastoma in vertebrae, flat bones, and small bones of the hands and feet. Young males are most commonly affected. Clinical features with rapid growth of the lesion and radiologic appearance of an osteolytic defect surrounded by an expanded and eroded cortex suggests a sarcoma. Extreme tenderness of the lesion is characteristic. Conservative wide local excision with preservation of adjacent uninvolved bone is the suggested treatment.

STAGMAN

The Influence of Tumor Dose Specification on the Early Clinical Results of Interstitial Radium Tongue Implants

Awwad HK, Burgers JMV, Marcuse HR: Radiology 110:177, Jan., 1974

The authors discuss the treatment of carcinoma of the tongue by radium implants. Clinical material, technique, dose calculations, clinical results, and statistical analysis of the data are presented.

Three tables, five figures and 18 references are included.

PAYNE

A Study of the Appearance of Early Asymptomatic Oral Squamous Cell Carcinoma

Mashberg A, Morrissey JB, Garfinkel L: Cancer 32:1436, Dec., 1973

The authors report a total of 158 asymptomatic malignant squamous cell lesions of the oral cavity in 125 patients. Location, color, size, surface configuration, bleeding, induration, local or distant metastasis are discussed. They note the rate of detection of early lesions to have increased from 2 in 1960 to 21 in 1971.

Four tables, five color photographs, six photomicrographs and 25 references are included.

PAYNE

Megavoltage Radiation Therapy for Supraglorric Carcinoma

Wang CC: Radiology 109:183, Oct., 1973

The author reviews the case histories of 184 patients, supraglottic with squamous cell carcinoma, treated by megavoltage radiotherapy. Therapeutic results are evaluated according to TNM Staging, and the surgical treatment of radiation failures is discussed.

Eight tables and 13 references are included.

PAYNE

The Radiotherapy of Nasopharyngeal Angiofibroma

Fitzpatrick PJ, Rider WD: Radiology 109: 171, Oct., 1973

The authors review a total of 39 patients seen between 1946 and 1971 at the Princess Margaret Hospital, Toronto, with the diagnosis of nasopharyngeal angiofibroma.

An excellent assessment of this rather rare tumor is provided including a discussion of the pathology, endocrinology, radiography, surgical treatment and radiotherapy as pertains the patient.

Ten figures, 12 radiographs, 2 photos and 21 references are included.

PAYNE

Accessory Lobe of the Submandibular Gland

Jafek BW, Strife JL: Radiology 109:75, Oct., 1973

Two case reports are presented for discussion of the differential diagnosis of masses within or adjacent to the submandibular gland. The embryology, anatomy, and developmental anomalies of the major salivary glands are described.

Sialography may aid in diagnosis and spare the patient surgical biopsy.

Three radiographs, 13 references are included.

PAYNE

The Frequency of Tonsillectomy and Appendectomy in Cancer Patients

Cassimos C, Sklavunu-Zurukzoglu S, Catriu D, et al: Cancer 32:1374, Dec., 1973

This report from the Pediatric Clinic, Thessaloniki, Greece, compares the incidence of tonsillectomy and appendectomy in 500 patients with varying forms of cancer and 500 "normals." The purpose of the study was to explore the hypothesis that tonsils and the appendix are vital in the immune mechanism and serve to protect against different antigens.

The authors discuss the relationship of tonsillectomy to the appearance of malignant disease and postulate that tonsils may sometimes favor the development of neoplasms.

Four figures, two tables, 16 references are included.

PAYNE

Role of Radiotherapy in the Treatment of Cancer of the Tongue

Vermund H, Gollin FF: Cancer 32:333, 1973

The authors discuss the indications for radiation therapy in the treatment of cancer of the tongue. A total of 154 patients seen during the period 1958 to 1968 are included. Tumor classification, treatment, results including factors affecting the results, lymph node metastases, complications, and the role of surgery are discussed.

Six tables, 11 figures, 7 color photographs and 25 references are included.

PAYNE

Esophageal Intramural Pseudodiverticulosis

Boyd RM, Bogoch A, Greig JH et al: Radiology 113:267, November, 1974

A case is presented to include radiologic, endoscopic, and autopsy findings with intramural esophageal diverticulosis. The literature is reviewed.

One table, four figures including micrographs, and 15 references are included.

PAYNE

Local Control and Site of Failure in Radically Irradiated Supraglottic Laryngeal Cancer

Ghossein NA, Bataini JP, Ennuyer A et al: Radiology 112:187, July, 1974

The authors present the results obtained in a total of 203 patients with supraglottic cancer after radical irradiation at the Fondation Curie in Paris. Local control, lymph node control, and incidence of major complications are discussed.

Seven tables, five figures, and 14 references are included.

PAYNE

Esophageal Intramural Pseudodiverticulosis

Lupovitch A, Tippins R: Radiology 113:271, November, 1974

The authors discuss a patient presenting with a five year history of dysphagia. The radiographic, endoscopic, and pathological, as well as histological findings, are described in an effort to show the evolution of the disease.

Six figures, including three micrographs, and five references are included.

PAYNE

Elective Neck Irradiation for T_xN_0 Squamous Carcinoma of the Oral Tongue and Floor of Mouth

Million RR: Cancer 34:149, July, 1974

The author discusses the use of elective neck irradiation in 43 patients with T_xN_0 (all T stages plus a clinically negative neck) squamous carcinoma of the oral tongue/floor of mouth treated at the University of Florida. Technic for concomitant irradiation of primary and neck are given. The advantages and disadvantages are enumerated.

Nine references, four tables, and six figures are presented.

PAYNE

NATIONAL AND INTERNATIONAL OTOLARYNGOLOGICAL SOCIETIES

American Academy of Facial Plastic and Reconstructive Surgery

President: Carl N. Patterson, M.D., Durham, North Carolina

Secretary: M. Eugene Tardy, Jr., M.D., Chicago, Illinois

Meeting: April 29-30, 1976, Palm Beach, Florida

American Academy of Ophthalmology and Otolaryngology

President: Frank W. Newell, M.D., Chicago, Illinois

Executive Secretary-Treasurer: C. M. Kos, M.D., Rochester, Minnesota

Meeting: September 21-25, 1975, Dallas, Texas

American Board of Otolaryngology

President: David D. DeWeese, M.D., Portland, Oregon

Secretary-Treasurer: Walter P. Work, M.D., Ann Arbor, Michigan

Certifying examination: November 15-21, 1975, Chicago, Illinois

American Broncho-Esophagological Association

President: Walter H. Maloney, M.D., Cleveland, Ohio

Secretary: Loring W. Pratt, M.D., Waterville, Maine

Meeting: April 27-28, 1976, Palm Beach, Florida

American Laryngological Association, Inc.

President: Stanton A. Friedberg, M.D., Chicago, Illinois

Secretary: John F. Daly, M.D., New York, New York

Meeting: April 24-25, 1976, Palm Beach, Florida

American Laryngological, Rhinological and Otological Society, Inc.

President: James A. Harrill, M.D., Winston-Salem, North Carolina

Executive Secretary: Richard L. Ruggles, M.D., Cleveland, Ohio

Meeting: April 27-29, 1976, Palm Beach, Florida

American Neurotology Society

President: Cecil W. Hart, M.D., Chicago, Illinois

Secretary-Treasurer: Jack L. Pulec, M.D., Los Angeles, California

Meeting: September 21-25, 1975, Dallas, Texas

American Otological Society, Inc.

President: Victor Goodhill, M.D., Los Angeles, California

Secretary-Treasurer: G. Dekle Taylor, M.D., Jacksonville, Florida

Meeting: April 25-26, 1976, Palm Beach, Florida

American Rhinologic Society

President: George H. Drumheller, M.D., Everett, Washington

Secretary-Treasurer: Pat A. Barelli, M.D., Kansas City, Missouri

Meeting: September 19, 1975, Dallas, Texas

American Society for Head and Neck Surgery

President: Emanuel Skolnik, M.D., Chicago, Illinois

Secretary: William M. Trible, M.D., Washington, D.C.

American Society of Ophthalmologic and Otolaryngologic Allergy

President: W. Leonard Draper, M.D., Houston, Texas

Secretary-Treasurer: Walter A. Ward, Jr., M.D., Winston-Salem, North Carolina

Meeting: September 19-20, 1975, Dallas, Texas

Association for Research in Otolaryngology

President: Jack Vernon, Ph.D.

Secretary-Treasurer: David Lim, M.D.

Meeting: September 19-20, 1975, Dallas, Texas

Barany Society

President: M. Morimoto, M.D., Kyoto, Japan

Secretary-General: M. Kitahara, M.D., Kyoto, Japan

Meeting: October 17-21, 1975, Kyoto, Japan

Canadian Otolaryngological Society

President: G. A. Badger, M.D.

Secretary: T. D. Briant, M.D.

Meeting: June 24-26, 1976, Vancouver, B.C.

Deutsche Gesellschaft Fur Hals-Nasen-Ohren-Heilkunde Kopf-Und Hals-Chirurgie

President: Professor Dr. R. Kirstein

Secretary: Professor J. Berendes, Weinheim, Germany

Meeting: May 30-June 3, 1976, Basel, Switzerland

Finish Otolaryngological Society

Chairman: Professor A. E. Kortekangas, Turku, Finland

Secretary: Jouko Suonpää, M.D., Turku, Finland

Irish Ear, Nose and Throat Society

President: M. O'Brien, F.R.C.S.

Secretaries: G. Fennell, F.R.C.S., and G. Smyth, F.R.C.S.

Meeting: June 23-26, 1976, Vancouver, British Columbia

Puerto Rico Medical Association, Section of Otolaryngology

President: Fernando Longo, M.D.

Secretary: Marco A. Berríos, M.D.

Society of Academic Chairmen of Otolaryngology

President: George T. Singleton, M.D., Gainesville, Florida

Secretary-Treasurer: George F. Reed, M.D., Syracuse, New York

Meeting: November 6, 1975, Washington, D.C.

Society of Military Otolaryngologists

President: Captain Tom Miller, MC, USN

Secretary-Treasurer: Col. Sonley R. LeMay, Jr., M.D., MC, USA

Meeting: September 24, 1975, Dallas, Texas

South African Society of Otorhinolaryngology

Chairman: W. F. Dickie-Clarke, M.D.

Secretary: Erich Kuschke, M.D.

Meeting: October 25-29, 1976, Durban, South Africa

INTERNATIONAL CONFERENCE ON CHOLESTEATOMA

May 26-29, 1976

DEPARTMENT OF OTOLARYNGOLOGY
AND MAXILLOFACIAL SURGERY
THE UNIVERSITY OF IOWA
IOWA CITY, IOWA 52242

CONFERENCE COCHAIRMEN

JACOB SADE, M.D.
MAXWELL ABRAMSON, M.D.
BRIAN F. MCCABE, M.D.

An in-depth consideration of the biology, pathophysiology, etiology, natural history, and management of Aural Cholesteatoma

CONTRIBUTORS

D. F. Austin	I. Friedberg	J. Lindsay	G. Shambaugh
S. H. Baron	V. Goodhill	W. B. Litton	J. Sheehy
R. J. Bellucci	L. A. Harker	G. Nager	G. D. Smyth
J. Bernstein	R. Hinchcliffe	T. Palva.	J. Thomsen
L. Bluestone	J. V. D. Hough	M. Paparella	J. Toller
W. H. Bradley	C. Jansen	D. Plester	B. Tool
D. T. Cody	C. M. Kos	F. N. Ritter	R. Trelstad
H. Diamant	S. Krane	S. Roth	W. K. Wright
A. Z. Eisen	E. Laurence	H. F. Schuknecht	S. H. Yuspa
I. Friedmann	D. G. Lim	B. H. Senturia	

Detailed program and registration
materials available upon request.

Ann Otol 85: 1976

SOME REFLECTIONS ON OUR SPECIALTY

JOHN J. CONLEY, M.D.

NEW YORK, NEW YORK

Otolaryngology has changed as much as any specialty in the past 50 years. These changes have occurred in the foundation and superstructure of the specialty and are associated with the outgrowths of medical and scientific discoveries, new operations, and socioeconomic developments. The dynamism in these growth patterns has created, in a sense, an evoluting and a new specialty. It is timely to assess these changes and ask some stimulating questions about this historical development and its future.

1. Is there need today for the specialty of Otolaryngology?

2. How should it be structured and organized?

3. What are its responsibilities?

There has not been the slightest suggestion from any sector that Otolaryngology should not exist, but there is strong debate about its area of activity. The reasons for this are not as complex as they are confused. In the evolution of one doctor taking care of one patient for all his ills on a one-to-one ratio to the contemporary status of empires, principalities, and regional territories, we have developed authorities, interests, and boundaries that are subject to change as a result of scientific discoveries, leadership personalities, training facilities, and administrative structuring. All of the specialties which have so far been recognized are still evoluting and this, understandably, causes friction. Perhaps some of this friction is a good thing, even though its primary roots may be associated with the ego, personal power, and economic factors. These human imperatives have become the ingredients of progress but have never been assayed in American medicine.

The structure and organization of Otolaryngology has been a mixture of a well-established foundation that has been amazingly successful and a superstructure that has accommodated new concepts and new discoveries. Some of the changes in otolaryngology have been spectacular. The original specialist was preoccupied with infections in the ear and mastoid, sinuses, and throat. Many of the conditions were both common and potentially fatal. The specialist who could handle them was preeminent. The specialty flourished. The great discoveries of antibiotics eliminated the vast majority of infections and fundamentally changed the involvement and the training of specialists in the area of otolaryngology. This occurred about 35 years ago and was a critical turning point in the life of otolaryngology. Those specialists were obligated to diversify their interests and their professional activity. Some became interested in allergy, some in plastic and cosmetic surgery, some in trauma and maxillofacial surgery, some in cancer of the head and neck, some in the restoration of hearing, some in laryngology and bronchoesophagology and some in general otolaryngology. These changes embraced several varieties of specialization within the original group. ENT was beginning to develop into regional specialties, with its own framework of specialization. Rules to restrict professional development which are in-

---

From the College of Physicians and Surgeons, Head and Neck Service, Columbia University, St. Vincent's Hospital Medical Center, New York, NY.

Presented at the meeting of the American Laryngological Association, Atlanta, Georgia, April 6-7, 1975.

consistent with responsibility and realism are unproductive.

There was nothing artificial about this trend, as otolaryngology was apparently the most logical starting point for all of these new developments. Natural "growing pains," territorial conflicts, and disputes regarding training and qualifications accompanied the metamorphosis. These understandable areas of differences of operation were debated, and many of the problems have been solved; others await historical assistance.

If regional and organ surgery are rational concepts and well-accepted principles for the practice of surgery, why shouldn't there be a regional surgeon in the area of the head and neck? This query is immediately answered by the fact that the original otolaryngologist was a regular surgeon, and this is complemented by the fact that two organ specialty groups practice in this area. They are the neurosurgeons and ophthalmologists, whose training and acceptance have long ceased to be a point of controversy. The other areas of the nasal cavity, oral and pharyngeal cavities, larynx and neck have been a part of Otolaryngology since its inception. It is quite natural to expand from this established orientation position to the adjacent structures in this area as new concepts and operations are developed.

One might claim that this is taking over other specialty prerogatives. As otolaryngologists we must recognize that we hold no sacred right or dictatorial control over these regions; neither is any other group so ordained. The general surgeon and his august role have been fractionalized by specialization, regional surgery, and organ surgery. He has not been excluded from the head and neck, however, when his interests persist in the thyroid gland, head and neck cancer, reconstructive surgery, and trauma. The general plastic surgeon is involved in all areas of the body, but many in that group are concentrating on congenital anomalies, maxillofacial problems, cosmetic surgery, trauma, and neoplasia. In many respects, this path is quite parallel to otolaryngology. Maxillofacial surgery, at one time, was quite active in the area of the oral cavity and made significant contributions. Unfortunately, in the United States and England their role was severely down graded by the general plastic surgeon, who wished to dominate this area. Recent attempts to resuscitate maxillofacial surgery by political and administrative maneuvering of the general plastic surgical group to serve their own purposes will hopefully give the maxillofacial group the opportunity they deserve to identify their need and their role. Oral surgeons, also, represent an area of specialization that is expanding and filling the deficiencies of their present structure.

It would appear logical that if regional surgery had any credence, the efforts of all of these specialists should be combined and coordinated within the framework of the head and neck surgeon. All of these various specialty groups would be relatively autonomous, would have combined meetings, overlapping interests, and an interdisciplinary relationship. Historically, the otolaryngologist has been the most involved specialist in this area. One may complain that in some instances his training has been deficient and that not all otolaryngologists are interested or equipped to cope with some of these problems, and this is true. But everyone must admit that he is a specialist who has received the basic training and exposure to the anatomy, physiology, pathology, and treatment of the various conditions in this area. The otolaryngologists are the specialists who, in their daily practice, are involved in the examination, diagnosis and treatment of these regions in the head and neck. No other specialist can claim this.

In one sense, otolaryngology is in the position that general surgery was in forty years ago. The intense interest in various regions and organs of the body led to the identity and then the autonomy of specialty groups in almost every region of the body. In most institutions, the wellspring of their background was general surgery. As these specialties became more identified, they rearranged their training programs, and none now requires the complete training in general surgery. This in no measure detracts from the value and enrichment of complete training in general surgery as preparation for any specialty. The majority of these specialties require one, two, or three years of training in general surgery, augmented by two, three, or four years of additional, specialized training. The variations in the number of years of preparation is determined by the specialty group to accommodate the minimum requirements of qualification. The thrust of the scientific expansion in specialization could not be contained within the framework of general surgery, and new societies proliferated to represent new interests. Perhaps, if the general surgeon had been more sensitive to these developments, he could have organized the movement and molded it within his own framework. It is interesting that, within the past two decades, the specialty societies have been developed within the structure of the American College of Surgeons and now comprise more than 50% of the membership.

There is such an opportunity for otolaryngologists at this moment. The question is whether we can recognize it and take the necessary steps to develop it. First, we must be aware that we are basically regional surgeons in the area of the head and neck, and that within this region are the specialties of general otolaryngology and medical otolaryngology, regional plastic and reconstructive surgery, head and neck cancer surgery, otology, trauma, cosmetic surgery, endoscopy, rhinology and laryngology, and maxillofacial and oral surgery. It is as impossible for the otolaryngologist to master all of the refinements in his region of activity as it is for the general surgeon to master all of the refinements of total body surgery and for the general plastic surgeon to master all of the plastic and reconstructive procedures of all of the regions of the body. His degree of excellence will be the product of his interest and his experience. Specialists in small communities understandably have a different involvement than those in large metropolitan areas and those in teaching and university centers. A general, broad involvement must be maintained, and upon this foundation superspecialization may be developed. In most instances, this is not determined during the general training period, but gradually formulates itself on the basis of professional growth and opportunity. It is indeed fortunate if a young doctor can determine which course he will follow during his residency program, so that he can have additional training at that time in a special branch of head and neck surgery. It is folly to believe that every otolaryngologist, every plastic surgeon, and every general surgeon can, or should, be trained to a high degree in all of these aspects of head and neck surgery. A broad spectrum of specialization, with overlapping and coordinating interests, would be the main objective of the structure of training and practice.

The biggest *external* problem in the above concept is the confrontation with other specialty groups that desire to not only participate in some aspects of this surgery, but actually to control it. The biggest *internal* problem is the recognition of the concept, then the taking of the necessary administrative measures to give it viability. In respect to the latter problem, we are faced with the reluctance to alter the *status quo*, the failure to provide leadership, and the difficulties of the struggles with vested professional interests. Otolaryngologists have been sluggish in many of these matters, and their basic program has consisted mainly of responding to a positive thrust of another society or to be led by the new specialty societies developing within their own house to accomplish change. This may be partially explained by a feeling of professional security and a tradition of superb leadership. There must be a plan and an objective, however, that is rational and correct, that we can approach in a professional manner, with dignity, in the highest traditions of our medical ethic.

The external problems are created by the response of other specialty societies to the developing role in otolaryngology. The response is a proclamation that otolaryngologists should not perform certain operations in the region of the head and neck. The reasons adduced for such a statement are that otolaryngologists are not suitably or well trained, and that other surgeons either do or would like to do these same operations without interference. The majority of training programs in otolaryngology that teach surgery in the area of the head and neck have both strong and weak points. Some are strong in cancer, some in otology, some in plastic and reconstructive surgery, some in maxillofacial surgery, some in cosmetic surgery, some in endoscopy, some in research, and some in general ENT. These situations fluctuate with the availability of material and the interest of the doctors. All other specialty groups that train surgeons in these areas have strong and weak points which are even more apparent. Some have glaring deficiencies, yet it may be claimed that because a young doctor has attained a certain type of specialty certificate, this proclaims him to be superior and competent. There are circumstances where this is totally false. It is hoped that the sincere leaders in the various specialty groups will recognize this fact and resist the ploy to manipulate this type of cynicism. A charade of this character can never prove professional competency.

The basic weakness, and strength, in most programs is that in their growth over the past four decades they have expanded upon the basis of local need, new operative techniques, leadership action, and competitive resistance. The first three are indigenous to otolaryngology, and the fourth is within the realm of other specialty groups practicing in the area of the head and neck. Many of our programs have failed to specifically identify the special role otolaryngology plays in cancer of the head and neck, facial plastic surgery, cosmetic surgery and trauma to the face, gullet, and airway. It is essential that their role in these subjects be fairly documented and taught in the finest manner, as these are the areas of competitive interests from other specialists. The leaders in otolaryngology are responsible for improvement in their training programs as this specialty evolves. The possibility of their doing this is not easy. One simple method would be some form of interspecialty cooperation. This is almost unheard of, because we are involved in a power struggle which is self-destructive and deceptive.

There must be a plan of organization to accompany this. Plans do not have to be exclusive, as new cooperative efforts may improve training and reduce friction. Interdisciplinary, cooperative efforts might prove very satisfactory, if attainable. A period of temporary transfer to a stronger program or a preceptorship may be the solution. Otology is unique in this analysis, being so highly specialized it enjoys a noncompetitive position and almost total autonomy.

Although the Residents Training Program has been very effective in maintaining minimum standards for training, there has been no national movement to improve weaknesses or to coordinate strengths.

We must give serious consideration to the qualities to be recognized as an otolaryngologist. In the past, a set of minimum standards were established, including academic and surgical training and formal examination. These well-founded requirements are not challenged, but need modification to accommodate other specialists with strong professional backgrounds who might wish to become otolaryngologists. Modifications should recognize the general otolaryngologist and the specialized otolaryngologist. There is no discrimination in this type of classification if it represents the truth.

One must admire the adaptation and improvisation of the general plastic surgeon in reducing the number of years of training in general surgery to three and giving three years' credit to the otolaryngologist and orthopedic surgeon entering into a plastic surgery training program. It was sagacious of them to rehabilitate and absorb the maxillofacial surgeon, whether we approve of their motives or their means. They are also addressing themselves to the role of the oral surgeon. Otolaryngology could have gained much by comparable adjustments and adaptations.

It is therefore time for otolaryngologists to reevaluate their training programs in respect to their future development and other specialty training programs. Our American Boards should consider adaptations and changes in respect to the broad scope of otolaryngology and the very sophisticated type of specialists within it. There should be a minimum set of qualifications and also specific qualifications for the various specialties within its framework. Neither should establish exclusive rights. The American Academy of Otolaryngology should be restructured to specifically represent the various specialties functioning inside general otolaryngology. It should also have representatives from the younger doctors and the general ENT specialists. These conglomerate specialty groups should be coordinated with the internal teaching program, with other specialty groups, and with the administrative aspects of the new "Federated Society." They should retain relative autonomy. Scientific meetings should be organized with the thought of embracing all aspects of surgery in the head and neck. There should be certification of competency for the specialists in otolaryngology who have spent extra time in training in one of the divisions of the specialty. There should be recertification every five years. Recognition should be given to the self-made specialist who gains competency outside of the residency program. In a sense, we are all self-made, and this driving force and motivation may be more productive than a residency. There must be a built-in flexibility rather than a built-in rigidity to the entire program. There must be a central authority that can coordinate socioeconomic, political, and legal activity. Fortunately, the American Council of Otolaryngology is moving in this direction.

It must be admitted that a number of the above suggestions are gradually taking place and are in the minds of the leaders. Accommodation, resistance, and some progress have been generated. There is, however, no overall plan projecting into the next five or ten years. This exposes otolaryngology to a potentially diminished role in this area in the future, and even to the possibility of being finessed out of the important aspects of head and neck surgery by more astute planners. If we fail in this, it could lead to restrictions in hospital appointments, limitations in the state and national societies, a control on insurance payments, and a loss of a most-favored position in the National Health Program. Such a chain of events would almost obliterate certain aspects of Otolaryngology.

A positive and coordinated program, consisting of a federation of all of the otolaryngological societies, academies, associations, councils, and committees in a cohesive and unified structure embracing the other specialty groups in the area of the head and neck, would create a small renaissance in the administrative capabilities of our specialty.

Ann Otol 85: 1976

FREY'S SYNDROME - A TECHNICAL REMEDY

ROY B. SESSIONS, M.D.

DAVID T. ROARK, M.D. BOBBY R. ALFORD, M.D.

HOUSTON, TEXAS

SUMMARY – The symptoms of Frey's syndrome are occasionally of sufficient magnitude to warrant curative treatment. In four patients, a fascia lata graft was placed under the involved skin in an attempt to offer permanent relief from the cutaneous discomfort suffered during eating. Two of these patients have excellent long-term results. The other two patients were lost to long-term follow-up but were asymptomatic several months following grafting.

Facial cervical gustatory sweating is relatively common following surgery or injury on or about salivary gland tissue but is usually not of sufficient magnitude to warrant surgical treatment. In a small percentage of patients, however, the flushing, sweating, and associated discomfort are of such intensity that curative treatment is desirable.[1] Herein is described a technique of symptom correction which has, thus far, proven reliable, effective, and lasting.

The symptoms of flushing, sweating, and cutaneous discomfort associated with mastication of food apparently were first described in 1757[2] in a patient in which the parotid gland had been injured. In the ensuing years, other reports of such an occurrence were made; and in 1923, Lucie Frey[3] pointed out that the sweating in such cases was confined to the area of distribution of the auriculotemporal nerve. The now well-known syndrome bears her name. Since that time, abnormal gustatory sweating has been noted following parotid and submaxillary gland surgery,[4] radical neck dissection,[5] and transposition of chest wall pedicle flaps to the lateral facial area.[6]

The neuroanatomy pertinent to this subject is somewhat involved but fairly well understood.[6] Anatomic alteration of autonomic nervous system relations is the basis by which abnormal gustatory sweating occurs. Preganglionic parasympathetic neurons which are destined to end in parotid gland tissue begin in the inferior salivatory nucleus of the brain stem. These fibers leave by way of the glossopharyngeal nerve, enter the tympanic plexus in the middle ear from whence they exit without synapse, then run in the middle cranial fossa as the lesser superficial petrosal nerve, and finally reach the otic ganglion by way of the foramen ovale. In the otic ganglion, they synapse with postganglionic parasympathetic fibers which then join the auriculotemporal nerve and leave this nerve during its course in the parotid gland. These postganglionic parasympathetic fibers are secretomotor to the glandular tissue of the parotid and in addition cause vasodilation of the blood vessels of the gland. This is a cholinergic system, i.e., the fibers liberate acetylcholine which acts on the glandular tissue as the chemical mediator of the nerve impulses.[6]

The sympathetic innervation of the parotid controls vasoconstriction of the

---

From the Department of Otorhinolaryngology and Communicative Sciences, Baylor College of Medicine, Houston, Texas.

Presented at the meeting of the American Laryngological Association, Atlanta, Georgia, April 6-7, 1975.

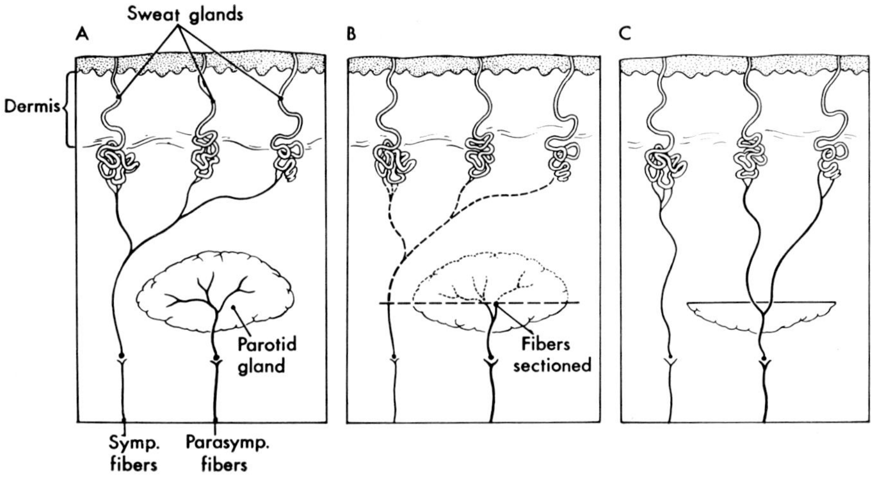

Fig. 1. A) Normal innervation of sweat glands. B) Surgery. C) Abnormal regeneration following surgery.

vessels of the glandular tissue. The preganglionic sympathetic fibers which ultimately affect the parotid gland originate in the spinal cord, in the first and second thoracic segments, in the lateral horn of white rami communicans, and go on to the cervical sympathetic ganglia where they synapse with postganglionic fibers. Most of these fibers join the internal and external carotid arteries and ultimately are carried with the auriculotemporal nerve to the parotid gland and sweat glands in the adjacent skin. Most postganglionic sympathetic fibers release noradrenaline or adrenalin rather than acetylcholine as is seen with parasympathetic fibers and are therefore adrenergic. The sympathetic fibers to the sweat glands are exceptions, however, and they release an acetylcholine-like substance which makes them functionally cholinergic.[6] It is this peculiarity in nerve physiology which allows the development of the abnormal neural regeneration which leads to gustatory sweating. Following parotid surgery or injury, both the sympathetic fibers to the sweat glands and the parasympathetic fibers to the parotid glandular tissue are injured. The most acceptable theory of development of gustatory sweating involves a misdirected regeneration of the injured parasympathetic fibers to the sweat glands of the adjacent skin[7] (Fig. 1A, B, and C). The fact that both the parotid parasympathetic and sweat gland sympathetic fibers are cholinergic allows this altered neural transmission. Thus, gustatory sweating is explainable both from a neurohumoral and an anatomic standpoint. With chewing of food, the parasympathetic secretomotor stimulation is directed to the sweat glands rather than the intended salivary gland tissue.

Laage-Hellman[8] demonstrated a very high incidence of subclinical gustatory sweating in persons who had undergone parotid surgery. That this occurs is not commonly recognized because the starch-iodine test is normally not performed on patients without symptoms. Myers and Conley[6] have made the distinction between normal and abnormal gustatory sweating. Normal gustatory sweating is seen on the lip area in some persons after looking at or smelling spicy foods.[9] Uprus, *et al*[10] pointed out that in persons with abnormal gustatory sweating the act of mastication was necessary and the mere presence of food in the mouth did not normally induce the symptoms. Also, Freedberg[11] noted that in patients with abnormal gustatory sweating, the chewing of a bland substance such as paraffin does not produce the phenomenon, whereas the chewing of food does.

TREATMENT

Various methods of treatment, some medical, most surgical, have been utilized in those patients with sufficient symptomatology to warrant therapy. Scopolamine hydrobromide cream (3%)[12] applied topically is often beneficial but its application is at times associated with blurring of vision, dry mouth, and urinary retention. Systemic atropine has also been recommended, but because of its annoying side effects, has been used only sparingly.

Section of the auriculotemporal nerve[13] is fraught with hazards to the nearby facial nerve because of the scarring from previous surgery. In addition, many patients have a recurrence of symptoms within 6-12 months following this procedure.[14,15]

Intracranial section of the glossopharyngeal nerve is apparently successful in relieving symptoms but seems too formidable a procedure for the symptoms. Excision of the involved skin offers only a temporary relief from the sweating and, in addition, is deforming.[16] Others[17] have advocated ablation of the sweat glands by radiation therapy. The dose level needed to accomplish this is high, and this method seems impractical.

Sectioning of the parasympathetic fibers in the tympanic plexus for the purpose of interrupting the secretory fibers to the parotid was first suggested by Hemenway.[18] Golding-Wood[19] later introduced the name "tympanic neurectomy" for this procedure. According to several reports since, this method is generally effective in treating gustatory sweating, although the symptoms are often not completely eliminated. Smith *et al*[1] summarized a collection of various data and stated that the results were "excellent" in 36% of the cases treated with tympanic neurectomy, "satisfactory" in 54% and "unsatisfactory" in 10%. The time of follow-up on these patients was not included in his writing.

Because of a possible connection between parasympathetic fibers in the chorda tympani nerve and the parasympathetic fibers in the otic ganglion, some authors have advocated combining excision of the chorda with tympanic neurectomy.[16]

The imperfections of past surgical efforts and a search for a more direct, reliable, effective, and longlasting method of eliminating the symptoms of Frey's syndrome led us to implanting fascia under the affected skin in four patients suffering from gustatory sweating in an effort to relieve their symptoms.

The following two case histories illustrate the benefits of this procedure.

CASE REPORTS

Case 1. A 29-year-old female underwent a left superficial parotidectomy for a benign tumor in 1965. Within months, the symptoms of gustatory sweating appeared over the operated site and in the following year increased to the extent that she had to mop her face with a towel during meals. Erythema and pain of the preauricular area also developed with mastication of food. The starch-iodine test was positive. Two years following surgery, she underwent a left tympanic neurectomy. Immediately following surgery she was free of symptoms, and no observable sweat was present in the skin during mastication of food. A starch-iodine test was not performed. Within three months following tympanic neurectomy, however, clinically apparent sweating recurred. In the fall of 1969, a facial flap was elevated along the line of previous parotid surgery; and a large piece of fascia lata which had been removed from the same patient's thigh was placed and sutured on to the tissue bed which corresponded to the undersurface of the affected skin. No symptoms have been noted in 5½ years since surgery, and the starch-iodine test remains negative.

Case 2. A 49-year-old male had a left superficial parotidectomy in July 1970 for a benign tumor. Two months later he developed cutaneous tenderness and

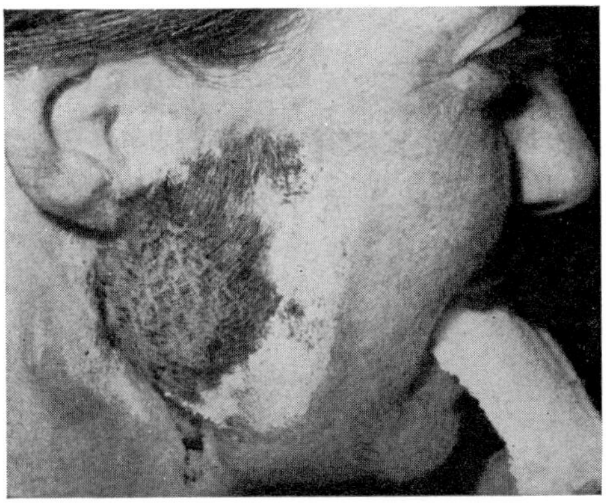

Fig. 2. Starch-iodine test demonstrating gustatory sweating.

sweating of the left cheek with mastication. The starch-iodine test was positive. In April 1971, a left tympanic neurectomy was performed with initial elimination of symptoms. Several months following the tympanic neurectomy, the symptoms of gustatory sweating reappeared in the same distribution as before surgery. In July 1972, a fascia lata graft was implanted beneath the involved skin, utilizing the previous parotidectomy incision. The elimination of all symptoms followed this procedure, and 2½ years later he is symptom-free and the starch-iodine test is negative.

SURGICAL TECHNIQUE

The area involved with gustatory sweating is carefully studied by the starch-iodine test method of demonstrating facial sweating (Fig. 2). The boundaries of the involved skin are tattooed with methylene blue on a needle point. At surgery, a thin skin flap, with a small amount of subcutaneous tissue attached, is designed. A large piece of fascia lata is removed from the lateral aspect of thigh. The fascia is then fashioned to the appropriate shape and size and is sutured to the subcutaneous and scar tissue bed from the previous surgery (Fig. 3A, B, and C). The facial skin flap is then returned, the incision

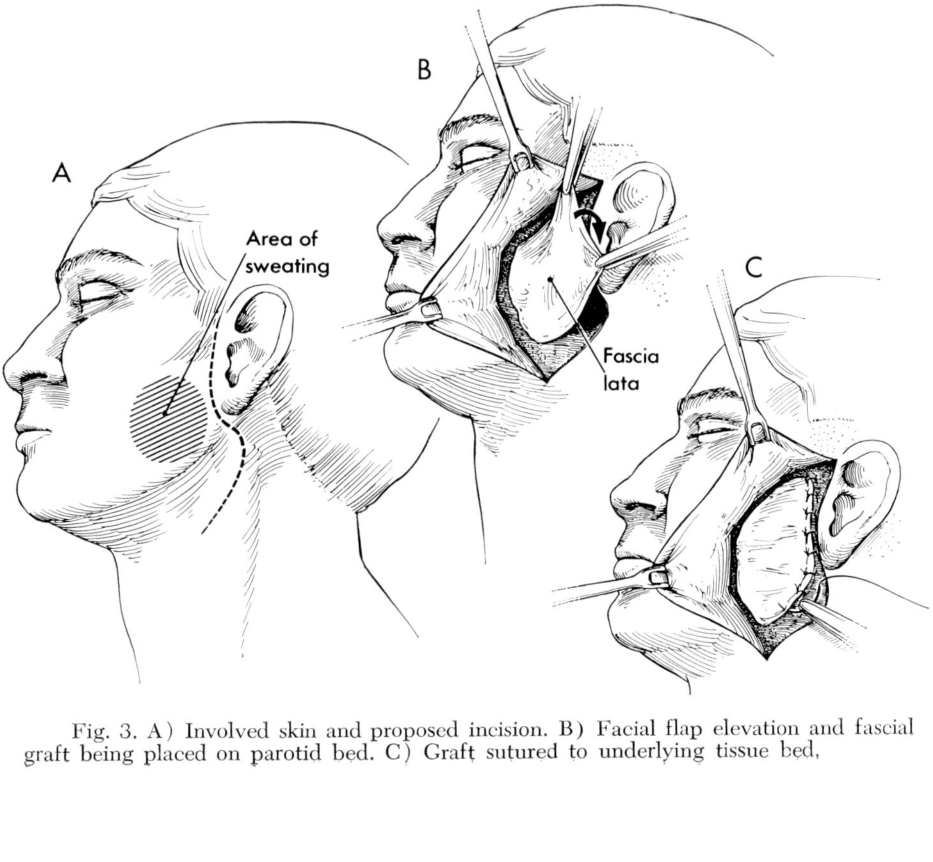

Fig. 3. A) Involved skin and proposed incision. B) Facial flap elevation and fascial graft being placed on parotid bed. C) Graft sutured to underlying tissue bed.

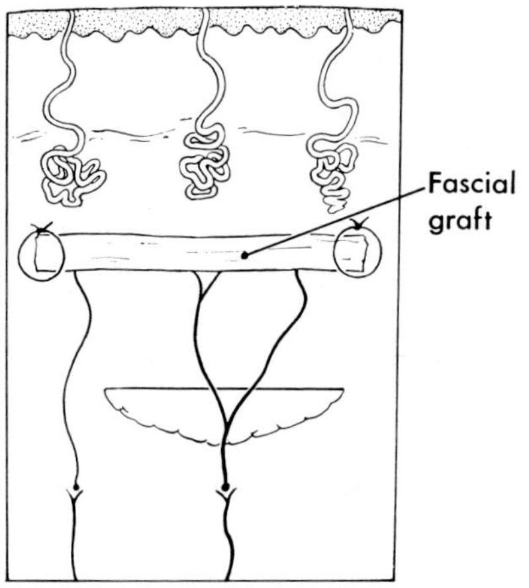

Fig. 4. Diagram showing placement level of graft and method of blocking abnormal regeneration of parasympathetic fibers.

closed, and a bulky dressing applied to insure hemostasis, flap security, and graft attachment to the overlying skin.

DISCUSSION

It seems sensible to interrupt the attachment of parasympathetic fibers to sweat glands at the most peripheral level, *i.e.* just beneath the skin, and to interfere with subsequent regrowth or reinnervation to the sweat glands (Fig. 4). To accomplish this safely and effectively, a material of a consistency that will prevent regrowth of nerves through it into the skin is required. Dermis would not fulfill this requirement and has some potentially undesirable sequelae (formation of cysts, *etc.*). The implantation of synthetic materials introduces the hazards of infection, skin slough, and rejection. Fascia, on the other hand, appears to provide a sufficient barrier and, in addition, is an autogenous material. Fascia lata is easily obtained, thicker than most fascial layers in the body, and its removal does not produce a significant disability to the patient. It should be removed from the lateral part of the thigh, for it is here that this fascia is the thickest.

It would seem important to avoid perforating the fascial graft so as not to allow penetration of nerve fibers. Also, it is obviously essential to implant one continuous piece of fascia which covers an area larger than the corresponding area of involved skin. Suturing the graft in place prevents sliding under the skin flap. The tough tissue to which the fascia is sutured offers a strong attachment site for the graft.

It is known that the ultimate results of treatment of gustatory sweating must be measured over a period of several years.[6] The two patients described above have been symptom-free and have also had negative starch-iodine tests for 5½ and 2½ years, respectively. Although recurrence of gustatory sweating seems unlikely at this late date, their outcome should be carefully followed. As noted, each had undergone a tympanic neurectomy with only temporary relief and had a recurrence of symptoms a few months later. In addition to these two patients, we have performed fascial implants on two additional patients with the same excellent result, but they were followed for only a few months before they were lost to follow-up.

CONCLUSION

We do not have sufficient experience with subcutaneous fascia lata grafting to advocate its use instead of either tympanic neurectomy alone or tympanic neurectomy in conjunction with chorda tympani neurectomy as standard treatment for abnormal gustatory sweating occurring after parotidectomy. The procedure is, however, reliable and safe; and if accumulated results follow the pattern seen thus far, it would seem to be the logical treatment of choice.

Request for reprints should be sent to Roy B. Sessions, M.D., Department of Otorhinolaryngology and Communicative Sciences, Baylor College of Medicine, Texas Medical Center, Houston, Texas.

REFERENCES

1. Smith RO, Hemenway WG, Stevens KM, et al: Jacobson's Neurectomy for Frey's Syndrome. Am J Surg 120:478-481, 1970

2. Duphenix cited by Spiro RH, Martin H.[5]

3. Frey L: Le syndrome du nerf auriculotemporal. Rev Neurol (Paris) 30:97-104, 1923

4. Young AG: A further report on the chorda tympani syndrome. Br Med J 5173: 620-621, 1960

5. Spiro RH, Martin H: Gustatory sweating following parotid surgery and radical neck dissection. Ann Surg 165:118-127, 1967

6. Myers EN, Conley J: Gustatory sweating after radical neck dissection. Arch Otolaryngol 91:534-542, 1970

7. Andre-Thomas: Le double reflex vasodilatateur et sudoral de la face consecutif aux blessures de la loge parotidienne; les parareflexes. Rev Neurol (Paris) 1:447-460, 1927

8. Laage-Hellman JE: Gustatory sweating and flushing after conservative parotidectomy. Acta Otolaryngol (Stockh) 48:234-252, 1957

9. List CF, Peet MM: Sweat secretions in man. Arch Neurol Psychiat 39:1228-1237, 1938

10. Uprus V, Gaylor JB, Carmichael EA: Localized abnormal flushing and sweating on eating. Brain 57:443-463, 1934

11. Freedberg AS, Shaw RS, McManus MJ: The auriculotemporal syndrome: A clinical and pharmacologic study. J Clin Invest 27: 669-678, 1948

12. Laage-Hellman JE: Treatment of gustatory sweating and flushing. Acta Otolaryngol (Stockh) 49:132-143, 1958

13. Coldwater KB: Surgical treatment of the auriculotemporal syndrome. Arch Surg 69:54-57, 1954

14. Glaister D, et al: The mechanism of postparotidectomy gustatory sweating. Br Med J 2:942-946, 1958

15. Chisa N, et al: Auriculo temporal syndrome. Arch Dermatol 90:457-459, 1964

16. Blumenfeld RJ, Friedman JE: Intratympanic Surgical Treatment of Frey's Syndrome. Arch Otolaryngol 86:28-33, 1967

17. Needles W: The auriculotemporal syndrome with suggestions regarding therapy. Arch Neurol Psychiatr 35:357-360, 1963

18. Hemenway WG: Gustatory sweating and flushing. Laryngoscope 70:84-90, 1960

19. Golding-Wood PH: Tympanic neurectomy. J Laryngol Otol 76:683-693, 1962

20. Friedman WH, Swerdlow RS, Pomarico JM: Tympanic neurectomy: a review and an additional indication for this procedure. Laryngoscope 84:568-576, 1974

NOTICE

The American Otological Society, Inc., notes with regret that its archives are not complete. The Council desires to remedy this insofar as possible and has directed the Editor-Librarian to seek replacement for volumes depleted from the library.

Accordingly, anyone in possession of any of the following volumes is earnestly requested to notify the Editor-Librarian. If recompense is desired, any fair price will be honored.

Vol. III, 1882-1887

Vol. XV, 1919-1921 (In some cases, these years may be in separate volumes)

Vol. XVIII, 1928

Vol. XXXIV, 1944

Vol. XLVI, 1958

Brian F. McCabe, M.D., Editor-Librarian, American Otological Society, Inc., University Hospitals, Iowa City, Iowa, 52242.

Ann Otol 84: 1975

PREOPERATIVE EMBOLIZATION OF JUVENILE ANGIOFIBROMAS OF THE NASOPHARYNX

JAMES D. PLETCHER, M.D. THOMAS H. NEWTON, M.D.

HERBERT H. DEDO, M.D. DAVID NORMAN, M.D.

SAN FRANCISCO, CALIFORNIA

SUMMARY – The juvenile nasopharyngeal angiofibroma is a vascular tumor. Careful and complete removal is challenging because of the brisk bleeding during surgery. The means applied to reduce this blood loss have included preoperative estrogens, ligation of feeding vessels, silicone embolization of feeding vessels, and cryosurgery. We have used preoperative Gelfoam® embolization of the internal maxillary artery in seven patients. Our clinical impression of significant reduction in loss of blood was confirmed by comparison with 16 previous patients. The average amount of blood lost in the embolized group was half that of the control group. A study of this type comprises many variables; however, the results do suggest that preoperative embolization of the internal maxillary artery is of advantage in the surgical treatment of juvenile angiofibromas.

The juvenile nasopharyngeal angiofibroma is a fibrovascular tumor that arises in the nasopharynx of young males. The treatment of choice is complete surgical removal. The location of the tumor, however, may cause difficulty in the surgical exposure, and the vascular nature of the lesion often results in massive intraoperative hemorrhage. The use of preoperative embolization in an attempt to reduce intraoperative bleeding and thus facilitate complete surgical removal, is here evaluated.

METHODS AND MATERIALS

Preoperative embolization of branches of the external carotid artery was employed in seven consecutive young male patients in whom juvenile angiofibroma was diagnosed. In two patients, in whom the tumor was supplied by both the right and left external carotid arteries, both external carotid arteries were embolized. Embolization was performed two to three hours before the surgical procedure in two patients; in the remainder, the embolization was employed on the afternoon preceding the surgical procedure.

The embolization was performed under local anesthetic by means of the transfemoral catheter technique.[1] After percutaneous puncture of the femoral artery, a polyethylene catheter (I.D. 0.045 inches; O.D. 0.065 inches) was advanced into the abdominal aorta by the Seldinger technique. With fluoroscopic control, the catheter was maneuvered into the common carotid artery. The catheter was then advanced into the external carotid artery under horizontal-beam fluoroscopy. Next, the catheter was further advanced into the vessel that had been identified on previous angiography to be the major blood supply to the tumor. In most instances, this vessel proved to be the internal maxillary artery. A selective, internal maxillary arteriogram was then obtained to define accurately the position of the catheter (Fig. 1A and B). Small fragments of Gelfoam®* (1 to 2 mm in diameter) were then injected through the catheter using saline as a bolus. The position of the catheter tip and the effect of embolization on the blood supply to the tumor were frequently checked fluoroscopically with injections of contrast media. Serial angiograms were obtained during the embolization procedure to determine the reduction of blood flow to the tumor. The procedure was terminated when angiograms showed obliteration or pronounced reduction in the vascularity of the tumor (Fig. 1C).

*Upjohn Company, Kalamazoo, Michigan.

From the Departments of Otolaryngology and Radiology, University of California, San Francisco, California.

Presented at the meeting of the American Laryngological Association, Atlanta, Georgia, April 6-7, 1975.

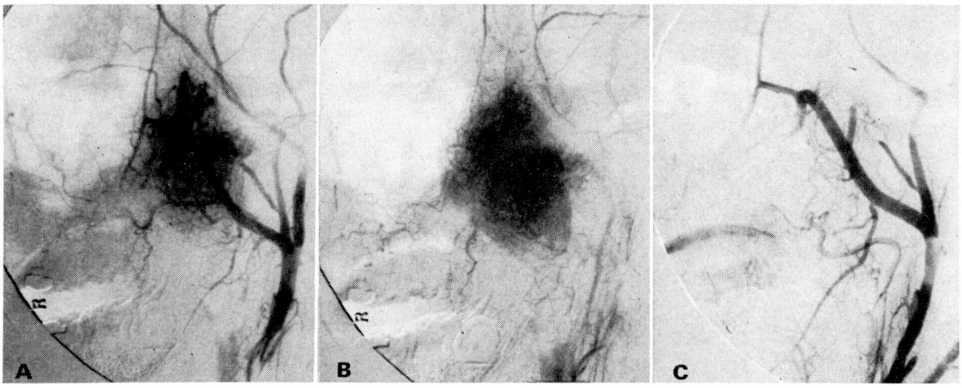

Fig. 1. Juvenile nasopharyngeal angiofibroma. Selective external carotid arteriogram, lateral projection. A) Early and B) late arterial phases before embolization. The highly vascular tumor in the nasopharynx is well shown. C) Postembolization arteriogram. The vascular neoplasm is no longer opacified.

TABLE I

SUMMARY OF 7 PATIENTS TREATED WITH PREOPERATIVE EMBOLIZATION

Case	*Age*	*Symptoms*	*Site of Tumor*	*Operative Approach*	*Estimated Blood Loss*
		Tumors Limited to Nasopharynx			
1	15	Nasal obstr., 4 mo	Nph.	Transp.	500 cc
2	19	Nasal obstr., 1 yr; intermittent epist., 3 mo	Nph.	Transp.	500 cc
3	15	Nasal obstr., 4 yr; severe epist. – 1 episode	Nph., nose	Transp.	670 cc
4	16	Nasal obstr.; intermittent epist., 1 yr	Nph., nose	Transp.	1275 cc
				Average:	736 cc
		Tumors Extending Beyond Nasopharynx			
5	17	Nasal obstr. and recurrent epist., 1 yr	Nph., sph.	Transp.	1500 cc
6	17	Nasal obstr., 2 yr	Nph., nose, sph., ptmax. space	Transp.	1300 cc
7	16	Nasal obstr., recurrent epist., 6 mo	Nph., sph., ptmax. space; max. sinus	Transp. Caldwell-Luc	2500 cc
				Average:	1767 cc

Obstr. – Obstruction.
Epist. – Epistaxis.
Nph. – Nasopharynx.
Transp. – Transpalatal.
Sph. – Sphenoid.
Ptmax. – Pterygomaxillary.
Max. – Maxillary.

TABLE II

SUMMARY OF 16 PATIENTS TREATED WITHOUT PREOPERATIVE EMBOLIZATION

Case	*Age*	*Symptoms*	*Site of Tumor*	*Operative Approach*	*Estimated Blood Loss*
		Tumors Limited to Nasopharynx			
1	13	Nasal obstr.	Nph.	Transp.	400 cc
2	13	Epist., left nasal obstr.	Nph.	Transp.	700 cc
3	17	Nasal obstr., 2 mo	Nph.	Transp.	800 cc
4	8	Recurrent epist., 1 yr	Nph., nose	Transp.	1000 cc
5	18	Recurrent epist.	Nph.	Transp.	1000 cc
6	15	Excessive bleeding following "polyp" removal	Nph.	Transp.	2000 cc
7	15	Epist.	Nph.	Transp.	2500 cc
				Average:	1200 cc
		Tumors Extending Beyond Nasopharynx			
8	17	Recurrent epist.	Nph., minimal sph. extension	Transp.	600 cc
9	17	Left nasal obstr.; left cheek swelling	Nph., left max. sinus; pterygomaxillary fossa	Transp. lip splitting incision, external carotid ligation	1000 cc
10	10	Recurrent epist.	Nph., nose, sph.	Transp.	1700 cc
11	14	Nasal obstr., 1 yr	Nph., sph.	Transp.	2000 cc
12	12	Nasal obstr., epist., foul nasal discharge	Nph., nose, sph.	Transp.	4000 cc
13	16	Nasal obstr.	Nph., sph., lateral pharyngeal space	Transp.	4500 cc
14	16	Nasal obstr., recurrent epist.	Nph., left max. antrum	Transp., lateral rhinotomy	4500 cc
15	17	Recurrent epist.	Nph., sph.	Transp.	5500 cc
16	14	Epist., nasal obstr. 6 wk	Nph., max. sinus; right cheek; floor of orbit	Transp.; Caldwell-Luc	6000 cc
				Average:	3311 cc

The age, presenting symptoms, site of tumor, operative approach, and estimated blood loss in the series of seven male patients are shown in Table I. In none of these patients had removal of the tumor been attempted previously. The tumor was limited to the nasopharynx and nose in four of the patients, and in three it had extended beyond these confines. The transpalatine surgical approach was employed in all patients. A Caldwell-Luc procedure also was needed in one patient to remove the extension of a tumor that filled the maxillary sinus.

An attempt was made to estimate carefully

the blood loss encountered during the operative procedure in the seven patients. The records of 16 patients with angiofibroma treated in this institution in the past 15 years were then reviewed to determine the estimated loss of blood in patients who had not been prepared with preoperative embolization. The estimated loss of blood as stated in the operative report was compared with the number of units of blood used in replacement transfusion. The loss was determined by the higher of the two figures. The anatomic extent, operative approach, and estimated blood loss in this group of patients are shown in Table II. The transpalatine exposure was the primary approach to the tumor in both groups of patients.

RESULTS

The average amount of blood lost during surgical removal in the seven patients was 1300 cc. In the four patients in whom the tumor was limited to the nasopharynx, the estimated blood loss averaged 736 cc. The amount lost during the exposure was estimated at 300 cc, and that during the closure as 200 cc. The average blood loss resulting from removal of the tumor was therefore estimated as only 236 cc. In the three patients in whom the tumor extended outside the confines of the nasopharynx and nose, the average blood loss increased to about 1767 cc. This increase was largely the result of oozing from the nasopharynx during the Caldwell-Luc procedure, and the antral and nasal bleeding during the closure of the palate.

The average total blood loss in the 16 patients who had undergone surgical removal of the tumor without preoperative embolization was about 2400 cc. In the seven patients of that group, in whom the tumor was limited to the nasopharynx, the loss of blood averaged 1200 cc. In the nine patients in whom the tumor extended beyond the nasopharynx, the blood was estimated as 3311 cc.

DISCUSSION

The juvenile nasopharyngeal angiofibroma is a highly vascular neoplasm typically found in pubescent males. It has been reported, however, in patients as early as eight years of age and as late as 50 years.[2] The origin of the tumor and the hormonal factors that may influence its activity have been discussed by previous authors.[3-5] These as yet undefined hormonal factors may account for the regression of a tumor, as occasionally observed in the postpubertal period.

Grossly, the tumor consists of a smooth, reddish or purple, nonulcerated, lobulated, firm mass which arises eccentrically from the roof of the anterior nasopharynx or from the posterior nasal fossa. Its base is usually rather broad, and it is not easily moved by the examining finger. This tumor must be distinguished from adenoid tissue, choanal polyps, nasopharyngeal cysts, nasopharyngeal carcinoma, and rhabdomyosarcoma. It may reach considerable size; its extensions tend to be polydirectional along natural foramina and fissures.[6] As the tumor enlarges, extensions from it project anteriorly into the posterior nares, laterally into the pterygomaxillary fossa, and superiorly into the sphenoid sinus. Particularly aggressive tumors may erode into the apex of the orbit or may extend intracranially through the base of the skull.

The usual presenting symptoms are those of nasal obstruction and epistaxis. The bleeding is intermittent and its control difficult, frequently requiring hospitalization and transfusions. Since the tumor is benign, pain is rarely an early symptom.

Roentgenograms of the sinuses and tomography of the skull base help to determine the extent of the tumor and the degree of bone involvement. Arteriography is essential to establish the diagnosis, to outline the blood supply to the tumor, and to demonstrate its anatomic extent. In the early stages of the disease, the blood supply to the tumor is almost exclusively from the ascending pharyngeal and internal maxillary branches of the external carotid artery. Selective external carotid arteriography shows dense contrast-medium staining of the tumor during the capillary phase of angiography. The maximum accumulation of contrast material in the tumor is usually seen three to six seconds after injection is begun. When the tumor ex-

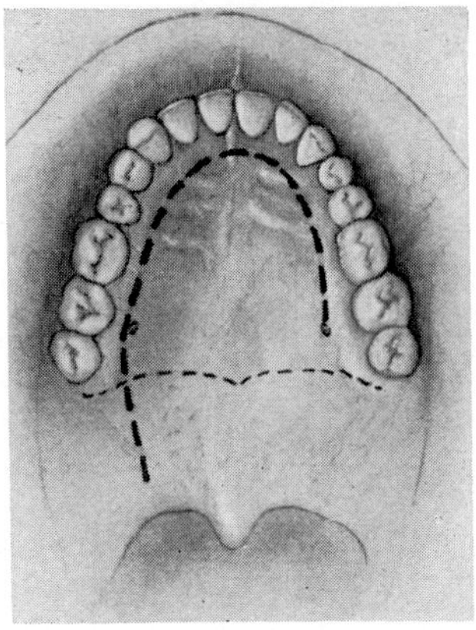

Fig. 2. Transpalatal incision with soft palate extension on one side to expose the nasopharynx.

tends intracranially, dural branches of the internal carotid artery and even cortical branches of the anterior or middle cerebral artery may contribute to the blood supply. Tumors that invade the ethmoid sinus or orbit may receive their blood supply in part from branches of the ophthalmic artery. Larger tumors may also receive contributions from the contralateral external or internal carotid arteries. Bilateral selective internal and external carotid arteriograms are advisable, therefore, in all patients with suspected nasopharyngeal angiofibromas. These studies are most easily accomplished by means of transfemoral catheter techniques. Magnification and subtraction techniques aid in the angiographic evaluation of these lesions.

The treatment of choice is complete surgical removal. Some authors[3,7] have recommended supportive measures until the tumor regresses spontaneously. Unfortunately, significant complications, such as life-threatening hemorrhage, infection, and intracranial extension of the tumor may precede spontaneous regression. Although Briant *et al*[8] recommended primary radiation therapy, we prefer to reserve such therapy for tumor recurrence or for those tumors which are inoperable because of intracranial extension.[9]

The transpalatine approach to the nasopharynx has provided good exposure, particularly when the incision is extended to the soft palate. The transpalatine incision starts just anterior to the greater palatine foramen on the side of the lesser tumor involvement. It curves around the dental arch, staying about 5 to 7 mm inside the gum line of the teeth continuing to the opposite greater palatine foramen (Fig. 2). The incision should pass lateral to this foramen since the vessels are divided on this side. From here the incision is extended posteriorly past the edge of the hard palate and 2 to 3 cm into the soft palate, stopping 1.5 to 2 cm from the free edge of the soft palate. This extension into the soft palate greatly improves the mobility of the palatal flap and is the key to excellent exposure of the entire nasopharynx. One of the greater palatine vessels is preserved to provide adequate blood supply to the flap. This transpalatine approach may be combined with an immediate or a delayed Caldwell-Luc procedure when the tumor has extended into the maxillary sinus. It may also be combined with a lateral rhinotomy in instances of extension into the ethmoid or pterygomaxillary fossae.

Despite adequate surgical exposure, however, the actual removal of the tumor is usually attended by brisk and often alarming hemorrhage. Such hemorrhage causes difficulty in the orderly, complete operation required to prevent recurrence. Many surgeons have attempted to reduce surgical blood loss by ligating the external carotid or internal maxillary arteries.[10] External carotid arterial ligation, however, has not proved to be particularly helpful because of the extensive collateral blood supply to the tumor. A hypotensive anesthetic with depression of the systolic blood pressure to 40 to 60 mm Hg may be of benefit.[11] Preoperative estrogen therapy has been advocated by several authors.[5,12,13] Angiograms showed decreased vascularity in three patients treated with estrogens.[13] Jafek *et al*[12] reported an average blood loss of 1970 cc in 9 patients treated with preoperative estrogen, compared to an average loss of 2960 cc in 25 patients not treated in this manner. Work *et al*[14] concluded that cryotherapy might be an effective adjunct to surgery but that it was not a substitute for standard surgical techniques. Cryotherapy might prove beneficial for small recurrences, but most tumors are too large for this technique.[15]

Embolization has proved to be a useful adjunct in the preoperative management of patients with juvenile angiofibromas. Roberson and coworkers[16] used barium-impregnated silastic spheres in the preoperative embolization of the internal maxillary artery in four patients with juvenile angiofibromas. Embolization must not be compared to proximal arterial ligation. The aim of embolization in these patients is to place the embolic material within the distal arterial branches or within the tumor itself. Gelfoam® has proved to be particularly suitable since it may be injected through the catheter in a compressed state. Soon after being exposed to blood, the injected fragments gradually swell to a larger size. Gelfoam®, therefore, has allowed the employment of relatively small catheters which can be introduced into the internal maxillary artery without causing arterial spasm. Reflux of the emboli into the cerebral circulation or inadvertent direct injection of emboli into the internal carotid artery represents the primary risk of this procedure. To avoid this complication, the catheter tip should be placed into the distal internal maxillary artery without obstructing its flow. Throughout the procedure, test injections with radiopaque contrast media are made to insure maintenance of the proper position of the catheter. Horizontal beam fluoroscopy is important to avoid rotation of the neck of the patient which could result in accidental displacement of the catheter. Small plugs of Gelfoam®, up to 100 or more, are injected to obstruct the small distal arterial branches that supply the tumor. The procedure is terminated when the circulation to the tumor has been obliterated or greatly diminished. Vigilance must be exercised toward the end of the procedure when flow in the internal maxillary artery is slowed, to prevent reflux of emboli into the internal carotid circulation. To date, we have had no complications from this procedure. Complications that involve the central nervous system remain a potential risk, especially when the embolization techniques are not applied carefully.

SUMMARY

Preoperative Gelfoam® embolization of the internal maxillary artery in seven male patients with juvenile nasopharyngeal angiofibroma is described. The average blood loss associated with removal of the tumor was reduced with this technique from an estimated 1200 cc to 736 cc when the tumor was limited to the nasopharynx. With tumors that extended beyond the confines of the nasopharynx, embolization reduced the average estimated blood loss from 3311 to 1767 cc. Preoperative embolization allows controlled surgical removal of the tumor and better visualization of its superior and lateral extensions.

Request for reprints should be sent to Herbert H. Dedo, M.D., Department of Otolaryngology, Room 495U, University of California, San Francisco, Third Avenue and Parnassus, San Francisco, California 94143.

REFERENCES

1. Newton TH, Kerber CW: Techniques of catheter cerebral angiography, Ch. 45, in Newton TH, Potts DG (eds): *Radiology of the Skull and Brain*. St. Louis, C. V. Mosby Co., 1974

2. Rosen L, Hanafee W, Nahum A: Nasopharyngeal angiofibroma: an angiographic evaluation. Radiology 86:103-107, 1966

3. Jereb B: Juvenile nasopharyngeal angiofibroma: a clinical study of 69 cases. Acta Radiol (Ther.) (Stockh) 9:302-310, 1970

4. Wilson WR: Juvenile nasopharyngeal angiofibroma. Laryngoscope 82(2):985-997, 1972

5. Schiff M: Juvenile nasopharyngeal angiofibroma. Laryngoscope 69:981-1016, 1959

6. Wilson GH, Hanafee WN: Angiographic findings in 16 patients with juvenile naso-

pharyngeal angiofibroma. Radiology 92:279-284, 1969

7. Martin H, Ehrlich HE, Abels JC: Juvenile nasopharyngeal angiofibroma. Ann Surg 127:513-536, 1948

8. Briant TDR, Fitzpatrick PJ, Book H: The radiological treatment of juvenile nasopharyngeal angiofibromas. Ann Otol Rhinol Laryngol 79:1108-1113, 1970

9. Ward PH, Thompson R, Calcaterra T, *et al*: Juvenile angiofibromas: A more rational therapeutic approach. Laryngoscope 84: 211-2194, 19874

10. Williams JD, Chisholm D: Internal maxillary artery ligation for the removal of juvenile nasopharyngeal angiofibroma. J Laryngol Otol 87(2): 1153-1158, 1973.

11. Daly J: Personal Communication.

12. Jafek BW, Nahum AM, Butler RM, *et al*: Surgical treatment of juvenile nasopharyngeal angiofibroma. Laryngoscope 83: 707-720, 1973

13. Christiansen TA, Duvall AJ, Rosenberg Z, *et al*: Juvenile nasopharyngeal angiofibroma. Trans Am Acad Ophthalmol Otolaryngol 78:140-147, 1974

14. Work WP, Boles R, Nichols RD: Angiofibromas: diagnosis and treatment including cryosurgery. Trans Am Acad Ophthalmol Otolaryngol 70:1108-1113, 1970

15. Conley J, Healey WV, Blaugrund SM, *et al*: Nasopharyngeal angiofibromas in the juvenile. Surg Gynecol Obstet 126:825-837, 1968

16. Roberson G, Biller H, Sessions R, *et al*: Pre-surgical internal maxillary artery embolization in juvenile nasopharyngeal angiofibroma. Laryngoscope 82(2):1524-1532, 1972

AMERICAN OTOLOGIC SOCIETY GUIDELINES FOR GRANTS

Our objective is clearly the problem of otosclerosis: its diagnosis and management, the possible causes and underlying conditions (such as the hereditary background), and an understanding of the disorder that may lead eventually to its prevention and cure.

Our present lack of understanding of the disorder and the absence, as far as known, of any similar condition in animals below man, makes research in this field particularly difficult. A direct attack on the disease is hardly feasible; therefore, it seems to be sound strategy to try circuitous approaches, such as the investigation of bone development, growth, and repair under various conditions, and the study of other diseases that show suggestive correspondence to this one. It is possible that directions of investigation that may seem initially somewhat remote from otosclerosis itself may provide insights that will eventually lead to success in reaching our goal. Therefore, our policy is to aid and encourage research in the immediate field of otosclerosis and also in adjoining fields if, in our considered opinion, there is a substantial promise that the results obtained will be of assistance in the ways just indicated and may lead to the attainment of our objective.

The Board of Trustees wishes to announce that funds are still available for suitable grants. Application forms may be obtained from the office of the Secretary of the Research Fund Trustees of the American Otologic Society. Write to Maurice Schiff, M. D., Secretary, 7255 Girard Ave., La Jolla, Calif. 92037.

Ann Otol 84: 1975

CLEFT LARYNX

A REPORT OF SEVEN CASES

SEYMOUR R. COHEN, M.D.

LOS ANGELES, CALIFORNIA

SUMMARY – The purpose of this paper is to familiarize the otolaryngologist with a difficult and frequently missed anomaly. It is hoped that this will increase the number of successfully managed patients with this affliction. Of the seven herein reported cases, four were posterior clefts limited to the cricoid lamina. Three were more extensive laryngotracheoesophageal clefts. Seven cases are thus added to the approximately 30 cases reported in the world literature. The limited cricoid lamina defect can only be diagnosed by endoscopic examination, and is treated medically. Feedings must be given by gastrostomy only. A tracheotomy is indicated only when oral secretions are aspirated into the tracheobronchial tree. The more extensive laryngotracheoesophageal cleft requires surgical repair through a lateral pharyngotomy approach. When the cleft is extensive and extends into the chest, surgery must include a thoracic approach. The occurrence of cleft larynx in association with tracheoesophageal fistulae, with or without atresia, may be more frequent than generally realized. A search should be made for this anomaly in patients who aspirate after atresia repair has been accomplished, before attributing this symptom to severe stricture formation, or recurrence of the fistula. The problem of aspiration in posterior cleft larynx is due to the lateral and posterior displacement of the arytenoids. This malposition is due to the absence or deficiency of the interarytenoidius muscle so that the posticus muscle is unopposed. The term "posterior cleft larynx" should be used only where the defect is limited to the cricoid lamina, while laryngotracheoesophageal cleft should be applied to the more extensive defect.

While laryngotracheoesophageal cleft is an uncommon anomaly, partial clefts limited to the cricoid lamina would appear rare. A review of the literature reports very few cases of posterior cleft larynx. Only 2 or possibly 3 of approximately 30 reported laryngotracheoesophageal clefts were limited to the larynx. Since the more extensive cleft is incompatible with life unless surgically repaired, the assessment of its occurrence in the general population may statistically be more accurate by clinical, surgical, or autopsy reports. Posterior cleft limited to the larynx is an anomaly compatible with life. Its occurrence, therefore, cannot be truly evaluated, since with careful medical management and with growth and development of the child, symptoms of this anomaly usually completely subside.

Since Shapiro and Falla reported the second successfully treated case of laryngotracheoesophageal cleft in 1966,[1] the number of reported cases of this anomaly has increased rapidly. Of the 30 reported cases, only 7 or 8 have been repaired successfully. This paper will deal with four cases of partial clefts, or posterior cleft larynx, without evidence of tracheoesophageal defect, and will also add three cases of laryngotracheoesophageal clefts which were repaired surgically. Two of the surgically treated children are alive, and the third, the first case seen by the author in 1962, succumbed from inadequate surgery done after central nervous system and lung damage had occurred. In all cases the diagnosis was made by endoscopic evaluation.

From the Division of Otolaryngology of the Children's Hospital of Los Angeles, University of Southern California, School of Medicine, Los Angeles, California.

Presented at the meeting of the American Laryngological Association, Atlanta, Georgia, April 6-7, 1975.

CLINICAL PICTURE

The chief presenting symptoms of a cleft larynx is aspiration, usually associated with some voice change. Where the defect is large and includes the tracheoesophageal septum, aspiration of secretions, especially when oral feedings are attempted, causes severe choking and cyanosis, followed by x-ray evidence of aspiration pneumonitis. When the cleft involves only the cricoid lamina, endogenous secretions may be handled fairly well, but feedings, being only liquids in the neonate, will produce choking and associated airway obstruction from aspirated secretions, and severe pneumonias. When solid or thickened feedings are added, they do not produce choking or aspiration.

While voice change is usually notable, it may not be severe enough to be clinically evident. Stridor, unless other lesions are present, is usually of the expiratory type, and is due to tracheobronchial obstruction from aspirated secretions. Laryngeal obstruction has not been a prominent presenting symptom in the cases herein reported.

Chest x-rays early show aspiration-type pneumonic infiltrates and hyperaeration. The cine-esophagram, best carried out by swallowing rather than injection through an indwelling catheter, will usually show spilling of contrast medium into the trachea, frequently interpreted as dyskinesis of swallowing. The study may be negative unless carefully performed.

The endoscopic examination must be depended upon to make the definitive diagnosis. While the literature indicates problems in diagnosis by either laryngoscopy, bronchoscopy, esophagoscopy, or by a combination of these procedures, failure to diagnose the lesion is due to inexperience or failure to observe what may be very esoteric changes within the larynx. This unusual anomaly and its extent cannot be diagnosed in any other way except by direct visualization.

DIFFERENTIAL DIAGNOSIS

Differential diagnosis of aspiration problems in the neonate is complex and involves many medical disciplines.

Central nervous system lesions associated with prematurity, abnormal development, hypoxia, or birth trauma may produce evanescent or permanent defects of the swallowing mechanism. Anatomic defects of the nose, nasopharynx, larynx, or esophagus and trachea, and laryngeal paralysis may produce aspiration by impairing the normal mechanism of deglutition. Diseases of the esophagus, such as cricopharyngeus spasm or patulous cricopharyngeal sphincter, nonsphincteric spasm of the esophagus, cardiospasm, or strictures, may produce aspiration. The latter are readily diagnosed by x-ray studies. Neuromuscular disorders such as myesthenia gravis, amyotonia congenita, and autonomic dysfunction of Riley-Day, must always be considered in aspiration problems. Prior to endoscopy, therefore, the pregnancy and birth history should be known. A complete physical examination including the neurological status of the patient should be performed. X-ray studies of the chest and of the swallowing mechanism with barium or other contrast media, followed by very careful endoscopic examination of the larynx, tracheobronchial tree, and esophagus, will yield the highest success rate in definitive diagnosis.

EMBRYOLOGY

One of the most important functions of the larynx is protection of the airway from foreign material. Any defect which prevents spasmodic closure of the larynx will produce severe dysfunction resulting in aspiration pneumonitis and failure to thrive. Since a cleft which involves the larynx alone or in conjunction with a defect of the tracheoesophageal septum can be a major problem resulting from faulty development of the larynx, it is appropriate to repeat the normal embryological development of this organ and indicate the abnormalities which result in this cleft type anomaly.[2-5]

Of primary interest in the developmental anatomy of the larynx are the visceral arches 3, 4, 5, and 6. The respiratory primordium, which will give rise to the larynx, trachea, and bronchi, starts as a ventromedian diverticulum of the foregut caudal to the pharyngeal pouches. The tracheobronchial groove appears in the 3 mm embryo at approximately 25 days. Lateral furrows develop on each side of the diverticulum, along the line of union of the groove and esophagus. As the furrows become deeper, eventually to join, the laryngotracheal tube is formed. The anterior and cranial bud of the tube develops into the primitive laryngeal additus or slit. The slit appears at about the 4 mm stage, and comes to be more definitely formed between the fourth and sixth branchial arches. The caudal end develops into the lung buds. Also, during this stage, the margin of the laryngotracheal groove begins to fuse in a caudocranial direction to form the tracheoesophageal septum. This separates the laryngotracheal tube from the esophagus.

During the fifth and sixth weeks, the laryngeal additus, or slit, is altered by the growth of the masses which are the primordia of the epiglottis (arches 3 and 4) and the two swellings of mesenchymal tissue that are the anlage of the arytenoid cartilages (arch 6) which, approximating each other medially, move towards the base of the tongue. This adds a transverse component to the top of the sagittal slit, and the additus becomes T-shaped. At the fifth to sixth weeks stage, the tracheoesophageal septum has developed to at least the first tracheal ring and the level of the future fusion of the posterior lamina of the cricoid cartilage. If the rostral advancement of the tracheoesophageal septum is arrested, preventing the dorsal fusion of the cricoid cartilage, a laryngotracheoesophageal cleft will result.[3]

Since the cricoid cartilage first develops as bilateral centers of cartilage fusing ventrally at about six weeks and dorsally at about seven weeks, the pathogenesis of the dorsal cleft will probably be found at the 9 mm stage. This cleft should not be confused with the large interarytenoid notch which persists even into the stage of three-month embryos.

The muscles of the larynx depend for their differentiation on the development and growth of the cartilage. The first muscle to develop into a recognizable form is the interarytenoid muscle which arises from the sixth arch at the 9 mm stage. Also, at this stage, the anlage of the cricoarytenoid muscle is visible. In clefts of the larynx, the interarytenoid notch remains deep, and the interarytenoid and posticus muscles are defective. It is apparent from the cases reported that failure or defects of posterior cricoid fusion may be an isolated defect not dependent on progression of closure of the tracheoesophageal septum.

CASE REPORTS

Case 1. A Caucasian female infant born on June 28, 1962, was admitted to the Children's Hospital of Los Angeles at six weeks of age. She had been treated elsewhere for pneumonia, with oxygen, penicillin, and Declomycin®.* The infant was suspected of having a tracheoesophageal fistula without atresia and was transferred for therapy. X-rays of the chest revealed displacement of the mediastinum to the right and diffuse infiltration of the right lung. A barium swallow showed barium to be present in both bronchi (Fig. 1).

The family history is sketchy since the mother had numerous marriages and divorces, and the infant had been put out for adoption. She was a product of a seven-month gestation, with a normal delivery, weighing 2.04 kg at birth. There was no distress immediately after her delivery, with no jaundice and no cyanosis. The infant was noted to cough and turn blue with her first feeding, and this was repeated after each attempt at oral feedings. She had recurrent aspiration pneumonias.

*Lederle Laboratories, Pearl River, N. Y.

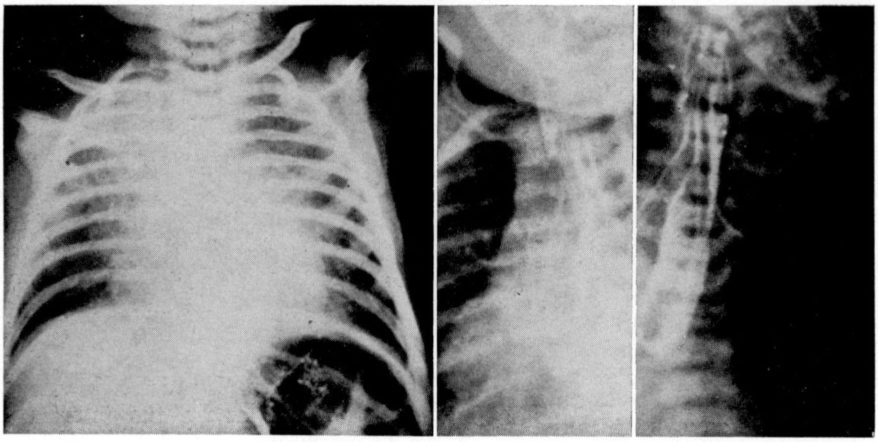

Fig. 1. Aspiration pneumonitis with barium esophagram showing high overflow of contrast medium into the trachea and esophagus.

On admission, the findings were relatively normal except for crackling rales in the right upper lung field, with no evidence of cardiomegaly or neurological deficit. With antibiotics she showed some improvement, and a gastrostomy was performed for feeding purposes. Additional studies with contrast media did not show evidence of a tracheoesophageal fistula. A feeding gastrostomy had been done, and while the infant had been admitted on August 9, 1962, endoscopic consultation had not been obtained until August 22, 1962. Direct laryngoscopy revealed the larynx to be defective posteriorly. In addition to the cricoid defect, the arytenoids were noted to hang from their anterior attachments like elephant ears. The larynx and esophagus could be examined through this defect at the same time, and a tracheoesophageal defect was noted.

On August 31, 1962, a tracheobronchogram was performed which showed a high division of the trachea in the neck, with an anomalous left mainstem bronchus (Fig. 2). Following bronchoscopy and the clearing of all secretions, she improved tremendously. She continued to have difficulty with secretions, and on September 7, 1962, after numerous episodes of apnea requiring artificial resuscitation, a tracheotomy was performed.

Immediately after tracheotomy, the child gradually improved, having fewer episodes of respiratory difficulty. Attempts to close the cricoid defect by injecting Teflon®* into the area were unsuccessful. Because of repeated apneic spells and failure to thrive, on July 24, 1963, a laryngofissure was performed, and closure of the large laryngotracheoesophageal cleft was attempted. Her immediate postoperative course was uneventful, but on the third postoperative day she expired. Autopsy diagnosis was chronic interstitial pneumonitis, tracheostomy, jejunostomy, congenital anomaly of the larynx and upper trachea, secretory inactivity of the adrenals, atrophy of the thymus, and acute bronchopneumonia.

The chief autopsy findings were limited to the larynx and lungs. The larynx was in normal position. On opening the esophagus posteriorly, a long, narrow defect (1.3 X 0.3 cm in size) of the posterior wall of the larynx and upper tracheoesophageal septum was noted. The larynx and esophagus communicated freely. The defect was located in the midline of the posterior wall, from the ligaments connecting the corniculate

*Ethicon Laboratories, Somerville, New Jersey.

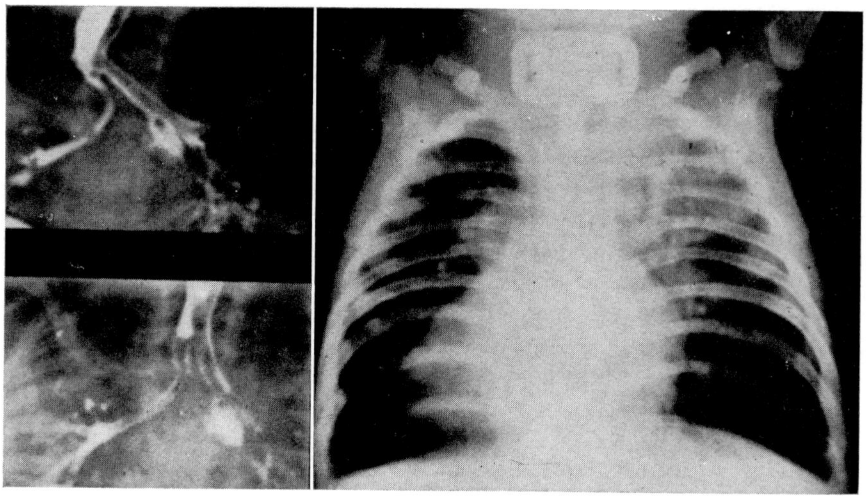

Fig. 2. Tracheobronchogram showing the trachea bifurcates in the neck and defective bronchi.

cartilages, extending downward through the ligaments connecting the arytenoid cartilage to the posterior portion of the cricoid cartilages. Silk sutures were seen in the margins, but the cleft was wide open, and the larynx and esophagus communicated freely through the defect. The vocal cord was not abnormal, and the larynx showed no evidence of stenosis or obstruction.

Case 2. An infant born on April 25, 1968, was admitted to the Children's Hospital of Los Angeles on March 10, 1969. The chief complaints were failure to thrive and recurrent pneumonia. The infant was a product of a nine-month gestation in a para 5 gravida 5 mother. Pregnancy was complicated by recurrent respiratory infections and dependent edema, and polyhydramnios. The infant breathed spontaneously but could not cry. She weighed 3.2 kg at birth. Because of difficulty in feeding and problems with oral secretions, the child was tube fed. At two months of age she had meningitis, and at three months of age she had a staphylococcal pneumonia. A second episode of pneumonia occurred at six months of age, and her third episode occurred at eight months of age. She had been treated for all these illnesses prior to her transfer. Noted on the chart was, "Has difficulty catching breath when drinking liquids. Occasionally will choke on her food." Her general development was slower than normal. Examination on admission showed an alert, but very thin and pale child, with a high pitched wheezing cry. She weighed 6.2 kg. There were suprasternal and substernal retractions, with an audible wheeze. The cry was weak, and there was a to-and-fro wheeze. The abdomen was soft, full, and protuberant. The impression was recurrent pneumonia of undetermined origin. Another esophagram still showed no evidence of abnormality, and a sweat chloride was found to be normal. An H-type tracheoesophageal fistula was suspected.

On March 12, 1969, direct laryngoscopy, bronchoscopy, and esophagoscopy revealed an H-type tracheoesophageal fistula. In addition, the laryngeal picture was one of an unusual anomaly. The arytenoids were displaced anteriorly, and on closure of the larynx there was a patent posterior cleft. The posterior cricoid lamina appeared abnormal. Interarytenoid closure was faulty (Figs. 3 and 4). On March 19, 1969, the tracheoesophageal fistula was closed. The child was discharged in good condition on April 12, 1969.

Direct laryngoscopy on May 7, 1973, showed the larynx to be normal other than the partial posterior cleft of the larynx. The vocal cords moved normally, and the posterior aspect of the larynx was elongated because of failure of fusion of the entire arytenoid to the cricoid cartilage. The cleft appeared to be well compensated for, and closure of the larynx was seen to be excellent. This patient's followup has been one worthy of note. She has had no problems feeding, no recurrent fistulae, no pneumonitis, and her development and growth has been excellent.

Case 3. A white male infant was admitted at five hours of age on April 22, 1969. He was the second of twins born by a delivery complicated by premature rupture of membranes. The amniotic fluid was meconium stained. Soon after birth, the child was noted to have marked increase in oral secretions. An esophagram showed a blind upper esophageal pouch, and he was transferred to the Children's Hospital of Los Angeles. The upper pouch was much narrower than is usually seen in atresia, and he was suspected of having an associated tracheoesophageal fistula with the upper pouch as well as the usual lower pouch fistula. Immediately after the infant was admitted to the hospital, a gastrostomy was performed under local anesthesia. At a later date, a small amount of contrast medium was introduced into the upper esophageal pouch, and the material was noted to immediately spill into the trachea. The significance of this was not recognized until the patient had undergone direct laryngoscopy and bronchoscopy on April 28, 1969, at which time a laryngotracheoesophageal cleft was visualized.

After treatment for seven days for pneumonitis, surgical correction of the esophageal atresia was performed. At thoracotomy, atresia with continuity of the esophageal muscle associated with two tracheoesophageal fistulas was found. The distal esophageal fistula and a fistula from the upper esophageal segment were interrupted, and an end-to-end esophagoesophagostomy was performed.

The postoperative course was complicated by right upper lobe atelectasis and episodes of respiratory distress. Two weeks after the operation, esophageal dilatations were begun, but because of repeated difficulties with aspirated secretions, a tracheostomy was performed four weeks after the thoracotomy.

On June 28, 1969, when the infant was nine weeks of age and weighed 3 kg, the laryngotracheoesophageal fistula was repaired by a lateral pharyngotomy route. The larynx was rotated anteriorly, and the cleft which extended through the cricoid cartilage and inferiorly through the third tracheal ring was repaired. The margins of the cleft were split and a double layer closure with 6-0 silk sutures was performed. The cleft was repaired to the level of the arytenoids. The larynx was replaced in its normal position, and the esophagus was then closed with interrupted silk sutures. The wound was drained and the skin was closed. The infant's postoperative course was uneventful, and feedings were continued via the gastrostomy, until healing occurred.

Direct laryngoscopy and esophagoscopy on October 8, 1969 (Fig. 5), revealed that closure of the tracheoesophageal cleft was complete, but another tracheoesophageal fistula was found immediately below the repaired cleft. Two weeks later, through a vertical cervical incision, the fistula was interrupted at its location at the level of the fourth tracheal ring. Again, the postoperative course was uneventful, and two weeks after the last surgery, direct laryngoscopy revealed closure of the cleft was intact. Oral feedings were begun, and esophageal dilatations were resumed.

The child was discharged from the hospital on January 3, 1970, at 8½ months of age, weighing 5.1 kg. Since then he has had regular esophageal dilatations for a narrowed anastomotic esophageal site, and repeated bronchoscopies for correction of lower tracheal and bronchial stenotic lesions. To the date of this writing, he still wears a tracheotomy tube, has developed normally, eats and drinks without choking, and it is anticipated that the tracheotomy tube will be removed when it is no longer necessary for tracheobronchial toilet after correction of the bronchial stenotic lesions.[6]

Case 4. A white male infant born November 11, 1969, was admitted to the Children's Hospital of Los Angeles on the sixth day of age. He was the product of a forty-five week gestation of a twenty-four-year-old gravida 2 para 1 mother. Membranes had ruptured at thirty-eight weeks, with leakage of fluid. There was no history of fever, labor was eight hours in duration, and delivery was by Frank breech presentation. The child cried weakly at birth, and weighed 2.4 kg. His Apgar was 8, with slight cyanosis and some respiratory difficulty. He was admitted with a diagnosis of atresia and tracheoesophageal fistula.

On November 17, the day of his admission, a gastrostomy was performed. On November 21, the esophageal atresia was corrected, and the tracheoesophageal fistula was interrupted. Leakage occurred at the site of anasthemosis, with episodes of apnea and some cyanosis on attempts to feed him. This was thought to be due to strictured esophagus.

On December 22, 1969, direct laryngoscopy was performed and a posterior cleft of the larynx was found (Fig. 6A, B, C). On December 30, 1969, a tracheotomy was performed after the child required intubation for an apneic spell. Bronchoscopy performed at that time showed lower tracheostenosis and severe bronchial stenosis.

Following the tracheotomy, the child improved gradually and steadily. He was discharged from the hospital on January 28, 1970, and to this date, he still has a tracheotomy tube for the purpose of tracheobronchial toilet. Repeated bronchial infections secondary to a stenotic trachea and left mainstem bronchus have required intensive antibiotic therapy. His most recent bronchoscopy revealed improvement in the status of the tracheobronchial tree, and it is anticipated that he will be decannulated soon. He eats and drinks normally, except when gulping liquids, which causes coughing.

Case 5. A white female infant was transferred to the Children's Hospital of Los Angeles on April 19, 1973, with the history of laryngeal obstruction. She was the product of a full term pregnancy, whose mother was a gravida 4 para 3. Labor was two hours, and delivery was accomplished with pudendal anesthesia. The Apgar was 5 at one minute without any spontaneous respirations. The patient was intubated in the delivery room, and remained pink after the tube was placed into the trachea. She then breathed without difficulty. The cry was extremely weak, and the larynx was noted to be abnormal. On admission to the Children's Hospital of Los Angeles, a nasotracheal tube was noted to be in place, and her examination, other than rhonchi in both sides of the chest, showed no evidence of abnormalities. An x-ray showed the endotracheal tube to be in place, and there was a right-sided pneumonic infiltrate.

On April 20, 1973, laryngoscopy and bronchoscopy were performed, and a cleft larynx with severe stenosis of the larynx and trachea were noted. The arytenoids were seen to be extremely edematous, and the endotracheal tube was seen to pass through a laryngotracheoesophageal cleft into the trachea. The immediate subglottic and upper trachea were severely stenosed, and a tracheotomy was performed on April 23, 1973. X-rays showed a normal esophagus without evidence of stricture. A gastrostomy was performed on April 24, 1973, and feedings were given with the infant gaining and doing well. The final diagnosis after endoscopy was laryngotracheal esophageal cleft with stricture of the esophagus. The esophagoscope could not be passed into the esophagus,

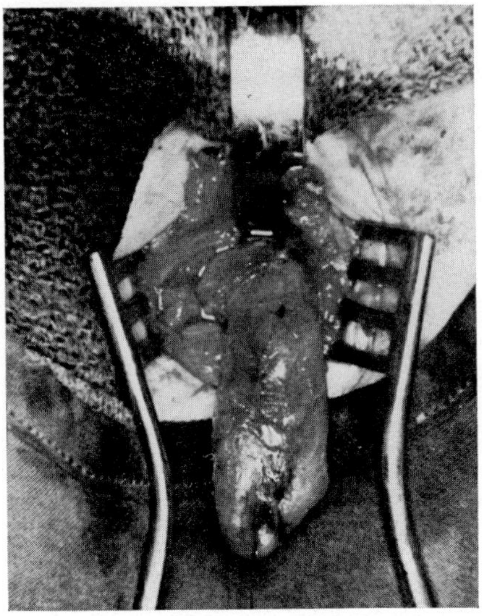

Fig. 7. Shows large diverticulum of esophagus which when opened revealed large laryngotracheoesophageal cleft.

and with a bronchoscope the cleft was seen.

On August 23, 1973, exploration of the neck showed a large esophageal diverticulum (Fig. 7) and a laryngotracheal esophageal cleft, and closure was accomplished. Her postoperative course was uneventful. An esophagram showed minor leaking of barium over the larynx but oral feedings were taken well. On October 3, 1973, she was discharged from the hospital and has returned periodically for esophageal and laryngeal dilatations. The laryngeal and upper tracheal stenosis was partly congenital and partly secondary to closure of the large tracheoesophageal cleft. On April 29, 1974, the gastrostomy was closed. The child eats and drinks well without aspiration. Her weight gain and development have been normal. It is anticipated that she will require a tracheostomy for a prolonged period of time and will return to the hospital for dilatations of the larynx and trachea.

Case 6. A three-year, six-month-old female Caucasian was first seen by the author on September 4, 1974, for closure of a persistent tracheocutaneous fistula. This child, birth date March 20, 1971, was the second born of a normal pregnancy and uneventful delivery, weighing 3 kg. From the first day, feeding was noted to cause choking and aspiration, and she was hospitalized with x-ray findings of an aspiration pneumonitis and airway obstruction from secretions. She was transferred to an Eastern Children's Hospital for diagnosis and correction of a suspected tracheoesophageal fistula, but exploration of the neck after numerous studies were done, failed to reveal the suspected fistula. Examination on April 15, 1971, after surgery, showed a bilateral vocal cord paralysis, and a tracheotomy was performed. A diagnosis of neuromuscular dysfunction of swallowing was made, and a feeding gastrostomy was performed. Her discharge

----

Fig. 3. A normal larynx for comparison.

Fig. 4. Shows persistent deep interarytenoid keyhole type defect seen even during spasmodic closure associated with partial laminal cleft.

Fig. 5. Arytenoids laterally displaced showing surgically repaired laryngotracheal cleft. The lamina of cricoid is defective with a healed fibrous septum. Esophagus is seen posteriorly.

Fig. 6. A) Deep interarytenoid cleft. Arytenoids appear laterally and posteriorly displaced. B) Closeup view of arytenoids. Larynx anteriorly dislocated by speculum of scope. Top opening larynx; posterior opening esophagus. C) Arytenoids separated and cricoid defect is noted — viewed is the caudal end of tracheoesophageal septum.

Fig. 8. A) Larynx on first inspection appears normal except for posterolateral position of arytenoids. B) Elevated anteriorly view of larynx showing deep interarytenoid cleft and fissure of cricoid. C) Separation of the arytenoids shows cleft and caudal end of tracheoesophageal septum (anteriorly).

Fig. 9. A) Top view of larynx. Note posteriolateral position of arytenoids. B) Larynx looks almost normal except for abnormal position of arytenoids (deep interarytenoid space). C) Part of the defect of cricoid is seen. D) Fibrous septum of defect of cricoid lamina comes into view on separating arytenoids. E) Cleft is visible and seen to be partial — separation connected by fibrous septum.

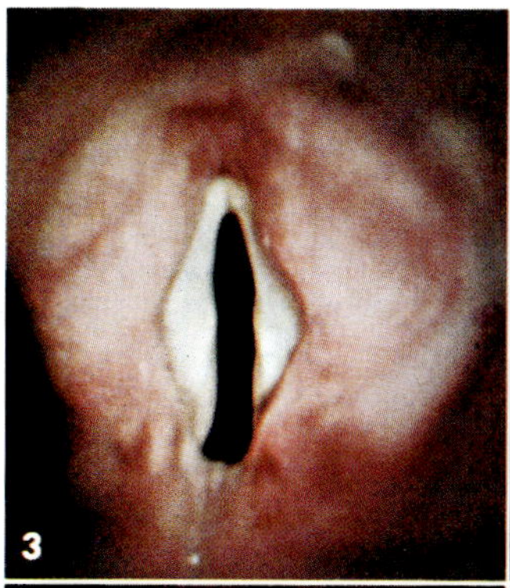
3

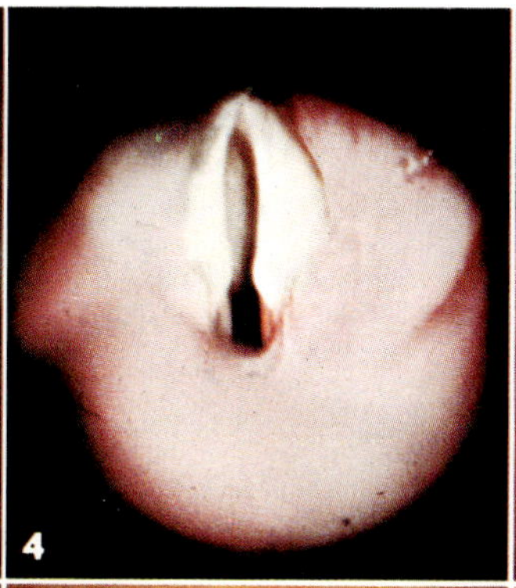
4

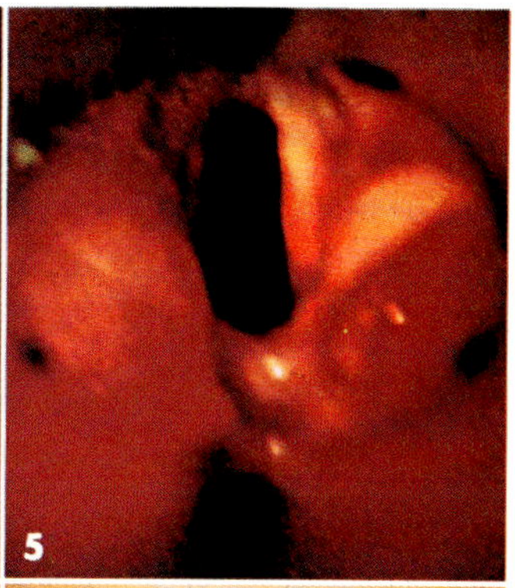
5

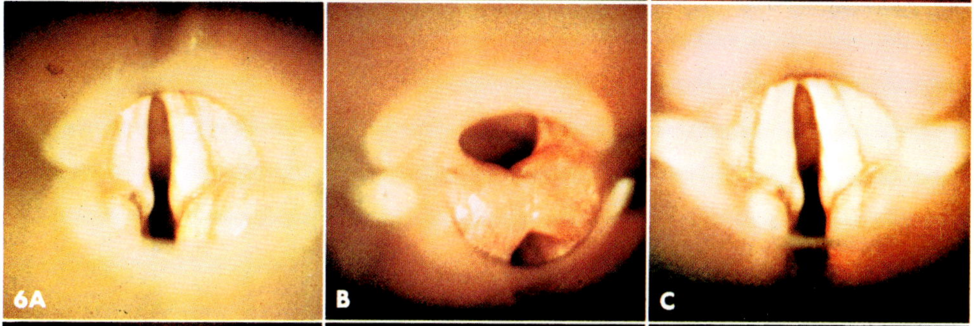
6A B C

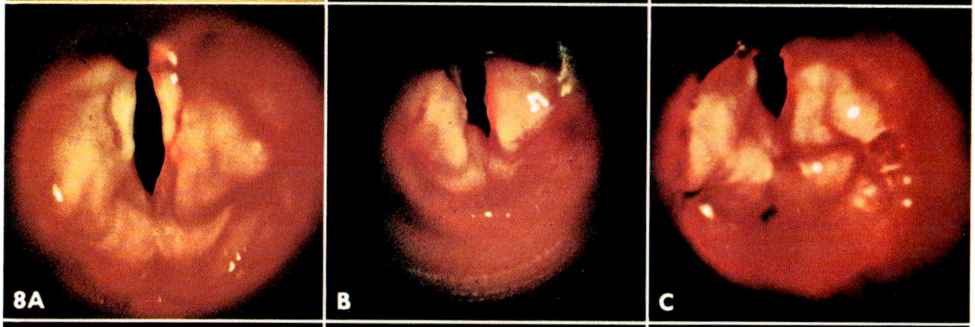
8A B C

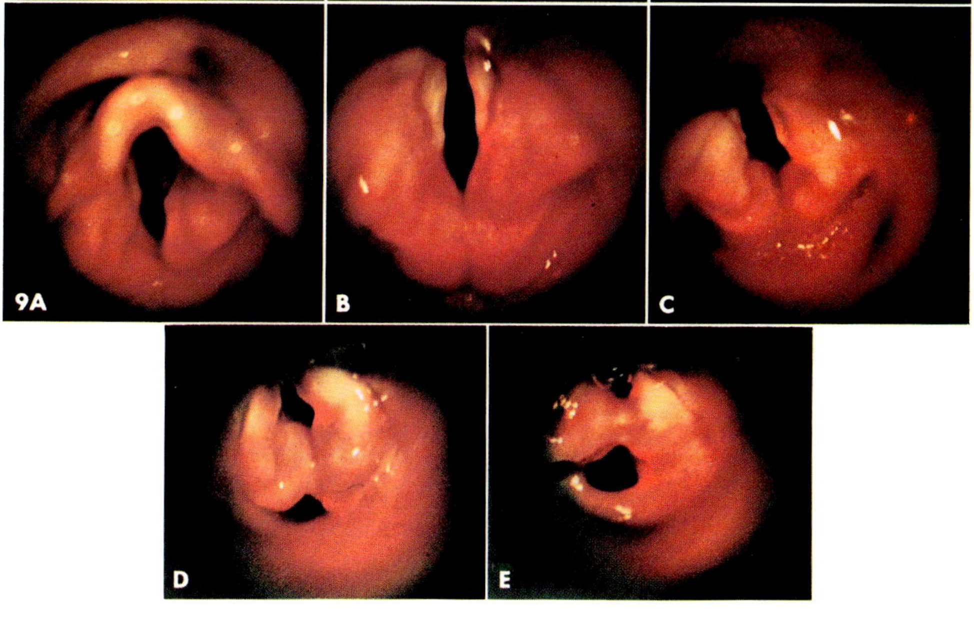
9A B C D E

from the hospital on May 24, 1971 was with the diagnosis of pseudobulbar palsy, with cricopharyngeal spasm and a left partial recurrent paralysis, and a right complete recurrent paralysis. All feedings were given by gastrostomy until 15 months of age, and on August 29, 1972, it was felt that her airway was adequate and she was extubated. It was noted that solids were taken well, but gulping liquid caused choking. On May 15, 1974, a laryngoscopy and bronchoscopy showed a good airway with a persistent tracheocutaneous fistula. The family then moved to the West Coast.

On October 27, 1974, as is usual prior to closure of a tracheocutaneous fistula, she was admitted to the Children's Hospital of Los Angeles for evaluation of the airway. Direct laryngoscopy showed a partial cleft of the posterior portion of the larynx (Fig. 8A, B, C). The esophagus was normal, and the tracheobronchial tree was normal. It is important to note that this child still chokes when she quickly gulps liquids but eats and drinks normally. On January 27, 1975, the tracheocutaneous fistula was excised, and the plastic repair of the defect was performed. Her postoperative course was uneventful.

Case 7. A female Caucasian born August 9, 1974, in Taiwan was admitted to the Children's Hospital of Los Angeles on September 10, 1974, with a history of trouble swallowing and aspiration immediately upon attempts to feed her. Persistent aspiration pneumonia was present. This patient weighed 3.2 kg at birth, tolerated her first feedings of 5 cc at eight hours of age, but at twelve hours, when given 30 cc, turned blue, choked, aspirated, and developed a pneumonitis. She was able to handle her own secretions well, and did not vomit. A barium esophagram was reported as normal. An x-ray of the chest showed bilateral pulmonary infiltrates. All attempts to feed the child produced cyanosis, gagging, and choking. Oral feedings were stopped, and gavage feedings were given and taken well. She was transferred to the Children's Hospital of Los Angeles for definitive diagnosis and treatment.

The child's delivery was normal and the mother's pregnancy was also normal. The family history is unremarkable. Examination on admission showed a normal infant with a nasogastric feeding tube in place. The cry was slightly weak, but she had a good suck and the moro and grasp reflex were normal. There were no abnormal neurological findings. A direct laryngoscopy was performed by four specialists in Taiwan, and only the pediatrician felt that the larynx was abnormal.

A direct laryngoscopy done at the Children's Hospital of Los Angeles revealed the larynx to be grossly abnormal with a cleft of the posterior larynx involving the cricoid (Fig. 9A, B, C). The arytenoids could be separated, revealing the tracheoesophageal septum, indicating a defect of the cricoid lamina. The larynx was somewhat edematous. Bronchoscopy showed the tracheobronchial tree to have inflammatory changes, and the mainstem bronchi were seen to be smaller than usual, interpreted as congenital cartilaginous defects. Esophagoscopy showed a normal esophagus, and diligent search for a tracheoesophageal fistula showed no such defect. The patient did well postoperatively, and had no problems with her secretions. She was fed by nasogastric feeding tube until a Stamm gastrostomy was done on September 20, 1974. The patient gained weight, and on October 3, 1974, she was discharged and returned to Taiwan.

Discharge diagnosis at the U. S. Naval facility in Taiwan was a term infant with congenital dysfunction of deglutition and aspiration pneumonitis.

The infant was again seen on February 21, 1975, at six months of age, weighing 5.4 kg and having no problems. Feedings were by gastrostomy. She still has a husky voice, and oral feedings will be withheld three more months, after which thickened feedings will be tried.

ASSOCIATED ANOMALIES

Of the cases reported, two (6 and 7) had no other anomalies. Two cases (3 and 4) had atresia of the esophagus and type C tracheoesophageal fistulae. Both of these cases also had associated bronchial stenosis and one (3) had multiple tracheoesophageal fistula. A severe laryngeal and tracheal stenosis and a large diverticulum were found in one case (5). One case (2) had an H type tracheoesophageal fistula. Tracheal and bronchial anomalies were found in one case (1), with the trachea bifurcating in the neck.

Request for reprints should be sent to Seymour R. Cohen, M.D., 1300 North Vermont Avenue, Los Angeles, California 90027.

REFERENCES

1. Shapiro MJ, Falla A: Congenital posterior cleft larynx. Ann Otol Rhinol Laryngol 75:961, 1966

2. Arey LB: *Developmental Anatomy*, ed 5, Philadelphia and London, W B Saunders Company, 1946, p 385

3. Blumberg JB, Stevenson JK, Lamire RJ, *et al*: Laryngotracheoesophageal cleft: The embryologic implications. Review of the literature. Surgery 57:559, 1965

4. Streeter GL: Developmental horizons in human embryos; Descriptions of age group XIII, embryos about 4 or 5 mm. long, and age group XIV, period of indentation of the lens vesicle. Contributions to Embryology 31: 27, 1945

5. Streeter GL: Developmental horizons in human embryos: Description of age groups XV, XVI, XVII, and XVIII. Contributions to Embryology 32:133, 1948

6. Mahour GH, Cohen SR, Wooley MM: Laryngotracheoesophageal cleft associated with esophageal atresia and multiple tracheoesophageal fistulas in a twin. J Thorac Cardiovasc Surg 65: No. 2:223, 1973

COSMETIC SURGERY OF THE NOSE AND FACE

The First Panamerican Course of Cosmetic Surgery of the Nose and Face, sponsored by the Panamerican Association of Otolaryngology will be held February 12-17, 1976 at the Intercontinental Hotel, Medellin, Colombia, South America. For further information write: Dr. Jaime Florez, 4220 Central Ave., St. Petersburg, Florida 33711.

Ann Otol 84: 1975

NONTRAUMATIC, NONNEOPLASTIC SUBGLOTTIC STENOSIS

MOHSEN DJALILIAN, M.D.
THOMAS J. MCDONALD, M.D. KENNETH D. DEVINE, M.D.
LOUIS H. WEILAND, M.D.
ROCHESTER, MINNESOTA

SUMMARY – During a 20-year period, 12 patients with nontraumatic, nonneoplastic subglottic stenosis were seen at the Mayo Clinic. The etiologic factors were relapsing polychondritis, amyloidosis, sarcoidosis, and Wegener's granulomatosis. Because of the diverse initial presentation of the disease, the clinician should consider that the stenosis is a manifestation of a systemic disorder and carry out an otolaryngologic and physical examination with the appropriate roentgenograms and blood and urine tests. Treatment, if a systemic disease is proved, consists of appropriate medication. Surgery may be necessary, depending on the nature of the lesion. Small strictures may not need to be treated.

Subglottic stenosis can be defined as any narrowing of the subglottic area. Its most common cause is use of cuffed tracheotomy tubes. Less common causes are external trauma to the larynx (for example, in automobile accidents), a high tracheotomy incision, and congenital stenosis, as in infants. Subglottic stenosis can also result from extension of neoplastic disease from other sites to the subglottic area.[1]

But what of subglottic stenosis in the adult or adolescent without preceding trauma? The diagnosis in such cases may be perplexing, and treatment is often difficult. The purpose of this report is to describe 12 cases of nontraumatic, nonneoplastic subglottic stenosis recorded during the last 20 years. The etiologic factors were: 1) relapsing polychondritis; 2) amyloidosis; 3) sarcoidosis; and 4) Wegener's granulomatosis. Features of each condition are illustrated in the case reports that form the basis of this report.

CASE REPORTS

RELAPSING POLYCHONDRITIS

Case 1. A 47-year-old female presented at the Mayo Clinic with a history of increasing shortness of breath for about 18 months. She stated that she had undergone bronchoscopy elsewhere and that her breathing had temporarily become easier. At the Mayo Clinic, indirect laryngoscopy revealed subglottic stenosis with mobile vocal cords, confirmed by tracheal tomograms. A saddle-nose deformity was noted. Results of screening blood tests, including serologic studies, were normal; the erythrocyte sedimentation rate (ESR) was 36 mm in 1 hour (Westergren). Tracheotomy followed by laryngoscopy was then performed. A 7 mm bronchoscope was passed through the area of subglottic stenosis, the diameter of which was 6 mm. The trachea below the stenotic area was normal. Representative biopsies were taken, and the area was injected with 1 ml of triamcinolone. Histopathologic examination produced evidence of chronic subepithelial inflammation with fibrosis. At follow-up examination 3 months later, the area of stenosis was found to be much smaller. At her next visit, 3 months later, she was again dyspneic, and recurrence of the stenosis was noted. She has continued to require a tracheotomy.

Case 2. A 26-year-old male had a two-year history of respiratory distress. Cortisone, given before he was seen at the Mayo Clinic, had given him no relief. His past history included intermittent episodes of conjunctivitis since childhood, particularly on the right side. Ophthalmic examination showed that his vision was normal, but chronic marginal corneal degeneration was noted bilaterally. Rhinolaryn-

From the Mayo Clinic and Mayo Foundation, Rochester, Minnesota.
Presented at the meeting of the American Laryngological Association, Atlanta, Georgia, April 6-7, 1975.

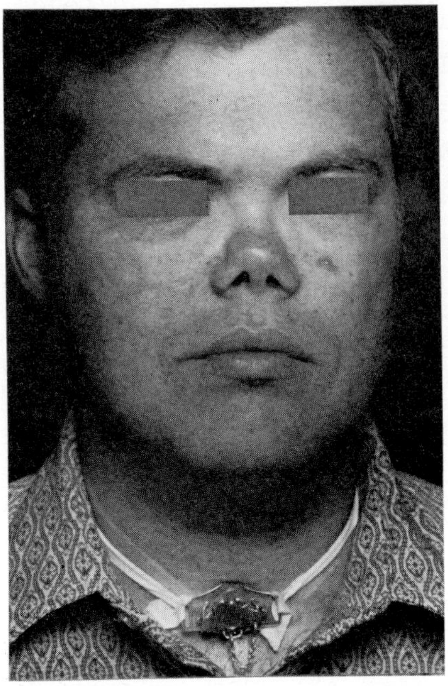

Fig. 1 (Case 2). Relapsing polychondritis. Note saddle-nose deformity and valved speaking tube.

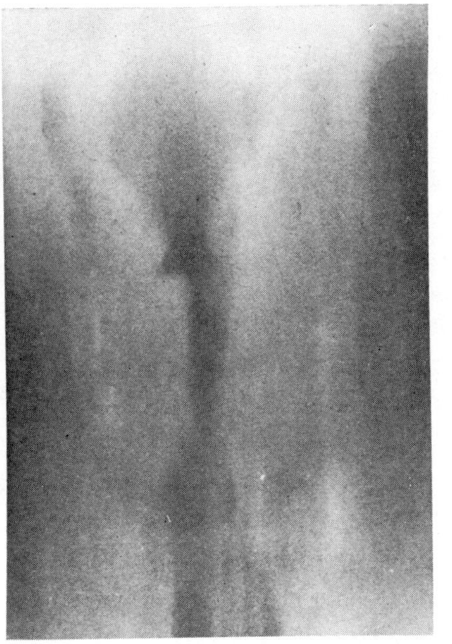

Fig. 2 (Case 2). Relapsing polychondritis. Note long area of subglottic narrowing.

gologic examination revealed a saddle deformity of the nose (Fig. 1) with mucosal crusting and, on indirect laryngoscopy, normal vocal cords with a narrowing of the subglottic area. Tracheal tomograms confirmed subglottic stenosis (Fig. 2). Results of screening blood tests, including serologic studies, and the ESR were normal. Direct laryngoscopy and bronchoscopy were followed by biopsy of the stenotic area; a mild, nonspecific fibroblastic reaction was reported. A speaking tracheotomy tube was inserted five days later; the portion of tracheal cartilage removed during this procedure disclosed inflammatory changes. The speaking tube was tolerated well.

Case 3. A 55-year-old female presented at the Mayo Clinic with recent progressive respiratory obstruction. A general medical examination revealed no abnormalities except a saddle-nose deformity, and results of screening blood tests, including serologic studies, and the ESR were normal. Indirect laryngoscopy showed subglottic stenosis, the upper limit of which was detected 1 cm below the true vocal cords; overall, the subglottic area was narrowed to about 4 mm. Tomograms of the trachea confirmed the subglottic narrowing. When she underwent tracheotomy and thyrotomy four months later, the stricture, at the level of the cricoid ring, was found to be formed chiefly by a band of scar supported by thick fibrous tissue on the posterior wall of the trachea; the 4 mm width of the subglottis noted earlier was confirmed. The scar tissue was removed and the denuded area (4 by 3 cm) was covered with a skin graft around a sponge rubber stent. This was removed by laryngoscopy, and decannulation three weeks later was easy. The airway since has been good.

Case 4. A 17-year-old male had noted a slowly progressive voice change and dyspnea on exertion for one year. Examination showed a saddle-nose deformity, a deformity of each external ear, and a dish-shaped deformity of the sternum. Tracheal tomograms showed narrowing from a point 2 cm below the true vocal cords to about the level of the clavicle. At the narrowest point, the diameter was about 6 mm. Results of screening blood tests, including serologic studies, and the ESR were normal. The larynx and subglottic region were opened through a vertical midline incision. The cricoid ring was incised and the cartilage outfractured in order to enlarge the airway. The new aperture was then skin grafted. Follow-up examination revealed much improved exercise tolerance and a good airway.

COMMENT

We believe that the lesions in these four patients were those of the quiescent phase of relapsing polychondritis. The term "relapsing polychondritis" was coined by Pearson, et al[2] in 1960, though

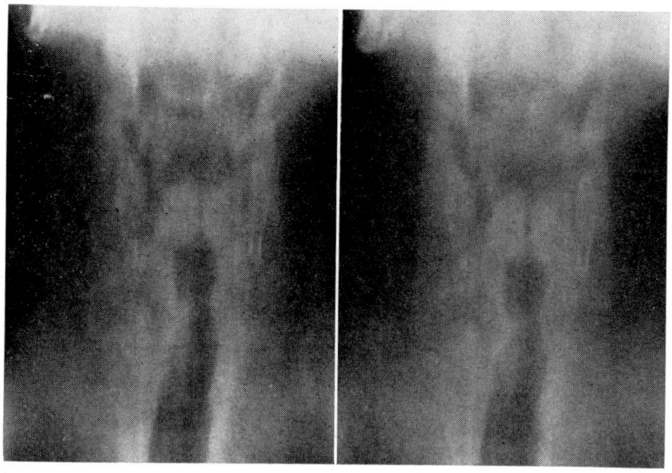

Fig. 3 (Case 5). Amyloidosis. Note focal narrowing of trachea about 3 cm below glottis.

Jaksch-Wartenhorst[3] in 1923 had described a condition, termed "polychrondropathy" by him, that was characterized by inflammatory changes in cartilages in different anatomic sites. Clinically, the usual sites of involvement are the cartilages of the external ear, the nasal septal cartilages, the larynx, and the tracheal bronchial tree. Cartilaginous involvement may occur simultaneously or at different times.

Even more interesting from an otolaryngologist's point of view are the audiovestibular manifestations of relapsing polychondritis. Daly[4] described these in one patient, and Cody and Sones[5] reviewed the records of 40 patients seen at the Mayo Clinic with relapsing polychondritis, among whom 11 had hearing loss due to the disease itself. The hearing loss may be either conductive or sensorineural.

The clinical picture in the acute phase is characterized by pain, swelling, redness, and tenderness of the external ear. The acute audiovestibular manifestations are those of tinnitus and dizziness; these are similar to the manifestations of endolymphatic hydrops of Ménière's disease or of Cogan's syndrome. With nasal involvement, the acute symptoms are pain, swelling, redness, and tenderness of the nose. Involvement of the tracheobronchial tree can lead to acute narrowing of the trachea with airway obstruction and possibly death. Ocular manifestations may also occur, including iritis, conjunctivitis, scleritis, and episcleritis.[6]

PATHOLOGY

Typically, inflammation causes fragmentation of the cartilage owing to necrosis and chondrolysis. In some areas, cartilage is separated by inflammatory cells; in others, cartilage is replaced by fibrous connective tissue.[7]

TREATMENT

In the acute phase, corticosteroids are of value; they may even be life saving, especially in cases with involvement of the tracheobronchial tree. Surgical intervention by "coring out" of the stenosed area and lining the area with skin or dilating it may or may not be necessary, depending on the degree of obstruction. A valved speaking tracheotomy tube is a useful compromise for those patients who do not want to undergo an operative procedure.

AMYLOIDOSIS

Case 5. A 54-year-old male complained of recurrent "colds" and progressive malaise. Despite normal results of a clinical otolaryngologic examination, tomograms of the trachea showed focal narrowing of the upper trachea at a point about 3 cm below the vocal cords (Fig. 3). Bronchoscopic examination revealed a subglottic mass that, on biopsy, proved to be amyloid. Results of the general medical examination were normal and a rectal biopsy was negative for amyloid tissue. He did not require a tracheotomy.

Case 6. A 49-year-old female had a one-year history of hoarseness. She had recently complained of dysphagia and hemoptysis. Indirect laryngoscopy revealed subglottic and upper tracheal stenosis. Results of screening blood tests, including serologic studies, and the ESR were normal. Tomograms of the larynx and trachea showed localized narrowing in the subglottic area. Biopsy showed amyloidosis. Coring out of as much tissue as possible at the center of the mass resulted in a good airway and improvement in the voice.

COMMENT

The term "amyloid" (starchlike) was coined by Virchow, who noted that amyloid treated by iodine and sulfuric acid turned blue-black, as did starch. The respiratory tract is the most common part of the body to be affected by localized amyloidosis; in the respiratory tract, the larynx is the most frequent site. The disease occurs most commonly in the fifth, sixth, and seventh decades of life, and men are afflicted more frequently than women (ratio, 2:1). Symmers[8] classified amyloidosis clinicopathologically as follows: 1) primary systemic amyloidosis not associated with known predisposing factors and affecting the heart, tongue, larynx, and skin; 2) generalized secondary amyloidosis usually associated with a predisposing disease, such as tuberculosis or lung abscess with empyema; 3) localized tumor-forming amyloid; and 4) amyloidosis associated with multiple myeloma.

In the larynx, the most common sites of amyloidosis are the ventricles, the false cords, the aryepiglottic fold, and the subglottic area, in that order.[9] The treatment of amyloidosis consists of removing the amyloid tumor if it causes obstruction. Although localized amyloid tumors are rarely associated with plasma-cell dyscrasias, the appropriate studies probably should be done to exclude multiple myeloma or solitary myeloma.

SARCOIDOSIS

Case 7. A 55-year-old male had a history of stridor. Indirect laryngoscopy revealed a smooth, slightly reddened symmetric bulge in the subglottic area. Biopsy material, taken after a tracheotomy had been performed, revealed inflammatory tissue only. Five months later, the larynx was explored through a thyrotomy incision; the subglottic thickening was excised, and a skin graft was applied to the denuded area. Pathologic examination of the excised tissue disclosed noncaseous granuloma consistent with sarcoidosis. Cultures for microorganism were negative. Decannulation later was easy; the airway was good. He died in 1958 with carcinoma of the kidney.

COMMENT

In this patient, biopsy on several occasions did not reveal the granulomatous nature of the disease in the larynx. It was not until the subglottic thickening was removed at an open operation that the true nature of the lesion in the subglottis became known. If this problem had been known before the open operation, intralaryngeal injection of cortisone acetate perhaps would have made thyrotomy and skin grafting unnecessary.[10] Judging from experience in this case, it is probably safe to excise as much of the offending tissue as necessary in order to improve the airway without fear that the operation will exacerbate the local disease.

WEGENER'S GRANULOMATOSIS

Case 8. A 45-year-old female gave a history of nasal obstruction for approximately three years. She had more recently complained of midfacial pain associated with nasal obstruction and bloody nasal drainage. Intranasal examination revealed crusting and granulation. Laboratory findings included the following: ESR, 80 mm in 1 hour (Westergren); hematuria; proteinuria, grade 3; and a normal chest roentgenogram. The histologic features of nasal biopsy material were consistent with those of Wegener's granulomatosis. She was treated with prednisone and cyclophosphamide and improved until she again presented with stridor three months later. Tomograms of the larynx showed definite narrowing of the upper trachea and subglottic area (Fig. 4). Direct laryngoscopy confirmed subglottic stenosis. Examination of the biopsy material revealed inflammatory tissue only. Her trachea was dilated at the same time and the condition of her airway was satisfactory thereafter. Therapy with

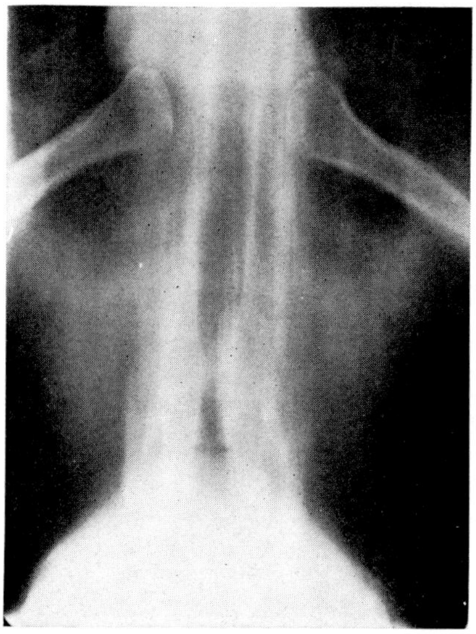

Fig. 4 (Case 8). Wegener's granulomatosis. Note narrowing of upper tracheal and subglottic areas.

cyclophosphamide and prednisone was continued; currently, she is doing well.

Case 9. A 50-year-old female required tracheotomy for upper airway obstruction. During a fissure operation, an ulcerative lesion involving the posterior two-thirds of the circumference of the trachea was excised; this lesion proved to consist of fibrous tissue only. The area was skin grafted, with a good result. At that time the ESR was 120 mm in 1 hour (Westergren), and hematuria was detected. Nearly two years later, she again presented with nasal pain, redness over the nasal dorsum, and nasal drainage but no diagnosis was then made. Then, six years later, she was found to have hemoptysis associated with a lesion in the right lung and also a nasal septal perforation with marked nasal atrophy and intranasal crusting. The diagnosis of Wegener's granulomatosis was made at that time by biopsy. The disease is currently controlled with steroids; the airway is satisfactory and the subglottis appears normal.

Case 10. A 53-year-old female had a five-year history of nasal crusting. Examination revealed an external saddle deformity, a large anterior cartilaginous septal perforation, and atrophy of both middle turbinates. Results of serologic studies were normal, as were the ESR and chest roentgenogram. She had noticed recent upper airway obstruction and she did have some degree of stridor. Indirect laryngoscopy revealed bulging of the tracheal wall below the cords with some impairment of the airway. Tomograms of the larynx and upper trachea showed no abnormalities. Laryngoscopy revealed extreme narrowing of the airway; it was almost impossible to pass an endotracheal tube through the subglottic region. The narrowing was due to a weblike thickening in the anterior subglottic region, a little more on the left than the right. The pink overlying mucosa was intact. Biopsied tissue consisted of inflammatory fibrosis only. Numerous pieces of tissue were also taken from the ethmoid area on both sides, around the septal perforation, and from the right maxillary antrum; histologic features of this tissue were consistent with those of Wegener's granulomatosis. Tracheostomy was unnecessary and no further treatment was started.

Case 11. A 24-year-old female, who was seen at the Mayo Clinic in 1973, had a history of removal of a left pseudotumor from the left orbit at the age of seven years, in 1956. In 1968 she had noticed the onset of dyspnea, which by 1970 had progressed to the point of acute airway obstruction that necessitated a tracheotomy, on which she continues to rely. Five repeated laryngoscopies had been done elsewhere and a biopsy report suggested the diagnosis of Wegener's granulomatosis. She had been treated with steroids and cyclophosphamide; she was receiving the latter when she presented at the Mayo Clinic.

Case 12. A 31-year-old female presented at the Mayo Clinic in 1972 with the following history: In 1956 a pseudotumor had been removed from the left orbit; she was treated with cortisone acetate. In 1960, the left eye was enucleated. She then had no symptoms for ten years when a pseudotumor developed in the right eye. The biopsy report on tissue taken from the right eye suggested the diagnosis of Wegener's granulomatosis. She was again treated with steroids. She was first seen in the Department of Otorhinolaryngology in 1970 with intranasal mucosal crusting, scales, and granulation tissue; the biopsy report gave a diagnosis of Wegener's granulomatosis. In 1972, she presented with a history of recurrent swelling of the right eye; at this point, she had stridor with hemoptysis. Indirect laryngoscopy revealed subglottic narrowing with a dry, crusty-looking subglottic mucosa. Narrowing was also revealed by tomograms (Fig. 5). Because of the adequacy of the airway, however, no biopsy was done and no treatment was considered necessary. She is now being observed for the diminishing vision in her remaining right eye.

COMMENT

These five patients with Wegener's granulomatosis who also had subglottic stenosis are part of a larger group of 52 patients with Wegener's granulomatosis seen at the Mayo Clinic whose cases were recently reported.[11]

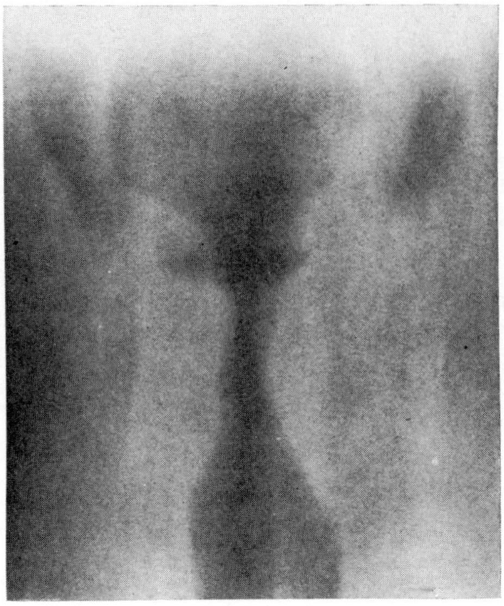

Fig. 5 (Case 12). Wegener's granulomatosis. Note subglottic narrowing.

PATHOLOGY

Wegener described the entity known as Wegener's granulomatosis in 1936[12] and again in 1939.[13] It has since been identified as a disease characterized by necrotizing granulomas and vasculitis of the upper and lower respiratory tract, focal necrotizing glomerulonephritis, and systemic angiitis. Among those patients who constituted the recent Mayo Clinic series, some were found to have necrotizing granulomas and vasculitis involving the respiratory tract, but without evidence of nephritis, and still others may have no evidence of involvement of the respiratory tract. This form of nonsystemic or localized Wegener's granulomatosis has been reported previously.[14] Among the 52 patients whose records were reviewed, 31 patients had nasal lesions, either alone or in combination with other sites. The five patients with subglottic stenosis whose cases are described in the present report are among these 31 patients with nasal involvement.

Despite the finding of only fibrous tissue on biopsy from the subglottic area in these five patients, it is reasonable to speculate that the fibrous tissue actually represents the end result of an inflammatory lesion as part of Wegener's granulomatosis possibly modified by previous treatment. If any of these five patients could have been seen in a so-called acute phase, biopsy at that time might well have revealed the evidence of vasculitis and necrotizing granulomas.

TREATMENT

Wegener's granulomatosis is a treatable disorder; steroids with or without cyclophosphamide are the treatment of choice. Since airway involvement is common, it is essential that the otolaryngologist remain alert to the possibility of this condition, because favorable prognosis depends on early recognition and treatment.

DISCUSSION

Much remains to be learned about connective tissue disorders. Despite recent and promising advances, we still do not understand the phenomena precipitating the complex biochemical, immunologic, and anatomic changes that manifest as these diseases. Initially, these diseases may present with signs and symptoms that mimic numerous otolaryngologic disorders. For instance, one of our patients who proved to have amyloidosis complained of recurrent head colds and another patient complained of a voice change. The initial symptom of one of our patients with proved Wegener's disease was unilateral proptosis. Moreover, all of the 31 patients with nasal involvement who constituted part of the group of 52 patients with Wegener's disease reported on recently[10] had "nasal obstruction" as the first and insidious symptom.

The clinician's obligation, therefore, when faced by a patient with subglottic stenosis of nonneoplastic, nontraumatic origin is to consider the stenosis as a possible manifestation of a systemic disorder. Consequently, a careful otolaryngologic examination is followed by a general examination, together with various investigations including chest and tracheal roentgenograms, a complete blood count, ESR, serologic studies, serum creatinine concentration, and urinalysis. Endoscopic examination of the larynx and trachea with biopsy then follows.

With respect to treatment, if systemic disease is proved, appropriate medication is initiated. The surgical management of the obstructed trachea depends not only on the nature of the lesion but also on the patient's wishes. For example, one of the patients with probable polychondritis elected to have the speaking tracheotomy tube rather than an operation.

For small strictures with adequate airway, treatment may not be necessary. For others, endoscopic dilatation may suffice. The "coring out" of a long stenotic area followed by a skin graft is very successful and has advantages over resection and end-to-end anastomosis.

Request for reprints should be sent to Thomas J. McDonald, M.D., Mayo Clinic and Mayo Foundation, Rochester, Minnesota 55901.

REFERENCES

1. Djalilian M, Beahrs OH, Devine KD, *et al*: Intraluminal involvement of the larynx and trachea by thyroid cancer. Am J Surg 128:500-504, 1974

2. Pearson CM, Kline HM, Newcomer VD: Relapsing polychondritis. N Engl J Med 263:51-58, 1960

3. Jaksch-Wartenhorst R: Polychondropathia. Wien Z Inn Med 6:93-100, 1923

4. Daly JF: Relapsing polychondritis of the larynx and trachea. Arch Otolaryngol 84: 570-573, 1966

5. Cody DTR, Sones DA: Relapsing polychondritis: audiovestibular manifestations. Laryngoscope 81:1208-1222, 1971

6. Purcelli FM, Nahum A, Monell C: Relapsing polychondritis with tracheal collapse. Ann Otol Rhinol Laryngol 71:1120-1129, 1962

7. Kaye RL, Sones DA: Relapsing polychondritis: clinical and pathologic features in fourteen cases. Ann Intern Med 60:653-664, 1964

8. Symmers WSC: Primary amyloidosis: a review. J Clin Pathol 9:187-211, 1956

9. Leroux RJ: Tumeurs amyloides du larynx. Ann Otolaryngol Chir Cervicofac 79: 249-270, 1962

10. Devine KD: Sarcoidosis and sarcoidosis of the larynx. Laryngoscope 75:533-569, 1965

11. McDonald TJ, DeRemee RA, Kern EB, *et al*: Nasal manifestations of Wegener's granulomatosis. Laryngoscope 84:2101-2112, 1974

12. Wegener F: Über generalisierte, septische Gefässerkrakungen. Verh Dtsch Ges Pathol 29:202-210, 1936

13. Wegener F: Über eine eigenartige rhinogene Granulomatose mit besonderer Beteiligung des Arteriensystems und der Nieren. Beitr Pathol 102:36-68, 1939

14. Carrington CB, Liebow AA: Limited forms of angiitis and granulomatosis of Wegener's type. Am J Med 41:497-527, 1966

COURSE IN NEUROTOLOGY

The Department of Otolaryngology of the Abraham Lincoln School of Medicine and the University of Illinois Hospital Eye and Ear Infirmary, University of Illinois at the Medical Center, will conduct a continuing education course in Neurotology, March 22-25, 1976.

The four day intensive course will offer a didactic and practical review of clinical neurotology under the direction of Nicholas Torok, M.D. It will be held at the Eye and Ear Infirmary and will include basic vestibular physiology and pathophysiology, commonly used testing methods applied in functional examination of the vestibular organ.

Enrollment is limited to 15. For application forms write: Department of Otolaryngology, 1855 West Taylor Street, Chicago.

Ann Otol 84: 1975

INJURIES TO THE NEONATAL LARYNX FROM LONG-TERM ENDOTRACHEAL TUBE INTUBATION AND SUGGESTED TUBE MODIFICATION FOR PREVENTION

ARTHUR S. HENGERER, M.D.
ROCHESTER, NEW YORK

MARSHALL STROME, M.D. BURTON F. JAFFE, M.D.
BOSTON, MASSACHUSETTS

SUMMARY – Since the early 1960's nasotracheal tubes have been used for neonates with primary respiratory diseases which necessitated positive pressure ventilation. This therapy may be required for extended periods of weeks to months meaning prolonged trauma to the neonatal larynx. The initial injury and long-term effects of the endotracheal tube in this age group have not been adequately investigated. The acute findings can be arytenoid and posterior commissure ulcerations and, in some cases, cartilage erosion. Long-term follow-up in these children to age 3.5 years showed a persistent arytenoid defect with chronic hoarseness. The consideration of a change in the structure of the endotracheal tube is suggested as a possible means of avoiding these injuries.

The first reported use of the endotracheal tube was by McEwen in 1880.[1] Since then its use in anesthesia and for support in airway problems has become common. One group of patients who require intubation are the premature infants born with respiratory distress syndrome. They require assisted ventilation with positive end expiratory pressure (PEEP) to maintain adequate respiratory function. It is the purpose of this paper to discuss the acute injuries that result from the prolonged intubation in this neonatal group and to report on the chronic changes that persist in some of the surviving children.

METHODS AND MATERIALS

A group of 17 newborns admitted to the neonatal division of the Children's Hospital Medical Center in Boston for treatment of respiratory distress were used in this clinical study. A period of nasotracheal intubation for the administration of positive pressure breathing was the only criterion used for inclusion in the study. In all cases 2.5 or 3.0 mm Portex tubes of the Magill shape were inserted, with no trauma, into the larynx. All the infants were classified as premature and suffered from respiratory distress syndrome. In addition, some had associated medical disorders.

Once a child was included in the study, he was followed until his discharge or death. After extubation, if any hoarseness persisted more than 24 hours, permission for a direct laryngoscopy without anesthesia was requested to assess the glottic and subglottic areas for injuries.

Three children with chronic hoarseness, who had required the above treatment regimen and were now one, two, and three and one-half years of age, underwent direct laryngoscopy to document the long-term changes.

The larynx from each child who expired and underwent an autopsy was removed and examined. The arytenoid cartilages were later removed and studied, using the dissection microscope.

From the University of Rochester School of Medicine, Rochester, New York, and Harvard Medical School, Boston, Massachusetts.

Presented at the meeting of the American Laryngological Association, Atlanta, Georgia, April 6-7, 1975.

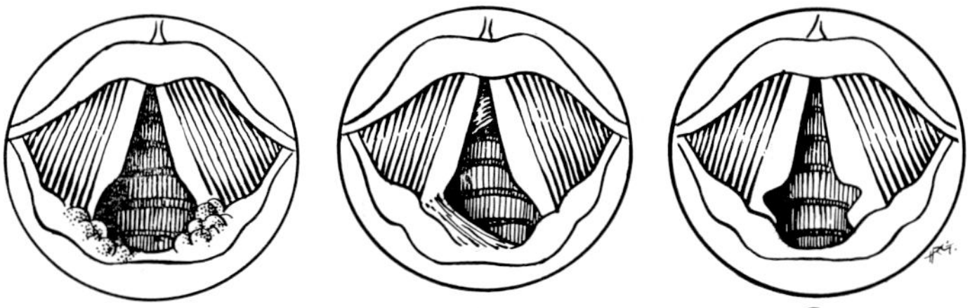

Fig. 1. Laryngeal findings of three patients in Group III: A) M.R. B) A.L. C) J.R.

RESULTS

The group of 17 infants can be separated into three distinct categories:

I. *Surviving Short-Term Intubations.* Five children were intubated for six days or less and when they were extubated had normal cries within 24 hours. Direct laryngoscopies were performed on three of these infants who had been intubated for three days and no abnormalities were found in the larynx.

II. *Surviving Long-Term Intubations.* This group is comprised of six infants who are survivors of long-term intubations. They are the most important subgroup in this study since four of these children manifest chronic laryngeal changes and hoarseness as a result of the treatment.

The first infant (M.R.) had Respiratory Distress Syndrome (RDS) and later manifested bronchopulmonary dysplasia which required intubation for 57 days with PEEP being used for 55 days. Aphonia was present for four days after extubation before he gradually developed a weak, hoarse cry that persisted until the time of a direct laryngoscopy at 2½ months of age (*i.e.*, 3 weeks after extubation). The operative findings showed granulations over the arytenoids with notching of the medial surface of the right arytenoid. There was fixation of the left true vocal cord from limited movement in the left cricoarytenoid joint. The subglottic area was normal (Fig. 1A). This child is now ten months of age and persists with a breathy cry that is slightly stronger than when he was examined.

The second infant (B.B.D.) with RDS is now six months old and was intubated for assisted ventilation with PEEP for a total of 38 days. Following extubation he required intermittent short term intubations for persistent bronchopulmonary dysplasia that has required continuous hospitalization. His cry following extubation was moderately hoarse but has been gradually improving in strength. A direct exam was performed at 5½ months of age after his pulmonary condition had stabilized. However, only a brief exam was possible without anesthesia because of rapidly developing cyanosis secondary to his pulmonary disease. The findings showed a normal larynx with mobile vocal cords and no arytenoid notching or granulation tissue. No anatomic cause for his hoarseness was found and further assessment was deferred.

The third child (A.L.) is 13 months old and required intubation for 44 days with PEEP for RDS and a patent ductus arteriosus that was ligated. When she was extubated, she remained aphonic for two days before a weak breathy cry developed. The child was discharged from the hospital, however, before a direct exam could be performed. After one year her voice remained weak and breathy, and a direct laryngoscopy under general anesthesia was recommended. The exam revealed bilateral arytenoid vocal process erosion giving the appearance of bowing of the posterior half of the true cords, resulting in incomplete glottic closure on adduction and phonation. There was decreased motion of the right true vocal cord with no cricoarytenoid joint fixation, and a scar band that extended across the posterior commissure to join the left vocal process. In the subglottic area a thin fibrous band had formed on the anterior wall (Fig. 1B).

The fourth patient (J.R.) is now 3½ years old. At birth he had RDS which required a nasotracheal tube for 27 days for assisted ventilation. When extubated he was severely hoarse, but no direct laryngoscopy was performed. Since then he has had a slow growth and development and his voice remained breathy without signs of improvement. For this reason a direct laryngoscopy was performed under general anesthesia. The exam revealed marked grooving of the medial surfaces of both the vocal processes from previous cartilage erosion, allowing significant air escape with the cords in full adduction. The anterior commissure and membranous true cords plus the subglottic area were normal as was the cord motion (Fig. 1C).

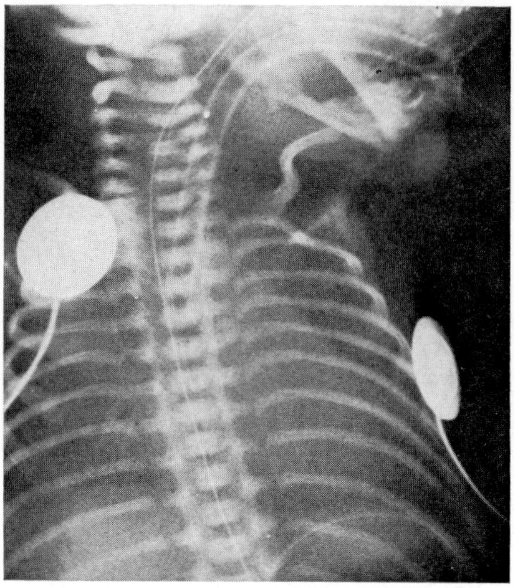

Fig. 2. X-ray of patient in supine position demonstrating lack of tube flexibility in laryngeal region.

The other two patients in this group were intubated for 15 days, respectively, and both had mild hoarseness when extubated. Now both are 18 months old, and one continues with mild inspiratory and expiratory stridor that is gradually improving. The second child is now asymptomatic. Neither of the children was examined, as their findings were disappearing with increasing age. This has been the usual finding in other studies regarding post-extubation hoarseness.

III. *Nonsurviving Intubations.* The remaining six children in the study expired during the neonatal period while still intubated and receiving assisted ventilation. Postmortem exams were performed on three of these patients, with the larynx removed for gross and microscopic examination. The first specimen was from a one-day-old infant intubated for 22 hours before death. The larynx showed no ulceration or erosion of the arytenoid vocal processes grossly, and minimal edema and reaction on microscopic sections.

The remaining two laryngeal specimens were from patients intubated 8 and 54 days, respectively. Grossly, both showed ulceration of the mucosa over the vocal processes and exposed cartilage which was grooved by erosion from the tube. The resulting glottic defect this created was the same found and described in the survivors. Further exam and dissection of the larynx with the operating microscope revealed that the cricoarytenoid joints had not fibrosed but remained freely mobile and normal. No microscopic sections of the cartilages were obtained as these changes have been well documented.

The three remaining cases had no autopsy; thus, findings could not be established.

DISCUSSION

During the past ten years the methods and knowledge of the neonatologists treating RDS have resulted in an increasing number of healthy, surviving infants, including the low birth weight group.[2,3] The usual criteria for using positive pressure ventilation in the treatment are a Pa02 of less than 40 mm Hg in 100% oxygen and/or apnea or slow gasping inadequate respirations. In order to deliver the assisted ventilation, the uniform method has become tracheal intubation with a thin walled Portex tube either by the nasal or oral passage. Initially, tracheotomy is not used or recommended.

Once intubation is required, the treatment regimen follows a program outlined in neonatal texts to maintain normal blood gases and pH. The endotracheal tubes require changing about twice weekly to maintain a secretion free lumen, which can usually be carried out with a minimum of laryngeal trauma.

At this hospital, intubation continues until pulmonary function warrants tube removal. There were no long-term intubations who were considered for a tracheotomy to replace the tube. As a result the length of intubation via the nasotracheal route varied from 1 to 57 days in these 17 patients. In adults, as the duration of intubation increases, the potential for problems in the glottic and subglottic areas rises. Previous studies in the adult have shown that intubation for 48-72 hours is usually tolerated without significant tissue damage to the larynx, after which the significance of vocal cord ulcerations, granulomas, webs, or stricture formation of the glottic and subglottic areas increase.[4-6] Thus, the usual practice is conversion to a tracheotomy for continued airway assistance after 72 hours.

The neonatal larynx responds differently to the effects of intubation as compared to the adult larynx and, as a result, the recommended duration of neonatal intubation can be extended. The neonate is often intubated for periods of up to one week with no significant findings of laryngeal injuries. However, this initial seven days may represent only the first stage of an intubation that may last many weeks as occurred in the cases presented. It is in these patients with prolonged laryngeal irritation that the consequences of intubation can become manifest. At present no definite length of time for the development of the laryngeal injuries with persisting hoarseness has been determined, as in adults.[3,6-9] The pediatric literature in general states that hoarseness immediately postextubation is associated with a normal direct laryngoscopy and virtually all the patients will have a normal cry by one month following extubation. This has not been the finding in the long-term intubations reported here.

It has been well established in the examination of postmortem specimens by Clement[10] and animal studies by Way[8] that the endotracheal tube rests in the posterior commissure of the glottis. The continuous pressure and tube movement due to PEEP and head motion causes changes to occur in the tissue of that area. The most marked finding has been ulceration and erosion of the medial surface of the arytenoid vocal process. There also may be thickening and granulation tissue formation of the interarytenoid region. It has been our experience with pathologic specimens, as well as surviving patients, that these changes occur in a significant number of neonates and do not always resolve completely as previously suggested.

The patients presented who remained hoarse after one year had significant laryngeal changes resulting from the neonatal period. These chronic changes as previously mentioned are located primarily in the posterior commissure and arytenoid region. In the four children with persistent hoarseness from six months to 3½ years postextubation, the consistent finding has been the residual grooving defect of the vocal process, leaving an incomplete glottic closure. One of these patients also had unilateral vocal cord paralysis with a mobile arytenoid, and another had unilateral arytenoid fixation. Both these problems were thought to be due to the prolonged intubation, but a congenital anomaly is still a possible explanation.

Although there was gradual improvement in the cry and voice production with increasing age, it was not completely normal in any of the long-term follow-ups that had been aphonic or severely hoarse at extubation. Thus, it appears that the degree of hoarseness at extubation may be an indication of the present damage and the future rate of recovery. If the patient is aphonic when extubated, the chance of finding significant laryngeal changes and long-term hoarseness is likely. Milder degrees of hoarseness show no significant laryngeal changes and tend to have faster and complete recovery. However, the duration of the intubation cannot be used as the lone indicator of what the eventual degree of injury and resulting voice production will be. The patient now 3½ years old who was intubated for 27 days still has a breathy voice with poor volume, while another intubated 38 days had less severe hoarseness at extubation and is showing steady improvement. In one study[6] of 57 infants (with 19 intubated longer than 72 hours), normal cries were present in all by one month postextubation although no mention was made of the sound of their cries initially. Another article[3] reported 2 of the 22 patients who were intubated for 11 and 45 days, respectively, were aphonic at extubation. Both these patients had direct laryngoscopy performed while neonates and the operative findings were reported as normal. Their hoarse-

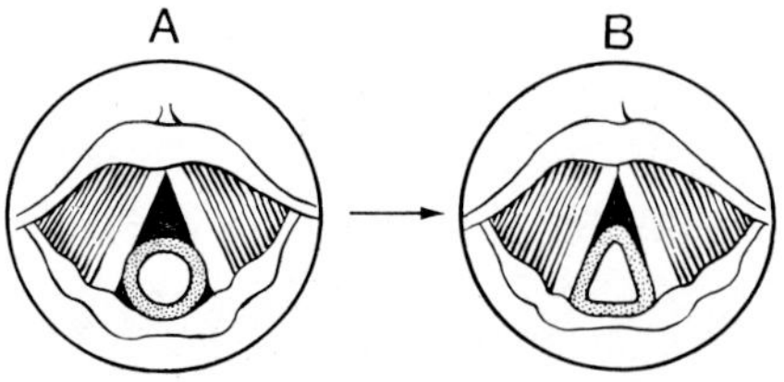

Fig. 3. Illustration of suggested tube change to decrease arytenoid pressure and ulceration.

ness had gradually cleared over a four-year period although the report did not say they now had normal voices. It is too early to say whether the group of patients we have followed will have the same successful recovery rate when they were aphonic or severely hoarse at extubation. The findings indicate that unless aphonia exists at extubation a direct laryngoscopy is not necessary, and the likelihood of a normal voice before one year of age can be anticipated. If aphonia is present after extubation, a direct exam should be performed when convenient to document the expected arytenoid changes so that the family can be advised that long-term voice problems are likely.

The complications from endotracheal tubes has been extensively analyzed, and the following causal factors were found: 1) The tube used has a gradually curving shape known as the Magill Design. This shape results in significant pressure on the posterior commissure from the weight of the tongue resting on the tube. Neck flexion also increases the posterior coiling of the tube against the posterior glottis in the supine patient. The tube wall stiffness can decrease the ability of the tube to bend and conform to the natural curves of the hypopharynx and larynx adding additional pressure (Fig. 2). 2) The posterior commissure and arytenoid area is a triangular anatomic space that is filled with a round tube. This inappropriate matching of shapes subjects several areas in the larynx to injury, especially the vocal processes of the arytenoids and the midline of the posterior commissure (Fig. 3). This effect is verified by the round grooves found in

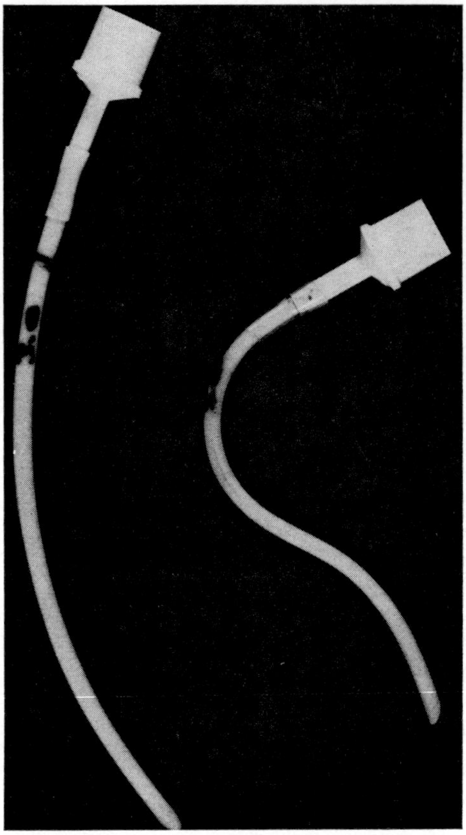

Fig. 4. Portex uncuffed endotracheal tubes, 3.0 mm. Left: Magill design in common use. Right: same tube with constant reverse curve alteration.

the vocal processes that lead to the incomplete glottic closure and breathy voice. 3) The usual method used in choosing the tube size may cause a problem. The size selected must easily pass through the glottis or be one size smaller in hopes of decreasing the degree of pressure.[11] The size of the tube has definitely been shown to influence the inflammation and eventual arytenoid ulceration.[8] However, in clinical practice the neonates usually require PEEP, and the resulting positive pressure is more effective if a fairly tight seal is created at the glottis. This is easily obtained by inserting a slightly larger tube than needed, which enhances the possibilities for irritation and ulceration.

These factors have led to the consideration of making two alterations in the shape of the present endotracheal tubes: 1) Change the shape of the tube from round to triangular over a 2 cm length that passes through the larynx, in an attempt to decrease the grooving of the vocal process. This change can be added to the present Magill design without affecting the ease of intubation or significantly decreasing the airway. 2) Add a reverse curve to the tracheal end of the present Magill tubes as described by Clement, *et al* in 1949[10] (Fig. 4). This change will permit the tube to conform more easily to the usual anatomic shape of the hypopharynx, thus resulting in less posterior laryngeal pressure that creates the chronic glottic defects. The latter alteration does have a drawback in that a stylet will be needed for insertion, making the intubation more difficult and increasing the possibility of laryngeal injuries if used improperly. For this reason this tube should not be considered for use in the initial stages of intubation but reserved for the latter stages of the long-term patients when the chronic injuries are likely. The incorporation of the triangular design into this new tube, plus all the presently used Portex tubes, may be of value. As yet no clinical experience has been obtained with the above described tubes, but future trials are planned.

CONCLUSIONS

During the past decade an increasing number of premature infants have survived because of diligent treatment and frequent use of respirators and endotracheal tubes. Although this management is becoming more successful, it is resulting in an increasing number of infants with potentially long-term laryngeal defects that to date have not been stressed. At present there is no definite means of preventing all these complications if we are to preserve life. However, the following regimen modifications could be used to decrease these complications: 1) The most important is the use of as soft and as small a tube as possible to minimize the glottic pressure. Taping the tube securely to limit the piston action transmitted from the respirator will also decrease the creation of ulcerations. 2) Adequate hydration to help prevent drying of the secretions in the tube and the membranes adjacent to it is necessary.[12]

In addition to these precautions, one should observe the sound of the cry while changing the tube, and if significant hoarseness or aphonia is noted, a smaller diameter tube (or eventually the alternative tube described in this paper) should be inserted.

No standard time interval for such a change can be given, but it will depend on each patient and the response of the patient's tissues to the intubation. The point to be stressed is that long-term intubation in the neonate is not innocuous. The above factors require constant supervision to avoid the chronic laryngeal injuries and breathy voices that can persist in some infants and children.

Request for reprints should be sent to Arthur S. Hengerer, M.D., The Rochester Otolaryngology Group, P.C., 1641 East Avenue, Rochester, N. Y. 14610.

REFERENCES

1. McEwen, cited by Dwyer CS, Krowenberg S, Saklad M: The endotracheal tube: a consideration of its traumatic effect with a suggestion for the modification thereof. Anesthesiology 10:714-728, 1949

2. Harrod JR, L'Heureux P, Wangensteen OD, *et al*: Long term follow-up of severe respiratory distress syndrome treated with IPPB. J Pediatr 84:277-286, 1974

3. Johnson JD, Malachowski NC, Grobstein R, *et al*: Prognosis of children surviving with the aid of mechanical ventilation in the newborn period. J Pediatr 84:272-277, 1974

4. Stetson JB: Prolonged endotracheal tube intubation. Brit J Anesth 40:712-713, 1968

5. Schlorf RA, Duvall AJ: Post intubation granulomas of the larynx. Minn Med 52:717-720, 1969

6. Lindholm C: Prolonged endotracheal intubation. Acta Anesthesiologica Scanda 13: (Suppl 33) 1-125, 1969

7. Coppel DL, Bennett EJ, Ahlgren EW, *et al*: The prophylactic use of a nasotracheal tube in infants under three months of age. Surgery 69:354-359, 1971

8. Way WL, Sooy, FA: Histologic changes produced by endotracheal intubation. Ann Otol Rhinol Laryngol 74:799-811, 1965

9. Davenport HT: Prolonged endotracheal intubation in children — A perspective. Int Anesthesiol Clin 8:909-924, 1970

10. Dwyer CS, Kronenberg S, Saklad M: The endotracheal tube: A consideration of its traumatic effects with a suggestion for the modification thereof. Anesthesiology 10:714-728, 1949

11. Slater EA: Endotracheal tube sizes for infants and children. Anesthesiology 16:950-961, 1955

12. Fearon B, MacDonald RE, Smith C, *et al*: Airway problems in children following prolonged endotracheal intubation. Ann Otol Rhinol Laryngol 75:975-986, 1966

FACIAL PLASTIC SURGERY: TELEVISION SEMINARS

A continuing education workshop devoted to all aspects of facial plastic surgery (including rhinoplasty) will be held February 1-5, 1976 on Key Biscayne, Miami, Florida.

Sponsored by the American Academy of Facial Plastic and Reconstructive Surgery, Inc. in cooperation with the Department of Otolaryngology, University of Miami, the workshop will include a broad interdisciplinary faculty of national prominence. Course directors are Robert Simons, M.D. and M. Eugene Tardy, Jr., M.D. For applications and reservations write: M. Eugene Tardy, Jr., M.D., 2800 Lake Shore Drive, Chicago, Illinois 60657.

SYMPOSIUM ON CONTROVERSIAL AREAS IN SURGERY OF HEAD AND NECK

The University of California at San Diego School of Medicine announces the Fifth Annual Symposium on Controversial Areas in Surgery of the Head and Neck, February 12-15, 1976 in San Diego, California.

For information write: Alan M. Nahum, M.D., University Hospital, 225 West Dickinson, San Diego, Ca. 92103.

Ann Otol 84: 1975

SECOND PRIMARY CANCER AFTER IRRADIATION OF LARYNGEAL CANCER

William Lawson, M.D.

Max Som, M.D.

New York, New York

SUMMARY – Thirty (5.6%) of 535 patients followed 5-25 years after treatment of cordal carcinoma (T1A,B) developed a second primary laryngeal carcinoma. When analyzed by treatment modality, 3.9% of operated cases and 9% of irradiated cases formed new laryngeal or laryngopharyngeal malignancies. An explanation by radiation-induced carcinogenesis for this statistically significant difference between the two groups is discussed. It is also suggested that supervoltage radiation directed to the laryngeal mucosa may produce the diminished latent period observed between the appearance of the second primary carcinoma.

While numerous studies cite the incidence of second primary tumors within the oropharynx, there is little published about their occurrence in the larynx. The therapy of cordal carcinoma by either irradiation or partial laryngectomy allows the whole or major part of the organ to remain for the various chemical, physical, and cellular factors as well as the genetic predisposition of the host to function in the development of a new growth. Additionally, comparison of the incidence of second primary malignancies in the surgical and radiotherapy groups may permit consideration of a possible etiologic role for radiation in carcinogenesis in the larynx.

RESULTS

Cordal carcinoma (T1A,B) is generally accepted to be equally curable by surgery or radiotherapy. We have found that lesions of the membranous portion of the true cord are eminently suitable for radiation therapy and have treated 225 patients in this way. One hundred ninety of these patients received supervoltage therapy, with the remaining 35 having conventional 250 kv orthovoltage.

Horseshoe lesions of the vocal cord or those extending onto the vocal process or the anterior face of the arytenoid itself are best treated by partial laryngectomy by either the hemilaryngectomy or anterior commissure technique. Cordectomy instead of radiotherapy was employed early in this period before the advent of supervoltage therapy and generally reserved as a prime modality in younger and more elderly patients, in diabetics, in verrucous cancer, or after radiation failure. We have treated 310 cases by hemilaryngectomy, anterior commissure technique, or cordectomy.

Among the 535 treated cases of cordal cancer followed from 5-25 years, second primary laryngeal carcinomas occurred in 30 (5.6%). In the group of 310 patients receiving surgery, 12 (3.9%) second laryngeal primaries occurred. Among the 225 patients receiving radiotherapy, 18 (8%) new laryngeal malignancies appeared. Six tumors occurred in 35 patients having orthovoltage, and 12 occurred in 190 patients receiving supervoltage. If two hypopharyngeal tumors developing within the field of radiation are included, the incidence rises to 9% (Table I). This difference in the inci-

---

From the Department of Otolaryngology, the Mount Sinai Medical Center, New York.

Presented at the meeting of the American Laryngological Association, Atlanta, Georgia, April 6-7, 1975.

TABLE I

INCIDENCE OF SECOND PRIMARY CARCINOMAS OF THE LARYNX
535 CORDAL LESIONS (T1a,b)

Cordectomy	71 (5)	Orthovoltage	35 (6)
Ant. comm. tech.	58 (1)	Supervoltage	190 (12)
Hemilaryngectomy	181 (6)		225 (18) (8%*)
	310 (12) (3.9%)		

*9% if 2 hypopharyngeal lesions in the field of radiation are included.

dence of second primary carcinomas in the radiotherapy and surgery groups was found to be statistically significant ($X^2 = 5.73$, $P = .017$).

The interval before the second laryngeal carcinoma appeared in the 12 operated cases was five to eight years in five and 9-14 years in seven. The latent period in the radiotherapy groups was five to eight years in 13 cases, 9-14 years in four cases and 21 years in one case (Table II).

TABLE II

LATENT PERIOD UNTIL APPEARANCE OF SECOND LARYNGEAL PRIMARY

	Surgery	*Radiotherapy*
5-8 Years	(5)	(13)
9-14 Years	(7)	(4)
15-25 Years	(0)	(1)
	(12)	(18)

Concerning the development of extra laryngeal malignancies, there were seven bronchogenic carcinomas, one adenocarcinoma of the prostate, and one melanoma in the surgery group. Among the radiotherapy patients there occurred three bronchogenic carcinomas, one adenocarcinoma of the rectum, one squamous cell carcinoma of the ear, and two carcinomas of the hypopharynx, yielding an incidence for malignant tumors occurring outside the larynx of 3% in both groups (Table III).

DISCUSSION

The ability of ionizing radiation to produce malignant neoplasms is a well-established phenomenon at such sites as the skin, thyroid gland, blood, bone and lung, with a causal relationship established by epidemiologic studies in susceptible human populations (*e.g.*, atomic bomb survivors, radiologists, and other occupational groups exposed to radiation and radioactive materials), as well as by the experimental induction in animals.[1-4] While radiation carcinogenesis is rare at mucosal sites, sufficient evidence has accumulated to support its existence within the larynx. By 1951 Goolden[5] had collected nine cases of malignant neoplasms of the larynx and hypopharynx (including four cases of his own) in patients previously radiated for benign disease.

TABLE III

INCIDENCE OF SECOND PRIMARY MALIGNANCIES OUTSIDE LARYNX

Surgery (310)		*Radiotherapy (225)*	
Lung	7	Lung	3
Prostate	1	Ear	1
Melanoma	1	Rectum	1
	9 (3%)	Hypopharynx	2
			7 (3%)

He proposed the following criteria for radiation induced carcinomas: 1) a history of irradiation for a benign condition; 2) the elapse of sufficient time for the development of the malignancy (latent period); 3) evidence of radiation injury (vascular or atrophic skin changes); and 4) histologic proof of the malignant character of the new tumor. In 1955 Som and Peimer[6] found 18 cases and by 1957 Goolden[7] reviewed 25 cases in the world literature of malignant tumors of the larynx, hypopharynx, or esophagus following radiation to the neck for benign conditions. We have discovered 20 additional cases recorded between 1957 and 1974.[8-17] Review of these 45 cases reveals that all were squamous cell carcinomas with the exception of two fibrosarcomas reported by Goolden[5] and Holinger and Rabbett.[18] The distribution of these lesions was 12 in the larynx, 33 in the hypopharynx, and two in the esophagus. Virtually all the patients received radiation for benign thyroid disease (goiter, thyrotoxicosis) or tuberculous cervical adenitis and showed telangiectasis or ulceration of the overlying skin as evidence of radiation damage. In five patients of this group multicentric malignant tumors developed. All three patients of McGraw and McKenzie[13] developed adenocarcinomas of the thyroid as well as squamous cell carcinoma of the hypopharynx, and one patient had a skin cancer within the portal of radiation as well. The patient of Cronin[17] developed carcinoma of both the larynx and the hypopharynx 30 years after irradiation for thyroid disease. In the case of Baker (1959), laryngeal and laryngopharyngeal malignancies developed 30 and 36 years after radiotherapy in addition to basal and squamous cell carcinomas in the irradiated skin. All the patients in this group received orthovoltage radiation with the latent period for the development of the second malignancy ranging from 8-51 years, averaging 27 years. In this group of patients were two children treated for laryngeal papillomatosis with radiotherapy who developed carcinoma of the hypopharynx 30 and 40 years later.[13,15] The ability of radiation to transform benign papillomas themselves into malignant tumors is another example of the oncogenetic effect of ionizing radiation directed to the larynx. Rabbett[19] accumulated nine instances of carcinoma of the larynx following orthovoltage radiation for juvenile laryngeal papillomatosis. The latent period for the development of a laryngeal malignancy ranged from 4-28 years, averaging 12 years.

The development of radiation-induced carcinomas of the larynx and laryngopharynx following therapeutic irradiation of the larynx for malignant disease was first recorded by Som and Peimer[6] who described two malignant tumors of the hypopharynx arising 17 and 20 years after such treatment. Thomas[20] reported three cases of laryngeal carcinoma recurring 12, 18, and 30 years after treatment (of which one patient had received surgery and the other two radiation) but acknowledged that the latter two tumors may have been radiation induced. Schindel and Castoriano[21] reported five cases of hypopharyngeal carcinoma occurring 7-12 years after the successful radiotherapy for an endo-laryngeal malignancy. They favored radiation induction as the histogenesis of these tumors rather than multicentricity because of the occurrence of all five lesions in the postcricoid area of males, an uncommon site of primary malignancies in this sex, but a region that was within the zone of radiation. All of these nine cases of a second primary carcinoma of the larynx and laryngopharynx arising in patients irradiated for a laryngeal malignancy received orthovoltage therapy, with a latent period of 7-30 years, averaging 15 years. We know of another case of a postcricoid lesion arising 12 years after radiotherapy with cobalt for a cordal carcinoma.

The five year survival of glottic carcinomas treated either by partial laryngectomy or radiation is quite good when compared to tumors arising at other laryngeal and hypopharyngeal sites. However, the advanced age of many of the patients precluded the protracted follow-up interval of 15-30 years generally regarded as the latent period of radiation-induced neoplasms. Consequently, we believe the increased incidence of second primary laryngeal carcinoma in the radiotherapy group to assume greater significance as many patients did not survive long enough to develop other tumors.

It may be argued that some of the lesions actually represent the delayed recurrence of the initial tumor. While in the head and neck area certain salivary gland tumors (adenocystic adenocarcinoma), papillary adenocarcinoma of the thyroid, and carotid body tumors may show an extremely indolent growth, a five year disease-free interval with squamous cell carcinoma virtually signifies cure, particularly with T1 lesions.

CONCLUSIONS

Reports of carcinoma of the larynx and hypopharynx developing after radiation to the neck for benign and malignant conditions have suggested an etiologic role for radiation in the histogenesis, but have not established a causal relationship. Baker and Weissman[22] (1971) treated seven patients with laryngeal malignancies who had received radiotherapy 5 to 25 years previously for another laryngeal carcinoma. This prompted them to suggest that radiation not be used in the treatment of laryngeal cancer in persons 45 years of age or less. Our study shows that second primary carcinomas arise spontaneously in the larynx at a low rate. However, the demonstration of a statistically significant increased incidence of second primary laryngeal carcinomas in the radiotherapy group definitely points to a role for ionizing radiation in the formation of some of these tumors. Although the latent period for the development of a laryngeal or hypopharyngeal carcinoma after orthovoltage therapy of benign disorders of the neck averaged 27 years, it dropped to 12 to 15 years when the beam was directed to the larynx itself in the treatment of papillomatosis or carcinoma. We have found in our material the average latent period for the development of a second laryngeal primary with supervoltage therapy to be seven years which may represent the enhanced radiobiologic effect of this form of ionizing radiation when directed to the laryngeal mucosa. Consequently, thought must be directed to the selection of the prime modality of treatment of cordal carcinoma. This decreased latent period of supervoltage therapy in the face of an increased life expectancy suggests that radiation be withheld in individuals under 50 years of age.

Request for reprints should be sent to Max L. Som, M.D., 121 East 60th Street, New York, New York 10021.

REFERENCES

1. Chisleag GH, Baran E, Petroveanu C: Radiation-induced tumours in man, in *Proceedings of a Symposium on Radiation-Induced Cancer.* Athens, 1969, International Atomic Energy Agency, Vienna, 1969, pp 459-467

2. Rosen VJ, Cole LJ: Radiation carcinogenesis: experimental and clinical aspects, in Berdjis CC (ed): *Pathology of Irradiation.* Baltimore, Williams and Wilkins, 1971, pp 120-145

3. Upton AC: Radiation carcinogenesis, in Dalyrymple GU, *et al* (eds) *Medical Radiation Biology.* Philadelphia, Saunders Co., 1973, pp 213-225

4. Prasad KN: *Human Radiation Biology.* Maryland, Harper and Row, 1974, pp 341-356

5. Goolden AW: Radiation cancer of the pharynx. Br Med J 2:1110-1112, 1951

6. Som ML, Peimer R: Postcricoid carcinoma as a sequel to radiotherapy for laryngeal carcinoma. Arch Otolaryngol 62:428-431, 1955

7. Goolden AW: Radiation cancer. A review with special reference to radiation tumours in the pharynx, larynx and thyroid. Br J Radiol 30:626-640, 1957

8. Lane N: Pseudosarcoma (polypoid sarcoma-like masses) associated with squamous cell carcinoma of the mouth, fauces, and larynx. Report of 10 cases. Cancer 10: 19-41, 1957

9. Baker DC: Pseudosarcoma of the pharynx and larynx. Ann Otol Rhinol Laryngol 68:471-477, 1959

10. Krahl P: Nil Nocere: Hypopharynx-und Larynx-Karzinoma als Spatfolge nach Röntgenbestrahlung Gutartiger Hautbzw. Lymphknotenerkrankungen im Halsgebiet. Munch Med Wochenschr 102:1911-1914, 1960

11. Wlodyka J: The cancerogenic effect of x-ray on the larynx. Arch Otolaryngol 76:372-376, 1962

12. Nehls K: Das Strahlentrauma als tumorauslosender Faktor. Z Laryngol Rhinol Otol 44:648-660, 1965

13. McGraw RW, McKenzie AD: Carcinoma of the thyroid and laryngopharynx following irradiation: A report of three cases. Cancer 18:692-696, 1965

14. Takahashi S, Kitabatake T: Skin and neck cancer following radiation therapy for benign disease. Tohoku J Exp Med 84:349-359, 1965

15. Piquet JJ, Dessaulty A, Decroix G: Les radio-cancers (A propos de deux observations). Ann Otolaryngol Chir Cervicofac 84: 125-129, 1967

16. Gerlings PG: Stralentrauma van pharynx en larynx (Stralencarcinoom en laryngitis radiotherapeutica). Ned Tijdschr. Geneeskd 113:1045-1050, 1969

17. Cronin J: Radiation-induced cancer of larynx and pharynx. J Laryngol Otol 85: 621-622, 1971

18. Holinger PH, Rabbett WF: Late development of laryngeal and pharyngeal carcinoma in previously irradiated areas. Laryngoscope 63:105-112, 1953

19. Rabbett WF: Juvenile laryngeal papillomatosis: the relation of irradiation to malignant degeneration in this disease. Ann Otol Rhinol Laryngol 74:1149-1163, 1965

20. Thomas R: Late recurrence of laryngeal cancer. J Laryngol Rhinol Otol 78:1123-1124, 1964

21. Schindel J, Castoriano IM: Late-appearing (radiation-induced) carcinoma. Arch Otolaryngol 95:205-210, 1965

22. Baker DC, Weissman B: Post irradiation carcinoma of the larynx. Ann Otol Rhinol Laryngol 80:634-637, 1971

MIDDLE EAR MICROSURGERY AND FLUCTUANT HEARING LOSS

The Shambaugh Fifth International Workshop on Middle Ear Microsurgery and Fluctuant Hearing Loss will be held at Northwestern University Medical School, Thorne Hall, March 1-6, 1976. Co-chairmen are George E. Shambaugh, Jr., M.D. and John J. Shea, M.D.

For further information write: American Hearing Research Foundation, Suite 2105, 55 East Washington Street, Chicago, Illinois 60602.

Ann Otol 84: 1975

EXPERIMENTAL GRANULOMA OF THE LARYNX

FERNANDO R. KIRCHNER, M.D.

KANSAS CITY, KANSAS

SUMMARY – This paper describes a series of experiments that were performed in dogs, attempting to reproduce in the laboratory a chronic granulomatous reaction of the larynx. The purpose of this work was to learn about the possible pathogenesis of these lesions and to find the reasons behind their chronicity and recurrence. The practical aspects of this research were to formulate and, hopefully, to develop reasonable diagnostic and therapeutical approaches that could be used in the treatment of patients. The positive and negative results of these experiments indicate that the granulomatous response is probably influenced not only by external factors, but also by intrinsic factors. Clinically these findings led to the concept of not circumscribing judgment to the peripheral changes only, but to the assessment of all facts surrounding each individual case.

The goals of moden laryngology are twofold: first and foremost, the eradication of the disease; and second, the preservation of function. These aims are best achieved through the individual assessment of the patient and knowledge of the fundamental facts behind the pathological process. Basic information about the larynx and the pathological conditions that may afflict this organ are, therefore, essential. Historically this information has been obtained from three main sources: clinical observations, examination of surgical and autopsy specimens, and from animal experiments.[1,2] All of these sources have contributed to advancement of the state of the art. In spite of this development there is still much to be learned about the health and diseases of the larynx. The studies in this report were prompted by a group of patients afflicted with different degrees of laryngeal impairment, in whom the outstanding finding was a persistent and recurrent granulomatous process. Experiments were carried out in dogs in an attempt to study and reproduce these chronic granulomas. The purpose of this work was to learn about the possible pathogenesis of these lesions and to find the reasons for their chronicity and recurrence. The practical aspects of this research were to formulate and, hopefully, to develop reasonable diagnostic and therapeutic approaches that could be used in the treatment of patients.

METHODS AND RESULTS

Anterior Commissure and Vocal Cords. In a representative group of animals, extensive studies were carried out about the possible induction of a chronic granulomatous process in the anterior commissure and vocal cords by: a) extensive epithelial denudation, b) reaction to surgical sutures, and c) artificially produced cartilaginous sequestra.

Superficial epithelial denudation of these structures was attempted in six mongrel dogs. In two of these animals this removal was performed mechanically with a cup forceps, in two other dogs with the thermocautery, and in the remaining two, by means of high frequency fulguration. The larynges of these animals were inspected directly every week with the operating microscope. At the end of five weeks all of these larynges appeared to be recovered by normal

From the Department of Otolaryngology, University of Kansas Medical Center, Kansas City, Kansas.

Presented at the meeting of the American Laryngological Association, Atlanta, Georgia, April 6-7, 1975.

epithelium. One animal that was treated by fulguration developed a small blunting of the anterior commissure. This dog's larynx was further inspected every week for two additional months. For three weeks no changes were observed, but on the fourth week a small exophytic granuloma was discovered arising from the superior aspect of the small anterior web. In the examination that was carried out six days later, no traces of the granuloma were encountered, and no other recurrences were observed up to the time that the dog was sacrificed. The histological examination of this larynx discovered a small sinus track of epithelium surrounded by the cicatricial tissue forming the webb. It is reasonable to assume from these findings that the transient granulomatous reaction was possibly produced by infection of debris entrapped in this epithelial sinus.

The production of granulomas in the anterior commissure by three suture materials, catgut, stainless steel wire, and braided silk, was studied in three animals. These sutures were purposely introduced through an external approach transversing the anterior commissure

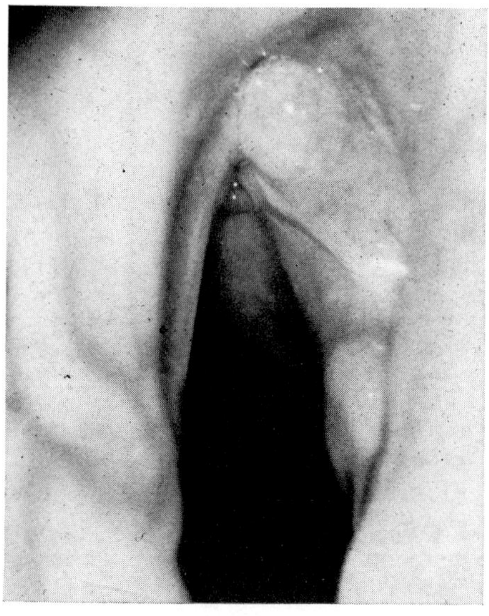

Fig. 1. Granuloma of the anterior commissure produced by a silk suture that was experimentally placed transversing the anterior commissure.

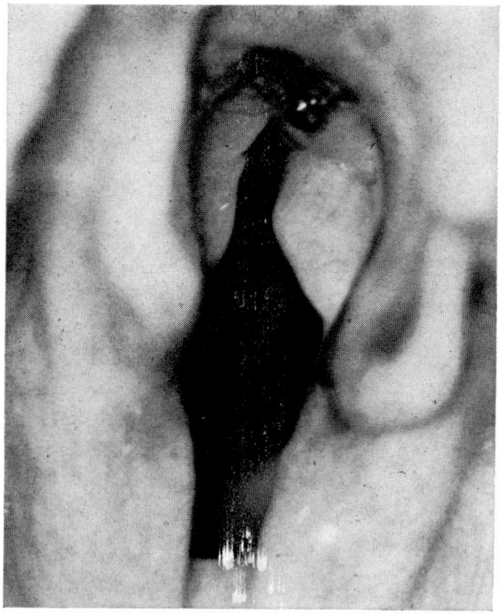

Fig. 2. Silk suture in the anterior commissure after the granulomatous reaction spontaneously subsided.

after drilling two holes in the thyroid cartilage. The larynges of these animals were also observed every week with the operating microscope. One of the animals was discarded in the first week because the catgut suture became extruded after becoming untied. Contrasting the lack of changes found in the larynx of the dog with the stainless wire suture during the full period of eight weeks of observation, the animal with the braided silk suture developed a granulomatous reaction concomitantly with a neck abscess almost immediately (Fig. 1). These two changes improved spontaneously, and at the end of two weeks the neck and larynx appeared to be well healed, in spite of the fact that the silk suture remained plainly visible on direct examination for the remaining eight weeks (Fig. 2).

The possible effect of an artifically produced cartilaginous sequestra implanted in the area of the anterior commissure was studied in one dog. In this animal the anterior keel of the thyroid cartilage was removed through an external approach. This segment of cartilage, measuring about 3 mm wide, was then fixed for one hour in a solution of 10%

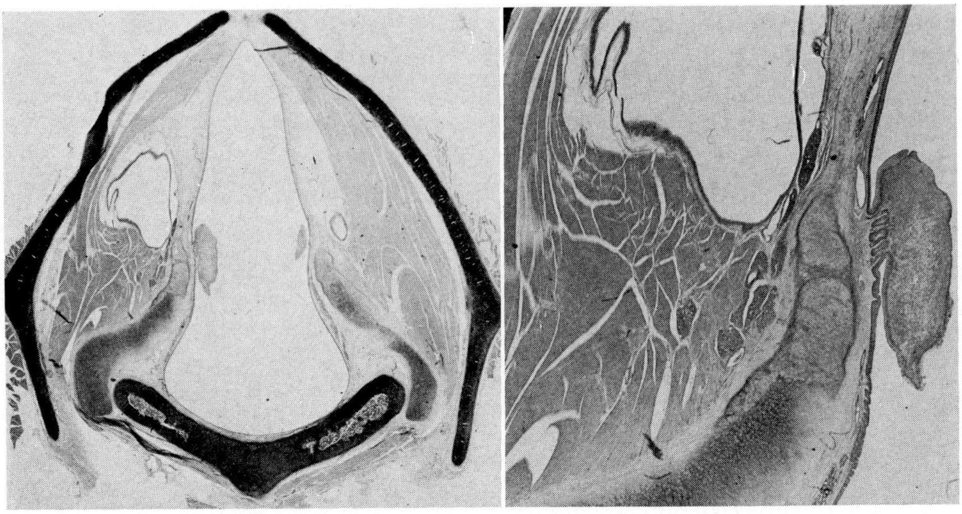

Fig. 3. A) Experimental granulomas arising at the level of the vocal process of the arytenoids during the stage of pediculation and spontaneous resolution. B) Experimental granuloma arising from an area of perichondritis in the vocal process of the arytenoid during the early stages of resolution. Notice the epithelium attempting to restore the normal contours of this portion of the posterior commissure.

formaldehyde. This piece of cartilage was then reimplanted into its original position and held in place by suturing the overlying strapped muscles. No changes were observed in the larynx of this animal at any time during the ensuing two months. The histological examination of this larynx demonstrated the complete replacement of this wedge of cartilage by connective tissue.

Posterior Commissure. The posterior commissures of eight animals were subjected to the following experimental conditions: a) pressure necrosis produced by stents made of Teflon®*, b) focal necrosis of the vocal process of the arytenoid cartilage with minimal epithelial denudation, and c) necrosis of vocal process of the arytenoid cartilage following extensive denudation.

Two dogs were used in the first experiments. In these animals a tubeless canine tracheostomy, as described by Miles,[3] was first instituted. With the airway secured in such a manner, tapering, shaped stents made of heavy Teflon® material were wedged in the posterior commissure against the vocal process of the arytenoids. The distal end of these implants was secured to the superior edge of the permanent tracheal stoma by means of wire sutures. These experiments were promptly discontinued because of failure to maintain the stents in the proper position.

Focal necrosis of the vocal process of the arytenoid cartilages, with minimal epithelial removal, was attempted in three animals. In two of these animals this structure was focally fulgurated. The other dog was subjected to submucosal injection of a 10% solution of lactic acid. Both of these techniques failed to produce a granulomatous reaction.

Three dogs were finally subjected to extensive denudation with the thermocautery of the epithelium covering the posterior one-third of the vocal cords, the vocal process, and the posterior commissure. The cartilage thus exposed was then deeply fulgurated. All of these animals developed large prominent granulomas in the third week. During

----

*E. I. du Pont de Nemours & Co., Inc., Wilmington, Del.

this stage one of the dogs was sacrificed, and its larynx was excised and processed for histological examination. The two other dogs were left alive and further examined with the dissecting microscope. On the seventh week the pedicle of the granulomas appeared less broad, and the bulkiness of these reactions was greatly reduced (Fig. 3A). At this stage a second dog was sacrificed. The third animal was sacrificed at the end of nine weeks when the larynx of this dog appeared to be grossly healed. The histological sections of these larynges were examined and the following results obtained.

The granulomas were composed of a core of fibroblasts intermingled with numerous neoformed vascular vessels. Some leukocytic infiltration was noticeable throughout the fibrous stroma.

The dog's larynx that was excised at the early stage of the experiment showed a prominent granuloma completely deprived of epithelial lining. This lining was found to be extending to the periphery of the lesions only. The granulomatous reaction was clearly arising from areas of necrotic cartilage of the vocal process of the arytenoid. Some differences were encountered in the examination of the second specimen. This granuloma was less bulky and had a clearly defined pedicle. This constriction was found to be formed by epithelium attempting to regenerate the normal contour of the adjacent laryngeal surfaces. The fibrous stroma was less exuberant and the areas of focal perichondritis less diffuse and more permeated by cicatricial tissue (Fig. 3B). In the third specimen only the cicatricial changes in the cartilage were evident.

DISCUSSION

These experiments support the observations made by several authors[4,5,6] about the pathogenesis of nonspecific granulomas of the larynx, particularly those encountered in the posterior commissure. The multifactor etiology of these lesions is strongly suggested by some of the positive, as well as negative, results obtained in these studies. The concept that, in the author's opinion, is quite outstandingly depicted in this work is the necessity in the clinical practice to appreciate and assess all circumstances, and not to circumscribe judgment only to the peripheral changes.

Representative of this concept are the following two clinical cases. These patients were referred because of persistent granulomas after undergoing, elsewhere, apparently adequate reductions of laryngeal fractures. In one patient a chronic granuloma arising from the anterior commissure obstructing the airway, was found to be produced by a surgical suture. The endoscopic removal of this stitch stopped the recurrence of this granuloma. The second patient was also afflicted with a recurrent granuloma located anteriorly in the subglottic space. Several inflammatory bouts and neck abscesses arising in this area led the referring physician to believe in a possible perichondritis. The histological examination of this granuloma revealed, however, epithelial cells and the typical clefts that are encountered when skin is displaced and entrapped into other tissues.[7] This granuloma ceased to recur after a tract of displaced epithelium was excised through a simple external approach.

CONCLUSIONS

Granulomas of the larynx appeared to be produced by a particular type of overgrowth of granulation tissue. The conclusions obtained from experiments conducted in dogs, attempting to reproduce these lesions, indicate that their responses appeared to be influenced by a variety of external factors. These studies also suggest the dependency of these lesions to still-unproven intrinsic factors.

Request for reprints should be sent to Fernando R. Kirchner, M.D., Department of Otolaryngology, University of Kansas Medical Center, Kansas City, Kansas 66103.

REFERENCES

1. Delahunty JE, Cherry J: Experimentally produced vocal cord granulomas. Laryngoscope 78:1941-1947, 1968

2. Biller HF, Harvey JE, Bone RC, et al: Laryngeal edema: an experimental study. Arch Otolaryngol 79:1084-1087, 1970

3. Miles WK: Tubeless canine tracheostomy for laryngeal experimentation. Arch Otolaryngol 92:124-127, 1970

4. Jackson C: Contact ulcer of larynx. Ann Otol Rhinol Laryngol 37:227-230, 1928

5. Jackson C: Contact ulcer granuloma and other laryngeal complications of endotracheal anesthesia. Anesthesiology (Philadelphia) 14: 425-436, 1953

6. Snow JC, Harano M, Balogh K, et al: Postintubation granuloma of the larynx. Anesth Analg (Cleve) 45:425-429, 1966

7. Hughes M, Kirchner JA, Branson RJ: A skin-lined tube as a complication of tracheostomy. Arch Otolaryngol 94:568-570, 1971

CONFERENCE ANNOUNCEMENT

The Second International Conference on the Diagnosis and Treatment of Craniofacial Anomalies will be held at the New York University Medical Center, New York, New York on May 3-5, 1976. The Conference is organized under the auspices of the Educational Foundation of the American Society of Plastic and Reconstructive Surgeons.

The Conference will focus on four major subject areas: orbitocephalic malformations, including orbital clefts and hypertelorism, craniofacial synostosis syndromes, mandibulofacial dyostosis (Treacher-Collins Syndrome) and craniofacial microsomia (maldevelopment of the first and second branchial arches). Emphasis will be placed on etiology, embryology, genetics, classification, pathology and the role of the different clinical specialties in the diagnosis and treatment of these anomalies. Special sessions will be devoted to associated speech and airway problems, helical deformities, audiology and middle ear surgery.

For detailed information please write: John Marquis Converse, M.D., Institute of Reconstructive Plastic Surgery, 550 First Avenue, New York, New York 10016.

Ann Otol 84: 1975

TRACHEAL INCISION AS A CONTRIBUTING FACTOR TO TRACHEAL STENOSIS

AN EXPERIMENTAL STUDY

Gary C. Lulenski, M.D.

John G. Batsakis, M.D.

Ann Arbor, Michigan

SUMMARY — Tracheostomies were performed on 25 mongrel dogs, employing either a vertical or inverted U flap incision in the trachea. Following cannulation for 14 days, the animals were maintained for three months and endolarygeal photographs were taken. At the time of autopsy, comparisons of the gross specimens were carried out, as well as histological sectioning through the tracheal stomal area. Both endolaryngeal examination and study of the gross specimens at autopsy revealed less distortion of the tracheal lumen following the flap versus vertical tracheostomy, especially in those animals having the flap of cartilage resewn to the trachea at the time of decannulation. Measurements of the cross sectional area at the tracheal stoma were also made. In animals having a flap tracheostomy, the stomal lumen was preserved, regardless of resuturing the flap. However, animals having a vertical tracheostomy lost an average of 18% of the tracheal area when compared with those having a flap incision. Histological examination revealed cartilaginous growth across the tracheostomy incision only in animals having the flap tracheostomy. Support for the flap tracheostomy is provided from animal experimentation.

Stenosis of the trachea, as a complication following endotracheal intubation or tracheostomy, has been the subject of considerable recent investigation.[1-3] Following tracheostomy, two sites of tracheal stenosis have been described: at the site of the stoma or tracheal incision and at the area of the tracheostomy tube cuff or tip.[4-6] Infection, excessive cuff pressure, and movement of the tracheostomy tube have been documented as contributing factors to the development of the latter stenotic area, but the factors leading to stomal narrowing are less clear.[1,6-8] This is true despite evidence that stenosis at the stoma may well be the more common injury.[1,9]

Some of the possible causative factors of tracheal stomal stenosis have been studied. Nelson indicates that intubation with uncuffed tracheostomy tubes will lead to significant stenosis if the tubes are left in place for ten days or longer.[10] The stenosis is accompanied by necrosis and deformity of the cartilaginous rings and replacement by fibrous connective tissue. The type of tracheostomy incision (vertical, cruciate, or window) did not appear to be significant in his study. Goldberg also found significant tracheal narrowing when uncuffed tubes were used. He suggests a lack of cartilage support and the size of the cannula as pertinent factors.[11] In this summary of the experimental findings, he states: "The defect at the stoma heals with fibrous tissue and the cartilage does not regenerate . . . therefore the dissolution of cartilage is a chronic process."

Refinements in the cuffed tracheostomy tube have produced low pressure systems allowing for reduction of steno-

From the Departments of Otolaryngology and Pathology, the University of Michigan Medical Center, Ann Arbor, Michigan.

Presented at the meeting of the American Laryngological Association, Atlanta, Georgia, April 6-7, 1975.

sis at the tracheostomy cuff site as the pressure delivered to the tracheal wall can be measured directly.[12] Reduction in the tracheal stomal stenosis awaits further explanation of its etiology.

The flap tracheostomy has been recently described and some evidence exists that it does not lead to tracheal stomal stenosis. An inverted V or U tracheal incision which can be sewn to the skin of the anterior neck has advantages in protecting the airway in the immediate postoperative period and in facilitating tracheal tube changing.[13,14] Strong recommendations have been made to replace this flap of cartilage at the time of decannulation. When done as a formal procedure in the operating room or at the bedside the flap tracheostomy has not led to stomal stenosis.[15,16] To date, the fate of the tracheal cartilage remains unclear and the necessity of replacing it at a formal surgical procedure is not supported by experimental data.

In the present report, we present morphological data derived from an experimental study designed to compare the influence on postoperative stomal stenosis of the flap tracheostomy incision and the time-honored, conventional, vertical tracheal incision.

METHODS AND MATERIALS

Twenty-six mongrel dogs, weighing 13 to 16 kilograms were used in this study. After appropriate inoculations, the animals underwent tracheostomy using pentobarbital and a combination of droperidol and fentanyl for anesthesia. One animal was used as a control and underwent no operative procedure.

TABLE I

EXPERIMENTAL GROUPS RELATING TRACHEAL INCISION TO TRACHEAL STENOSIS

Group	*No. of Experimental Dogs*	*No. of Dogs Surviving*	*Tracheal Incision*
I	9	7	flap (flap resewn)
II	9	7	flap (flap not resewn)
III	7	6	vertical

The test animals were divided into three groups (Table I) according to the type of tracheal incision used for tracheostomy: vertical versus a flap. In each animal a No. 6 tracheostomy tube* was inserted after the low pressure cuff had been removed by sharp dissection, and left in place for 14 days. The cuff was removed because a pilot study had shown that animals would die from respiratory obstruction, being unable to breathe around the outer cannula if the cuff were present and the inner cannula were to become obstructed. To obviate this problem further, the inner cannula was changed twice daily during the period of cannulation. The vertical incision was made through the least number of tracheal rings required to allow insertion of the tube. In nearly all instances this involved three tracheal rings. The flap tracheostomy was based inferiorly and was made through two rings, and the flap of cartilage was sewn to the skin of the anterior back above the suprasternal notch.

The animals in Groups I and II underwent flap tracheostomy with the following differences: Group I animals had the flap of cartilage freed at the time of decannulation under anesthesia and reapproximated to the anterior trachea with 3-0 chromic sutures; Group II animals had their cannulae removed, and the flap of cartilage was simply left in the granulating wound.

In the period following decannulation (30 or 60 days following tube removal) selected photographs of the animals' tracheae were taken using the Brubaker-Holinger camera. Additional gross photographs were taken at the time of necropsy (90-95 days following decannulation) when the stomal area and an adjacent area of the trachea were excised. This area was then processed, mounted in celloidin, and 10 micron sections made for microscopic examination.

Measurement of the tracheal lumens were made at the midstomal point and at a point removed from the tracheostomy incision by at least two tracheal rings. Measurements taken were the anteroposterior and lateral diameters and the cross-sectional area. The latter was calculated using a planimeter, with three separate measurements taken of each area in each animal and averaged.

RESULTS

Five of the 26 animals in the study expired in the immediate postoperative

*Shiley Laboratories, Inc., Santa Ana, Calif.

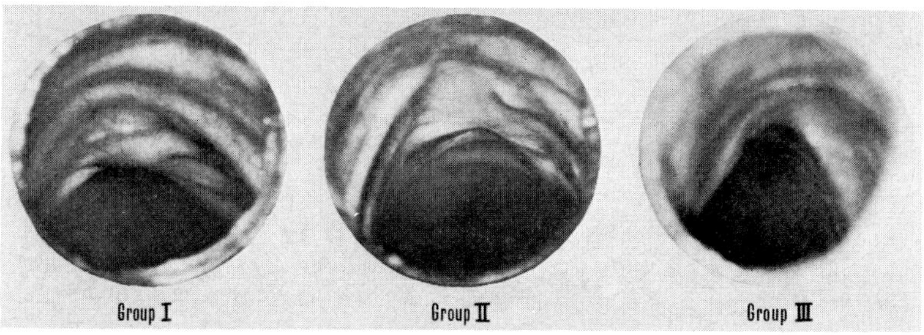

Fig. 1. Endotracheal appearance of the stomal area one month following decannulation. Group I animals underwent flap tracheostomy with the flap resewn; in Group II the flap was not resewn; and in Group III a vertical incision was done.

period, despite antibiotic therapy and changing of the inner cannula twice daily. Mechanical obstruction of the airway appeared to be the cause of death and confirms the problem found in this type of research by others.

The endolaryngeal photographs of selected animals in each study group demonstrated rather striking findings. As shown in Figure 1, animals from the two Groups (I and II) who had flap tracheostomies did not manifest significant distortion of their tracheae at the stomal area. Animals who had vertical tracheostomies (Group III) exhibited a loss of the anterior concavity of the trachea. This was not an isolated observation, as can be seen when comparing typical gross specimens from necropsy (Fig. 2) in which the animals are different from the three depicted in Figure 1.

Measurements of the tracheal stomas are summarized in Table II. A definite loss of the lateral diameter of the tracheae at the stoma was found in the Group III (vertical incision) animals. Compared

TABLE II

AVERAGE TRACHEAL STOMAL MEASUREMENTS

Group	*A-P Diameter (mm)*	*Lateral Diameter (mm)*	*Cross Sectional Area (cm^2)*
I	14.8	16.3	2.13
II	14.7	16.4	2.12
III	15.0	12.5	1.76

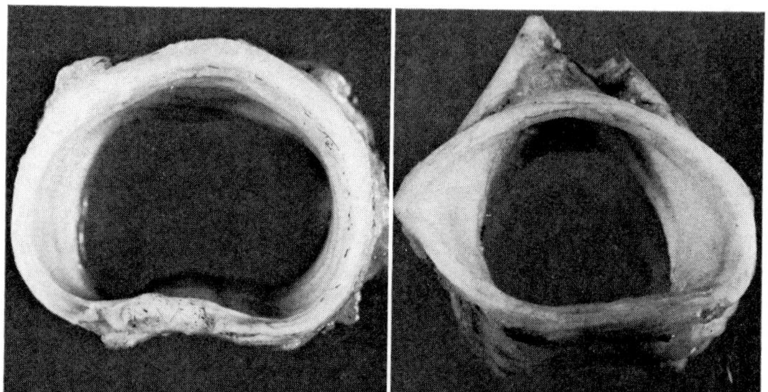

Fig. 2. A) Representative gross specimen of the tracheal stomal area from an animal in Group I. B) Similar area from an animal in Group III, showing distortion of cartilage (See Table I for description of groups).

with the flap tracheostomy Groups (I and II), this Group exhibited an 18% decrease in cross-sectional area. In addition, these animals undergoing vertical tracheostomy also had a reduced lateral tracheal diameter at a point at least two cartilaginous rings removed from the tracheal stoma (15.4 versus 16.3).

The tracheal measurements of the control animal were similar to the mean of those found in Groups I and II, an anteroposterior measurement of 15.0 mm and a lateral measurement of 16.4 mm.

MICROSCOPIC EXAMINATION

Each of the three Groups was histologically separate with an overlap of change occurring only between Groups II and III.

Tracheae from the Group I animals manifested the least histological abnormality (Fig. 3) and, in contrast to

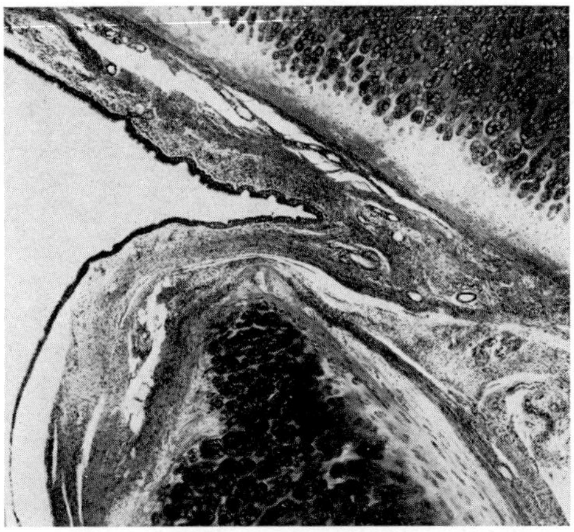

Fig. 3. Prototype appearance of Group I tracheae. Note the virtual absence of scarring and perichondrial reaction. The overlying cartilage is hyperplastic, yet normal in configuration (H. and E., X65).

Groups II and III, exhibited no stromal, vascular, perichondral, or cartilaginous changes. The cartilage of the flap and the nearby tracheal ring are clearly viable.

The predominant histological abnormality found in the Group II tracheae

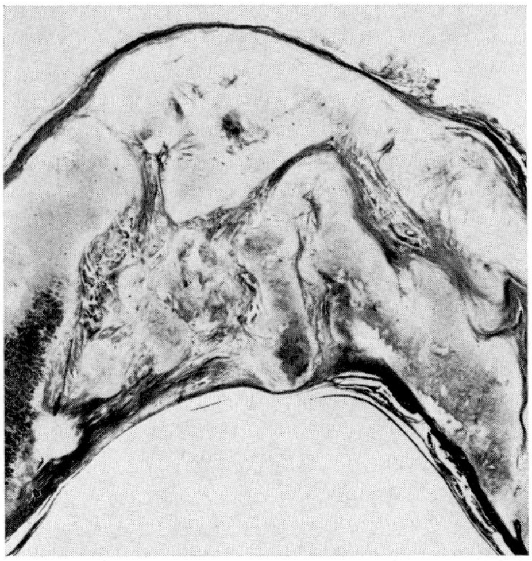

Fig. 4. Marked, disorderly proliferation of cartilage produces bulbous distortion of the tracheal wall. This histological appearance typified the reaction seen in Group II tracheae (H. and E., X65).

was a reactive deformity of the tracheal cartilage. This was present in all sections examined and in several instances was pronounced (Fig. 4). The tracheal lumen, however, was not significantly altered.

Group III animals responded to the vertical incision by a proliferation of soft tissue (vascular connective tissue) and submucosal scarring with perichondrial proliferation (Fig. 5). Two animals also manifested the cartilaginous overgrowth that typified Group II animals. In this Group III alone was there evidence of a subacute inflammatory reaction in the peritracheal soft tissue.

DISCUSSION

Three points of consideration may be derived from this study: the effect of the type of tracheal incision on the development of tracheal narrowing, the mechanism of healing at the site of tracheostomy, and the temporal management of the flap tracheostomy.

Tracheal Incisions and Stomal Stenosis. Only the vertical tracheal incision was associated with tracheal narrowing in this study. The flap tracheostomy in-

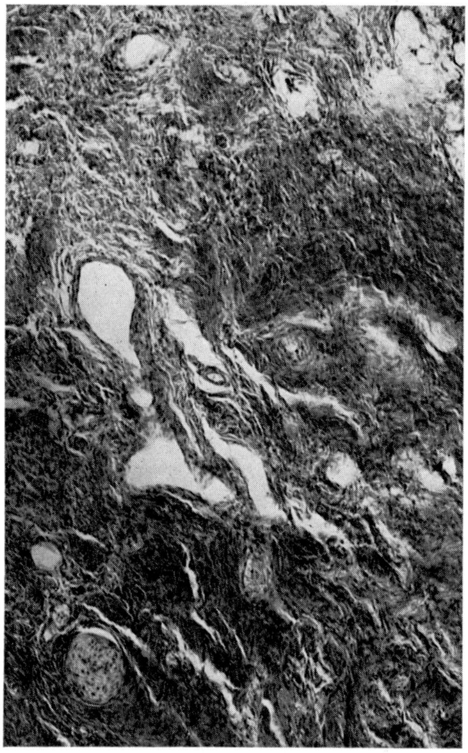

Fig. 5. Vascularized connective tissue with entrapped nerve and fibroadipose tissue represented the tissue response in Group III. This tissue was interposed between cartilage and in some instances extended into the lumen of the trachea (H. and E., X100).

cision, inferiorly based, did not result in any tracheal stenosis. In the vertical tracheostomy there was narrowing at the tracheal stoma as well as distal to the stoma, and the findings were consistent.

Healing at the Tracheal Stoma. The interpretation of results in previous studies concerning healing at the tracheal stoma are not supported by our data. Our studies indicate that gross and microscopic difference in the healing process are related to the type of incision used for tracheostomy. Distortion of cartilage as well as interposition of inflammatory tissue between margins of the remaining cartilage are consistently found following vertical tracheal incisions. This is contrasted to the rather smooth healing of the cartilage defect following the flap incision. The flap of cartilage remained viable despite a two-week period of cannulation, stomal infection, and a three-month period following decannulation. This was true even if the flap of cartilage was not returned to its original position. The lack of inflammatory reaction about the cartilage suggests that pressure against the cartilage inhibits normal healing. By necessity, the vertical incision results in the tracheostomy tube forcibly opening the tracheal rings. This is minimized by the somewhat circular opening of the flap tracheostomy and constitutes one of the major differences between the two incisions. Gross examination clearly shows the adverse effects of pressure upon the tracheal cartilage (Fig. 2).

Management of the Flap Tracheostomy. The recommendation has previously been given that the flap of cartilage raised to form the tracheostome should be resewn at the time of decannulation as a formal operative procedure. This recommendation is said to offer a better alignment of the anterior wall of the trachea, but it insures the risks of an operative procedure, and on the basis of the tracheal measurements in this study may not be warranted. Resuturing does, however, promote a smoother contour of the trachea. Further investigation by the present authors is focusing on the feasibility of a bedside procedure of releasing the flap of cartilage in promoting this more normal healing process. Another factor being studied in the management of the flap tracheostomy is the time necessary for skin healing, dependent on the handling of the flap at the time of decannulation.

SUMMARY

The morphological changes at tracheostomy stomas were investigated in this study. The only variable was the type of tracheal incision. Both in terms of preservation of the tracheal lumen and the healing at the stoma, it was demonstrated that the inferiorly based flap tracheostomy provided functional advantages over the more typically used vertical incision.

Request for reprints should be sent to Gary C. Lulenski, M.D., Department of Otolaryngology, University of Michigan Medical Center, Ann Arbor, Michigan 48104.

REFERENCES

1. Andrews MH, Pearson FG: The incidence and pathogenesis of tracheal injury following cuffed tube tracheostomy with assisted ventilation — An analysis of a three year prospective study. Ann Surg 173:244-263, 1971

2. Davidson IA, Cruickshank AM, Duthei WH, *et al*: Lesions of the trachea following tracheostomy and endotracheal intubation. Proc R Soc Med 64:886-891, 1971

3. Freeman GR: A comparative analysis of endotracheal intubation in neonates, children, and adults: complications, prevention, and treatment. Laryngoscope 82:1385-1398, 1972

4. Pearson FG, Goldberg M, De Silva AJ: Tracheal stenosis complicating tracheostomy with cuffed tubes. Arch Surg 97:380-394, 1968

5. Grillo HC, Cooper JD, Griffin B, *et al*: A low pressure cuff for tracheostomy tubes to minimize tracheal injury. A comparative clinical trial. J Thorac Cardiovasc Surg 62:898-907, 1971

6. Cooper JD, Grillo HC: The evolution of tracheal injury due to ventilatory assistance through cuffed tubes. A pathologic study. Ann Surg 169:334-348, 1969

7. Cooper JD, Grillo HC: Experimental production and prevention of injury due to cuffed tracheal tubes. Surg Gynecol Obstet 165:1235-1241, 1969

8. Bryant LR, Trinkle JK, Dubilier L: Reappraisal of tracheal injury from cuffed tracheostomy tubes. JAMA 215:625-628, 1971

9. Gibson P: Aetiology and repair of tracheal stenosis following tracheostomy and intermittent positive pressure respiration. Thorax 22:1-6, 1967

10. Nelson TC: *Tracheostomy: A Clinical and Experimental Study*. Baltimore, Williams and Wilkins, 1958

11. Goldberg M, Pearson FG: Pathogenesis of tracheal stenosis following tracheostomy with a cuffed tube — an experimental study in dogs. Thorax 27:678-691, 1972

12. Cheng NP, Ayres SM, Paegle RP, *et al*: The contribution of cuff volume and pressure in tracheostomy tube damage. J Thorac Cardiovasc Surg 62:402-410, 1971

13. Acuna PT: Tracheostomy: A simplified technique. Ann Otol Rhinol Laryngol 75:826-829, 1966

14. Bjork VO: Partial resection of the only remaining lung with the aid of respiratory treatment. J Thorac Cardiovasc Surg 39:179-188, 1960

15. Dukes HM: Tracheostomy. Thorax 25:573-576, 1970

16. Chew JY, Cantrell RW: Tracheostomy. Arch Otolaryngol 96:538-545, 1972

EUROPEAN SYMPOSIUM

A European Symposium, Neurophysiology of Hearing: Interpretation of Human Electrophysiological Data, sponsored by the European Economic Community (Medical Research Committee: Ad hoc Working Group on Deafness) and organized by M. Portmann and J. M. Aran, will be held May 20-22, 1976, in Bordeaux, France. Registration fees: 350.00 F.F. For further information write: M. Portmann, 114 Avenue d'Ares, 33000 Bordeaux, France.

Ann Otol 84: 1975

CHARACTERIZATION OF TUMOR ANTIGEN IN EPIDERMOID CARCINOMA

CHARLES J. KRAUSE, M.D.

JOHN NYSATHER BRIAN F. MCCABE, M.D.

IOWA CITY, IOWA

SUMMARY — Tumor antigens have been isolated from nine epidermoid carcinomas of the head and neck. The most strongly reactive antigens have a molecular weight of $\simeq$ 25,000-50,000 daltons, though other antigens weighing $\simeq$ 120,000-400,000 daltons were noted in six of the tumors. The most strongly reactive antigens from three of the tumors were further purified by isoelectric focusing. Each of these antigens had a pI between 8.36 and 8.40. The cross reactivity of these antigens will be studied next. It is hoped that the purified tumor antigen will be useful in the development of an immunodetection system for epidermoid carcinoma.

The growth of knowledge about immunobiologic processes has brought about a better appreciation of the complex interaction between the host immune system and a neoplasm. Methods are being sought to effectively monitor a patient's immunosurveillance system for early evidence that a malignancy is present. Such a system might be useful as a screening method for cancer, and most certainly would increase the accuracy of posttherapeutic detection of residual cancer.

An immunodiagnostic method might assay for either circulating tumor specific antigens (TSA) or for antitumor antibodies. TSA appear to be released into the general circulation but in such minute quantities that detection is difficult. Radioimmunoassays (RIA) have been developed which are capable of demonstrating nanogram/ml levels of fetal antigens. The two major circulating fetal antigens which have been found to be associated with carcinomas are carcinoembryonic antigen (CEA) and alphafetoprotein (AFP). Unfortunately, these antigens are not specific for cancer and have been found in a variety of benign, as well as malignant, conditions.

Both humoral and cellular-fixed antitumor antibodies are demonstrable in cancer patients. Difficulty in detecting antitumor antibodies in patients with early lesions and lack of specificity of the antibodies continues to be a problem which limits the general usefulness of such techniques.

This study was designed to purify and characterize tumor specific antigens from epidermoid carcinoma arising in the head and neck. The purified tumor antigens will then be utilized to develop an RIA capable of detecting circulating tumor antigens or assay techniques for antibody titers directed against the specific tumor antigens. Such an immunoassay system would provide an early detection method so important for effective cancer control.

Considerable evidence now exists that specific antigens are present on the cell membranes of cancer cells which are different from antigens present on normal cells. These TSA have been isolated

From the Department of Otolaryngology and Maxillofacial Surgery, University of Iowa Hospitals, Iowa City, Iowa 52242.

Presented at the meeting of the American Laryngological Association, Atlanta, Georgia, April 6-7, 1975.

from a variety of tumors in animals[1-4] and man[5-7] alike. Billings and Terasaki[8] found purified tumor antigens isolated from human lymphomas to have a molecular weight of $\simeq$ 27,000.

Early studies[9,10] suggested that tumor antigens found in chemically-induced solid tumors were different from those in other similarly induced tumors. However, more recently Ankerst and his associates[11] demonstrated cross reactivity in chemically induced rat mammary fibroadenomas, as did Steel and Sjogren[12] in rat colon cancer.

Cross reactivity of some solid tumors in man has also been found. The Hellstroms[13] demonstrated very nicely that lymphocytes from patients with various types of cancer will destroy not only their own cancer cells but also cells from cancers of the same histologic type found in other patients. Utilizing the same cytotoxicity method, Kennedy[14] working in our department found that lymphocytes from 12 patients with epidermoid carcinoma of the head and neck destroyed cells in culture from a single epidermoid carcinoma of the larynx, whereas nonsensitized lymphocytes from control patients did not. Of interest, cell mediated antibody was present in one additional female patient who had no recurrence of her head and neck cancer, but did have epidermoid cancer of the cervix. This finding suggested that cross reactivity existed between the epidermoid carcinoma of the cervix and that of the head and neck.

Gold and Freedman[15] isolated an antigen from adenocarcinomas of the colon that is normally found in the human fetus but not in the normal adult. This glycoprotein, called carcinoembryonic antigen (CEA), could be identified within the general circulation of most patients with colon carcinoma. However, CEA has also been found in a variety of other gastrointestinal tract malignancies and benign conditions as well.

Another circulating antigen associated with fetal development, as well as with carcinoma, is AFP, which was described by Tatarinov.[16] This globulin is normally produced by the fetal liver but disappears from the general circulation shortly after birth. Though most commonly associated with hepatomas, levels of circulating AFP have been demonstrated in a variety of malignant and nonmalignant conditions. With both of these fetal antigens, lack of specificity has limited their usefulness in the immunodiagnosis of cancer.

Antibody response to these tumor antigens is extremely complex. The response of the host T-lymphocyte system appears to be of paramount significance in tumor destruction. Sensitized lymphocytes which destroy specific tumor cells remain in the peripheral circulation for about 24 months[14] after removal of a tumor, then disappear unless a recurrence of the tumor develops.

Humoral antibodies against tumor antigens are associated with B-lymphocytes. High antibody titers directed against the Epstein-Barr virus have been found in patients with nasopharyngeal carcinoma as well as with some other head and neck carcinomas.[17] These elevated antibody titers rapidly fall to normal in patients who are free of tumor after treatment.[18] Hollinshead, *et al*[19] demonstrated elevated antibody titers against herpes simplex virus nonvirion antigens in a series of patients with head and neck cancer.

The role of antibody in the rejection of tumor is at present poorly understood. In some situations it appears that antibodies or antigen-antibody complexes may actually impair or block the action of sensitized lymphocytes against the tumor cells.

METHODS AND MATERIALS

A block of fresh tumor cells is removed from the specimen core at the time of surgical resection of head and neck epidermoid carcinoma. The remaining specimen is processed in standard fashion to obtain H. and E. slides for histologic identification. The tumor specimen is minced and the protein and glycoprotein molecules enzymatically cleaved from the cell surface utilizing 2.5% solution of trypsin.[20]

After centrifugation of the specimen at

TABLE I

SUMMARY OF DATA ON INDIVIDUAL PATIENTS WITH EPIDERMOID CARCINOMA

Sex	*Age*	*Tumor Site*	*Protein Fractions Yielding Positive Skin Tests (Molecular Weight – Daltons)*
F	66	Neck	200,000 42,000
M	55	Floor of mouth	34,500 25,000
F	73	Buccal mucosa	260,000
F	88	Gingivo-buccal sulcus	40,000 32,000
F	58	Pyriform sinus	200,000 34,000
M	58	Floor of mouth	140,000 26,500
M	55	Alveolar ridge	400,000 30,000
F	41	False vocal cord	34,000
F	80	Tongue	400,000 42,000 29,000

2,000 rpm for 15 minutes, the supernatant is mixed with an equal volume of a saturated solution of ammonium sulfate (SAS) and centrifuged for 30 minutes at 15,000 rpm at 2 C.

The supernatant is discarded, and the tumor extract thus precipitated is suspended in an aliquot of PBS and dialyzed exhaustively against PBS at 2 C. The crude tumor extract is then applied to the Biogel A-1.5 m column. Protein concentrations as measured by optical density at 280 nm are plotted versus molecular weight, resulting in a curve as illustrated in Figure 1.

Fractions from each peak are dialyzed exhaustively against normal saline solution at 2 C, and adjusted to 250 μg protein/0.05 ml.

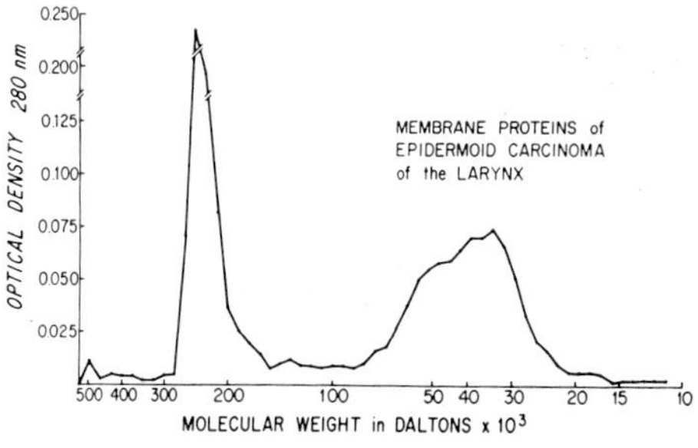

Fig. 1. Typical protein concentration curve following passage of crude tumor extract through Biogel A-1.5m column.

The fractions are then sterilized via membrane filtration (pore size 0.22μ), and 0.05 cc is injected intradermally into the volar aspect of the forearm. An area of erythema 5 mm in diameter or greater at 48 hours is considered a positive reaction.

Those fractions which resulted in a positive skin test reaction are then applied to an isoelectric focusing column resulting in a separation of protein complexes relative to their isoelectric point (pI). The fractions thus separated are then dialyzed against normal saline solution and the concentration adjusted to 250 μg/0.05 cc. Each specimen is sterilized via membrane filtration as before, and 0.05 cc is injected intradermally. The reaction is read at 48 hours. Those portions to which the patient demonstrates a positive skin test are thought to represent highly purified tumor antigens.

RESULTS

Preparation of Tumor Extract. Epidermoid carcinoma specimens from nine patients were processed. Table I lists the patients' age, sex, tumor site, and molecular weight of antigenic fractions. Trypsin was utilized to cleave antigens from the cell membranes resulting in a crude tumor extract containing a variety of antigens.

Gel Filtration. Initial purification of

the tumor extract utilized passage through a Biogel A - 1.5m column. The results of this method were remarkably consistent with each tumor, showing a high peak at ≃ 200,000 - 280,000 daltons and lesser peaks at ≃ 25,000 - 50,000 daltons.

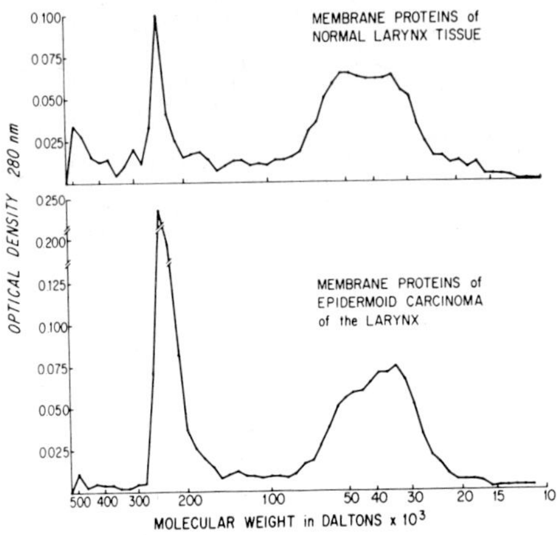

Fig. 2. Comparison of curves produced by tumor and normal tissue extracts in the same patient. Greater concentration of protein in the tumor extract at ≃ 220,000 and 34,000 represents tumor antigens.

When normal tissue extracts were compared with tumor extracts from the same patient (Fig. 2), major peaks appeared at similar molecular weights. However, the protein concentration at two of the major peaks was considerably greater in the tumor extract suggesting that these two peaks contain normal antigens as well as tumor antigens.

Skin Tests. If the patient is capable of mounting a hypersensitivity skin reaction, he should develop no reaction when normally occurring autochthonous antigens (such as HL-A) are injected intradermally but should react with a secondary response (within 48 hours) to injected tumor antigens.[21] Preparations from each individual peak were sterilized and injected intradermally into the host. Table I lists the molecular weight of each fraction to which positive skin tests (5 mm diameter at 48 hours) oc-

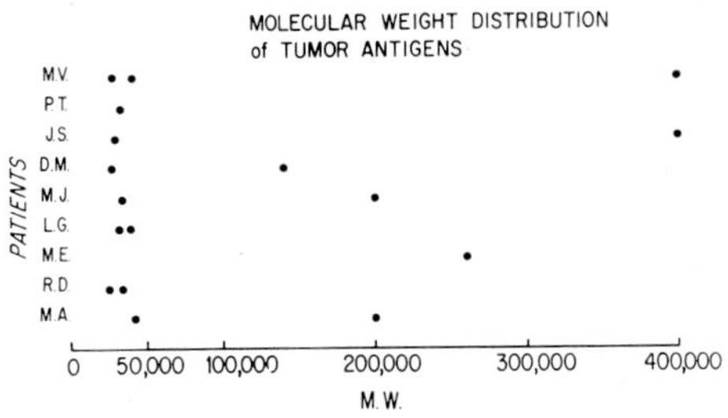

Fig. 3. Molecular weight of protein fractions to which each patient developed a positive delayed hypersensitivity skin reaction. These fractions contain tumor antigens.

curred. In eight of the nine patients a strongly positive reaction developed to antigens with molecular weights in the 25,000 - 50,000 dalton range. Six of the patients also had secondary reactions to antigens in the 120,000 - 400,000 dalton range, though less strongly so (Fig. 3). None of the patients developed positive reactions when skin tested with extracts from normal tissue. Interestingly, three patients were skin tested initially before

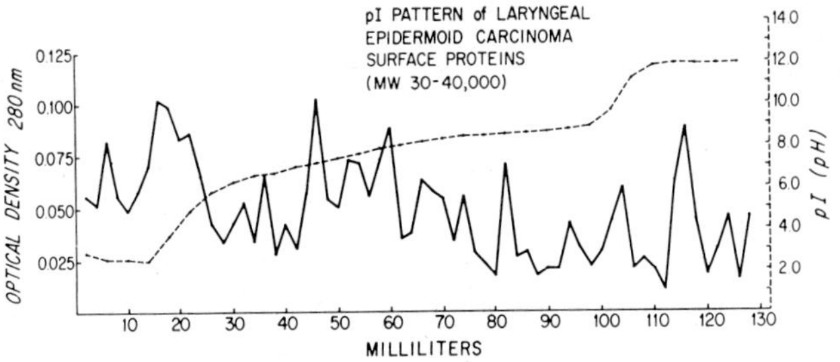

Fig. 4. Typical isoelectric pattern of surface antigens with molecular weight in the range of 30,000-40,000. Fraction from each peak was injected intradermally in three patients.

surgical removal of the tumor. None of the patients developed positive skin reactions. Each of these patients was again skin tested after removal of the primary tumor and developed a positive skin test which appears to indicate immunosuppression by the tumor.

Isoelectric Focusing. In three patients the most strongly antigenic extracts (26,500 - 34,000) have been further purified utilizing an isoelectric focusing column (Fig. 4). Again, individual peaks were adjusted for concentration and injected intradermally. All three patients reacted only to fractions with a pI of 8.36 to 8.40 (Fig. 5), which is within the limits of accuracy for the technique.

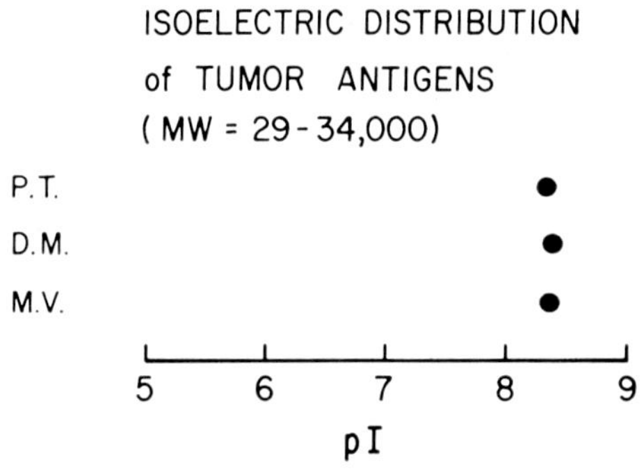

Fig. 5. Positive skin test reaction occurred in each of the three patients to a fraction with isoelectric point between 8.36 and 8.40.

DISCUSSION

This is a report of some early information obtained about tumor antigens found in epidermoid carcinoma of the head and neck. Though only a small number of tumors have been processed, the results are strikingly consistent, suggesting that this will prove to be a very effective method of obtaining highly purified tumor antigens. The most strongly reactive antigens appear to have a molecular weight in the range of $\simeq$ 25,000 to 50,000 daltons and to have a pI of about 8.4. Other tumor antigens may be present in the molecular weight range of $\simeq$ 120,000 - 400,000, though these appear to be less strongly antigenic.

The cross reactivity of these tumor antigens is now being studied. These purified antigens will be used to develop sensitive immunoassays for circulating tumor antigen and antitumor antibody titers in patients. It is hoped that such a method of immunodetection will be capable of identifying cancer when it is still quite small and readily curable.

Request for reprints should be sent to Charles J. Krause, M.D., Department of Otolaryngology and Maxillofacial Surgery, University of Iowa Hospitals, Iowa City, Iowa 52242.

REFERENCES

1. Kolb JP, Poupon MF, Lespinats G: Tumor-associated antigen (TAA) and antibodies in the serum of BALB/c mice with plasmacytomas. J Natl Cancer Inst 52:723-727, 1974

2. Jones DB, Moore M: Antigens of tumours induced by naturally occurring murine sarcoma virus (MSV-FBJ). I. Detection of group and type specific antigens by complement fixation. Br J Cancer 29:21-30, 1974

3. Bystryn JC, Schenkein I, Baur S, *et al*: Partial isolation and characterization of antigens associated with murine melanoma. J Natl Cancer Inst 52:1263-1269, 1974

4. Baldwin RW, Glaves D, Harris JR: Tumor specific antigens associated with aminozo-dye induced rat hepatomas. Transplant Proc 3:1189-1190, 1971

5. Lewis MG: Proceedings: Tumor specific antigens in melanoma. Proc Natl Cancer Conf 7:77-83, 1973

6. Nordquist RE: Specific antigens in human alveolar carcinoma. Cancer Res 33: 1790-1795, 1973

7. Edynak EM, Hirschaut Y, Old LJ, *et al*: Antigens of human breast cancer. Proc Am Assoc Cancer Res 12:75, 1971

8. Billings R, Terasaki PI: Human leukemia antigen. II. Purification. J Natl Cancer Inst 53:1639-1643, 1974

9. Foley EJ: Antigenic properties of methylcholanthrene-induced tumors in mice of the strain of origin. Cancer Res 13:835, 1963

10. Prehn RT, Main JM: Immunity to methylcholanthrene-induced sarcomas. J Natl Cancer Inst 18:769, 1957

11. Ankerst J, Steel G, Sjogren HO: Cross-

reacting tumor-associated antigens of adenovirus type 9-induced fibroadenomas and a chemically induced mammary carcinoma in rats. Cancer Res 34:1794, 1974

12. Steel G, Sjogren HO: Cross-reacting tumor-specific transplantation antigens in chemically induced rat colon carcinomas. Cancer Res 34:1801, 1974

13. Hellstrom I, Hellstrom KE, Sjogren HO, *et al*: Demonstration of cell-mediated immunity to human neoplasms of various histological types. Int J Cancer 7:1, 1971

14. Kennedy JT: *A Search for Common Tumor Specific Antigen and Serum Blocking Factor in Head and Neck Epidermoid Carcinomas*, thesis. University of Iowa, Iowa City, 1973

15. Gold P, Freedman SO: Demonstration of tumor-specific antigens in human colonic carcinomata by immunological tolerance and absorption techniques. J Exp Med 121:439, 1965

16. Tatarinov YS: Content of embryo-specific alpha-globulin in fetal and neonatal sera and sera from adult humans with primary carcinoma. Fed Proc (Transl Suppl) 25:344, 1966

17. Henle W, Henle G, Ho H, *et al*: Antibodies to Epstein-Barr virus in nasopharyngeal carcinoma, other head and neck neoplasms and control groups. J Natl Cancer Inst 44: 225-231, 1970

18. Henle W, Ho HC, Henle G, *et al*: Antibodies to Epstein-Barr virus related antigens in nasopharyngeal carcinoma. Comparison of active cases with long term survivors. J Natl Cancer Inst 51:361, 1973

19. Hollinshead AC, Chretien PB, Rawls WE, *et al*: Antibodies to herpesvirus nonvirion antigens in squamous carcinomas. Science 182:713, 1973

20. Slimowska V, Kawiak J: Liberation of cell surface material by the insoluble trypsin derivative. Acta Biochim Pol 20:113-118, 1973

21. Herberman RB: Delayed hypersensitivity skin reaction to antigens on human tumors. Cancer 34:1469-1473, 1974

CALL FOR ABSTRACTS FOR THE SCIENTIFIC FORUM OF THE AMERICAN COLLEGE OF SURGEONS

The 1976 Clinical Congress of the American College of Surgeons will be held in Chicago October 11-15. A special session of the Surgical Forum will be devoted to otorhinolaryngology. The Forum is designed to provide young investigators an opportunity to present their clinical and basic research work at a national level to an interested and critical audience. It is not necessary for the authors to be Fellows of the American College of Surgeons in order to participate in the Forum.

The deadline for the submission of abstracts to the Surgical Forum Committee is March 11, 1976. The abstracts must be mailed to the College Office, 55 East Erie Street, Chicago, Illinois 60611. The specific instructions are published in the January issue of the *Bulletin of the American College of Surgeons.* It is imperative that the instructions in the *Bulletin* be followed to the letter. Be sure to mark abstracts "Otorhinolaryngology" as directed.

Accepted abstracts will be published in longer form in the *Surgical Forum.* The author may publish the material elsewhere after the presentation at the Clinical Congress.

Ann Otol 84: 1975

PYRIFORM SINUS CANCER: A CLINICAL AND LABORATORY STUDY

JOHN A. KIRCHNER, M.D.

NEW HAVEN, CONNECTICUT

SUMMARY — In our patient population, cancer of the hypopharynx arose 19 times as often in the pyriform sinus as in the postcricoid space (152:8). Most of the growths were far advanced when first seen (90% T3), and enlarged cervical nodes were present in 66% of the patients. Three year survival rates free of disease were as follows: primary surgical treatment (laryngectomy, radical neck dissection) (8/28) 29%; primary radiotherapy (2/55) 4%; and combined preoperative radiation (12/33) 36%. Serial section studies of 51 surgical specimens indicate that T1 and T2 lesions, especially those confined in the medial wall, are probably curable by radiotherapy. Larger lesions invade deeply into the larynx and resemble transglottic growth in their pattern of spread. Conservation surgery would have been inadequate for all but perhaps one growth in this series of 51 lesions, because of the high rate of invasion by cancer into and through the thyroid cartilage and cricoid ring (22/51). Although surface presentation of this group of pyriform sinus cancers rarely reflected the extent of invasion, each of the 22 growths that invaded portions of the thyroid or cricoid cartilages was characterized by clinical involvement of the apex and lateral wall of the pyriform sinus on laryngoscopy or barium swallow.

It is sometimes difficult to determine the starting point of a hypopharyngeal cancer if it has spread beyond its point of origin to invade adjoining structures. This study includes only those growths whose major bulk occupied the pyriform sinus or those in which the pyriform sinus contained an ulcerating neoplasm with induration extending into the larynx or base of tongue. Epiglottic lesions have not been included nor have those originating in the lateral pharyngeal wall or postcricoid area.

The period of study starts in 1958 when supervoltage radiation equipment was acquired at Yale New Haven Hospital and ends in 1971 to provide a minimum three year follow-up period. All diagnoses were confirmed histologically.

The patient population comprises those admitted to the Yale New Haven Hospital and another group admitted to the USVA Hospital at West Haven. Radiation therapy for the two institutions was given at Hunter Radiation Center at Yale New Haven Hospital. Surgery was performed by members of the otolaryngology staff of the Yale New Haven Hospital.

Of the 152 pyriform sinus cancers seen at the Yale New Haven Hospital between 1958 and 1971, 36 were not included in this study for the following reasons: treatment incomplete (19); first treatment elsewhere (16); and treated with ortho-voltage radiation[1] (Table I).

Survival rates have been calculated on the basis of a three-year period with no evidence of disease. Other status categories have been listed as follows:

Died Free of Disease. Patients were free of discernible disease at the time of death from other causes, usually in less than three years.

From the Department of Surgery, Section of Otolaryngology, Yale University School of Medicine, New Haven, Connecticut.

Supported by USPHS 9 RO1-NS-10551-08.

Presented at the meeting of the American Laryngological Association, Atlanta, Georgia, April 6-7, 1975.

TABLE I

PYRIFORM SINUS CANCER
1958-1971

Total No. Cases		152
Not included		36
Incomplete treatment	(19)	
First treatment elsewhere	(16)	
250 KV	(1)	
Case Material		116

Died of Other Causes. This includes one group of patients who died of other causes at intervals varying from a few weeks after operation up to seven months. Another group died of a second cancer three years or more after treatment.

Died with Disease. Death resulted from the original cancer, usually in a period of less than three years.

TABLE II

PYRIFORM SINUS CANCER (116)

Primary Surgery		28
T1	(2)	
T2	(2)	
T3	(24)	

Each tumor was originally staged according to the American Joint Commission (A.J.C.) classification available at the time. For the present report, the original staging of each tumor was expressed according to the 1973 supplement to the TNM classification of the International Union Against Cancer (I.U.A.C.) and A.J.C.[1]

Although there are as many small lesions as large ones in each of the three treatment categories (surgery, radiotherapy, and combined treatment), an element of selection must be allowed for in assessing results in treatment as with any retrospective study (Tables II, III, IV).

TABLE III

PYRIFORM SINUS CANCER (116)
1958-1971

Radiotherapy		55
T1	(2)	
T2	(2)	
T3	(51)	

TABLE IV

PYRIFORM SINUS CANCER (116)

Combined Treatment		33
T1	(2)	
T2	(1)	
T3	(30)	

CASE MATERIAL

During the period 1958-1971 when 152 cases of pyriform sinus cancer were seen at Yale New Haven Hospital and USVA Hospital, eight cases of postcricoid cancer were also seen (Table V). This results in a 19:1 ratio of pyriform sinus to postcricoid cancer, in striking contrast to the distribution in northern Europe where postcricoid cancer forms a much higher percentage of hypopharyngeal growths. Harrison's group of 67 hypopharyngeal cancers, for instance, included 40 postcricoid growths, 60% of the total. This may not reflect incidence rates precisely, as Harrison points out, but rather a degree of artificial selection related to the particular interest of his group in the surgical management of postcricoid cancer.[2] Jacobsson's series, however, shows a similar distribution among patients treated at Radiumhemmet in Stockholm.[3]

TABLE V

CANCER OF HYPOPHARYNX

Pyriform sinus	152
Postcricoid	8
Posterior wall	17

If the 152 cases of pyriform sinus cancer, 143 were in men. Unlike the sex distribution in northern Europe, six of the eight postcricoid cancers were in men (Table VI).

Most pyriform sinus cancer is diagnosed only after the disease is far advanced. Of the 116 cases making up this

TABLE VI

CANCER OF HYPOPHARYNX
1958-1971

	Male	*Female*
Pyriform sinus (152)	143	9
Postcricoid (8)	6	2
Posterior wall (17)	14	3

TABLE VII

PYRIFORM SINUS CANCER
1958-1971

Total No. Cases		116
T1	6	
T2	5	
T3	105	

study, 105 were in the most advanced category (T3) at the time of diagnosis (Table VII). Seventy-seven of the 116 patients had palpably enlarged cervical lymph nodes on admission, and in 19 others histologically positive nodes developed after treatment by surgery or radiation (Table VIII).

TABLE VIII

PYRIFORM SINUS CANCER

Total Number of Cases		116
Palpable Cervical Nodes (35/49 pos.) – 74%	77	
No Nodes Palpable (9/20 pos.) – 45%	20	
Nodes Not Sectioned	19	

Lymph node metastasis showed little if any relation to the stage of the primary tumor. Of six T1 lesions, three were associated with palpably enlarged nodes, of which two cases were histologically positive. Of five T2 lesions, three had regional metastasis and of 105 T3 lesions, 55 were shown histologically to have lymph node metastasis among 63 neck specimens available for study. Many of the remaining 42 cases were treated by radiotherapy and never had a neck dissection or biopsy of the neck nodes (Table IX).

For the same reason, the relationship

TABLE IX

PYRIFORM SINUS CANCER (116)

Primary	*Nodes Palpable*	*Nodes Pos.*
T1	3/6	2/3
T2	2/5	3/3*
T3	72/105	55/63

*One N-O.

between cervical node metastasis and histological differentiation of the primary tumor is not entirely reliable (Table X).

TABLE X

PYRIFORM SINUS CANCER (116)
GRADED (85)
LYMPH NODE METASTASES

Primary	*No. Cases*	*Pos. Nodes*	*%*
Well differentiated	30	15	50
Mod. differentiated	21	9	43
Poorly differentiated	34	13	38

TREATMENT AND RESULTS

Primary surgical treatment was employed in 28 cases and consisted of laryngectomy and radical neck dissection. Of these 28 patients, nine survived three years or more free of disease. Fourteen died of disease, including ten who had been treated by postoperative irradiation. Of the other five, three died of other causes, one is alive with cancer, and one died at three years with no evidence of disease. There were thirteen local or regional recurrences among these 28 patients (Table XI).

TABLE XI

PYRIFORM SINUS CANCER (116)

Primary Surgery			(28)
N.E.D.* > 3 years		(9)	
Alive with disease		(1)	
Died		(18)	
with disease	(14)		
other causes	(3)		
N.E.D.* 3 years	(1)		

*N.E.D.: No evidence of disease.

Supervoltage radiation therapy was used as the primary treatment in 55 cases. Of these, there were only two survivors after three years. Forty-four patients died with disease; nine died of other causes within three to twenty-eight months after treatment. One T1 and one T3 made up the survivors. Seven patients had laryngectomy for uncontrolled disease after radiotherapy, but none survived. There were 28 local or regional recurrences in this group of 55 (Table XII).

TABLE XII

PYRIFORM SINUS CANCER (116)

Primary Radiotherapy			(55)
N.E.D. > 3 years		2	
Died		53	
with disease	(44)		
other causes	(8)		
CVA* at 4 mo.	(1)		

*Cerebro-vascular accident.

Combined therapy was employed in 33 cases and consisted of planned preoperative irradiation, usually 4,000 rads in four weeks followed by laryngectomy and radical neck dissection in four to eight weeks (15 patients). Eighteen patients had other irradiation doses: ten were below 4,000 rads, averaging 3,600, and eight above, between 5,000 and 5,600 rads.

TABLE XIII

PYRIFORM SINUS CANCER (116)

Combined Treatment			(33)
N.E.D. > 3 years		12	
N.E.D. < 3 years		1	
Died		20	
with disease	(16)		
N.E.D. 3 years	(4)		

Of the 33 patients, twelve survived three years or more free of disease. This group includes both of the two patients with T1 and ten with T3. One patient with T2 and fifteen with T3 died with disease; five other patients with T3 died of other causes. There were six local or regional recurrences among these 33 patients (Tables XIII, XIV, XV).

TABLE XIV

PYRIFORM SINUS CANCER (116)

Local Recurrence After Treatment		(66)
Primary Surgery	13/28	46%
Primary Radiotherapy	42/55	76%
Combined	11/33	33%

Serial Section Studies. Fifty-one of the pyriform sinus cancers removed by laryngectomy and radical neck dissection were studied by whole organ serial section of the larynx. It was our intention to find answers to such questions as the following: Are there any predictable patterns of growth and spread of cancer from the pyriform sinus? Are there any characteristics of the primary growth that indicate likelihood of invasion of the thyroid cartilage, cricoid cartilage, or thyroid gland? How reliable is the gross appearance of a pyriform sinus cancer in estimating safe margins for resection?

TABLE XV

PYRIFORM SINUS CANCER (116)

	No. Cases	*N.E.D.*	*Surv. Rate*
Primary Surgery	28	8	29%
Primary Radiotherapy	55	2	4%
Combined	33	12	36%

How safe would "conservation surgery" have been in this group?

These 51 cases were treated as follows: primary surgery, 26; preoperative radiation, 19; and surgery for radiation failure, 6.

In the nonirradiated group there was very little about the gross appearance of any one of these 26 pyriform sinus cancers that indicated its potential for local or regional spread. This is due largely to the advanced stage in which most of these lesions were first seen. Of the 26 specimens serially sectioned, 24 had been staged in the most advanced group, T3, so that the exact point of origin within the pyriform sinus could not be determined. In the remaining 25 specimens, the growth pattern as observed in serial sections was distorted by preoperative radiotherapy.

Of the six radiation failures, two had no identifiable cancer on serial section beyond the biopsy site. Of the 19 combined treatment cases, ten had identifiable residual cancer; five showed a few small nests of "burned out" cells that probably represented the original disease and in four there was no identifiable cancer. On the other hand, most of these 19 cases still had positive cervical nodes.

There was an opportunity of studying the accuracy of lymph node staging in all but four of these 51 cases. In over half the cases in which the nodes were clinically negative, (N0, N1a, N2a) cervical metastasis was found histologically (13/22) (Table XVI).

TABLE XVI

FIFTY-ONE SERIALLY SECTIONED SPECIMENS. CERVICAL NODE INVOLVEMENT

	Number	*Histologically Positive*	*Unknown*
Clinically Negative	22	13	3
Clinically Positive	29	21	1

Of the 29 clinically positive necks, 21 were proven histologically. The other cases were among those treated by radiotherapy or preoperative irradiation so that the disease in the nodes may have been cured or masked.

Pyriform sinus cancer may spread medially into the larynx, displacing and fixing the lateral wall of the larynx so as to suggest a transglottic cancer, particularly one that may have arisen in the ventricle (Fig. 1). Vocal cord immobility may also be due to infiltration of the posterior crico-arytenoid muscle by cancer, to invasion of the crico-arytenoid joint, or to invasion of the recurrent laryngeal nerve trunk by cancer.[4] These

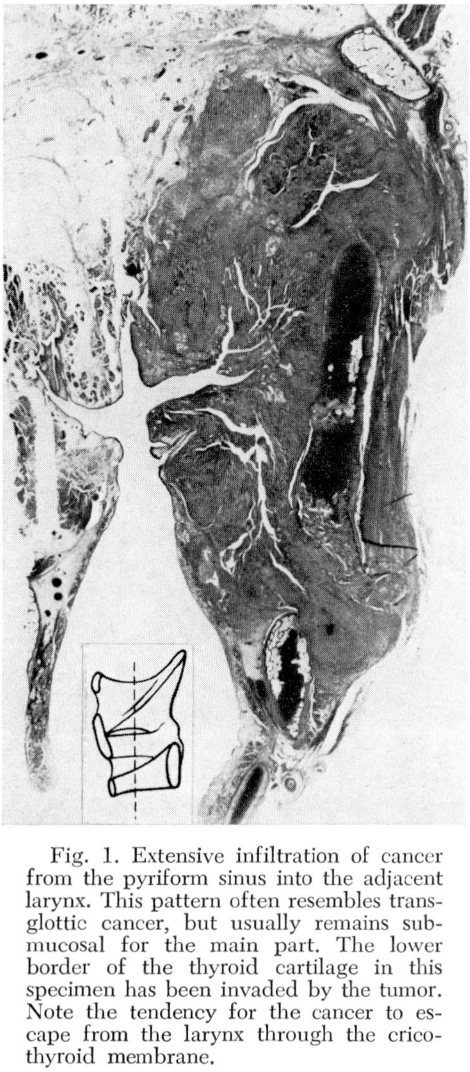

Fig. 1. Extensive infiltration of cancer from the pyriform sinus into the adjacent larynx. This pattern often resembles transglottic cancer, but usually remains submucosal for the main part. The lower border of the thyroid cartilage in this specimen has been invaded by the tumor. Note the tendency for the cancer to escape from the larynx through the cricothyroid membrane.

latter three patterns are usually associated with considerable invasion of the thyro-arytenoid muscle. Olofsson and vanNostrand have made similar observations.[5]

Larger growths may extend from the pyriform sinus on to the lateral or posterior walls of the hypopharynx or in the opposite direction across the upper postcricoid area to involve the opposite pyriform sinus.

Next in frequency to the pattern of spread into the adjacent supraglottic

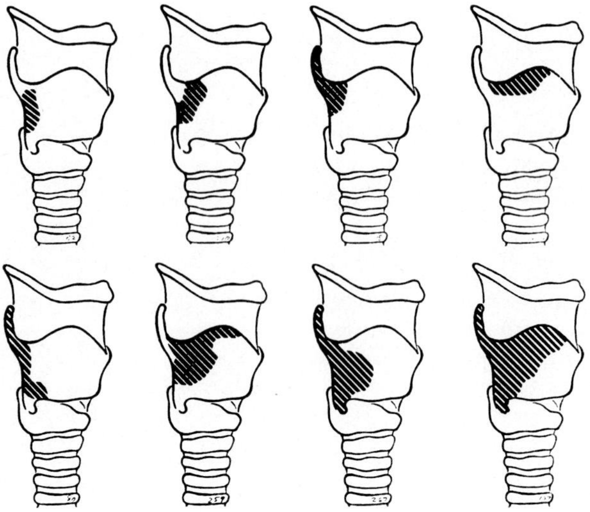

Fig. 2. Pattern of invasion by pyriform sinus cancer into the thyroid cartilage. Twenty specimens showed invasion of the thyroid and/or thyroid and cricoid cartilages.

larynx, and probably more ominous, is upward spread into the base of the tongue. Downward spread into the cervical esophagus has not been the pattern in this material. In three specimens showing involvement of this latter area, one was a postcricoid cancer, and the other two appeared to have arisen in the cervical esophagus and involved the pyriform sinus by upward extension.

In nine specimens the bulk of the neoplasm occupied mainly the medial wall of the pyriform sinus. Obviously none of these nine invaded the thyroid cartilage. Seven had been treated by preoperative irradiation, and growth patterns distorted. Three, however, showed no residual cancer. In four, small nests of "burned-out" tumor cells were seen. One nonirradiated specimen showed tumor cells close to the arytenoid cartilage and the other case recurred at the margin of resection after a partial laryngopharyngectomy.

By contrast, the 22 specimens which showed invasion or destruction of the thyroid or cricoid cartilage on serial section had all shown involvement of the lateral wall of the pyriform sinus at laryngoscopy and in the gross specimen.

Pyriform sinus cancer eroded the thyroid cartilage in 20 of 51 specimens, usually along the posterior edge, although the cricoid cartilage alone was invaded in two of 51 specimens. Cricoid invasion is usually observed as an extension of the same process in the thyroid ala. The risk of direct invasion of the superior lobe of the thyroid gland in these cases is obvious (Figs. 2, 3).

Preoperative irradiation appeared to have no destructive action on the laryngeal framework. Among 25 specimens which had been irradiated before operation, 13 showed dissolution limited to the postero-lateral portion of the thyroid ala or cricoid ring, the same pattern as seen in the nonradiated cases (10/26), where the destruction was obviously caused by cancer. It would appear, then, that the portion of the thyroid ala or cricoid ring that had been invaded by cancer simply disappeared under radiation therapy.

The thyroid lobe on the involved side was usually not removed if it did not appear to be near tumor or if there was no induration palpable in the superior lobe. However, the pattern of erosion of the thyroid and cricoid cartilages indicates that this is not a safe practice, even when the superior lobe can be

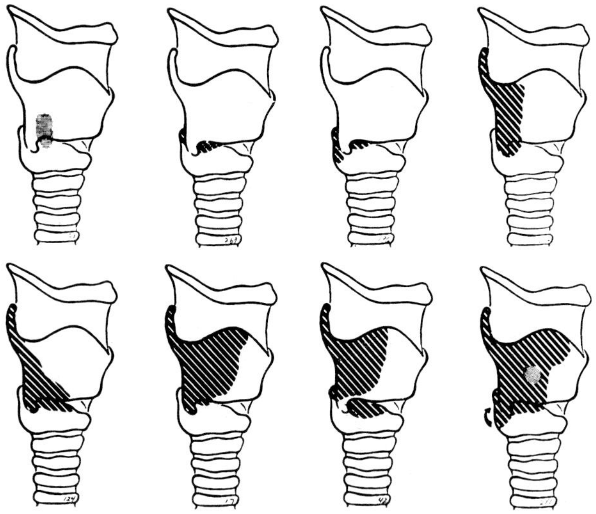

Fig. 3. Patterns of invasion in those specimens in which the cricoid cartilage was involved. Two specimens showed invasion limited to the cricoid cartilage. In one of the latter, both pyriform sinuses contained cancer. The specimen represented in the upper left corner diagram showed erosion only on the inner cortex of the thyroid and cricoid cartilages.

easily displaced off the larynx, and when there is no obvious involvement of the laryngeal framework by the growth.

Ogura observed that the gland may be invaded even if the cancer has not eroded through the thyroid cartilage. In addition to lymphatic tumor emboli, he demonstrated a case showing tumor within vascular channels of the gland.[6] This would suggest that involvement of the thyroid gland or the adjacent paratracheal nodes may have been responsible for the 14 local and regional recurrences among the 22 cases with invasion of the laryngeal framework. The same could be true of the 13 recurrences among the remaining 29 uninvaded cases (Fig. 4).

Histological Differentiation. Of the 22 growths which invaded the laryngeal framework, the degree of differentiation was estimated at 17. Six were well differentiated, four moderately, and seven poorly.

Cervical Node Metastasis. In 38 of the 51 growths, the degree of differentiation was reported by the pathologist. Of 16 well differentiated primary growths, eight had proven metastasis. Of eight moderately well differentiated growths, six had proven metastasis. Of fourteen poorly differentiated growths, seven had proven metastasis.

The metastatic rate is probably higher than indicated by these figures since, in many of these cases, the neck had been included in the field of preoperative irradiation or radiotherapy.

Peripheral Growth Pattern. A pushing edge was seen in five of the 51 specimens. In four there was no invasion of the laryngeal framework. In the fifth, the cancer spilled over the top and presented as a palpable mass under the skin (Fig. 5). Further posteriorly, this tumor destroyed the thyroid cartilage (Fig. 6). Despite their relatively benign appearance on section, this feature did not insure a good prognosis. Two of the five patients died within two years with primary recurrence.

CONSERVATION SURGERY

Serial section studies indicate that pre-

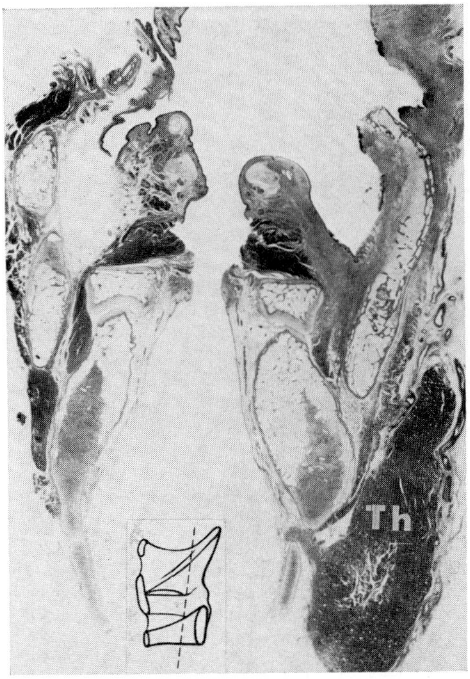

Fig. 4. Relation of superior lobe of thyroid gland to cricothyroid membrane. Cancer escaping from the lower larynx could invade the gland by direct extension. This specimen had been given 5,600 rads five weeks before laryngectomy.

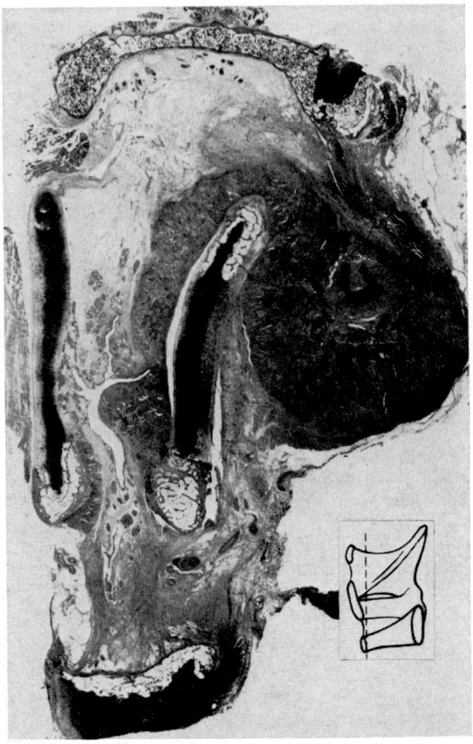

Fig. 5. This growth, characterized by a "pushing edge" escaped through the thyrohyoid membrane and presented as a mass under the skin of the neck. The pyriform sinus apex was clinically invaded by the tumor, and there was extensive destruction of the posterior portion of the thyroid cartilage, as shown in Figure 6.

operative irradiation disqualifies a pyriform sinus cancer for conservation surgery. This is not so much because of the healing problems caused by the scar tissue resulting from irradiation, but rather because of the unpredictable extent of invasion into the larynx and other surrounding structures. Surface presentation of a pyriform sinus cancer rarely reflects the exact extent of invasion even before irradiation. After treatment, not only is the tumor smaller, but also the surrounding normal tissues are shrunken and distorted so that the surgical procedure is hampered by unidentifiable margins. In this regard, Ogura's series of 28 pyriform sinus cancers treated by partial laryngopharyngectomy did not include any cases subjected to preoperative irradiation.[7]

In his 1960 report on partial laryngopharyngectomy for pyriform sinus cancer, Ogura set forth certain criteria for selecting cases suitable for conservation surgery. These included the caution that there must be no involvement of the apex of the pyriform sinus and that the thyroid cartilage must be free of tumor.[8] The present study confirms the validity of these criteria and illustrates their histological rationale.

Of the 40 growths which involved the lateral wall of the pyriform sinus on laryngoscopy or barium studies, 22 invaded the thyroid cartilage, cricoid ring, or both. The apex of the pyriform sinus was clinically involved by the growth in each of these 22 cases.

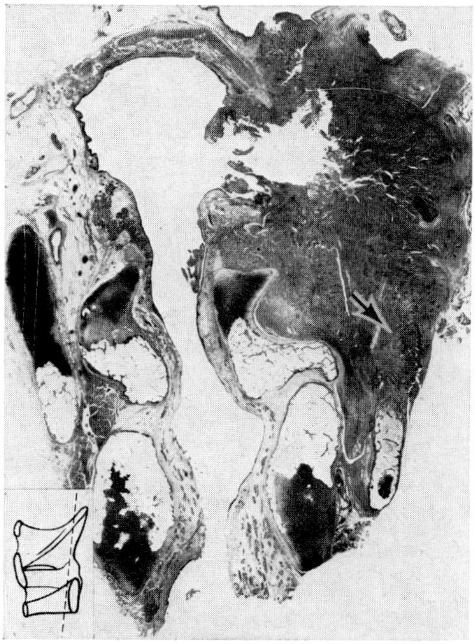

Fig. 6. Destruction of the upper two-thirds of the thyroid ala (arrow) by cancer invading from the pyriform sinus. The tumor was classified as "well differentiated," but the patient died six weeks after operation with pulmonary metastases.

In the remaining 18 cases there was no invasion of the thyroid or cricoid cartilage, and clinical involvement of the pyriform sinus apex was minimal or incidental (Fig. 7). It can be said of our material, then, that every case in which thyroid or cricoid cartilage invasion was found in serial sections had exhibited involvement of the pyriform sinus apex clinically (Table XVII).

TABLE XVII

LATERAL WALL INVOLVED CLINICALLY (40)

↓	↓
Framework Invaded (22)	Framework Not Invaded (18)
↓	↓
Pyriform Sinus Apex Involved	Pyriform Sinus Apex Involved
|	|
Always	Rarely

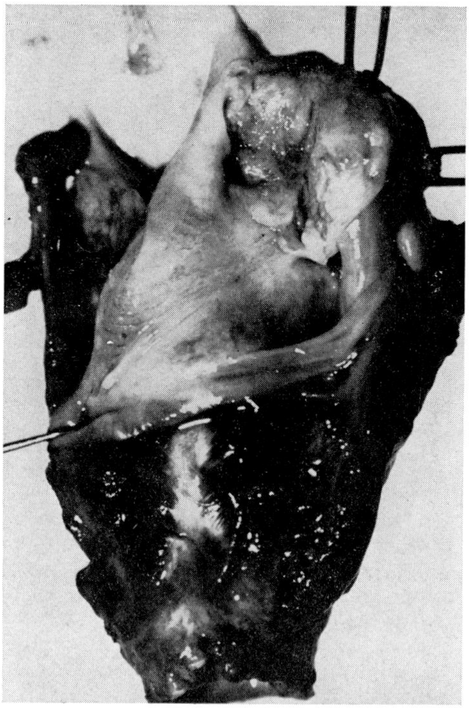

Fig. 7. Cancer of the upper portion of the pyriform sinus with no involvement of the apex. In serial section studies, growths of this type never invaded the thyroid cartilage. It was only among those growths showing clinical involvement of the lateral wall and apex that invasion of the laryngeal framework was frequently observed histologically.

Even though the destruction was usually confined to the posterior portion of the thyroid ala and the upper edge of the cricoid ring, this pattern varied considerably and the extent of invasion could not have been predicted on the basis of surface presentation. Conservation surgery, therefore, would have been entirely inappropriate in any one of these 40 cases with involvement of the lateral wall and apex of the pyriform sinus. In many of our specimens, the saw cut would have traversed cancer in the thyroid ala (Fig. 8).

Of the 47 T3 lesions sectioned, no other feature of the primary growth, such as histological differentiation, appeared to influence the tumor's tendency to in-

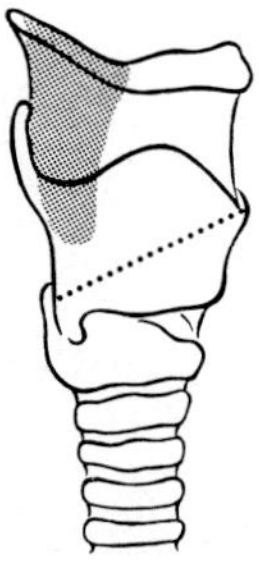

Fig. 8. Stippled area on diagram shows position of pyriform sinus. The dotted line shows the saw cut, usually employed in partial laryngopharyngectomy, which in most of our specimens would have passed through, or very close to the cancer. Clinical involvement of the apex of the pyriform sinus is therefore a contraindication to conservation surgery for cancer in this area.

vade the laryngeal framework. None of the T1 and T2 lesions invaded the thyroid or cricoid cartilages.

Small growths on the medial wall of the pyriform sinus that appeared to be possible candidates for conservation surgery appeared on histological examination to have responded well to irradiation. In the smallest lesion there was infiltration of the soft tissue around the arytenoid cartilage so that the mandatory arytenoidectomy would have been oncologically unsafe.

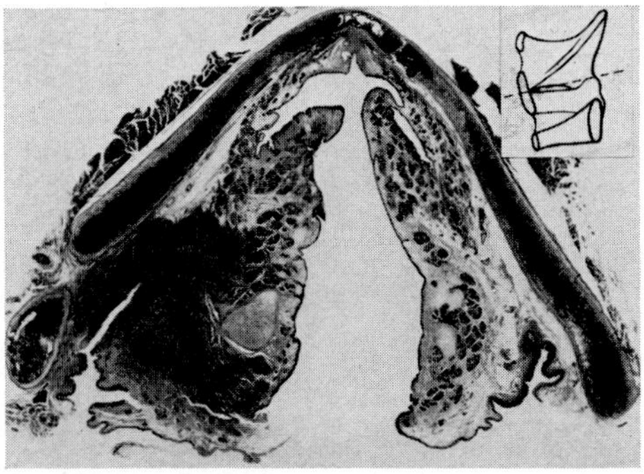

Fig. 9. Horizontal section of specimen in Figure 7 (right side of specimen is on left of picture). Cancer has partly surrounded the arytenoid cartilage and infiltrated the submucosal portion of the false cord.

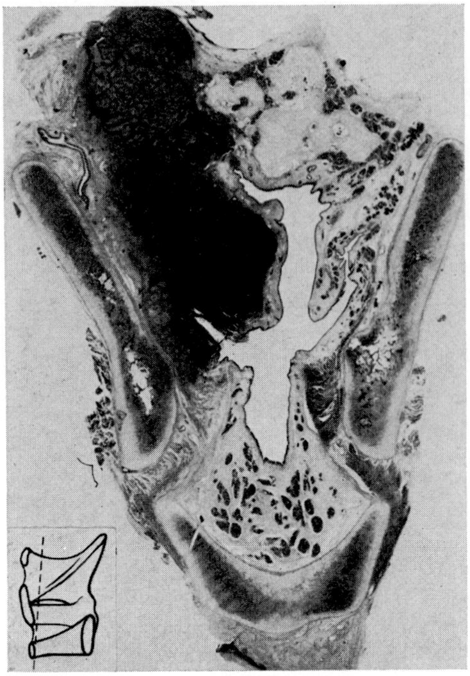

Fig. 10. Cancer invading the false cord and extending downward, lateral to the ventricle. Further extension of this type produces fixation of the true vocal cord, resembling a transglottic growth in this respect. Note the intact mucous membrane of the false cord.

Larger growths on the medial and anterior walls showed a significant degree of deep infiltration by cancer cells into the supraglottic larynx (Fig. 9). Cancer invading this region does not follow the usual pattern of supraglottic cancer, but invades downward within the paraglottic space, extending below the level of the ventricle and resembling a transglottic growth in this respect (Fig. 10). It tends to escape from the larynx via the cricothyroid membrane where it may invade the lower border of the thyroid cartilage and the upper border of the cricoid.

Request for reprints should be sent to John A. Kirchner, M.D., Professor and Chief, Department of Surgery/Otolaryngology, Yale University School of Medicine, 333 Cedar Street, New Haven, Connecticut 06510.

REFERENCES

1. *U.I.C.C. and A.J.C. Supplement to TNM Classification of Malignant Tumors.* Geneva, G. de Buren S. A., rev. 1973

2. Harrison DFN: Pathology of hypopharyngeal cancer in relation to surgical management, J Laryngol Otol 84:349-367, 1970

3. Jacobsson F: Carcinoma of the hypopharynx, Acta Radiol [Diagn] (Stockh) 35: 1-21, 1951

4. Kirchner JA: One hundred laryngeal cancers studied by serial section. Ann Otol Rhinol Laryngol 78:689-709, 1969

5. Olofsson J, vanNostrand AWP: Growth and spread of laryngeal and hypopharyngeal carcinoma with reflections on the effect of preoperative irradiation: 139 cases studied by whole organ serial sectioning, Acta Otolaryngol [Suppl] (Stockh) 308:1-84, 1973

6. Ogura JH: Surgical pathology of cancer of the larynx. Laryngoscope 65:867-926, 1955

7. Ogura JH, Mallen RW: Partial laryngopharyngectomy for supraglottic and pharyngeal carcinoma. Trans Am Acad Ophthalmol Otolaryngol 69:832-845, 1965

8. Ogura JH, Jurema AA, Watson RK: Partial laryngopharyngectomy and neck dissection for pyriform sinus cancer: conservation surgery with immediate reconstruction, Laryngoscope 70:1399-1417, 1960

Ann Otol 84: 1975

RADIATION FAILURES IN CANCER OF THE LARYNX

EMANUEL M. SKOLNIK, M.D.

LAWRENCE MARTIN, M.D. KING F. YEE, M.D.

MICHAEL A. WHEATLEY, M.D.

CHICAGO, ILLINOIS

SUMMARY — Overwhelming statistics have been published regarding the success of radiation therapy in the management of laryngeal carcinoma. The fate of those patients whose cancers are not controlled by radiotherapy is often left to speculation. An analysis is made of 61 patients with early and advanced laryngeal cancer treated initially with radiation therapy and subsequently operated upon because of recurrent or persistent tumor. Frequently, diagnosis of recurrence is difficult or delayed. Preservation of voice can only be accomplished when recurrence of T_1 and T_2 lesions is detected early and strict criteria are followed. Conservation surgery is not feasible for early lesions which progress after radiation failure. Advanced T_3 and T_4 lesions which become radiation failures also require laryngectomy for salvage. In cancer of the larynx, there is a definite, identifiable group of patients in whom surgery would be advisable as the initial therapy.

Radiation therapy for cancer of the larynx, and especially the glottic region, is receiving increased emphasis today. Its contribution in the management of laryngeal cancer is well known. However, like its surgical counterpart, it is not without its share of failures. But, unlike its surgical counterpart, delay in diagnosis of recurrent tumor after radiation therapy failure is common.

In early vocal cord cancer, the cure rates have been reported to be 80-96%. In Till's report of larynx cancer end results (10,989 patients), presented at the Centennial Conference on Laryngeal Cancer, the initial treatment was radiation therapy for cure in the majority of cases.[1] However, the crude five-year survival for 3,296 T_1N_0 glottic patients was only 72%, and the same survival for 637 T_1N_0 supraglottic patients was only 55%. These crude five-year survival rates do not reveal the status or quality of the voice following therapy. Only cure is reported, and patient survival may not reflect the reliability of the primary treatment method. Often salvage surgery is required after radiation therapy has failed. Survival, then, does not always correlate with voice preservation.

Both radiotherapists and surgeons would concur that the first opportunity is the best opportunity for cure in cancer of the larynx. The advantages of radiation therapy in preserving laryngeal function have been well outlined by Lederman[2] who has treated large numbers of patients with early and advanced lesions of the larynx. Unfortunately, the microscopic characteristics of a tumor from a biopsy specimen offer no prediction as to the response of the tumor to radiotherapy.

During the past twenty years, other laryngologists have advocated conservation surgery of the larynx while preserving laryngeal function. The voice in these partial procedures is certainly adequate, and the surgery is not incapacitating. There is a definite group of patients who are best advised to have sur-

From the Department of Otolaryngology, Abraham Lincoln School of Medicine, College of Medicine, University of Illinois at the Medical Center.

Presented at the meeting of the American Laryngological Association, Atlanta, Georgia, April 6-7, 1975.

TABLE I

CRITERIA FOR PARTIAL LARYNGECTOMY[5] FOLLOWING RADIATION FAILURE

1. The cancer must have been localized originally
2. Regional lymph node metastasis should not be a dominant feature of the disease
3. The original extent of the cancer should be circumscribed by the surgical procedure

gery as the initial therapy. These patients will be identified later. Lederer's classic article on laryngic descriptive discrepancy would support the advantage of having a surgical specimen to examine following initial therapy.[3] The confusion and discrepancy of indirect and direct laryngoscopy by different examiners is solved when the entire specimen is in hand. Macroscopic and microscopic correlations can be made. Analysis of the

TABLE II

CRITERIA FOR HEMILARYNGECTOMY[6] FOLLOWING RADIATION FAILURE

1. No opposite cord tumor except anterior commissure
2. No arytenoid involvement except vocal process
3. No subglottic extension >5 mm
4. No cartilage involvement
5. No cord fixation
6. Recurrence should correlate with original tumor

specimen offers prognostic information at once regarding the fate of the patient. This opportunity is lost when radiation therapy is used as the initial treatment.

Radiation failures of T_1 and T_2 laryngeal lesions can be treated by partial laryngectomy with voice preservation. In 1951, Som first reported four cases of radiation failure managed by partial laryngectomy.[4] Other laryngologists have reported similar success, and Ballantyne and Fletcher (1966)[5] and Biller, *et al* (1968)[6] have outlined the criteria for partial procedures following radiation therapy (Tables I and II). However,

TABLE III

LOCATION BY TNM STAGING SUPRAGLOTTIC (11 Pts.)

	N_0	N_1	N_2	N_3	*Total*
T_1	2	0	0	0	2
T_2	2	0	0	1	3
T_3	2	1	0	0	3
T_4	1	0	1	1	3

these early cord lesions can progress to large tumors when recurrence is not detected early, thus making conservation surgery impossible. For various reasons, T_3 and T_4 lesions best treated with surgery initially are occasionally given radiotherapy for cure. Only total laryngectomy can salvage these patients after radiation failure.

Ideally, the well-trained laryngologist would: a) avoid failure by choosing the

TABLE IV

LOCATION BY TNM STAGING GLOTTIC (49 Pts.)

	N_0	N_1	N_2	N_3	*Total*
T_1	15	2	0	0	17
T_2	9	0	0	0	9
T_3	15	2	0	0	17
T_4	2	4	0	0	6

appropriate initial therapy, b) detect failure early, and c) manage and salvage these failures by using the appropriate surgical therapy.

METHODS AND MATERIALS

Sixty-three patients were evaluated by the otolaryngology staff as radiation failures of the larynx during 1955-1974. Two patients were excluded from the report because they developed epidermoid carcinoma in a different site at 84 months (supraglottic primary) and at 79 months (glottic primary) after initial radiation therapy. This development was considered to be evidence for a second primary carcinoma of the larynx. There were 11 supraglottic, 49 glottic, and 1 subglottic cases for analysis. The location by TNM staging is shown in Tables III and IV for the supraglottic and glottic groups, respectively. The lone sub-

TABLE V

STATUS OF SUPRAGLOTTIC RADIATION FAILURES (11 Pts.)

Patients	*Status*
5	A $\bar{s}$ D
0	A $\bar{c}$ D
1	D $\bar{s}$ D
5	D $\bar{c}$ D
Average recurrence	5.3 Mo
Average survival	42 Mo

A $\bar{s}$ D – Alive without disease.
A $\bar{c}$ D – Alive with disease.
D $\bar{s}$ D – Dead without disease.
D $\bar{c}$ D – Dead with disease.

glottic carcinoma was staged T_3N_0. There were no glottic carcinoma *in situ* patients. There were 56 males and only five females in the series. Age range was from 39 to 80 years. A history of excessive tobacco and alcohol was elicited in more than 80% of the patients.

Reasons for radiation therapy as the initial treatment are not individualized. Patients with early, as well as advanced, lesions had refused surgery originally and were treated with radiotherapy for cure. Several patients were referred as radiation failures. Radiation therapy had been deemed the best treatment initially by the referring physician and/or radiotherapist. Diagnosis of recurrence was made and institution of surgical treatment was then done in our department. All patients were originally treated for cure by ^{60}Co (Cobalt) with at least 6,000 R over a 6 to 7 week period.

Detection of recurrence or persistent disease was usually made by direct laryngoscopy and biopsy. Laryngogram, xeroradiogram, and tomograms were helpful in assessing the extent of recurrence prior to endoscopy. Often, repeat biopsies were necessary to confirm the diagnosis. Occasionally, microscopic laryngoscopy with supravital staining was needed. Thyrotomy or laryngofissure was also used in order to obtain sufficient tumor for analysis.

On two occasions, patients presented with aspiration due to fixed vocal cords and pain due to perichondritis. In both instances, biopsies were insufficient for diagnosis of recurrence. In the first patient, tracheotomy had to be done prior to repeated endoscopy so as not to compromise the airway. Laryngectomy without positive biopsy was considered in the second patient until deeper sections of the first biopsy revealed cancer.

TABLE VI

SURGICAL PROCEDURES FOR SUPRAGLOTTIC RADIATION FAILURE (11 Pts.)

Supraglottic laryngectomy	1
Supraglottic laryngectomy RND	1
Laryngectomy	3
Laryngectomy RND	4
Laryngopharyngectomy and RND	1
Contralateral RND	1

RESULTS

Each of the three distinct regions of the larynx is analyzed separately.

Supraglottic. The status of the 11 radiation failures is shown in Table V. All failures occurred within nine months; the average recurrence was at 5.3 months, and the average survival after initial therapy was 42 months.

Table VI indicates the surgical procedures for the supraglottic patients. Table VII reveals salvage by initial site and if a partial procedure was successful in preserving the voice. Salvage by surgery overall was 6/11 (55%). Only two patients had partial procedures; the others required at least laryngectomy, except for one patient who underwent contralateral radical neck dissection only. The T_4N_0 patient remains free of disease seven years after supraglottic laryngectomy and radical neck dissection. Residual dis-

TABLE VII

SUPRAGLOTTIC SALVAGE BY SITE AND VOICE PRESERVATION

	Pts.	*Salvage*	*%*	*P.P.**
T_1	2	1/2	50	0
T_2	3	2/3	67	1
T_3	3	1/3	33	0
T_4	3	2/3	67	2
	11	6/11	55	3

*P.P. – Partial procedure successful in preserving voice. (Patient had a contralateral neck dissection only.)

TABLE VIII

SUPRAGLOTTIC RADIATION FAILURES (11 Pts.) COMPLICATIONS AFTER SURGERY

	Pts.	*%*
Fistula	2	18
Carotid Blowout	2	18
Postop. bleeding	1	9
Wound infect./dehis.*	5	45

*Infection/dehiscence

ease was detected at three months after radiation therapy, however. The T_2N_0 (epiglottic) patient has required a permanent tracheotomy following supraglottic laryngectomy. She is 80 years old. The T_4N_3 patient has had a contralateral radical neck dissection after control of the primary lesion and ipsilateral neck with radiation therapy. Her follow-up is limited to 13 months.

TABLE IX

STATUS OF GLOTTIC RADIATION FAILURES (49 Pts.)

Patients	*Status*
15	A $\bar{s}$ D
0	A $\bar{c}$ D
7	D $\bar{s}$ D
25	D $\bar{c}$ D
2	LTF
Average recurrence	13.5 Mo
Average survival	39.2 Mo

Complications for the supraglottic group are noted in Table VIII. Two patients expired with carotid artery blowout.

Glottic. The status of the 49 radiation failures is shown in Table IX. All failures occurred within 42 months; the average recurrence was 13.5 months, and the average survival after initial therapy was 39.2 months.

Table X indicates the surgical procedures for the glottic patients. Table XI reveals salvage by initial site and if

TABLE X

SURGICAL PROCEDURES FOR GLOTTIC RADIATION FAILURES (49 Pts.)

Cordectomy	2
Hemilaryngect. (vert.)	4
Laser(s)	1
Laryngectomy	25
Laryngectomy and RND	16
Laryngopharyngectomy and RND	3
Contralateral RND	4

a partial procedure was successful in preserving the voice. Salvage by surgery, overall, was 22/49 (45%). Only five patients could be salvaged by partial laryngectomy. Two patients had successful cordectomies by thyrotomy. Four patients underwent (vertical) hemilaryngectomy for salvage, but one patient (T_2N_0) ultimately underwent laryngectomy and staged bilateral radical neck

TABLE XI

GLOTTIC SALVAGE BY SITE AND VOICE PRESERVATION

	Pts.	*Salv.*	*%*	*P.P.**
T_1	17	8/17	47	5
T_2	9	6/9	67	0
T_3	17	7/17	41	0
T_4	6	1/6	17	0
	49	22/49	45	5

*P.P. — Partial procedure successful in preserving voice. (Patient had a contralateral radical neck dissection only.)

dissection to control persistent disease. He remains free of disease at 54 months.

A 69-year-old male initially had radiotherapy for cure for an early cord lesion (T_2N_0). Recurrence developed at 16 months after several biopsies were taken on different occasions. Transoral laser surgery was utilized for the recurrence, but he ultimately required laryngectomy. He died at 22 months from pulmonary metastases due to bronchogenic carcinoma.

TABLE XII

GLOTTIC RADIATION FAILURES (49 Pts.) COMPLICATIONS AFTER SURGERY

	Pts.	%
Fistula	7	14
Carotid blowout	0	0
Postop. bleeding	2	4
Wound infec./dehis.	5	10
Slough	4	8
Stomal recurrence	4	8

Four patients had contralateral radical neck dissection for control of neck recurrence. The aforementioned first patient (T_2N_0) underwent (vertical) hemilaryngectomy for recurrence at 24 months; at 36 months he required laryngectomy and radical neck dissection; and at 48 months, he underwent contralateral radical neck dissection. He is free of disease at 54 months. The second patient (T_4N_0) is free of disease at 24 months after undergoing laryngectomy and staged bilateral radical neck dissection. The third patient (T_4N_1) required laryngopharyngectomy and staged bilateral radical neck dissection for recurrence at four months. Multiple reconstructions were necessary for partial neck flap slough before this patient expired after 24 months with disease. The fourth patient (T_1N_0) died with stomal disease at 53 months following laryngectomy and staged bilateral radical neck dissection for recurrence detected at 41 months.

Complications are noted in Table XII, including stomal disease. A total of four patients had stomal recurrence, and two of these patients had original T_1N_0 lesions. Five patients had partial neck flap slough requiring further surgery including the use of regional pedicle flaps.

Subglottic. The lone subglottic patient (T_3N_0) failed at ten months and died with disease after 24 months. Extensive recurrence was noted and the patient developed a fistula and a wound infection/dehiscence postoperatively.

DISCUSSION

Failure rates in carcinoma of the larynx vary with the extent of the tumor and the anatomical site of origin. Supraglottic cancer is less responsive to radiation and more apt to develop metastases than glottic cancer. Fifty-five percent of the supraglottic patients were salvaged by surgery, but only three patients have voice preservation. At least five patients had lesions amenable to supraglottic laryngectomy initially.

Salvage after radiation therapy is well documented for early glottic lesions. Excellent salvage with voice preservation for early glottic lesions (T_1 and T_2) has been reported by Biller, *et al*[6] in 14 of 18 patients. Norris also reported similar results[7] for ten of 12 comparable patients. These patients were obviously well followed and recurrence detected early. Biller, *et al* also advocate hemilaryngectomy as the treatment of choice for true vocal cord cancer extending beyond the confines of the membranous cord; they report a three-year tumor control rate of 77% with hemilaryngectomy when strict criteria are maintained.[8]

Only 14 of 26 T_1 and T_2 patients in the present series were salvaged by surgery, and the voice was preserved in only five of these patients. We can only speculate what the outcome for these patients with early cord lesions might have been had they not been given radiation therapy.

Salvage for advanced glottic radiation failures is not well documented. Only 8 of 23 T_3 and T_4 patients were salvaged in this series. Nineteen of these patients required radical neck dissection with laryngectomy. Four patients ultimately required contralateral radical neck dissection. Microscopic node metastases may occur during the course of radiation therapy, but clinical evidence may not become apparent until much later.

Early cord lesions are not commonly seen in our department. Most of the patients present with advanced laryngeal lesions. We are concerned about identifying the patients who are likely to become radiation failures. This group can be selected for conservation or ablative laryngeal surgery. Many of our patients are from the lower socioeconomic class and have abusive tobacco and alcohol habits. It is difficult to explain to these patients the nature of their cancerous process and to turn them from their "suicidal habits." These same patients are unreliable in receiving radiation therapy and follow-up appointments. Relentlessly, they continue their habits during and even after treatment. Often, they present several months after receiving radiation therapy with fungating tumors, neck metastases, and complications such as fistula and aspiration pneumonia. True, frequently these patients initially refuse surgery and are given radiation therapy as an alternative. However, this group of patients and their families need to be informed and even strongly urged that surgery may be the best initial therapy.

Another group of patients, usually referred to a university hospital for laryngeal cancer, are mental patients and inmates of penal or correctional institutions. For security and other logistic reasons, these patients are best treated with conservation surgery for early lesions and laryngectomy for advanced lesions.

Financial assistance is often required for transportation and accommodation by patients undergoing six weeks of radiation therapy. State and national health coverage is not available in this country to provide these funds for transportation and accommodation. Frequently, the radiation center is miles from the patient's home. Often the cancer victim is the breadwinner of a large rural family, and the time and expense involved with daily therapy may be exorbitant. Definitive surgery for these patients may be the treatment of choice. The family is often relieved to know that the entire tumor was removed by surgery.

Elderly patients seem to do better with surgery as primary therapy for laryngeal cancer. Thirty-five of the patients in the series were 60 years of age or older. There were no operative deaths,

TABLE XIII

POSTRADIATION COMPLICATIONS[10]

1. Laryngeal edema
2. Perichondritis
3. Cartilage necrosis
4. Changes in irradiated skin

and two octogenarians are free of disease at 48 months and 53 months.

Regular follow-up at close intervals is mandatory for all patients who have undergone radiation therapy for laryngeal malignancy. Brewer has detailed the signs and symptoms of early laryngeal disease in a recent report.[9] These subtle changes may be of aid in the diagnosis of recurrent cancer, and they should be investigated thoroughly when present.

The effects of radiation therapy may mask early recurrence and make diagnosis both difficult and delayed. Lederman noted four postradiation complications in 1970:[10] 1) laryngeal edema, 2) perichondritis, 3) cartilage necroses, and 4) changes in irradiated skin (Table XIII). Protracted postradiation edema is the most common factor responsible for the delay in diagnosis of recurrence. Ward, *et al*[11] found a high incidence of residual cancer in patients who had persistent edema six months after completion of radiotherapy. In their series of 43 cases who met this criteria, 23 patients had recurrent carcinoma. Many of these patients had original T_1 and T_2 lesions. Only six of these patients were salvaged, and no conservation procedures with voice preservation were done.

With this in mind, repeat biopsies at 6- to 8-week intervals are recommended when the index of suspicion for recurrence is high. Deep biopsy is usually required in the postradiation state for the mucous membrane overlying the residual tumor may be normal except for the edema. Multiple biopsies are usually necessary because the recurrence may be present in tiny nests of cells. Multiple biopsies are discouraged when evaluating a recurrence for possible conservation surgery because the tumor margin may become indistinct.

At times we have had to resort to microlaryngoscopy with supravital staining under general anesthesia and thyrotomy for definitive diagnosis of recurrence. Toluidine blue will only identify residual surface cancer; however, tumor deep in the laryngeal musculature will not be stained. Thyrotomy or laryngofissure offers direct vision, and this technique can be a good diagnostic tool when recurrence is suspect. Frozen section can be obtained, and, if applicable, hemilaryngectomy can then be done. Consent should also be obtained for total laryngectomy when this procedure is considered.

On occasion, laryngectomy without a positive biopsy has been considered when the larynx becomes a functionless organ and is hazardous to the patient's health. Fixed cords causing aspiration and sepsis and occasionally perichondritis with actual cartilage necrosis may be enough evidence of recurrence to warrant laryngectomy. In these unfortunate patients, aspiration will not cease until the larynx is removed.

Late recurrence is not unusual in glottic carcinoma treated initially with radiation therapy. Four glottic failures in the series did not occur until 36 months or later. Follow-up every three months (or sooner if symptoms warrant) is recommended even three years after the initial therapy. Long term follow-up may reveal a second primary carcinoma of the larynx. Both patients excluded from the study because of the development of a new primary lesion continued to smoke and imbibe alcohol. The role of radiation therapy in this sequence is unknown.

Modern training in otolaryngology and facial plastic and reconstructive surgery includes the principles of regional pedicle flaps. Not infrequently, multiple flaps were used to reconstruct the hypopharynx, cervical esophagus, and cervical neck defects after radiation failure. Expertise in the use of these flaps in heavily radiated tissue is essential. If the radiotherapist and the laryngologist are not aware of the potential reconstructive problems, it may be wise to refer the patient where a definitive initial procedure may be done. Only a well-trained, creative surgeon utilizing pedicle flaps can reconstruct these patients.

CONCLUSIONS

From the findings and implications in this series of patients who have been radiation failures in cancer of the larynx, several points can be made.

Total patient consideration is necessary in planning the initial therapy. There is an identifiable group of patients who do better with conservative or ablative surgery of the larynx. Surgery offers a surgical specimen which can be analyzed to better evaluate a patient's prognosis.

Survival rates in cancer of the larynx following radiation therapy should not be interpreted to mean that the voice is always preserved. Close follow-up after radiation therapy is mandatory. Recurrence may not be evident until after 36 months. Laryngeal edema persisting longer than six months after the initial radiotherapy may indicate recurrent tumor. Repeat biopsies at 6- to 8-week intervals are necessary when recurrence or persistence of tumor is suspected. Deep biopsies are emphasized since tumor cell nests may be present in the submucosal tissue. Microlaryngoscopy and thyrotomy occasionally are necessary in order to diagnose recurrence.

Laryngectomy without positive biopsy is indicated when the larynx becomes a functionless, hazardous organ. The laryngologist must be willing to accept and undertake the reconstructive problems that arise in radiation failures of cancer of the larynx.

Request for reprints should be sent to Emanuel M. Skolnik, M.D., Department of Otolaryngology, Abraham Lincoln School of Medicine, College of Medicine, University of Illinois at the Medical Center, Chicago, Illinois 60680.

REFERENCES

1. Till JE, Bruce WR, Elwan MA, *et al*: A preliminary analysis of end results for cancer of the larynx. Laryngoscope 85:259-275, 1975

2. Lederman M: Radiotherapy of cancer of the larynx. J Laryngol Otol 84:867-896, 1970

3. Lederer FL: Laryngic descriptive discrepancy. Ann Otol Rhinol Laryngol 72:396-415, 1963

4. Som ML: Limited surgery after failure of radiotherapy in the treatment of carcinoma of the larynx. Ann Otol Rhinol Laryngol 60: 695-703, 1951

5. Ballantyne AJ, Fletcher GH: Preservation of the larynx in the surgical treatment of cancer, recurrent after radiation therapy. Am J Roentgenol Radium Ther Nucl Med 99:336-339, 1967

6. Biller HF, Barnhill FR Jr, Ogura JH, *et al*: Hemilaryngectomy following radiation failure for carcinoma of the vocal cords. Laryngoscope 80:249-253, 1968

7. Norris CM, Peale AR: Partial laryngectomy for irradiation failure. Arch Otolaryngol 84:558-562, 1966

8. Biller HF, Ogura JH, Pratt LL: Hemilaryngectomy for T_2 glottic cancers. Arch Otolaryngol 93:238-243, 1971

9. Brewer DW Sr: Early diagnostic signs and symptoms of laryngeal disease. Laryngoscope 85:499-515, 1975

10. Lederman M: Radiotherapy of cancer of the larynx. J Laryngol Otol 84:867-896, 1970

11. Ward PH, Calcaterra TC, Kagan AR: The enigma of postradiation edema and recurrent or residual carcinoma of the larynx. Laryngoscope 85:522-529, 1975

Ann Otol 84: 1975

REHABILITATION OF THE SHOULDER AFTER RADICAL NECK DISSECTION

W. H. SAUNDERS, M.D.

E. W. JOHNSON, M.D.

COLUMBUS, OHIO

SUMMARY — After classical radical neck dissection with removal of the sternocleidomastoid muscle and division of the spinal accessory nerve, there are certain disabling or disagreeable musculoskeletal defects. This paper describes the muscular deficiencies and gives a set of exercises which can be counted on to minimize the problems.

After classical radical neck dissection with excision of the sternocleidomastoid muscle and division of the spinal accessory nerve supplying the trapezius muscle, there is weakness and deformity, and often pain of the shoulder.

To avoid these postoperative difficulties, some surgeons have advocated grafting between the cut ends of the spinal accessory nerve using the greater auricular nerve. While not a common practice, this procedure does afford adequate neural supply to the trapezius muscle in most instances. Others have performed various types of modified neck dissections in which both the sternocleidomastoid muscle and the nerve supply to the trapezius are spared. Bocca* saves even the internal jugular vein, removing only the fascial compartments around muscles, vessels, and nerves.

Most surgeons still prefer the classical operation to the various modified or conservative procedures. Intent on removal of the patient's malignancy and with consideration for a reasonable cosmetic result, they are apt to ignore the functional deformity resulting from neck dissection. It is for these patients, some with bilateral radical neck dissections, that we present the following rehabilitative program designed to relieve postoperative pain, early and late, and to restore as much function as possible to the shoulder.

The Normal Trapezius. The trapezius is an important stabilizer of the scapula. It has three parts, upper, middle, and lower, and is a large muscle, extending inferiorly farther than is commonly realized. It resembles a fan, attaching at one end to the vertebrae and at the other to the scapular spine. Its function includes hugging the scapula tightly to the posterior thoracic cage during movements of the arm, rotating the scapula upward and downward, and retracting it. Participating muscles which compensate for loss of the trapezius are the levator scapulae and the rhomboids (Figs. 1-2).

The usual test for trapezius function, having the patient shrug his shoulder against resistance, tests chiefly the upper trapezius. A better test, or an additional one, is to have him hold both arms in full abduction above his head while the examiner pulls each arm downward laterally against resistance (Fig. 3). The

*Bocca E: Personal communication.

From the Departments of Otolaryngology and Physical Medicine, The Ohio State University College of Medicine, Columbus, Ohio.

Presented at the meeting of the American Laryngological Association, Atlanta, Georgia, April 6-7, 1975.

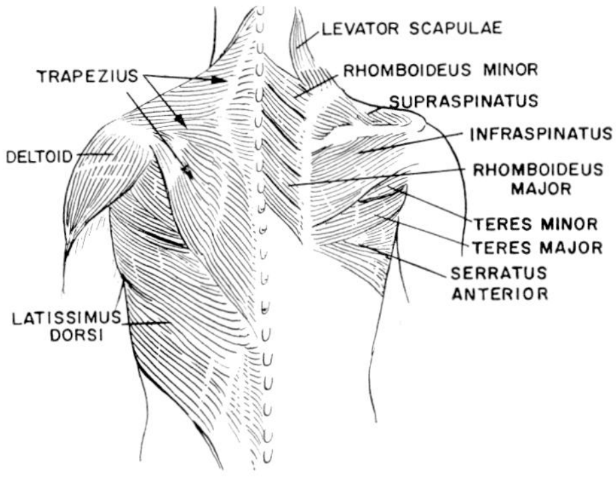

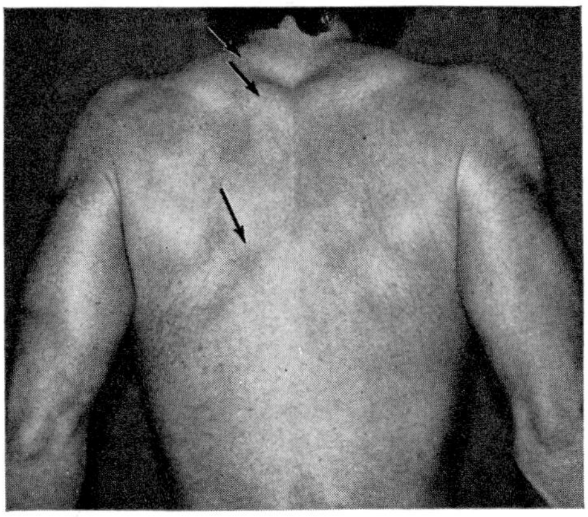

Fig. 1. Muscles of back.
Fig. 2. Trapezius, indicating its three parts.

weakened middle and lower trapezius muscles are demonstrated as one arm is brought down easily while the other is not. Even better testing for the middle and lower segments is done with the patient lying prone, arms outstretched laterally, and thumbs pointed upward in the "hitchhiking" position. Having him raise his arms in the direction of the upward extended thumbs brings these muscles into prominence.

Effects of Paralysis. The major antagonist of the trapezius may be considered to be the serratus anterior which moves the scapula forward and downward when the trapezius is paralyzed. In paralysis, the vertebral border of the scapula becomes flared, particularly inferiorly and laterally (Fig. 4), and this flaring is accentuated when the arm is abducted from the side against resistance. Futhermore, since the scapula must be stabilized and synergistically moved in concert with the humerus (scapulohumeral joint), abduction of the shoulder is apt to be limited. In ten consecutive patients tested by electromyography, all three parts of the trapezius showed complete denervation. Patients with marked loss of shoulder abduction, 70° or less, characteristically try to compensate by contralateral flexion of the trunk (Fig. 5). Even though the trapezius is paralyzed, the shoulder forward flexors may elevate the arm

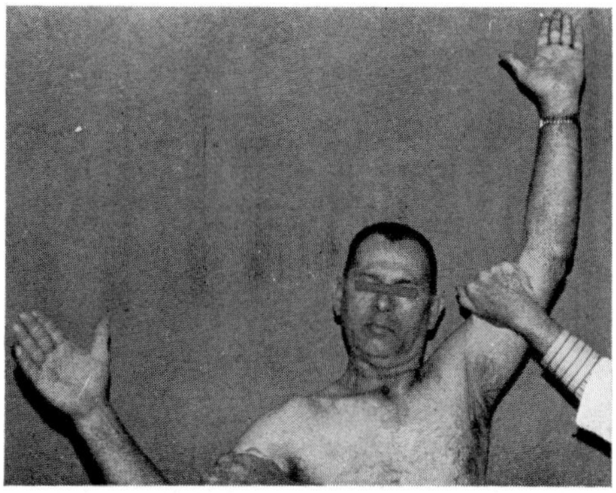

Fig. 3. Demonstration of how one arm can be pulled downward against resistance, while the other cannot. (Paralysis of the trapezius.)

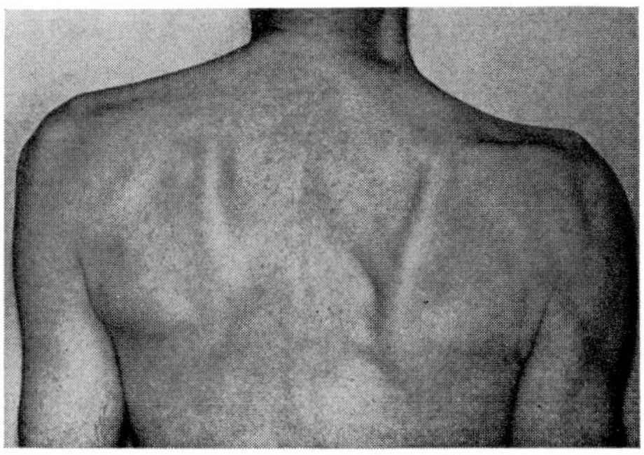

Fig. 4. Prominent vertebral border of scapula in patient with paralyzed trapezius. Also note atrophy of upper portion of the muscle.

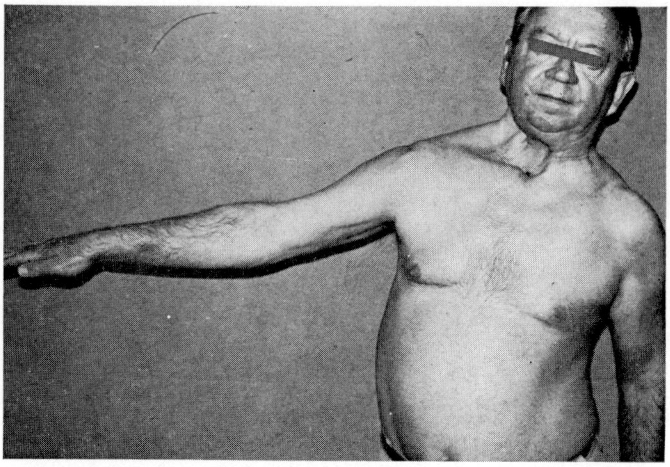

Fig. 5. Maximum abduction patient could achieve. Note compensatory contralateral flexion of trunk. (Compare to Fig. 6.)

180° since the serratus anterior can stabilize the scapula with the arm in forward flexed position (Fig. 6). Thus, it may appear that the patient is abducting the arm, while in reality he is using forward flexors to raise the arm above the head.

Since rotation of the shoulder joint must accompany abduction, the extremes of external rotation generally are lost because of disuse. Additionally, pain associated with the surgery, at least in the early postoperative weeks, may limit extremes of shoulder motion. The scapulohumeral joint tends to lose motion and in some cases develops a condition best described as periarthritis or adhesive capsulitis of the shoulder. The characteristic postoperative position of the scapulohumeral complex is forward and downward (Fig. 7).

Functional limitations after neck dis-

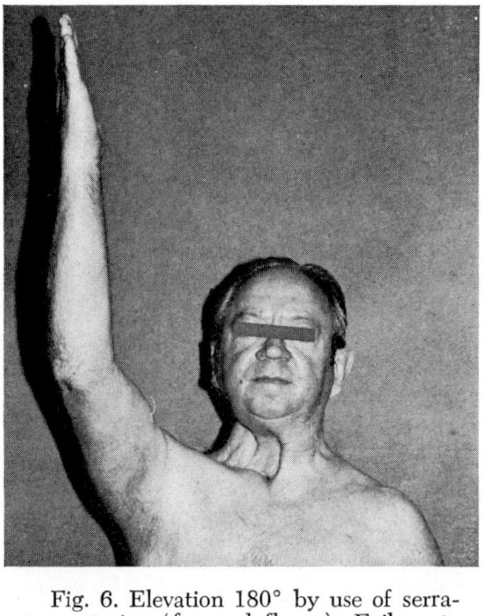

Fig. 6. Elevation 180° by use of serratus anterior (forward flexor). Failure to note this alternate mechanism for raising arm may confuse examiner regarding trapezius paralysis. (Compare to Fig. 5.)

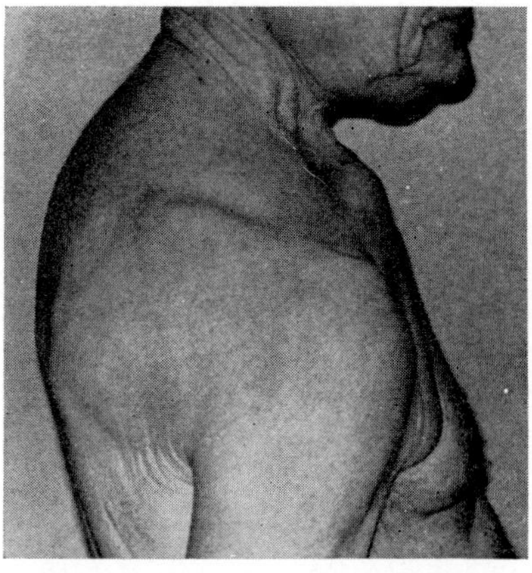

Fig. 7. Characteristic downward and forward position of shoulder complex after neck dissection.

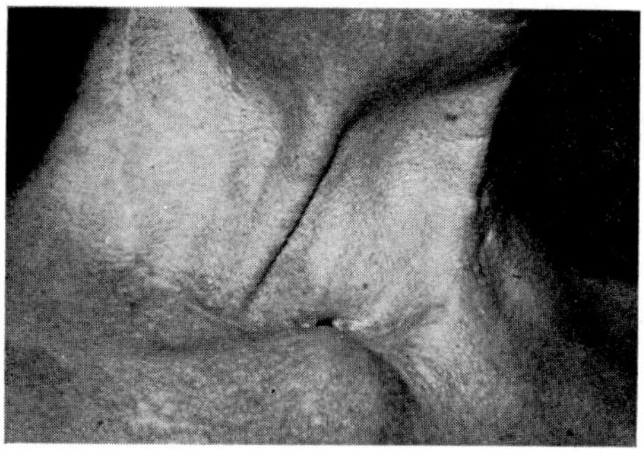

Fig. 8. Osteoarthritis of sternoclavicular joint, one cause of postoperative pain.

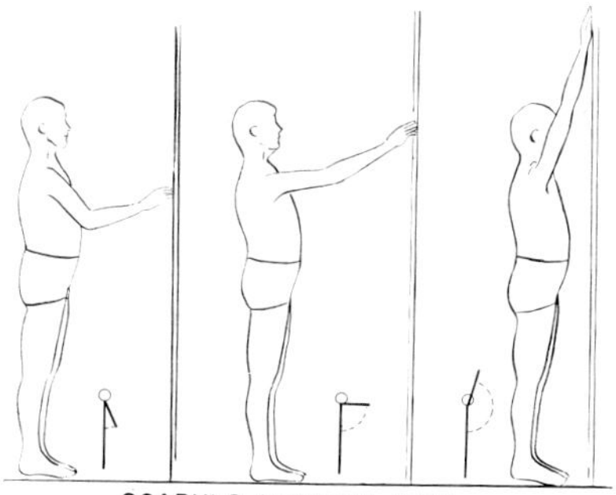

Fig. 9. Exercises recommended for patients after radical neck dissection.

section are imposed by: 1) painful motion of the scapulohumeral joint (periarthritis), and 2) inability fully to abduct the shoulder because of loss of scapular stability.

Cosmetic considerations include the forward and downward displacement of the shoulder complex. Loss of the sternocleidomastoid muscle produces abnormal contour at the junction of the neck and shoulder as well as a flatness of one side of the neck. Atrophy of the trapezius is particularly evident in its upper portion.

Pain is imposed by stretching of the chief scapular retractor (rhomboids) and the elevator (levator scapulae), initiated by the now unbalanced pull of the serratus anterior. Periarthritis of the scapulohumeral joint also is a factor in some patients. A relatively infrequent cause of pain is osteoarthritis of the sternoclavicular joint on the side of the paralysis (Fig. 8). This may occur as the result of long standing stress imposed by the unbalanced scapulohumeral complex.

Physical treatment is directed at: 1) pain, using infrared luminous 250 watt lamp at home, 2) strengthening the scapular retractors and elevators, using regressive resistance technique: first ten repetitive exercises at maximum effort, then 8, and finally 5 (Fig. 9), 3) range of motion exercises to increase scapulohumeral joint motion (Fig. 10), and 4)

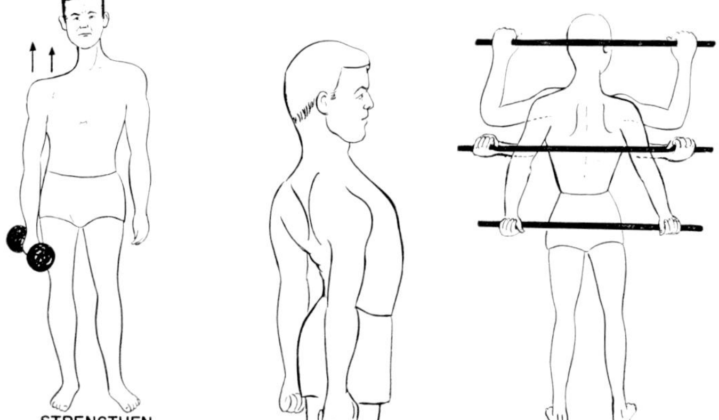

Figs. 10, 11, and 12. Exercises recommended for patients after radical neck dissection.

active stretch of the shortened scapular protractor (serratus anterior) (Figs. 11, 12).

The patient is instructed in two or three sessions by the physical therapist, then checked every three to four weeks to insure progress. 35 mm color photographs are useful to demonstrate cosmetic improvement, especially the position of the shoulder complex.

The usual result of treatment is relief of pain, then an improvement in posture, and finally functional improvement of the arm as shoulder motion increases.

Request for reprints should be sent to W. H. Saunders, M.D., Department of Otolaryngology, The Ohio State University College of Medicine, 456 Clinic Drive, Columbus, Ohio 43210.

Ann Otol 84: 1975

CARCINOMA OF THE NASOPHARYNX IN CHILDREN

JAMES B. SNOW, JR., M.D.
PHILADELPHIA, PENNSYLVANIA

SUMMARY – Seven children with carcinoma of the nasopharynx have been treated and followed for five years. In this group of patients there were no cranial nerve palsies or radiographic evidence of destruction of the base of the skull. Four of the seven patients are living and well. The development of lymphoepithelioma in two siblings is of great interest from an environmental and genetic point of view. The older sibling developed the clinical manifestations of the tumor at 12 years of age and four years later the younger sibling developed them at 14 years of age. The possible etiologic relationship of carcinoma of the nasopharynx to the Epstein-Barr virus is discussed. The good survival rate in these patients under 21 years of age suggests that the prognosis in carcinoma of the nasopharynx is better in the younger age group than in adults. The management of these patients illustrates that carcinoma of the nasopharynx should be managed as a regional rather than a systemic disease. Systemic drug therapy is sometimes advocated because of confusion over the name lymphoepithelioma on the assumption that these tumors are more related to lymphomas and lymphosarcomas than carcinomas. It is clear that lymphoepitheliomas should be managed as carcinomas.

Carcinoma of the nasopharynx is more common in adults than in children. Seven patients under 21 years of age were treated for carcinoma of the nasopharynx at the University of Oklahoma Health Sciences Center during the ten-year period between 1962 and 1972.

In children, carcinoma of the nasopharynx is often composed of large epitheloid cells with characteristics of malignant cells and normal appearing lymphocytes and is often designated lymphoepithelioma although most authorities consider lymphoepitheliomas to be squamous cell carcinomas.

HISTORICAL ASPECTS

Skull lesions in an Egyptian mummy circa 3000 BC, an ancient Peruvian skeleton, and a medieval English skeleton indicate that carcinoma of the nasopharynx is a very old disease.[1] Bosworth, in 1889, reviewed the literature and added a sixth case of his own.[2] Durand-Fardel, in 1837, reported the first case.[3] Jackson, in 1901, added eight cases and condemned the use of surgery in the treatment of carcinoma of the nasopharynx.[4]

Dobson's 1924 letter to the editor of the *China Medical Journal* is a landmark in the history of thought regarding the etiology of carcinoma of the nasopharynx.[5] In this letter he calls attention to the nasopharynx in cases of malignant enlargement of the cervical glands and suggests that the cause of these tumors is exposure to the smoke of candles, kerosene and peanut oil lamps, tobacco, and incense, as well as dry grass and poor quality wood cooking fires. Similar conditions were described by Clifford more recently in Kenya.[6]

INCIDENCE

The incidence of carcinoma of the nasopharynx is low in Caucasian populations and high among the Chinese. Carcinoma of the nasopharynx accounts for 18% of all malignant neoplasms in some reports from China.[7] Nasopharyngeal cancer comprises 0.25% of all malignan-

From the Department of Otorhinolaryngology and Human Communication, University of Pennsylvania School of Medicine, 3400 Spruce Street, Philadelphia, Pennsylvania.

Presented at the meeting of the American Laryngological Association, Atlanta, Georgia, April 6-7, 1975.

cies in Caucasian populations and has an incidence of 2 per 100,000 population per year.[8] In nonwhite populations in the United States (90% Negro), the rates are slightly higher. In Caucasian populations 5.5% of cancers of the head and neck are primary in the nasopharynx, while in Chinese, 82% of the cancers of the head and neck are primary in the nasopharynx.[9]

In nearly every series of carcinoma of the nasopharynx, there are more males than females. The sex ratio is approximately two to one in all races.[10]

The clinical manifestations of carcinoma of the nasopharynx occurs at relatively young ages. In Caucasian populations 6% of nasopharyngeal carcinomas occur before the age of 30 years, and 30% occur before the age of 50 years.[8] The youngest patient with carcinoma of the nasopharynx is a four-year-old girl reported by Lederman.[10] Females contract the disease at an earlier age than males. Chinese patients tend to be younger than patients of other ethnic groups.

ETIOLOGIC FACTORS

The inhalation of known potent carcinogens such as 3, 4- benzpyrene contained in smoke and soot from poorly ventilated cooking fires, incense and tobacco, and the sniffing of snuff have long been considered possible etiologic factors.[11] Snuffing by the Bantu appears to increase the risk of carcinoma of the nose and paranasal sinuses but not of the nasopharynx.[12] Industrial exposure to nickel, chromium, arsenic, isopropyl alcohol, and radioactive dusts increase the risk of carcinoma of the nose and paranasal sinuses. The role of incense smoke may be very limited in view of Ho's report from Hong Kong that of 2,000 patients there were only one Taoist temple attendant and one Buddhist nun.[13]

The high incidence among the Chinese probably results from a combination of genetic and environmental factors. Zippin, *et al*, in 1962, reported a high incidence of carcinoma of the nasopharynx in young immigrant Chinese males in the United States. The risk was somewhat less among older immigrant Chinese males and among Chinese males born in the United States.[14] In Kenya, the incidence appears to relate to environmental factors and not to racial factors.

Herrold has induced in rodents squamous cell carcinomas from the nasal cavities to the bronchi experimentally with subcutaneously injected diethylnitrosamine.[15] Dawe has induced nasopharyngeal neoplasms in mice with the polyoma virus, but these tumors are not lymphoepitheliomas or squamous cell carcinomas.[16] Spontaneous neoplasms of the upper respiratory tract in wild and domestic animals occur occasionally in the nose and paranasal sinuses but only rarely in the nasopharynx.[17] It is of interest that nasal carcinomas often occur endemically in horses, cattle, sheep, and pigs. Liang's serological study of carcinoma of the nasopharynx in Chinese suggests that infection with adenoviruses 7 and 12 may be significant.[18]

Immunologic similarities exist in patients with Burkitt's lymphoma, nasopharyngeal carcinoma, and infectious mononucleosis. The virus of infectious mononucleosis remained unclassified until recently but has now been placed in the Herpes virus group of the DNA viruses.[19] The evidence that the Epstein-Barr virus (EBV) is the etiologic factor in infectious mononucleosis is that antibodies to the virus appear during the course of the illness, the virus can regularly be recovered from leukocyte cultures of patients with the illness, the heterophile antibody of infectious mononucleosis has been reproduced in monkeys inoculated with the EBV, and immunity to the illness is associated with the presence of the EBV antibodies.[20] In lower socioeconomic circumstances, primary EBV infections as evidenced by seroconversions occur earlier in childhood.[21] The EBV transforms human and simian blood leukocytes into continuous cell lines.[20]

The EBV is suspected to be etiologic in Burkitt's lymphoma and carcinoma of the nasopharynx. The EBV was originally isolated from cultured cell lines from patients with Burkitt's lymphoma. Elevated titers of anti-EBV antibodies have been found in patients with Burkitt's lymphoma and nasopharyngeal carcinoma.[22] Although significantly high antibody titers to EBV are present in only 45% of patients with Stage I carcinoma of the nasopharynx, the titers are elevated in 100% of patients with Stage V lesions.[23] Treated patients without evidence of recurrence have lower titers. Elevated titers occur in patients with squamous cell carcinoma and lymphoepithelioma.[24] The role of the EBV in the etiology of Burkitt's lymphoma and carcinoma of the nasopharynx is obscured by the fact the virus can persist in lymphoid tissue for long periods as a latent infection. Therefore, its presence in these diseases may be on the basis of a previous EBV infection. Although the EBV may not be the etiologic agent in Burkitt's lymphoma and carcinoma of the nasopharynx, it appears to be a necessary factor for Burkitt's lymphoma and carcinoma of the nasopharynx. There is apparently some other unidentified necessary factor.

PATHOLOGIC CHARACTERISTICS

Squamous cell carcinomas consist of epitheloid cells with pleomorphic and hyperchromatic nuclei, prominent nucleoli, and a relatively large cytoplasmic to nuclear ratio. Intercellular bridges, individual cell keratinization, and epithelial pearls are characteristics. In children and young adults, tumors lack these characteristics. The cells may be large with pale staining nuclei, prominent and multiple nucleoli, and poorly defined cytoplasm, and the stroma may contain numerous lymphocytes. Under these circumstances, the term lymphoepithelioma is appropriate.

Regaud introduced the term lymphoepithelioma in 1921 to describe highly radiosensitive tumors composed of a syncytium of anaplastic epithelial cells surrounded by lymphoid cells.[25] Schmincke described a similar tumor in the same year.[26] The possibility that the tumor originates from lymphocytes as well as epithelial cells is still debated. The presence of lymphocytes in the metastases tends to support the concept of the mixed origin of the tumor. The presence of the lymphocytes in the primary and the metastases is probably evidence of the immunologic response of the host to the tumor.

CLINICAL MANIFESTATIONS

Carcinoma of the nasopharynx arises from the lateral wall in 37% of patients and from the roof in 32%.[10] It arises from the posterior wall in only 15%. The fossa of Rosenmüller is the site of prediction in the lateral wall. Carcinoma may infiltrate rapidly into the parapharyngeal space, cranial cavity, and orbit.

Eustachian tube obstruction with serous otitis media and a conductive hearing loss was the presenting complaint in 17% of Lederman's patients, and nasal obstruction with rhinorrhea and epistaxis occurred in 38%. Cranial nerve paralysis and lymph node metastases are common presenting complaints. Trotter's triad of unilateral hearing loss, fixation of the soft palate, and neuralgia or anesthesia of the third division of the trigeminal nerve is occasionally seen as the presenting symptom complex. These findings can be explained by invasion of the prestyloid compartment of the parapharyngeal space through the anterior, inferior aspect of the fossa of Rosenmüller through the fascial space surrounding the levator veli palatini muscle.

Mechanism of Spread. The fossa of Rosenmüller is directly adjacent to the parapharyngeal space. It is separated from the parapharyngeal space by the internal lamina of the parapharyngeal fascia. The parapharyngeal space is divided into three compartments by the styloid process and its muscles and fascial attachments as well as the fascia of the carotid sheath: the prestyloid compartment, the retrostyloid compartment, and the retropharyngeal compartment. The prestyloid compartment has as its roof the greater wing of the sphenoid with its foramen spinosum and foramen ovale.

The retrostyloid compartment contains the carotid sheath, the cervical sympathetics, and cranial nerves IX, X, XI, and XII. The retropharyngeal compartment separates the nasopharyngeal mucous membrane and superior pharyngeal constrictor muscle from the prevertebral fascia and muscles, and it contains lymph nodes, in particular a laterally placed node known as the node of Rouviere.

Invasion of the prestyloid compartment of the parapharyngeal space may cause neuralgia, anesthesia, or paresthesia of the mandibular division of the trigeminal nerve and paralysis of the muscles of mastication. The pterygoid muscles may be invaded, and trismus may be produced. The tumor may extend as far as the stylomastoid foramen and cause paralysis of the VII cranial nerve.

Invasion of the retrostyloid compartment of the parapharyngeal space may cause paralysis of cranial nerves IX, X, XI, and XII and Horner's syndrome. From this compartment, tumor can follow the internal jugular vein through the jugular foramen and the internal carotid artery through the carotid canal to gain access to the parasellar area occupied by cranial nerves III, IV, and VI and the ophthalmic and maxillary divisions of the trigeminal nerve and to produce diplopia and neuralgia, anesthesia, and paresthesia of the trigeminal divisions.

Invasion of the cranial cavity through the foramen lacerum, foramen rotundum, and foramen ovale, though rare, may cause paralysis of cranial nerves II, III, IV, and VI (Jacod's syndrome). The VI cranial nerve is vulnerable because of its enclosure in Durello's canal which is relatively inflexible. Often the VI cranial nerve is involved first, then the III, V, IV, and II.[10] In contrast to the situation with orbital invasion, there is no proptosis.

The V cranial nerve is most frequently involved (16%) according to Lederman, but others have found the VI to be most frequently involved. The nerves of the extraocular muscles and the trigeminal are most frequently affected as a group, and the last four cranial nerves are next most frequently involved as a group. The olfactory nerve is least frequently involved, and the VII and VIII cranial nerves are rarely involved.[10]

Invasion of the pituitary fossa is rare and usually does not result in hypopituitarism. The tumor gains access to the pituitary fossa through the sphenoid sinus, and there is usually concurrent involvement of cranial nerves II, III, IV, and VI.

In order for the tumor to reach the orbit, it must invade the nasal cavity and then gain access to the orbit through the maxillary and ethmoid sinuses. This sequence of events is rare. When it occurs, proptosis and paralysis of the nerves of the extraocular muscles may be produced.

Metastases. Carcinoma of the nasopharynx metastasizes early to cervical lymph nodes. Eighteen percent of Lederman's series presented with lymph node enlargement.[10] Clinically evident metastases to cervical lymph nodes were present in 70% of his patients and bilateral in 39%. Primary tumors arising in the roof of the nasopharynx tend to metastasize bilaterally. Males are more likely to present with cervical lymph node metastases than females, and cervical metastases are more likely to be present initially in children than in adults.[10]

Metastasis occurs more readily from the roof and lateral wall as compared with the posterior wall. Metastases are often bilateral because the tumor is centrally placed; but even if the primary is distinctly unilateral, the metastases may occur on the contralateral side as well as the ipsilateral side. The route of the cervical metastasis is to the lateral retropharyngeal nodes of Rouviere and then to the superior deep cervical nodes. The superior deep cervical nodes of the jugular chain lie deep to the superior portion of the sternocleidomastoid muscle and are usually the first to enlarge sufficiently to become clinically detectable in carcinoma of the nasopharynx. Metastasis to the node of Rouviere can be suspected when there is paralysis of cranial nerves IX, X, XI, and XII.

In Lederman's series of those who had enlarged cervical nodes, 70% had jugulodigastric nodes, 66% had superior posterior cervical triangle nodes, 34% had jugulo-omohyoid nodes, 28% had spinal accessory nodes, and 20% had inferior cervical nodes.[10] Submaxillary nodes are rarely involved and indicate spread of the tumor to the oropharynx, soft palate, or parapharyngeal space. Direct extension to the parotid compartment and the submaxillary triangle may occur from the prestyloid space.

It is to be emphasized that enlarged lymph nodes in the superior part of the posterior cervical triangle should raise suspicion that the primary site of the lesion is in the nasopharynx.

Metastases may appear in the viscera, skeleton, lung, and central nervous system (CNS). Lederman demonstrated distant metastases in 26 of 218 patients on initial evaluation. Nine were to the viscera, seven were to the skeleton, five were to the lung, two were to the CNS and three were to other sites.

Staging. The staging of carcinoma of the nasopharynx by the American Joint Committee for Cancer Staging and End Results Reporting is adopted from the TNM system of classification of the International Union Against Cancer.[27] The sites for the nasopharynx are the posterior superior wall (vault) and the lateral wall. The posterior superior wall extends from the superior border of the choanae to the level of the free border of the soft palate and is limited laterally by the groove between the lateral wall and the base of the skull. The lateral wall extends from the base of the skull to the level of the free border of the soft palate. The size and extent of the primary tumor is described by three "T" categories. The T_1 category describes tumor limited to one site in the nasopharynx. The T_2 category describes tumor extending into two sites in the nasopharynx. The T_3 category describes tumor extending beyond the nasopharynx into the nasal cavities or oropharynx, into or through bone, to the brain, or into the pterygopalatine fossa.

The presence or absence of lymph node metastasis is described by three "N" categories. The N_0 category indicates no palpable cervical lymph nodes. The N_1 category describes clinically palpable cervical lymph node(s) that are not fixed in which metastasis to the node(s) is suspected. The N_2 category describes clinically palpable cervical lymph node(s) that are fixed in which metastasis to the node(s) is suspected.

The presence or absence of distant metastasis is described by two "M" categories. The M_0 category indicates no distant metastasis. The M_1 category describes clinical and/or radiographic evidence of metastasis other than to cervical lymph nodes. Radiographic evidence of bone erosion at the base of the skull or clinical signs of intracranial extension should be considered as evidence of distant metastasis (M_1).

Patients with carcinoma of the nasopharynx are designated as Stage I who are categorized as T_1 N_0 M_0. Stage II consists of those patients who are categorized as T_2 or T_3 N_0 M_0. Stage III consists of those patients who are categorized as T_1 or T_2 or T_3 N_1 M_0. Stage IV consists of those patients who are categorized as T_1 or T_2 or T_3 N_2 M_0 and T_1 or T_2 or T_3 N_0 or N_1 or N_2 M_1.

DIAGNOSTIC FEATURES

Clinical Evaluation. Carcinoma of the nasopharynx becomes clinically apparent in diverse ways and should be suspected in patients with serous otitis media, nasal obstruction, rhinorrhea, epistaxis, cervical lymphadenopathy (particularly in the superior part of the posterior cervical triangle), and any cranial nerve paralysis.

On physical examination, a granular mass or ulcer may be seen through the nasal cavity. The palate may be deformed by the bulk of the nasopharyngeal mass or its mobility may be limited by paralysis of the levator veli palatini. With visualization of the nasopharynx by mirror or nasopharyngoscope, the carcinoma characteristically appears as a granular mass. It may be quite bulky or there may be an ulcer instead of a mass. The tumor may spread deep to the mucous membrane and appear as a slight fullness, while the mucous membrane may appear normal. Because of this tendency of carcinoma of the nasopharynx, biopsy through apparently normal mucous membrane is frequently diagnostic.

General anesthesia is necessary to palpate the extent of the primary lesion. The biopsy is also facilitated by general anesthesia. Carcinoma in the nasopharynx produces a firm mass which stands out from any remaining adenoid tissue. If there is no definite mass, the removal of the adenoid tissue in children as in an adenoidectomy is likely to provide the diagnosis.

Roentgenographic Evaluation. Roentgenographic evaluation ordinarily includes a lateral view of the nasopharynx, a submental-vertex view of the base of the skull and tomographs of the orbits, paranasal sinuses, and petrous pyramids. In the lateral view of the nasopharynx, soft tissue masses are contrasted with the air column of the nasopharynx. In children, a soft tissue density projecting from the posterior wall and the roof of the nasopharynx is normally produced by the adenoid tissue. A similar density in an adult raises the possibility of a neoplasm. Normally the air column of the nasopharynx has in the submental-vertex view bilateral convex lateral borders. In obese individuals these convexities disappear. In patients with nasopharyngeal tumors, the air column may become asymmetrical since the tumor may cause a loss of these convexities. The submental-vertex view also provides evidence of destruction of the base of the skull which can be demonstrated in approximately 30% of patients with carcinoma of the nasopharynx.[10] The foramen lacerum, carotid canal, greater wing of the sphenoid bone, and hypophyseosphenoidal area are particularly likely to be sites of bone destruction. The tumor may enter the carotid canal and thereby the foramen lacerum. The tumor may reach the greater wing of the sphenoid bone intracranially but extradurally through the carotid canal or by direct invasion of the prestyloid compartment of the parapharyngeal space. The foramen ovale and foramen spinosum may become indistinct on the submental-vertex view as destruction of the greater wing of the sphenoid bone occurs. The tumor may destroy the tip of the petrous pyramid through the same intracranial but extradural route. This destruction can be demonstrated particularly well with tomographs of the petrous pyramids. In patients with carcinoma of the nasopharynx who have cranial nerve paralyses, destruction of the base of the skull occurs five times more frequently than in patients without cranial nerve paralyses.[28] Carcinoma tends to be more destructive of the base of the skull than are lymphomas and sarcomas.[10]

DIFFERENTIAL DIAGNOSIS

In children lymphomas and sarcomas are the lesions most likely to require differentiation from carcinoma. Other possibilities for differentiation include benign tumors such as the juvenile angiofibromas, cysts of the nasopharynx, and the infectious granulomata. The differential diagnosis is based on biopsy of the primary lesion. Neck masses should not be biopsied until the nasopharynx has been inspected and palpated and any suspicious lesion has been biopsied because biopsy of the metastases violates the integrity of the block of tissue that must be removed if radical neck dissection is required. A biopsy of the neck mass may result in implantation of the tumor in the skin and subcutaneous tissue. Even if a histologic diagnosis is obtained from biopsy of the cervical metastases, it is necessary to demonstrate the tumor in the nasopharynx by biopsy prior to the initiation of therapy.

TREATMENT

Radiation Therapy. Radiation therapy is the treatment of choice for carcinoma of the nasopharynx. The full extent of the primary lesion must be determined as accurately as possible to include all areas involved with the tumor in the treatment fields. Such determinations ordinarily include careful physical examination, the outlined radiographic studies, and examination of the nasopharynx under anesthesia. The radiation should be delivered to all areas bearing the primary tumor and to both sides of the neck whether there is clinically evident metastasis or not. The therapy should be delivered from a supervoltage source and be fractionated at a rate of 150 to 200 rads per day for a total dose of 7,000 rads to the primary lesion and 5,000 rads to each side of the neck.

Surgery. Surgical therapy in the form of a radical neck dissection should be considered for patients in whom cervical metastases remain clinically palpable following radiation therapy. Likewise, patients who develop neck masses subsequent to radiation therapy should be considered for a radical neck dissection. As a general rule, radical neck dissection is indicated only if there is evidence that the primary lesion has been controlled. Clinical and radiographic evidence of control of the primary is usually all that is appropriate; however, if the nasopharynx has a suspicious appearance, biopsy of the nasopharynx should be repeated prior to the radical neck dissection.

Chemotherapy. Chemotherapy is of value in certain symptomatic patients in whom radiation therapy or surgery have failed to control the tumor. Since there is no specific and reliably effective agent for squamous cell carcinoma, chemotherapy is not ordinarily appropriate as the primary form of therapy. In investigative therapy, chemotherapeutic agents are in use in conjunction with radiation therapy and surgery. In patients experiencing pain or other distressing symptoms in which radiation therapy and appropriate surgery have been utilized, Methotrexate®,* blenomycin, and Adriamycin®** benefit a small percentage of such patients. Methotrexate appears to be the most reliable and has an acceptable ratio of benefits to complications.

Cryosurgery. Cryosurgery may occasionally be of benefit in the patient in which the primary lesion in the nasopharynx persists following radiation therapy, there is no evidence of local extension beyond the nasopharynx, and there is no evidence of uncontrolled local or distant metastases. In this situation, the persisting tumor may be frozen through a transpalatal approach. This rather aggressive form of treatment may result in palliation and an occasional cure. Relative contraindications to cryosurgery are radiographic evidence of destruction of the base of the skull, cranial nerve palsies, and trismus.

PROGNOSIS

The prognosis for patients with carcinoma of the nasopharynx is adversely affected by cranial nerve paralyses and destruction of the base of the skull. The five-year survival rate for radiation therapy ranges from 76% for Stage I lesions of the vault to 17% for Stage IV lesions of the lateral wall.[29] Although Lederman reports an overall five-year survival rate of 13%, the generally accepted overall five-year survival is 35%.[10] The outcome is very similar whether there are clinically evident cervical metastases or not, apparently because failure results from persistence of the primary tumor in both instances. Female patients have a higher survival rate than male patients. Younger patients have a higher survival rate than older patients. The survival rate according to the American Joint Commission is higher among patients with posterior superior wall lesions as compared to patients with lateral wall lesions.[27] The five-year survival rate of Lederman's patients with posterior wall lesions was 26%, while the patients with lateral wall lesions had a 12% five-year survival rate.

* Lederle Laboratories, Pearl River, New York.

** Adria Laboratories, Inc., Wilmington, Delaware.

CASE REPORTS

Seven patients under 21 years of age were treated for carcinoma of the nasopharynx at the University of Oklahoma Health Sciences Center between 1962 and 1972. These patients ranged in age, at the time of diagnosis, from nine to 17 years. Two of the patients were girls, and five were boys. Three of the patients were Negro and four were Caucasian. Four are living and free of disease, and three are dead. The five-year survival rate in this group of patients is 57%.

Case 1. A 12-year-old Caucasian male presented with a right cervical mass in September 1963. A right radical neck dissection was performed, and the histopathologic diagnosis of lymphoepithelioma was made. Subsequently the nasopharynx was biopsied, and the lymphoepithelioma was demonstrated again. He received radiation therapy to the nasopharynx and to both sides of the neck from September to November 1963. He is living and well 11 years after the diagnosis was made.

As a general rule in evaluating cervical masses, the primary lesion should be sought and biopsied rather than biopsying the metastasis.

Case 2. A 12-year-old Negro male presented in November 1963 with complaints of headache, epistaxis, and frequent tonsillitis for one year and with a 2 cm by 2 cm nontender node in the superior part of the right posterior cervical triangle. A tonsillectomy and adenoidectomy was performed in December 1963. The right cervical mass increased in size, and in February 1964 histopathologic reexamination of the adenoid tissue demonstrated a lymphoepithelioma. Radiation therapy to the nasopharynx and to both sides of the neck was carried out from March to May 1964. The patient is now living and well 11 years after the diagnosis was made.

This patient's history demonstrates the essentiality of careful histopathologic study of all tonsillar and adenoid tissue.

Case 3. A 14-year-old Negro male, the younger brother of Case 2, presented in July 1967 with bilateral posterior cervical triangle lymphoadenopathy and a mass in the nasopharynx. The nasopharyngeal mass proved to be a lymphoepithelioma on biopsy. From August to October 1967 the patient received radiation therapy to the nasopharynx and to both sides of the neck. A right radical neck dissection was performed for a persistent right cervical mass in December 1967. The patient developed a staphylococcal wound infection with massive necrosis of the cervical skin flaps and exsanguinated from carotid artery rupture. No tumor was found in the surgical specimen.

The development of the lymphoepithelioma in two siblings is of great interest from an environmental and genetic point of view. The older sibling developed the clinical manifestations of the tumor at 12 years of age, and four years later the younger sibling developed them at 14 years of age. None of the previously proposed environmental etiologic factors could be elicited in this family, and no new factors came to light.

Case 4. A 15-year-old Caucasian male presented with a large left cervical mass in September 1966. The mass in the left side of the neck was biopsied, but the biopsy was not diagnostic. A mass was found in the nasopharynx, and the nasopharyngeal biopsy demonstrated a lymphoepithelioma. Radiation therapy was given to the nasopharynx and to both sides of the neck from September to November 1966. A left radical neck dissection was performed for a persistent left cervical mass in January 1967. No tumor could be demonstrated in the surgical specimen. In March 1967 the proximal portion of the left fibula was resected because of pain in the leg and a radiolucent defect in the fibula. The tissue removed was similar to the primary tumor in the nasopharynx. He remained free of clinically apparent tumor for five years and died in February 1973 of carcinomatosis.

This patient demonstrates the exceptional circumstance in which surgical control of a distant metastasis proved to be beneficial.

Case 5. A 10-year-old Caucasion male presented with sore throat, bilateral lymphadenopathy, fever, and malaise in June 1967. The diagnosis of lymphopithelioma was established by biopsy of the nasopharynx. He was treated with intravenous Cytoxan®* with a good clinical response. Radiation therapy was given to the nasopharynx and to both sides of the neck from August to October 1967. A left radical neck dissection was performed for a persistent mass in the left side of the neck in December 1967. No tumor could be demonstrated in the surgical specimen. A right radical neck dissection was performed for a persistent right cervical mass in April 1968. No tumor could be demonstrated in the surgical specimen. On the third postoperative day, the patient developed sudden upper respiratory obstruction apparently due to edema of the hypopharynx and larynx and had a cardiac arrest. Following resuscitation there was persistent hypotension, and the patient died on the sixth postoperative day.

In spite of clear indications for the radical

* Mead Johnson Laboratories, Evansville, Indiana.

neck dissections, no tumor was found in the surgical specimens. Such aggressive management of carcinoma of the nasopharynx merits continued evaluation.

Case 6. A nine-year-old Caucasian female presented with bilateral cervical lymphadenopathy in April 1969. During the previous seven months, she had had multiple nondiagnostic biopsies of the cervical masses and multiple incisions and drainages of what were thought to be cervical abscesses. In June 1969 a cervical node biopsy demonstrated lymphoepithelioma. Examination of the nasopharynx, oropharynx, hypopharynx, and larynx under general anesthesia failed to demonstrate a primary lesion. The tonsils and adenoids were removed, but no tumor was demonstrated in the specimens. Nevertheless, it was elected to radiate the nasopharynx as well as both sides of the neck. She is now living and well six years after the diagnosis was made.

Case 7. A 17-year-old Negro female presented with a right cervical mass in June 1970. A biopsy of the nasopharynx demonstrated a lymphoepithelioma. The patient received radiation therapy to the nasopharynx and to both sides of the neck from June to August 1970. She is living and well five years after the diagnosis was made.

DISCUSSION

The five-year survival rate in this group of patients under 21 years is 57% and is very good compared to the more usual five-year survival rate of 35% for all age groups. The prognosis for patients with carcinoma of the nasopharynx appears to be better in the younger patient. None of these patients had cranial nerve palsies or roentgenographic evidence of destruction of the base of the skull which have an adverse effect on prognosis.

The high survival rate in these patients illustrates that carcinoma of the nasopharynx in children should be managed as a regional disease rather than a systemic one. Systemic drug therapy is occasionally advocated rather than regional radiation therapy because of confusion over the name lymphoepithelioma. The assumption is sometimes made that these tumors are more related to lymphomas and lymphosarcomas than carcinomas.

No serious complication of radiation therapy has so far been encountered in this group of patients.

Five radical neck dissections (RND) were performed in four patients. One of these was performed prior to radiation therapy. Two mortalities in this group of young patients were directly related to RND. The RND's following radiation therapy were clearly indicated by the persistence of a cervical mass. The operative mortality of the RND's following radiation therapy was 50%. Although failure to demonstrate tumor in a surgical specimen does not exclude its existence, no tumor could be demonstrated in any of the postradiation neck dissection specimens. The value of RND in this age group following radiation therapy for carcinoma of the nasopharynx merits further critical review.

Request for reprints should be sent to James B. Snow, Jr., M.D., Department of Otorhinolaryngology and Human Communication, University of Pennsylvania School of Medicine, 3400 Spruce Street, Philadelphia, Pennsylvania 19104.

REFERENCES

1. Muir CS: Nasopharyngeal cancer — a historical vignette, in Muir CS, Shanmugaratnam K (eds): *Cancer of the Nasopharynx*. New York, Medical Examiners Publishing Co, 1967

2. Bosworth FH: *A Treatise on Diseases of the Nose and Throat*. New York, Wm Wood Co, 1889, vol 1, pp 612-616

3. Durand-Fardel J: Cancer de pharynx — ossification dans la substance musculaire du coeur. Bull Soc Anat (Paris) 12:73-80, 1837

4. Jackson C: Primary carcinoma of the nasopharynx: a table of cases. JAMA 37:371-377, 1901

5. Dobson WH: Cervical lymphosarcoma (letter to editor). China Med J 38:786-787, 1924

6. Clifford P: Malignant diseases of the nasopharynx and paranasal sinuses in Kenya, in Muir CS, Shanmugaratnam K (eds): *Cancer of the Nasopharynx*. New York, Medical Examiners Publishing Co, 1967

7. Digby KH, Fook WL, Che YT: Naso-

pharyngeal carcinoma. Br J Surg 28:517-537, 1941

8. Bailar JC: Nasopharyngeal cancer in white populations – a worldwide survey, in Muir CS, Shanmugaratnam K (eds): *Cancer of the Nasopharynx*. New York, Medical Examiners Publishing Co, 1967

9. Martin H, Quan S: The racial incidence (Chinese) of nasopharyngeal cancer. Ann Otol Rhinol Laryngol 60:168-194, 1951

10. Lederman M: *Cancer of the Nasopharynx – Its Natural History and Treatment*, Springfield, Charles C Thomas Publishing Co, 1961

11. Falk HL, Steiner PE: The identification of aromatic polycyclic hydrocarbons in carbon blacks. Cancer Res 12:30-39, 1952

12. Keen P, DeMoor NG, Shapiro MP, *et al*: The aetiology of respiratory tract cancer in South African Bantu. Br J Cancer 9:528-538, 1955

13. Ho HC: Nasopharyngeal carcinoma in Hong Kong, in Muir CS, Shanmugaratnam K (eds): *Cancer of the Nasopharynx*. New York, Medical Examiners Publishing Co, 1967

14. Zippin C, Tekawa IS, Bragg KU, *et al*: Studies on heredity and environment in cancer of the nasopharynx. J Natl Cancer Inst 29: 483-490, 1962

15. Herrold KM: Induction of olfactory neuroepithelial tumors in Syrian hamsters by diethylnitrosamine. Cancer 17:114-121, 1964

16. Dawe CJ: Neoplasms induced by polyoma virus in the upper respiratory tracts of mice, in Muir CS, Shanmugaratnam K (eds): *Cancer of the Nasopharynx*, New York, Medical Examiners Publishing Co, 1967

17. Cotchin E: Spontaneous neoplasms of the upper respiratory tract in animals, in Muir CS, Shanmugaratnam K (eds): *Cancer of the Nasopharynx*, New York, Medical Examiners Publishing Co, 1967

18. Liang D: Virus as the cause of rhinopharyngeal carcinoma. Acta Otolaryngol (Stockh) 67:190-199, 1969

19. Snow JB: The classification of respiratory viruses and their clinical manifestations. Laryngoscope 79:1485-1493, 1969

20. Miller G, Niederman JC, Andrews LL: Prolonged oropharyngeal excretion of Epstein-Barr virus after infectious mononucleosis. N Engl J Med 288:229-232, 1973

21. Henle W, Henle G: Epstein-Barr virus and infectious mononucleosis. N Engl J Med 288:263-264, 1973

22. Klein G, Geering G, Old LJ, *et al.*: Comparison of the anti-EBV titre and the EBV-associated membrane reactive and precipitating antibody levels in the sera of Burkitt lymphoma and nasopharyngeal carcinoma patients and controls. Int J Cancer 5:185-194, 1970

23. Henle W: Elevated antibody titers to Epstein-Barr virus in nasopharyngeal carcinoma, other head and neck neoplasms and control groups. J Natl Cancer Inst 44:225-231, 1970

24. Miller D, Goldman J, Goodman M: Etiologic study of nasopharyngeal cancer. Arch Otolaryngol 94:104-108, 1971

25. Regaud C: Discussion of paper by Reverchon L, Coutard H: Lymphoepitheliome de l'hypopharynx traite par le roentgentherapie. Bull Soc franc, Oto-rhino-laryngol 34: 209-214, 1921

26. Schmincke A: Ueber lymphoepitheliale Geschwülste. Beitr Pathol 58:161-170, 1921

27. *Clinical Staging System for Carcinoma of the Pharynx (Nasopharynx, Oropharynx, and Hypopharynx)*, in American Joint Committee for Cancer Staging and End Results Reporting. American College of Surgeons, 1965

28. Godtfredsen E: Opthalmologic and neurologic symptoms at maligant nasopharyngeal tumors. Acta Psychiatr Scand (Suppl) 34, 1944

29. Smith RR, Frazell EL, Caulk R, *et al*: The American Joint Committee's Proposed Method of Stage Classification and End Results Reporting applied to 1,320 pharynx cancers. Cancer 16:1505-1520, 1963

Ann Otol 84: 1975

OBSERVATIONS ON THE PRIMATE HYOEPIGLOTTIC COMPLEX

GABRIEL TUCKER, JR., M.D.

JOHN A. TUCKER, M.D.

PHILADELPHIA, PENNSYLVANIA

SUMMARY – In the species presented, the orifice to the subhyoid air sac is found at the tuberculum (when the epiglottis attaches at the level of the ventricle); here also is noted the presence of a cartilaginous island(s) just anterior to the duct. When seen in coronal section along the axis of the duct, the glandular elements cluster around the sac in the anterior supraglottic subhyoid wedge, in preference to the area around the ventricles.

The analogy between laryngocele[1] in the human larynx and various primate ventricular air sacs[2] is indeed not new. Less frequently discussed are those air sacs termed "subhyoid" by Negus.[3] The hyoid bone in such animals is found to be thin and concave. The concavity embraces the anterosuperior aspect of the thyroid ala and is separated from it by the neck of the air sac. Indeed Negus suggested that the concave hyoid "protected" the neck of the sac which in turn he postulated to be a secondary organ of respiration.

Negus schematized a number of subhyoid air sacs.[3] Such schema nicely demonstrate the relationship between the hyoid bone, the anterior portion of the thyroid "notch" and the "subhyoid" air sac.

Nèmai[4] (quoted by Kelemen[5]) schematized a sagittal section which suggested that the air sac in the cercopithecus monkey might have its orifice in the region of the epiglottic tuberculum.

LABORATORY STUDIES

In the spring of 1974, we were privileged to review the primate laryngeal collection of Dr. George Kelemen. This collection, accumulated over at least four decades, was comprised of some 41 specimens representing 15 species. Most of the specimens had been split in the midsagittal plane before imbedding, thus making it possible to section the mirror halves of any one larynx in two different planes.

Dr. Kelemen's tracer series were studied in his laboratory at the Ear Research Institute. The unstained sections of 33 primate larynges were forwarded to the laboratory of the Institute of Laryngology and Human Communications at Hahnemann for staining and further study. It is from this latter material that those sagittal sections published herein were obtained.

To Dr. Kelemen's material has been added coronal sections processed through the cooperation of the Armed Forces Institute of Pathology. This material was prepared to complement the prior sections by providing coronal sections perpendicular to an intact midsagittal plane. Our current efforts are directed toward the processing of whole, unsplit,

From the Department of Laryngology and Broncho-esophagology, Temple University Health Sciences Center, and the Institute of Laryngology and Human Communications, The Hahnemann Medical College, Philadelphia, Pa.

Presented at the meeting of the American Laryngological Association, Atlanta, Georgia, April 6-7, 1975.

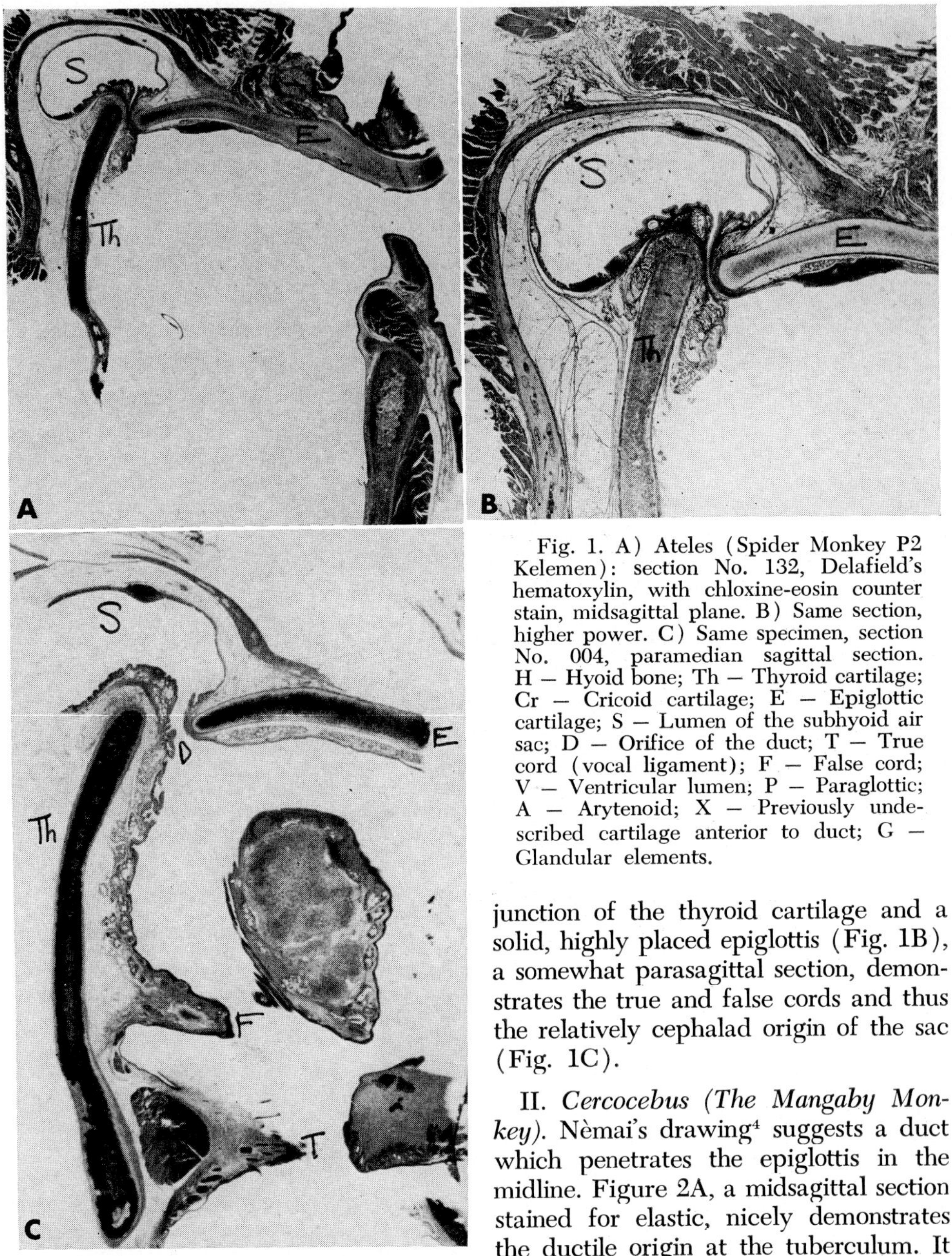

Fig. 1. A) Ateles (Spider Monkey P2 Kelemen): section No. 132, Delafield's hematoxylin, with chloxine-eosin counter stain, midsagittal plane. B) Same section, higher power. C) Same specimen, section No. 004, paramedian sagittal section. H — Hyoid bone; Th — Thyroid cartilage; Cr — Cricoid cartilage; E — Epiglottic cartilage; S — Lumen of the subhyoid air sac; D — Orifice of the duct; T — True cord (vocal ligament); F — False cord; V — Ventricular lumen; P — Paraglottic; A — Arytenoid; X — Previously undescribed cartilage anterior to duct; G — Glandular elements.

primate larynges in all three planes of section.

OBSERVATIONS

I. *Ateles (The Spider Monkey).* Midsagittal section (Fig. 1A) demonstrating a subhyoid air sac; the orifice is at the junction of the thyroid cartilage and a solid, highly placed epiglottis (Fig. 1B), a somewhat parasagittal section, demonstrates the true and false cords and thus the relatively cephalad origin of the sac (Fig. 1C).

II. *Cercocebus (The Mangaby Monkey).* Nèmai's drawing[4] suggests a duct which penetrates the epiglottis in the midline. Figure 2A, a midsagittal section stained for elastic, nicely demonstrates the ductile origin at the tuberculum. It also demonstrates a separate previously undescribed cartilage (Fig. 2B, higher power) anterior to the duct. Also to be noted is the hyoepiglottic ligament extending from the trailing edge of the concave hyoid. Figure 2C, a paramedian sagittal section, demonstrates the inter-

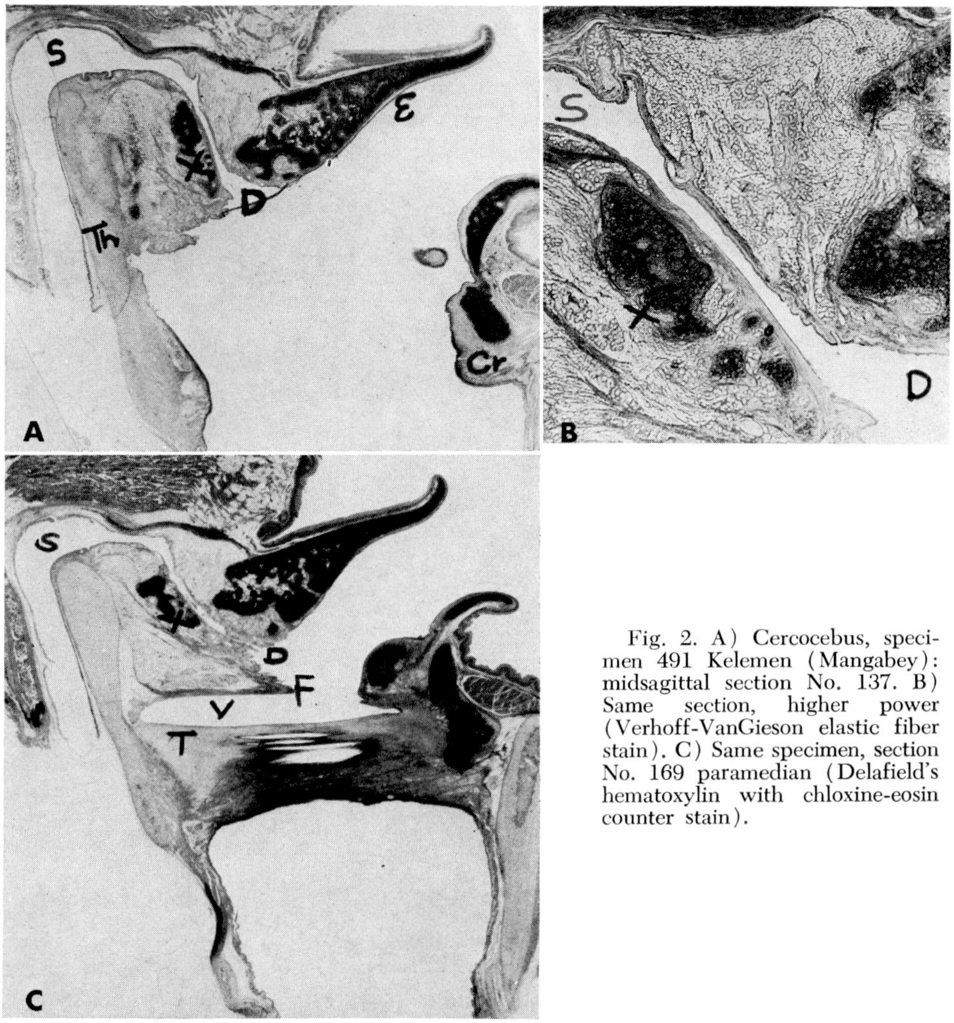

Fig. 2. A) Cercocebus, specimen 491 Kelemen (Mangabey): midsagittal section No. 137. B) Same section, higher power (Verhoff-VanGieson elastic fiber stain). C) Same specimen, section No. 169 paramedian (Delafield's hematoxylin with chloxine-eosin counter stain).

position of the false cord between the ventricle and the duct.

III. *Lutong (The Purple Faced Langur).* Figure 3A demonstrates the larynx in which the proportions are somewhat varied (*i.e.*, the epiglottis is foreshortened, forward tipping of the arytenoid, *etc.*), yet there is the same basic pattern. Duct is better seen at higher power in Figure 3B.

IV. *Macaca Mulatta.* Similar pattern (Fig. 4) X indicates cartilage anterior to the duct.

V. *Baboon.* This specimen was processed and photographed at the A.F.I.P. and is indeed similar to the human larynx. Close inspection reveals an orifice at the epiglottic tuberculum (Fig. 5). In the coronal section (Fig. 6), the lumen of the duct can be traced from the orifice at the epiglottic tuberculum up into the sac under the body of the hyoid.

DISCUSSION

The parallel between tumor spread from the tuberculum into the preepiglottic space[6] is naturally intriguing. A firm conclusion in this regard would seem premature.

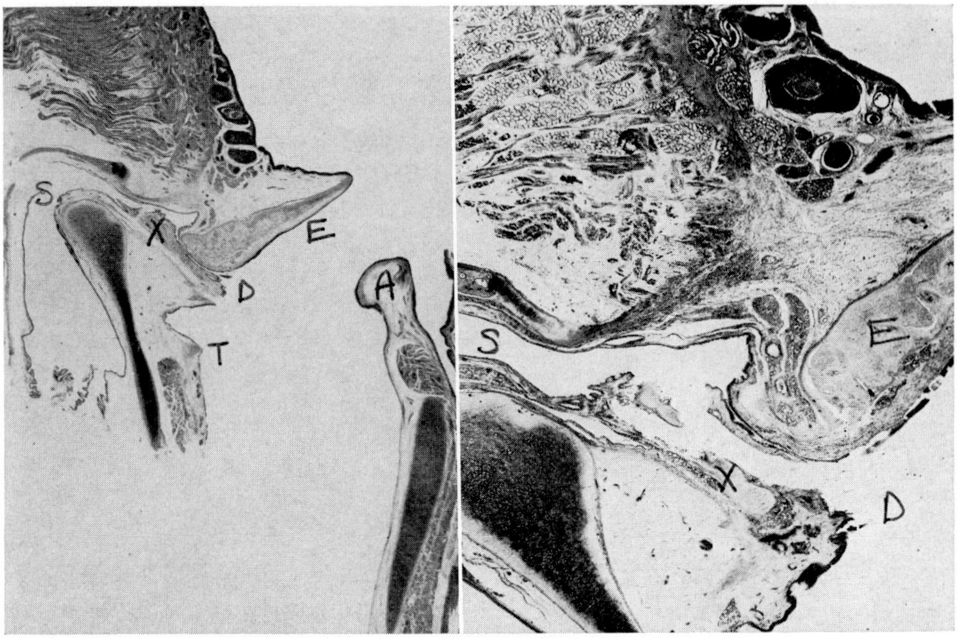

Fig. 3. A) Lutong P94A Kelemen (the purple faced Langur): section No. 316, midsagittal. B) Higher power, same section.

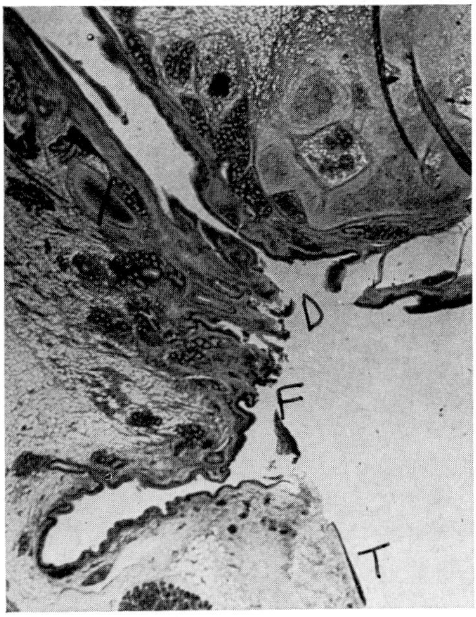

Fig. 4. *Macaca mulatta,* No. 2 Kelemen: section No. 53, midsagittal section, high power.

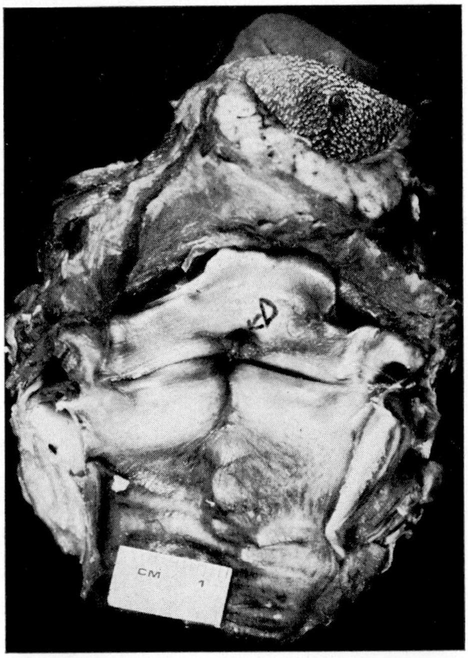

Fig. 5. Baboon (A.F.I.P.): specimen photographed conventional posterior split.

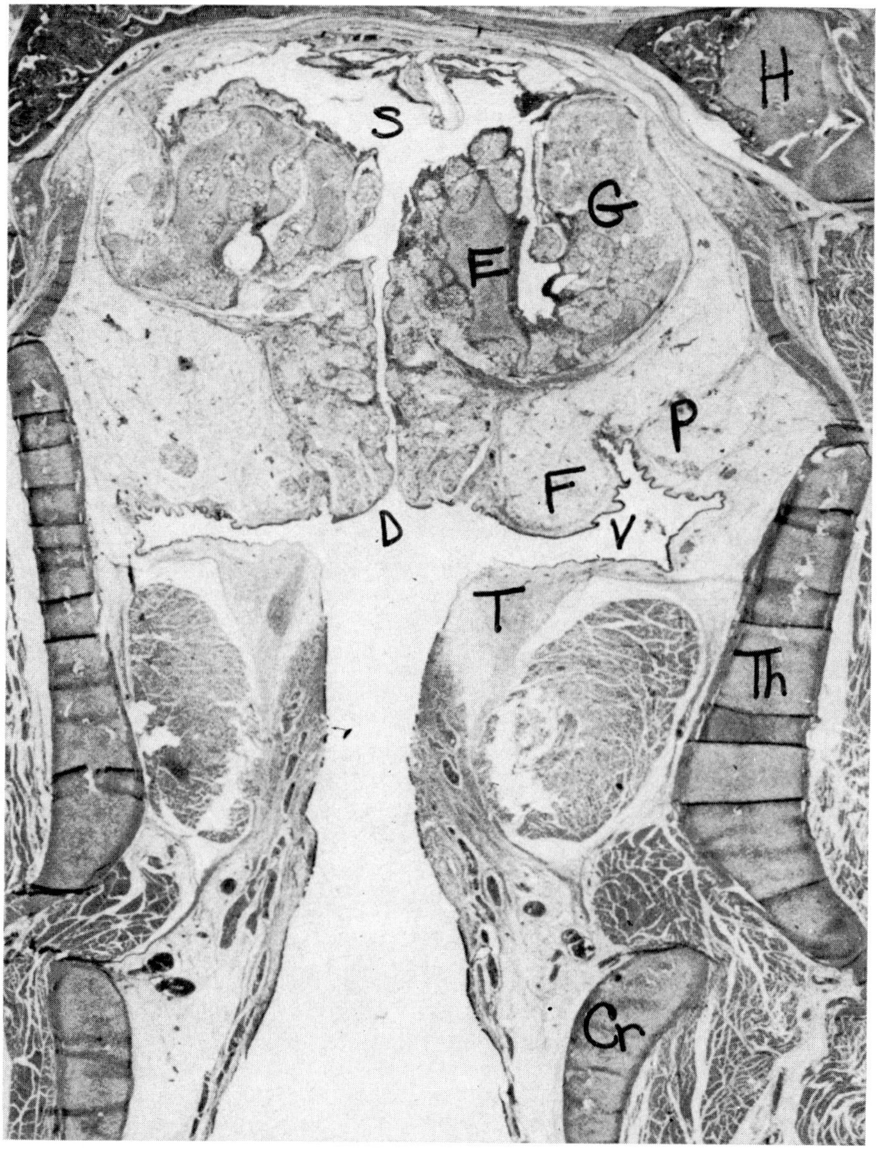

Fig. 6. Delafield's hematoxylin with chloxine-eosin counter stain. Coronal midcord section.

The preliminary studies reported herein suggest the possible value of comparative primate histologic studies in furthering our understanding of the human larynx.

The developmental sequence of air sac formation of the primate if similar to the human would approximate the later stages of the embryonic period and during the early portion of the fetal development.[7]

CONCLUSION

The above studies suggest a more complex arrangement between the hyoid and the conventional "larynx" in other primates than is usually assumed for the human.

Such observations would tend to reinforce the suggestion that the hyoid be included in our conceptualization of the larynx rather than as a separate entity.

Request for reprints should be sent to Gabriel Tucker, Jr., M.D., Children's Memorial Hospital, 2300 Children's Plaza, Chicago, Ill. 60614.

Acknowledgement — This study would have been impossible without the outstanding help and generosity of Dr. George Kelemen of the Los Angeles Foundation of Otology in giving to the authors precious unstained material collected over many years and in making available for study his stained tracer series of the same material. Mary Lou Gregory HT (ASCP), Research Assistant at the Institute of Laryngology, stained sections selected from the material donated by Dr. Kelemen. Frances Schoppy, from the laboratory of the ENT Branch of the A.F.I.P., prepared, sectioned, and stained the baboon larynx reported herein. Photography credits: Whole baboon specimen — A.F.I.P. Histologic sections: Hahnemann and Temple Medical Schools, Departments of Photography.

REFERENCES

1. Broyles EN: Anatomical observations concerning the laryngeal appendix. Ann Otol Rhinol Laryngol 68:461-470, 1959

2. Negus VE: *The Comparative Anatomy and Physiology of the Larynx.* New York, Grune and Stratton, 1949

3. Negus VE: *The Mechanism of the Larynx.* St. Louis, C. V. Mosby, 1929

4. Nèmai J: Das Stimmorgan der Primaten. Z Anat Entwickslungs Gesch 81:657-672, 1926

5. Kelemen G: Comparative anatomy and performance of the vocal organ in vertebrates, in Busnel RG (ed): *Acoustic Behavior of Animals.* New York, Elsevier Publ. Co., 1964, chap 18

6. Tucker GF: The anatomy of laryngeal cancer. Can J Otolaryngol 3:417-431, 1974

7. Tucker J, Tucker G: Some aspects of fetal laryngeal development. Ann Otol Rhinol Laryngol 84:49-55, 1975

Ann Otol 84: 1975

INCIDENCE, PREDISPOSING FACTORS AND OUTCOME OF PHARYNGOCUTANEOUS FISTULAS COMPLICATING HEAD AND NECK CANCER SURGERY

DOUGLAS D. DEDO, M.D.

WILLIAM A. ALONSO, M.D. JOSEPH H. OGURA, M.D.

ST. LOUIS, MISSOURI

SUMMARY — A major complication of head and neck cancer surgery following radiation and extensive resection is pharyngocutaneous fistula. A retrospective analysis of 36 fistula patients out of 376 major head and neck procedures between January 1971 and July 1973 revealed certain guidelines for improved clinical management. Since a large discrepancy existed in the incidence of fistulas between the different surgical procedures, each operative group was examined separately. The incidence, predisposing factors, and methods of treatment for this complication following composite jaw-neck resections and various laryngeal procedures are analyzed and discussed.

INTRODUCTION

Oro- and pharyngocutaneous fistulas complicating head and neck cancer surgery significantly increase patient morbidity and mortality. A retrospective study of this complication on the Head and Neck service from January 1971 to July 1973 was undertaken. The incidence, predisposing factors, and outcome of these fistulas were reviewed in order to establish criteria for improved management. The following guidelines were introduced: 1) preoperative identification of the high risk patient likely to develop a fistula; 2) prediction of spontaneous fistula closure or the need for surgical reconstruction; 3) alteration of the proposed surgical procedure to include primary reconstruction; and 4) prevention of future fistulas.

METHODS AND MATERIALS

Charts from January 1971 to July 1973 were reviewed of all major head and neck cancer patients whose courses were complicated by the development of a fistula. As summarized in Table I, a total of 50 immediate and delayed fistulas complicated 376 primary resections for an incidence of 13.3%. Nine fistulas were created primarily at the time of resection and five developed spontaneously more than six weeks after surgery. Omission of these 14 cases reduces the incidence of fistulization to 9.6%. The major head and neck procedures under study included composite jaw-neck resections, partial laryngopharyngectomies (PLP), subtotal supraglottic laryngectomies (SSL), and total laryngectomies. It does not include hemilaryngectomies since none were complicated by a fistula. A significant difference in the incidence of fistulas was noted among the various surgical procedures (Table I). Each surgical category was analyzed separately to account for this discrepancy and to identify any factors that might be unique to each procedure.

RESULTS

One hundred twenty composite jaw-neck dissections were performed. Twelve patients (10%) developed a fistula. Three of the 12 cases developed late fistulas and all were related to persistent carcinoma. The site of the primary tumor

From the Department of Otolaryngology, Washington University School of Medicine, St. Louis, Missouri.

Supported in part by NIH Training Grant No. 5T01 NSO 5190-15 from NINDS.

Presented at the meeting of the American Laryngological Association, Atlanta, Georgia, April 6-7, 1975.

TABLE I

INCIDENCE OF FISTULAS WITH RESPECT TO SURGICAL TREATMENT OF PRIMARY TUMOR

	No. of Cases	*Total No. Fistulas*	*No. Fistulas Complicating Surgery*
Jaw neck dissection	120	12 (10 %)	9 (7.5%)
Partial laryngopharyngectomy (and radical neck dissection)	72	17 (23.6%)	15 (20.8%)
Subtotal supraglottic laryngectomy (and radical neck dissection)	60	5 (8.3%)	5 (8.3%)
Total laryngectomy	117	9 (7.6%)	7 (5.9%)
Total laryngopharyngectomy with surgical reconstruction	7	7 (100 %)	0 —
Totals	376	50 (13.3%)	36 (9.6%)

correlated with the location of the fistula in the remaining nine cases (7.5%). In seven of the nine patients the tumor involved the posterior oropharynx (base of tongue, tonsil, lateral pharyngeal wall, *etc.*). In all of these patients the fistula developed at the trifurcation in the skin, overlying the lateral pharyngeal suture line. In contrast, two patients with a floor of the mouth cancer developed fistulas in the submental triangle.

TABLE II

FACTORS CONTRIBUTING TO FISTULAS FOLLOWING JAW NECK DISSECTION

Large T_3 lesions*	9
Fluid accumulation under cervical flaps	7
Necrosis of cervical flaps	5
Dosage of preop irradiation >3,000 rads	4
Recurrent carcinoma	
Local	1
Distant	4
Systemic disease	3
Hemorrhage requiring reexploration	2
Osteomyelitis of mandible	2
Previous rhytidectomy	1

*Classification according to UICC.

It is difficult to single out a specific etiology for each of the nine fistulas. Numerous factors influence the pharyngocutaneous breakdown (Table II). All nine patients had advanced T_3 lesions. Seven patients required counter drainage of their wounds after fluid accumulation under the flaps. Five of the nine patients had partial necrosis of their cervical flaps. Four of the patients with fistulas received more than the usual dose of 3,000 rads preoperatively. Five cases were subsequently treated for local persistence (1) or distant metastases (4). Two patients had diabetes mellitus and a third developed hepatic failure postoperatively. Two patients required reexploration of a wound hematoma. Osteomyelitis of the mandible developed at the margin of resection in two other cases. These were successfully treated with debridement. Another patient, with a rhytidectomy prior to composite jaw-neck resection, was treated with 5,000 rads preoperatively. Postoperatively the cervical flaps were noted to be very atrophic. High dose preoperative irradiation combined with the face lift played a major role in her wound dehiscence.

Analysis of these nine cases reveals certain predisposing factors which contributed to fistula formation. Four patients received high dose preoperative irradiation for large T_3 lesions, two involving the lateral pharyngeal wall. After resection with an adequate margin and primary closure, the hypopharyngeal suture line was under excessive tension. An irradiated suture line under tension is susceptible to ischemia, necro-

TABLE III

OUTCOME OF THE FISTULAS COMPLICATING JAW AND NECK DISSECTION

	No. of Cases	*Avg. No. Days from 1° Resection to Closure*	
Closed spontaneously without any surgical manipulation	3	120	(22-180)
Closed spontaneously without surgical reconstruction	3	45.6	(34- 53)
Closed with surgical reconstruction	1	105	
Never closed	2	7 6	mo mo

sis, and fistula formation. Disruption of the normal healing process by fluid, flap necrosis, or counter drainage in an irradiated neck further predisposes to fistula formation.

The five remaining patients received low dose preoperative irradiation. Their postoperative course was complicated by two or more local wound disruptions. This included reexploration for hemorrhage (2), flap necrosis (3), fluid accumulation (3), and osteomyelitis of the mandible (2). In addition, three patients had disabling systemic disease.

Preoperative identification of three of these high risk patients (high dose irradiation, pharyngeal wall involvement, alteration of cervical skin) might have decreased the incidence of spontaneous fistula by 33%. Subsequent alteration of the surgical procedure in these three patients to include immediate reconstruction or a controlled pharyngostome would have decreased morbidity.

Table III summarizes the outcome of these nine fistulas. Three small fistulas closed spontaneously after an average of 120 days (22-180) from the day of primary resection. They were treated conservatively with daily dressing changes. Two of the three were followed on an outpatient basis. Three moderately sized fistulas also closed spontaneously after an average of 45 days (34-53). The principal difference between these two groups of patients is the fact that the latter three fistulas were debrided in the operating room and had a Bakamjian chest flap staged. The three largest fistulas required multiple surgical procedures for closure. One patient was successfully reconstructed by the 105th postoperative day. Another fistula remained open, and the patient died of distant metastases seven months following the primary resection. The third case had been draining for six months and was terminated by the end of the study.

The highest incidence of postoperative fistulas was seen after PLP. Seventeen patients (23.6%) developed fistulas out of a total of 72 PLP's. Two control fistulas were created at primary resection, reducing the postoperative incidence to 20.8%. The remaining 15 fistulas developed within six weeks of surgery and are considered a complication of a PLP.[1]

Hypopharyngeal tumors involving the pyriform sinus, vallecula, or pharyngeal walls are treated with a PLP. Closure of the hypopharynx after a PLP is dependent upon the amount of mucosa remaining after primary tumor resection. When the lateral wall of the pyriform sinus is free of disease, closure of the neopharynx can be accomplished without difficulty. However, in large tumors extending to the lateral and/or posterior pharyngeal walls, the mucosal closure may be compromised. As a result, the approximation of perichondrium to mucosa may be placed under excessive tension. Necrosis and separation of the lateral pharyngeal suture line can occur. Sixteen of the 17 patients in this group had large T_3 or T_4 lesions. Fourteen of the 17 involved the pyriform fossa with extension to the lateral (9) and/or posterior pharyngeal walls (4).

Several factors involved in the development of these fistulas are summarized in Table IV. In seven patients split thickness skin grafts and Negus stents were used following resection to close the pharynxes. Six patients developed fluid

TABLE IV

FACTORS RESPONSIBLE FOR POST PLP FISTULAS

Large T_3 or T_4 lesions	16
Use of Negus stent and STSG for closure of neopharynx	7
Fluid accumulation	6
Necrosis of cervical flaps	4
Persistent carcinoma	
Local	1
Distant	3
Dosage of preop irradiation (>3,000 rads)	3
Suture abscess	2
Created surgically	2
Multiple operations for post PLP glottic insufficiency	1
Improper feeding	1
Omission of prophylactic antibiotics	1

under the flaps. Necrosis and partial slough of the cervical flaps occurred in four cases. One patient had residual tumor at the margin of the resection and three developed distant metastases during fistula treatment within a year of surgery. Three of the 17 patients received greater than 3,000 rads preoperatively. Four attempts were made on one patient with persistent aspiration to restore glottic competence. After the fourth open procedure, the patient developed a fistula which drained for two weeks. Against medical advice, one patient fed herself on the fourth postoperative day and resisted attempts to curtail her oral intake. One patient did not receive prophylactic antibiotics. Two patients developed fistulas on the 34th and 37th days postoperatively. Both had been decannulated and had good oral intake. Exploration revealed silk suture abscesses along the base of the tongue-perichondrial suture line.

The outcome in this group of 17 fistulas is summarized in Table V. Two were classified as small fistulas and closed spontaneously with conservative therapy after an average of 41.5 days (23-60). Three patients were prepared for surgical reconstruction with a staged Bakamjian chest flap, but the fistula

TABLE V

RESOLUTION OF FISTULAS FOLLOWING A PLP

	No. of Cases	*Avg. No. Days from 1° Resection to Closure*
Closed spontaneously without any surgical manipulation	2	41.5
Closed spontaneously without surgical reconstruction	3	92
Closed with surgical reconstruction	11	116
Never closed	1	

closed spontaneously after an average of 92 days (29-210). Eleven patients (including seven repaired with split thickness skin grafts and Negus stents, and two with controlled pharyngostomes) required surgical reconstruction for closure. An average of 3.9 months (23 days to 14 months) from the day of tumor resection to fistula repair was required. Two patients with a controlled pharyngostome were successfully closed 23 and 36 days following resection with return of the chest flaps. One patient died of a carotid artery rupture while being prepared for surgical reconstruction of the fistula.

Preoperative identification of the high risk patient likely to develop a fistula following a PLP is largely related to two factors. First, large T_3 or T_4 tumors of the pyriform sinus are associated with a high incidence of postoperative fistulas (16 of 17). Secondly, tumor involvement of the lateral or posterior pharyngeal wall markedly complicates suitable primary closure of the neopharynx following extensive resection (13 of 17).

An SSL was performed on 60 patients. Five patients in this series developed a pharyngocutaneous fistula for an incidence of 8.3%.

In all five cases fistulas were traced to a breakdown at the perichondrial-base of tongue suture line. Table VI summarizes the factors responsible for

TABLE VI

FACTORS RESPONSIBLE FOR POSTOPERATIVE SSL FISTULAS

Suture abscess	3
Necrotic thyroid cartilage	2
Liver failure	1

wound dehiscence in this group of patients. Three patients required incision and drainage (I and D) for localized abscesses. At the core of each abscess was a mass of silk suture. In two patients fragments of necrotic cartilage were debrided after the fistulas were exteriorized. Liver failure complicated wound healing in another patient.

Two of three fistulas discovered after I and D of a suture abscess closed spontaneously within 38 days of surgery (Table VII). The third case closed spontaneously 51 days after primary resection and staging of a Bakamjian chest flap. These three cases were staged as T_2 or T_3 lesions. By comparison, the two cases requiring surgical closure were T_4 lesions. Successful surgical rehabilitation required 90 days and five months, respectively.

TABLE VII

OUTCOME OF THE POST SSL FISTULAS

	No. of Cases	*Avg. Day Postop*
Closed spontaneously without any surgical manipulation	2	38
Closed spontaneously without surgical reconstruction	1	51
Closed with surgical reconstruction	2	120

The lowest incidence (7.6%, or nine out of 117 patients) of postoperative fistulas occurred after total laryngectomy. Two of the nine fistulas appeared two and five years following primary resection. The remaining seven or 5.9% represent the true incidence of fistula as a surgical complication.

TABLE VIII

FACTORS INVOLVED IN POST TOTAL LARYNGECTOMY FISTULAS

High dose irradiation >3,000 rads	4
Persistent carcinoma (1 delayed)	3
Extension to posterior pharyngeal wall	3
Systemic disease	3
Foreign body granuloma, 1 delayed	2
Postsurgical persistence	2

The most frequent sites of fistula drainage were either through carcinoma (3), or adjacent to the tracheostoma. Table VIII summarizes the factors involved in the development of the seven fistulas. Four patients received 4,000-8,000 rads prior to surgery. Two were radiation failures. Three had tumor extending into the lateral and posterior pharyngeal walls. Two patients required excision of foreign body granulomas. (One granuloma developed more than five years postoperatively.) Two patients required a total laryngectomy for residual tumor after hemilaryngectomy and SSL, respectively. In three patients, systemic disease such as diabetes mellitus or chronic obstructive pulmonary disease (COPD) complicated their clinical course.

Patients with a high risk of fistula formation after total laryngectomy are those who are radiation or surgical failures. Cancer involvement of the lateral and posterior pharyngeal walls or serious systemic disease are additional factors which modify the clinical course. A controlled pharyngostome followed by secondary reconstruction should be considered in these cases.

Results of fistula repair and survival were poor in this group of patients. There were no spontaneous fistula closures (Table IX). One fistula closed after debridement 70 days after tumor resection. Another fistula was closed surgically following excision of a granuloma and fistula tract with primary closure of the defect. The remaining seven cases never closed. Six patients (66%) died within six months after recognition

TABLE IX

OUTCOME OF FISTULAS COMPLICATING TOTAL LARYNGECTOMIES

	No. of Cases	*Avg. No. Days from 1° Resection to Closure*
Closed spontaneously	0	—
Closed spontaneously after surgical manipulation	1	70
Surgical closure without reconstruction	1	21
Never closed	7	—

of a fistula. The causes of death were uncontrolled primary (3), bronchopneumonia (2), and severe COPD with multiple spontaneous pneumothoraces (1). Poor survival rates in this group of patients was in part related to the large size of the tumors. Chronic debilitation and poor nutrition also contributed to their demise despite vigorous supportive care.

For purposes of discussion, seven patients with primary chest flap reconstruction at the time of total laryngopharyngectomy will be analyzed. Four patients received 6,000 rads preoperatively and three received 3,000 rads. Three patients were treated for a postsurgical or postirradiation cancer persistence. Table X summarizes the outcome in these cases.

Four of five patients with unilateral chest flap reconstruction were successfully rehabilitated after an average of 50 days (28-90). Although the pedicle flaps were usually returned to the donor site within 25 days of primary resection, drainage often continued for two additional months at the inferior suture line. Two patients requiring multiple flaps for reconstruction required seven months to close. Of seven patients, 50% developed a recurrence within six months of the original surgery.

DISCUSSION

The period January 1971 through July 1973 was chosen for study for two reasons. First, by reviewing relatively recent years, established techniques of primary resection and reconstruction could be analyzed and compared. Second, povidone-iodine ointment[2] was added to the regimen of local fistula care in November 1972. Our clinical impression was that the fistulas were healing more rapidly with povidone-iodine than with the other nonsurgical local treatments. In order to design a laboratory model and test the efficacy of this local wound management, accumulation of more clinical information about fistula formation was necessary.

The 9.6% total incidence of spontaneous fistulization compares favorably with other studies.[3-6] Lavelle[7] reported a 37% and Smits, *et al*[8] a 36% incidence of fistulas following total laryngectomy. We have a 5.6% fistula rate for 117 total laryngectomies. The 20% rate of spontaneous fistulization following PLP will decrease as the Negus stent is being replaced by other modes of reconstruction. Recent use of controlled pharyngostomes in PLP's and other extensive resections to decompress the neopharyngeal suture line has been successful in reducing spontaneous, uncontrolled fistulas.

TABLE X

FOLLOW-UP OF SEVEN CASES OF TOTAL LARYNGOPHARYNGECTOMY

	No. of Cases	*Avg. No. Days Before Closure*	*Recurrent Carcinoma*
Reconstruction using a single chest flap	5	50* (28-90)	3
Reconstruction using more than 1 pedicle flap	2	7 mo (5-9)	1

*Does not include one patient cut off by end of study who had been draining for 77 days.

The combined incidence (15%) of fistulas following conservation laryngeal surgery is two and one-half times greater than the incidence for total laryngectomies. We consider this an acceptable risk in exchange for better patient function and quality of life.

Common predisposing factors to fistula formation among the various surgical procedures allows the preoperative identification of high risk patients. In general, patients with a systemic disease (diabetes mellitus, COPD, *etc.*) will have a complicated clinical course. Large T_3 and T_4 tumors requiring resection of large amounts of the lateral and posterior pharyngeal walls may be difficult to close primarily. Patients requiring large surgical resections for postirradiation or postsurgical tumor persistence may require staged reconstruction. While there is controversy regarding the dose of irradiation which significantly impairs wound healing, it is generally recognized[8-11] that as higher doses of irradiation (4,500-8,000 rads) are employed, neopharyngeal dehiscence is more likely to occur. Two or more of these common factors combined with local wound disruption will predispose the majority of patients to a cutaneous fistula.

Technical weaknesses inherent in each surgical procedure contribute to the development of a fistula. For example, in a composite jaw-neck resection, inadequate removal or cover of the resected mandible can result in osteomyelitis and drainage. When a PLP is utilized for large pyriform sinus tumors extending to the posterior pharyngeal wall, the neopharyngeal suture line can break down if not primarily reconstructed or decompressed with a controlled pharyngostome. Careful elevation of the perichondrial flap and gentle handling of the thyroid cartilage during the saw cuts are necessary to avoid cartilage necrosis and subsequent drainage in both SSL's and PLP's.

The pharyngeal mucosa was closed with silk sutures in all cases except after total laryngectomies. After 14 days, the silk suture acts as an impediment to wound healing. This was amply demonstrated after exteriorizing the fistulas. A large number of silk sutures was always removed from the sloughed area of the pharyngeal or thyroid cartilage suture lines. Not only does the silk act as a nidus for infection, but its mucosal holding properties are dissipated within two weeks. A study is currently underway to compare the various suture materials for closure of the pharynx.

The results of the management of these 36 fistulas may be summarized as follows: seven (19.4%) closed spontaneously, eight (22.2%) required some form of surgical manipulation before closing spontaneously, 13 (36%) required surgical closure, and eight (22.2%) failed to close. Prediction of spontaneous or surgical fistula closure is largely related to the operation performed. Following a composite jaw-neck resection, debridement in the operating room within ten days of fistula development is recommended to decrease prolonged morbidity. Concomitant staging of the chest flap for future use during debridement will save time, especially if the size of the fistula is large. A PLP complicated by a fistula has an 80% probability of requiring surgical manipulation for closure. Therefore, shortly after the diagnosis of a fistula, debridement and staging of a chest flap should be completed. Fistulas developing after SSL's for small lesions will close spontaneously following removal of necrotic cartilage and silk sutures. A fistula following a total laryngectomy is an ominous sign. In addition to vigorous supportive care, debridement and staging of a chest flap for moderate to large fistulas will be necessary.

Preoperative planning of the surgical procedure to include staged reconstruction in the high risk patient should be considered to lessen patient morbidity and expensive postoperative stays. In two PLP's with primary chest flap reconstruction, wound closure was achieved an average of 29 days after resection. This is in marked contrast to an average of 3.9 months required for closure of the nine uncontrolled PLP fistulas. The five cases of total laryngopharyngectomies with single chest flap reconstruction were closed an average of 50 days from the day of resection. The decrease in number of hospital days for those patients reconstructed at the time of initial tumor resection justifies a more frequent use of chest flaps and controlled pharyngostomes in head and neck extirpative surgery.

Over 70% of the fistulas reported were diagnosed within three weeks following surgery. Frequently, the patients were eating and decannulated when their wounds drained. Since an average wound does not reach its maximum breaking strength for six weeks,[12] an irradiated wound would be expected to be delayed even longer. Swallowing and coughing subject the neopharyngeal suture line to significant stress. To prevent fistulas and encourage wound healing, we delay decannulation and oral intake for three weeks in high risk patients. In addition, any patient who displays abnormal wound healing postoperatively (*e.g.*, cellulitis, edema, fluid accumulation) is placed on high dose IV antibiotics until the complication is resolved. Decannulation and peroral feeding are similarly delayed for three weeks to encourage further wound healing.

SUMMARY

A retrospective analysis of 36 fistulas which complicated 376 major head and neck resections between January 1971 and July 1973 was made to establish guidelines for improved clinical management and prevention of this complication.

Criteria for the preoperative identification of the high risk patient was based upon the predisposing factors and outcome of these 36 fistulas. In general, the size of the lesion, dosage of irradiation, presence of systemic disease, and failure of prior treatment modalities (surgery or irradiation) are the common factors which predispose the majority of patients to a cutaneous fistula. Prediction of spontaneous or surgical closure is dependent upon the tumor site and operation performed. Prevention of spontaneous fistulization postoperatively may be accomplished by delaying peroral feeding for at least three weeks in the high risk patient and/or a more frequent use of controlled pharyngostome to decompress the neopharyngeal suture line.

REFERENCES

1. Ogura JH, Mallen RW: Partial laryngopharyngectomy for supraglottic and pharyngeal carcinoma. Trans Am Acad Ophthalmol Otolaryngol 69:832-845, 1965

2. Connell JF, Rousselot LN: Povidone-iodine, extensive surgical evaluation of a new antiseptic agent. Am J Surg 108:849-851, 1964

3. Rolandez TL, Everts EC, Shumrick DA: Carcinoma of the tonsil: a planned combined therapy approach. Laryngoscope 81: 1199-1207, 1971

4. Constable WC, Marks RD, Robbins JP, *et al*: High dose preoperative radiotherapy and surgery for cancer of the larynx. Laryngoscope 82:1861-1868, 1972

5. Goldman JL, Silverstone SM, Roffman JD, *et al*: High dosage preoperative radiation and surgery for carcinoma of the larynx and laryngopharynx – a 14 year program. Laryngoscope 82:1869-1882, 1972

6. Wang CC, Schulz MD, Miller D: Combined radiation therapy and surgery for carcinoma of the supraglottic and pyriform sinus. Laryngoscope 82:1883-1890, 1972

7. Lavelle RJ, Maw AR: The aetiology of post-laryngectomy pharyngocutaneous fistulae. J Laryngol Otol 86:785-793, 1972

8. Smits RG, Krause CJ, McCabe BF: Complications associated with combined therapy of oral and pharyngeal neoplasms. Ann Otol Rhinol Laryngol 81:496-500, 1972

9. Myers EN: The management of pharyngocutaneous fistula. Arch Otolaryngol 95:10-17, 1972

10. Peacock EE Jr, Van Winkle, W Jr: *Surgery and Biology of Wound Repair*. Philadelphia, Saunders, 1970

11. Dingman RO: Factors of clinical significance affecting wound healing. Laryngoscope 83:1540-1554, 1973

12. Levenson SM, Geever EF, Crowley LV, *et al*: The healing of rat skin wounds. Ann Surg 161:293-298, 1965

REPRINTS: 517 S. Euclid, St. Louis, Mo. 63110 (Dr. Dedo).

Ann Otol 84: 1975

VERTIGO OF DELAYED ONSET AFTER SUDDEN DEAFNESS

Joseph B. Nadol, Jr., M.D.

Alfred D. Weiss, M.D. Stephen W. Parker, M.D.

Boston, Massachusetts

SUMMARY – An entity of episodic true vertigo of delayed onset following sudden and profound sensorineural hearing loss is described. Data on 12 patients and three case reports are presented. The latency between sudden deafness and the onset of the vertigo varied from 1 to 68 years. The vestibular symptoms are identical to the vestibular symptoms of Ménière's disease, and there is some evidence that endolymphatic hydrops in the previously deafened ear represents at least part of the labyrinthine pathology. Labyrinthectomy in the deaf ear was curative. Tentatively, this entity is best considered a variant of Ménière's disease.

Episodic vertigo with progressive sensorineural hearing loss is typical of Ménière's disease.[1] However, otogenic episodic vertigo following many years after sudden and profound hearing loss has not been reported previously. Twelve patients are presented in whom true vertigo with delayed onset occurred from 1 to 68 years after sudden and profound sensorineural hearing loss. The episodic vertigo in these patients is indistinguishable from the vertiginous episodes of Ménière's disease. In two patients, diagnostic labyrinthotomy suggested endolymphatic hydrops as the underlying pathophysiology of the vertigo, and in another patient, histological examination of the stapes extracted at labyrinthectomy showed membranous labyrinth adherent to the medial surface of the footplate, also suggesting endolymphatic hydrops. Labyrinthectomy was performed on the deaf ear of ten patients, and all were cured of their vertigo.

CASE REPORTS

The symptoms and signs of 12 patients are summarized in Tables I-III. Three illustrative cases are presented in detail.

Case 1. This 60-year-old male experienced the onset of vertigo at the age of 56 years. The episodes of vertigo lasted from 30 to 60 minutes each and were accompanied by nausea, vomiting, and an increase in tinnitus in his right ear. During one episode his internist noted horizontal nystagmus. The episodes became more frequent over the four-year period, and during the three months prior to surgery, he suffered daily vertiginous episodes despite treatment with meclizine hydrochloride. He suffered a sudden and profound hearing loss in his right ear with tinnitus but without any vertiginous symptoms at the age of 50 years, while eating breakfast. This loss was ascribed to a viral labyrinthitis.

Examination at the age of 60 showed normal tympanic membranes, essentially normal hearing in the left ear and an SRT of 100 dB with 4% discrimination in the right ear. Hallpike calorics as recorded by electronystagmography showed right vestibular hypofunction. Neurological examination was normal.

A transcanal diagnostic labyrinthotomy and labyrinthectomy were performed. Analysis of the inner ear fluid showed protein, 209 mg%; sodium, 7 mg%; potassium, 136 mg%; this was consistent with normal endolymph. Post-

From the Department of Otolaryngology and Division of Otoneurology of the Massachusetts Eye and Ear Infirmary, 243 Charles Street, Boston, Massachusetts.

operatively there were no further episodes of vertigo over a period of four years. An ice water caloric test performed five months after surgery showed no response in the right ear.

Case 2. A ten-year-old white female suffered the onset of episodic vertigo at seven years of age. This was characterized by nausea, vomiting, and pounding tinnitus in the left ear. Each episode lasted from 20 to 90 minutes at intervals of one to four weeks over a three-year period prior to surgery. At six years of age she experienced a sudden and profound hearing loss in her left ear coincident with a well documented episode of mumps. Vertigo accompanied her hearing loss and resolved completely over the ensuing one week. She experienced no vertigo after the acute episode until one year later. Examination at the age of ten revealed normal tympanic membranes. The neurological examination and electroencephalogram were normal. An audiogram showed a profound sensorineural hearing loss in the left ear and normal cochlear function on the right. Hallpike calorics as recorded by electronystagmography were interpreted as normal bilaterally. The morphology of the internal auditory canals as studied by laminography was normal. A transcanal labyrinthectomy of the left ear was performed at the age of ten years. There was no further episode of vertigo in a follow-up period of two years.

Case 3. A 28-year-old female suffered the onset of episodic vertigo at 25 years of age, beginning during a pregnancy. These episodes lasted approximately one hour, once every three days, and were accompanied by nausea and vomiting, tinnitus, and pressure in her left ear. Her episodes grew steadily more severe despite medical treatment with meclizine hydrochloride, phenobarbital, and chlordiazepoxide hydrochloride. She had a profound sensorineural hearing loss in her left ear, presumably since birth and documented by audiogram at the age of three years.

Examination at age 28 revealed normal tympanic membranes, and an audiogram showed normal hearing in her right ear and an SRT of 96 dB and a discrimination of 0% in the left ear. Ice water calorics (Kobrak) revealed a hypoactive left vestibular response. Neurological examination was normal. X-rays of the internal auditory canals were normal.

At age 28 she underwent a diagnostic labyrinthotomy and labyrinthectomy of the left ear. Analysis of the inner ear fluid revealed protein, 226 mg%; sodium, 21 mg%; potassium, 159 mg%; these findings were consistent with endolymph. There were no further episodes of vertigo in a four-year follow-up period.

DISCUSSION

A clinically observed entity of episodic vertigo, delayed in onset after sudden sensorineural hearing loss in 12 patients is described. In each patient the profound sensorineural hearing loss was sudden and related to a variety of causes, some clearly traumatic, some probably viral, and others of unknown cause. A few patients had coincident involvement of the vestibular apparatus with transient vertigo, while most patients had no history of vestibular symptoms at the time of the sudden loss of hearing. Each patient subsequently developed episodic true vertigo, and the presumed otogenic source of the vertigo was corroborated by the fact that each operated patient was cured of his vertigo by labyrinthectomy of the deaf ear, and otoneurological evaluation and symptoms suggested a peripheral source of the vertigo.

The nature of the inner ear pathology responsible for the episodic vertigo in these patients is speculative. The vertiginous characteristics of the episodes are indistinguishable from Ménière's disease. The symptoms include episodic true vertigo, nausea, vomiting, tinnitus, and pressure in the previously deafened ear, and in one patient, documentation of spontaneous horizontal nystagmus during an episode of vertigo. Neurological examinations were uniformly normal, as was the radiographic morphology of the internal auditory canals.

TABLE I

CHARACTERIZATION OF SUDDEN PROFOUND UNILATERAL HEARING LOSS PRECEDING THE ONSET OF EPISODIC VERTIGO

Case No.	*Age/Sex*	*Ear*	*Etiology Age at Onset (Yrs)*	*Evidence for Coincident Involvement of Vestibular Labyrinth*	*Audiological Data*
1	60/M	R	?Viral labyrinthitis 50	None	L - N R - SRT 100 dB Discr - 4%
2	10/F	L	Mumps 6	1 wk. of slowly improving vert.	L - No function R - N
3	28/F	L	Congenital or neonatal	None	L - SRT 96 dB Discr - 0% R - N
4	27/M	L	Basilar skull fracture 4	None	L - No function R - N
5	42/F	R	URI 2	None	L - N R - No function
6	37/M	L	Congenital	None	L - Profound loss R - N
7	22/F	L	Head trauma or mumps 8	None	L - Profound loss R - N
8	45/M	L	Trauma 3	None	L - SRT 96 dB Discr - 0% R - N
9	74/F	R	Diphtheria 3	None	L - Mild S-N loss, N discr R - No function
10	50/M	R	URI - bilat. deafness 3	None	L & R, Profound S-N loss, Discr - 0%
11	30/M	R	β. strep. mastoiditis and labyrinthitis 8	2° nystagmus and vert., 1 wk. No response to air calorics R ear.	L - N R - Profound loss Discr - 0%
12	54/M	R	Mumps 8	None	L - N R - SRT 88 dB Discr - 0%

S-N - Sensorineural; N - Normal; Vert. - Vertigo; URI - Upper respiratory infection

In most patients, unilateral vestibular hypofunction was demonstrated in the deaf ear. In addition, in two patients (Cases 1 and 3), diagnostic labyrinthotomy confirmed the diagnosis of endolymphatic hydrops, and in another patient (Case 10, Tables I-III) histological study of the extracted stapes demonstrated membranous labyrinth attached to the medial surface of the footplate, also suggesting endolymphatic hydrops. The discussion of this patient has been the subject of a separate report.[2] However, in three patients, (Cases 4, 7, and 10, Tables I-III), diagnostic labyrinthotomy yielded inner ear fluid consistent with normal perilymph. This does not, however, rule out hydrops, but proves

TABLE II

CHARACTERIZATION OF EPISODIC VERTIGO

Case No.	*Age at Onset (yr)*	*Latency Betw. Hearing Loss and Vert. (yr)*	*Avg. Interval Betw. Episodes (days)*	*Symptoms During Episodes/Duration of Episodes*	*Calorics*	*Laminograms of IAC*	*Other*
1	56	6	2	N & V. Increased Tin. L/½ - 1 hr	R Hypo. (ENG)	—	Nystagmus during attack. Lab.: Na 7 mg%, K 136 mg%
2	7	1	14	N & V. Tin. & pressure L/1 hr	Norm. (ENG)	Norm.	EEG - Norm.
3	25	25	4	N & V. Tin. & pressure L/½ - 1 hr	L Hypo. (Kobrak)	Norm.	Lab.: Na 21 mg% K 159 mg%
4	27	23	1	N & V. Fullness & Tin. L/10 min to 6 hr	L Hypo. (ENG)	Norm.	Positional test norm. Lab.: Na 221 mg%; K 9.5 mg%
5	42	40	4	N & V./2 hr	No response 0° R	Norm.	—
6	31	31	2	N & V./1 hr	L Hypo. (Kobrak)	Norm.	—
7	10	2	15	N. & V. Objective clockwise vert.	L Hypo. (Kobrak)	—	Lab.: Na 128 mg% K 6 mg%
8	42	39	30	N & V. Increased Tin. L/5 - 30 min	L Hypo. (ENG)	—	—
9	71	68	14	N & V. Frequent falls/½ - 3 hr	R Hypo. (ENG)	Norm.	—
10	48	45	4	N & V. Tin. & fullness R/½ - 2 hr	R Hypo. (ENG)	Norm.	Lab. perilymph
11	30	22	4	N & V./2 hr	R Hypo. (ENG)	—	—
12	37	30	14	N & V./5 min	R Hypo. (ENG)	Norm.	—

EEG - Electroencephalogram; ENG - Electronystagmography; Hypo. - Hypofunction; IAC - Internal auditory canals; K - Potassium; Kobrak - Minimal caloric; Lab. - Labyrinthotomy; L - Left ear; R - Right ear; N - Nausea; Na - Sodium; Norm. - Normal; Tin. - Tinnitus; V - Vomiting; Vert. - Vertigo.

TABLE III

TREATMENT OF EPISODIC VERTIGO

		Medical Treatment		*Surgical Treatment (Transcanal Labyrinthectomy)*	
Case No.	*Duration of Vertigo (Mo)*	*Medication*	*Treatment Effect*	*Effect*	*Multiple of avg. interval between episodes before surgery*[14]
1	48	Meclizine HCl	None	No vert. 4 yr	730 X
2	36	–	–	No vert. 2 yr	56 X
3	36	Phenobarb. meclizine chlordiaz-epoxide	None	No vert. 4 yr	448 X
4	3	–	–	No vert. 1 yr	365 X
5	12	–	–	No vert. 1 yr	112 X
6	72	Meclizine HCl	None	No vert. 4 yr	672 X
7	144	–	–	No vert. 1 yr	24 X
8	36	–	–	No vert. 9 yr	108 X
9	36	–	–	No vert. 1 yr	112 X
10	24	–	–	No vert. 1 yr	112 X
11	3	–	–	Spontaneous remission No surgery	
12	192	Dimenhydrinate promethazine	None	Declined surgery	

Vert. - Vertigo

only that the membranous labyrinth was not in contact with the footplate either at the site, or at the time, of footplate puncture. Silverstein[3] has suggested that the incidence of false negative taps for Ménière's disease is approximately 7% (3 out of 41 patients), where the hydrops has been long standing. The examination[4] of serial sections of 25 temporal bones of patients with long standing Ménière's disease from the collection of the Massachusetts Eye and Ear Infirmary, showed that in only 12 (48%) was there juxtaposition of the membranous labyrinth with the footplate over part or all of its medial surface, the presumed prerequisite for a positive tap for endolymph.

The delay of one to 68 years between the sudden onset of hearing loss and the later onset of ipsilateral otogenic vertigo is puzzling. In all patients the onset of the vertigo was clearly distinguishable from the acute episode which had destroyed the cochlear function. If indeed, the pathophysiology of the vertigo in these patients is related to endolymphatic hydrops, the observations of Schuknecht and Kimura[5,6] are of interest. In the guinea pig, endolymphatic hydrops followed within weeks of obliteration of the vestibular aqueduct, whereas in the cat, three years were required to develop the hydropic change. It is conceivable that in man a longer average interval is required between obstruction and the development of hydrops, and that interval is represented by the latency between hearing loss and the onset of vertigo in our patients.

The etiology of sudden hearing loss in these 12 patients was probably viral in five, bacterial in two, traumatic in two, and unknown in three. Schuknecht and others[7,8] have suggested that viral labyrinthitis is the likely etiology of idiopathic, sudden hearing loss. However, endolymphatic hydrops is a rare finding in documented viral labyrinthitis.[7-12] Furthermore, the presence of endolymphatic hydrops does not necessarily result in any vestibular symptoms, as demonstrated in a case reported by Schuknecht and Wright[13] of profound congenital deafness with endolymphatic hydrops, presumably secondary to fibrous obliteration of the endolymphatic duct, but with no vestibular symptoms.

It is also possible that we are observing the fortuitous coincidence of two separate otological diseases, that is, a Ménière-like syndrome developing in ears that had been deafened years previously from a variety of causes. We, however, would prefer to interpret this as one pathological process, that is, progressive inner ear degeneration after sudden deafness from a variety of causes, resulting in episodic otogenic vertigo. This process may involve endolymphatic hydrops. Tentatively, this would best be considered a third variant of Ménière's disease, grouped with the cochlear and vestibular variants,[14] since the vestibular symptoms are indistinguishable.

REPRINTS: Joseph B. Nadol, Jr., M.D., Dept. of Otolaryngology, Massachusetts Eye and Ear Infirmary, 243 Charles St., Boston, Mass. 02114.

REFERENCES

1. Schuknecht HF: Correlation of pathology with symptoms of Ménière's disease. Otolaryngol Clin North Am 1:433-440, 1968

2. Nadol JB: Positive fistula sign with an intact tympanic membrane. Clinical report of three cases and histopathological description of vestibulofibrosis as the probable cause. Arch Otolaryngol 100:273-278, 1974

3. Silverstein H: Labyrinthine tap as a diagnostic test for acoustic neurinoma. Otolaryngol Clin North Am 6:229-244, 1973

4. Antoli-Candela F: Ménière's disease. II. Volumetric studies. Acta Otolaryngol 1974. In press

5. Kimura RS, Schuknecht HF: Membranous hydrops in the inner ear of the guinea pig after obliteration of the endolymphatic sac. Pract Otorhinolaryngol (Basel) 27:343-354, 1965

6. Schuknecht HF, Northrop C, Igarashi M: Cochlear pathology after destruction of the endolymphatic sac in the cat. Acta Otolaryngol 65:479-487, 1968

7. Schuknecht HF, Kimura RS, Naufal PM: The pathology of sudden deafness. Acta Otolaryngol 76:75-97, 1973

8. Schuknecht HF, Benitz J, Beekhuis J, *et al*: The pathology of sudden deafness. Laryngoscope 72:1142-1157, 1962

9. Lindsay J R, Davey PR, Ward PH: Inner ear pathology in deafness due to mumps. Annals Otorhinolaryngologica 69:918-935, 1960

10. Lindsay JR, Hemenway WG: Inner ear pathology due to measles. Ann Otol Rhinol Laryngol 63:754-771, 1954

11. Schuknecht HF: *Pathology of the Ear.* Boston, Harvard University Press, 1974

12. Nager FR: Beiträge zur Histologie der erworbenen Taubstummheit. Zeitschrift fur ohrenheil-kunde 54:217-244, 1907

13. Schuknecht HF, Wright JL: Pathology in a case of profound congenital deafness. J Laryngol Otol 87:947-955, 1973

14. Barber HO, Pennington C, Pulec JL, *et al*: Report of subcommittee on equilibrium and its measurement. Ménière's Disease: criteria for diagnosis and evaluation of therapy for reporting. Trans Am Acad Ophthalmol Otolaryngol 76:1462-1464, 1972

Ann Otol 84: 1975

RATES OF ION MOVEMENT FROM PLASMA TO ENDOLYMPH IN THE DOGFISH

THOMAS H. MAREN, M.D.

ERIK R. SWENSON, A.B. ALBERT D. F. ADDINK, PH.D.

GAINESVILLE, FLORIDA

SUMMARY – The rates of movement of Na^+, Rb^+, Cl^- and HCO_3^- from plasma to endolymph were studied in the elasmobranch fish, *Squalus acanthias*, by use of the appropriate isotopes. Rb^+ was used as a marker for K^+. The half-times to equilibrium for Na^+, Rb^+ and Cl^- were about 100 hours; for HCO_3^- it was 6 hours. The equilibrium ratios, endolymph/plasma, are Na^+ 0.87, K^+ 26, Cl^- 1.37, HCO_3^- 1.47. Carbonic anhydrase inhibition decreased the rate of HCO_3^- accumulation, suggesting that the process is actually the formation of endolymphatic HCO_3^- from plasma or tissue CO_2. Increase in plasma pCO_2 elevates endolymph HCO_3^- concentration. The secretory tissue contains carbonic anhydrase and Na-K-ATPase. These and other data suggest that a dominant feature of endolymph chemistry may be HCO_3^- formation linked in some fashion with K^+ transport, through rates catalyzed by these two enzymes.

This study gives the electrolyte physiology of the endolymph in the elasmobranch fish, *Squalus acanthias*, in terms of both concentrations and rates of accession. There has been no previous work of this type in any species, in which the movements of the four major ions have been compared under identical conditions.

S. acanthias, the spiny dogfish, is particularly suitable for this work because of the accessibility of the endolymph and the relatively large (0.2 - 0.3 ml) volume of fluid. Figure 1 shows the anatomy of the internal ear in this species. Further advantages lay in the fact that the general electrolyte physiology of this species is very well known, and we have already made similar studies on the cerebrospinal fluid.[1]

Murray and Potts[2] have studied and summarized data on the labyrinthine fluids of several elasmobranch species. They showed that these fish share with mammals (and presumably all other vertebrates) the characteristic of high concentration of potassium in the endolymph. Our own preliminary work showed that there was carbonic anhydrase in the sacculus wall of the inner ear of *S. acanthias*, in agreement with the finding of this enzyme in several regions of the inner ear of the cat.[3] More recent work on the electrolyte physiology of endolymph has been reviewed by Johnstone[4] and by Maren.[5]

The following topics are presented in this paper: 1) a note on the histology of the tissues of the inner ear; 2) normal ion composition of the endolymph and perilymph; 3) effect of hypercapnia on the ion composition; 4) carbonic anhydrase activity of inner ear tissues; 5) effect of acetazolamide (carbonic anhydrase inhibition) upon ion composition; 6) effect of ethacrynic acid on ion composition; 7) rates of transfer of Na^+, Cl^-, Rb^+ (for K^+) and CO_2/HCO_3^- from plasma to endolymph; 8) effect of acetazolamide upon these transfer rates;

From the Department of Pharmacology and Therapeutics, University of Florida College of Medicine, Gainesville, Florida, and Mount Desert Island Biological Laboratory, Salisbury Cove, Maine.

This investigation was supported by NIH grant GM 16934 and NSF grant GM 28139.

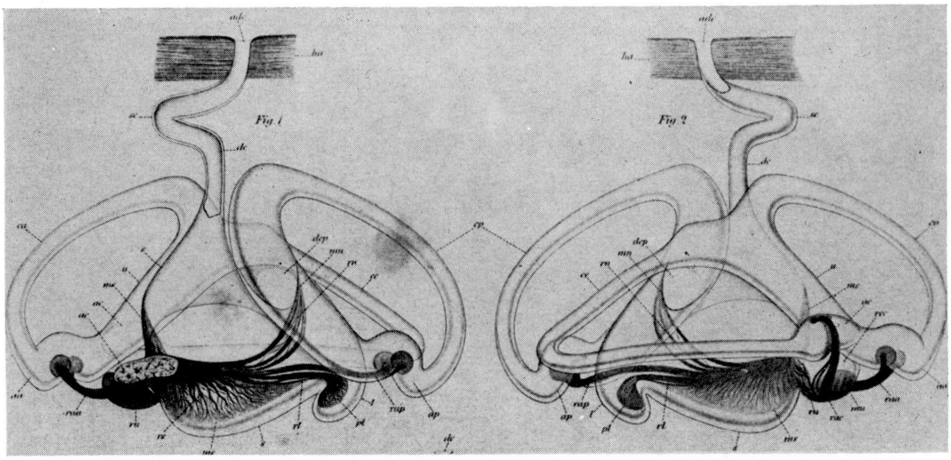

Fig. 1. The right internal ear of S. *acanthias* viewed from the inner (left) and outer (right) side (Retzius, G: Das Gehörorgan der Wirbelthiere. *Morphologisch-histologische Studien*, vol I, Stockholm, Samson & Wallin, 1881.

u - Utriculus, rec - Recessus utriculi, aa - Ampulla anterior, ae - Ampulla externa, ap - Ampulla posterior, ca - Canalis m. anterior, ce - Canalis m. externus, cp - Canalis m. posterior, dcp - Ductus can. posterioris, s - Sacculus, de - Ductus endolymphaticus, se - Saccus endolymphaticus, ade - Apertura duct. endolymph. ext., l - Lagena cochleae, mu - Macula ac. recessus utriculi, ms - Macula ac. sacculi, mn - Macula ac. neglecta, pl - Papilla ac. Lagenae, ac - Acusticus, ru - Ramulus rec. utriculi, raa - Ramulus amp. anterioris, rae - Ramulus amp. externae, rap - Ramulus amp. posterioris, rs - Ramulus sacculi, rn - Ramulus neglectus, rl - Ramulus lagenae.

and 9) relation among rates and concentration of newly formed fluid.

METHODS AND MATERIALS

Animal Procedures and Sampling. Fish were caught by trawl line in Frenchman's Bay, Salisbury Cove, Maine, during the summer months of 1972. Before and during experiments they were generally kept in live cars under the dock, freely swimming. They were brought to the laboratory for sampling, at which point they were perfused through the spiracles with cold oxygenated sea water at a rate of 1-2 liters/minute. The animals were gently restrained in a trough, and covered with wet towels to prevent drying.

Certain experiments were carried out with the fish in this laboratory situation, rather than in the live car. These included very short term protocols (less than 20 minutes) and those involving hypercapnia. For this purpose 5% CO_2 was admitted to the perfusate.

Injections of isotopes and drugs were made intravenously through the tail vein. Care was taken to flush isotopes cleanly into the blood stream. Sampling of blood was also done through a tail vein; at least 2 ml were taken for each sample. These procedures were usually done with the animal almost fully immersed in water. We have fully described these various techniques.[1]

Endolymph was taken, following dissection, from the dorsal surface of the head. A small needle attached to a 0.5 ml syringe was introduced into the sacculus, and 0.1 to 0.2 ml of endolymph was withdrawn. Perilymph was taken from the dorsal space above the sacculus. Exact measurement of these samples was done by weighing. The sampling procedure took 10-15 minutes, during which time perfusion was continued, as noted above.

Chemistry and Isotope Counting. Sodium and potassium concentrations were determined by flame photometry, chloride by titration with mercuric nitrate, and total CO_2 by microgasometry (Kopp-Natelson) or Conway microdiffusion procedure. The latter was more suitable for endolymph. ^{22}Na was measured in a deep-well gamma counter. $H^{14}CO_3$, ^{36}Cl and ^{86}Rb were measured in a liquid scintillation counter. The latter isotope was used as a marker for K^+. All samples (0.1 ml) were counted for ten minutes. The samples were prepared and counted as previously described.[1]

Carbonic anhydrase was measured by the changing pH method, as scaled down to volume of 0.8 ml.[6] In the present case we used barbital buffer and bromthymol blue indicator.

A unit is the amount of enzyme that doubles the reaction rate. The units reported here apply to this micro-method; in this system human red cells contain about 25,000 units/ml and those from S. *acanthias* about 600 units/ml. These activity units are converted into our older "standard" units[7] using a macromethod and carbonate buffer, by dividing by

TABLE I

ELECTROLYTE CONCENTRATION IN EAR FLUIDS OF S. *ACANTHIAS*(*mM*)

	Na^+	K^+	Cl^-	CO_2	*Urea*	*n*
			Endolymph			
Mean	223	107	314	11.2	282	7-14
±S.E.	4	3	4	0.8	3	
			Perilymph			
Mean	253	3.3	264	10.5		5-9
±S.E.	5	0.3	5	0.5		
			Plasma			
Mean	256	4.1	230	7.6	350	10-15
±S.E.	2	0.1	3	0.6	5	

20. This reference[7] also gives the molar equivalent of carbonic anhydrase for these units.

Na-K-ATPase was measured by the standard technique of liberating inorganic phosphate from MgATP, in the presence of Na^+ and K^+, and measuring the portion inhibited by ouabain. Details are given by Jampol and Forrest.[8]

Calculations. Plasma decay curves were obtained for all four of the isotopes. For sodium, chloride, and rubidium, the radioactivity of 0.1 ml of plasma 18 minutes after the injection was assigned a value of 100. For bicarbonate the same convention was used, but at three minutes. These times were selected to allow reasonable distribution of isotopes in the fish. All further measurements during an experiment were related to these standard values. The rate constant k_{in} was obtained by dividing the rate of increase of isotope in endolymph, over a given time, by the isotopic concentration in plasma at the midpoint of the period. This has been discussed previously.[1] For this to correspond to the formally derived k_{in} as used by Davson,[9] two restrictions are necessary. Early phases of the curves (less than about 40% toward equilibrium) must be used, and the plasma concentration should be reasonably constant. The latter is only approximated in these experiments.

A useful term which may be extracted from these data is the time for the various ions to equilibrate between plasma and endolymph. The following expression is used, derived from the kinetics of opposing first order reactions:

$$\ln \frac{100}{100-x} = \frac{k_{in} \cdot t}{r}$$

where k_{in} is the rate constant, r is the equilibrium ratio (from Table I) and t is the time for the injected isotope to reach a given percent (x) of the equilibrium value r. This equation is used to generate curves for accession of the ions, under the conditions of constant plasma concentration. The treatment is analogous to that of Davson for cerebrospinal fluid.[9]

Drugs. Acetazolamide (80 mg/kg) was administered as the sodium salt, 24 hours before isotope injection, except for special experiments, as noted, with labeled HCO_3^-, in which the inhibitor was given 30 minutes before isotope. Based on the amount given, the plasma half-life (about 1.5 days), and the physiological effects previously observed,[10] this dose will inhibit essentially all carbonic anhydrase in the body for at least four, and probably six, days.

Ethacrynic acid was given at a dose of 30 mg/kg by vein, and sampling of endolymph was carried out at later intervals as described below. This drug was used because of the findings of Cohn *et al*[11] and Bosher *et al*[12] that endolymph K^+ in the dog and rat respectively, was markedly decreased after its use.

RESULTS

Histology of Inner Ear. Dr. W. L. Doyle[13] studied the structure of these tissues with the following findings:

"Preliminary electron microscopic survey of the lateral wall of the sacculus of *Squalus* reveals a bilayered epithelium supported on an interdigitating fibrous basement membrane. The basal cells have abundant smooth endoplasmic reticulum and clear vacuoles with relatively few mitochondria. The superficial layer exhibits cells in two stages. In some areas, patches of superficial cells are filled apically with large clear vacuoles and in many of these cells the apical cell membranes were ruptured. In most areas, the superficial cells were characterized by complex interdigitation with basal cells, elaborate development of Golgi areas and abundant distended smooth endoplasmic reticulum.

Granular endoplasmic reticulum was sparse and mitochondria only moderately abundant. The nuclei were irregular in contour and scattered cells of this type displayed large intranuclear single crystalloids. The general morphology of the epithelium is consistent with moderately active secretion of fluid. Further study is required but there is reasonable correspondence in cell structure to that of the stria vascularis of higher forms. As yet we have found no intraepithelial capillaries in the wall of the sacculus but some are present in the semicircular canals where the epithelium is nonsecretory."

Normal Ion Composition. Table I shows the concentration of ions in the endolymph and perilymph of S. *acanthias,* compared to plasma. The striking characteristics of endolymph are high K^+, Cl^-, and HCO_3^-. Note that the data show good stoichiometry, in that $Na^+ + K^+ = Cl^- + HCO_3^-$. Endolymph contains more charged particles than plasma; this is balanced by a urea deficit of some 70 mM. The osmolar concentration of the five measured solutes of endolymph is 937 mOsm. That for plasma is 848 mOsm, but an unmeasured solute is trimethylamine oxide, which is present in plasma at a concentration of some 90 mM. In the absence of further data, we suppose that endolymph is approximately isotonic with plasma, but contains little trimethylamine oxide. Perilymph has the same approximate composition as CSF,[1] except that total CO_2 is about 20% higher.

Effect of Elevated pCO_2 upon Ionic Composition of Endolymph and Other Fluids. Table II shows a representative (of six) experiment in which 5% CO_2 was admitted to the fluid perfusing the gills. This raised the pCO_2 of plasma from 4 mm Hg to about 18 mm Hg; the procedure was sustained for three hours. As we have shown previously,[1] there was a striking elevation of total CO_2 (essentially HCO_3^-) in CSF. However, this was not seen in the endolymph or in the other fluids. The reason for this (with respect to endolymph)

TABLE II

EFFECT OF THREE HOURS HYPERCAPNIA ON TOTAL CO_2 OF BODY FLUIDS†

	Na^+	*K^+*	*Cl^-*	*CO_2*
	(expressed in mM)			
Plasma	264	4.9	230	9
Endolymph	213	96	313	10
CSF*				22
Perilymph*				7
Aqueous*				11
Cranial fluid*				6

† 5% CO_2 was bubbled through water perfusing the gills
* Normal values 6-10 mM

will be apparent below, when it will be shown that the turnover of fluid and accumulation of HCO_3^- is too slow to result in a concentration change in three hours.

Carbonic Anhydrase and Na-K-ATPase Activity of Inner Ear Tissues. Six samples of the wall of the sacculus were analyzed for carbonic anhydrase activity, and yielded 11-105 units/g. Seven samples of the semicircular canals yielded 14-105 units/g; this was surprising, since the canals did not appear to have a secretory structure (see above). The activity of both sacculus and canals was abolished by 10^{-4} M methazolamide. The range of enzyme activity is significant although somewhat less than we have found for other secretory tissues of this species, ciliary process and choroid plexus being about 400 units/g on this scale.[7,10] It should be emphasized that falsely high values are impossible (except by gross contamination), while low values could be artifactitious if samples contain relatively high amounts of nonsecretory tissue. The endolymphatic duct contained enzyme only in the doubtful range of activity.

The sacculi of four fish were taken for assay of Na-K-ATPase. The mean value was 1.9 μmoles PO_4/mg protein per hour, close to what Jampol and Forrest[8] found for the ciliary process

TABLE III

EFFECT OF ACETAZOLAMIDE (80 mg/kg) ON HCO_3^- CONCENTRATION OF ENDOLYMPH*

	Plasma CO_2 mM	Plasma pH	Plasma pCO_2 mmHg	Endolymph CO_2 mM	CSF CO_2 mM
Control	7.6	7.62	5	11.2	8.6
1 hr	8.0	7.10	16	11.6	13.3
16 hr	13.0	7.15	25	15.3	20.0
19 hr	13.5	7.20	21	17.1	18.3
24 hr	14.0	—	—	22.3	20.5
48 hr	15.2	—	—	19.8	17.8

* These data were from one fish at each of the times noted. The endolymph data are the average of measurements from the two ears.

in this species.

Effect of Acetazolamide upon Ion Concentration of Endolymph. Carbonic anhydrase was inhibited *in vivo* by the intravenous injection of 50-80 mg/kg acetazolamide. Electrolytes were measured, in individual fish, at intervals from 1-48 hours. Three fluids were compared: endolymph, cerebrospinal fluid (CSF), and plasma. There were no changes in the concentration of Na^+, K^+, or Cl^-, in any of the fluids, in the time intervals observed. This agrees with previous data on plasma and CSF.[11]

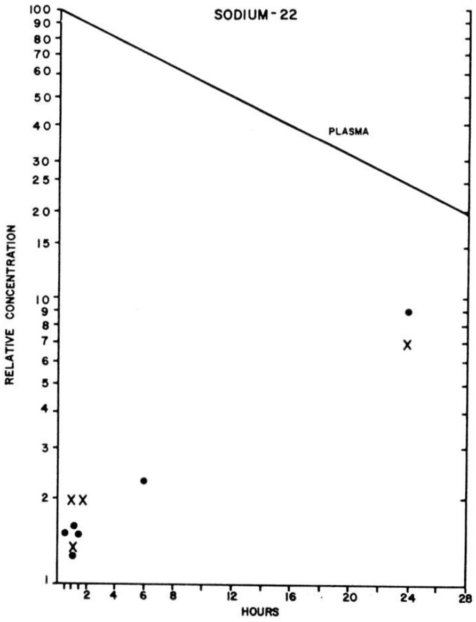

Fig. 2. Accession of ^{22}Na to endolymph in normal fish and following carbonic anhydrase inhibition. Line shows decay in plasma, composite data acquired from approximately 25 experiments in 1971-1973. Normal and inhibited fish give same plasma data[1] ● gives control concentration in endolymph. X gives concentration in endolymph 24 hours after i.v. injection of 80 mg/kg acetazolamide.

Table III shows the changes in HCO_3^- concentration (and pH of plasma) of the three fluids. It will be seen at once that acetazolamide induces a striking respiratory acidosis. At one hour, this does not elevate plasma HCO_3^- but does elevate CSF HCO_3^-.[11] The reason for this is quite clearly that the elevated CO_2 "drives" the production of CSF HCO_3^- even when carbonic anhydrase is inhibited.[1] At one hour, endolymph HCO_3^- is normal, and we have already seen (Table II) that, even at three hours of hypercapnia, endolymph HCO_3^- is still normal. Acetazolamide, however, enables us to maintain hypercapnia for any length of time. Now we make the critical observation that at 16 hours, endolymph HCO_3^- is elevated, and by 24 hours it is twice normal and as high as CSF (Table III). Thus the same process we have described for CSF seems to be at work, except that it is much slower. It

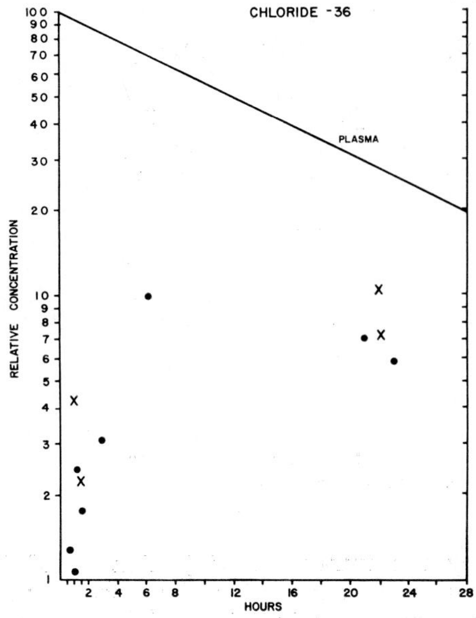

Fig. 3. Accession of ^{36}Cl to endolymph. See legend for Figure 2.

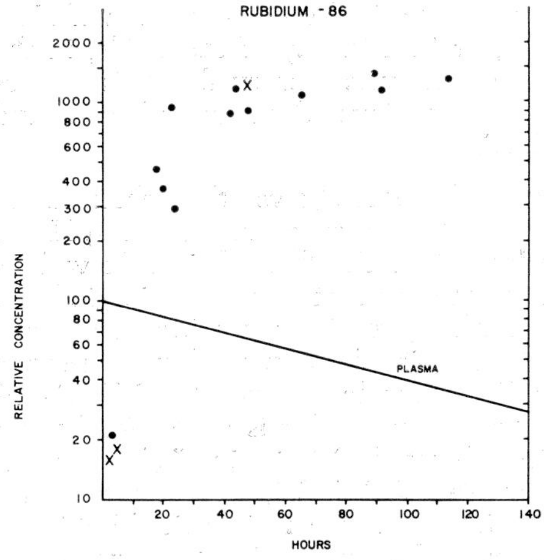

Fig. 4. Accession of ^{86}Rb to endolymph. Plasma curve based on 13 experiments. See legend for Figure 2.

will be shown below that all the ionic and fluid movements of endolymph are slower than that of CSF, by factors of at least tenfold.

Effect of Ethacrynic Acid Upon Ion Concentration. Thirty mg/kg was given intravenously to two dogfish, and endolymph was sampled at 2, 4, and 21

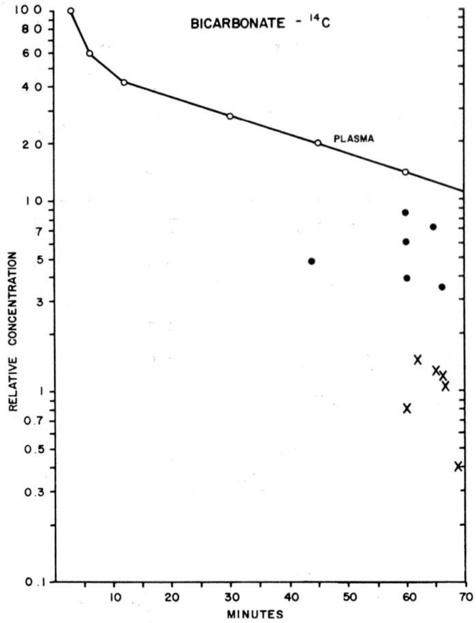

Fig. 5. Accession of $H^{14}CO_3$ to endolymph. See legend for Figure 2. In this case three of the inhibited fish were given acetazolamide 30 minutes before isotope, and three 24 hours before.

hours. There was no change in concentration of electrolytes (not shown).

Rates of Transfer of Ions and Fluid from Plasma to Endolymph. These will be discussed in terms of the individual ions and graphed in Figures 2-6.

Sodium. Figure 2 shows the accession of sodium to the endolymph. The process is rather slow, so that all the points from 1-24 hours are well before equilibrium and can be used to calculate a rough rate constant, which is 0.0062 hr^{-1} (Table IV). This means that the time for turnover of half the sodium is 100 hours, and for 90% equilibration is 333 hours (Fig. 6).

Chloride. Figure 3 shows the accession of chloride to the endolymph. The kinetics closely resemble those for sodium. All eight points are used to calculate the rate constant k_{in}, which is 0.0084 hr^{-1} (Table IV). The half-time for turnover is then 118 hours, and for 90% equilibrium, 394 hours (Fig. 6).

Rubidium. Figure 4 shows the ac-

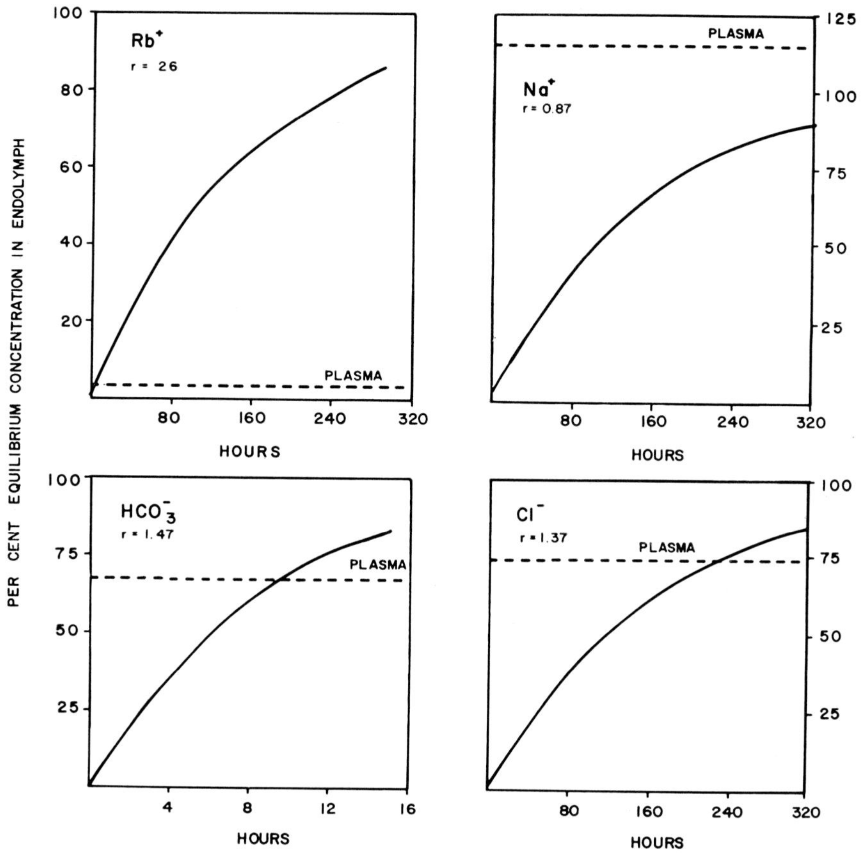

Fig. 6. Curves for accession of ions to endolymph in S. *acanthias*. See Calculations part of Methods and Materials section.

cession of rubidium to the endolymph, as a marker for potassium. [It is most important to note that the chemical equilibrium ratio for potassium (Table I) between endolymph and plasma, 26, is within limits of experimental error, the same as the ratio of ^{86}Rb approached in these fluids toward the end of the experiment. Thus, it seems reasonable to use Rb^+ as a marker here, as has been done in a variety of other biological systems.] The data of Figure 4 suggest that a rate constant may be obtained from the 20-hour accession data; this yields for k_{in} the value of 0.17 hr^{-1}. Calculation is also made for the period 20-44 hours, whence $k_{in} = 0.20\ hr^{-1}$. Figure 6 shows generation of an ideal curve for access of rubidium (or potassium) in which 50% equilibrium between the two fluids is achieved in 105 hours, and 90% equilibrium in 350 hours.

Bicarbonate. Figure 5 shows the accession of HCO_3^-, which is far more rapid than that of the other ions. The rate constant, 0.17 hr^{-1}, is the same as for rubidium, but because of the much lower equilibrium concentration in endolymph (compared to rubidium) HCO_3^- reaches equilibrium much more rapidly, 90% in 20 hours (Fig. 6). The rate constant 0.17 hr^{-1} is calculated on the basis of isotopic $HC0_3^-$ concentration, to facilitate comparison with the other ions. However, we believe the process is not that of ionic movement but plasma $CO_2 \rightarrow$ endolymph HCO_3^-. On the basis of isotopic plasma CO_2, the rate constant would be some 24 times greater, 4.1 hr^{-1}. The accession

TABLE IV

KINETICS OF ION MOVEMENT FROM PLASMA TO ENDOLYMPH IN NORMAL DOGFISH (C) AND FOLLOWING CARBONIC ANHYDRASE INHIBITION (I)*

	Plasma mM	*Plasma t ½ hrs*	*k_{in}, hr^{-1} ±S.E.† (n)*		*Accession Rate mM hr^{-1} Col. 1 x Col. 3*		*k_{out}, hr^{-1} Col. 4 ÷ Endo. conc.‡*	
			C	I	C	I	C	I
Na^+	256	12	0.0062 0.0013 (5)	0.0087 0.0019 (3)	1.6	2.2	0.0071	0.010
Cl^-	230	12	0.0084 0.0016 (5)	0.0070 0.0015 (3)	1.9	1.6	0.0061	0.005
Rb^+	4.1	75	0.17 0.03 (13)	0.21 (2)	0.7	0.9	0.0065	0.0084
HCO_3^-	7.3	0.6	0.17 0.02 (6)		1.2		0.11	
	8.0**			0.075 0.004 (3)		0.6		0.043
	14			0.063 0.024 (3)		0.9		0.50

* By 80 mg/kg acetazolamide 24 hrs before the isotope test, except in the HCO_3^- experiment denoted by **, in which 50 mg/kg was given 30 minutes before isotope.

† First line gives mean and second line, S.E. mean.

‡ From Table I.

rate, 1.2 mM hr^{-1}, remains the same whether the calculation is based on plasma HCO_3^- or CO_2.

Fluid. Table IV shows that accession rates (k_{in} • conc. plasma) of the four ions are all the same order of magnitude. Rates of k_{out} for Na^+, Cl^- and Rb^+ are approximately the same. Since $[Cl^-] \cong [Na^+ + K^+]$ and is so much greater than any other anion, it is reasonable to assume that k_{out} for Cl^- approximates the k_{out} ($= k_{in}$) for fluid turnover itself. If this be the case, the half-time for fluid turnover is 100 hours. We may then calculate fluid formation rate $= k_{in}$ (.0071 hr^{-1}) • volume (0.3 ml) $= 2$ µl/hr.

Effect of Acetazolamide upon Transfer Rates of the Ions. Figures 2-5 include data showing the effect of large doses of acetazolamide upon the entry of the ions. In the cases of Na^+, Cl^- and Rb^+ there was no effect; in the case of HCO_3^- (Fig. 5) the entry was decreased about three-fold by the carbonic anhydrase inhibitor. Table IV shows the calculated rate constants and accession rates during inhibition. Using the standard errors for k_{in} as a guide, it is again clear that the drug produced no effect upon the transport of N^+, Cl^- or Rb^+. However, there is clearly a significant effect upon HCO_3^- entry. Note that k_{in} is reduced to some 40% of control values, in both the cases where isotope was given 0.5 and 24 hours after acetazolamide.

TABLE V

HALF-TIMES OF ION ACCESSION TO ENDOLYMPH, AND CONCENTRATION IN NEWLY FORMED FLUID

	*Endolymph** *mM*	*t½†* *Pl → Endo.* *hrs*	*Accession Rate*** *mM hr⁻¹*	*Conc. New Fluid* ‡ *mM*
Na^+	223	100	1.6	240
Cl^-	314	118	1.9	286
K^+ (Rb^+)	107	105	0.7	105
HCO_3^-	11.2	6	1.2	180
				59***

* Table I
† Fig. 6
** Table IV
‡ Accession rate x $\frac{\text{vol. endolymph (0.3 ml)}}{\text{endolymph flow (0.002 ml/hr)}}$
*** Calculated from $Na^+ + K^+ - Cl^-$

Relation among Rates, and Concentration of Newly Formed Fluid. Table V makes it possible to compare the movement of the various ions. Of particular importance is the last column, giving the concentration of ions in the newly formed fluid, according to principles previously described for cerebrospinal fluid.[1]

This allows an analysis of some of the factors involved in ionic and fluid movement. Since the concentrations in newly formed fluid of sodium and potassium are the same as those in measured fluid, it may be assumed that there is little or no back-flux of these ions — the same as has been found for sodium with respect to cerebrospinal fluid.[9] Chloride ion appears in newly formed fluid at slightly lower concentration than in endolymph, but this may not be significant. Bicarbonate is clearly much higher, but the value shown (180 mM) cannot be the real concentration, since this would yield a large excess of anions in the fluid. It must be assumed that a considerable amount of HCO_3^- measured in this way is involved in back-flux to plasma; the real amount accumulated may be judged by the values of $Na^+ + K^+ - Cl^- = 59$ mM. (A similar situation showing back-flux has been described for cerebrospinal fluid in the cat[14] and for aqueous in S. acanthias.[15]) Thus, endolymph as formed does have high HCO_3^- concentration, just as previously found in S. *acanthias* for CSF[1] and aqueous humor.[15]

DISCUSSION

This is the first study of the rates of entry of all the major ions from plasma to endolymph. Before summarizing the characteristics of entry, we may inquire whether these data, from an elasmobranch fish, are applicable to those of other vertebrates, including man. We believe that they are in the broad sense, because numerous characteristics of endolymph and its secretory tissue in this fish are similar to those in mammals. These include high K^+ concentration, and the presence of carbonic anhydrase and Na-K-ATPase in the epithelia. Differing points from the mammalian situation are the chloride excess (over plasma) in the fish, and the sodium concentration, which is almost as high as plasma. However, the need for very high osmolarity in the fluids of the shark family make it almost inevitable that they contain considerable Na^+ and Cl^-. An important datum, as yet unmeasured, is HCO_3^- concentration of mammalian endolymph.

Table VI compares endolymph, aque-

TABLE VI

FLOW AND VOLUME RELATIONS AMONG ENDOLYMPH, AQUEOUS HUMOR AND CEREBROSPINAL FLUID IN S. *ACANTHIAS*

	Endolymph	*Aqueous**	*CSF†*
Volume, ml	0.3	0.25	1.6
Formation rate constant, k_{in} hr^{-1}	0.006	0.4	0.18
Formation rate, μl/hr	2	108	280

* From Maren *et al*[15]

† From Maren[1]

ous humor and cerebrospinal fluid in *S. acanthias*. A striking feature of the endolymph is its slow turnover; this also seems to be true of the fluid in mammals. For instance, using Choo and Tabowitz'[16] data on K^+ entry in the cat, we may calculate a turnover rate constant of 0.00037 min^{-1}, which is about 1/40 that of our value for CSF in the same species.[14] Table VI shows a fraction of 1/26 for the relation between endolymph and CSF turnover in the dogfish.

The kinetic characteristics of the entry of the ions may be gauged in two ways: by the accession rate (mM hr^{-1}, Table IV) and by the half-time to equilibrium. Table IV shows that the accession rates among the four ions are not greatly different, ranging from 0.7 for K^+ to 1.9 for Cl^-. What occurs is that the two ions in high concentration in plasma (Na^+ and Cl^-) have low inward rate constants and the two that have low concentrations (K^+ and HCO_3^-) have high rate constants. Thus, within a two to three-fold range, the four ions move in at roughly the same magnitude. Figure VI shows the approach to equilibrium, using curves generated as described in the Methods and Materials section. For HCO_3^- the half-time to equilibrium is relatively rapid (6 hours); for the other ions it is about 100 hours. Thus, although potassium moves in rapidly, equilibrium takes much longer, because the equilibrium concentration in endolymph relative to plasma is 26.

Endolymph potential in the elasmobranch sacculus relative to plasma or perilymph is —3mV[4]. Thus, for passive distribution, the ratio of cations in endolymph to the surrounding fluids should be about 1.1, and for anions 0.9. Clearly this is not the case (Table I), and all the ions must be "pumped," as they are in mammals.[4]

The data on carbonic anhydrase inhibition (Table IV and Fig. 5) certainly suggest that HCO_3^- enters the endolymph, not from plasma HCO_3^- but from plasma CO_2, which is enzymatically hydroxylated in the secretory tissue to yield HCO_3^-.[1] When this process is diminished by acetazolamide, the rate of HCO_3^- accession is reduced, but apparently not enough to influence Na^+ or Rb^+ accession within the limits of our measurements. The reason seems clear, since in this species, plasma HCO_3^- and CO_2 are very low compared to their concentration and relation to the other ions in mammals. For instance, Na^+/HCO_3^- concentration is 6 in man, and 34 in elasmobranchs. Thus, HCO_3^- would not be expected to influence cation movement to any large degree. This has also been our finding for CSF[1] and aqueous humor[15] in dogfish.

It may be presumed that Na-K-ATPase plays a central role in the entry of K^+ to endolymph in vertebrates.[17] A test of this point *in vivo* is difficult, since ouabain is relatively toxic to most species. It is not possible to keep a dogfish alive at doses exceeding 50 μg/kg for the relatively long duration of an experiment of the type of Figure 4. However, the role of Na-K-ATPase is clearly indicated by experiments on the excised inner ear of the frog, which secretes K^+ into endolymph; the process is inhibited by 10^{-4} M ouabain, a concentration difficult to achieve *in vivo*.[18] Our view of endolymph secretion is the same as put forward for other epithelia: HCO_3^- formation from CO_2 is coupled in some fashion to cation transport, which for Na^+ or K^+ is linked to Na-K-ATPase.[19]

Finally, the data in this study may be used to consider the similarities and differences among the processes responsible for formation of endolymph, aqueous humor, and CSF; this has not been done before in one species. The differences in rate of fluid formation have already been mentioned; of greater interest is the chemistry of the fluids as they are formed. As a broad overall view, we perceive the following similarities. In each case, HCO_3^- formation is the most rapid of the ionic processes, and the results following acetazolamide or methazolamide indicate that HCO_3^- does not arrive at the fluid as a result of transfer from plasma, but by formation in the secretory cell from $CO_2 + OH^-$. In addition to carbonic anhydrase, there is Na-K-ATPase in the secretory tissue for all three fluids. The presumption is that the first of these enzymes makes an anion, HCO_3^-, rapidly available, and that the second does the same for either sodium or potassium. In some way not yet understood, the formation of HCO_3^- is linked to the transport of cation and to the flow of fluid.

Request for reprints should be sent to Thomas H. Maren, M.D., the J. Hillis Miller Health Center, University of Florida, Gainesville, Florida 32610.

REFERENCES

1. Maren TH: Bicarbonate formation in cerebrospinal fluid: role in sodium transport and pH regulation. Am J Physiol 222:885-899, 1972

2. Murray RW, Potts WTW: The composition of the endolymph, perilymph and other body fluids of elasmobranchs. Comp Biochem Physiol 2:65-75, 1961

3. Erulkar SD, Maren TH: Carbonic anhydrase and the inner ear. Nature 189:459-460, 1961

4. Johnstone BM: Ion fluxes in the cochlea, in Bittar EE (ed), *Membranes and Ion Transport,* New York, Wiley-Interscience, 1971, vol 3, pp 167-184

5. Maren TH: The cerebrospinal fluid, with notes on aqueous humor and endolymph, in Mountcastle VB (ed): *Medical Physiology,* ed 13 St. Louis, Mosby Company, 1974, pp 1116-1141

6. Maren TH: A simplified micromethod for the determination of carbonic anhydrase and its inhibitors. J Pharmacol Exp Ther 130: 26-29, 1960

7. Maren TH: Carbonic anhydrase: chemistry, physiology, and inhibition. Physiol Rev 47:595-781, 1967

8. Jampol LM, Forrest JN Jr: Aqueous humor formation in fish: the role of sodium-potassium-activated adenosine triphosphatase in the dogfish *(Squalus acanthias)* eye. Exp Eye Res 13:315-319, 1972

9. Davson H: *Physiology of the Cerebrospinal Fluid,* Boston, Little, Brown and Company, 1967

10. Maren TH: Ionic composition of cerebrospinal fluid and aqueous humor of the dogfish, *Squalas acanthias.* II. Carbonic anhydrase activity and inhibition. Comp Biochem Physiol 5:201-215, 1962

11. Cohn ES, Gordes EH, Brusilow SW: Ethacrynic acid effect on the composition of cochlear fluids. Science 171:910-911, 1971

12. Bosher SK, Smith C, Warren RL: The effects of ethacrynic acid upon the cochlear endolymph and stria vascularis. Acta Otolaryngol (Stockh) 75:184-191, 1973

13. Doyle WL: (Personal communication)

14. Vogh BP, Maren TH: Sodium, chloride and bicarbonate movement from plasma to cerebrospinal fluid in cats. Am J Physiol 228: 673-683, 1975

15. Maren TH, Wistrand P, Swenson ER, *et al*: The rates of ion movement from plasma to aqueous humor in the dogfish, *Squalus acanthias.* Invest Ophthalmol. To be published

16. Choo YB, Tabowitz D: The formation

and flow of the cochlear fluids. Ann Otol Rhinol Laryngol 74:140-145, 1965

17. Bonting S: Sodium-potassium activated adenosinetriphosphatase and cation transport, in Bittar EE (ed), *Membranes and Ion Transport*, New York, Wiley-Interscience, 1970, vol. 1, pp 257-363

18. Simon EJ, Hilding DA, Kashgarian M: Micropuncture studies of the mechanism of endolymph production in the frog. Am J Physiol 225:114-118, 1973

19. Maren TH: The relation between renal acidification and bicarbonate reabsorption. A view of CO_2-mediated secretion in renal and other epithelia, in Callingham BA (ed), *Drugs and Transport Processes*, Baltimore, University Park Press, 1974, pp 73-93

Ann Otol 84: 1975

GRAND ROUNDS: PARANASAL SINUS INFECTION UNIVERSITY OF IOWA DEPARTMENT OF OTOLARYNGOLOGY AND MAXILLOFACIAL SURGERY

BRIAN F. MCCABE, M.D., CHAIRMAN

PARTICIPANTS

KENNETH D. DOLAN, M.D.

MAXWELL ABRAMSON, M.D.

LEE A. HARKER, M.D.

RESIDENTS AND STUDENTS

Dr. Brian McCabe: This week the sole subject of grand rounds will be paranasal sinus infection, to include diagnosis and especially treatment, and covering as widely as time permits the spectrum of the disease.

Dr. Donald Eagles: The patient is a 42-year-old white male with the chief complaint of several aching teeth in the left maxilla of two days' duration, and a nonpainful spongy area on the left hard palate. He has a subsiding nose cold contracted about a week ago. He has noted neither nasal obstruction nor discharge but has been taking an antihistamine regularly for his cold. He saw his dentist and the complete dental examination including radiography was negative. His past medical history is not significant, his general health has been excellent, and he has had no other recent illnesses except another nose cold about a month ago. He is unaware of any allergies.

Physical examination demonstrated a well developed white male in mild distress. Both nasal chambers were erythematous but there was no pus even after thorough shrinkage of the mucosa in the left middle meatus. The nasopharynx and choanae were also free of pus. The orbits were normal. There was no edema of the preantral soft tissues, but there was a nontender spongy area of mucosa on the left hard palate 1.0 x 1.5 cm that was suggestive of a small amount of subperiosteal fluid. The remainder of the examination was normal. All laboratory tests were normal except for a WBC of 12,400.

Dr. McCabe: What is your diagnosis at this point?

Dr. Eagles: The most likely would seem to be an acute suppurative process of the maxillary sinus (antrum).

Dr. McCabe: And your next step?

Dr. Eagles: Paranasal sinus films were ordered.

Dr. Kenneth Dolan: The most revealing radiograph on the patient is the Waters view. Note the diffuse groundglass appearance of the left antral cavity (Fig. 1A). This is compatible with exudate. The cavity does not have the opacity one sees with marked lining thickening of a cavity filled with polyps (Fig. 1B), no airfluid level and so we cannot say from

---

From the Department of Otolaryngology and Maxillofacial Surgery, University of Iowa Hospitals and Clinics, Iowa City, Iowa.

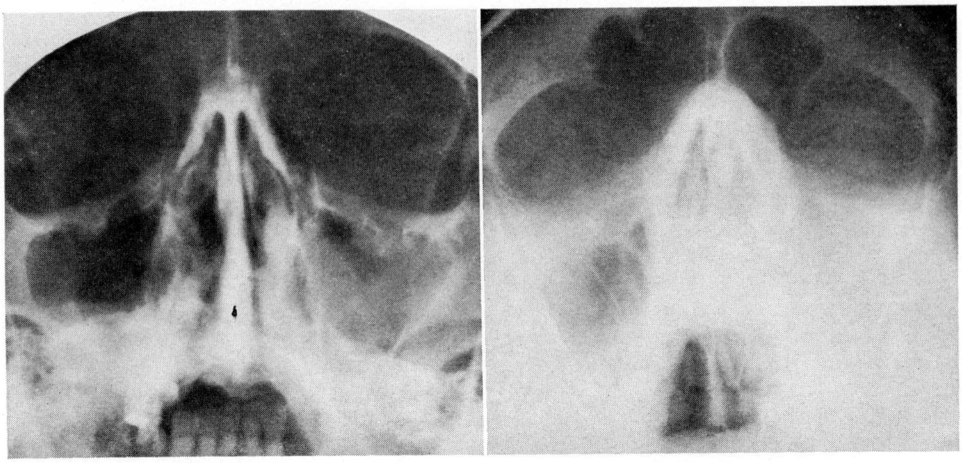

Fig. 1. A) Waters view. The diffuse, ground glass appearance of the left antrum suggests the presence of exudate rather than tissue. B) Waters view. The marked opacification of the left antrum suggests tissue, such as a sinus filled with infected polyps.

the radiographic appearance alone whether this represents active disease, or, let us say, old healed disease with mild diffuse submucosal scarring. This is why the clinical correlation is important. There is no evidence of destruction of any of the walls of the sinus on any of these conventional radiographs, but of course laminography by linear or preferably hypocycloidal technique would be necessary to rule it out, and should be done if this is an important consideration in this case.

Dr. McCabe: You have brought out well the importance of the radiologist and the clinician in concert interpreting the importance of radiographs.

Dr. Dolan: Particularly important here, I think, is the question of bone destruction. Do you think this is critical to the next step in care of the patient? We do not want to subject the patient to the cost of extensive radiodiagnostic studies if it is not of significance to patient care. You have to tell us.

Dr. McCabe: Good point. We come now to a matter of judgment. Dr. Harker, so far, do you see a need for input from laminograms?

Dr. Lee Harker: Hard to say. Without the patient in front of me it is most difficult. My guidelines would be the degree of symptomatology. Here I just don't have enough to go on. Generally, I don't order laminograms on cases of acute suppurative disease.

Dr. Maxwell Abramson: I agree with Dr. Harker. I am bothered a bit by the oral symptoms and findings, but I do agree that laminograms would not be the next logical step. We have here all the concomitants of acute suppurative disease of a sinus except pus. The next step would be to establish or disprove this, and that would be to needle and aspirate the sinus, and irrigate if necessary.

Dr. McCabe: He happened to be my patient, and this is exactly what we did. Cannulation of the natural ostium being virtually a lost art and not in my armamentarium, an inferior meatus needling was carried out. Aspiration was tried but nothing could be brought into the syringe, not even air. It was as though the needle tip were in solid tissue. Some gentle attempts at irrigation were carried out without the sinus accepting any irrigant. The procedure was then abandoned.

Dr. Leopold (Res): What magnitude of positive and negative pressures did you use?

Dr. McCabe: The barrel of the

syringe is drawn back to the 3-5 cc mark. The negative pressure thus created is the adequate test. The positive pressure level is harder to quantify, and is probably best measured in terms of discomfort levels. When it begins to hurt and no return is evident, quit.

Dr. Harker: It is important in both aspiration and irrigation to vary the traverse of the needle to ascertain that the tip is not in the submucosa or imbedded in a polyp. It is sometimes difficult to find the lumen of a diseased sinus.

Dr. Spelvin (Res): If you couldn't get any return on saline irrigation, why not inject some air to more gradually express any exudate which is present?

Dr. McCabe: Ever since the 30's, when two deaths from air emboli were reported, this has been interdicted. Never inject air during a sinus puncture.

Dr. George (Res): Could it be that suppurative sinusitis isn't the problem at all? Maybe this is a red herring. I have never performed a sinus irrigation that was not rewarding. Were other possibilities followed up with other things in mind such as eosinophilic granuloma, mucormycosis, systemic diseases like lupus, regional diseases like sphenopalatine neuralgia, atypical facial neuralgia, and the like? Have we had test results of C-reactive protein, lymphocyte transformation test, anaerobic as well as usual cultures, Klebsiella cultures, and hypocycloidal polytomes? What about internal medicine, neurology, and infectious disease consultations? Until we have these, can we really go further?

Dr. McCabe: Doctor, I am glad you asked that question. I am also glad you are still in training. The answer to your last question is – yes, we can ourselves go further, and moreover, yes, we should. The reason for not distributing referral requests and shotgunning laboratory tests are twofold: 1) In this age of sharply escalating medical costs, tests and referrals should be limited to those definitely indicated. The patient may ask how long he can afford to have you as his doctor; and, 2) What is the next most logical step in view of the total clinical picture that would be most likely of great yield?

Dr. George: To find out, somehow, what is in that antrum.

Dr. McCabe: To make a long story short, we did just that in the most direct way.

Dr. Roberts: The patient was taken to the operating room and under local anesthetic a sublabial incision was made and the left antrum entered. As soon as the cavity was opened with a gouge, pus under pressure was encountered.

Dr. McCabe: And so the diagnosis was made. What was it, Dr. Roberts?

Dr. Roberts: Acute suppurative disease of the antrum.

Dr. McCabe: Acute empyema. Pus under pressure in a natural cavity. That defines empyema.

Dr. Katz (Res): How does one handle a sinus empyema definitively? I realize it is surgical, but we see this disease so seldom in our residency it would be helpful to have some general guidelines.

Dr. McCabe: In this particular situation, the disease was adjudged subacute on the basis of the time course of symptoms and the appearance of the mucosa. The former seemed likely to have been present for weeks rather than months or years. The mucosa was measured at 2-3 mm thickness rather uniformly without mucosal ulceration, polyps, or granulation tissue; there was no evidence of bone disease as manifested by soft bone in any area, infected granulation tissue on bone, ulceration with exposed bone, or severely hyperplastic mucosa in any area. Thus, without any of these conditions present, the mucosal disease was deemed reversible, and an antromeatal window was made without removal of the antral lining or thorough curettage of the bony surfaces, as we would do in a Caldwell-Luc. This was followed

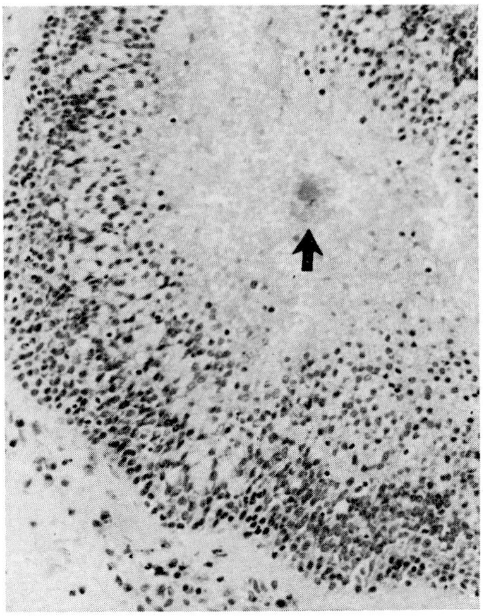

Fig. 2. A microabscess in the submucosa of surgical specimen from a chronically infected antrum. Arrow points to center of abscess filled with degenerating leucocytes.

by daily irrigations of the antrum through the surgical window. The patient rapidly recovered.

The guiding principle in the immediate management of any acute empyema is incision and drainage. In the case of the maxillary sinus it is an antromeatal window. I would advise it transantrally rather than endonasally. Then it can be determined whether it is an acute exacerbation of a chronic sinusitis; and in the latter situation, a Caldwell-Luc should be performed on the spot. In the case of the frontal sinus, it is a trephination of the floor of the sinus with placement of a short tube into the sinus. The tube should have a lumen of at least 5 mm so that not only can regular irrigation be carried out but the character of the mucosa can be inspected directly. If either the lining infection does not resolve or the patency of the nasofrontal duct does not reestablish itself, a more radical operation is indicated; at least an external frontoethmoidectomy or an osteoplastic flap. If the latter is preformed, every scrap of infection must be removed or matters will simply be made worse. In the case of the sphenoid sinus, it implies a sphenoidostomy by wide removal of the sphenoid rostrum.

Dr. Abramson: This last type is, incidentally, the hardest to diagnose. In the case of frontal or maxillary sinus, we have edema to tip us off. In this patient, the subperiosteal fluid on the hard palate was the tipoff; more usual is edema of the lateral wall of the nose. It is extremely difficult to recognize edema of the sphenoid rostrum. The most constant finding is pain. This may be bitemporal or fore-and-aft, like a tension headache. The pain may be bizarre, however: we had a case of isolated sphenoid empyema last month in which the pain was referred to the neck, near the angle of the mandible! The pain ceased rather dramatically in the operating room immediately after the sinus was opened.

Dr. McCabe: Pain localization in sinus disease is interesting. There was a study done in which balloons were placed into the various sinuses and inflated to above pain threshold, and the pain was quite localized to the facial area of the sinus: to the cheek in the case of the maxillary, to the forehead in the case of the frontal, and paranasally in the case of the ethmoid. In the sphenoid it was quite variable, however. The more common location was bitemporal but often occurred behind the eye, suboccipital, in the forehead, or even in the throat or neck.

Dr. McGuirt (Res): You mentioned both external frontoethmoidectomy and osteoplastic flap operations as treatment for chronic frontal sinus disease. What are the indications for one or the other?

Dr. Harker: The indications are rather straightforward. If you have disease isolated to the frontal sinus (except for neoplasm), the operation of choice is an osteoplastic flap. The ideal lesion is a non-functional nasofrontal duct, such as with a frontal mucocele. A marginal lesion for this operation is chronic frontal sinus osteomyelitis,

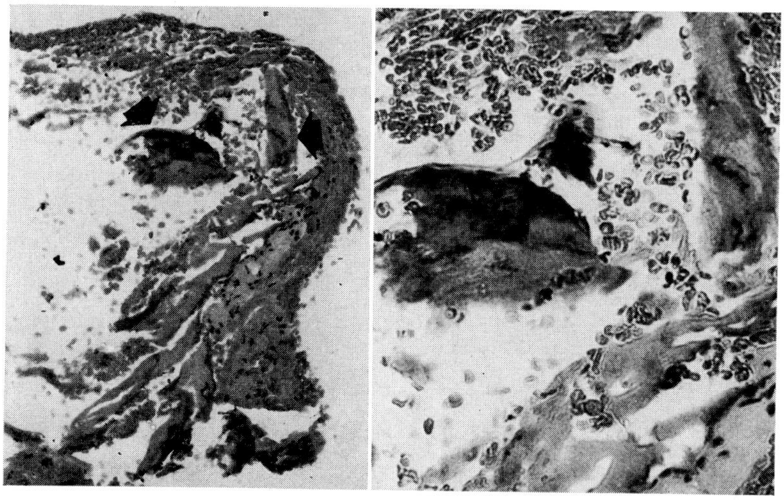

Fig. 3. A) Another specimen from chronic sinusitis. Arrows point to bony spicules in soft tissue (microsequestrae). B) High power view of Fig. 3A. Note the empty lacunae in the bone.

where one must be absolutely certain infection has been ablated, and quite frankly, this takes a pretty good surgeon. When on the other hand both the frontal and the ethmoids are diseased, a frontoethmoidectomy is the operation of choice. I see very few if any indications for a combined osteoplastic flap and intranasal ethmoidectomy. Perhaps benign polypoid disease might be one; or a combination of frontal mucocele and ethmoid polyposis; but I question this because the reason for the mucocele is likely to be polypoid disease of the nasofrontal duct, which is almost invariably coincident with suppurative disease. I should add here that the technique of external frontoethmoidectomy – whether by the Lynch, Killian, or Riedel surgical approach – is such a demanding one that the occasional operator should not undertake it any more than the occasional mastoidectomy surgeon. The complications of the one (blindness, diplopia, chronic epiphora, hyphema, glaucoma, and recurrent frontal disease) are just as real as in the other (facial paralysis, total deafness, labyrinthitis, etc.).

Dr. Roberts (Res): You mentioned different types of frontoethmoidectomies. How do they differ?

Dr. Harker: Essentially, all types seek to do the same thing, and that is to communicate the resulting frontal sinus cavity widely with the nasal chamber. This is done through wide removal of the anterior ethmoid, nasofrontal duct, lachrymal bone, and surrounding bone, including the medial aspect of the nasal bone, the ascending process of the maxilla in its upper portion, and descending orbital process of the frontal bone in its orbital and nasofrontal portions. The variations that go by name refer actually to the frontal sinus portion of the operation. The least extensive is the Lynch, wherein the above is accomplished with removal of only the floor of the frontal sinus. This is feasible if the sinus is not tall, let us say around 2.5 cms or less. If taller, removal of a window of the frontal wall may also be necessary so that one may reach the vault for removal of all mucosal and bony disease. In this latter technique, called the Killian, the window of the anterior table reaches the vault but spares a 1 cm bar of bone, or bridge, between the inferior approach and the anterior window. This "2.5 cm rule" is of course a function of the character of the disease and the skill of the surgeon.

Dr. Abramson, who trained with Dr. Robert L. Goodale and Dr. William W. Montgomery who pioneered the osteoplastic flap operation, may feel differently.

Dr. Abramson: I don't believe that the osteoplastic flap operation is the only operation for frontal sinus disease. Certainly in isolated frontal disease it is likely to be the operation of choice, especially when the nasofrontal duct is occluded. It is particularly useful where the frontal sinus is large or in revision surgery. However, disease surrounding the frontal must be considered and dealt with. This may preclude an osteoplastic flap operation. When that is the case, one must have these other techniques in his armamentarium; if he does not he is unable to serve his patient well.

Dr. McCabe: I would second these comments.

Dr. Kuenster (Res. Family Practice): You have considered the indications for surgical intervention in the frontal and ethmoid sinuses, but how about the maxillary sinus? Isn't that the more commonly infected sinus?

Dr. Harker: It is commonly thought so, but actually the ethmoid is without doubt the more commonly infected. The reason is because the ethmoid communicates more widely with the nose, where the infection begins; it also has much more "square footage" of lining tissue. Since it is very cellular, it is estimated that there is twice the lining mucosa of the antrum, a sinus which occupies much more volume. It may well be true, however, that the antrum produces more problems, in terms of chronicity, than the ethmoid.

Dr. McCabe: That, of course, is because the antrum has its drainage point into the nose high on the medial nasal wall, while this is less so in the case of the other sinuses. It reminds me of an old wives' tale in sinus disease. Bemember hearing that if we were quadrupeds, which we were when the paranasal sinuses were designed, we wouldn't be having so much sinus disease because the antra could drain better? That overlooks of course the fact that quadrupeds hold their heads in no different posture than bipeds, that is, upright. The alignment of the thoracic and lower vertebrae is the only difference. How then, in the two, could the incidence of sinus disease be affected by gravity? Not at all.

This, of course, doesn't answer Dr. Kuenster's question. What are your indications for what kind of management in chronic maxillary sinusitis? Let us say you have established the diagnosis, pus chronically at the maxillary ostium, and you have on x-ray a picture of a cloudy antrum, but not really opaque as compared with the surrounding bone.

Dr. Abramson: In this case after culture and sensitivities I would try an antibiotic for 10 to 14 days.

Dr. McCabe: If it fails? By that, I mean at two weeks you see no pus, but at four weeks the condition has recurred, then what?

Dr. Abramson: Then I would probably do an antromeatal window.

Dr. Harker: I would do at least an A-M window at the first sitting, chronicity established.

Dr. McCabe: I would tend to agree more with Dr. Harker. There would appear to be no place for systemic antibiotics in well established chronic suppurative sinusitis, considering the nature of the disease. In the greatly thickened mucosa there are multiple microabscesses (Fig. 2) usually in the form of sheets of purulent exudate containing organisms, infection of deep mucous glands, and breaks in the periosteum with microscopic bone destruction and even microsequestrae (Fig. 3). Abscesses, deep glandular infection, and sequestrae are conditions calling for surgical measures, and hence the management of chronic suppurative sinusitis is surgical.

REPRINTS: Brian F. McCabe, M.D., Dept. of Otolaryngology and Maxillofacial Surgery, University Hospitals, Iowa City, Iowa 52242.

X-RAY OF THE MONTH

LYMPHOEPITHELIOMA OF THE NASOPHARYNX

Saadoon Kadir, M.D.
Alfred L. Weber, M.D.
Boston, Massachusetts

PATIENT

The patient is a 17-year-old Chinese male who presents with a two-month history of recurrent epistaxis, anosmia and right superior rectus paresis. Three months prior to admission the patient's mother died from a metastatic undifferentiated carcinoma of the nasopharynx.

RADIOGRAPHS

The films reveal a large, midline nasopharyngeal mass, which extends anteriorly to the choana and posteriorly to the C1-C2 vertebrae. There is involvement of the posterior ethmoids and sphenoid sinuses with destruction of the floor of the sphenoid sinus, basisphenoid and part of the basiocciput (Fig. 1A). The sella is poorly defined with partial destruction of the floor and posterior wall. A common carotid angiogram reveals encasement of the internal carotid artery, with slight stretching and narrowing (Fig. 1B).

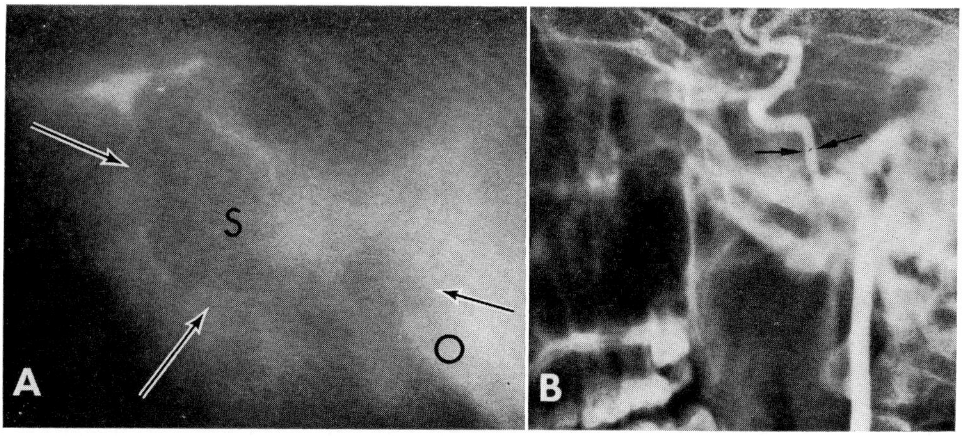

Fig. 1. A) Lateral tomogram showing the destruction of the floor and anterior walls of sphenoid sinus (S) and the basiocciput (O). B) Abnormal left carotid arteriograms showing narrowing of the artery (arrows) by the tumor.

From the Department of Radiology, Massachusetts Eye and Ear Infirmary, Boston, Massachusetts.

DIAGNOSIS

Biopsy was done and revealed a lymphoepithelioma. Subsequently, the patient was treated with radiation.

DISCUSSION

The Chinese, living in their native country or abroad, show a marked predilection for cancer of the nasopharynx. The incidence of nasopharyngeal cancer in Hong Kong, for example, represents approximately 18% of all malignant neoplasms as compared to about 2% in New York.[1] Lymphoepithelioma was first described by Schmincke and Regaud in 1921.[2] Histologically, the tumor consists of an undifferentiated squamous cell carcinoma, interspersed with a non-neoplastic lymphocytic component. Clinically, cancer of the nasopharynx tends to appear at an earlier age than other forms of adult cancer; average age being in the late 40's. Clinical symptoms are caused by either nasal obstruction with or without epistaxis, serous otitis media, local invasion with neurological symptoms or metastases.[3] Infiltration into the cranial cavity occurs in advanced cases and can be assessed by angiography, pneumoencephalography or computerized axial tomography. Most cancers of the nasopharynx are avascular or show poor vascularization, as opposed to the angiofibroma.

REFERENCES

1. Martin H, Quan S: The racial incidence (Chinese) of nasopharyngeal cancer. Ann Otol Rhinol Laryngol 60:168, 1951

2. Schmincke A: Uber Lympho-epitheliale Gaschwulste. Beitr Pathol Anat Allg Pathol 68:161, 1921

3. Lederman M: *Cancer of the Nasopharynx: Its Natural History and Treatment.* Springfield, Illinois, C. C. Thomas, 1961

COMMUNICATIONS

To The Editor: Re: "Large Tracheal Papillomas: A Difficult Anesthetic Problem and an Apparent Cure." Edward Carden, FRCP(C), George B. Ferguson, M.D. Ann Otol Rhinol Laryngol 84:233-237, 1975.

We have been successfully using a similar technique for ventilating patients undergoing microlaryngoscopy and laryngeal surgery to that quoted by Edward Carden and George Ferguson in the March-April 1975 number of the *Annals*.

The complication we encountered was a pneumothorax. The tension in the pneumothorax was high enough to cause surgical emphysema and mediastinal shift.

The cause was an obstruction of the upper airways for which the patient was undergoing microlaryngoscopy. Inspiration was not impeded but expiration was, resulting in a progressive increase in intrapulmonary pressure. Initially alveolar rupture with interstitial emphysema, tracking towards the hilum, was the probable mechanism. An additional factor may have been poor tissue quality as the patient is 75 years old.

Preventing this problem in patients with upper airways obstruction could be approached in two ways. One would be to decrease the driving pressure but this could impair ventilation. The other would be the insertion of a second cannula alongside the first, to act as a blow-off valve, and prevent the build up of excessive intra-pulmonary pressure.

D. G. Fenwick, FFARACS
R. Baker, FRACS

Department of Anesthesia
Royal Adelaide Hospital
Adelaide, South Australia 5000

Dear Editor:

The letter of Drs. Fenwick and Baker has brought forward a most important facet which must be taken into consideration when ventilating patients with jets placed below the cords. In order to obviate problems which they have obviously run into, it is imperative that the anesthesiologist continually monitor the excursion of the patient's chest when ventilating the patient. He must blow gas into the patient's lungs and then wait for the chest to resume its original deflated position prior to giving the next ventilation to the patient. This point has been made in some of the papers published on the subject.[1-3]

When this type of anesthesia is being given to patients under my care, the chest of the patient is never draped and the excursion of the chest is continually monitored. While the blood pressure is being taken, or for any other reason the eyes are not on the patient's chest, then ventilation is curtailed until such time as the excursion of the chest can again be monitored. In the 350 or so cases which I have done, I have not had this problem.

Complications of this sort have occurred in the past, but they have not been publicized. Drs. Fenwick and Baker's letter will, hopefully, make people more aware of the inherent complications in this technique.

Edward Carden, FRCP(C)

Veterans Administration
Wadsworth Hospital Center
Wilshire and Sawtelle Blvds.
Los Angeles, CA 90073

REFERENCES

1. Carden E, Crutchfield W: Anaesthesia for microsurgery of the larynx: A new method. Can Anaesth Soc J 20:378-389, 1973

2. Carden E, Ferguson GB, Crutchfield WM: A new silicone elastomer tube for use during microsurgery on the larynx. Ann Otol Rhinol Laryngol 83:360-364, 1974

3. Carden E, Vest HR: Further advances in anesthetic technics for microlaryngeal surgery. Anesth Analg (Cleve) 53:584-587, 1974

ABSTRACTS OF CURRENT ARTICLES

Acute Leukemia Presenting as Laryngeal Obstruction

Ti M, Villafuerte R, Chase PH et al: Cancer 34:427, August, 1974

The authors present a case report of a 68-year-old woman who was admitted with severe respiratory stridor to the Jewish Hospital in Brooklyn. A diagnosis of leukemia was made only after the tracheotomy had been performed. A review of ten cases in the literature is included.

Three figures and seven references are presented.

Payne

Oral Monilia Study on Patients with Head and Neck Cancer During Radiotherapy

Chen TY, Webster JH: Cancer 34:246, August, 1974

The authors discuss the incidence of oral *Candida albicans* in a total of 101 patients with head and neck cancer receiving radiation therapy.

The results of the double-blind randomized program are described in relation to age distribution, location of tumor, source of radiation, field arrangement, the period of maximum reaction during treatment, and the relation of culture results to the severity of maximum acute radiation reaction.

Eight references and seven tables are presented.

Payne

Tumors of the Nasopharynx in Tunisia

Cammoun M, Hoerner GV, Mourali N: Cancer 33:184, January, 1974

The authors present an anatomic and clinical study of 143 patients seen at the National Cancer Institute in Tunisia. Malignancies of the nasopharynx constitute the most commonly encountered tumor in Tunisia. Incidence, presenting symptoms, clinical findings, histopathological findings, and geographical distribution are discussed.

Eighteen references, two tables, eight figures, including seven photomicrographs, are presented.

PAYNE

Clinical and Immunologic Response to Bacteria Isolated from Tracheal Secretions Following Tracheostomy

Espinoza, Hernan, et al: J Thorac Cardiovasc Surg 68:432, 1974

Bacteriologic and immunologic data from six patients who developed pneumonia after tracheostomy were compared with data from six patients who developed pneumonia after tracheostomy. *Pseudomonas aeruginosa* or *Proteus mirabilis* predominated in patients who developed pneumonia. In contrast, patients with tracheobronchitis had a much wider range of infecting organisms. Immunoglobulin content and antibody titers of tracheal secretions were similar in the two groups and did not rise. Serum antibody titers increased significantly in all patients with pneumonia, but did not rise significantly in patients with tracheobronchitis. These studies lend some support to a possible future role of Pseudomonas vaccines in preventing Pseudomonas pneumonia.

FRIEDBERG

Laryngo-tracheoplasty

Evans JNG, Todd GB: J Laryngol Otol 58: 589, 1974

A new technique for the surgical correction of refractory subglottic stenosis in infants is presented.

The thyroid cartilage is split in the midline and the incision is carried in a step-wise fashion through the cricoid and, if necessary, the upper tracheal rings. The mucosa of the larynx and upper trachea is incised at the same time and the stenotic mass is excised in a submucosal plane between the mucosa and surrounding cartilage. Silastic sheeting, curled upon itself, is inserted into the upper trachea and through the glottis. The cartilaginous interdigitations are retracted and sutured in their new position with wire. The teflon roll is held in position by a transfixion suture. The wound is then closed in layers.

The skeletal framework is thus held open externally by the wire sutures and internally by the silastic roll which has a constant tendency to uncurl and exerts gentle pressure upon the tracheal mucosa obliterating any dead space and allowing mucosal regeneration to occur. The silastic sheeting is removed endoscopically in six weeks and decannulation is usually performed two weeks later.

Five children, ages nine months to two years, were all successfully decannulated. The average length of stay in the hospital prior to laryngo-tracheoplasty was 14 months. The average number of endoscopic procedures prior to laryngo-tracheoplasty was 15. There were no serious complications and all have remained free of symptoms for a period of one and one-half to two years. Whether long-term complications, as regards to laryngeal growth, will develop has yet to be assessed.

HUTCHINSON

Pharyngeoesophageal Dysphagia and Recurrent Laryngeal Nerve Palsy

Henderson RD, et al: J Thorac Cardiovasc Surg 68:507, 1974

This report concerns 15 patients with recurrent laryngeal nerve paralysis from intrathoracic involvement by bronchogenic carcinoma or from deliberate resection at pneumonectomy. Eleven patients developed dysphagia with significant aspiration symptoms and three required pharyngeoesophageal myotomy for relief of potential lung damage. Twenty pneumonectomy patients with intact recurrent laryngeal nerves did not have dysphagia. Five autopsy dissections with microscopy revealed branches of the recurrent laryngeal nerve to the proximal esophagus and to the cricopharyngeus muscle.

FRIEDBERG

Adenocarcinoma Involving the Esophagus

Hankins John R, et al: J Thorac Cardiovasc Surg 68:148-158, 1974

The records of 20 patients with adenocarcinoma of the esophagus and esophagogastric junction were compared with those of 255 patients with epidermoid carcinoma of the esophagus observed in the same period. The survival rate for patients with adenocarcinoma, as a group, was as poor as that for those with epidermoid cancer. The authors found the lowest average age and poorest survival in patients with primary adenocarcinoma of the esophagus. Adenocarcinoma associated with hiatus hernia was characterized by the oldest average age and best survival. Intermediate average age and survival occurred in patients with adenocarcinoma of the esophagogastric junction. Evidence is accumulating that the columnar-lined esophagus is a premalignant lesion.

FRIEDBERG

Tracheoesophageal Fistula Following Blunt Chest Trauma

Antkowiak JG, et al: Arch Surg 109:529, 1974

Two patients with tracheoesophageal fistula following blunt chest trauma (automobile) are discussed. Both were cured by surgical division of the fistula. A review of the literature revealed 28 additional cases of tracheoesophageal fistula following blunt chest trauma. The most frequent mechanism of production involved the driver of the car being thrown against the steering wheel. All reported patients were males, usually relatively young.

Rib fractures frequently are not present. Cervical subcutaneous emphysema is almost always present. Medistinal air, with or without pneumothorax, is frequent. The symptom complex of cough immediately after swallowing begins three to four days after the accident. Bronchoscopy, esophagoscopy, and contrast studies confirm the diagnosis. The typical fistula is located just above the carina. Treatment is surgical division of the fistula.

HUTCHINSON

The Epidemiology and Etiology of Esophageal Cancer in North China — A Preliminary Report

The Coordinating Group for Research on Etiology of Esophageal Cancer in North China: Chinese Medical Journal 1:167-183, May 1975

The incidence and mortality rates of esophageal cancer, including cancer of the gastric cardia, are high in certain areas of North China, where in some counties it ranks first as cause of death in the total mortality rate. Since 1959, a series of epidemiologic surveys has been made, the last being from 1969 to 1971, which covered 181 counties and cities with a total population of nearly 50 million.

The epidemiologic survey gave the following results: the average crude mortality rate of cancer of the esophagus 37.39/100,000, highest adjusted rate 139.80/100,000 and lowest adjusted rate 1.43/100,000. In Linhsien County, the trend of mortality rates of esophageal cancer showed little change from 1941-1970. The average age-sex adjusted incidence rate was 108.56/100,000 and mortality rate 99.76/100,000. Trace elements in the soil and drinking water, nitrosamines, secondary amines, nitrites and nitrates contained in food items, and fungus contamination were analysed for comparative values in high and low incidence areas. Extensive cytologic examination of esophageal mucosa in the high risk areas revealed a high frequency of epithelial hyperplasia in the adult population. On the basis of these new data, practical measures to block or inhibit carcinogenic factors and to treat the disease at its earliest stage are being given clinical trials.

SENTURIA

Evaluation of University of Florida Split-Course Technique for Various Head and Neck Squamous Cell Carcinomas

Million RR, Zimmerman RC: Cancer 35: 1533-1536, 1975

Retrospective nonrandomized study and evaluation was made of 260 patients with squamous cell carcinoma of the head and neck as relative values of split-course versus continuous radiation techniques. Study included patients with carcinoma arising in oral tongue, floor of mouth, tonsil, base of tongue, soft palate, posterior pharyngeal wall, pyriform sinus epiglottis, and nasopharynx treated at the university between October 1964 and December 1971. Split course was introduced in 1967 and has been used in almost all cases since 1968. The authors intend to return to continuous course therapy.

Although the authors urge cautious appraisal of the results obtained because of the two-year minimum follow up, they state split-course radiation seems to be safe for early lesions, but results suggest poorer control of the local lesion and poorer two-year survival in moderately advanced lesions. At the sacrifice of local control, a decrease in major complications were noted.

Six tables, one figure, 11 references presented.

PAYNE

Carcinoma of the Oral Tongue and Floor of Mouth: Fifteen Years' Experience with Linear Accelerator Therapy

Gilbert EH, Goffinet DR, Bagshaw MA: Cancer 35:1517, 1975

The authors present a total of 114 patients with carcinoma of the tongue and of the floor of the mouth treated at Stanford University from 1956 to 1970. Five year survival for T lesions, 73%; T_2 lesions 37%; and T_3 lesions 19-25% was recorded when treated with high-dose megavoltage radiation.

Results are tabulated by the methods of treatment: interstitial radiation, external radiation alone, or in combination dosages of treatment. Local control of primary achieved in 26 of 56 oral tongue, whereas local control of the primary floor of mouth lesions was obtained in 28 of 56 patients. Control of neck disease, metastatic disease complications and prophylactic irradiation are discussed.

Seven figures, six tables and 14 references are included.

PAYNE

ANNALS OF OTOLOGY, RHINOLOGY AND LARYNGOLOGY
CALENDAR OF EVENTS
1976

Jan. 4-10
WORKSHOP — 9th Annual Otolaryngology Postgraduate Workshop. Kingston 10, Jamaica, W.I.

Jan. 19-23
COURSE — Surgery of the Paranasal Sinuses. The Page and William Black Postgraduate School of Medicine, Mount Sinai School of Medicine (CUNY), New York, New York 10029

Jan. 25-30
COURSE — Septorhinoplasty by the External Approach. University of Toronto and American Academy of Facial Plastic and Reconstructive Surgery. University of Toronto, Toronto, Ontario, Canada.

Jan. 26-30
COURSE — Clinical Neurotology. Instituto Mexicano Del Seguro Social Sociedad Mexicana de Otorrinolaringologia. Hospital General del Centro Medico Nacional, Av Cuauhtemoc No. 330, Mexico 7, D.F.

Jan. 31 - Feb. 4
SEMINAR—Facial Plastic Surgery. University of Miami School of Medicine, Miami, Florida 33152

Feb. 1-5
WORKSHOP — Facial Plastic Surgery. American Academy of Facial Plastic and Reconstructive Surgery, Inc. and Department of Otolaryngology, University of Miami, Key Biscayne, Miami, Florida

Feb. 1-7
SEMINAR—Florida Midwinter Seminar of Ophthalmology and Otolaryngology. University of Miami School of Medicine, Miami, Florida 33152

Feb. 2-13
COURSE—Bronchoesophagology. Department of Laryngology and Broncho-Esophagology, Chevalier Jackson Clinic, Philadelphia, Pa. 19140

Feb. 7-13
COURSE—Second Postgraduate Course in Clinical Allergy for the Otolaryngologist. University of Miami School of Medicine, Key Biscayne, Miami, Florida.

Feb. 12-15
SYMPOSIUM — Controversial Areas in Surgery of Head and Neck. University of California at San Diego School of Medicine, San Diego, California 92103

Feb. 12-17
COURSE—First Panamerican Course of Cosmetic Surgery of the Nose and Face. Panamerican Association of Otolaryngology, Medellin, Colombia, South America.

Feb. 14-21
WORKSHOP — Electronystagmography. Miami Hearing and Speech Center, Montego Bay, Jamaica.

Feb. 22-28
SYMPOSIUM—Nose and Cosmetic Facial Surgery. General Rose Memorial Hospital, Denver, Colorado 80209

Feb. 28 - March 1
SYMPOSIUM—Mardi Gras Otolaryngology Symposium. Department of Otolaryngology and Maxillofacial Surgery, Tulane University School of Medicine, New Orleans, Louisiana 70112

Feb. 29 - March 3
COURSE—Otolaryngological Allergy. Department of Otolaryngology and Maxillofacial Surgery, University of Tennessee, Memphis, Tennessee 38104

March 1-6
WORKSHOP — Shambaugh Fifth International Workshop on Middle Ear Microsurgery and Fluctuant Hearing Loss. Northwestern University Medical School, Chicago, Illinois.

March 14-17
COURSE — Basic Principles of Rhinoplasty. Department of Otolaryngology and Maxillofacial Surgery, University of Tennessee, Memphis, Tennessee 38163

March 14-21
MEETING — American Decibel and Diopter Society. San Diego, California.

March 22-25
COURSE — Neurotology. Department of Otolaryngology, Abraham Lincoln School of Medicine and University of Illinois Hospital Eye and Ear Infirmary, University of Illinois at the Medical Center, Chicago, Illinois.

March 25-27
COURSE—Clinical Neuro-otolaryngology. Eye and Ear Hospital of Pittsburgh, Pittsburgh, Pennsylvania 15213

April 8-10
COURSE—Rubin Fifteenth Annual Electronystagmography Course. New Orleans, Louisiana 70002

April 19-23
COURSE—Tympanoplasty Course. Brooklyn Eye and Ear Hospital, Brooklyn, New York 11238

April 22-23
COURSE—Occupational Hearing Loss and Hearing Conservation. American Council of Otolaryngology. Palm Beach, Florida.

April 24-25
MEETING—American Laryngological Association. Palm Beach, Florida.

April 25-26
MEETING—American Otological Society, Inc. Palm Beach, Florida.

April 27-28
MEETING — American Broncho-Esophagological Association. Palm Beach, Florida.

April 27-29
MEETING — American Laryngological, Rhinological and Otological Society, Inc. Palm Beach, Florida.

April 29-30
MEETING—American Academy of Facial Plastic and Reconstructive Surgery. Palm Beach, Florida.

May 3-5
CONFERENCE — Second International Conference on Diagnosis and Treatment of Craniofacial Anomalies. New York University Medical Center, Institute of Reconstructive Plastic Surgery, New York, New York 10016

May 9-16
COURSE—Head and Neck Oncology. University of Iowa, Iowa City, Iowa 52242

May 10-12
SEMINAR — Head and Neck Surgery. Columbia University College of Physicians and Surgeons, New York, New York 10032

May 14-15
SYMPOSIUM—Oral and Pharyngeal Disorders. Department of Otolaryngology and Maxillofacial Surgery, University of Tennessee, Memphis, Tennessee 38163

May 20-22
SYMPOSIUM—Neurophysiology of Hearing: Interpretation of Human Electrophysiological Data. European Economic Community (Medical Research Committee, Ad hoc Working Group on Deafness). Bordeaux, France.

May 26-29
CONFERENCE—First International Conference on Cholesteatoma. Department of Otolaryngology and Maxillofacial Surgery, University of Iowa, Iowa City, Iowa 52242

June 11-14
COURSE—Pediatric Otolaryngology. University of Pittsburgh School of Medicine, Pittsburgh, Pennsylvania 15213

June 24-26
MEETING — Canadian Otolaryngological Society. Vancouver, British Columbia, Canada.

July 1-11
COURSE—Microsurgery of the Ear. Portmann Foundation and E.N.T. Department of the University of Bordeaux II (France).

July 5-11
SYMPOSIUM — Fifth Symposium on Middle Ear Surgery. Theodor Heuss Academy and Municipal City Hospital, Gummersbach (Cologne), West Germany.

July 12-23
COURSE—61st Annual Course Head and Neck Anatomy and Clinical Otolaryngology. Indiana University School of Medicine, Indianapolis, Indiana 46202

Aug. 9-13
SYMPOSIUM — Fourth International Symposium on Facial Nerve Surgery. Zurich, Switzerland.

Oct. 6-10
MEETING—American Academy of Ophthalmology and Otolaryngology, Las Vegas, Nevada.

Oct. 18-21
CONGRESS — Thirteenth International Congress of Audiology, International Society of Audiology, Florence, Italy.

Oct. 24-29
CONGRESS—Pan American Medical Association Golden Anniversary Congress. Hollywood, Florida.

Oct. 27-20
CONGRESS — Brazilian Federation of Otolaryngology. Rio de Janeiro, R.J. Brazil.

Oct. 29-31
COURSE—Fundamentals of Clinical Otology II. Department of Otolaryngology and Maxillofacial Surgery, University of Tennessee, Memphis, Tennessee 38163

Nov. 7-11
CONGRESS—15th Pan American Congress of Otolaryngology and Bronchoesophagology. New Orleans, Louisiana 70112

Nov. 12-14
SYMPOSIUM—Infection and Allergy of the Nose and Paranasal Sinuses International Symposium. Tokyo, Japan.

Every effort is made to insure that this information is accurate. However, no responsibility is assumed for errors in this listing.

AUTHOR INDEX

ABRAMSON, A. L., 102
Abramson, M., 158, 250, 425
Addink, A. D. F., 847
Adour, K. K., 433
Agarwal, A. K., 359
Akitaya, T., 344
Alford, B. R., 734
Alonso, W. A., 833
Andrus, W. S., 56
Antoli-Candela, F., 145
Antoli-Candela, F., Jr., 145
Applebaum, E. L., 379, 384
Arslan, M., 256
Asarch, R. G., 425

BABIN, R., 473
Batsakis, J. G., 327, 781
Beagley, H. A., 297
Becker, G. D., 401
Beery, Q., 56, 333
Behrens, H. W., 607
Bergstrom, L., Suppl. No. 21
Berkowitz, W. P., 576
Bhatia, P. L., 359
Black, F. O., 174
Bluestone, C. D., 56, 333
Bobbin, R. P., 192
Boles, R., 327, 513
Britton, B. H., 364
Brinton-Darnell, M., 607
Brody, S., 544
Brownson, R. J., 152
Burgio, P. A., 499

CALCATERRA, T. C., 473
Cantekin, E. I., 333
Cantrell, R. W., 627
Carden, E., 233, 631
Carrera, G. F., 719
Castell, D. O., 569
Castor, W. R., 107
Cenzi, M., 256
Ciralsky, R., 73
Cohen, S. R., 747
Compagno, J., 308
Conley, J. J., 729
Cummings, C. W., 182
Cunningham, C. D., 125

DAVIS, H., 297
Davis, W. E., 213
De Cozar, F. A., 145
Dedo, D. D., 833
Dedo, H. H., 740
Devine, K. D., 758
Diehl, W. H., Jr., 152
Dirks, D., 80
Djalilian, M., 758
Don, A., 187
Donnelly, W. H., Jr., 174
Doty, H. E., 433
Dix, R. C., 683
Durrant, J. D., 88
Duvall, A. J., III, 657

EASON, R. L., 102
Enriquez, P., 125

FALBE-HANSEN, J., JR., 315
Fee, W. E., 80
Ferguson, G. B., 233
Ferguson, R. J. L., 379
Filipo, R., 544
Finnegan, D. A., 643
Fontana, R. S., 583
Fried, M. P., 152

GACEK, R. R., Suppl. No. 18
Gaug, O., 218
Gelot, R., 238
Glasscock, M. E., III, 530
Glazebrook, G. A., 107
Gondra, M. I., 192
Good, R. A., 607
Goodman, M. L., 182
Gould, W. J., 206
Graham, M. D., 483
Gupta, I. M., 359
Gupta, O. P., 359
Guzowski, J., 657

HANSON, D. G., 459
Hays, J. W., 530
Hengerer, A. S., 764
Henkin, R. I., 672
Herndon, J. W., 218
Hilsinger, R. L., Jr., 433
Holinger, P. H., 619
Hoppe, W., 94
Horowitz, M. J., 218
House, W. F., 493
Huang, C. C., 158
Hutchinson, J. L., 17
Hyams, V. J., 308
Hyatt, R. E., 635
Hybels, R., 513

INGELSTEDT, S., 198
Izumi, S., Suppl. No. 21

JAFFE, B. F., 764
Johnson, B., 198
Johnson, E. W., 812
Joseph, D. J., 213
Joyner, L. R., 596

KADIR, S., 865
Kahn, A. R., 2
Kamio, T., 483
Karmody, C. S., 179
Kashima, H. K., 643
Keim, R. J., 223
Kerby, G. R., 602
Kiang, N. Y. S., 2, 164
Kimm, J., 368
Kimura, R. S., 271
Kirchner, F. R., 776
Kirchner, J. A., 344, 793
Kitajima, K., 206
Koike, Y., 117
Konak, S., 203
Konrad, H. R., 473
Krause, C. J., 787
Kurdziel, S., 384

LALANI, A. S., 11
Lapidot, A., 238
Larson, A. L., 672
Lawrence, M., 499
Lawson, W., 771
Leiberman, A., Suppl. No. 21
Lentle, B. C., 107
Lichti, E. L., 213
Lindsay, J. R., 37, 174, 350
Linthicum, F. H., Jr., 11, 187, 544
Litton, W. B., 250, 425
Lulenski, G. C., 781
Lynes, T. E., 218
Lyons, G. D., 614

MAC LEAN, J. M., 368
Maisel, R. H., 627
Makishima, K., 391
Maren, T. H., 847
Markel, J., 117
Marr, E. M., 164
Marsh, B. R., 624
Martin, L., 804
McCabe, B. F., 130, 260, 787, 859
McDonald, T. J., 758
Megighian, D., 256
Megill, N. D., 2
Merzenich, M. M., 494
Messer, E. J., 102
Michelson, R. P., 494
Modinari, G., 256
Mogi, G., Suppl. No. 20
Montandon, P. B., 2, 164
Morgan, D. E., 80
Morioka, W. T., 627
Mozzo, W., 256
Murphy, J. P., 530
Muzaffar, K., 245

NADOL, J. B., JR., 841
Nager, G. T., Suppl. No. 22
Newman, A., 344
Newton, T. H., 740
Nichols, R. D., 245
Noffsinger, D., 384
Norman, D., 740
Nuttall, A. L., 499
Nysather, J., 787

OGATA, J., 391
Ogura, J. H., 73, 152, 576, 833

PALVA, A., 112
Palva, T., 112
Pant, G. C., 359
Paparella, M. M., 459
Paradise, J. L., 333
Parker, S. W., 841
Pascoe, D. P., Suppl. No. 23
Peacor, D. R., 22
Peake, W. T., 2, 164
Perkins, R., 518
Pierce, G., 602
Pletcher, J. D., 740
Powell, R. D., 672
Proctor, D. F., 589
Proctor, L. R., 683
Pryor, W. H., 102
Pulec, J. L., 483

QUICK, C., 94, 607

RAJ, P. P., 631
Rao, K. N., 459
Rhea, J., 558
Rhee, T. R., 238
Rhodes, M. L., 650
Rice, D. H., 513
Richter, H. J., 327
Roark, D. T., 734
Rolnick, M. I., 662
Ronis, M. L., 88
Rontal, E., 662
Rontal, M., 662
Roper, C. L., 576
Rosen, G., 203
Ross, M. D., 22
Rubin, W., 541
Ruffini, G., 256
Rundcrantz, H., 198
Ruth, W. E., 602

SACHS, G. B., 223
Sadé, J., 695
Salome, R. G., 158
Samant, H. C., 359
Sanderson, D. R., 583
Sando, I., Suppl. No. 21
Sasaki, C. T., 344
Sataloff, J., 527
Saunders, W. H., 812
Scheinhorn, D. J., 596
Schenck, N. L., 65
Schild, J. A., 619
Schilling, R. W., 158
Schindler, D. N., 494
Schindler, R. A., 494
Schneider, E. A., 228
Schuknecht, H. F., 271, 704
Senturia, B. H., 1
Sessions, D. G., 152, 576
Sessions, R. B., 734
Shepard, N. T., 164
Singleton, G. T., 125
Skolnik, E. M., 804
Smith, C. A., 287, 443
Smith, M. F. W., 552
Smith, R. O., 125
Smith, T. W., 627
Snow, J. B., Jr., 817
Som, M., 771
Spector, G. J., 73, 576
Spector, M., 374
Ste-Marie, P., 308
Stitik, F. P., 589
Strome, M., 764
Suga, F., 37
Swenson, E. R., 847

TAKEMORI, S., 318
Tanabe, M., 206
Taub, S., 45
Tucker, G., Jr., 49, 827
Tucker, J. A., 49, 827

ULVESTAD, R., 459

WARD, P. H., 473
Weber, A. L., 558, 719, 865
Weiland, L. H., 758
Weiss, A. D., 841
Weymuller, E., Jr., 182
Wheatley, M. A., 804
Williams, P. S., 339
Wong, M. L., 643
Wood, R. P., II, Suppl. No. 21
Work, W. P., 513
Wright, D. N., 17

YEE, K. F., 619, 804

ZAJTCHUK, J. T., 350
Zavala, D. C., 650
Zehnder, P. R., Jr., 614

SUBJECT INDEX

ACOUSTIC Neuroma Surgery, Complications in. M. E. Glasscock III, J. W. Hays, J. P. Murphy, 530.

Acrocephalosyndactyly (Apert's Syndrome): Temporal Bone Findings. J. R. Lindsay, F. O. Black, W. H. Donnelly, Jr., 174.

Adenoidectomy and Tonsillectomy, Workshop on. Suppl. No. 17.

Adult Medulloblastoma: Neurotologic Manifestations. B. H. Britton, 364.

Air Bypass Voice Prosthesis for Vocal Rehabilitation of Laryngectomies. S. Taub, 45.

Airway Lesions, Major, Evaluation Using Flow-Volume Loop. R. E. Hyatt, 635.

Aminooxyacetic Acid, Intracochlear Effect of, on Cochlear Potentials and Endolymph Composition. R. P. Bobbin, M. I. Gondra, 192.

Anesthesia, Local, in Otolaryngology. A Re-Evaluation. N. L. Schenck, 65.

Anesthetic Problem and Apparent Cure, Large Tracheal Papillomas. A Case Report. E. Carden, G. B. Ferguson, 233.

Angiofibroma, Juvenile, of Nasopharynx, Radionuclide Angiography in. W. R. Castor, B. C. Lentle, G. A. Glazebrook, 107.

Angiofibromas, Juvenile of Nasopharynx, Preoperative Embolization of. J. D. Pletcher, T. H. Newton, H. H. Dedo, D. Norman, 740.

Angiography, Radionuclide, of Juvenile Angiofibroma of Nasopharynx. W. R. Castor, B. C. Lentle, G. A. Glazebrook, 107.

Antigen, Tumor, Characterization in Epidermoid Carcinoma. C. J. Krause, J. Nysather, B. F. McCabe, 787.

Apert's Syndrome (Acrocephalosyndactyly): Temporal Bone Findings. J. R. Lindsay, F. O. Black, W. H. Donnelly, Jr., 174.

Application of Inverse Filtering for Detecting Laryngeal Pathology. Y. Koike, J. Markel, 117.

Artifact in Electronystagmography—ENG of Month. B. F. McCabe, 130.

Auditory Canal, Internal, Transvestibular Approach to. F. Antoli-Candela, Jr., F. A. De Cozar, 145.

Auditory-Nerve Potentials from Ear Canals of Patients with Otologic Problems. P. B. Montandon, N. T. Shepard, E. M. Marr, W. T. Peake, N. Y. S. Kiang, 164.

Auditory-Nerve Potentials, Recording of as an Office Procedure. P. B. Montandon, N. D. Megill, A. R. Kahn, W. T. Peake, W. Y. S. Kiang, 2.

Auditory Tests, Special, Value of in Latero-Medial Inferior Pontine Syndrome. D. Noffsinger, S. Kurdziel, E. L. Applebaum, 384.

Aural Cholesteatoma, Experimental, Causing Bone Resorption. M. Abramson, R. G. Asarch, W. B. Litton, 425.

Avian Tectorial Membrane, Structure of. K. Tanaka, C. A. Smith, 287.

BENIGN Granular Cell Tumors of Larynx: Review of 36 Cases with Clinicopathologic Data. J. Compagno, V. J. Hyams, P. Ste-Marie, 308.

Benign Paroxysmal Positional Vertigo: A Clinical Study. J. W. Herndon, O. Gaug, M. J. Horowitz, T. E. Lynes, 218.

Bone Resorption, Experimental Aural Cholesteatoma Causing. M. Abramson, R. G. Asarch, W. B. Litton, 425.

Brain Stem Tumor and Otoneurologic Manifestations: Report of Case with Autopsy. K. Makishima, J. Ogata, 391.

Breathing Pattern, Effect of Microaerosol Inhalation. C. T. Sasaki, A. Newman, T. Akitaya, J. A. Kirchner, 344.

Bronchofiberscope, Clinical Experience in Pleuroscopy. G. R. Kerby, G. Pierce, W. R. Ruth, 602.

Bronchoscope, Fiberoptic, New Role for Foreign Body Removal. D. C. Zavala, M. L. Rhodes, 650.

Bronchoscopy, Fiberoptic, Special New Low Resistance to Flow Tube and Endotracheal Tube Adapter for Use During. E. Carden, P. P. Raj, 631.

Burns, Severe Lye of Esophagus, Surgical Management of by Colon Interposition. W. P. Berkowitz, C. L. Roper, D. G. Sessions, G. J. Spector, J. H. Ogura, 576.

Burns, Upper Digestive Tract, Caused by Denalan® Denture Cleanser Powder. A. L. Abramson, R. L. Eason, W. H. Pryor, E. J. Messer, 102.

CALORIC Stimulation of Vestibular Receptor, New Approach to. L. R. Proctor, R. C. Dix, 683.

Cancer of Larynx, Radiation Failures in. E. M. Skolnik, L. Martin, K. F. Yee, M. A. Wheatley, 804.

Cancer of Lung, Early, Detection and Localization. D. R. Sanderson, R. S. Fontana, 583.

Cancer, Pyriform Sinus: Clinical and Laboratory Study. J. A. Kirchner, 793.

Cancer, Radiologically Occult, Delayed Clearance of Tantalum. F. P. Stitik, D. F. Proctor, 589.

Cancer, Second Primary, After Irradiation of Laryngeal Cancer. W. Lawson, M. Som, 771.

Cancer Surgery, Head and Neck, Incidence, Predisposing Factors and Outcome of Pharyngocutaneous Fistulas Complicating. D. D. Dedo, W. A. Alonso, J. H. Ogura, 833.

Carcinoma and Juvenile Papillomatosis. P. R. Zehnder, Jr., G. D. Lyons, 614.

Carcinoma, Epidermoid Characterization of Tumor Antigen in. C. J. Krause, J. Nysather, B. F. McCabe, 787.

Carcinoma, Epidermoid, of Oral Cavity and Larynx, Collagenase Activity in. M. Abramson, R. W. Schilling, C. Huang, R. G. Salome, 158.

Carcinoma, Follicular, of Hürthle Cell Type as Cause of Hemoptysis. C. W. Cummings, E. Weymuller, Jr., M. L. Goodman, 182.

Carcinoma of Nasopharynx in Children. J. B. Snow, Jr., 817.

Carcinoma, Primary Oat-Cell of Head and Neck. R. Gelot, T. R. Rhee, A. Lapidot, 238.

Cerebellar Lesions, Visual Suppression of Vestibular Nystagmus after. S. Takemori, 318.

Cervical Metastasis from Unknown Primary. M. P. Fried, W. M. Diehl, R. J. Brownson, D. G. Sessions, J. H. Ogura, 152.

Cervical Vertigo Patients, ENG of The Month. B. F. McCabe, 260.

Characterization of Tumor Antigen in Epidermoid Carcinoma. C. J. Krause, J. Nysather, B. F. McCabe, 787.

Cholesteatoma, Experimental Aural, Causing Bone Resorption. M. Abramson, R. G. Asarch, W. B. Litton, 425.

Chordomas: Nasopharyngeal Presentation and Atypical Long Survival. H. J. Richter, Jr., J. G. Batsakis, R. Boles, 327.

Cleft Larynx. A Report of Seven Cases. S. R. Cohen, 747.

Cleft Palate, Eustachian Tube Ventilatory Function in Relation to. C. D. Bluestone, Q. C. Beery, E. I. Cantekin, J. L. Paradise, 333.

Clinical Experience with Pleuroscopy Utilizing Bronchofiberscope. G. R. Kerby, G. Pierce, W. E. Ruth, 602.

Clinical Pathological Conference. Grand Rounds. H. F. Schuknecht, 704.

Clinical Use of Electrocochleography, Survey of. D. E. Crowley, H. Davis, H. A. Beagley, 298.

CNS Disease, Electronystagmographic Findings in. M. Spector, 374.

CNS Lesions, Known, Disconjugate Eye Movements During ENG Testing in Patients with. J. Kimm, J. M. MacLean, 368.

Cochlea of Guinea Pig, Innervation of by Use of Golgi Stain. C. A. Smith, 443.

Cochlear Implant: Current Status. W. F. House, (Abstract) 493.

Cochlear Microcirculation, Effect of Histamine on, Contribution to Physiology of Perilymph. Part IV. E. Schneider, 228.

Cochlear Otospongiosis, Sensorineural Hearing Loss Due to, Theoretical Considerations of Etiology. F. H. Linthicum, Jr., R. Filipo, S. Brody, 544.

Cochlear Potentials and Endolymph Composition, Effect of Intracochlear Aminooxyacetic Acid on. R. P. Bobbin, M. I. Gondra, 192.

Cochlear Potentials and Oxygen Associated with Hypoxia. M. Lawrence, A. L. Nuttall, P. A. Burgio, 499.

Cochlear Prosthesis, Present Status and Future Development of. R. P. Michelson, R. A. Schindler, M. M. Merzenich, D. N. Schindler, 494.

Collagenase Activity in Epidermoid Carcinoma of Oral Cavity and Larynx. M. Abramson, R. W. Schilling, C. Huang, R. G. Salome, 158.

Colon Interposition, Surgical Management of Severe Lye Burns of Esophagus by. W. P. Berkowitz, C. L. Roper, D. G. Sessions, G. J. Spector, J. H. Ogura, 576.

Complications in Acoustic Neuroma Surgery. M. E. Glasscock III, J. W. Hays, J. P. Murphy, 530.

Congenital Osteogenesis Imperfecta and Tarda, Temporal Bone Report. J. T. Zajtchuk, J. R. Lindsay, 350.

Conservation of Hearing, Industrial and Otology. J. Sataloff, 527.

Conservative Management of Ménière's Disease: Furstenberg Regimen Revisited. R. Boles, D. H. Rice, R. Hybels, W. P. Work, 513.

Contribution to Physiology of Perilymph. Part IV: Effect of Histamine on Cochlear Microcirculation. E-A. Schneider, 228.

DEAFNESS, Genetic Sensorineural in Adults. M. M. Paparella, D. G. Hanson, K. N. Rao, R. Ulvestad, 459.

Deafness, Permanent, Associated With Furosemide Administration. C. Quick, W. Hoppe, 94.

Deafness, Sudden, Vertigo of Delayed Onset After. J. B. Nadol, Jr., A. D. Weiss, S. W. Parker, 841.

Delayed Clearance of Tantalum by Radiologically Occult Cancer. F. P. Stitik, D. F. Proctor, 589.

Denture Cleanser Powder (Denalan®) As Cause Of Upper Digestive Tract Burns. A. L. Abramson, R. L. Eason, W. H. Pryor, E. J. Messer, 102.

Desmoplastic Fibroma of Mandible. A Case Report. C. D. Cuningham, R. O. Smith, P. Enriquez, G. T. Singleton, 125.

Diagnosis and Management of Primary Tumors of Petrous Apex. R. R. Gacek, Suppl. No. 18.

Digestive Tract, Upper, Burns Caused by Denalan® Denture Cleanser Powder. A. L. Abramson, R. L. Eason, W. H. Pryor, E. J. Messer, 102.

Disconjugate Eye Movements During ENG Testing in Patients with Known CNS Lesions. J. Kimm, J. M. MacLean, 368.

Doppler Ultrasonic Flowmeter, Use of for Pedicle Flaps. W. E. Davis, E. L. Lichti, D. J. Joseph, 213.

Dysgeusia, Hyposmia, Hypogeusia, and Dysosmia Following Influenza-Like Infection. R. I. Henkin, A. L. Larson, R. D. Powell, 672.

Dysosmia, Hypogeusia, Dysgeusia, and Hyposmia Following Influenza-Like Infection. R. I. Henkin, A. L. Larson, R. D. Powell, 672.

EAR, Guinea Pig, Surgical Anatomy of. R. Asarch, M. Abramson, W. B. Litton, 250.

Ear Surgery, Reconsrtuctive, Grafting Materials and Methods in. R. Perkins, 518.

Early Lung Cancer Detection and Localization. D. R. Sanderson, R. S. Fontana, 583.

Editorial. B. H. Senturia, 1.

Effect of Fistulae on Endolymphatic Hydrops. R. S. Kimura, H. F. Schuknecht, 271.

Effect of Intracochlear Aminooxyacetic Acid on Cochlear Potentials and Endolymph Composition. R. P. Bobbin, M. I. Gondra, 192.

Effect of Microaerosol Inhalation on Pattern of Breathing. C. T. Sasaki, A. Newman, T. Akitaya, J. A. Kirchner, 344.

Effusion, Middle Ear, Gas Tension and pH in. S. Ingelstedt, B. Johnson, H. Rundcrantz, 198.

Effusions, Middle Ear, Tympanometric Pattern Classification in Relation to. Q. Beery, W. S. Andrus, C. D. Bluestone, 56.

Electronystagmography, Artifact in—ENG of Month. B. F. McCabe, 130.

Electrocochleography, Survey of Clinical Use of. D. E. Crowley, H. Davis, H. A. Beagley, 298.

Electronystagmographic Findings in CNS Disease. M. Spector, 374.

Electronystagmography: Review of 17 Years Experience. W. Rubin, 541.

Embolization of Juvenile Angiofibromas of Nasopharynx, Preoperative. J. D. Pletcher, T. H. Newton, H. H. Dedo, D. Norman, 740.

Endolymph Composition and Cochlear Potentials, Effect of Intracochlear Aminooxyacetic Acid on. R. P. Bobbin, M. I. Gondra, 192.

Endolymph in Dogfish, Rates of Ion Movement from Plasma to. T. H. Maren, E. R. Swenson, A. D. F. Addink, 847.

Endolymphatic Hydrops, Effect of Fistulae on. R. S. Kimura, H. F. Schuknecht, 271.

Endotracheal Tube Adapter and Special New Low Resistance, Flow Tube for Use During Fiberoptic Bronchoscopy. E. Carden, P. P. Raj, 631.

Endotracheal Tube Intubation, Long-Term, Suggested Tube Modification for Prevention of Injuries to Neonatal Larynx. A. S. Hengerer, M. Strome, B. F. Jaffe, 764.

ENG of Month. G. D. Becker, 401.

ENG of Month, Artifact in ENG. B. F. McCabe, 130.

ENG of Month. Cervical Vertigo Patients. B. F. McCabe, 260.

ENG Testing in Patients with Known CNS Lesions, Disconjugate Eye Movements During. J. Kimm, J. M. MacLean, 368.

Epidermoid Carcinoma, Characterization of Tumor Antigen in. C. J. Krause, J. Nysather, B. F. McCabe, 787.

Epidermoid Carcinoma of Oral Cavity and Larynx, Collagenase Activity in. M. Abramson, R. W. Schilling, C. Huang, R. G. Salome, 158.

Esophageal Sphincter, Lower, Physiology and Pathophysiology of. D. O. Castell, 569.

Esophagus, Surgical Management of Severe Lye Burns, by Colon Interposition. W. P. Berkowitz, C. L. Roper, D. G. Sessions, G. J. Spector, J. H. Ogura, 576.

Eustachian Tube Function, Tympanometric Pressure Swallow Test for Assessment of. P. S. Williams, 339.

Eustachian Tube Lymphatics. J. L. Pulec, T. Kamio, M. D. Graham, 483.

Eustachian Tube Ventilatory Function in Relation to Cleft Palate. C. D. Bluestone, Q. C. Beery, E. I. Cantekin, J. L. Paradise, 333.

Evaluation of Major Airway Lesions Using Flow-Volume Loop. R. E. Hyatt, 635.

Experimental Aural Cholesteatoma Causing Bone Resorption. M. Abramson, R. G. Asarch, W. B. Litton, 425.

Experimental Granuloma of Larynx. F. R. Kirchner, 776.

External Otitis, Predisposed, Prophylaxis of. J. L. Hutchinson, D. N. Wright, 17.

Extracochlear Recordings, Remote Versus Intracochlear Recordings in Guinea Pig. J. D. Durrant, M. L. Ronis, 88.

Extraluminal Foreign Bodies (Coins) in Food and Air Passages. K. F. Yee, J. A. Schild, P. H. Holinger, 619.

Eye Movements, Disconjugate, During ENG Testing in Patients with Known CNS Lesions. J. Kimm, J. M. MacLean, 368.

FACIAL Nerve Reconstruction and its Prognosis. J. Sadé, 695.

Facial Paralysis, Idiopathic, Pregnancy, and the Menstrual Cycle. R. L. Hilsinger, Jr., K. K. Adour, H. E. Doty, 433.

Fate of Cartilage Grafts for Ossicular Reconstruction in Tympanoplasty. A. Don, F. H. Linthicum, Jr., 187.

Fetal Laryngeal Development, Some Aspects of. J. Tucker, G. Tucker, 49.

Fiberoptic Bronchoscope, New Role for Foreign Body Removal. D. C. Zavala, M. L. Rhodes, 650.

Fiberoptic Bronchoscope, Transbronchial Lung Biopsy Through in Diffuse Lung Disease. L. R. Joyner, D. J. Scheinhorn, 596.

Fiberoptic Bronchoscopy, Special New Low Resistance to Flow Tube and Endotracheal Tube Adapter for Use During. E. Carden, P. P. Raj, 631.

Fibroma, Desmoplastic of Mandible. A Case Report. C. D. Cunningham, R. O. Smith, P. Enriquez, G. T. Singleton, 125.

Fistulae, Effect of on Endolymphatic Hydrops. R. S. Kimura, H. F. Schuknecht, 271.

Fistulas, Pharyngocutaneous, Complicating Head and Neck Cancer Surgery, Incidence, Predisposing Factors and Outcome of. D. D. Dedo, W. A. Alonso, J. H. Ogura, 833.

Flow-Volume Loop, Evaluation of Major Airway Lesions, Using. R. E. Hyatt, 635.

Follicular Carcinoma of Hürthle Cell Type as Cause of Hemoptysis. C. W. Cummings, E. Weymuller, Jr., M. L. Goodman, 182.

Foreign Bodies (Coins), Extraluminal in Food and Air Passages. K. F. Yee, J. A. Schild, P. H. Holinger, 619.

Foreign Bodies, Unexpected Radiographic Findings Related to. W. T. Morioka, R. H. Maisel, T. W. Smith, R. W. Cantrell, 627.

Foreign Body Removal: New Role for Fiberoptic Bronchoscope. D. C. Zavala, M. L. Rhodes, 650.

Frequency Responses of Hearing Aids and Their Effects on Speech Perception of Hearing-Impaired Subjects. D. P. Pascoe, Suppl No. 23.

Frey's Syndrome – A Technical Remedy. R. B. Sessions, D. T. Roark, B. R. Alford, 734.

Furosemide Administration, Permanent Deafness Associated With. C. Quick, W. Hoppe, 94.

Furstenberg Regimen Revisited: Conservative Management of Ménière's Disease. R. Boles, D. H. Rice, R. Hybels, W. P. Work, 513.

GAS Tension and pH in Middle Ear Effusion. S. Ingelstedt, B. Johnson, H. Rundcrantz, 198.

Gelatin and Silastic Film Sheeting in Tympanoplasty. J. Falbe-Hansen, M. Tos, 315.

Genetic Sensorineural Deafness in Adults. M. M. Paparella, D. G. Hanson, K. N. Rao, R. Ulvestad, 459.

Giant Cell Tumor of Sphenoid Bone. I. M. Gupta, O. P. Gupta, H. C. Samant, P. L. Bhatia, A. K. Agarwal, G. C. Pant, 359.

Glomus Tumors in Head and Neck: III Analysis of Clinical Manifestations. G. J. Spector, R. Ciralsky, J. H. Ogura, 73.

Golgi Stain, Innervation of Cochlea of Guinea Pig by Use of. C. A. Smith, 443.

Grafting Materials and Methods in Reconstructive Ear Surgery. R. Perkins, 518.

Grafts, Cartilage, for Ossicular Reconstruction in Tympanoplasty, Fate of. A. Don, F. H. Linthicum, Jr., 187.

Grand Rounds at Padova Otorhinolaryngological Clinic. M. Arslan, G. Modinari, D. Megighian, W. Mozzo, Mario Cenzi, G. Ruffini, 256.

Grand Rounds. Clinical Pathological Conference. H. F. Schuknecht, 704.

Grand Rounds: Paranasal Sinus Infection. B. F. McCabe, 859.

Granular Cell Tumors of Larynx, Benign: Review of 36 Cases with Clinicopathologic Data. J. Compagno, V. J. Hyams, P. Ste-Marie, 308.

Granuloma of Larynx, Experimental. F. R. Kirchner, 776.

Granuloma, Thorotrast (Thorium Dioxide) of Neck: Surgical Considerations. K. Muzaffar, R. D. Nichols, 245.

Guinea Pig Ear, Surgical Anatomy of. R. Asarch, M. Abramson, W. B. Litton, 250.

HEAD and Neck Cancer Surgery, Incidence, Predisposing Factors and Outcome of Pharyngocutaneous Fistulas Complicating. D. D. Dedo, W. A. Alonso, J. H. Ogura, 833.

Hearing Aids, Frequency Responses of and Their Effects on Speech Perception of Hearing-Impaired Subjects. D. P. Pascoe, Suppl. No. 23.

Hearing Conservation, Industrial and Otology. J. Sataloff, 527.

Hearing-Impaired Subjects, Frequency Responses of Hearing Aids and Their Effects on Speech Perception of. D. P. Pascoe, Suppl. No. 23.

Hearing Loss, Sensorineural, Due to Cochlear Otospongiosis: Theoretical Considerations of Etiology. F. H. Linthicum, Jr., R. Filipo, S. Brody, 544.

Hemoptysis, Follicular Carcinoma of Hürthle Cell Type as Cause of. C. W. Cummings, E. Weymuller, Jr., M. L. Goodman, 182.

Histamine, Effect of on Cochlear Microcirculation, Contribution to Physiology of Perilymph, Part IV. E. Schneider, 228.

Histochemistry of Mucosa in Secretory Otitis. T. Palva, A. Palva, 112.

Hürthle Cell Type Follicular Carcinoma as Cause of Hemoptysis. C. W. Cummings, E. Weymuller, Jr., M. L. Goodman, 182.

Hydrops, Endolymphatic, Effect of Fistulae on. R. S. Kimura, H. F. Schuknecht, 271.

Hyoepiglottic Complex, Primate, Observations on. G. Tucker, Jr., J. A. Tucker, 827.

Hyoid Autograft Repair of Chronic Subglottic Stenosis. D. A. Finnegan, M. L. Wong, H. K. Kashima, 643.

Hyperlucent Lung: Swyer-James Syndrome, Cause of. J. Guzowski, A. J. Duvall III, 657.

Hypogeusia, Dysgeusia, Hyposmia, and Dysosmia Following Influenza-Like Infection. R. I. Henkin, A. L. Larson, R. D. Powell, 672.

Hyposmia, Hypogeusia, Dysgeusia, and Dysosmia Following Influenza-Like Infection. R. I. Henkin, A. L. Larson, R. D. Powell, 672.

Hypoxia, Cochlear Potentials and Oxygen Associated with. M. Lawrence, A. L. Nuttall, P. A. Burgio, 499.

IDIOPATHIC Facial Paralysis, Pregnancy, and the Menstrual Cycle. R. L. Hilsinger, Jr., K. K. Adour, H. E. Doty, 433.

Immunoglobulin A, Secretory, in Oral and Respiratory Passages in Man. G. Mogi, Suppl. No. 20.

Implant, Cochlear, Current Status. W. F. House, (Abstract) 493.

Incidence, Predisposing Factors and Outcome of Pharyngocutaneous Fistulas Complicating Head and Neck Cancer Surgery. D. D. Dedo, W. A. Alonso, J. H. Ogura, 833.

Industrial Hearing Conservation and Otology. J. Sataloff, 527.

Influenza-Like Infection, Hypogeusia, Dysgeusia, Hyposmia, and Dysosmia Following. R. I. Henkin, A. L. Larson, R. D. Powell, 672.

Injuries to Neonatal Larynx from Long-Term Endotracheal Tube Intubation and Suggested Tube

Modification for Prevention. A. S. Hengerer, M. Strome, B. F. Jaffe, 764.
Innervation of Cochlea of Guinea Pig by Use of Golgi Stain. C. A. Smith, 443.
Internal Auditory Canal, Transvestibular Approach to. F. Antoli-Candela, Jr., F. A. De Cozar, 145.
Intracochlear Recordings, Remote Versus Extracochlear Recordings in Guinea Pig. J. D. Durrant, M. L. Ronis, 88.
Inverse Filtering for Detecting Laryngeal Pathology, Application of. Y. Koike, J. Markel, 117.
Ion Movement, Rates of, from Plasma to Endolymph in Dogfish. T. H. Maren, E. R. Swenson, A. D. F. Addink, 847.
Irradiation of Laryngeal Cancer, Second Primary Cancer After. W. Lawson, M. Som, 771.
JUVENILE Angiofibromas of Nasopharynx, Preoperative Embolization of. J. D. Pletcher, T. H. Newton, H. H. Dedo, D. Norman, 740.
Juvenile Papillomatosis and Carcinoma. P. R. Zehnder, Jr., G. D. Lyons, 614.

LABYRINTHITIS Ossificans Due to Chronic Otitis Media. F. Suga, J. R. Lindsay, 37.
Labyrinthitis, Viral—An Experimental Study. C. S. Karmody, 179
Large Tracheal Papillomas: Difficult Anesthetic Problem and Apparent Cure. A Case Report. E. Carden, G. B. Ferguson, 233.
Laryngeal Cancer, Radiation Failures in. E. M. Skolnik, L. Martin, K. F. Yee, M. A. Wheatley, 804.
Laryngeal Cancer, Second Primary Cancer After Irradiation of. W. Lawson, M. Som, 771.
Laryngeal Development, Fetal, Some Aspects of. J. Tucker, G. Tucker, 49.
Laryngeal Pathology, Application of Inverse Filtering for Detecting. Y. Koike, J. Markel, 117.
Laryngeal Phonatory Reflex. Effect of Anesthetization of Internal Branch of Superior Laryngeal Nerve: Acoustic Aspects. M. Tanabe, W. J. Gould, 206.
Laryngectomies, Vocal Rehabilitation of, Air Bypass Voice Prosthesis for. S. Taub, 45.
Larynx and Oral Cavity, Collagenase Activity in Epidermoid Carcinoma of. M. Abramson, R. W. Schilling, C. Huang, R. G. Salome, 158.
Larynx, Benign Granular Cell Tumors of: Review of 36 Cases with Clinicopathologic Data. J. Compagno, V. J. Hyams, P. Ste-Marie, 308.
Larynx, Cleft. A Report of Seven Cases. S. R. Cohen, 747.
Larynx, Experimental Granuloma of. F. R. Kirchner, 776.
Larynx, Neonatal, Injuries to, from Long-Term Endotracheal Tube Intubation and Suggested Tube Modification for Prevention. A. S. Hengerer, M. Strome, B. F. Jaffe, 764.
Larynx, Papillomatosis of, Treatment with Transfer Factor. C. A. Quick, H. W. Behrens, M. Brinton-Darnell, R. A. Good, 607.
Latero-Medial Inferior Pontine Syndrome. E. L. Applebaum, R. J. L. Ferguson, 379.
Latero-Medial Inferior Pontine Syndrome, Value of Special Auditory Tests in. D. Noffsinger, S. Kurdziel, E. L. Applebaum, 384.
Local Anesthesia in Otolaryngology. A Re-Evaluation. N. L. Schenck, 65.
Lung Biopsy, Transbronchial, Through Fiberoptic Bronchoscope in Diffuse Lung Disease. L. R. Joyner, D. J. Scheinhorn, 596.
Lung Cancer, Early, Detection and Localization. D. R. Sanderson, R. S. Fontana, 583.
Lung Disease, Diffuse, Transbronchial Lung Biopsy Through Fiberoptic Bronchoscope. L. R. Joyner, D. J. Scheinhorn, 596.
Lye Burns, Severe of Esophagus, Surgical Management of by Colon Interposition. W. P. Berkowitz, C. L. Roper, D. G. Sessions, G. J. Spector, J. H. Ogura, 576.
Lymphoepithelioma of Nasopharynx: X-Ray of Month. S. Kadir, A. L. Weber, 865.
Lympthatics, Eustachian Tube. J. L. Pulec, T. Kamio, M. D. Graham, 483.

MACROGLOBULINEMIA, Positional Nystagmus in Association with. R. J. Keim, G. B. Sachs, 223.
Mandible, Desmoplastic Fibroma of. A Case Report. C. D. Cunningham, R. O. Smith, P. Enriquez, G. T. Singleton, 125.
Mastoidectomy Ear, Open Reconstruction of: Six Year Progress Report. M. F. W. Smith, 552.
Medulloblastoma, Adult: Neurotologic Manifestations. B. H. Britton, 364.
Ménière's Disease, Conservative Management of: Furstenberg Regimen Revisited. R. Boles, D. H. Rice, R. Hybels, W. P. Work, 513.
Menstrual Cycle, Pregnancy and Idiopathic Facial Paralysis. R. L. Hilsinger, Jr., K. K. Adour, H. E. Doty, 433.
Metastasis, Cervical from Unknown Primary. M. P. Fried, W. M. Diehl, R. J. Brownson, D. G. Sessions, J. H. Ogura, 152.
Microaerosol Inhalation, Effect on Pattern of Breathing. C. T. Sasaki, A. Newman, T. Akitaya, J. A. Kirchner, 344.
Midle Ear Effusion, Gas Tension and pH in. S. Ingelstedt, B. Johnson, H. Rundcrantz, 198.
Middle Ear Effusions, Tympanometric Pattern Classification in Relation to. Q. Berry, W. S. Andrus, C. D. Bluestone, 56.
Middle Ear Muscle Reflex, Nonacoustical Stimulation of. W. E. Fee, D. Dirks, D. E. Morgan, 80.
Mucosal Histochemistry in Secretory Otitis. T. Palva, A. Palva, 112.
Muscle Reflex, Nonacoustic Stimulation of Middle Ear. W. E. Fee, D Dirks, D. E. Morgan, 80.

NASOPHARYNGEAL Presentation and Atypical Long Survival of Chordomas. H. J. Richter, Jr., J. G. Batsakis, R. Boles, 327.
Nasopharynx Carcinoma in Children. J. B. Snow, Jr., 817.
Nasopharynx, Lymphoepithelioma of: X-Ray of Month. S. Kadir, A. L. Weber, 865.
Nature and Crystal Growth of Otoconia in Rat. M. D. Ross, D. R. Peacor, 22.
Neck Dissection, Radical, Shoulder Rehabilitation After. W. H. Saunders, E. W. Johnson, 812.
Neonatal Larynx, Injuries to, from Long-Term Endotracheal Tube Intubation and Suggested Tube Modification for prevention. A. S. Hengerer, M. Strome, B. F. Jaffe, 764.
Nerve, Facial, Reconstruction and its Prognosis. J. Sadé, 695.
Nerve, Internal Branch of Superial Laryngeal, Effect of Anesthetization of: Acoustic Aspects. M. Tanabe, W. J. Gould, 206.
Nerve, Laryngeal: Laryngeal Phonatory Reflex, Effect of Anesthetization of Internal Branch of Superior. M. Tanabe, W. J. Gould, 206.
Nerve Potentials, Auditory, from Ear Canals of Patients with Otologic Problems. P. B. Montandon, N. T. Shepard, E. M. Marr, W. T. Peake, N. Y. S. Kiang, 164.
Neurectomy, Tympanic, Scanning Evaluation of Parotid Gland after. G. Rosen, S. Konak, 203.
Neuroma Surgery, Acoustic, Complications in. M. E. Glasscock III, J. W. Hays, J. P. Murphy, 530.
Neurotologic Manifestations of Adult Medulloblastoma. B. H. Britton, 364.
New Approach to Caloric Stimulation of Vestibular Receptor. L. R. Proctor, R. C. Dix, 683.
Nonacoustic Stimulation of Middle Ear Muscle Reflex. W. E. Fee, D. Dirks, D. E. Morgan, 80.
Nontraumatic, Nonneoplastic, Subglottic Stenosis. M. Djalilian, T. J. McDonald, K. D. Devine, L. H. Weiland, 758.
Nystagmus, Positional, in Association with Macroglobulinemia. R. J. Keim, G. B. Sachs, 223.
Nystagmus, Vestibular, after Cerebellar Lesions, Visual Suppression of. S. Takemori, 318.
OAT-CELL Carcinoma, Primary of Head and Neck. R. Gelot, T. R. Rhee, A. Lapidot, 238.

Obituary, B. J. Anson, 131.
Objective Evaluation of Vocal Pathology Using Voice Spectrography. E. Rontal, M. Rontal, M. I. Rolnick, 662.
Observations on Primate Hyoepiglottic Complex. G. Tucker, Jr., J. A. Tucker, 827.
Operative Treatment of Surgical Lesions with Objective Tinnitus. P. H. Ward, R. Babin, T. C. Calcaterra, H. R. Konrad, 473.
Oral and Respiratory Passages in Man, Secretory Immunoglobulin A in. G. Mogi. Suppl. No. 20.
Oral Cavity and Larynx, Collagenase Activity in Epidermoid Carcinoma of. M. Abramson, R. W. Schilling, C. Huang, R. G. Salome, 158.
Ossicular Reconstruction in Tympanoplasty, Fate of Cartilage Grafts for. A. Don, F. H. Linthicum, Jr., 187.
Osteogenesis Imperfecta Congenita and Tarda: Temporal Bone Report. J. T. Zajtchuk, J. R. Lindsay, 350.
Otitis Externa, Predisposed, Prophylaxis of. J. L. Hutchinson, D. N. Wright, 17.
Otitis Media, Chronic, Labyrinthitis Ossificans due to. F. Suga, J. R. Lindsay, 37.
Otitis, Secretory, Mucosal Histochemistry in. T. Palva, A. Palva, 112.
Otoconia in Rat, Nature and Crystal Growth of. M. D. Ross, D. R. Peacor, 22.
Otolaryngology, Some Reflections on. J. J. Conley, 729.
Otologic Problem Patients, Auditory-Nerve Potentials of. P. B. Montandon, N. T. Shepard, E. M. Marr, W. T. Peake, N. Y. S. Kiang, 164.
Otology and Industrial Hearing Conservation. J. Sataloff, 527.
Otoneurologic Manifestations and Brain Stem Tumor: Report of Case with Autopsy. K. Makishima, J. Ogata, 391.
Otosclerosis, Unilateral, Sensorineural Impairment in. F. H. Linthicum, A. S. Lalani, 11.
Otospongiosis, Cochlear, Sensorineural Hearing Loss Due to: Theoretical Considerations of Etiology. F. H. Linthicum, Jr., R. Filipo, S. Brody, 544.
Oxygen and Cochlear Potentials Associated with Hypoxia. M. Lawrence, A. L. Nuttall, P. A. Burgio, 499.
PADOVA Otorhinolaryngological Clinic, Grand Rounds at. M. Arslan, G. Modinari, D. Megighian, W. Mozzo, Mario Cenzi, G. Ruffini, 256.
Paget's Disease of Temporal Bone. G. T. Nager, Suppl. No. 22.
Papillomas, Tracheal: Difficult Anesthetic Problem and Apparent Cure. A Case Report. E. Carden, G. B. Ferguson, 233.
Papillomatosis, Juvenile and Carcinoma. P. R. Zehnder, Jr., G. D. Lyons, 614.
Papillomatosis of Larynx, Treatment of with Transfer Factor. C. A. Quick, H. W. Behrens, M. Brinton-Darnell, R. A. Good, 607.
Paranasal Sinus Infection: Grand Rounds. B. F. McCabe, 859.
Parotid Gland, Scanning Evaluation of after Tympanic Neurectomy. G. Rosen, S. Konak, 203.
Paroxysmal Vertigo, Benign Positional: A Clinical Study. J. W. Herndon, O. Gaug, M. J. Horowitz, T. E. Lynes, 218.
Pathophysiology and Physiology of Lower Esophageal Sphincter. D. O. Castell, 569.
Pedicle Flaps, Use of Doppler Ultrasonic Flowmeter for. W. E. Davis, E. L. Lichti, D. J. Joseph, 213.
Perilymph, Contribution to Physiology of. Part IV: Effect of Histamine on Cochlear Microcirculation. E-A. Schneider, 228.
Permanent Deafness Associated with Furosemide Administration. C. Quick, W. Hoppe, 94.
Petrous Apex, Primary Tumors of, Diagnosis and Management of. R. R. Gacek, Suppl. No. 18.
Pharyngocutaneous Fistulas Complicating Head and Neck Cancer Surgery, Incidence, Predisposing Factors and Outcome of. D. D. Dedo, W. A. Alonso, J. H. Ogura, 833.
Phonatory Reflex, Laryngeal. Effect of Anesthetization of Internal Branch of Superior Laryngeal Nerve: Acoustic Aspects. M. Tanabe, W. J. Gould, 206.
Physiology and Pathophysiology of Lower Esophageal Sphincter. D. O. Castell, 569.
Physiology of Perilymph, Contribution to. Part IV: Effect of Histamine on Cochlear Microcirculation. E-A. Schneider, 228.
Pin, Open Safety, Problem of. B. R. Marsh, 624.
Plasma in Dogfish, Rates of Ion Movement to Endolymph. T. H. Maren, E. R. Swenson, A. D. F. Addink, 847.
Pleuroscopy Utilizing Bronchofiberscope, Clinical Experience with. G. R. Kerby, G. Pierce, W. E. Ruth, 602.
Pontine Syndrome, Latero-Medial Inferior. E. L. Applebaum, R. J. L. Ferguson, 379.
Pontine Syndrome, Latero-Medial Inferior, Value of Special Auditory Tests in. D. Noffsinger, S. Kurdziel, E. L. Applebaum, 384.
Positional Nystagmus in Association with Macroglobulinemia. R. J. Keim, G. B. Sachs, 223.
Pregnancy, Menstrual Cycle and Idiopathic Facial Paralysis. R. L. Hilsinger, Jr., K. K. Adour, H. E. Doty, 433.
Preoperative Embolization of Juvenile Angiofibromas of Nasopharynx. J. D. Pletcher, T. H. Newton, H. H. Dedo, D. Norman, 740.
Present Status and Future Development of Cochlear Prosthesis. R. P. Michelson, R. A. Schindler, M. M. Merzenich, D. N. Schindler, 494.
Primary Oat-Cell Carcinoma of Head and Neck. R. Gelot, T. R. Rhee, A. Lapidot, 238.
Primate Hyoepiglottic Complex, Observations on. G. Tucker, Jr., J. A. Tucker, 827.
Problem of Open Safety Pin. B. R. Marsh, 624.
Progress Report, Six Year on Reconstruction of Open Mastoidectomy Ear. M. F. W. Smith, 552.
Prophylaxis of Predisposed Otitis Externa. J. L. Hutchinson, D. N. Wright, 17.
Prosthesis, Cochlear, Present Status and Future Development of. R. P. Michelson, R. A. Schindler, M. M. Merzenich, D. N. Schindler, 494.
Pyriform Sinus Cancer: Clinical and Laboratory Study. J. A. Kirchner, 793.
RADIATION Failures in Cancer of Larynx. E. M. Skolnik, L. Martin, K. F. Yee, M. A. Wheatley, 804.
Radiographic Findings, Unexpected, Related to Foreign Bodies. W. T. Morioka, R. H. Maisel, T. W. Smith, R. W. Cantrell, 627.
Radionuclide Angiography in Juvenile Angiofibroma of Nasopharynx. W. R. Castor, B. C. Lentle, G. A. Glazebrook, 107.
Rates of Ion Movement from Plasma to Endolymph in Dogfish. T. H. Maren, E. R. Swenson, A. D. F. Addink, 847.
Reconstructive Ear Surgery, Grafting Materials and Methods in. R. Perkins, 518.
Reconstruction, Facial Nerve and its Prognosis. J Sadé, 695.
Reconstruction of Open Mastoidectomy Ear: Six Year Progress Report. M. F. W. Smith, 552.
Recording Auditory-Nerve Potentials as an Office Procedure. P. B. Montandon, N. D. Megill, A. R. Kahn, W. T. Peake, W. Y. S. Kiang, 2.
Rehabilitation of Shoulder after Radical Neck Dissection. W. H. Saunders, E. W. Johnson, 812.
Remote Extracochlear Versus Intracochlear Recordings in Guinea Pig. J. D. Durrant, M. L. Ronis, 88.
Respiratory and Oral Passages in Man, Secretory Immunoglobulin A in. G. Mogi, Suppl. No. 20.
Review of 17 Years Experience with Electronystagmography. W. Rubin, 541.
SAFETY Pin, Open, Problem of. B. R. Marsh, 624.
Scanning Evaluation of Parotid Gland after Tympanic Neurectomy. G. Rosen, S. Konak, 203.
Second Primary Cancer After Irradiation of Laryngeal Cancer. W. Lawson, M. Som, 771.

Secretory Immunoglobulin A in Oral and Respiratory Passage in Man. G. Mogi, Suppl. No. 20.
Secretory Otitis, Mucosal Histochemistry in. T. Palva, A. Palva, 112.
Sensorineural Deafness, Genetic, in Adults. M. M. Paparella, D. G. Hanson, K. N. Rao, R. Ulvestad, 459.
Sensorineural Impairment in Unilateral Otosclerosis. F. H. Linthicum, A. S. Lalani, 11.
Sensorineural Hearing Loss Due to Cochlear Otospongiosis: Theoretical Considerations of Etiology. F. H. Linthicum, Jr., R. Filipo, S. Brody, 544.
Shoulder Rehabilitation after Radical Neck Dissection. W. H. Saunders, E. W. Johnson, 812.
Silastic and Gelatin Film Sheeting in Tympanoplasty. J. Falbe-Hansen, M. Tos, 315.
Sinus Infection, Paranasal: Grand Rounds. B. F. McCabe, 859.
Some Aspects of Fetal Laryngeal Development. J. Tucker, G. Tucker, 49.
Some Reflections on our Specialty. J. J. Conley, 729.
Special New Low Resistance to Flow Tube and Endotracheal Tube Adapter for Use During Fiberoptic Bronchoscopy. E. Carden, P. P. Raj, 631.
Spectrography, Voice, Use in Objective Evaluation of Vocal Pathology. E. Rontal, M. Rontal, M. I. Rolnick, 662.
Speech Perception of Hearing-Impaired Subjects, Frequency Responses of Hearing Aids and Their Effects on. D. P. Pascoe, Suppl. No. 23.
Sphenoid Bone, Giant Cell Tumor of. I. M. Gupta, O. P. Gupta, H. C. Samant, P. L. Bhatia, A. K. Agarwal, G. C. Pant, 359.
Stenosis, Chronic Subglottic, Hyoid Autograft Repair of. D. A. Finnegan, M. L. Wong, H. K. Kashima, 643.
Stenosis, Subglottic, Nonneoplastic, Nontraumatic. M. Djalilian, T. J. McDonald, K. D. Devine, L. H. Weiland, 758.
Stenosis, Tracheal, Tracheal Incision as Contributing Factor to. Experimental Study. G. C. Lulenski, J. G. Batsakis, 781.
Structure of Avian Tectorial Membrane. K. Tanaka, C. A. Smith, 287.
Subglottic Stenosis, Chronic, Hyoid Autograft Repair of. D. A. Finnegan, M. L. Wong, H. K. Kashima, 643.
Subglottic Stenosis, Nonneoplastic, Nontraumatic. M. Djalilian. T. J. McDonald, K. D. Devine, L. H. Weiland, 758.
Surgical Anatomy of Guinea Pig Ear. R. Asarch, M. Abramson, W. B. Litton, 250.
Surgical Management of Severe Lye Burns of Esophagus by Colon Interposition. W. P. Berkowitz, C. L. Roper, D. G. Sessions, G. J. Spector, J. H. Ogura, 576.
Survey of Clinical Use of Electrocochleography. D. E. Crowley, H. Davis, H. A. Beagley, 298.
Swallow Test, Tympanometric Pressure, for Assessment of Eustachian Tube Function. P. S. Williams, 339.
Swyer-James Syndrome: Cause of Hyperlucent Lung. J. Guzowski, A. J. Duvall III, 657.
TANTALUM, Delayed Clearance of by Radiologically Occult Cancer. F. P. Stitik, D. F. Proctor, 589.
Tectorial Membrane, Avian, Structure of. K. Tanaka, C. A. Smith, 287.
Temporal Bone Histopathological Findings in Trisomy 13 Syndrome. I. Sando, A. Leiberman, L. Bergstrom, S. Izumi, R. P. Wood II, Suppl. No. 21.
Temporal Bone, Paget's Disease of. G. T. Nager, Suppl. No. 22.
Temporal Bone Report, Osteogenesis Imperfecta Congenita and Tarda. J. T. Zajtchuk, J. R. Lindsay, 350.
Thorium Dioxide (Thorotrast) Granuloma of Neck: Surgical Considerations. K. Muzaffar, R. D. Nichols, 245.
Thorotrast (Thorium Dioxide) Granuloma of Neck: Surgical Considerations. K. Muzaffar, R. D. Nichols, 245.
Tinnitus, Objective, Operative Treatment of Surgical Lesions with. P. H. Ward, R. Babin, T. C. Calcaterra, H. R. Konrad, 473.
Tonsillectomy and Adenoidectomy, Workshop on. Suppl. No. 17.
Tracheal Incision as Contributing Factor to Tracheal Stenosis. Experimental Study. G. C. Lulenski, J. G. Batsakis, 781.
Tracheal Papillomas, Large: Difficult Anesthetic Problem and Apparent Cure. A Case Report. E. Carden, G. B. Ferguson, 233.
Transbronchial Lung Biopsy Through Bronchoscope in Diffuse Lung Disease. L. R. Joyner, D. J. Scheinhorn, 596.
Transfer Factor, Treatment of Papillomatosis of Larynx with. C. A. Quick, H. W. Behrens, M. Brinton-Darnell, R. A. Good, 607.
Transvestibular Approach to Internal Auditory Canal. F. Antoli-Candela, Jr., F. A. De Cozar, 145.
Treatment of Papillomatosis of Larynx with Transfer Factor. C. A. Quick, H. W. Behrens, M. Brinton-Darnell, R. A. Good, 607.
Trisomy 13 Syndrome, Temporal Bone Histopathological Findings in. I. Sando, A. Leiberman, L. Bergstrom, S. Izumi, R. P. Wood II, Suppl. No. 21.
Tumor Antigen, Characterization in Epidermoid Carcinoma. C. J. Krause, J. Nysather, B. F. McCabe, 787.
Tumor, Brain Stem, and Otoneurologic Manifestations: Report of Case with Autopsy. K. Makishima, J. Ogata, 391.
Tumor, Giant Cell, of Sphenoid Bone. I. M. Gupta, O. P. Gupta, H. C. Samant, P. L. Bhatia, A. K. Agarwal, G. C. Pant, 359.
Tumor, Primary, of Petrous Apex, Diagnosis and Management of. R. R. Gacek, Suppl. No. 18.
Tumors, Glomus, in Head and Neck: III. Analysis of Clinical Manifestations. G. J. Spector, R. Ciralsky, J. H. Ogura, 73.
Tumors of Larynx, Benign Granular Cell: Review of 36 Cases with Clinicopathologic Data. J. Compagno, V. J. Hyams, P. Ste-Marie, 308.
Tympanic Neurectomy, Scanning Evaluation of Parotid Gland after. G. Rosen, S. Konak, 203.
Tympanometric Pattern Classification in Relation to Middle Ear Effusions. Q. Beery, W. S. Andrus, C. D. Bluestone, 56.
Tympanometric Pressure Swallow Test for Assessment of Eustachian Tube Function. P. S. Williams, 339.
Tympanoplasty, Fate of Cartilage Grafts for Ossicular Reconstruction in. A. Don, F. H. Linthicum, Jr., 187.
Tympanoplasty, Silastic and Gelatin Film Sheeting in. J. Falbe-Hansen, M. Tos, 315.
UNEXPECTED Radiographic Findings Related to Foreign Bodies. W. T. Morioka, R. H. Maisel, T. W. Smith, R. W. Cantrell, 627.
Use of Doppler Ultrasonic Flowmeter for Pedicle Flaps. W. E. Davis, E. L. Lichti, D. J. Joseph, 213.
VALUE of Special Auditory Tests in Latero-Medial Inferior Pontine Syndrome. D. Noffsinger, S. Kurdziel, E. L. Applebaum, 384.
Ventilatory Function of Eustachian Tube in Relation to Cleft Palate. C. D. Bluestone, Q. C. Beery, E. I. Cantekin, J. L. Paradise, 333.
Vertigo, Cervical, ENG of Month. B. F. McCable, 260.
Vertigo of Delayed Onset After Sudden Deafness. J. B. Nadol, Jr., A. D. Weiss, S. W. Parker, 841.
Vertigo, Positional Benign Paroxysmal: A Clinical Study. J. W. Herndon, O. Gaug, M. J. Horowitz, T. E. Lynes, 218.
Vestibular Nystagmus after Cerebellar Lesions, Visual Suppression of. S. Takemori, 318.
Vestibular Receptor, New Approach to Caloric Stimulation of. L. R. Proctor, R. C. Dix, 683.
Viral Labyrinthitis—An Experimental Study. C. S. Karmody, 179.
Visual Suppression of Vestibular Nystagmus after Cerebellar Lesions. S. Takemori, 318.
Vocal Pathology, Objective Evaluation of Using Voice Spectrography. E. Rontal, M. Rontal, M. I. Rolnick, 662.
Vocal Rehabilitation of Laryngectomies, Air Bypass Voice Prosthesis for. S. Taub, 45.
Voice Prosthesis Air Bypass, for Vocal Rehabilitation of Laryngectomies. S. Taub, 45.
WORKSHOP on Tonsillectomy and Adenoidectomy. Suppl. No. 17.
X-RAY of Month. G. F. Carrera, A. Weber, 719.
X-Ray of Month. J. Rhea, A. L. Weber, 558.
X-Ray of Month: Lymphoepithelioma of Nasopharynx. S. Kadir, A. L. Weber, 865.

INTERNATIONAL CONFERENCE ON CHOLESTEATOMA

May 26-29, 1976

DEPARTMENT OF OTOLARYNGOLOGY
AND MAXILLOFACIAL SURGERY
THE UNIVERSITY OF IOWA
IOWA CITY, IOWA 52242

CONFERENCE COCHAIRMEN

Jacob Sade, M.D.
Maxwell Abramson, M.D.
Brian F. McCabe, M.D.

An in-depth consideration of the biology, pathophysiology, etiology, natural history, and management of Aural Cholesteatoma

CONTRIBUTORS

M. Abramson
D. F. Austin
S. H. Baron
R. J. Bellucci
J. Bernstein
C. Bluestone
W. H. Bradley
D. T. Cody
E. Derlacki
H. Diamant
A. Z. Eisen
I. Freedberg
I. Friedmann
V. Goodhill
L. A. Harker
R. Hinchcliffe
J. V. D. Hough
C. Jansen
C. M. Kos
S. Krane
C. Krause
E. Laurence
D. G. Lim
J. Lindsay
W. B. Litton
I. Mackenzie
B. F. McCabe
G. Mundy
G. Nager
T. Palva
M. Paparella
G. Peck
D. Plester
F. N. Ritter
S. Roth
J. Sadé
H. F. Schuknecht
B. H. Senturia
L. Severeid
G. Shambaugh
J. Sheehy
G. D. Smyth
C. Tschopp
J. Thomsen
J. Toller
B. Tool
R. Trelstad
W. K. Wright

Detailed program and registration materials available upon request.

DIAGNOSIS AND MANAGEMENT OF PRIMARY TUMORS OF THE PETROUS APEX

RICHARD R. GACEK, M.D.

BOSTON, MASSACHUSETTS

SUMMARY – Five patients with primary tumors of the petrous apex were diagnosed and treated between the years 1968 to 1974; two had congenital epidermoids, two had chondromyxosarcomas and one had neurofibroma. The embryological development of the foramen lacerum and the pattern of expansion of these primary tumors support the contention that these three categories of tumors arise in the foramen lacerum. Knowledge of the structures surrounding the foramen lacerum can provide a guide to early diagnosis of petrous apex tumors. Since these tumors cannot be completely removed, the goal of surgery is to obtain histological diagnosis and to produce permanent fistulization of the petrous apex. Although there are several recommended surgical approaches to the petrous apex, the transmastoid-translabyrinthine procedure was used in this series.

Primary neoplasms of the petrous apex are rarely encountered in otological practice. The lack of familiarity with tumors in this area is a handicap to early diagnosis and management. Since these tumors occur infrequently and are located in an inaccessible region of the skull, they are usually not diagnosed until they reach considerable size and cause multiple cranial nerve deficits or intracranial complications. The present study constitutes an evaluation of five patients with the signs and symptoms of three types of tumor (congenital epidermoid, chondromyxosarcoma and neurofibroma) that may arise at the petrous apex. A discussion of the origin and development of these tumors is given with suggested guidelines for early diagnosis and effective surgical management of these neoplasms.

CASE REPORTS

CASE ONE

Congenital Epidermoid Cyst. A thirty-two-year-old female was first seen in April 1968 with a complaint of a hearing loss in the right ear for four to five months. The hearing loss followed an upper respiratory infection and despite decongestants and myringotomy, there was only temporary improvement in her serous otitis media. Otolaryngological examination was normal except for a blue-appearing right ear drum and a conductive hearing loss on the right. Following myringotomy with insertion of a pressure equalizing tube, the conductive hearing loss was eliminated. Despite this initial improvement, the patient continued to have some discomfort in the right ear and had a brownish mucoid discharge through the pressure equalizing tube, which persisted for two months. Because of increased pain in the right ear, x-rays of the mastoid cell system were taken in early June 1968 and revealed destruction of cell partitions.

A course of antibiotic therapy failed to improve the symptoms, and therefore in June 1968 a simple mastoidectomy was performed. Granulation tissue with flecks of keratin which filled the mastoid cells was removed. Histological examination showed cholesterol granuloma. Improvement in symptoms continued until February 22, 1969 when she was seen in the emergency room with severe right-sided temporal parietal headaches and pain in the lower jaw and teeth. X-rays (Fig. 1A) revealed an osteolytic lesion in the petrous apex which was present on previous x-rays but was not identified at that time. The patient was

From the Massachusetts Eye and Ear Infirmary, Harvard Medical School, 243 Charles St., Boston, Mass.

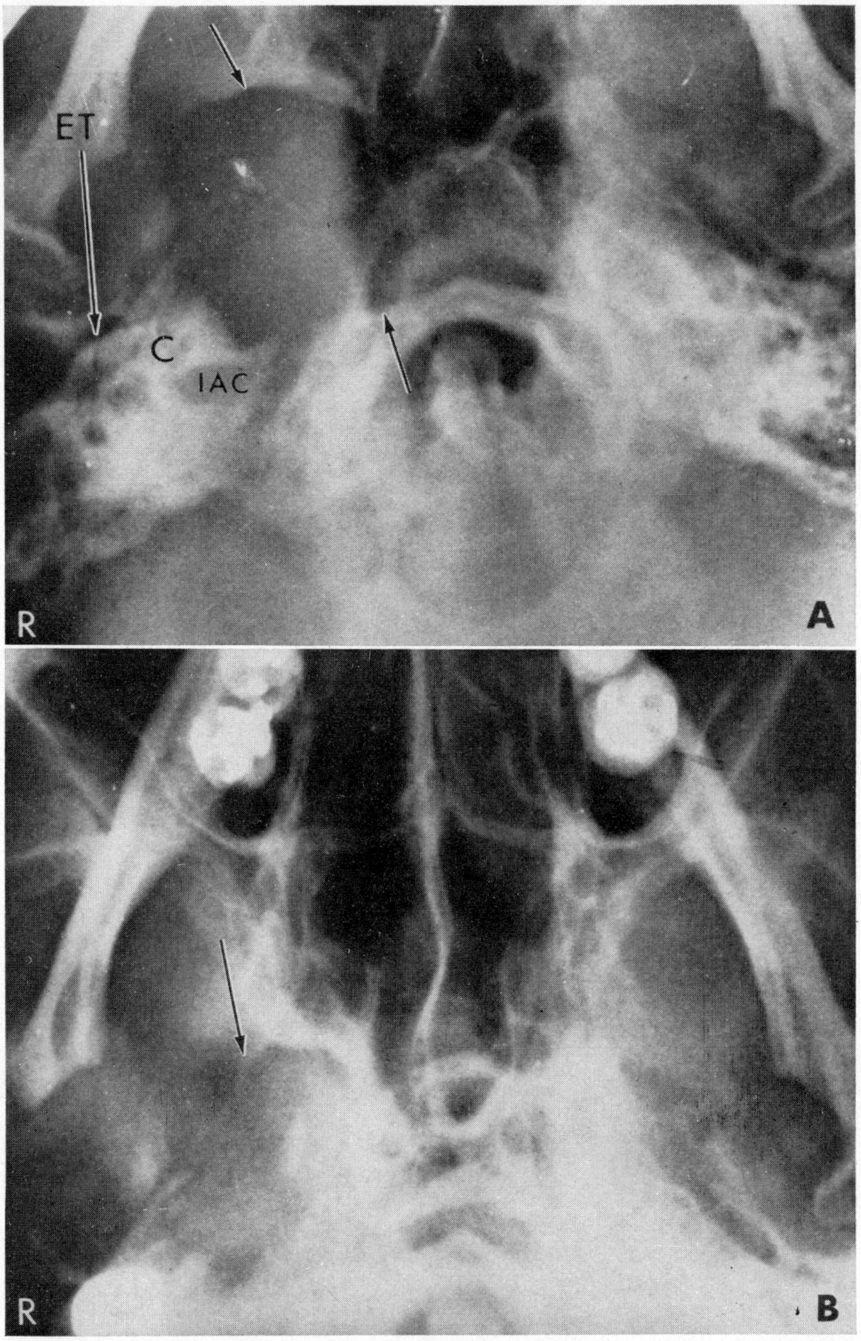

Fig. 1. A) Case 1. X-ray view of the base of the skull showing the osteolytic epidermoid cyst (small arrows) at the petrous apex. The cochlea (C) and the internal auditory canal (IAC) are not involved but the Eustachian tube (ET) is compressed. B) Postoperative x-ray taken one year after successful fistulization of the cyst. Note reduction in size of cyst as evidenced by the recalcification of bony margin of foramen ovale (arrow).

then admitted to the hospital for a complete work-up including an arteriogram, pneumoencephalogram and brain scan. These studies revealed an extradural avascular mass in the petrous apex which displaced the internal carotid artery laterally.

In order to establish a diagnosis, the middle cranial fossa was explored on April 11, 1969 and a cystic lesion containing xanthochromic fluid and keratin material was identified and evacuated. The wall of the cyst was adherent to the internal carotid artery and surrounding structures, and therefore could not be removed. Pathological examination of the aspirate revealed old blood and amorphous keratin material. Postoperatively the patient experienced complete relief from her headaches until May 11, 1969 when she was again admitted as an emergency case because of severe headaches and blurred vision. At this time the mandibular condyle was removed and a radical mastoidectomy was performed in order to fistulize the cyst into the ear canal. The fistula was created anterior to the carotid canal in an effort to preserve labyrinthine function. The fistulous tract was lined with skin grafts and a silastic tube was inserted to hold them in place. This tube extruded after five months and the fistula closed spontaneously. The "exploding type" headache and blurred vision recurred. Therefore, in December 1969 a revision mastoidectomy and a labyrinthectomy were performed to create a wider fistulous tract into the cyst. The bone removal included the medial wall of the middle ear, from the carotid canal anteriorly to the descending portion of the facial canal posteriorly and inferiorly to the level of the jugular bulb. This opening was lined with split-thickness skin grafts. Complete relief from headaches and eye symptoms occurred and recovery from the effects of labyrinthine destruction was sufficient to permit discharge from the hospital after five to six days. The patient has remained completely free of headaches to the present date, a period of 4½ years. Radiological evaluation one year after the last operation has revealed a decrease in size of the cyst as revealed by recalcification of bony landmarks such as the foramen ovale (Fig. 1B).

CASE TWO

Congenital Epidermoid Cyst. A twenty-seven-year-old male was first seen in January 1973 with a complaint of short lasting episodic dizziness for ten weeks. He also complained of fluctuating hearing loss and a blocked sensation in the left ear for several months. Numbness over the left dental area and the lower left cheek was also noted for six months, and headache around the left ear was present for one month. The ear, nose and throat examination was entirely normal. Neurological evaluation was also within normal limits except for a slightly diminished left corneal reflex. Audiometric testing revealed bilateral high tone sensorineural loss at 4,000 Hz and normal speech discrimination scores. No conductive hearing loss was found. Electronystagmography revealed a slightly diminished response in the left ear and a type II positional nystagmus which was attributed to a possible brain stem lesion. Conventional and tomographic x-rays of the mastoids and base of the skull revealed an osteolytic lesion of the left petrous apex (Figs. 2 and 3A). Brain scan, arteriography and pneumoencephalography revealed an avascular petrous apex mass with a middle fossa extension. The internal carotid artery was displaced laterally in the region of the petrous apex. The preoperative diagnosis was primary cholesteatoma of the petrous apex, and on February 13, 1973 radical mastoidectomy and fistulization of the petrous apex was performed through the region of the labyrinth. A wide opening into the keratin filled cyst was created after removal of bone from the carotid canal to the vertical portion of the facial nerve canal and from the middle fossa dura to the jugular bulb. Split-thickness skin grafts were placed in the fistula after evacuation of a large amount of keratin debris from the cholesteatoma cyst. The patient was discharged four days following surgery, having made striking improvement from the effects of the labyrinthectomy. He

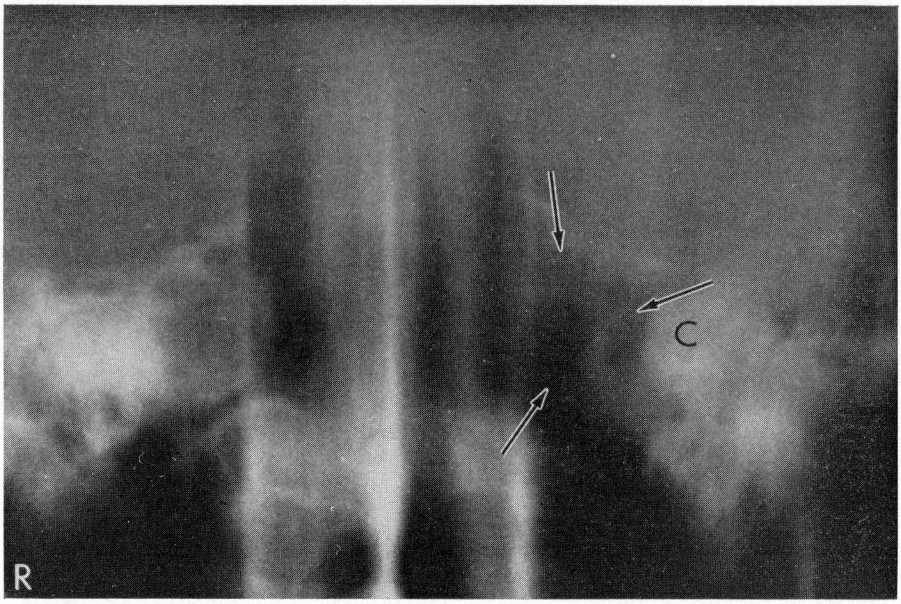

Fig. 2. Case 2. Frontal tomograms of the petrous apices demonstrating a complete destruction of the left petrous apex by the epidermoid cyst (arrows). C — Cochlea.

has been completely free of headaches except for one severe headache episode and an elevated temperature one month following surgery which occurred in association with a profuse cerebrospinal fluid leak from the left ear. Hematological and cerebrospinal examinations were normal. Symptoms gradually subsided on nonspecific therapy and there was gradual cessation of the cerebrospinal fluid otorrhea. The cholesteatoma remained marsupialized (Fig. 3B) and the patient has been free of symptoms for 16 months.

CASE THREE

Neurofibroma. A seventy-three-year-old white female was first evaluated otologically in January 1962 for hearing loss and tinnitus in the left ear of two years duration. No complaints of vertigo, headache or facial pain were elicited. Complete otolaryngological examination was normal except for a left serous otitis media. Needle paracentesis of the left middle ear produced thin amber fluid and marked improvement in hearing. Following this, audiometric evaluation showed normal hearing in the right ear and a flat sensorineural hearing loss of about 50 dB with complete recruitment and 56% speech discrimination score in the left ear. Tone decay was normal. Caloric response was present but somewhat reduced in the left ear. Radiological evaluation of the base of skull showed a questionable area of destruction of the floor of the middle fossa. It was felt that no relationship existed between the serous otitis media, sensorineural hearing loss, and questionable x-ray abnormalities. No further therapy was instituted and the patient was instructed to return in six months.

The patient next returned in January 1969 with a history of increasing symptoms during the preceding 6-12 months; the left-sided hearing loss was now complete, pulsating tinnitus continued, horizontal diplopia was present, and a vague unsteadiness occurred from time to time. Examination revealed a "blue" drum on the left (brownish fluid on paracentesis), a slight left VI nerve weakness, profound left hearing loss, and markedly reduced caloric response in the left ear. No headache, facial pain or facial weakness were present. Radiological evalua-

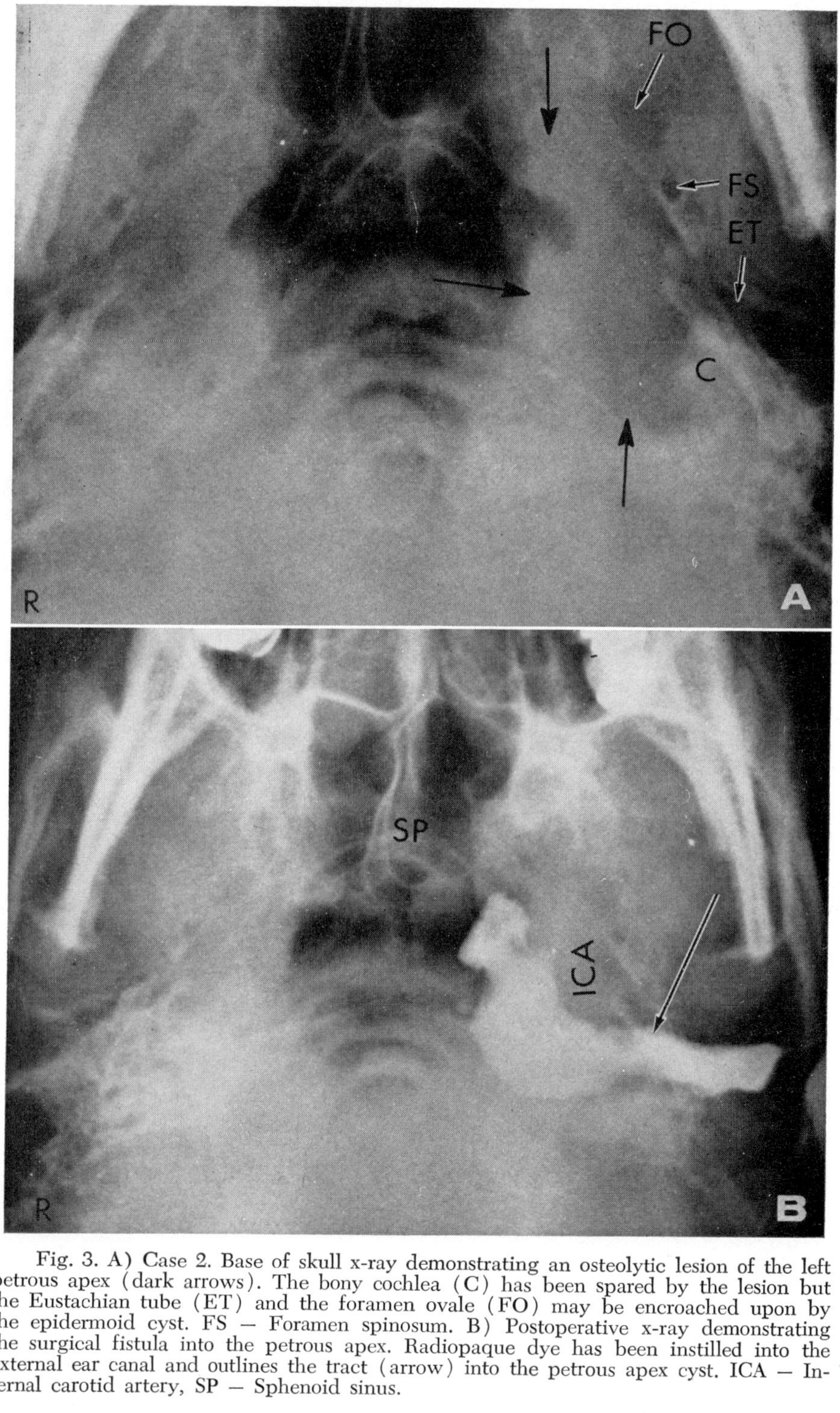

Fig. 3. A) Case 2. Base of skull x-ray demonstrating an osteolytic lesion of the left petrous apex (dark arrows). The bony cochlea (C) has been spared by the lesion but the Eustachian tube (ET) and the foramen ovale (FO) may be encroached upon by the epidermoid cyst. FS — Foramen spinosum. B) Postoperative x-ray demonstrating the surgical fistula into the petrous apex. Radiopaque dye has been instilled into the external ear canal and outlines the tract (arrow) into the petrous apex cyst. ICA — Internal carotid artery, SP — Sphenoid sinus.

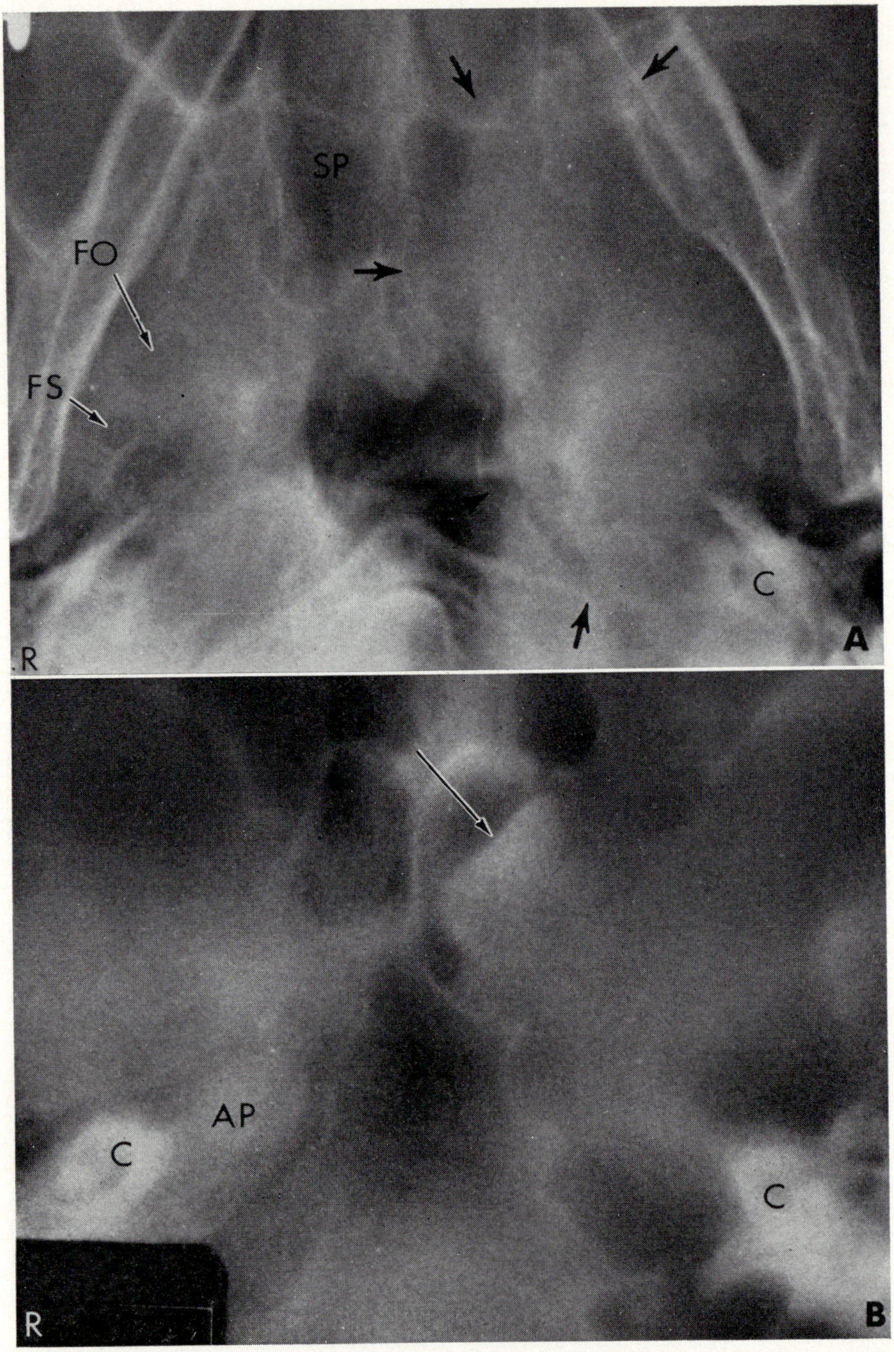

Fig. 4. A) Case 3. Conventional x-ray demonstrating a very extensive lesion (dark arrows) which has destroyed the petrous apex, the foramen ovale and the foramen spinosum. The tumor has extended into the sphenoid sinus (SP). C — Cochlea. Note normal foramen ovale (FO) and foramen spinosum (FS) on the right side. B) This tomogram clearly shows the extension into the left sphenoid sinus (arrow). C — Cochlea. Note normal petrous apex (AP) on the right.

tion revealed a definite osteolytic lesion of the left petrous apex and floor of the middle cranial fossa. Carotid arteriography demonstrated marked lateral displacement of the internal carotid artery in the region of the petrous apex. The diagnosis of primary petrous epidermoid cyst was made and surgery recommended.

The patient refused surgery and was followed over the next five years. There was no essential progression in symptoms and no new signs appeared. An intermittent discharge of brownish fluid from the left ear provided relief from the pressure and tinnitus during these years. In June 1974 a follow-up radiological examination revealed an extensive area of destruction involving the petrous apex and the sphenoid bone, with extension into the left sphenoid sinus (Figs. 4A and B). Because of the increase in size of the tumor, the patient was referred to the author for surgical management to prevent intracranial complications (meningitis) and further neurological deficits.

In November 1974 exploration of the left petrous apex was performed. After a wide field radical mastoidectomy, the carotid canal was identified anteriorly and the bone over the cochlea was removed between the internal carotid artery and the vertical portion of the facial nerve. A solid tumor mass was encountered in the petrous apex. Several biopsies were taken of the firm avascular mass. The area was skin grafted and packing inserted into the cavity. The patient had an uneventful postoperative course. Histological examination of the biopsy material revealed neurofibroma.

Surgical removal of this tumor was not attempted because of the risk associated with extirpation of such a large tumor in an elderly patient. Unless signs or symptoms of critical nature occur, no surgical procedure is contemplated in the future.

CASE FOUR

Chondromyxosarcoma. A twenty-seven-year-old female was first seen in November 1971 with a complaint of headache, unsteadiness and a progressive right hearing loss. Otological examination two years previously revealed a right serous otitis media which was treated by the introduction of a middle ear pressure equalizing tube. Six months later, after the tube had extruded, the hearing loss recurred and a second pressure equalizing tube was introduced. After the second tube extruded, the patient had recurrence of hearing loss, unsteadiness with falling to the right and weakness of the right arm. The patient was then referred for consultation. Otological examination at this time showed a right serous otitis media, a reddish mass behind the inferior part of the right tympanic membrane, and a pure conductive hearing loss of 40-50 dB on the right and normal hearing in the left ear. Caloric tests with 5 cc of 26.6 C water revealed bilaterally symmetrical responses of normal duration. There was weakness of the right sternocleidomastoid and trapezius muscles, hemiparesis and hyperreflexia of the right arm and leg, right facial weakness, complete paralysis of the right vocal cord, and deviation of a fasciculating tongue to the right. Radiological studies of the mastoid and skull revealed increased density with destruction of the right petrous apex extending to the region of the jugular foramen. Exploration of the middle ear was carried out under general anesthesia and biopsy of the mass revealed chondromyxosarcoma.

Since there were signs of increasing brain stem compression, partial removal of the intracranial component of the tumor was performed neurosurgically. However, the patient followed a progressive downhill course following surgery and died from bronchopneumonia twelve days after surgery.

Autopsy revealed a multilobulated encapsulated tumor mass which involved the right sphenoid and petrous portion of the temporal bone. The tumor extended into the basiocciput as far as the articular cartilage of the first cervical vertebra, and herniated into the middle and posterior cranial fossae, enveloping

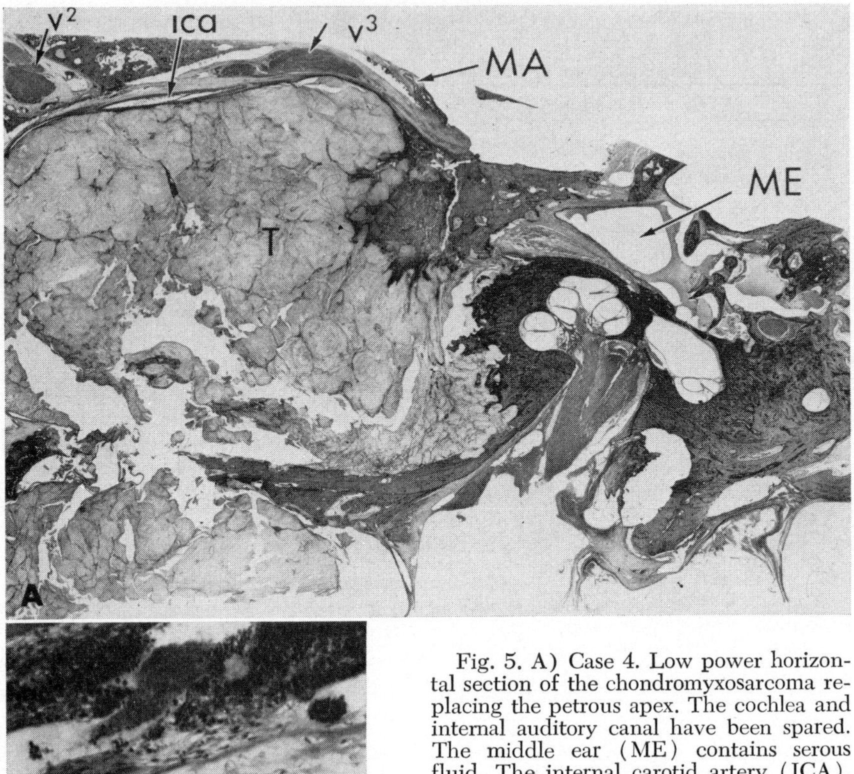

Fig. 5. A) Case 4. Low power horizontal section of the chondromyxosarcoma replacing the petrous apex. The cochlea and internal auditory canal have been spared. The middle ear (ME) contains serous fluid. The internal carotid artery (ICA), the mandibular division of the trigeminal nerve (V^3) and the middle meningeal artery (MA) are compressed by the tumor (T) which has also extended into the posterior fossa. V^2 – Second division of trigeminal nerve. (Reproduced from Figure 1 in "Primary Sarcomas of the Temporal Bone" by Pierre Naufal, reprinted from the *Archives of Otolaryngology,* July, 1973, Volume 98:44-50, Copyright 1973, American Medical Association.) B) High power photomicrograph (195X) of the tumor showing the cartilage tumor cells of chondrosarcoma.

the right III to XII cranial nerves. The temporal bones were removed for study, and the right temporal bone revealed a massive solid tumor which replaced the petrous bone with extension into the middle and posterior cranial fossae (Figs. 5A and B). The tumor extended through the infralabyrinthine cell tract into the hypotympanum, where it was visible on otoscopy. The internal carotid artery and mandibular division of the trigeminal nerve were displaced markedly in an

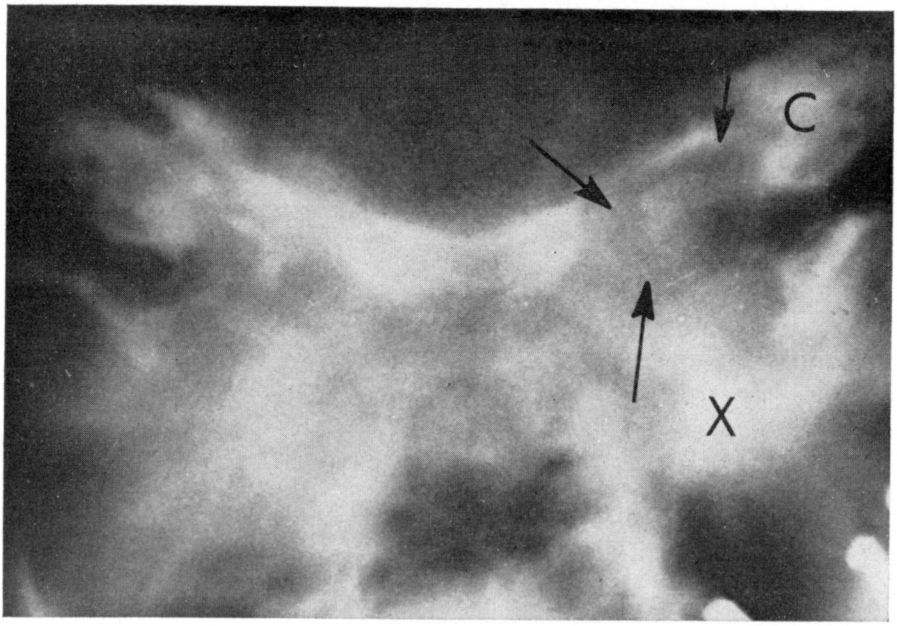

Fig. 6. Case 5. Frontal tomogram of petrous apices demonstrating the typical osteolytic lesion (arrows) of the apex which spares the cochlea (C). X – Indicates extension of the tumor into the infratemporal fossa.

anterolateral direction. The carotid artery was compressed to the point of occlusion. The lumen of the bony and cartilaginous portions of the Eustachian tube was also compressed by tumor. However, the bony labyrinth capsule was intact; the sensory areas of the cochlea and the vestibular organs were normal.

CASE FIVE

Chondromyxosarcoma. A thirty-one-year-old female was first seen in May 1971 with the complaint of difficulty in speaking and swallowing; a left paralyzed vocal cord was found. An examination including arteriogram was performed in October 1971, but no abnormality was discovered. In November 1971 she developed left-sided headaches. A diagnostic work-up which included polytomography, arteriography, and pneumoencephalography was performed at another hospital. As a result of these studies, the patient underwent a transmastoid exploration of the left jugular foramen and cartilaginous material was removed which was diagnosed histologically as "normal cartilage." The patient noted some improvement in symptoms postoperatively but continued to have a pulsating feeling in the left ear. She was then reasonably well until November 1972 when she noted blurring of vision on turning her head, and in January 1973 experienced intermittent diplopia. This became constant by February 1973 and at that time it was noted that a left VI nerve palsy was present. In May 1973 she experienced the onset of intermittent tingling over the left mandible. At this time she was seen at the MEEI where a paralyzed left vocal cord, asymmetric elevation of the palate, and a questionable slight weakness of the left shoulder muscles were noted. The tongue was normal in appearance and movement. No extremity weakness was noted. Manual examination revealed a fullness inferior and deep to the left tympanic bone. Hearing evaluation and vestibular testing were normal bilaterally. No evidence of brain stem compression was found on this examination. Polytomography performed in April 1973 revealed a large erosive lesion extending from the petrous apex back to the jugular fora-

TABLE I

SUMMARY OF SYMPTOMS AND SIGNS IN PATIENTS WITH PRIMARY TUMORS OF THE PETROUS APEX

Tumor	*Patient*	*Headache*	*V Nerve Signs*	*Eustachian Tube Obstruction*	*Int. Carotid Artery Compression*	*Other Cranial Nerves*
Congenital epidermoid cyst	32F	+	+	+	+	none
	27M	+	+	±	+	none
Neurofibroma	73F	—	—	+	—	VI, VIII
Chondromyxosarcoma	24F	+	+	+	+	III, VI, VII, IX, X, XI, XII
	31F	+	+	±	+	IV, VI, IX, X, XI

± = incomplete Eustachian tube obstruction

men and as far posteriorly as the foramen magnum (Fig. 6). Carotid arteriography revealed anterolateral displacement and compression of the petrosal segment of the internal carotid artery. A diagnosis of primary cholesteatoma of the petrous apex or a chondroid tumor was entertained. Surgical exploration of the petrous apex was performed through a mastoid and middle ear approach. In the middle ear a small extension of tumor was noted protruding into the anterior hypotympanum between the exposed internal carotid artery anteriorly and the basal turn of the cochlea posteriorly. This area was enlarged by removing sufficient bone to create a fistula into the petrous apex without injuring the labyrinth. Solid and degenerated bluish cartilaginous material was removed for biopsy purposes. A large amount of degenerated tumor was then aspirated and the bony fistula was lined with split-thickness skin grafts to maintain a permanent tract into the petrous apex. Histologically this was diagnosed as a low-grade chondromyxosarcoma. The patient recovered from the surgery uneventfully and after the ear was completely healed, radiation therapy was administered on the 160 MeV proton beam machine to a dose of 6,125 rads. The patient tolerated radiation therapy well and experienced relief from headaches. Some improvement in the VI nerve palsy was noted. Deficits of cranial nerves IX, X, and XI remain unchanged.

Table I summarizes the findings in these five patients with petrous apex tumors. Except for one patient, these patients were all females and in a young age group. Significantly, four out of five patients experienced severe headaches, signs of involvement of the third division of the trigeminal nerve, and signs of internal carotid compression. While three out of five patients showed signs of complete Eustachian tube obstruction (serous otitis media), the remaining two patients had complained of ear blockage which was interpreted as incomplete tubal obstruction. These findings are associated with the early stage of development of petrous apex tumors. Only when the tumors reached extensive proportions were other cranial nerves involved as demonstrated by the last three cases in the table.

DISCUSSION

Although this report discusses an almost equal number of patients with each of these primary tumors of the petrous apex, chondromyxosarcomas and neurofibromas are extremely rare in this area. In an extensive review of the literature on primary sarcomas of the temporal bone, Naufal[1] found one chondrosarcoma reported by Tucker[2] and added a second case (Case 4). There are numerous reports describing congenital cholesteatoma arising in the middle ear[3-8] and in the petrous apex.[9-18]

Clinical Features. Patients with congenital epidermoid cysts and patients with chondromyxosarcoma are usually in the young adult age group; they ranged in age from 24-32 years in this series. Other reports on congenital epidermoids of the petrous apex consistently report a young adult age group prevalence with these tumors.[1,3-7,9-19] Neurofibromas can occur in almost any part of the body and have been reported in all age groups.

Headache was one of the most prominent symptoms in these patients and was described as a severe headache usually ineffectively treated with medication. The headache pain was usually located in the side of the ear affected, although in Case 1 the patient's headache was sometimes described as a deep exploding headache located in the center of the head. Headache is probably an indication of dural stretching by an expanding tumor at the petrous apex. Another common symptom was involvement of the *mandibular division of the trigeminal nerve.* Involvement of the third division of the V cranial nerve produced either pain, parasthesia or anesthesia over the distribution of this nerve. Very likely this indicated compression of the mandibular division of the V cranial nerve in the foramen ovale. Varying degrees of *occlusion of the Eustachian tube were also found* in these patients. In three patients (Cases 1, 3 and 4), complete obstruction of the Eustachian tube produced serous otitis media. In the other two patients (Cases 2 and 5), serous otitis media was not present but the patients complained of some form of blockage of the ear which could be interpreted as incomplete Eustachian tube obstruction. In the patients with complete Eustachian tube obstruction, conductive hearing loss was documented by audiometry.

Symptoms related to internal carotid artery compression were also common. Slow compression of the internal carotid artery in young patients probably does not produce hemiparesis. Therefore, in Case 4 the right hemiparesis was probably due to direct brain stem compression by the extensive tumor. However, lesser symptoms described as blurring of vision on turning of the head (Cases I and 5), or as dizziness (Case 2) may be ischemic effects from internal carotid artery compression. More significant symptoms occurred in the patients with a solid malignant tumor (chondromyxosarcoma) as compared to patients with a cystic tumor (congenital epidermoid) or a slow growing benign tumor (neurofibroma) which probably exert a less compressive effect on the artery.

The two patients with chondromyxosarcoma presented with a more extensive involvement of the base of the skull. In these patients the nerves of the jugular foramen (IX, X and XI), and the hypoglossal foramen (XII) were involved. Other nerves compressed by anterior extension at the base of the skull were III, IV and VI. While these multiple cranial nerve deficits were more common with solid malignant tumors as chondromyxosarcoma, it is also possible that extensive benign tumors of the petrous apex may involve these cranial nerves (Case 3).

Aside from the cranial nerve deficits associated with very extensive tumors, the otolaryngological examination was either normal (Cases 2 and 5), or revealed merely serous otitis media if the tumor was large enough to compress the Eustachian tube (Cases 1, 3 and 4). Only when the tumor is massive may it present otologically (Case 4).

In four of these patients both auditory and vestibular labyrinthine function was normal. This was true even in the cases of chondromyxosarcoma where there was extensive destruction of the petrous bone. The preservation of labyrinthine function underlines the resistance of the bony labyrinth to tumor erosion. However, extensive tumors may eventually destroy the bony labyrinth wall and cause loss of auditory and vestibular function as in Case 3.

Radiological Findings. While conventional routine x-rays of the petrous bone

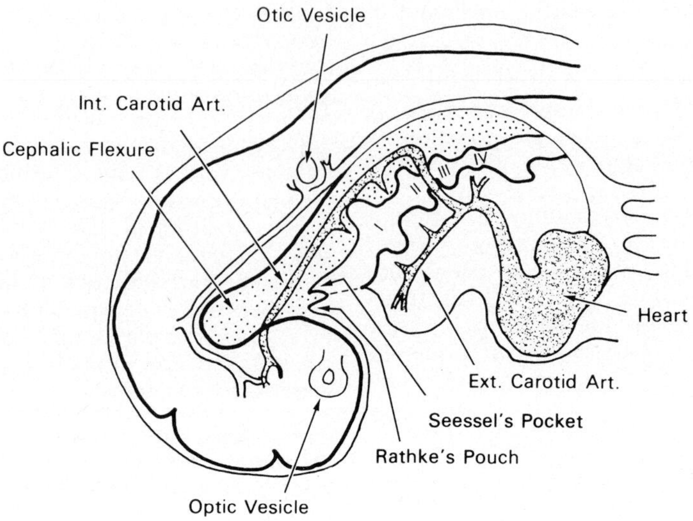

Fig. 7. Drawing of the cephalic flexure and relationship to the internal carotid artery at the one-month embryo stage. Note the location of Seessel's pocket and Rathke's pouch adjacent to the stomodeal plate (broken line). Roman numerals I-IV identify branchial pouches. (Redrawn from Figure 74 in Patten, B. M., *Human Embryology*, McGraw-Hill, 1953. Used with permission of McGraw-Hill Book Company.)

and the base of the skull may occasionally provide clear evidence of an osteolytic lesion at the petrous apex, frequently when the tumor is small the findings on plain views are equivocal and confirmatory evidence may be obtained with polytomography and arteriography. In all cases in this series, there was radiological evidence of bone destruction at the petrous apex. Plain views and tomograms of the petrous bone demonstrated this radiologic defect. In the extensive tumors, the area of bone destruction extended posteriorly to include the jugular foramen and the hypoglossal canal and anteriorly to involve the sphenoid sinus. Arteriography in all cases consistently showed lateral displacement of the petrous segment of the internal carotid artery by an avascular mass. Pneumoencephalography showed these tumors to be extradural in location.

Origin of Tumors. It seems likely that these tumors of the petrous apex arose from the foramen lacerum. The foramen lacerum is the name given to the space (occupied by the basal fibrocartilage) with jagged margins between the pars basilaris of the occipital bone and the temporal wing of the sphenoid bone on the one hand, and the apex of the petrous segment of the temporal bone on the other.

Several reasons may be given as support for the hypothesis that these tumors arose from the foramen lacerum.

1. The foramen lacerum normally contains fibrocartilage, a mesenchymal derivative of embryonic development. This fibrocartilage appears the most likely source for the origin of chondroid tumors, although other cartilage rests are located in the enchondral bone layer of the bony labyrinth. However, if the cartilage tumors arose in the enchondral layer, loss of labyrinthine function would be an expected early sign.

2. While no structures pass through the foramen lacerum, there are two types of structures that course across the foramen. These are the internal carotid artery and the nerves which merge to form the vidian nerve (greater superficial petrosal and deep petrosal). Therefore, tumors of neural origin can arise in the foramen lacerum with little or no ob-

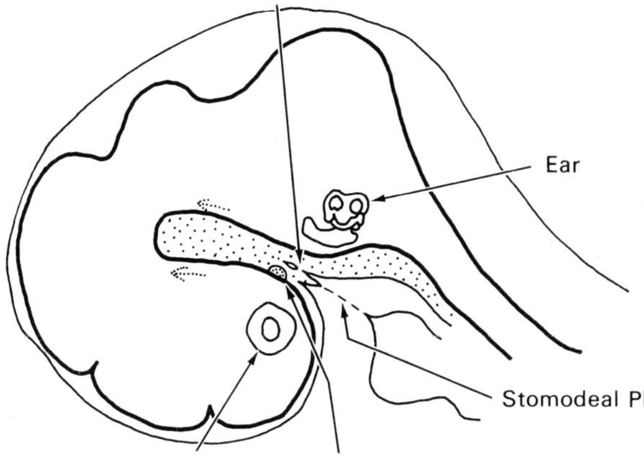

Fig. 8. This drawing illustrates the proposed mechanism whereby epithelial rests from Seessel's pocket are trapped in the mesenchyme (stippled area) of the cephalic flexure. Dotted arrows indicate the deepening of the cephalic flexure which promotes the entrapment of epithelial rests.

vious signs or symptoms related to the involved nerve.

3. The foramen lacerum appears to be a likely area for epithelial remnants to be trapped during embryonic development and then develop later into congenital epidermoid cysts.

Early in embryonic development one of the important changes occurring is flexion of the embryo from a straight to a semicircular shape in order to conform to the limited space in utero.[20] Bending of the ectodermal tube which will form the central nervous system produces the cephalic flexure (Fig. 7). In a one-month embryo the internal carotid artery, which ascends through the cephalic flexure, is recognizable after absorption of the intersegmental arterial branches between pharyngeal pouches. An invagination at the stomodeum reaches toward the primitive gut to the point where a stomodeal plate is formed marking the transition between ectodermal and entodermal epithelium. Resorption of this stomodeal plate occurs early in embryonic development. Concomitant with the resorption of the stomodeal plate is the lengthening of the cephalic flexure and an associated shift of the mesenchyme filling the flexure. Accompanying this movement is a withdrawal of the epithelium adjacent to the stomodeal plate into the cephalic flexure. The most external of these epithelial invaginations is Rathke's pouch and the internal one is Seessel's pocket (Fig. 7).

As these two epithelial invaginations are drawn up into the mesenchymal tissue filling the cephalic flexure, isolated epithelial remnants of Rathke's pouch or Seessel's pocket may remain. Epithelial remnants derived from Rathke's pouch in the midline form a portion of the adult hypophysis. It seems possible that isolated epithelial islands from the lateral recesses of a deep Seessel's pocket may also remain trapped in condensing mesenchyme at the base of the cephalic flexure (Fig. 8). While most of the mesenchyme in the cephalic flexure undergoes resorption, a small portion at the base forms the fibrocartilage filling the foramen lacerum. Support for the contention that the base of the cephalic flexure is identical with the foramen lacerum is shown in Figure 9, where the trigeminal ganglion can be seen stretching across from the petrous apex to the mandibular region, and in Figure 10,

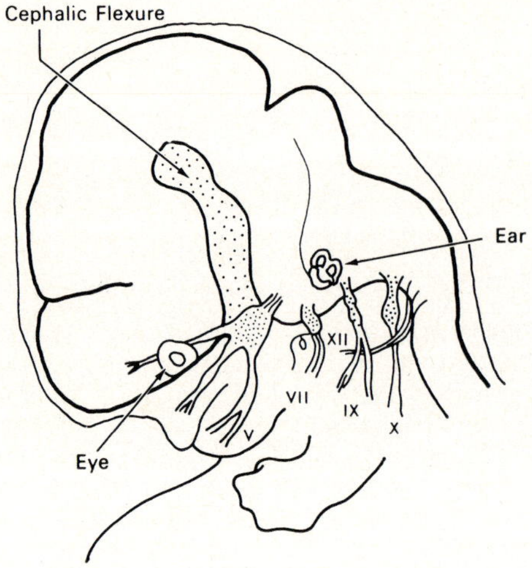

Fig. 9. Drawing which shows the relationship of the trigeminal nerve and ganglion to the cephalic flexure, the eye and the ear, and the other cranial nerves. Note how the ganglion is located anterolateral to the base of the flexure, indicating that this area is located at the apex of the petrous pyramid. (Redrawn from Figure 66 in Patten, B. M., *Human Embryology*. McGraw-Hill, 1953. Used with permission of McGraw-Hill Book Company.)

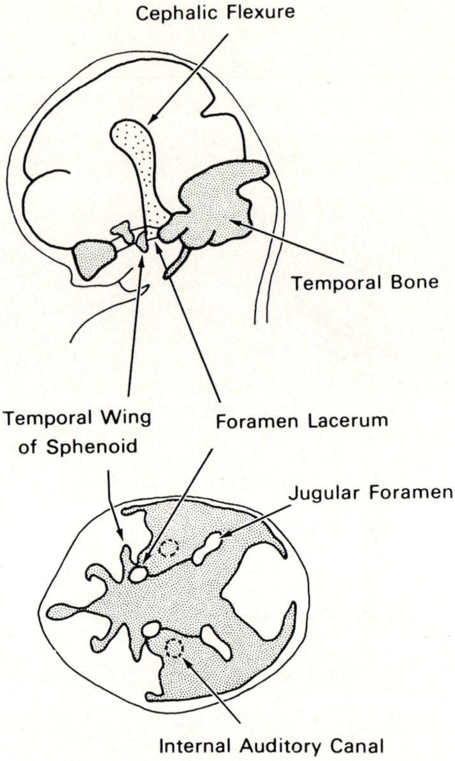

Fig. 10. Drawing of the ossification of the bones at the base of the skull (heavy stipple) and their relationship to the cephalic flexure. Note how the base of the flexure is located between the apex of the petrous bone and the temporal wing of the sphenoid bone. The mesenchyme in the cephalic flexure (light stipple) forms the cartilage in the foramen lacerum. Upper drawing represents side view, lower drawing is a base view of the skull. (Redrawn from Figure 165 in Patten, B. M., *Human Embryology*, McGraw-Hill, 1953. Used with permission of McGraw-Hill Book Company.)

where the ossification of bones at the base of the skull in the embryo can be seen. The ossification of the temporal bone and the temporal wing of the sphenoid surrounds the base of the cephalic flexure. Incomplete fusion of these ossification centers and retention of mesenchyme as fibrocartilage form the adult foramen lacerum. Retained epithelial remnants of Seessel's pocket may be entrapped in this fibrocartilage and give rise to congenital epidermoid cysts or cholesteatomas later in life.

4. Finally, the pattern of expansion and involvement of structures surrounding the base of the skull suggests that these primary tumors of the petrous apex arise from the foramen lacerum. Figure 11 demonstrates the relationship of the foramen ovale, Eustachian tube, and the internal carotid artery to the foramen lacerum. Expanding tumors from the foramen lacerum would most likely involve these structures before other structures at the base of the skull. Tumors arising in more distant areas such as the jugular foramen or the middle ear would involve other structures such as the tympanic membrane, the facial nerve or the nerves of the jugular foramen before involving structures at the petrous apex. Lateral displacement of the internal carotid artery by tumors in this region would argue against epithelial rests from the Eustachian tube (branchial pouch I) as the source of congenital cholesteatoma of the apex. If the epidermoid arose from Eustachian tube elements, the internal

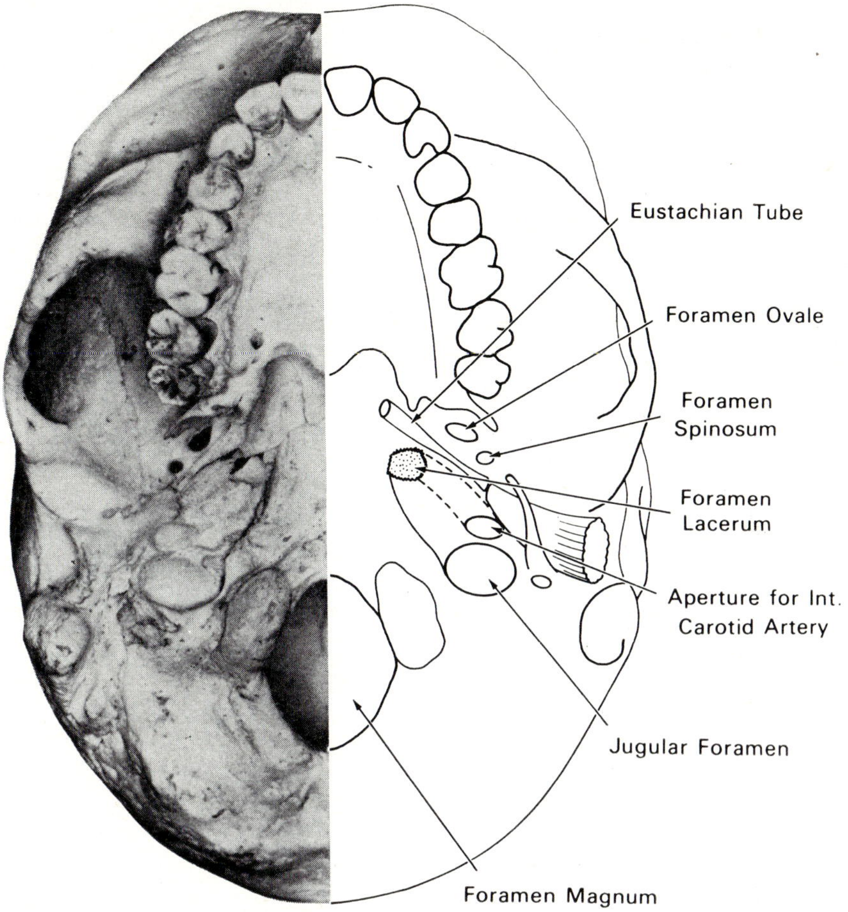

Fig. 11. Half photograph and half drawing of structures at the base of the skull. Note relationship of Eustachian tube, foramen ovale, and internal carotid artery to the foramen lacerum.

carotid artery would be displaced medially.

Stages in Growth of Tumor. In the otological and neurosurgical literature, primary epidermoids of the petrous apex have been described in three clinical forms.

1. Olivecrona[19] and Revilla[13,14] have emphasized the association of mandibular division of the trigeminal nerve signs along with normal VIII and VII nerve function in patients with primary epidermoid of the petrous apex. Normal radiological and neurological examinations were also usually present. It is likely that these patients are seen primarily by the neurosurgeon because of the large number of patients with tic douloureaux treated by this specialty.

2. In the otological literature the characteristic clinical presentation of primary petrous apex epidermoid consists of VII and VIII nerve deficits either with or without cholesteatoma in the middle ear or mastoid.[9-11,17] This association is undoubtedly related to the presence of otological functional deficits at the time of diagnosis. Otological reports of patients with petrous apex congenital cholesteatoma having normal VII and VIII nerve function are rare.[12]

3. Primary epidermoids are included

in the classifications of cerebellopontine angle tumors when there is encroachment of the nerves in the internal auditory canal by a mass lesion which is usually located anterior to the VII and VIII nerves in the posterior cranial fossa. Trigeminal nerve involvement is sometimes used to differentiate clinically epidermoid from other cerebellopontine angle tumors. This description of primary epidermoid is present in both the neurosurgical[13,14,19] and otological[15,16,18] literature.

An analysis of the patients described in this report and in the literature points to a common pattern of expansion in the petrous apex. The bone of the apex contains marrow spaces and would more likely allow for expansion of a tumor than the other solid bony components of the skull. Knowledge of the structures surrounding the foramen lacerum provides a guideline for early detection of expanding tumors in this area.

Based on the involvement of surrounding structures at the base of the skull, primary tumors at the petrous apex may be divided clinically into three stages which more or less correspond to the clinical types described in the literature.

Stage I. Tumors at this stage involve those structures in the immediate vicinity of the foramen lacerum. These are: the middle or posterior fossa dura attached to the petrous apex, the mandibular division of the trigeminal (V) nerve, the Eustachian tube, and the internal carotid artery. Symptoms resulting from encroachment on these structures are: headache, pain, anesthesia or paresthesia in the distribution of the third division of the V nerve, hearing loss or a blocked feeling in the ear, and various complaints related to cerebral ischemia such as blurred vision or faintness.

At this stage only one or two of these structures may be clinically involved and otolaryngological examination including evaluation of labyrinthine function may be entirely normal. Therefore, a high index of suspicion is necessary in order to make the diagnosis of tumor at the petrous apex. Careful radiological evaluation of the base of the skull is the simplest and most informative diagnostic study to carry out. Failure to suspect a lesion at the petrous apex at this early stage may lead to unnecessary surgical treatment for Eustachian tube obstruction (myringotomy with insertion of ventilating tubes, simple mastoidectomy) and potentially dangerous delays in diagnosis.

Stage II. As the tumors enlarge, extension is usually in a posterior or anterior direction because the bone in these areas at the base of the skull offers the least resistance. Compression of the VII and VIII nerves at the internal auditory meatus, cranial nerves IX, X and XI in the jugular foramen, and the XII nerve in the hypoglossal foramen may occur with posterior extension. Cranial nerves III, IV, and VI may become involved with anterior extension of the tumor toward the cavernous sinus. These neurological deficits make the diagnosis of petrous apex tumor more apparent.

Stage III. Further extension of an expanding neoplasm at the petrous apex may involve a region where the tumor mass can be detected by clinical examination. These areas are: the nasopharynx, the middle and posterior cranial fossae, the middle ear, or the infratemporal fossa. Detection of tumor in such areas may be by direct visualization and palpation (nasopharynx, middle ear or neck) or by the effects of tumor compression on vital structures such as the brain stem (the posterior cranial fossa). When such extension involves the posterior fossa, a cerebellopontine angle tumor mass is present.

The bony labyrinth resists erosion from the enlargement of these tumors.[21] Therefore, normal labyrinthine function is frequently found on clinical evaluation. However, this resistance is not absolute and with extensive erosion, loss of labyrinthine function and facial paralysis may occur. Seventh and VIII cranial nerve function may be impaired by direct compression of the nerves as they course toward the brain stem or by erosion of the bony labyrinth wall. When

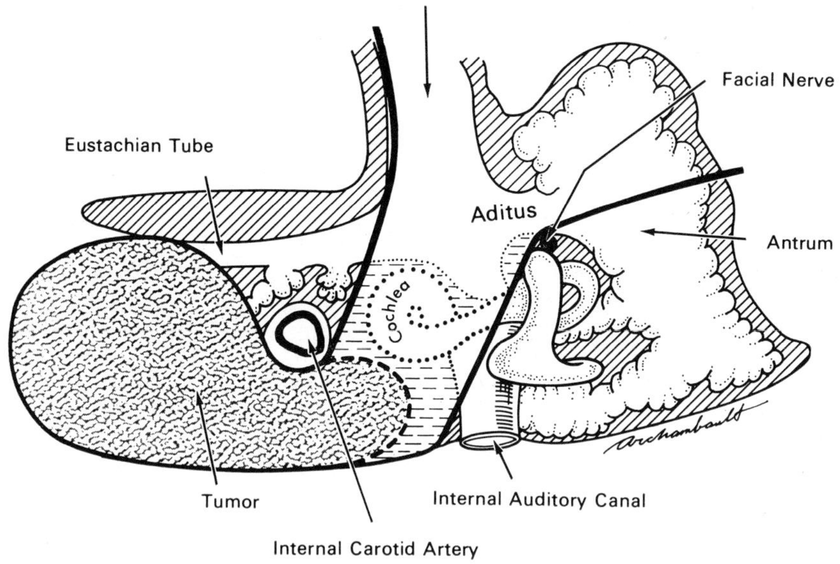

Fig. 12. Drawing of the temporal bone showing the otologic approach to fistulize (heavy solid lines) a tumor located in the petrous apex. Areas surrounding the cochlea (dashed + dotted lines) indicate bone removal necessary to reach the tumor after exposure with radical mastoidectomy.

these signs are present they are late indications of a petrous apex tumor.

DIAGNOSIS

Since tumors at the petrous apex are inaccessible to direct clinical detection, early diagnosis must rest on a high index of suspicion based on recognition of the early signs and symptoms of expanding tumors at the petrous apex. When there is an indication of involvement of the dura of the cranial fossae, the mandibular division of the V cranial nerve, the Eustachian tube, or the internal carotid artery, then conventional radiological views and tomography of the petrous apices and the base of the skull should be obtained. If no abnormality is found, then careful follow-up examination at five to six month intervals should be carried out if symptoms persist.

If an area of bone destruction at the petrous apex is detected, then pneumoencephalography, brain scan, and carotid arteriography are the most helpful diagnostic studies that may be performed. These studies along with a complete otolaryngologic and neurologic examination are usually sufficient to rule out other entities in the differential diagnosis such as petrositis, metastatic nasopharyngeal carcinoma, metastatic carcinoma from a distant primary (such as breast, thyroid and prostate), glomus jugulare tumor, meningioma, internal carotid artery aneurysm, and eosinophilic granuloma. If the lesion is one of the primary neoplasms of the foramen lacerum discussed in this study, the diagnostic studies would demonstrate an avascular extradural mass lesion at the petrous apex which displaces the internal carotid artery laterally.

SURGICAL MANAGEMENT

Delay in diagnosis of petrous apex tumors resulted in no treatment (Case 5) or in treatment for a relatively benign condition secondary to tumor growth such as serous otitis media (Cases 1, 3 and 4). This delay can probably be attributed to a lack of awareness of the early signs and symptoms of these tumors and as a result inadequate radiological evaluation of the petrous apex of the temporal bone.

Once the radiological diagnosis of a destructive lesion at the petrous apex was made, exploration of the petrous apex was carried out in Cases 1, 2 and 5. It was clear from the experience with Case 1 that simple exploration and evacuation of the primary epidermoid cyst of the petrous apex does not result in permanent relief of symptoms. Permanent fistulization was then the goal in the treatment of congenital cholesteatomas of the petrous apex. A conservative approach to fistulizing the congenital epidermoid in Case 1 met with failure. In this patient, a fistula into the cyst was created anterior to the carotid canal and skin grafted with preservation of labyrinthine function; the fistula closed eventually because it was not wide enough. The successful operation in Case 1 consisted of complete labyrinthectomy and removal of the bony labyrinth from the internal auditory canal to the internal carotid artery (Fig. 12) and lining the bony fistula with split-thickness skin grafts. The effectiveness of this approach was again demonstrated in Case 2 where, at the initial surgical procedure, the transmastoid and translabyrinthine fistulization of the congenital cholesteatoma was successful.

Surgical exploration of the petrous apex tumor in Case 3 was carried out to prevent the occurrence of complications from rupture of an extensive primary epidermoid cyst. Instead, exploration and biopsy via the translabyrinthine route revealed a solid benign tumor which was too extensive to remove safely. The surgical procedure in this case served a diagnostic purpose.

In Case 4 the chondromyxosarcoma was too extensive at its initial recognition to permit effective surgical or radiotherapeutic management. The surgical procedures performed provided 1) histological diagnosis and 2) neurosurgical decompression of the expanding tumor. The patient eventually died from an intracranial complication of the primary tumor. In Case 5 where the tumor was diagnosed histologically, following the approach to the petrous apex through a large infralabyrinthine cell tract, a drainage procedure was accomplished by fistulizing the tumor mass. Radiation therapy has been administered.

SURGICAL APPROACHES TO THE PETROUS APEX

Because of the inaccessible location of the tumors in the petrous apex, complete extirpative surgery is usually not possible. Therefore, the surgical management consists of diagnostic exploration and fistulization of the expanding mass. Biopsy is necessary to obtain tissue diagnosis; fistulization either may form the definitive treatment, as in the case of primary epidermoid cysts, or may act as a drainage procedure for necrotic tumor cells following radiation therapy for chondromyxosarcoma. There are several surgical approaches to the petrous apex.

Middle Fossa Extradural. This approach to the petrous apex via the middle cranial fossa can serve to reach the tumor for diagnostic purposes. Biopsy of a solid tissue mass or aspiration of a cystic lesion may be accomplished via this route but permanent fistulization is not possible. Thus in the case of primary epidermoid cysts, recurrence is frequently the case as demonstrated in Case 1 in the present series. An advantage of this procedure is that labyrinthine function may be preserved.

Posterior Fossa Craniotomy. The morbidity associated with this approach limits its usefulness to those tumors of the cerebellopontine angle where the neoplasm may be intracranial in origin, thus requiring intracranial removal. This approach may also be necessary as a decompression procedure where intracranial extension of a petrous apex tumor may produce signs of brain stem compression (as in Case 4). However, some neurosurgical reports have described complete or near complete removal of epidermoids using this approach.

Transethmoidosphenoid. This approach through the ethmoid and sphenoid sinus to the petrous apex has been described to successfully fistulize congenital epidermoid cysts at the petrous apex.[12] While this can be accomplished via this route, the space limitation may add difficulty to the maintenance of a permanent fistula into the cyst. It is not possible to apply skin grafts to the fistula, and one must depend on the opening of the fenestra in the sphenoid sinus to maintain a fistula. Furthermore, the risk of an ascending infection into the permanently fistulized lesion from a potentially contaminated area such as the nasopharynx must be considered. The difficulty of evacuating a keratin filled mass through the nasal cavity may also be a minor disadvantage of this procedure. On the other hand, the preservation of labyrinthine function is a major advantage of this approach to the petrous apex.

Transmastoid - Translabyrinthine. In this approach, a wide field mastoidectomy and removal of the cochlea is essential in order to expose the tumor. Meticulous removal of all vestibular sensory tissue is also necessary to assure complete elimination of all vestibular function and a satisfactory recovery from the labyrinthectomy. Purposeful destruction of the cochlear and vestibular labyrinth is justified in order to successfully expose a life-threatening lesion at the apex of the temporal bone. A wide bony fistula into the petrous apex is created by exenterating the bone from the carotid canal anteriorly to the descending facial nerve posteriorly and from the jugular bulb inferiorly to the middle cranial fossa superiorly (Fig. 12). As the petrous apex is exposed, solid tissue may be obtained for biopsy or the contents of an epidermoid cyst may be evacuated completely. The bony fistula is then lined with split-thickness skin grafts that are held in place with packing. Packing for 10-14 days is sufficient to allow for the implantation of skin grafts. After a large fistulous tract into the petrous apex has been created, the cystic space can be easily aspirated on an outpatient basis and little chance of ascending infection is present. The most significant disadvantage of this procedure is the loss of labyrinthine function. However, this is justifiable in order to achieve relief of symptoms and the complete control of a potentially life-threatening tumor. In the case of solid tumors as chondromyxosarcoma, a wide fistulous opening may provide satisfactory drainage of necrotic tumor following radiation therapy.

Factors Influencing Choice of Surgical Approach. Regardless of approach, the fundamental aim of surgery is to reach the tumor and to form a permanent fistula into it. Since a lesion at the petrous apex cannot be marsupialized via the middle or posterior fossa route, the effective choice is either the nasal or the middle ear approach. This choice can be guided by several factors.

Preference of the Surgeon. Familiarity with the anatomical variations and surgical technique associated with sphenoid or middle ear surgery must be considered by the surgeon. Experience with surgical anatomy and its variations are essential to approaching the petrous apex safely and the surgeon should choose the route with which he feels most confident.

The otologic approach is favored over the rhinologic one in this report for several reasons: 1) The middle ear route is more direct and the working distance to the apex is less. Therefore, the contents of the cholesteatoma or solid tumor can be aspirated more easily. 2) Split-thickness skin grafts may be applied to the bony fistula by means of the middle ear route. 3) There is less chance for ascending infection from the middle ear into a fistulized cyst as compared to the nasopharynx.

Degree of Labyrinthine Function in the Involved and Uninvolved Ear. If the hearing on the side with tumor is profoundly depressed, the otologic approach is clearly indicated. However, if the involved ear represents an only-hearing ear, then the nasal approach to fistulize the petrous apex tumor through the sphenoid sinus should be considered.

Additional Incidental Factors. If both ears have normal inner ear function, then other anatomical and pathological factors guide the decision. These may be real or potential factors. The presence of a sclerotic sphenoid sinus or of chronic sinusitis would contraindicate the nasal approach. Even the potential risk of ascending infection into a fistulized cyst may favor the otologic approach. The sacrifice of labyrinthine function in one ear is justified by the serious nature of an expanding cholesteatoma or solid tumor in the petrous apex. In petrous apex tumors that have extended outside the apex (Stage III), the extension into the sphenoid sinus or middle ear may dictate the logical approach.

Massachusetts Eye and Ear Infirmary, 243 Charles St., Boston, Mass. 02114.

REFERENCES

1. Naufal PM: Primary sarcomas of the temporal bone. Arch Otolaryngol 98:44-50, 1973

2. Tucker WN: Cancer of the middle ear. Cancer 18:642-650, 1965

3. Day KM: A primary cholesteatoma of the middle ear. Ann Otol Rhinol Laryngol 64: 161-163, 1955

4. Derlacki EL, Clemis JD: Congenital cholesteatoma of the middle ear and mastoid. Ann Otol Rhinol Laryngol 74:706-727, 1965

5. Derlacki EL: Congenital cholesteatoma of the middle ear and mastoid. Arch Otolaryngol 97:177-182, 1972

6. House HP: An apparent primary cholesteatoma. Laryngoscope 63:712-713, 1953

7. Kerr AG, Smyth GD: Congenital cholesteatoma of the temporal bone. Laryngoscope 77:86-88, 1967

8. Sheehy JL: True cholesteatoma. Arch Otolaryngol 69:57-60, 1959

9. Brookler KH, Pulec JL and Hallberg OE: Congenital cholesteatoma of the temporal bone. Arch Otolaryngol 90:71-74, 1969

10. Cawthorne E, Griffith A: Primary cholesteatoma of the temporal bone. Arch Otolaryngol 73:252-261, 1961

11. Cawthorne T: Congenital cholesteatoma. Arch Otolaryngol 78:248-252, 1963

12. Cole TB, McCoy G: Congenital cholesteatoma of temporal bone and sphenoid sinus. Arch Otolaryngol 87:576-579, 1968

13. Revilla AG: Tic douloureaux and its relationship to tumors of the posterior fossa. J Neurosurg 4:233-239, 1947

14. Revilla AG: Differential diagnosis of tumors at the cerebellopontile recess. Bull Johns Hopk Hosp 83:187-212, 1948

15. Hitselberger WE, House WF: Tumors of the cerebellopontine angle. Arch Otolaryngol 80:720-731, 1964

16. House WF, Doyle JB Jr: Early diagnosis and removal of primary cholesteatoma causing pressure to eighth nerve. Laryngoscope 72:1053-1062, 1962

17. Jefferson G, Smalley AA: Progressive facial palsy produced by intratemporal dermoids. J Laryngol Otol 53:417, 1938

18. Lewis ML, Echols DH: Pearly tumor of the cerebellopontine angle. Report of a case with reversible deafness. Laryngoscope 61: 1123-1125, 1951

19. Olivecrona H: Cholesteatomas of the cerebellopontine angle. Acta Psychiat et Neurol 24:639-643, 1949

20. Patten BM: *Human Embryology,* ed. 2. New York, McGraw-Hill, 1953

21. Proctor B, Lindsay JR: Tumors involving the petrous pyramid of the temporal bone. Arch Otolaryngol 46:180-194, 1947

PARTICIPANTS IN THE WORKSHOP ON TONSILLECTOMY AND ADENOIDECTOMY

Charles D. Bluestone, M.D., Workshop Chairman, Professor of Otolaryngology, University of Pittsburgh School of Medicine, Director of the Department of Otolaryngology, Children's Hospital of Pittsburgh, 125 DeSoto Street, Pittsburgh, Pennsylvania 15213.

Leona Baumgartner, M.D., Visiting Professor, Department Social Medicine, Harvard Medical School, 10 Shattuck Street, Boston, Massachusetts 02115.

Virgil M. Howie, M.D., Pediatrician, 2345 Whitesburg Drive, South, Huntsville, Alabama 35801.

Peter Hurst, M.D., Department of Pediatrics, Kaiser Permanente, 5055 North Greeley Avenue, Portland, Oregon 97217.

Geza J. Jako, M.D., Research Professor, Otolaryngology, Boston University School of Medicine, Director, Otolaryngology Research, University Hospital, 750 Harrison Avenue, Boston, Massachusetts 02111.

Edward H. Kass, M.D., William Ellery Channing Professor of Medicine, Harvard Medical School, Director, Channing Laboratory, 774 Albany Street, Boston, Massachusetts 02118.

Jerome O. Klein, M.D., Associate Professor Pediatrics, Harvard Medical School, Associate Director Pediatrics, Boston City Hospital, Channing Laborary, 774 Albany Street, Boston, Massachusetts 02118.

George Lamb, M.D., Associate Professor, Preventive and Social Medicine, Harvard Medical School, Chief, Division of Community Child Health, Children's Hospital Medical Center, Boston, Massachusetts 02115.

Jere Mead, M.D., Professor of Physiology, Harvard School of Public Health, 665 Huntington Avenue, Boston, Massachusetts 02115.

Abraham Morag, M.D., Professor, Department of Pediatrics and Microbiology, The Children's Hospital, 219 Bryant Street, Buffalo, New York 14222.

Hughlett L. Morris, Ph.D., Professor of Speech Pathology, University of Iowa School of Medicine, Director, Division of Speech and Hearing, University Hospital, Iowa City, Iowa 52242.

Pearay L. Ogra, M.D., Professor, Departments of Pediatrics and Microbiology, University of Buffalo, The Children's Hospital, 219 Bryant Street, Buffalo, New York 14222.

Joseph H. Ogura, M.D., Professor and Head, Department of Otolaryngology, Washington University School of Medicine, 517 So. Euclid, St. Louis, Missouri 63110.

Arthur Oleinick, M.D., Head, Epidemiology Studies Section, Kaiser Foundation Hospitals, Health Services Research Center, 4610 S.E. Belmont, Portland, Oregon 97215.

Jack L. Paradise, M.D., Associate Professor of Pediatrics and Community Medicine, School of Medicine, University of Pittsburgh; Director, Ambulatory Services, Children's Hospital of Pittsburgh, Pittsburgh, Pennsylvania 15213.

Donald F. Proctor, M.D., Professor, Laryngology and Otology, Johns Hopkins School of Medicine, Professor, Environmental Medicine, Johns Hopkins School of Hygiene and Public Health, 615 North Wolfe Street, Baltimore, Maryland 21205.

Samuel Pruzansky, D.D.S., Director, Center for Craniofacial Anomalies, University of Illinois Medical Center, P. O. Box 998, Chicago, Illinois 60680.

Buckminster Ranney, M.D., Extramural Programs, National Institute of Neurological Diseases and Stroke, Westwood Building, Room 7 A 16, 53333 Westbard Avenue, Bethesda, Maryland 20014.

Bernard Rosner, Ph.D., Instructor Preventive Medicine, Harvard Medical School, Lecturer on Statistics, Harvard University, Channing Laboratory, 774 Albany Street, Boston, Massachusetts 02118.

Asher H. Shapiro, Sc.D., Professor and Head, Department of Mechanical Engineering, Massachusetts Institute of Technology, Room 3174, Cambridge, Massachusetts 02139.

Philip Sprinkle, M.D., Professor and Chairman, Division of Otolaryngology, West Virginia University, School of Medicine, Morgantown, West Virginia 26506.

Norman S. Stearns, M.D., Associate Dean for Continuing Education, Tufts University School of Medicine, 136 Harrison Avenue, Boston, Massachusetts 02111.

Sylvan E. Stool, M.D., Associate Professor, Otolaryngology, University of Pennsylvania, Children's Hospital of Philadelphia, 1740 Bainbridge Street, Philadelphia, Pennsylvania 19146.

J. Daniel Subtelny, D.D.S., Chairman, Orthodontics Department, Eastman Dental Center, 800 Main Street, Rochester, New York 14612.

Floyd H. Taylor, Sc.D., Associate Research Professor of Community Medicine, School of Medicine, University of Pittsburgh, Pittsburgh, Pennsylvania 15261.

Stanley Walzer, M.D., Career Investigator, National Institute of Mental Health, Assistant Professor, Psychiatry, Harvard Medical School, Senior Associate in Genetics, Children's Hospital Medical Center, Judge Baker Guidance Center, 295 Longwood Avenue, Boston, Massachusetts 02115.

Louis Weinstein, M.D., Visiting Professor of Medicine, Harvard Medical School; Physician, Peter Bent Brigham Hospital, Boston, Massachusetts 02115.

TABLE OF CONTENTS

PAGE

CHAPTER I. BACKGROUND AND OBJECTIVES OF THE CONFERENCE 7

CHAPTER II. STATE OF THE ART AND CURRENT PROBLEMS. 8

CHAPTER III. FORMAL PAPERS. 15

Pittsburgh Tonsillectomy and Adenoidectomy Study: Differences from Earlier Studies and Problems of Execution. Jack L. Paradise, M.D., Pittsburgh, Pennsylvania. 15

Collaborative Studies. Edward H. Kass, M.D., Boston, Massachusetts. 20

Involvement of a Prepaid Health Plan in Prospective Studies on Tonsillectomy and Adenoidectomy. Peter L. Hurst, M.D., Portland, Oregon. 22

Criteria for the Diagnosis of Adenotonsillitis. Philip M. Sprinkle, M.D., Morgantown, West Virginia. 25

Microbiology of Diseases of Tonsils and Adenoids. Jerome O. Klein, M.D., Boston, Massachusetts. 30

Diseases of the Tonsils and Adenoids in Adults. Louis Weinstein, M.D., Boston, Massachusetts. 34

Immunologic Aspect of Tonsils. Abraham Morag, M.D., Pearay L. Ogra, M.D., Buffalo, New York. 37

Obstructive Adenoids in Relation to Otitis Media. Charles D. Bluestone, M.D., Pittsburgh, Pennsylvania. 44

Effect of Upper Airway Obstruction on the Lower Airway and Cardiovascular System. Joseph H. Ogura, M.D., St. Louis, Missouri. 49

Effect of Diseases of Tonsils and Adenoids on Dentofacial Morphology. J. Daniel Subtelny, D.D.S., Rochester, New York. 50

Roentgencephalometric Studies of Tonsils and Adenoids in Normal and Pathologic States. Samuel Pruzansky, D.D.S., Chicago, Illinois. 55

The Speech Pathologist Looks at the Tonsils and the Adenoids. Hughlett L. Morris, Ph.D., Iowa City, Iowa. 63

Natural History of Otitis Media. Virgil M. Howie, M.D., Huntsville, Alabama. 67

Diseases of the Tonsils and Adenoids in Relation to Rhinitis and Sinusitis. Sylvan E. Stool, M.D., Philadelphia, Pennsylvania. 73

CHAPTER IV. REPORTS OF SUBCOMMITTEES. 75

CHAPTER V. CONCLUSIONS AND RECOMMENDATIONS. 78

This Workshop was supported in part by Grant No. 1 R13 NS 12042-01 awarded by the National Institute of Neurological Diseases and Stroke, DHEW.

CHAPTER I

BACKGROUND AND OBJECTIVES OF THE CONFERENCE

I. Background: Origin of the Conference

Early in 1973 an *Ad Hoc* Committee on Tonsillectomy and Adenoidectomy was formed in an attempt to define "state of the art" and to arrive at a consensus on management. The Committee members were selected on the basis of their clinical and research interests and represented divergent opinions on the subject. The Committee consisted of the following members:

Charles D. Bluestone, M.D., Chairman.

Virgil M. Howie, M.D.
Jerome O. Klein, M.D.
Alexander D. Langmuir, M.D.
Arnold G. Maran, M.D., F.R.C.S.
Pearay L. Ogra, M.D.
Jack L. Paradise, M.D.
Philip M. Sprinkle, M.D.
Sylvan E. Stool, M.D.
Floyd H. Taylor, Sc.D.
Louis Weinstein, M.D.

The Committee met on October 7 and 8, 1973, in Toronto, and on March 1, 1974, in Pittsburgh. They defined the problems as the following:

1. Inadequate Knowledge.

2. Inadequate Communication and Education.

3. Lack of Concern in Finding Solutions.

4. Socioeconomic Considerations.

The Committee concluded its initial report and recommended that high priority consideration be given to the initiation of prospective investigations, the purpose of which would be to define as specifically as possible, optimal methods of management of the diseases of the tonsils and adenoids. The Committee also suggested studies leading to better understanding of epidemiology, pathogenesis, and pathophysiology.

In January, 1974, a formal request for a Workshop on Tonsillectomy and Adenoidectomy was submitted to the National Institutes of Neurological Diseases and Stroke section of the National Institutes of Health. In April, 1974, the grant request was approved and the Workshop was convened on June 12-14, 1974, at the Marriott Motor Hotel in West Newton, Massachusetts.

II. Objectives of the Conference

The objectives of the Conference were the following:

1. To decide whether or not a nationwide collaborative prospective controlled study of tonsillectomy and adenoidectomy is indicated.

2. Determine the feasibility of such a prospective study of tonsillectomy and adenoidectomy.

3. Discuss the planning phase if such a study is found to be both indicated and feasible.

4. Define research questions related to epidemiology, pathogenesis and pathophysiology, diagnosis and management of the diseases of the tonsils and adenoids.

5. Determine the best possible methods of solution of these research questions related to either a prospective study or separate concurrent investigations, or both.

6. Determine the best manner in which to disseminate the information and conclusions of the Conference.

CHAPTER II

STATE OF THE ART AND CURRENT PROBLEMS*

Nine participants in the Workshop on Tonsillectomy and Adenoidectomy were members of the *Ad Hoc* Committee on Tonsillectomy and Adenoidectomy and prepared this report.

The purpose of the Committee was to examine available knowledge of diseases of the tonsils and adenoids and not to examine the performance of tonsillectomy and adenoidectomy in the individual patient. The state of the art and current problems are summarized in the following outline.

THE PROBLEM

Inadequate Knowledge. The information present in the literature is not adequate to answer certain pertinent questions (see literature review).

1. What are the clinical and microbiological criteria for the diagnosis of tonsillitis and adenoiditis?

2. What is the pathogenesis of the diseases of the tonsils and adenoids?

3. What is the pathophysiology of the diseases of the tonsils and adenoids?

4. What are the characteristics of the populations affected by the diseases of the tonsils and adenoids?

5. What are the criteria for treatment of diseases of the tonsils and adenoids?

6. What are the most effective surgical and nonsurgical methods of treatment?

7. How do these disorders and their management affect health?

Inadequate Communication and Education. Neither health professionals nor the public have sufficient information concerning the nature of the problem. Inadequate communication exists among members of the health profession. Preconceived ideas rather than scientific data frequently determine the method of treatment.

Lack of Concern in Finding Solutions. Neither practitioners, investigators, nor funding agencies have shown much interest in exploring the problem.

"*Socioeconomic Considerations.* It is well known that wide divergencies in practice regarding tonsillectomy and adenoidectomy exist between nations, geographic areas, systems of health care delivery, and medical and surgical specialties. These differences, in turn, reflect differences among individual physicians in a variety of factors, including nature of training, quality of judgment, vulnerability to parental pressure, method of remuneration, and sensitivity to financial incentives when such exist."**

In the past, more children in higher socioeconomic groups have received the operation than in lower. In the United Kingdom, four times as many children in private schools have had tonsillectomy by age 14 as those in public schools. In the United States, ten times as many children receiving care from private physicians had tonsillectomies as those who went to clinics. It is estimated that about 1,000,000 tonsillectomies and adenoidectomies and adenotonsillectomies are performed in the United States each year which would make the operation a 375-500 million dollar health industry. In the United Kingdom there were 200,000 procedures performed at an estimated cost of £3,000,000 in 1969, perhaps £5,000,000 in 1973, for which the

*Certain modifications and deletions were made by the Editor with the approval of the Executive Committee of the Workshop.

**Quotation from an article by Paradise JL: Clinical Trials of Tonsillectomy and Adenoidectomy: Limitations of Earlier Studies, and a Latter-Day Design. Submitted for publication.

Department of Health bears the cost. However, the cost effectiveness is unknown.

LITERATURE REVIEW[1*]

There exists a general feeling among critical observers that the majority of these procedures may be unnecessary or actually harmful, but even thoughtful and conscientious physicians maintain divergent attitudes and practices on the matter. Thus, some of them, cognizant of potential anesthetic, immunologic, and psychologic risks, and of widely publicized condemnations of the procedure, almost routinely refuse to consider tonsillectomy for any of their patients; others, having cared for patients who appear to have been helped — sometimes dramatically — by tonsillectomy or adenoidectomy or both, continue to recommend surgery for selected patients. A recent poll conducted among physicians in general practice and in various specialties attests to appreciable disagreements among them also with regard to tonsil and adenoid surgery.[2]

These differences in practice may to some extent reflect disagreements among authorities, or lack of specificity in their advice. For example, one current, standard, pediatric textbook[3] questions whether any indications for tonsillectomy exist, whereas several others recommend the procedure for "repeated" or "recurring" episodes of sore throat, and in various other circumstances.[4-7] Less disagreement exists concerning adenoidectomy; most authorities advocate surgery for children with recurrent or chronic otitis media and for those with adenoid hypertrophy of such degree as to interfere with nasal breathing. Other possible indications for adenoidectomy, e.g., recurrent or chronic nasopharyngitis or sinusitis, have not received general agreement.

Inquiry as to the reasons for disagreement among experts leads quickly to the realization that, despite an immense clinical literature, conclusive studies of the indications for, and results of, tonsillectomy and adenoidectomy are lacking. Relevant publications have tended to fall into one of four categories:

1. Discussions of the indications for surgery, based on the experience or opinions of the authors.[8,9]

2. Reviews of published studies or reports, often without adequate analysis of their statistical shortcomings, by authors who have not themselves participated in the studies.[10-12] Such "vicarious" publications tend to contain some of the strongest, and in turn, most frequently quoted, condemnations of tonsillectomy and adenoidectomy.

3. Comparisons made, prospectively or retrospectively, of certain aspects of the health status of two population groups — those who have received tonsillectomies and adenoidectomies, and those who have not. If, as is usually the case, no difference in favor of the operated group is found, the value of the procedure is impugned.[13-15] These studies have not been controlled; however, there is no reason to believe that the operated and unoperated groups were similar before surgery was undertaken. Such studies are of very limited value since the intent of surgery in the first place was to convert, as nearly as possible, those in the operated group (whose health status prior to surgery had presumably been unsatisfactory) to the status of those in the unoperated group (whose health status was presumably so satisfactory that surgery was not deemed advisable). If surgery had accomplished the desired effect completely, no difference ought to be found; even a difference in favor of the unoperated group would not rule out the possibility of partial improvement in the operated group.

4. Controlled studies in which candidates for surgery, having been identified on the basis of certain indications, are divided into operated and control groups, and their postoperative courses compared.[16-20] Only such studies can

---

*This section is an excerpt from an article by Jack L. Paradise, M.D., entitled "Why T & A Remains Moot" and published previously in *Pediatrics*.[1] Reprinted with permission of the publisher.

hope to provide valid and generally applicable results, but, ironically, none has been reported in the United States since Kaiser's pioneering study[16] undertaken fifty years ago. Kaiser's, moreover, was the only controlled study in the English language literature until 1963, when McKee[17,18] reported his careful and comprehensive studies in England. Since then, only two other controlled studies, both similar to McKee's, have been reported – one in England, and one in New Zealand.[20]

Unhappily, the findings of all five of these studies are open to question, since each of them suffers from most if not all of the following limitations or flaws in experimental design:

1. The selection of patients for surgery was not random.[16]

2. Adenoidectomy, tonsillectomy, and adenotonsillectomy were not considered as separate procedures with separate indications and separate results.[16,17,19,20]

3. It is unclear to what extent clinical severity might have varied within, and between, the operated and control groups.[16-18,20]

4. The indications for surgery were not stringent, so that it is doubtful whether the cumulative disability from illness in some patients exceeded that which might be expected from the operative procedure itself.[16-20]

5. Children who appeared to the authors to be most in need of surgery (but whose numbers and indications for surgery were not stated) were excluded from the study and operated on, as it was considered "unethical" not to do so. This left for evaluation only those children in whom the indications appeared less compelling, or even doubtful.[17-20]

6. There was apparently limited clinical sophistication in the recognition and treatment of middle ear disease. Thus, methods for assessing the presence or severity of otitis media were not described,[17-20] or consideration was limited to patients with purulent otorrhea.[16] Throughout, there was no mention of serous otitis media, myringotomy, or tympanostomy tube insertion.[16-20]

7. Postoperative evaluation was based not on direct examination of the children, but only on information obtained from parents.[16-18,20]

8. The study lacked, as additional controls, a group of children not deemed appropriate candidates for tonsil or adenoid surgery.[16-19]

TERMINOLOGY

Members of the Committee found it difficult to agree and arrived at what they think is presently the most acceptable classification of terminology and definitions.

I. Obstructive diseases of the tonsils or adenoids or both
   - A. Tonsils obstructive to airway
     Tonsils obstructive to food passage
   - B. Adenoids obstructive to airway
     Adenoids obstructive to Eustachian tube

II. Inflammation
   - A. Tonsillitis
     1. Acute
     2. Chronic
     3. Recurrent acute
   - B. Adenoiditis
     1. Acute
     2. Chronic
     3. Recurrent acute
   - C. Adenotonsillitis
     1. Acute
     2. Chronic
     3. Recurrent acute
   - D. Pharyngotonsillitis
     1. Acute
     2. Chronic
     3. Recurrent acute

III. Trauma
   - A. Tonsils
   - B. Adenoids

IV. Neoplasia
  A. Benign
    1. Tonsils
    2. Adenoids
  B. Malignant
    1. Tonsils
    2. Adenoids

Complications and conditions associated with diseases of the tonsils and adenoids.

I. Common
  A. Peritonsillar cellulitis
  B. Peritonsillar abscess
  C. Retropharyngeal abscess
  D. Parapharyngeal abscess
  E. Cervical lymphadenitis
  F. Rhinitis
  G. Paranasal sinusitis
  H. Otitis media
  I. Abnormalities of dentition
  J. Abnormalities of speech
  K. Impairment of hearing
  L. Disorders of olfaction
  M. Fetor oris
  N. Weight loss or failure to gain weight

II. Uncommon
  A. Tonsillar abscess
  B. Hemorrhage
  C. Gangrene of tonsils
  D. Congestive heart failure

DEFINITIONS

1. Acute tonsillitis/adenoiditis — acute inflammation of the tonsils or adenoids.

2. Acute pharyngitis — acute inflammation of the pharynx which may or may not involve the tonsils or adenoids or both.

3. Acute sore throat — acute sore throat is a symptom, not a discretely definable illness. Acute sore throat has been cutomarily thought of as an illness in which tonsillitis or pharyngitis is the predominant or main feature.

PATHOGENESIS

1. Obstruction due to adenoids or tonsils or both — tonsils or adenoids may obstruct the food and air passages (including the Eustachian tube) and cause abnormalities of breathing, speaking, feeding, hearing or facial development.

2. Acute tonsillitis and adenoiditis or adenotonsillitis — a variety of microorganisms may be etiologically involved in acute tonsillitis, adenoiditis, or adenotonsillitis. Most of these are viruses. Among bacteria, *Streptococcus pyogenes* or *C. diphtheria* are recognized as important agents. Evidence concerning the involvement of other bacteria is wanting.

3. Chronic tonsillitis and adenoiditis are poorly understood conditions in which the pathogenetic mechanisms have yet to be defined.

TREATMENT

I. MEDICAL

Acute Tonsillitis, Adenoiditis and Pharyngotonsillitis. Treatment of these conditions should be guided mainly by the results of the culture. It is presently recommended by the authorities in the field of infectious disease that in bacteriologically confirmed infections due to Group A, B-hemolytic streptococcus, treatment with penicillin G or V is indicated. Supportive management should also be instituted. If the patient is allergic to penicillin, then a penicillin substitute should be used, e.g., erythromycin, clindamycin, or oral cephalosporin.

Chronic Tonsillitis, Adenoiditis and Pharyngotonsillitis. Treatment should be guided in the same manner as for acute. However, a trial of antibiotic management may be instituted even when the culture is negative.

Recurrent Acute Tonsillitis, Adenoiditis and Pharyngotonsillitis. Each bout should be treated as outlined under acute tonsillitis. However, in certain patients with recurrent tonsillitis, adenoiditis, and pharyngotonsillitis, a trial period of prophylactic penicillin may be warranted.

Noninflammatory Obstructive Disease. Watchful waiting, with education and reassurance of the patient, parents, and health professionals, frequently remains the preferred management.

Complications of Medical Treatment. Untoward effects varying in severity may be associated with the use of any antimicrobial agent.

II. Surgical Treatment

Indications for surgery have been arbitrarily divided into three groups:

Group A. Conditions in which indications for the procedure listed are clear and unquestionable.

Group B. Conditions in which the indications are not supported by evidence. Experienced clinicians are divided, some in favor and some against, in their attitude concerning the efficacy of the procedure. More investigation is necessary to address the problem satisfactorily.

Group C. Conditions for which the procedure listed is not indicated.

Obstructive Disease. When inflammation is present and causes obstructive disease of the tonsils or adenoids or both, an appropriate and adequate treatment trial of antibiotics would appear to be indicated. In the rare case in which the tonsils are obstructive to the digestive tract, causing dysphagia, weight loss or failure to gain weight for six or more months, tonsillectomy is *certainly* indicated. Likewise, cor pulmonale can be the result of tonsillar and adenoidal obstruction of the airway. For this rare condition, adenotonsillectomy is certainly indicated. When adenoids persistently obstruct the nasal airway, causing abnormalities of breathing, speech or dental occlusion, or when obstructive adenoids are associated with recurrent, acute, or chronic rhinitis or sinusitis, the patient should be considered a *possible* candidate. When adenoids appear obstructive to the nasal airway, Eustachian tube, or both, with associated middle ear disease, adenoidectomy *may* be indicated. Obstructive tonsils may be associated with altered speech or dental abnormalities which are ill-defined, and for which the procedure should be considered *possibly* indicated.

Inflammation. For patients with recurrent episodes of acute tonsillitis or pharyngotonsillitis, (three or more per year for at least two consecutive years) tonsillectomy is of possible benefit. Similarly adenotonsillectomy should be considered as a possible procedure for patients with recurrent episodes of acute adenotonsillitis. For patients with chronic tonsillitis and pharyngotonsillitis, tonsillectomy is possibly indicated, as is adenotonsillectomy for chronic adenotonsillitis.

Surgical Indications. There are certain conditions in which the indications for the procedures are clear and unquestionable — and others where the operation is clearly not indicated. On the other hand, some patients are considered *possible* candidates for surgery, but until the body of knowledge is broadened, surgery should be approached with caution. In order to be more certain about the indications, especially when the history is unreliable, the physician may elect to:

1. Obtain the patient's past medical records.

2. Personally follow the patient for an extended trial period.

3. Evaluate the patient for the possible existence of allergy.

4. Obtain laboratory studies, i.e., nose and throat cultures, nasal smear for eosinophils, or immunologic function.

5. Obtain roentgenograms, i.e., lateral soft tissue films of the neck for adenoid size, tele- or cinefluoroscopy in patients who have velopharyngeal insufficiency, and sinus films, when sinusitis and rhinitis are associated conditions.

6. If otitis media is present, obtain serial audiometric and tympanometric testing.

7. Consult with specialists in speech,

TABLE I

TONSILLECTOMY AND ADENOIDECTOMY: MORTALITY AND MORBIDITY[23]

Number of Deaths	*Average*	*Percent*
	1/16,381	0.006
Cause		
Anesthetic	1/44,429	0.002
Cardiac arrest	1/48,627	0.002
Hemorrhage	1/55,637	0.002
Nonfatal Bleeding		
Carotid ligation		
Immediate	1/12,253	0.008
Delayed	1/ 4,128	0.02
Transfusions		
Five or more	1/11,479	0.009

allergy, hematology, or infectious disease, when indicated.

Contraindications. When velopharyngeal insufficiency is present, adenoidectomy is contraindicated. The operation is also contraindicated in patients with certain types of blood dyscrasia associated with abnormality of clotting.

Complications of Surgery. In 1968, the Commission on Professional and Hospital Activities[21] reported an average of one death per 16,207 tonsillectomies, adenoidectomies, or both. Ranger[22] in 1968 reported seven deaths a year in England from tonsillectomies and adenoidectomies, or one in 27,000 operations. Table I is information obtained from a survey of practicing otolaryngologists by Pratt, in 1970.[23]

UNANSWERED QUESTIONS

The Committee recommends that high priority consideration be given to the initiation of prospective investigations, the purpose of which will be to define, as specifically as possible, approaches to the optimal management of diseases of the tonsils and adenoids. It is the opinion of the Committee that further studies of pathogenesis, pathophysiology and epidemiology of these disorders will be required to define basic mechanisms, an understanding of which it considers critical in the solution of the therapeutic problems.

REFERENCES

1. Paradise JL: Why T & A remains moot. Pediatrics 49:648-651, 1972

2. Poll on Medical Practice. Modern Medicine 37:77, 1969

3. Einhorn AH: In Barnett HL (ed): *Pediatrics,* ed 14. New York, Appleton-Century-Crofts, 1968, pp 1675-1677

4. Eichenwald HF, McCracken GH Jr: In Nelson WE, Vaughan CV III, McKay RN (eds): *Textbook of Pediatrics,* ed 9. Philadelphia, W B Saunders Co, 1969, pp 895-897

5. Shore S: In Gellis SS, Kagan BM (eds): *Current Pediatric Therapy,* ed 4. Philadelphia, W B Saunders Co, 1970, pp 162-164

6. Hughes JG: *Synopsis of Pediatrics,* ed 3. St. Louis, C V Mosby Company, 1971, pp 375-376

7. Proctor DF: In Cooke RE (ed): *The Biologic Basis of Pediatric Practice.* New York, McGraw-Hill Book Company, 1968, p 279

8. Reid JM, Donaldson JA: The indications for tonsillectomy and adenoidectomy. Otolaryngol Clin North Am 3:339, 1970

9. Haggerty RJ: Diagnosis and treatment: tonsils and adenoids — a problem revisited. Pediatrics 41:815, 1968

10. Bakwin H: The tonsil-adenoidectomy enigma. J Pediatr 52:339, 1958

11. Evans HE: Tonsillectomy and adenoidectomy: review of published evidence for and against the T & A. Clin Pediatr (Phila) 7:71, 1968

12. Bolande RP: Ritualistic surgery — circumcision and tonsillectomy. N Engl J Med 280:591, 1969

13. Paton JHP: Tonsil-adenoid operation in relation to health of a group of schoolgirls. Q J Med 12:119, 1943

14. McCorkle LP, Hodges RG, Badger GF, et al: A study of illness in a group of Cleveland families. VIII. Relation of tonsillectomy to incidence of common respiratory disease in children. N Engl J Med 252:1066, 1955

15. Chamovitz R, Rammelkamp CH, Wannamaker LW, et al: The effect of tonsillectomy on the incidence of streptococcal respiratory disease and its complications. Pediatrics 26: 355, 1960

16. Kaiser AD: Results of tonsillectomy; a

comparative study of 2,200 tonsillectomized children with an equal number of controls three and ten years after the operation. JAMA 95:837, 1930

17. McKee WJE: A controlled study of the effects of tonsillectomy and adenoidectomy in children. Br J Prev Soc Med 17:49, 1963

18. McKee, WJE: The part played by adenoidectomy in the combined operation of tonsillectomy with adenoidectomy; second part of a controlled study in children. Br J Prev Soc Med 17:133, 1963

19. Mawson SR, Adlington P, Evans M: A controlled study evaluation of adenotonsillectomy in children. J Laryngol Otol 81:777, 1967

20. Roydhouse N: A controlled study of adenotonsillectomy. Arch Otolaryngol 92:611, 1970

21. Commission on Professional and Hospital Activities; Memorandum Report, T & A Study, Private Communication to Thayer Hospital, Waterville, Maine (March, 1969)

22. Ranger D: Tonsillectomy and adenoidectomy. Lancet 1:1205, 1968

23. Pratt LW: Tonsillectomy and adenoidectomy: mortality and morbidity. Trans Am Acad Ophthalmol Otolaryngol 74:1146-1154, 1974

CHAPTER III. FORMAL PAPERS

PITTSBURGH TONSILLECTOMY AND ADENOIDECTOMY STUDY: DIFFERENCES FROM EARLIER STUDIES AND PROBLEMS OF EXECUTION

JACK L. PARADISE, M.D.
PITTSBURGH, PENNSYLVANIA

At the Children's Hospital of Pittsburgh we have been engaged in a prospective study of indications for tonsillectomy and adenoidectomy for almost three years, but the program has been in full operation only since June, 1973 when it was funded by NIH. Our study was designed in an effort to overcome certain flaws in the only four controlled studies previously published, not one of which, by the way, was carried out in the United States. Each of those four studies had in common with ours a fundamental element of design, that is, candidates for surgery were identified, and randomly divided into surgical and control groups. I have previously mentioned in the literature[1] the deficiencies in design of the previous studies, but will itemize them and indicate how we are hoping to avoid them in our study. Three of the four previous studies were reported from England, two by McKee,[2,3] and one by Mawson and his colleagues,[4] and the fourth was reported from New Zealand by Roydhouse[5] and was patterned almost identically after McKee's first study. The first problem with all the studies was that, except in the case of McKee's second study, adenoidectomy, tonsillectomy, and adenotonsillectomy were not considered separate procedures with separate indications and separate results. In our study, we are dealing with them individually.

Another problem with the earlier studies was that indications for surgery were not stringent, and in the Mawson[4] study, not even explicitly defined. Accordingly, patients with lesser degrees of difficulty must have predominated over those with greater degrees, and it is therefore possible that the results of surgery in the severely affected patients were obscured by less striking results in the larger number of less severely affected patients. We have attempted to meet this problem by establishing rather stringent criteria for surgery, so that we should be able to examine results in patients with significant degrees of illness or disability.

Another serious problem in design of the earlier studies, and one compounding the problem just mentioned, was the exclusion from those studies of children who appeared to the authors to be most seriously affected and most urgently in need of surgery. Since it was considered unethical to withhold surgery from such children, they were all operated on, leav-

---

From the Departments of Pediatrics and Community Medicine, University of Pittsburgh School of Medicine, and the Ambulatory Care Center of the Children's Hospital of Pittsburgh, Pittsburgh, Pa.

Supported in part by a grant from the Dr. E. R. McCluskey Memorial Research and Program Fund of the Children's Hospital of Pittsburgh, and by a research grant (HDO 7403) from the National Institute of Child Health and Human Development.

ing for evaluation only the children in whom the indications appeared less compelling, the so-called "routine cases." Unfortunately also, we know only in general terms, or not at all, what constituted those urgent indications; we do not know what proportion of the total number of patients had them, and we know nothing about the results of surgery in those patients. In the Pittsburgh study we have attempted to meet this problem by limiting our criteria for "urgent surgery" to those quite unusual circumstances in which children are manifestly uncomfortable or handicapped because of tonsil- and adenoid-related problems. Furthermore, we are counting these children with "urgent" indications, and keeping close track of what happens to them postoperatively.

Another problem in earlier studies was the inadequacy with which middle ear disease was recognized and dealt with. In none of the earlier studies was there mention of secretory otitis media, myringotomy, or tympanostomy tube insertion. We have developed very precise methods of evaluating middle ear disease, including routine pneumatic otoscopy, impedance testing, and audiometry, and I do not believe that there should be much equivocation about the continuing middle ear status of our patients.

Yet another problem with earlier studies was the method of obtaining postoperative evaluation. In the McKee and Roydhouse studies,[2,3,5] information was obtained from parents at intervals of two months by public health nurses who made home visits but did not examine the children. In the Mawson study[4] the children were examined at two-month intervals by the authors, but interim information was necessarily limited.

In our study we are maintaining two separate information tracks. The objective track consists of direct examination at six-week intervals, and also at the time of any intervening respiratory illness. The subjective track consists of information obtained by telephone at intervals of 14 days, with a standardized list of questions looking into minor symptoms which would ordinarily not serve to bring a child to the doctor's office, but which are to one degree or another troublesome. Such symptoms include minor cough, rhinorrhea, sore throat, reduced physical activity, and the like. By using these parallel tracks, we believe that we will be able to obtain a very comprehensive continuing evaluation of the patients' status with respect to the aspects of health that concern us.

Finally, only the study of Roydhouse[5] incorporated a comparison group of patients not considered candidates for tonsil or adenoid surgery because they failed to meet the criteria established. We are also including in our study a large group of such patients who have been referred to us for consideration of surgery, but who have failed to meet our criteria. If our criteria have validity, the children assigned to the "no-surgery" group should ultimately develop much more tonsil- and adenoid-related illness than those children considered not to be suitable candidates for surgery.

Having mentioned briefly how we hope to overcome some of the difficulties of earlier studies, I will review some of the problems that we have encountered, both in instituting our study and since it has gotten underway. These problems seem to fall into about five general categories, which might be termed problems of design, problems related to process, diagnostic difficulties, practical obstacles, and problems related to our particular local situation.

Problems of Design. First of all, the design problems. Of these, the most difficult is the problem of eliminating observer bias — bias on the part of both parent and physician. By the nature of the situation, it is impossible to mount either a double-blind or single-blind study. Thus we must depend on observations which will, of necessity, be influenced to some extent by knowledge of foregoing events. We have not been able to think of any way in which this apparently inherent problem can be overcome.

A second problem in design has to do with arriving at criteria on the basis of which children originally assigned to a "no-surgery" category would be transferred to a surgical category on the basis of difficulties which have continued or become worse. In the case of children who develop criteria which we have arbitrarily established as "urgent" there is no problem. However, there is an intermediate group of children who do not have urgent indications, but who continue to be appreciably affected, or whose difficulties become worse. How severely affected must they be over how long a period of time before we decide to relent on our original decision not to operate? Parents, of course, can influence this process by electing to have surgery done, since we have already advised them that surgery is a reasonable undertaking to consider. However, we have found that most parents are willing to go along with whatever we request, and so we are faced with the judgmental question as to where to draw the line. We have some ideas on this matter, but have not really resolved it to our satisfaction and developed a systematic way of dealing with it. This is one of the decisions which we will have to come to in the very near future.

A third design issue has to do with the duration of follow-up of patients. Originally we had thought in terms of a three-year follow-up, but many questions will be left unanswered by follow-up limited to that period. For example, some experts have the impression that there is an upsurge of recurrent sore throat among adolescent girls, and are concerned that this problem will be exaggerated if tonsillectomy is withheld during earlier years. In order to study this aspect of natural history, it will of course be necessary to follow certain patients at least through adolescence. Other processes may undergo spontaneous change in one direction or another over somewhat shorter periods of time, but without an adequate observation period, which should perhaps extend into adulthood, the information to be gained will be limited.

Problems of Process. Next are problems of process. The first of these is the unreliability of histories. We have come to feel increasingly strongly as the study has progressed that we cannot rely on history as a basis for classifying children, no matter how reliable the parent *seems* to be. There are just too many subjective considerations, and even when we obtain previous records from other physicians, it is impossible to know very much about the severity or exact nature of the illnesses described. Because of this unreliability, we no longer accept history as face value unless the documentation in our or other records is overwhelming. Instead, we place patients into an "observe" category, and advise parents that we must follow the children for some time ourselves in order to decide whether or not our criteria for surgery have been met.

The second process-related problem is that of inter-observer standardization. Tonsils which are "large" to one observer may seem "moderate" in size to another. Eardrums which are "dull and thick" to one observer may seem to another "within normal limits" because mobility is not appreciably impaired. The nasal mucous membrane may appear "inflamed" to one observer whereas another would describe it as "bluish and edematous." Voice quality in a single subject may be described by different observers as "nasal," "hyponasal," or "markedly hyponasal." In order to maintain meaningful clinical data, observers must call things by the same name, and use standardized conceptual definitions. We have attempted to meet this problem in two ways. First of all we have kept the number of professionals involved in the study to a minimum, and secondly we have instituted and maintained a system in which all new patients and many return patients are seen independently by two or more observers, with the findings being recorded independently before being checked against each other. This kind of continuing effort has enabled us to reach and sustain a high degree of inter-observer reliability.

A third problem related to process is

the construction of forms for the recording of clinical information. Since we began the study we have been through countless revisions of our various forms in order to meet the variable kinds of requirements imposed by the study design. At the same time, of course, forms have had to be designed with an eye to the computer so that information will be readily retrievable. It may be, in fact, that a study of the type we are attempting would have been practically impossible to consummate without the assistance of the computer. We have a form which will enable us to record on one sheet results of any or all of the various laboratory, x-ray, and other diagnostic procedures which we carry out on these children. As we have revised our forms, we have had to delay our keypunching until such time as we arrive at a final version of the form which appears entirely satisfactory. Information can then be transferred from all previous versions to this final one.

Yet another problem within the category of process has to do with the delegation of professional tasks. The amount of clinical follow-up required in the study imposes formidable needs for professional time. We would have considered it a practical impossibility to mount this study had we relied entirely on physicians for all the observations necessary. We have faced this problem by training a pediatric nurse-practitioner to acquire a high degree of observational and diagnostic skill in diseases of the ears, nose, and throat, and she sees most of the children for their follow-up visits without direct consultation. If there is doubt about a particular child's status, or if he is ill, one of the physicians directly involved in the study consults, but it is rare that the nurse-practitioner's judgment requires adjustment. Her skills are such that medical students are routinely assigned to work with her, and members of the house staff ask her for advice in assessing other patients of their own. Similarly, we have trained two highly intelligent lay persons to do the routine telephone follow-up data collecting.

A final problem in the category of process has been the need to obtain informed parental consent before subjecting children to randomization. I was initially fearful that parents would be generally unwilling to have the decision for or against surgery depend on random assignment. We have learned, however, to our gratification, that an overwhelming majority of parents have agreed to allow this after experiencing our initial evaluation, the explanations which accompanied it, and a discussion of the goals and design of the study.

Diagnostic Difficulties. The third category of problem we face has to do with precision of diagnosis. It is not always easy to differentiate simple upper respiratory infection accompanied by sore throat from isolated pharyngitis. Similarly, we do not feel that we can always differentiate nasal obstruction due to allergic rhinitis from that caused by enlarged adenoids. Sometimes the two seem to occur together, while at other times the one simulates the other. We sometimes have difficulty in sorting out the relative extent to which maxillofacial or dental abnormalities rather than enlarged adenoids cause mouth breathing. In this we obtain assistance from our dental colleagues, but uncertainties sometimes remain. Necessarily, some of the diagnostic judgments must be in part subjective.

I should mention in connection with diagnostic issues, the routine studies which we have recently instituted in study patients in order to detect allergy and to measure aspects of immunological competence. We are now doing a standard battery of skin tests on each new patient, and also obtaining determinations of their circulating immunoglobulins, eosinophils, B-lymphocytes and T-lymphocytes. These latter studies will be repeated at six-month intervals, and so we hope to shed some additional light on both natural history and possible immunologic effects of removing tonsils and adenoids.

Practical Obstacles. The fourth category of problem can be described quite simply, but the problems are not so readily solved. The first of these is finding enough patients to meet our criteria for surgery. Despite continuing education of our house staff, many of the patients referred to us do not meet our criteria. As an example, during the past eight working months we have seen about 125 new patients. Within that same period six patients have been considered urgent candidates for adenoidectomy, twenty have satisfied criteria for adenoidectomy and have been randomized, and only one has met criteria for tonsillectomy. Patients who have histories of repeated episodes of tonsillitis seem almost invariably to stop having them once we start to observe them. (We have, of course, put many patients into an "observe" category who will probably eventually meet our criteria). Part of the problem lies in the limitations of our drawing population, and there may be ways to enlarge this as we go along.

A somewhat related, practical problem has to do with the occasional loss of patients to follow-up, or with patients occasionally slipping out of the system for care by family physicians. Some of our patients come appreciable distances, and while every effort is made to have the patient seen by us for every respiratory or related illness, this is not invariably possible. Under such circumstances we must rely on the observations of others, and this is never entirely satisfactory. Our "no-show" rate, incidentally, is much lower than usually published rates for teaching hospital out-patient departments, and much lower than rates for our other clinics. Recently it has averaged just under 14%.

Local Problems. The last category of problems has to do with our own local situation. The overwhelming majority of the patients in our study come from lower socioeconomic strata, as this is a reflection of the general hospital clinic clientele. While these are patients who may be more at risk than those in higher socioeconomic groupings, nonetheless it represents a skewed sample of the population in general, and as such has distinct limitations. We are hoping to be able to alter this as the study progresses, but we have no guarantee that this will occur.

So much for some of the major problems which we have encountered. There are other minor mechanical problems having to do with scheduling, the arrangement of various procedures, and a host of other more or less petty but sometimes nettlesome problems that can be readily imagined.

I would like to consider briefly some special problems that I would foresee in a collaborative study. Aside from the problems of standardization which I have described, one would be faced with the necessity to monitor widely separated programs in order to ensure uniformity at every level. The problem of turnover of personnel in a long-term study would be difficult, as institutional affiliations are not necessarily lasting. I do not believe that funding alone can guarantee the availability of personnel who are both capable of carrying on such a study and motivated to do so with the kind of care that we would consider necessary. This is not to say that exploratory efforts in this direction are not worthwhile, but only to suggest that the task would be formidable, not only to begin but to sustain.

REFERENCES

1. Paradise JL: Why T & A remains moot. Pediatrics 49:648-651, 1972

2. McKee WJE: A controlled study of the effects of tonsillectomy and adenoidectomy in children. Br J Prev Soc Med 17:49, 1963

3. McKee WJE: The part played by adenoidectomy in the combined operation of tonsillectomy with adenoidectomy; second part of a controlled study in children. Br J Prev Soc Med 17:133, 1963

4. Mawson SR, Adlington P, Evans M: A controlled study evaluation of adeno-tonsillectomy in children. J Laryngol Otol 81:777, 1967

5. Roydhouse N: A controlled study of adeno-tonsillectomy. Arch Otolaryngol 92: 611, 1970

COLLABORATIVE STUDIES

EDWARD H. KASS, M.D.

BOSTON, MASSACHUSETTS

Some collaborative studies in the past have been highly successful while others have proven to be so cumbersome that they have not been fully productive. An example of a successful study was the nationwide poliomyelitis vaccine trial. However, the perinatal study attempted to answer too many questions and not all of them could be answered effectively with the design that was used. The nationwide hypertension study now in progress is a good example of a collaborative study that has been carefully designed and appears to be operationally sound.

The problems of design of a prospective study of tonsillectomy and adenoidectomy have been identified by Dr. Paradise from his experience with the Pittsburgh study. One of these appears to be the socioeconomic aspect of the problem. The diseases of the tonsils and adenoids as well as infectious diseases of the upper respiratory tract, in general, appear to be more common in the lower socioeconomic groups but surgery of the tonsils and adenoids is more common in the upper. The Paradise study is heavily weighted toward the lower socioeconomic groups since the participants are entered from the clinic population. However, involvement of the patients from private practice could increase the cost since there may not be enough patients to study. Therefore, there may have to be loading toward the lower socioeconomic groups. Cooperation in such studies has been better in the lower socioeconomic groups than the higher.

There may be social problems attached to such loading. In the hypertension study some purposeful loading toward black participants was used with design since hypertension is twice as common in the black than in the white population. Lower socioeconomic groups could resent this type of loading, but on the other hand, are also aware that emphasis on diseases that are particularly a problem in certain groups may lead to more effective preventive or therapeutic activity. In the case of the study of diseases of tonsils and adenoids, it might be useful to include all socioeconomic strata, but to load the population more heavily toward those at highest risk of sequelae of the disease.

VALUE OF COLLABORATIVE STUDIES

Standardization of Clinical Approach. Criteria are standardized, the observer becomes disciplined, and there is an elimination of looseness. This often helps to make clinical practice more rigorous outside the collaborative study.

Identification of Weaknesses Within a Health Care System. An example of this is the experience with the hypertension study. Blood pressures were being recorded by "rounding off" to the nearest tenth. This could introduce a significant bias unless the personnel recording the findings standardize their technique. Similar standardization of chemical methods for determination of plasma lipids and plasma cholesterol, or of radiological methods have been of substantial value.

Improved Technology. Collaborative studies frequently result in the development of new instruments, e.g., an objective method to determine the amount of airway obstruction in the nose and nasopharynx.

Maximization of Personnel. If the study reveals that many adenotonsillectomies performed today are not indicated, then this could allow personnel currently involved in this part of health care to perform other duties.

Involvement of Paraprofessionals. Studies of this nature frequently demonstrate that personnel other than physicians can perform many duties.

Maximal Care Versus Routine Care. Studies such as the one in question usually result in a better definition of maximal health care as opposed to routine care.

Related Research. By looking at a large population carefully, other observations become apparent, and provide opportunities for "spin-off" of other related research.

Availability of a Large Population for Study. One of the most important advantages of a collaborative study is the availability of a large number of patients for study that would not be possible in one center alone.

PROBLEMS OF COLLABORATIVE STUDIES

Commitment. One of the biggest problems encountered in the past has been sustained commitment of the centers throughout the entire study period. Frequently everyone wants to be in at the beginning, but as time passes, commitment lags. Centers must be chosen that can prove commitment will be sustained.

Enrollment. It is often difficult to enlist the enthusiastic cooperation of a proposed population. There are concerns and suspicions that must be met openly and honestly.

Difficulties in Coordination. When more than one research center is involved in a project, coordination becomes a major problem, and this in turn may affect the analysis of the data.

Developing Criteria for People at Risk. The criteria for identification of the population at risk could be difficult. Not all clinical definitions of risk are reliable, and many identify only a small proportion of those at actual risk.

End-Point Criteria. It may be difficult to establish prior to the study the point at which the data should be analyzed. If the data are looked at too frequently during the course of the study this could influence the data analysis.

A nationwide prospective, collaborative controlled study of tonsillectomy and adenoidectomy similar to the one currently being conducted in Pittsburgh appears to be indicated since this is the only manner in which some of the questions regarding management can be answered. Reduction of even 10% of the estimated half billion dollars spent on tonsillectomy and adenoidectomy in this country could be a 50 million dollar saving per year and a value to society. What we should know is the cost benefit of this procedure.

INVOLVEMENT OF A PREPAID HEALTH PLAN IN PROSPECTIVE STUDIES ON TONSILLECTOMY AND ADENOIDECTOMY

PETER L. HURST, M.D.

PORTLAND, OREGON

General Considerations. Kaiser-Permanente has been cited as a prototype health maintenance organization.[1] The Oregon region has a current membership of slightly under 200,000, located in the metropolitan area of Portland-Vancouver and comprising about 15% of the total population. The medical group of 190 physicians includes all major and most subspecialties. There are 24 pediatricians, four pediatric nurse practitioners, four ENT surgeons. The membership is served by one 250 bed hospital with another under construction, plus five outlying clinics to provide easily accessible primary care. Patient continuity with the same primary care physician is encouraged, although not always achieved.

An important adjunct to the medical care program is the Health Services Research Center. Established in 1964, with contributions from the Community Services Program of the Bess Kaiser Hospital, it was funded in 1968 by the National Center for Health Services Research and Development as one of eight regional Health Services Research Centers. The Kaiser-Permanente system, with its well characterized health plan population, has served as laboratory for the Center in studies of medical care organization, utilization parameters, medical sociology, biometry, pharmacy administration, epidemiology, and clinical investigation. The work at the Center is carried out by permanent investigators representing various disciplines, as well as by physicians from the medical group. Supporting personnel furnish expertise in research administration, health planling, systems analysis, computer sciences, and technical editing.

Kaiser-Permanente offers the following advantages for clinical research:

1. Integration of clinical research with ongoing medical care would avoid duplication of facilities and personnel and would reduce the drop-out rate because of member stability. The opportunity to participate in a clinical study in the usual medical care setting could enhance patient participation.

2. The well defined health plan population is demographically and socioeconomically representative of the community, and therefore, offers a ready-made study group.

3. Each health plan member has a single in- and outpatient record, centrally stored and available at all times. In addition, 1,500 poor families (7,000 individuals) and a simple random sample of 8,000 plan members have had all their medical encounters abstracted and stored on magnetic tape since 1967.

4. Referrals within the medical group and frequent contact among the physicians tend to promote cooperation, a prerequisite for combined studies.

5. Since the medical group contracts with the health plan on the basis of a capitation per health plan member and not on the basis of amount or type of service rendered, randomization of treatment in a prospective research project is of no monetary consequence to the medical group.

6. The Research Center offers a valu-

able resource in the collection and processing of data.

Tonsillectomy and Adenoidectomy at Kaiser-Permanente, Oregon: Present State of the Art. Dr. Harvey Klevit, pediatrician and endocrinologist, and Dr. Arthur Oleinick, pediatrician and chief epidemiologist at the Research Center, analysed data on the 1,433 T & A's performed in the period 1965 to 1969.[2] Pre- and postoperative morbidity among T & A patients was compared to that of a control group with acute appendicitis. The age adjusted (0-14 years) rate for all procedures decreased from 125 per 10,000 in 1965 to 53 per 10,000 in 1969. Since then, it has decreased even further: 36 per 10,000 in 1973, compared to a nation-wide age adjusted rate of about 150 to 200 per 10,000. During 1968-1969, 40% of all procedures were T & A's, 14% were adenoidectomies, 10% were tonsillectomies, and 36% were T & A's with myringotomies. The most frequent indication (not mutually exclusive) was recurrent tonsillitis (59%), followed by serous otitis (46%), recurrent otitis (38%), hearing loss (29%), airway obstruction (20%), and peritonsillar abscess (10%). In the unselected T & A groups, there was a suggestion that otitis media, streptococcal throat infection, and undifferentiated upper respiratory tract infection had a rate decline in the first year following the procedure other than for medical or social reasons. The demographic distribution of the T & A group compared with the appendectomy group showed the following: 1) fathers of the T & A group were more likely to be unskilled, semiskilled or unemployed; 2) there are more children in the families of the T & A group; and 3) there was no correlation between the T & A group and the employment status of the mother. The demographic analyses are at variance with the customary observation that T & A's are more commonly performed among the prosperous.

Reflections on Study Design. With our diminishing T & A rate, criteria for the procedure have become more stringent and its necessity more urgent, at least as perceived by the referring and operating physician. Randomization under these circumstances as well as under circumstances of lowering criteria in order to satisfy a study design may, therefore, raise ethical problems. And yet, strict randomization and fixed criteria (plus long-term follow-up) are prerequisites for conclusive results and have been absent in previous T & A investigations. Criteria for surgery must be sufficiently stringent to minimize useless surgery, but not so stringent as to exclude surgery when it might prove to be useful.

It is difficult to envision a single investigation to answer the seven questions posed by the *Ad Hoc* Committee in the Report of April, 1974.[3] Number 1 is a matter of consensus; 2 and 3 are complex problems in microbiologic and pathophysiologic basic research, unlikely to be solved statistically; 4 is an epidemiologic problem and could be resolved either retrospectively or prospectively; 5, 6, and 7 are questions which lend themselves to long-term, prospective clinical research, as proposed by Paradise.[4]

Question 4 asks, What are the characteristics of the populations affected by the diseases of the tonsils and adenoids? This would appear to be a suitable project. Material for such a project could be obtained from magnetic tapes containing all medical encounters, demographic data, outpatient visits and diagnoses, phone calls, correspondence, and hospital admissions on about 7,000 individuals on the poverty program, plus a randomized 5% sample of the regular health plan membership. These data have been collected for the past seven years and continue being collected. Our group's epidemiologist is Dr. Arthur Oleinick.

As a second study, independent of the above, we would favor the topic of "Adenoidectomy and Otitis Media" along lines set forth by Bluestone, Wittel, Paradise, and Felder.[5] The aim of assessing the effectiveness of adenoidectomy in chronic and recurrent otitis media would be achieved through the following objectives:

1. The establishment of fixed criteria, such as number of attacks per year, duration of unresolved disease, size of air-bone gap, Eustachian tube function, adenoid size, and tonsil size.

2. The selection of two study groups — the first to consist of patients whom the participating pediatricians consider to be candidates for adenoidectomy on the basis of a preliminary screen; they will then undergo final screening. The preoperative observation period of this group will be short. About 70 to 100 children per year will participate in the final randomization of the treatment program. A second study group would be composed of those children who, by non-stringent criteria (e.g., two attacks of otitis per year), could become candidates for adenoidectomy. These patients can be identified by the participating pediatricians as they come through the clinic.[6] Out of this group an additional 30 to 40 children will eventually meet the stringent requirements for adenoidectomy; and their preoperative observation period is long.

3. Referral to ENT of patients who have met stringent criteria.

4. Randomization into three subgroups: myringotomy and tubes; myringotomy, tubes and adenoidectomy; myringtotomy, tubes, T & A.

5. Postoperative assessment of hearing and Eustachian tube function.

6. Long-term follow-up, at least five years and preferably longer.

7. Correlation of short and long-term postoperative clinical status with mode of treatment.

It is suggested that the medical management of otitis media, antibiotics, and decongestants be standardized for all patients on the study. Children with dysphagia due to large tonsils and with compromized pulmonary circulation due to large adenoids are to be excluded. Airway obstruction and nasal speech should have pre- and postoperative dental consultation, as well as volume flow spirometry, to be done at our pulmonary function lab.

In order to assure a sufficient number of patients for the study, patients are to be enrolled for three consecutive years, yielding about 300 to 400 patients. Attrition from the health plan over a seven year period will reduce this number to about 250.

The above outline should lend itself to integrating the investigation at Kaiser-Permanente, Oregon with a nation-wide project.

REFERENCES

1. Somers AR (ed): *The Kaiser-Permanente Medical Care Program.* New York, The Commonwealth Fund, 1971

2. Klevit HD, Oleinick A: The decline of tonsillectomy in a prepayment practice. Read at the International Congress of Pediatrics, Vienna, 1971

3. Ad Hoc Committee on Tonsillectomy and Adenoidectomy, Am Council of Otolaryngology, April, 1974

4. Paradise JL: Why T & A remains moot. Pediatrics 49:648-651, 1972

5. Bluestone CD, Wittel RA, Paradise TL, et al: Eustachian tube function as related to adenoidectomy for otitis media. Trans Am Acad Ophthalmol Otolaryngol 76:1325-1339, 1972

6. Hurst PL, Greenlick NR: Illness after health supervision visits. Pediatrics 46:427, 1970

CRITERIA FOR THE DIAGNOSIS OF ADENOTONSILLITIS

PHILIP M. SPRINKLE, M.D.

MORGANTOWN, WEST VIRGINIA

The purpose of this paper is to present a new concept of adenotonsillitis. This concept enables more of the known facts regarding adenotonsillitis to be included in the practicing clinician concept of the illness as it occurs naturally.

How Did the T & A Operation Become So Popular? We are questioning the efficacy of an operative procedure which had been accepted by the medical profession throughout the world, to the extent that it became the most common operation performed on the human pediatric population. The tonsil and adenoid (T & A) operation now may be secondary in frequency only to the insertion of ventilation tubes through the tympanic membrane to correct secretory otitis media.

In an effort to determine if there was a lasting physiologic effect from the T & A operation, Dr. Robert Veltri and I undertook an evaluation of the total microbiologic flora of children with recurrent tonsillitis and otitis media before and after the operation. This work has become fairly well known.[1-3] Matanoski[4] had previously reported similar findings with regard to the *Streptococcus pyogenes* in a controlled family study of rheumatic fever patients.

The results of our research showed marked qualitative and quantitative changes in the oropharyngeal microflora after operation on those children carrying large numbers of bacteria associated with disease processes prior to T & A. The most consistent change was the reduction in the number of children who carried *Streptococcus pyogenes* in their oropharynx subsequent to T & A. These changes of the oropharyngeal microflora toward a more physiologic state have been consistent for up to five years. An update of all data from our computer again shows consistent data.

When considering the problems that faced the practicing clinician in the preantibiotic era of the 1930's, the number of clinical syndromes associated with streptococcal disease was legend. The only tool that the practicing clinician had in this preantibiotic era, (as well as today), to convert an abnormal oropharyngeal microflora back to more nearly normal, with the elimination of *Streptococcus pyogenes* being the most consistent result, was the operation adenotonsillectomy. It is no small wonder that the operation became so popular, became so widely used and subsequently became misused. Similar use and misuse of popular antibiotics, whose effect is so dramatic at times, is a too frequent occurrence today.

If elimination of bacterial pathogens from the oropharynx is a goal in the treatment of tonsillitis and/or otitis media, then T & A is an effective means of realizing that end. Similarly, bacterial infections of the sinuses, viral-bacterial and bacterial-bacterial synergistic infections may also be reduced by the T & A operation in such a patient sample. However, there is no substantive data to show that elimination of bacterial pathogens from the oropharynx by means of a T & A reduces the incidence or severity of recurrent infections of the oropharynx or ears of children.

The clinical research at West Virginia University Medical Center has been limited primarily to those children who have recurrent exudative tonsillitis. Acute sore throat is a symptom, not a discretely, definable illness. While sore throat has been customarily thought of as an illness in which tonsillitis or pharyngitis is the predominant feature, our studies have been limited to a specific definable group of patients from the broad category of sore throat.

In the broadfield microbiologic and immunologic study of the pediatric patient sample with documented recurrent exudative tonsillitis, the analysis has shown specific microbiologic and immunologic characteristics that have better enabled us to make a more objective definition of exudative tonsillitis.

Microbiologically,[1,3] these children carry an ecological microflora different from normal. This flora is characterized by multiple bacterial species that have been associated with disease processes. A normal child may become transiently colonized with a pneumococcus or *Streptococcus pyogenes*. Recurrent exudative tonsillitis has been characterized by the persistent presence of multiple bacterial and fungal species commonly seen with disease processes of the head and neck, notably: *Streptococcus pyogenes, Pneumococcus sp, Staphylococcus aureus, Hemophilus influenzae, Candida albicans*, as well as many Gram negative enteric aerobes and anaerobes. Typically, we have been able to identify three to five species present in the oropharynx and nasopharynx at the time of a single microbiologic sampling. The presence of multiple species of potentially pathogenic bacteria associated with clinical disease has better enabled us to define recurrent exudative tonsillitis in a microbiologic fashion.

Immunologically,[2] the general characteristic of the pediatric sample with recurrent exudative tonsillitis has been the statistically significant presence of hypergammaglobulinemia. This presence of adult or higher than adult levels of IgG and IgA in the children with recurrent tonsillitis suggests that they have been subject to numerous infections. Removal of tonsils and adenoids has shown that the level of IgG and IgA in these children returns to normal after the operation. The normal levels of IgG and IgA occur gradually over many months after the operation, and continued sampling of IgG and IgA levels over a period of years has shown them to remain stable at normal levels.

TABLE I

FACTORS WHICH MODIFY ORAL MICROFLORA

Intrinsic	*Extrinsic*
Secretory IgA	Radiation
Secretory IgE	Some disease states
Salivary enzymes	Antibiotics
Interferon	T & A
Antibiosis	
Aging	
Dentition	

Pathogenesis of Tonsil and Adenoid Disease. Before I discuss the criteria of adenotonsillitis, I must give you some background of what we believe to be the pathogenesis of adenotonsillitis. The most difficult part of microbiology to comprehend is a broadfield understanding of the ecological aspects of the human oropharynx, nasopharynx and upper respiratory tract. Each of us is again cautioned that any conclusion drawn must be regarded as tentative. Isolated well-done bits of research data may be misinterpreted when viewed alone and not within the scope of all the factors that affect or modify the microflora of the upper respiratory tract.

Until such broadfield microbiological, immunological and serological data are available on specific definable disease processes of the upper respiratory tract, no conclusion can be considered final.

A list of intrinsic and extrinsic factors that also may affect or modify the ecological system present in the upper respiratory tract in the human host is shown in Table I.

The limitations of treating, as well as diagnosing, the cause of tonsillitis based on the results of a throat culture are real. It is obvious that the throat culture, as it is routinely used in clinical practice, is not sophisticated enough, in and of itself, to base all decisions upon regarding whether or not to treat tonsillitis with antibiotics. The throat culture in its

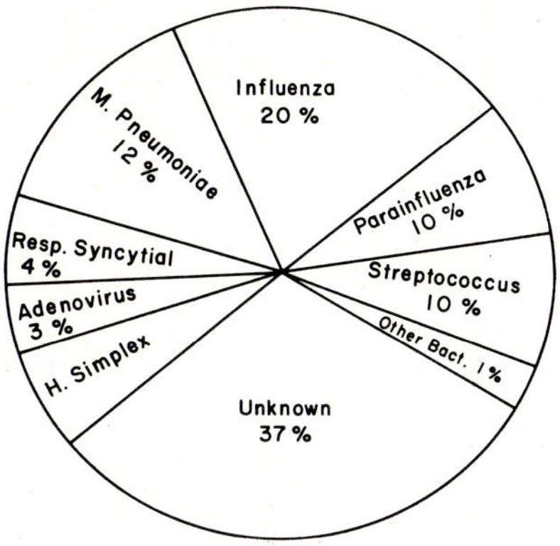

Fig. 1. Etiological spectrum for respiratory infections in Wisconsin students (data for several years). (With permission of the World Health Organization, Vol. 36, No. 3 and Otolaryngologic Clinics of North America 7:909-925, 1974.)

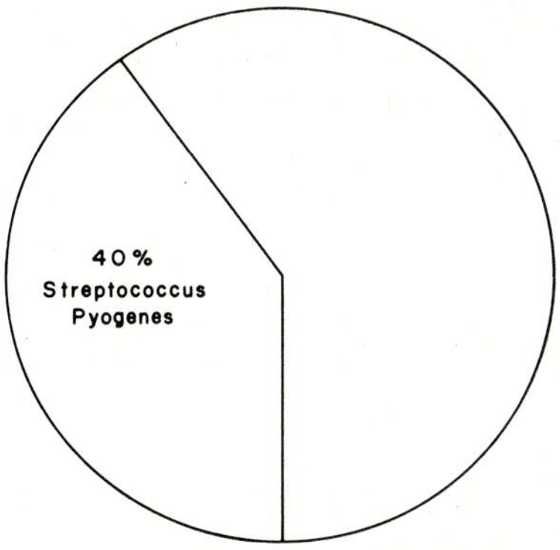

Fig. 2. Incidence of *Streptococcus pyogenes* in patients with recurrent tonsillitis and otitis media in West Virginia University Medical Center study. (With permission of Otolaryngologic Clinics of North America 7:909-925, 1974.)

present form also falls far short of the mark in categorizing an etiological agent as the cause of adenotonsillitis.

However, as tissue culture techniques for virology improved and as immunologic techniques improved, a large scale study was done on a group of Wisconsin students. The results of this study are shown in Figure 1. This was one of the first studies from which conclusions were drawn that 90% of all cases of acute tonsillitis were due to virus infections and that T & A was of no value in viral illness.

The majority of otolaryngologists later fell into the trap and accepted that study as complete fact without analyzing it. Let us look more critically at this data.

It is evident from the report, that all types of sore throat were studied and further, that no attempt was made to analyze one specific type of sore throat. It is our opinion that sore throat is a symptom and not a diagnosis.

If all the cases of exudative tonsillitis were removed from the Wisconsin students and studied separately, other facts become more obvious. It would be possible that all exudative tonsillitis would have entirely different microbiologic characteristics than the mean or average of all sore throats when lumped together for reporting purposes.

This is exactly what we have reported when we studied recurrent exudative tonsillitis. The incidence of *Streptococcus pyogenes* in recurrent tonsillitis is shown in Figure 2 and is seen to be 40%.

However, when we show the evidence of associated viral disease in Figure 3, the picture becomes much more complex. We have recently reported evidence of Epstein-Barr viral infections (without mononucleosis) in the sera

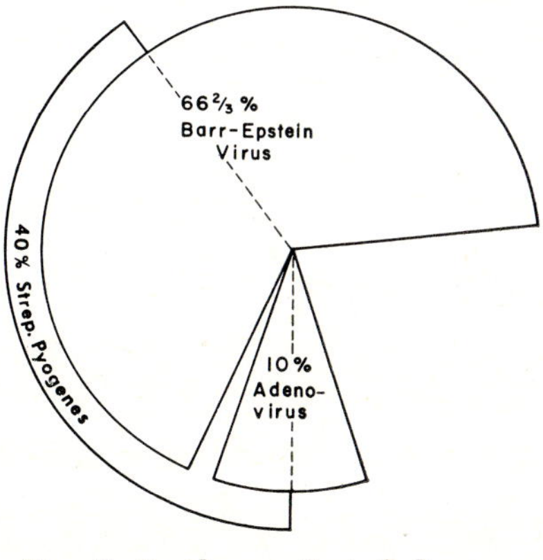

Fig. 3. Incidence of viral disease and associated *Streptococcus pyogenes* infection. (With permission of Otolaryngologic Clinics of North America 7:909-925, 1974.)

from our original patients with recurrent exudative tonsillitis.[5]

It would appear that the *Streptococcus pyogenes* "infections" or rather, presence in the tonsils, is probably opportunistic, or certainly shows direct evidence suggestive of a bacterial-viral cause of recurrent exudative tonsillitis. This work is complex, difficult technically and needs to be repeated in many other laboratories before being considered final. However, it is an extremely exciting report with many, many clinical considerations.

An example of the clinical considerations that are suggested by our report of the bacterial-viral etiology of recurrent exudative tonsillitis is seen when one remembers that Epstein-Barr virus is a herpes-like virus. These viruses remain in the body for long periods of time and clinical disease may be activated by nonspecific environmental factors that are thought to play a part in clinical disease.

Also, rheumatic fever which is caused, at least in part, by streptococcal infections could be better understood. The production of rheumatic fever by *Streptococcus pyogenes* does not meet Koch's postulates. Since the augmentation systems, notably complement, are involved in the disease process of rheumatic fever, it is interesting to see how the bacterial-viral relationship shown in Figure 3 might activate the complement system and produce, or at least contribute to, rheumatic fever.

However cogent, the above speculation is far from proven and further illustration would be more idle speculation.

Criteria for the Diagnosis of Adenotonsillitis. Recurrent adenotonsillitis is defined as a bacterial-viral illness. Microbiologically, these patients carry an abnormal nasopharyngeal and oropharyngeal microflora. Typically, this flora is characterized by the persistent presence of two to five bacterial species which are most frequently associated with clinical infections of the head and neck. *Streptococcus pyogenes, Staphylococcus aureus, Hemophilus influenzae, Pneumococcus sp, Candida albicans,* and the enteric Gram negative aerobes and anaerobes. The viruses present are adenoviruses and Epstein-Barr virus.

Immunologically, patients with recurrent adenotonsillitis typically have hypergammaglobulinemia. The elevated IgA contains the antibodies to viruses and the elevated IgG contains the antibodies to the Gram positive bacteria. As antibiotics compromise or reduce the immunologic response to *Streptococcus pyogenes,* for example, one wonders how high these might go if antibiotics were withheld or not available.

Clinically, recurrent adenotonsillitis may be associated with exudative tonsillitis, recurrent suppurative otitis media and recurrent or persistent secretory otitis media. It is possible that simple hypertrophy without appreciable clinical disease is the usual presentation of adenotonsillitis. It is also possible that a bacterial-viral adenotonsillitis may be clinically activated by nonspecific environmental factors, such as chilling, sunburn, etc.

Advantages of This Concept of Adenotonsillitis. 1) This concept brings attention to the limitation of treating as well as diagnosing the cause of tonsillitis based on the results of a throat culture as it is routinely used in clinical practice. The throat culture in its present form falls short of the mark in categorizing an etiological agent as the cause of adenotonsillitis. 2) This view of adenotonsillitis could lead the clinician to a more thorough immunologic and microbiologic analysis of his patient prior to initiating therapy, be it medical or surgical. 3) This concept of adenotonsillitis is more consistent with what is seen in nature as the natural illness evolves; rather than one person's concept of the fitness of things. This concept allows freedom to bring in many specific as well as nonspecific factors affecting illness in the human host; rather than one person's preconceived ideas, based on isolated well-done bits of research data that may have been misinterpreted when viewed alone. 4) Finally this concept of adenotonsillitis appears consistent with what limited data are available.

In closing, it would appear more prudent to find the cause, then possibly treat or modify the disease process, rather than evaluate two methods of treatment, i.e., medical or surgical.

Costly nationwide prospective studies of appropriate urban and rural population, geographically placed, would appear to be an option that would be difficult to implement. Besides the cost and years of study, the ethical problems associated with treating or not treating such children seem too complex to surmount in today's medical environment.

REFERENCES

1. Veltri RW, Sprinkle PM, Keller SA, et al: Ecological alterations of oral microflora subsequent to tonsillectomy and adenoidectomy. J Laryngol Otol 86:893-903, 1972

2. Veltri RW, Sprinkle PM, Keller SA, et al: Immunoglobulin changes in pediatric otolaryngic patient sample subsequent to T & A. J Laryngol Otol 86:905-916, 1972

3. Sprinkle PM, Veltri RW: Quantitative alterations in the ecology of the oropharyngeal microflora subsequent to tonsillectomy and adenoidectomy. Trans Am Acad Ophthalmol Otolaryngol 78:60-63, 1974

4. Matanoski GM: The role of the tonsils in streptococcal infections: a comparison of the tonsillectomized children and sibling controls. Am J Epidemiol 95:278-291, 1972

5. Veltri RW, Sprinkle PM, McClung, JE: Epstein-Barr virus as an etiological agent of exudative tonsillitis without infectious mononucleosis sequelae. Abstracts of the annual meeting of the American Society for Microbiology, 1974

MICROBIOLOGY OF DISEASES OF TONSILS AND ADENOIDS

JEROME O. KLEIN, M.D.

BOSTON, MASSACHUSETTS

A variety of infectious agents have been implicated in diseases of the tonsils and adenoids[1-3] (Table I). The association of these microorganisms with disease may be considered in the following categories:

1. Microorganisms that are well documented causes of pharyngotonsillitis or adenoiditis.

The group A beta hemolytic streptococci are the predominant bacterial cause of pharyngotonsillitis and exudative tonsillitis.

The adenoviruses are responsible for a syndrome of pharyngoconjunctival fever and are also associated with exudative tonsillitis.

The Epstein-Barr virus (the etiologic agent of infectious mononucleosis) is a major cause of acute pharyngitis or exudative tonsillitis in adolescents and young adults.

The group A coxsackieviruses are associated with herpangina and acute lymphonodular pharyngitis and occur in epidemic patterns in the summer and fall.

Candida albicans produces thrush in the young infant, the immuno-compromised host, and the patient who has received broad spectrum antimicrobial therapy for a prolonged period.

Primary *Herpesvirus hominis* infection is usually associated with lesions in the anterior mouth but extensive disease may also involve the oropharynx.

Neisseria gonorrhoeae is now a frequent cause of pharyngitis in promiscuous adults who participate in oral sexual acts.

Staphylococcus aureus is not a major cause of pharyngotonsillitis but is a cause of suppurative adenoiditis. Although abscess in the adenoid tissue is now seen infrequently, it may be a cause of prolonged and undetected fever. In addition, an oropharyngeal focus is the source of suppurative cervical adenitis due to this organism.

2. Microorganisms that are frequent causes of diffuse upper respiratory infection including pharyngotonsillitis.

Mycoplasma pneumoniae and the respiratory viruses, including the rhinoviruses, the respiratory syncytial virus, and the parainfluenza and influenza viruses are responsible for various upper respiratory signs and symptoms including those of pharyngotonsillitis.

3. Microorganisms that now occur infrequently in this country in association with tonsillitis and adenoiditis but whose relationship to these diseases is well established.

Diphtheria is now uncommon but still occurs as a cause of pharyngotonsillitis in unimmunized populations.

Tuberculosis and syphilis produce pharyngotonsillitis but these manifestations are now infrequently recognized.

Anaerobic bacteria have been isolated from tonsillar and peritonsillar abscesses. Technical improvements in isolation and identification of these fastidious organisms may result in increased interest in their role in infection and disease of the oral cavity.

4. Microorganisms of importance in disease in contiguous areas but of limited importance as causes of pharyngotonsillitis.

TABLE I

MICROORGANISMS ASSOCIATED WITH PHARYNGOTONSILLITIS AND ADENOIDITIS

Bacteria	*Viruses*	*Mycoplasma*	*Mycoses*
Streptococcus pyogenes	Adenoviruses	*M. pneumoniae*	*Candida albicans*
Staphylococcus aureus	*Epstein-Barr virus*	*M. hominis*	
Haemophilus influenzae	Coxsackievirus A		
Diplococcus pneumoniae	*Herpesvirus hominis*		
Corynebacterium diphtheriae	Rhinoviruses		
Neisseria gonorrhoeae	Parainfluenza viruses		
Mycobacterium tuberculosis	Respiratory syncytial virus		
Treponema pallidum	Influenza viruses		
Bacterial variants (L-forms)			
Anaerobic bacteria			

Haemophilus influenzae and *Diplococcus pneumoniae* are major causes of otitis media and sinus infection but are uncommon as pathogens associated with simple pharyngotonsillitis.

Diseases of the oral cavity, including Vincent's infection (associated with fusiform bacilli and oral spirochetes), Noma (due to fuso-spirochetes and possibly oral streptococci and staphylococci) and apthous stomatitis (the etiology remains uncertain) usually do not involve the tonsils or adenoids.

5. Microorganisms responsible for systemic disease which may include inflammation of the tonsils and pharynx.

A wide variety of agents such as the measles, hepatitis, varicilla and echoviruses, *Neisseria meningococcus, Toxoplasma gondii* and *Listeria monocytogenes* may produce pharyngotonsillitis as part of a generalized illness.

6. Microorganisms that have been suggested as causes of pharyngotonsillitis but whose relationship to disease is equivocal.

Experimental infection of human subjects with *Mycoplasma hominis* resulted in exudative tonsillitis in some participants.[4] There is no evidence, however, that natural infection with this organism produces a similar illness.

Recent studies[5] suggest that cell wall defective bacteria (L-forms) may be associated with pharyngotonsillitis but the data are insufficient to establish an etiologic role for these organisms.

FACTORS ASSOCIATED WITH ISOLATION OF MICROORGANISMS FROM PATIENTS WITH PHARYNGOTONSILLITIS

Various factors must be considered in evaluating studies of the microflora of the respiratory tract and the etiologic role of specific organisms in pharyngotonsillitis.

Identification of the Study Patients. The patient population may be defined by various criteria and some investigators have chosen a narrow definition (exudative tonsillitis) whereas others have used very general criteria (complaint of sore throat or local inflammation). The microorganisms isolated in one study may have little pertinence to the second.

Control Group. Since many of the microorganisms are prevalent in healthy individuals, the inclusion of a matched control group evaluated by the same methods as the study patients is necessary in considering the etiologic role of a microorganism. The control group must be carefully selected and should include subjects of comparable age, sex, socioeconomic status and potential exposure to the infectious agents.

Microbiologic Techniques. The results

of microbiologic isolation and identification studies must be appraised according to the adequacy of the techniques used. Viruses, mycoplasma, and anaerobic bacteria require special conditions for culture. If these methods are not considered, the study will be defective in failing to recognize the role of those microorganisms.

Differences in technique may also affect the rate of isolation of group A beta hemolytic streptococci from the oropharynx. A single pharyngeal culture employing a cotton swab will result in a lower incidence of streptococcal isolates than two or four cultures from the same patient. Inoculation of the swab directly into nutrient broth and then onto agar (after a six-hour incubation period) will result in a higher yield of streptococci than direct inoculation onto agar. Surface cultures of the tonsil may fail to isolate streptococci revealed when minced tonsillar tissue obtained at operation is cultured.

Epidemiologic Factors. The oropharyngeal pathogens may produce different signs and symptoms during various age periods. Thus, the signs of streptococcal infection in the young child, under three years of age, are likely to include rhinorrhea and other upper respiratory manifestations rather than exudative tonsillitis. Infectious mononucleosis is unlikely to cause exudative tonsillitis in the preschool age child but is a frequent cause of this sign in adolescents and young adults.

The time of the year is important in the pattern of infectious agents in the community and studies should be planned to include all seasons.

Since most of the respiratory pathogens spread by droplet nuclei from the oropharynx, the degree of crowding in living and working areas is an important variable and the control group should be selected from similar background.

Environmental pollution is now being examined more closely for possible relation to upper respiratory infection and patients and controls should be chosen from similar geographic areas.

Host Factors. Defects in normal host defense mechanisms against respiratory infection include anatomic, immunologic or physiologic abnormalities and these factors must be considered in selecting the study and control groups. Other host factors include history of allergy or hypersensitivity to various microbial and nonmicrobial antigens, prior infection and immunity to specific microorganisms, and the effect of various habits, including smoking and gum chewing.

ASSOCIATION OF INFECTION AND DISEASE

It is clear that there is an extensive microflora of the tonsils and adenoids and ample opportunity for the chance isolation of one or more organisms from the oropharynx of patients with disease. The occurrence of an infectious agent does not necessarily implicate it as a cause of the patient's disease. Koch developed a set of postulates to define the steps of proof required to establish the etiology of infectious agents. The recognition of many new organisms, mostly viruses, prompted Huebner[6] to reevaluate the criteria needed to identify a microorganism as the causative agent of a disease. It is apparent that very few of the organisms associated with diseases of the tonsils and adenoids (Table I) would satisfy the postulates of Koch or Huebner.

Although we are accustomed to consider an infectious disease as caused by a single microorganism, it is also possible that disease may result from the interaction of two or more agents or the combined effect of a noninfectious condition (allergy, smoking, environmental pollution) with an infectious agent. The nature of chronic disease may be particularly difficult to describe since the causative events took place sometime in the past and few clues may remain to identify the agent. These relationships will not yield easily to investigation, but it is critical that we understand the pathogenesis and microbiology of disease of the tonsils and adenoids before considering a program of medical and surgical treatment.

REFERENCES

1. Evans AS, Dick EC: Acute pharyngitis and tonsillitis in University of Wisconsin Students. JAMA 190:699-708, 1964

2. Glezen WP, Clyde WA Jr, Senior RJ, et al: Group A streptococci, mycoplasmas, and viruses associated with acute pharyngitis. JAMA 202:455-460, 1967

3. Moffet HL, Siegel AC, Doyle HK: Nonstreptococcal pharyngitis. J Pediatr 73:51-60, 1968

4. Mufson MA, Ludwig WM, Purcell RH, et al: Exudative pharyngitis following experimental *Mycoplasma hominis* type 1 infection. JAMA 192:1146-1152, 1965

5. Sprinkle PM: Current status of mycoplasmatales and bacterial variants in chronic otolaryngic disease. Laryngoscope 82:737-747, 1972

6. Huebner RJ: The virologist's dilemma. Ann N Y Acad Sci 67:430-438, 1957

DISEASES OF THE TONSILS AND ADENOIDS IN ADULTS

LOUIS WEINSTEIN, M.D.

BOSTON, MASSACHUSETTS

The infectious disorders of the upper respiratory tract of adults and children differ very little etiologically. However, certain features of the diseases produced present problems in adults that rarely supervene in children.

Hemophilus Influenzae. Although *H. influenzae* is a common cause of pharyngitis in children, it has been thought to produce upper respiratory infection only rarely in adults. However, recent experience indicates an increasing frequency of this type of disease in older individuals. Some of the infections in this age group are produced by type B organisms, while others are due to strains that are unencapsulated and untypable. While the syndrome in children is characterized by redness, edema and injection of blood vessels in the pharynges and occasionally even the presence of exudate on the pharynx and tonsils in the young age group, the clinical manifestations in adults are strikingly few. Examinations of the throat may reveal no more than very mild injection of the blood vessels with very little redness of the mucosa, but patients complain bitterly of pain so severe that they have great difficulty even in swallowing saliva. Ampicillin is the therapy of choice for this form of pharyngitis; for adults, the dose is 2 grams orally per day. It must be emphasized, however, that ampicillin resistant strains of type B *H. influenzae* have been reported recently.

Staphylococcus Aureus. Staphylococcus aureus, rarely, if ever, is a primary agent in the etiology of pharyngitis in either children or adults. This organism may, however, produce disease of the pharynx in the severely immunosuppressed individual, in patients with severe leukopenia and in those receiving antimicrobial agents to which this organism is not sensitive over a long period of time; even this type of disease is rare in adults.

Mycoplasma Pneumoniae. Although it has been suggested that this organism, the etiologic agent of so-called primary atypical pneumonia, may be etiologically involved in sore throat, this has been uncommon in my experience. However, it must be pointed out that studies carried out in human volunteers many years ago in which this organism was inoculated via the upper respiratory tract, indicated that it could produce acute pharyngitis as an isolated lesion or as the prodrome of pneumonia.

Infectious Mononucleosis. Although this disease is known to occur in children, it is most common in young adults. However, older individuals may rarely acquire this infection. Extensive studies now indicate that the Epstein-Barr virus, a member of the herpesvirus group, is responsible for this disease. Acute pharyngitis has always been considered an integral feature of infectious mononucleosis. It must be emphasized that, although many patients with this disorder experience moderate to severe sore throat at the beginning and through a good part of the clinical course, an appreciable number do not have this symptom at any time. Others may have no pharyngeal discomfort at the beginning of the illness and develop it only later in the course. Examination of the pharynx often reveals marked redness, swelling of all of the lymphoid tissue and marked injection of the blood vessels. In some instances, a considerable collection of yellow exudate may be present on the posterior pharyngeal wall and tonsils. In patients with severe leukopenia, secondary invasion of the throat may take place by members of the normal bacterial flora. In these cases, fusobacteria are involved and produce the typical Plaut-Vincent angina, the features of which are collections of dark grey exudate, ulceration and a characteristic anaerobic odor to the breath. When group A streptococci (beta-hemolytic streptococci) are secondary invaders, pharyngeal discomfort may be very severe; the physical findings are those characteristic of streptococcal sore throat. In a few patients with infectious mononucleosis, the physical findings in the pharynx are highly suggestive of diphtheria because of the presence of a typical pseudomembrane; the writer has studied ten patients who had serologically-documented infectious mononucleosis from whose pharynges toxigenic strains of *C. diphtheriae* were isolated.

Neisseria Gonorrhaeae. The incidence of pharyngitis due to this organism has increased strikingly over the last few years. Unfortunately, the physical findings in the pharynx are not specific enough to suggest the etiology. Because of the epidemic nature of gonorrhea in this country and the changes in sex habits, the possibility of gonorrheal pharyngitis must be considered in any instance in which venereal contact is known. The gonococcus will not grow on the media commonly used for the etiologic diagnosis of pharyngitis. For this reason, in any suspected case, throat cultures should be carried out on Thayer-Martin medium.

Treponema Pallidum. Acute pharyngitis is a manifestation of the secondary stage of syphilis in some patients. In addition, the throat may also be the site of the primary chancre; this lesion presents as a single nonpainful ulcer. The pharyngeal lesions in the secondary stage of the disease are the mucous patches which are also present on the buccal mucosa and tongue; they are teeming with spirochetes and highly contagious. Diagnosis is established by examination of the lesions with the dark-field microscope and serological test.

Viruses. A number of viral agents may be responsible for varying degrees of sore throat. This may be the sole manifestation of the infection or constitute the prodrome or clinical course of the disease. Adenovirus may produce a pharyngitis of moderate severity in which there is exudate on the pharyngeal wall and tonsil; this is often confused with streptococcal pharyngitis. One of the manifestations of viral influenza is often a sore throat. This is undoubtedly due to infection of the pharyngeal mucosa. The mild sore throat of the so-called common cold, due primarily to rhinoviruses, is another example of a primary viral pharyngitis. Among the pharyngitides associated with systemic viral infections are those associated with measles, chicken pox (typical vesicles are present in the pharynx), poliomyelitis (prodrome), Australia antigen-positive infectious hepatitis and disease due to Coxsackie and Echo viruses.

Candida Albicans. Although thrush is a common finding in newborn children, infection of the pharynx by *Candida albicans* is rare in normal children or adults. This occurs most often in immunosuppressed individuals and in those receiving antimicrobial agents, especially those with so-called broad-spectrum activity. The lesions are patchy, white in color and, when the exudate is removed, a shallow reddish ulcer is revealed. Diagnosis is established by demonstrating the typical yeast forms in stained smears and by culture.

Tumors. Adults, unlike children, occasionally present the difficult differential diagnosis of tumor when they present with a complaint of sore throat. Sharply localized pain, sometimes with no alteration in the appearance of the pharynx but more often with local areas of swelling, especially of a single tonsil, should suggest the possibility of tumor, the diagnosis of which is established by biopsy. In our experience, the most common lesions have been lymphoma, Hodgkin's disease and carcinoma involving the tonsil.

Tonsillectomy and Adenoidectomy. Although it has been suggested for a long time that tonsillectomy is indicated when recurrent sore throats, especially those due to group A streptococci, become a problem, valid statistically-significant data in support of this procedure are not available. In fact, some published experiences suggest that this operation is without benefit in preventing recurrences. It is obvious that this therapeutic and prophylactic modality requires further strictly controlled study and statistical validation of the results.

IMMUNOLOGIC ASPECT OF TONSILS

ABRAHAM MORAG, M.D.
PEARAY L. OGRA, M.D.
BUFFALO, NEW YORK

The involvement of external mucosal surfaces in the mechanism of defense against pathogenic microorganisms has recently attracted much attention. Many infectious agents gain access to the human body through the mucosa of nasopharynx, respiratory, genitourinary or lower gastrointestinal tracts. The immunocompetent lymphoid tissue in the mucosal portal of entry plays an important role in the mucosal immune system. The nasopharyngeal mucosa, tonsils and adenoids are replete with immunocompetent tissue. Because of their strategic anatomic location these tissues are in a relatively intimate and constant contact with the external environment, and constitute the primary sites of initial exposure to inhaled or ingested antigens. In addition to the "gatekeeper" site and function of the tonsils and adenoids, the tonsillar lymphoid tissue may also be involved in the overall development of the human immune system. This review will briefly focus on the immunologic consideration of the nasopharynx and tonsils, and examine the possible role of tonsils in the mechanisms of local immunity.

DEVELOPMENT AND STRUCTURE OF TONSILS

The complex of lymphoid tissue encircling the pharynx is referred to as Waldeyer's ring. This includes two faucial tonsils (tonsils), pharyngeal tonsil (adenoids), lymphoid tissue at the base of the tongue (lingual tonsil), and the lymphoid tissue on the posterior wall of the pharynx. The tonsils develop from the second pharyngeal pouch in close proximity to developing embryonic thymus. Lymphoid cells appear near the epithelial surface during the third month of gestation and organize as follicles after the sixth month. A schematic representation of the structure of mature tonsil is shown in Figure 1. It has been suggested that tonsillar tissue may be more reactive immunologically than other developing lymphoid tissue in early weeks of life.[1] Recent studies on fetal development of tonsils in experimental animals have indicated that lymphopoiesis in this tissue may be similar to thymus, and when tonsillar tissue is implanted in thymectomized animals, its actions appear to be somewhat similar to those observed after transplantation of thymus in thymectomized animals.[2,3]

Electronmicroscopic studies of normal human tonsils have shown that its cell population consists of lymphoid cells (80-90%) in various stages of development, plasma cells (5-20%), and a small number of monocytes and polymorphonuclear leukocytes.[4] Two populations of lymphocytes can be identified: The bone marrow derived or (bursa equivalent) thymic independent (B) lymphocytes, and thymic dependent (T) lymphocytes.[5,6,7] The B cells of tonsils range in diameter from 4-8 μ. The cells are generally spherical with numerous long microville, some B cells appear to be indulated with a relatively smooth sur-

---

From the Departments of Pediatrics and Microbiology, State University of New York at Buffalo, and Division of Virology, Children's Hospital, Buffalo, New York.

Supported in part by grants from National Institute of Allergy and Infectious Diseases (AI32522) (AI42511), National Institute of Arthritis Metabolism and Digestive Disease (AMI7050), National Institute of Child Health and Human Development (HDO6321) and Clinical Research Center Grant (RR628) from the U. S. Public Health Service.

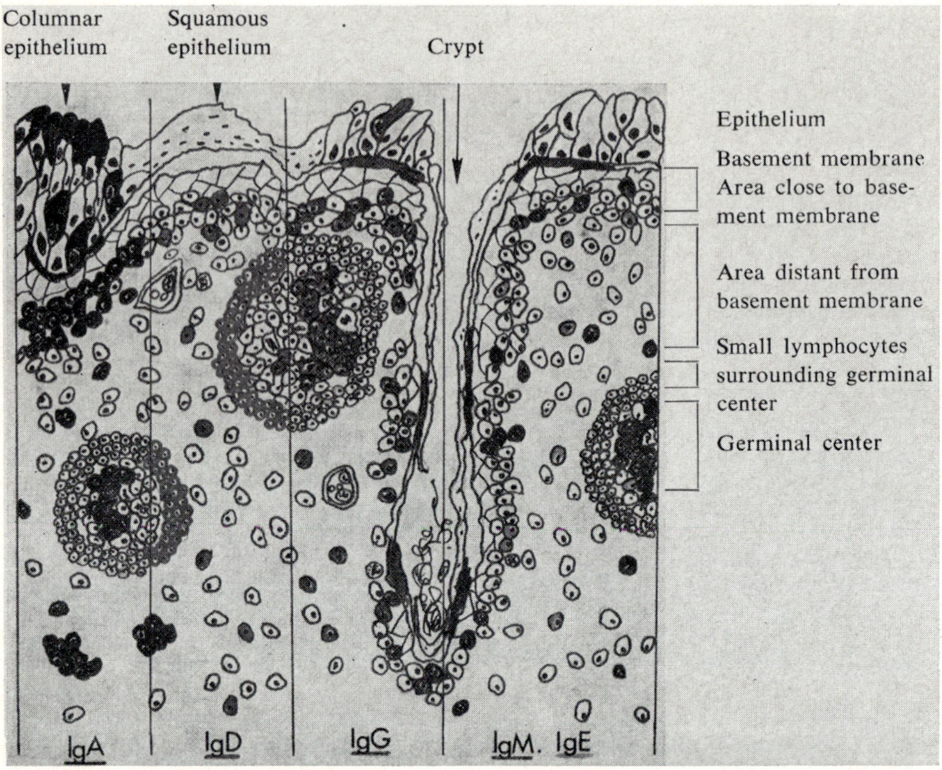

Fig. 1. Diagrammatic drawing of the distribution of immunoglobulins in tonsils. IgA: most of the IgA was seen in columnar epithelium, basement membrane, the cells closer to basement membrane and in many of the germinal centers. IgD: most of the IgD-containing cells (most likely, small lymphocytes) were seen in the mantle zone surrounding the germinal centers. IgG: the IgG-containing cells were scattered throughout the lymphoid tissues. Most of the germinal centers contained IgG. IgM: the IgM was seen in basement membrane, in single cells scattered throughout the tissue and in many of the germinal centers. IgE: single cells containing IgE were seen throughout the tissue. (Reprinted with permission of the authors and S. Karger, Basel.)

face harboring few short microville.[8] The B-lymphocytes can be recognized by the presence of membrane immunoglobulin and complement fixing receptors and by their ability to form rosettes with sheep erythrocytes in the presence of amboceptor and complement (EAC-rosette). The T-lymphocytes are spherical in shape and range from 3-5 μ in diameter. Usually their surface is smooth with a few stud-like microvilli. These cells can be identified in the tonsils by their ability to form rosettes with sheep red cells directly (E-rosette).[7] The T-cells do not seem to possess surface receptors for immunoglobulin and complement fixation. Although the ratio of B-lymphocytes to T-lymphocytes in the tonsils may vary from one individual to another,[4] studies carried out in our laboratory on tonsils obtained from children suggest that approximately 14-47% of the tonsillar lymphocytes appear to be thymus derived as identified by rosette formation with sheep red blood cells.[9] Other investigators have reported that approximately 30-40% of the tonsillar lymphocytes can be identified as T-cells.[10]

The localization and relative number of immunoglobulin containing cells in the tonsillar tissue has been the subject of several recent studies.[11-14] In a detailed study, Gitlin and Sasaki[11] have estimated IgG, IgA and IgM immunoglobulin in single cells obtained from the tonsils. The IgG containing cells were represented in a larger number than the IgA or IgM bearing cells. However, the average amount of immunoglobulin produced per cell was IgG, 0.46 pg; IgA, 2.6 pg; and IgM, 1.7 pg. Recently, IgD and IgE containing cells have also been observed in the tonsils.[12-15] It appears that of the various lymphoid tissues studied, the tonsils contain the largest number of IgE producing cells.[12] The relative distribution of major immunoglobulin producing plasma cells in the tonsils is schematically shown in Figure 1. The vast majority of IgA forming cells are found close to the basement membrane of the tonsil, the glandular tissue in the epithelium, and in the germinal centers. IgG and IgM containing cells are scattered throughout the lymphoid tissue, including the germinal centers. Most of the IgD bearing cells are seen in the mantle zone surrounding the germinal centers, while cells containing IgE are seen frequently scattered throughout the tissue.[13] IgA immunoglobulin found in tonsillar tissue appears to be of mostly secretory (11S) type, although appreciable amounts of 7S IgA are also detectable.

TONSILS AND SECRETORY IMMUNE FUNCTION

The current concept of local immunity defines the mechanism of secretory immune system as the local, and generally independent response of immunocompetent lymphoid cells in mucosal surfaces to locally available antigens. The development and the intensity of such response seems to be related to the type of antigen (replicating vs nonreplicating), route of administration (local vs parenteral), the ability of the mucosal tissues to capture the antigen, the type of immunocompetent cells available locally, and the degree of prior exposure or sensitization with the specific antigen (primary vs reinfection).

The tonsils, because of their location at the portal of entry for many microorganisms, have often been considered as the first line of defense against respiratory infections. Microbial antigens present in the environment are constantly being applied to the surface of the tonsils.[16] The ability of tonsils to capture such antigens has been recently demonstrated,[17,18] and it seems that the tonsils may act as both regional and nonregional lymph nodes and serve as an initial trapping mechanism for a variety of antigens.[17,19]

As indicated earlier, antibody producing cells of all major classes of immunoglobulin are found within the tonsils. Recent studies have clearly demonstrated that tonsillar tissue is capable of synthesizing various types of immunoglobulins and specific antibodies *in vivo* and *in vitro* states.[1,11,14,19-22] Sloyer et al[23] cultured lymphocytes from human tonsils *in vitro* with poliovirus and observed synthesis of specific antibody in the tissue cultures. The production of the antibody was dependent on DNA synthesis in the cultured lymphocytes. Other investigators have demonstrated the production of specific antibodies by tonsillar lymphocytes when cultured *in vitro* with such antigens as sheep red blood cells and tetanus toxoid, etc.[19,24] Further, few fragmentary pieces of evidence suggest that in addition to their ability to function locally, the tonsils might be a source of immunologic messengers responsible for propagating the induction of immune response in remote lymphoid organs.[19]

A variety of soluble mediators are elaborated by lymphocytes which have been activated by nonspecific mitogens or by antigens to which the donor is previously sensitized. The production of such mediators can be demonstrated by *in vitro* lymphocyte transformation (LTF), inhibition of macrophage migration, lymphocytoxicity and several other assays. These assays are currently acceptable as the *in vitro* correlates of cellular immunity (CMI), and possibly reflect the function of T-lymphocytes.

The initial studies with cultured tonsillar lymphocytes and their response to mitogens and antigens were carried out by Oettgen et al in 1966.[25] They demonstrated that tonsillar lymphocytes are stimulated *in vitro* by phytohemagglu-

TABLE I

MEAN MIGRATION AND STIMULATION INDICES OF TONSILLAR LYMPHOCYTES EXPOSED *IN VITRO* TO RUBELLA VIRUS ANTIGEN AFTER PRIOR IMMUNIZATION OR INFECTION WITH RUBELLA VIRUS

Group	*Migration Index*	*Stimulation Index*
Seronegative	0.94 (0.78-1.04)	1.09 (0.33- 2.65)
Natural infection	<u>0.64</u> (0.54-0.66)	<u>8.12</u> (3.60-14.31)
HPV-77 DE/5 S.C.	0.84 (0.59-1.05)	1.72 (0.42- 3.41)
RA27/3 I.N.	<u>0.70</u> (0.59-0.90)	<u>5.80</u> (2.12-20.21)

( ) = The values represent the range observed in each experimental group.
___ = Statistically significant.
S.C. = Subcutaneous immunization.
I.N. = Intranasal immunization.

tinin (PHA), poliovirus, *Bordetella pertussis*, and tetanus and diphtheria toxoids. The stimulation by the antigens occurred when the tonsillar lymphocytes were obtained from children who were previously immunized with these antigens. In addition to their blastogenic response to mitogens, tonsillar lymphocytes have been found to undergo transformation when cultured *in vitro* with allogenic lymphoid cells.[26] Recently we have conducted a prospective study on the CMI of tonsillar lymphocytes to rubella and mumps viruses.[27,28] Employing the assays of *in vitro* lymphocyte transformation and migration inhibitory factor activity, the development of CMI in circulating and tonsillar lymphocytes was studied in groups of children who underwent tonsillectomy at varying intervals after natural rubella infection, subcutaneous immunization with HPV-77 DE/5 or intranasal inoculation with RA27/3 live attenuated rubella virus vaccines. Development of specific CMI in tonsillar lymphocytes was regularly observed after natural infection and intranasal immunization. However, CMI response in tonsils was conspicuously absent after subcutaneous immunization (Table I). Similarly induction of specific CMI in tonsillar lymphocytes was also observed after natural infection with mumps virus. These observations suggest the induction of local CMI in tonsillar lymphoid cells after local nasopharyngeal infection with rubella or mumps virus. Stimulation with a nonspecific mitogen (phytohemagglutinin) generally results in blastogenesis of both B and T- cells, as has been shown in a number of recent studies.[9,29] This raises the question of specificity of LTF responses as a function of T-cell activity. However, a combined technique of E-rosette formation and autoradiography after specific stimulation of tonsillar lymphocytes with rubella antigen has recently demonstrated that the majority of rubella induced lymphocyte transformation is a function of E-rosette forming T-cells (Fig. 2).

MUCOSAL IMMUNITY AND TONSILLECTOMY

The question whether the removal of the tonsils might compromise the microbial defense or local immunologic functions of the host is the focus of a long standing controversy surrounding the surgical removal of tonsils and adenoids. Although tonsillar lymphoid tissue appears to be immunologically active, its role in local mucosal defense and its contribution to the maturation of total immune system remains to be determined. A few investigations have attempted to examine the effects of tonsillectomy on the nasopharyngeal reinfection with viruses and bacteria. In a recent study, levels of specific secretory IgA antibody to poliovirus in the nasopharynx were examined before and after tonsillectomy.[30] After poliovirus immunization, and before tonsillectomy, all the children studied had specific secretory IgA antibody. However, the level of such antibody decreased significantly

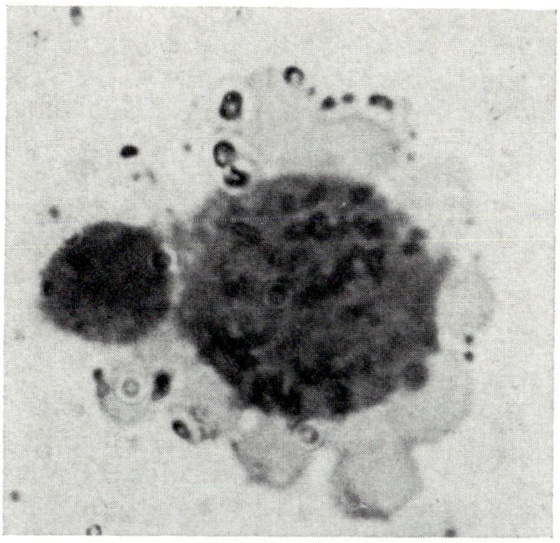

Fig. 2. *In vitro* rubella-antigen-induced transformation of tonsillar lymphocytes. The blast cell (as indicated by incorporation of 3H thymidine) form a rosette with sheep red blood cells.

after surgery, particularly in young children. In subsequent studies it was found that the nasopharyngeal antibody response to poliovirus was significantly higher in children with intact tonsils than those whose tonsils had been previously removed.[30]

Earlier epidemiologic studies have clearly demonstrated an increased incidence of paralytic poliomyelitis following tonsilloadenoidectomy. In view of the immunologic information presented, the possibility that removal of tonsils in young children may impair the anti-polio defense mechanism in the respiratory tract, and maturation of γA immunoglobulin system must therefore be entertained. Impairment of local immune mechanism may conceivably increase the risk of the spread of poliovirus from nasopharynx to central nervous system via the nerve roots.

The development and participation of cell-mediated immune responses in the tonsils and respiratory tract has been recently demonstrated. However, its functional role in the mechanism of mucosal defense remains to be clearly delineated. Little or no information is available regarding the effects of tonsillectomy on nasopharyngeal cell-mediated immune responses. In one study, it has been suggested that the incidence of Hodgkin's disease may be higher among tonsillectomized individuals.[31] The mechanism underlying this association is not clear, although change in cellular immune responses secondary to tonsillectomy may be a contributing factor. On the other hand, other well controlled epidemiologic studies have failed to discern such an association.[32,33] Until additional immunologic and epidemiologic data are available, it is difficult to develop any meaningful association between tonsillectomy, malignancy and any alterations in the immune system.

ADENOIDS AND IMMUNE SYSTEM

Since adenoidectomy is almost always carried out in conjunction with tonsillectomy, little or no information which specially relates to adenoids relative to the clinical, immunologic and epidemiologic aspects of adenoidal disease is available. Despite the paucity of available information, it would seem that the degree to which adenoids are exposed to exogenous antigens is similar to that of tonsils. Adenoids appear to be immunologically reactive. Approximately 25-30% of adenoidal lymphocytes are T-cells which manifest cell-mediated immune function in response to specific antigens. The contribution of adenoids in local antibody response has not been carefully examined. Preliminary data from our laboratory suggest that adenoids may participate only minimally in the local immune response, and the effects of adenoidectomy on nasopharyngeal immune response may not be as pronounced as after tonsillectomy.

DISCUSSION

The observation summarized in the preceding sections suggests that tonsils are immunologically reactive lymphoid organs, which manifest specific antibody, and B and T-cell activity in response to a variety of antigens. The immunologic system of the external mucous membranes appears to function as a first line of defense against pathogens for which primary portal of entry is the mucosa of nasopharynx and respiratory and alimentary tracts.

Developmental studies of human immunoglobulin production have indicated that normal newborn infants are essentially agammaglobulinemic at birth, with the exception of transplacentally acquired maternal γG immunoglobulin. However, after birth, and subsequent to mucosal colonization with bacteria and exposure to other antigens, the immune system begins to mature rapidly, particularly for γM and γG immunoglobulin and T-cell function. The γA immune system appears to mature late, and adult levels of serum and secretory γA are generally attained several years after birth. It is therefore conceivable that during early years of life, all available immunocompetent lymphoid tissue may be necessary for optimal maturation and development of immunoglobulins, particularly of γA class in the serum and secretory sites. Tonsils and, to a small extent, adenoids, may contribute to the normal immunologic developmental process, and their removal during the growth period may compromise subsequent local nasopharyngeal immunological responses, and overall immunity against infections in the respiratory tract.

It is obvious that this summation is based on fragmentary pieces of information, and raises more questions without providing any answers about tonsils and tonsillectomy. Carefully controlled studies need to be undertaken to explore some of these questions in more detail. For example, it is crucial to learn the underlying state of host defense and nasopharyngeal immunity in patients who suffer from recurrent sore throats and who eventually undergo tonsillectomy and/or adenoidectomy. Recently it has been suggested that patients who undergo tonsillectomy may have a relative immunodeficiency of T-cell function and antibody activity, which may be the primary contributing factor for recurrent tonsillitis in these children.[34] Unfortunately, a careful postoperative immunological evaluation was not carried out in this study. Prospective studies need to be undertaken to evaluate functional parameters of immunologic system before and after tonsillectomy. The exact nature of the immune response elicited by the tonsils and adenoids, and its contribution to the local immune system needs to be carefully evaluated. The role of tonsils in the protection or pathogenesis of allergic disorders merits special investigation, since tonsils are very rich in γE producing cells. Finally, the effect of tonsillectomy, adenoidectomy or both on the immune response in the nasopharynx and the effect of such surgery on subsequent resistance against pathogenic viruses and bacteria need to be studied in some detail.

REFERENCES

1. Godrick EA, Patt GR: A comparison of the immune response of tonsils with the appendix and spleen in neonatal rabbits. Acta Otolaryngol 71:357, 1971

2. Harrison BH, Patt D, Albright JT: Cellular development in the palatine tonsil of the fetal rabbit, with special emphasis on lymphoiesis. Tissue and Cell 2:1, 1970

3. Harrison BH: Tonsillar tissue implants in neonatally thymectomized mice. J Immunol 105:38, 1970

4. Zucker-Franklin D, Berney S: Electron microscopy study of surface immunoglobulin bearing human tonsil cells. J Exp Med 135: 533, 1972

5. Rabellino E, Grey HM: Immunoglobulins on the surface of lymphocytes. III. Bursal origin of surface immunoglobulins on chicken lymphocytes. J Immunol 106:1418, 1971

6. Unanue ER, Grey HM, Rabellino E, et al: Immunoglobulins of the surface of lymphocytes. II. The bone marrow as the main source of lymphocytes with detectable surface-bound immunoglobulins. J Exp Med 133:1188, 1971

7. Lay WH, Mendes NF, Bianco C, et al: Binding of sheep red blood cells to a large population of human lymphocytes. Nature (Lond) 230:531, 1971

8. Sun Lin P, Cooper AG, Wortis HH: Scanning electron microscopy of human T-cell and B-cell rosettes. N Engl J Med 289:548, 1973

9. Morag A, Morag B, Beutner KR, et al: Development of in-vitro correlates of cell-mediated immunity in human tonsils after natural or induced rubella virus infection. In press

10. Hurtado RC, Rola-Pleszczynski M, Menda MA, et al: The immunologic role of

tonsillar tissues in local cell-mediated immune responses. Pediatr Res (Abstr) 8:140, 1974

11. Gitlin D, Sasaki T: Immunoglobulins G, A and M determined in single cells from human tonsils. Science 164:1532, 1969

12. Tada T, Ishizaka K: Distribution of IgE forming cells in lymphoid tissue in human and monkey. J Immunol 104:377, 1970

13. Wicher K, Ishikawa T, Arbesman CE: Direct immunofluorescent staining of IgE containing cells in tissues of human and monkey. Abstr Excerpta Med Int Congr Ser 211:17, 1970

14. Ishikawa T, Wicher K, Arbesman CE: Distribution of immunoglobulins in palatine and pharyngeal tonsils. Int Arch Allergy Appl Immunol 43:801, 1972

15. vanBoxel JA, Paul WE, Terry WD, et al: IgD bearing human lymphocytes. J Immunol 109:648, 1972

16. Veltri RW, Sprinkle PM, Keller SA, et al: Ecological alterations of oral microflora subsequent to tonsillectomy and adenoidectomy. J Laryngol Otol 86:893, 1972

17. Surjan L, Surjan L Jr, Surjan M: Further investigations into the immunological role of the tonsils. Acta Otolaryngol 73:222, 1972

18. Merler E, Silberschmidt M: Uptake of antigen by human lymphocytes. Immunology 22:821, 1972

19. Surjan L, Surjan M: Immunological role of human tonsils. Acta Otolaryngol 71: 190, 1971

20. Ogra PL, Karzon DT: Formation and function of poliovirus antibody in different tissues. Progr Med Virol 13:156, 1971

21. Burtin P, Buffe D: Synthesis of human immunoglobulins in germinal centers of lymphoid organs. J Immunol 98:536, 1967

22. Pesak V: The localization of IgA and IgE globulins in the palatinal tonsils, nasal mucous membrane and nasal polypi. Folia Microbiol (Praha) 16:323, 1971

23. Sloyer JL, Veltri RW, Sprinkle PM: In-vitro IgM antibody synthesis by human tonsil-derived lymphocytes. J Immunol 111:183, 1973

24. Hoffman MK, Schmidt D, Oettgen HF: Production of antibody to sheep red blood cells by human tonsil cells in-vitro. Nature 243:408, 1973

25. Oettgen HF, Silber R, Miesher PA, et al: Stimulation of human tonsillar lymphocytes in-vitro. Clin Exp Immunol 1:77, 1966

26. Schwartz MR: Response of thymus and other human lymphoid tissues to PHA, PWN and genetically dissimilar lymphoid cells. Proc Soc Exp Biol Med 125:701, 1967

27. Morag A, Bernstein JM, Beutner K, et al: Development and characteristics of viral induced cell-mediated immune responses in upper respiratory tract. Pediatr Res 8:141, 1974

28. Beutner KR, Morag A, Bernstein JM, et al: Local and systemic immune response to mumps virus in man. Presented in the 74th Annual Meeting, American Society for Microbiology, Chicago, Ill., May 12-17, 1974

29. Merler E, Silberschmidt M: Separation of antibodies from subcellar components of lymphocytes. Immunology 22:813, 1972

30. Ogra PL: Effect of tonsillectomy and adenoidectomy on nasopharyngeal antibody response to poliovirus. N Engl J Med 284:59, 1971

31. Vianna NJ, Greenwald P, Daview JNP: Tonsillectomy and Hodgkin's disease: The lymphoid tissue barrier. Lancet 1:431, 1971

32. Johnson SK, Johnson RE: Tonsillectomy history in Hodgkin's disease. N Engl J Med 287:1122, 1972

33. Ruuskanea O, Vanha-Perttula T, Kouvalainen K: Tonsillectomy, appendectomy and Hodgkin's disease. Lancet 1:1127, 1971

34. Donovan R, Soothill JF: Immunological studies in children undergoing tonsillectomy. Clin Exp Immunol 14:347, 1973

OBSTRUCTIVE ADENOIDS IN RELATION TO OTITIS MEDIA

CHARLES D. BLUESTONE, M.D.

PITTSBURGH, PENNSYLVANIA

Recurrent acute otitis media and chronic middle ear effusions are common problems in childhood, and adenoidectomy is frequently undertaken in an effort to ameliorate them. However, the efficacy of the operation has yet to be shown. In 1930 Kaiser[1] reported a lower incidence of purulent otorrhea in a large group of children who had received adenotonsillectomy as compared with a control group. In 1963 McKee[2,3] reported two controlled studies of tonsillectomy and adenoidectomy. Entry into the study was based on a history of three or more sore throats during the previous year. He concluded that tonsillectomy did not seem to alter the course of otitis media but found a reduction in ear disease following adenoidectomy. In two similar studies, Roydhouse[4] also found a decreased incidence of otitis media but Mawson[5] did not.

Unfortunately, in all of these studies the methods for assessing the presence or severity of otitis media were not described and secretory otitis media, myringotomy, tympanostomy tube insertion or hearing evaluations were not mentioned. Prospective controlled studies of adenoidectomy for otitis media have not been reported.

CURRENT STUDIES

In an attempt to improve preoperative selection of patients for adenoidectomy, Bluestone et al[6] studied the Eustachian tube roentgenographically before and after adenoidectomy in a group of children who had recurrent or chronic otitis media. The nasopharynx and the nasopharyngeal portion of the Eustachian tube were visualized after the instillation of radiopaque material into the nasopharynx through a nasal catheter. In some instances it was also possible thereby to visualize the middle ear and protympanic portion of the Eustachian tube. If not, and if a tympanostomy tube had previously been inserted, contrast medium was instilled transtympanically into the middle ear. Using these techniques, it was possible to evaluate not only structure but function, as manifested by the flow of contrast medium, at both ends of the Eustachian tube. Adenoid size was also estimated roentgenographically. Three types of abnormal Eustachian tube function were found: retrograde obstruction, retrograde reflux, and prograde obstruction. An additional abnormality, manifested by the positive roentgenographic Toynbee test was described. Normal retrograde function and prograde clearance were both present in 5 of 44 children (11%) before adenoidectomy and in 23 of 33 children (70%) following adenoidectomy (Table I). Thirteen of the 33 children (39%) developed otitis media within a period of nine months or less following adenoidectomy, and the results were considered failures. Eight of these children developed more severe ear disease than had been present before adenoidectomy. Favorable otologic results were maintained following adenoidectomy in 20 of the 33 children (61%) (Table II). Eight of these had normal prograde clearance, normal retrograde function, and a negative roentgenographic Toynbee test following adenoidectomy. The remaining 12 (and also two "failures") had normal prograde clearance and retrograde function, but their roentgenographic Toynbee test was positive. The effectiveness of adenoidectomy in preventing otitis media appeared to be correlated, to a considerable degree, with the preadenoidectomy roentgenographic findings: In 19 of the 27 children (70%) who had retrograde obstruction the results were successful, whereas

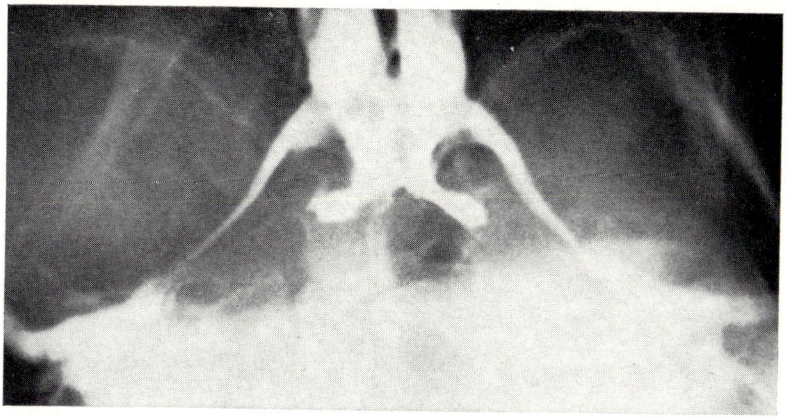

Fig. 1. Postadenoidectomy roentgenogram of a child who demonstrated retrograde reflux. (By permission of the *Laryngoscope* 82:1654-1670, 1972.)

in two of the three (67%) with normal retrograde function and in all three with reflux the results were failures (Fig. 1). Allergic rhinitis was associated with a high failure rate; in only two of ten allergic children (20%), as compared with 18 of 23 nonallergic children (80%), the results were considered successful. Adenoid size was not necessarily predictive of Eustachian tube function, although most children with large adenoids had retrograde obstruction.

In an effort to develop a more simple and accurate method to identify children in whom adenoidectomy might prevent otitis media, Bluestone, et al[7] assessed the ventilatory function of the Eustachian tube by a manometric technique. Nasal pressures during swallowing were also determined in some. The study group consisted of 23 children with otitis media in whom tympanostomy tubes had been inserted. All were judged clinically and roentgenographically to have prominent adenoids. Inflation-deflation Eustachian tube ventilation studies were obtained in 36 ears that remained intubated, aerated, and dry both before and eight weeks after adenoidectomy. Fifteen of the 36 (42%) ears had improvement in Eustachian tube ventilatory function postadenoidectomy which was attributed to relief of extrinsic mechanical obstruction of the tube. In the remaining 21 (58%) ears in whom Eustachian tube function was not improved, mechanical obstruction was not apparent preoperatively. The effect of nasopharyngeal pressures on a pliant Eustachian tube (Toynbee phenomenon) due to obstruction of the posterior nasal choanae by the adenoid mass was sug-

TABLE I

PRE- AND POSTADENOIDECTOMY ROENTGENOGRAPHIC ASSESSMENT OF RETROGRADE EUSTACHIAN TUBE FUNCTION IN 33 CHILDREN WITH PREVIOUS CHRONIC OR RECURRENT OTITIS MEDIA

		Adenoidectomy (No. of Children) After		
Before	*N*	*Obstructed*	*Normal*	*Reflux*
Obstructed	27	3	21	3
Normal	3	1	2	0
Reflux	3	0	0	3

TABLE II

OTITIS MEDIA BEFORE AND AFTER ADENOIDECTOMY IN 33 CHILDREN

	Adenoidectomy (No. of Children)	
Otitis Media	*Before*	*After*
Present	33 (100%)	13 (39%)
Absent	0	20 (61%)

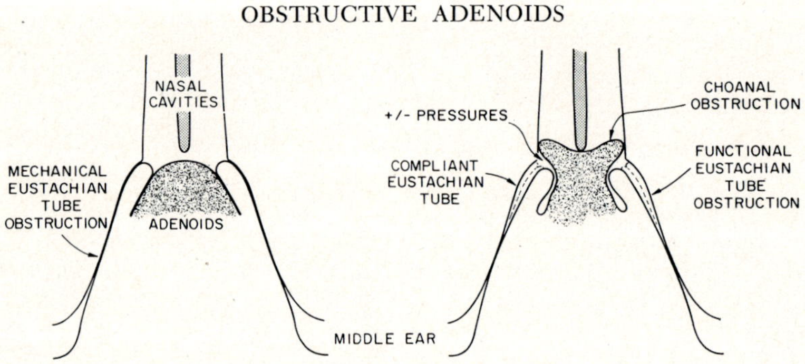

Fig. 2. Author's conception of mechanical and functional obstruction of the Eustachian tube caused by obstructive adenoids.

gested as a possible cause of functional Eustachian tube obstruction (Fig. 2). In several instances in which preadenoidectomy mechanical obstruction of the Eustachian tube was not demonstrated, the tube appeared to have been made more pliant by the operation. This increase in compliance of the Eustachian tube was attributed to loss of adenoid support of the tube in the fossa of Rosenmüller (Fig. 3).

UNANSWERED RESEARCH QUESTIONS

Unfortunately, many basic questions remain unanswered. The following is a list of some of these questions.

Epidemiology.

What are the population characteristics of otitis media in relation to adenoids?

Pathogenesis and Pathophysiology.

Do the adenoids mechanically obstruct the Eustachian tube?

If so, where? In the fossa of Rosenmüller? At the nasopharyngeal orifice? To what degree?

How does this obstruction affect the protective, clearance, and ventilation functions of the tube?

What effect does inflammation (allergy or infection) of the adenoids have on tubal function?

Does intrinsic inflammation of the tube play a role?

Is the compliance of the tube a factor? The geometry of the nose and nasopharynx?

Do the adenoids obstruct the posterior nasal choanae?

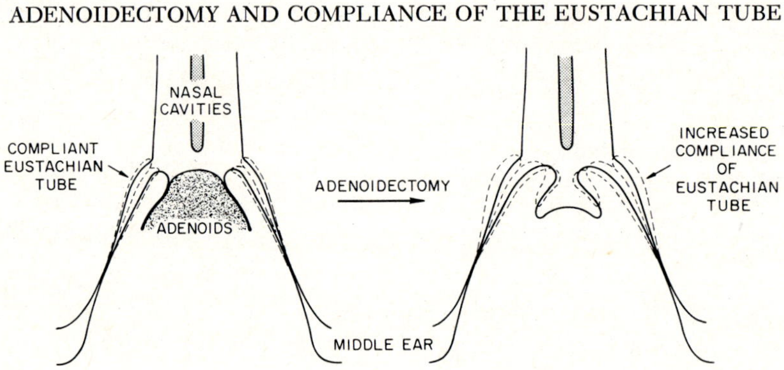

Fig. 3. Author's conception of increased compliance of Eustachian tube following adenoidectomy.

If so, how, when, where, and to what degree?

What role does inflammation play? Is the geometry of the nose and nasopharynx (craniofacial morphology) a factor? Is age a factor?

What effect does nasal obstruction have on the function of the Eustachian tube?

What are the nasopharyngeal pressures during tubal opening?

When does the tube open?

Can functional Eustachian tube obstruction result?

Is the compliance of the tube a factor?

Is velopharyngeal function important?

What factors contribute to the compliance of the Eustachian tube? Amount and consistency of the cartilage support? Muscle tension or vector? Craniofacial morphology?

Does the mucus blanket of the Eustachian tube play a role?

Which technique is best for evaluation of the adenoids in relation to the nasal airway and Eustachian tube, e.g., roentgenographic, manometric, tympanometric? When should the test be performed, e.g., during periods of inflammation or between episodes, or both?

MEDICAL MANAGEMENT OF OBSTRUCTIVE ADENOIDS.

What is the effect of medical treatment of the adenoids in relation to otitis media?

What are the effects of nasal decongestants, antihistamines, and antibiotics on adenoids that are obstructive to the posterior nasal choanae or Eustachian tube, or both?

SURGICAL MANAGEMENT OF ADENOIDS.

Does adenoidectomy alter the course of acute otitis media or chronic middle ear effusions?

What is the effect of adenoidectomy on the function of the Eustachian tube?

Does the compliance of the Eustachian tube change?

Which method of evaluation of the nasopharynx and Eustachian tube is best?

Which technique of adenoidectomy is best? When should the adenoids be removed from the fossa of Rosenmüller?

At what age is adenoidectomy indicated? Should a myringotomy be performed or tympanostomy tubes inserted into the tympanic membrane when effusion is present in the middle ear? When should the tympanostomy tubes be removed?

METHODS OF FINDING THE ANSWERS TO THE RESEARCH QUESTIONS

EPIDEMIOLOGY.

Determine the population characteristics of otitis media (suppurative and nonsuppurative) in relation to adenoids.

PATHOGENESIS AND PATHOLOGY.

Define the normal physiology of the nose-nasopharynx-palate-Eustachian tube-middle ear-mastoid system.

Study the effect of adenoids on the "system" in relation to otitis media.

Study the effect of inflammation on the system.

Study the effect of surgical and nonsurgical management on the system.

Develop techniques to evaluate the system including the following:

Roentgenography.

Static-lateral and basalar cephlometrics; dynamic-video and cine basalar and lateral projections, contrast media.

Manometry.

Tympanometry.

Audiometry.

Electromyography.

Studies of craniofacial morphology as related to the adenoids within the system.

Special studies of the Eustachian tube as related to structure and function.

Studies of the histopathology, biochemistry, rheology of the system.

Studies of middle ear effusions.

Develop an animal model to study the system.

Studies of normal physiology and induced pathophysiologic states.

MANAGEMENT.

Design a prospective controlled study to determine the best surgical and nonsurgical methods of management of otitis media when associated with obstructive adenoids. The following should be included in the design:

Entry into the study should be based on objective criteria.

Objective evidence of otitis media by tympanometry, audiometry, and objective otoscopy.

Objective evidence of obstructive adenoids to the nose or Eustachian tube or both by manometry or roentgenographic techniques.

Complete work-up including immunologic status.

Determine the pathophysiologic changes in the "system" prior to management.

Accurate documentation of the technique employed when surgery is selected.

Follow-up should include evaluation of the system by objective methods, i.e., tympanometry, audiometry, and objective otoscopy.

Documentation of all other surgical procedures performed both before and after management, i.e., myringotomy, tympanostomy tube insertion.

CONCLUSION

A prospective, controlled study of the best surgical vs the best nonsurgical management of adenoids in relation to otitis media appears indicated. Studies leading to better understanding of the population characteristics, pathogenesis and pathophysiology of otitis media in relation to adenoids will also be necessary.

REFERENCES

1. Kaiser AD: Results of tonsillectomy: A comparative study of 2,200 tonsillectomized children with an equal number of controls three and ten years after operation. JAMA 95:837, 1930

2. McKee WJE: A controlled study of the effects of tonsillectomy and adenoidectomy in children. Br J Prev Soc Med 17:49, 1963

3. McKee WJE: The part played by adenoidectomy in the combined operation of tonsillectomy with adenoidectomy; Second part of a controlled study in children. Br J Prev Soc Med 17:133, 1963

4. Roydhouse N: A controlled study of adenotonsillectomy. Arch Otolaryngol 92:611, 1970

5. Mawson SR, Adlington P, Evans M: A controlled study evaluation of adeno-tonsillectomy in children. J Laryngol Otol 81:777, 1967

6. Bluestone CD, Wittel RA, Paradise JL, et al: Eustachian tube function as related to adenoidectomy for otitis media. Trans Am Acad Ophthalmol Otolaryngol 76:1325-1339, 1972

7. Bluestone CD, Cantekin EI, Beery QC: Certain effects of adenoidectomy on Eustachian tube ventilatory function. Laryngoscope 85:113-127, 1975

EFFECT OF UPPER AIRWAY OBSTRUCTION ON THE LOWER AIRWAY AND CARDIOVASCULAR SYSTEM

JOSEPH H. OGURA, M.D.

ST. LOUIS, MISSOURI

During the past twenty years we have been interested in obstructive disease of the upper airway. This interest stemmed from the acknowledgment that little is known of the area. The following is an outline of past studies conducted in our laboratories.

Observations Between Nose and Pulmonary System. Patients were studied employing a standard body plethysmograph, cathode ray oscilloscope, ink writer, computer and write-out system. An esophageal balloon was also utilized. Investigations involving patients with deviated septa were studied and their compliance and resistance assessed. When the nose was obstructed, nasal resistance increased and lung compliance went down.

The effect of nasal obstruction on the pulmonary mechanics of the dog was studied. Unilateral nasal obstruction in the dog was compensated; however, when bilateral obstruction was induced, pulmonary airway resistance was persistently increased and there was a compliance change throughout a five-month observation period.

The conclusion of these experiments is that nasal obstruction alters the total pulmonary resistance in human and animal experiments.

Arterial Gas Changes in Animals with Laryngeal Obstruction. Experiments in dogs revealed that laryngeal obstruction resulted in an elevated PCO_2 and decrease in PO_2. The combination of modest hypercapnia and a more marked hypoxia in these experiments suggest that the changes occur at the ventilation perfusion ratio, the degree of changes of arterial hypoxia correlate well with the degree of increase in the expiratory laryngeal resistance. The decline of the PO_2 values was found to correlate most linearly with the expiratory laryngeal resistance.

Laryngeal resistance surgically created by severing both recurrent laryngeal nerves resulted in an arterial blood gas decrease in PO_2. Increased laryngeal obstruction was associated with an increase in pulmonary resistance. Therefore, neuroanatomic changes in larynx can influence changes in the airway.

Experiments in Humans with Nasal Packing for Epistaxis. The observation that some patients who had nasal packing for epistaxis suddenly died, prompted an investigation into the pathogenesis of this phenomenon. Studies revealed arterial blood gas changes in the PO_2 and PCO_2 in such patients. The PO_2 changes were observed when the nose was packed even though the subject was breathing through his mouth. After the nasal packs were removed the PO_2 returned to normal. This suggests a reflex relationship between the nose and the tracheobronchial tree probably mediated through the maxillary nerves. In conclusion then, complete nasal obstruction can result in increased pulmonary resistance.

EFFECT OF DISEASES OF TONSILS AND ADENOIDS ON DENTOFACIAL MORPHOLOGY

J. Daniel Subtelny, D.D.S.

Rochester, New York

For many years past, it has been believed that the nasorespiratory area plays an important role in dentofacial development and in the developing facial configuration. One has only to peruse the literature to find frequent reference to the so-called "adenoid-type" face. In essence, it is descriptive of a particular facial expression, supposedly typifying individuals with a super abundance of adenoid tissue and a resulting mouthbreathing habit. In individuals with a mouthbreathing habit, of course, the mouth characteristically stays open, the upper lip may appear short, the lower lip may be somewhat everted in posture and if the face manifests a certain degree of narrowness the individual is supposedly afflicted with an adenoid type face. Since adenoid tissue and/or excessive hypertrophy of this tissue may affect facial conformity, much interest has been engendered in gathering information pertaining to adenoid tissue and its surrounding nasopharyngeal spaces and in investigating its influence on facial development.

To this end, many orthodontists have utilized oriented cephalometric x-rays to investigate the location, configuration, and growth of the adenoid tissue and to evaluate its influence on the postural relationships of structures closely associated with the nasal-oral-pharyngeal complex. Soft tissue structures as well as hard tissue structures are readily visible on a cephalometric radiograph. It is entirely possible to examine the oronasopharyngeal areas radiographically and to appraise the soft tissues inside as well as outside of the oral-nasal cavities. Unfortunately, adenoid tissue cannot be radiographically visualized as a three-dimensional object but certainly much information has and can be gained from a radiographic registration representative of the midsagittal plane. On the lateral radiograph, adenoid tissue located in the nasopharyngeal area may be visualized as a somewhat convex prominence facing the superior or nasal surface of the soft palate. Its attachment to the roof of the nasopharynx may extend anteriorly as far forward as the posterior nasal choanae, from which the anterior border of the adenoid tissue may be observed to extend downward, approaching the soft palate to varying degrees. The inferior border of the adenoid tissue is then observed to extend posteriorly to join and blend into the posterior pharyngeal wall, at the approximate level of the anterior tubercle of the atlas. It has been observed that the adenoid tissue may occupy varying amounts of the nasopharyngeal cavity. In some instances the inferior border of this tissue may be far removed from the nasal surface of the soft palate. In other instances, it may be in close approximation with the nasal surface of the soft palate.

In studying the growth of adenoid tissue, serial cephalometric x-rays taken on the same individual indicate that the nasopharyngeal lymphatic tissue follows a specific growth cycle. From all indications, adenoid tissue seems to have a specific growth potential of its own upon which may be superimposed the hypertrophic reactions of nasorespiratory infections and allergies. During the early years of life, as evidenced by the radiographic registrations, the increase in the mass of adenoid tissue seemed quite rapid and, by approximately three years of age, was seen to occupy a sizable portion of the nasopharyngeal cavity. In some individuals, it was observed that as much as one-half of the nasopharyngeal cavity was occupied by lymphatic tissue. Subsequent radiographs indicated that the adenoid tissue continues to grow, predominantly in a downward and forward direction, but at a somewhat retarded rate until its peak of growth or greatest bulk is attained. In the sample studied, the peak mass was observed to occur somewhere between 10 to approximately 14 to 15 years of age. After the peak of adenoid growth was attained, the growth process seemed to reverse itself. The adenoid tissue was observed to progressively decrease in mass and regress away from the nasal aspect of the soft palate, towards the bony roof of the nasopharynx. By adulthood, the adenoid tissue had atrophied and the greatest dimension to the nasopharyngeal airway space was established.

It is of upmost importance to recognize that this tissue is growing within a constantly changing environment. Not only is the nasopharyngeal cavity continuously growing and changing in configuration, but the whole craniofacial complex itself is concomitantly growing and changing in configuration. It is the differential timing of growth as well as the differential amounts of growth of all of the involved structures that may actually affect dentofacial development. In considering the influence of differential growth on facial configuration, one concept must be kept in mind. Different parts of the human body grow at different rates and at different times. During overall body growth, one can readily substantiate the concept of disproportional growth. At the time of birth, the head measures approximately one-quarter of total body length. With progression of time into maturity, the head may proportionately measure approximately one-eighth of total body length. This does not mean the head has not been growing; it simply means that the head has been growing disproportionately relative to other parts of the human body. This is also true within the craniofacial complex; different parts of the human head grow at different rates and at different times. One has only to understand the progressive development of the soft tissues and skeletal tissues of the craniofacial complex to understand the significance of this observation relative to facial configuration.

In most instances, growth of the adenoid tissue and growth of the nasopharyngeal area seems to strike a fine state of equilibrium. During the early years, the adenoid tissue may be growing rapidly but the upper face is concomitantly growing at a rapid pace permitting the maintenance of an adequate airway space in the sense that the distance between the nasal surface of the resting soft palate and the inferior surface of adenoid tissue is sufficiently open for nasorespiratory needs. In most instances, this state of equilibrium persists until the peak of adenoid growth is reached. Subsequently, of course, the airway space may become larger as the adenoid commences to atrophy. At times, there may be a disturbance in this delicate balance and this equilibrium in differential growth may be disrupted as the adenoid tissue can be observed to increase in mass at a faster rate than the increase in the dimensions of the nasopharyngeal cavity. Whether this is a result of excessive adenoid growth or a reaction to infectious or allergic agents resulting in excessive hypertrophy of the lymphatic tissue is difficult to determine. However, in any case an approximation or a near approximation of the adenoid tissue with the nasal surface of the soft palate will create a blockage of the nasopharyngeal cavity causing difficulty in nasal breathing and the development of a mouth-breathing habit. Oral respiration necessitates numerous changes in the postural relationships of the structures involved. The lips, in repose, part, and the tongue moves downward and forward away from the soft palate with an accompanying depression in the posture of the mandible. Quite recently, this relationship of parts has been shown to have an influence on the configuration of the developing face, in a study conducted by Sten Linder-Aronson. In his Ph.D. study, Linder-Aronson used cephalometric radiography to evaluate 81 children who were selected for an adenoidectomy by an otolaryngologist. He compared these individuals with a comparable control group of children of the same age and sex who seemed to have no nasal-respiratory problems. In the group scheduled for adenoidectomies, 26% of the children were judged to have what has been called an adenoid face, whereas this was true in only 4% of the control subjects. In evaluating the facial morphology of the youngsters scheduled for adenoidectomy, he found them to have a longer and narrower face than the control group. The height of the face below the level of the anterior nasal spine seemed to be greater, there was a greater steepness to the lower border of the mandibular jaw which might indicate a more open gonial angle in the experimental group, there seemed to be a greater tendency for a retrusion of the maxillary and mandibular jaws as well as a smaller sagittal depth to the nasopharynx. In comparing the occlusion of the youngsters scheduled for an adenoidectomy with those in the control group, he found a narrower upper arch, a tendency towards an anterior open bite and a retroinclination of the upper and lower incisor teeth in the experimental group. On the cephalometric radiographs, taken at rest, he found a lower tongue position in the so-called "adenoid" subjects which might be coincidental with the mouthbreathing habit. Thus, it seems that excessive adenoid tissue which may require a mouthbreathing habit may cause an alteration in the developing dentofacial form.

Interestingly enough, these same cases were evaluated over a five-year postoperative period in order to ascertain changes incident to the removal of the mouthbreathing habit and a reinitiation of nasal respiration. Upon evaluation of the progressive cephalometric radiographs some interesting features were reported. There was an increase in the sagittal depth of the bony nasopharynx and, with growth, changes in the facial skeleton and in the dentition seem to occur in the direction of the control group so that these subjects more closely resembled that group after a period of time. With continued growth and the change to nasal respiration there seemed to be a proportional decrease in the lower facial height with a concomitant reduction in the angulation or steepness of the lower border of the mandible relative to the palatal plane or the roof of the mouth. Linder-Aronson calls this a "normalization" in skeletal relationships. When the dentition was evaluated, he noted an increase in the width of the upper dental arch in the region of the molars and an increase in the proclination of the upper and lower incisor teeth. Tongue position was raised with the elimination of the mouthbreathing habit and, of course, lips could approximate each other. Nasal respiration seemed to be more conducive to good facial dental development with increment in age.

Objective and subjective determinations can be made from lateral cephalometric roentgenograms, so that the presence and amount of adenoid tissue can be substantiated and quantified, as well as evaluated in its positional relationship to contiguous structures. Linder-Aronson suggests that under certain conditions adenoids be removed to enhance nasal respiration and permit proper dentofacial development. It should be emphasized that not all children with adenoid tissue will develop a mouthbreathing habit causing improper facial development. The nasopharyngeal air passage must be obstructed to the extent that nasal respiration is substituted by oral respiration. It is equally true that most children who are mouthbreathers because of enlarged adenoids will probably outgrow the habit. With continued growth and development, the adenoid tissue will atrophy, but this transformation may occur too late to prevent any of the developing dentofacial problems. Unfortunately, a good proportion of craniofacial growth and development will have occurred by the time the adenoid tissue commences to atrophy. It must also be remembered that adenoid growth reaches a peak mass long before facial growth is complete. The adenoid tissue may reach its peak mass prior to the timing of the prepubertal growth spurt in many individuals.

During early stages of craniofacial development, other lymphatic tissue in the naso-oral-pharyngeal respiratory tract may be present and may have an influence on dentofacial development. Even if adenoid tissue is not creating a naso-respiratory blockage, tonsillar tissue located between the faucial pillars could be a problem. Grossly enlarged tonsillar tissue can create an obstruction in the oropharyngeal area posterior to the root of the tongue. Unfavorable tongue postures have been noted in some subjects with grossly enlarged tonsils. If the obstruction is severe enough, the tongue may be forced to posture considerably forward to its normal position because of the physiologic need to maintain an adequate oropharyngeal space for respiration and for the passage of food. Clinically, the tongue may be observed to rest between the anterior teeth incident to the forward posturing of the tongue. In such instances, forward tongue posturing must be considered in relation to the stage of facial growth and development. At birth, and for a significant number of years subsequent to birth, the tongue is disproportionately large relative to the oral cavity, in that it occupies a disproportionately large part of the oropharyngeal cavities. At early ages, because of its relative size, the tongue may posture in a protruded position relative to the dentoalveolar complex. This postural relationship will usually change as a function of time. In most instances, changes will usually occur in the relative disproportion because of continued maxillary and mandibular growth and a comparative reduction in the amount of tongue growth. Eventually, and usually, jaw growth will be adequate to contain the tongue within the confines of the upper and lower jaw structures. To a degree, this can explain the spontaneous closure of open bite malocclusions incident to time and growth, as is sometimes observed at later age levels. However, during prepubertal age levels, the mandible may still not have grown sufficiently to encompass the tongue mass. In the late deciduous dentition and the early transitional dentition period, it is not unusual to observe youngsters suffering with enlarged tonsils. In essence, this adds insult to injury. The large tonsillar masses may cause a still comparatively large tongue to be postured excessively forward, keeping the root of the tongue and the tonsillar tissue away from the posterior pharyngeal wall to maintain an open port posteriorly for respiratory purposes. The tonsils, in conjunction to some comparative largeness to the tongue, may necessitate an anterior tongue posture, some depression of the mandibular jaw, and may be instrumental in causing an open bite deformation. Furthermore, the mandibular jaw is still growing and during the early and rapid growth phases it would seem that the mandible may be subject to some deformation. With anterior tongue posturing and with some degree of openness of the mandibular jaw relative to the roof of the mouth, it is conceivable that increment in the steepness of the lower border of the mandibular jaw may occur with continued growth and development. This, in conjunction with potential eruption of posterior teeth, may lead to increased facial dimension between the level of the palate and the lower aspect of the chin. That is, increased lower facial height, much as was seen in the adenoid cases studied by Sten Linder-Aronson. In essence, at times, the removal of the enlarged tonsillar tissue may be desirable. This concept may be illustrated by longitudinal cephalometric roentgenograms obtained on patients with anterior open bite malocclusion and excessive oro-pharyngeal lymphatic tissue. In many instances after surgical removal of enlarged tonsillar masses, a change in tongue posture and occlusion can be observed. A retropositioning of the tongue, more posteriorly into the oral cavity, can be observed and further eruption of anterior teeth can be noted. At times, an anterior open bite may self-correct incident to the judicious removal of tonsillar tissue and with continued growth and development of the jaws.

Once again, it is stressed that these oropharyngeal and nasopharyngeal obstructions may occur before and during the prepubertal growth spurt stage of development. During these ages, the skeletal jaws are continuously growing. At present, an interesting concept has been put forward relative to the mechanism of growth of the craniofacial structures, generally called the "functional matrix theory." In essence, it is hypothesized that craniofacial growth is closely associated with the functional activities carried out by different components of the head and neck area and the soft tissues involved in these functions. Respiration is one such functional element, while mastication and deglutition would be examples of other functional elements carried out in the head and neck area. Considering this doctrine of functional matrices, if there are obstructions in the nasorespiratory and ororespiratory area, some influence may be exerted on the direction of growth of the skeletal structures of the face incident to the need for continued reposturing of soft tissue and skeletal structures. We should be cognizant of this potential influence on facial configuration since it may be possible to prevent maldevelopment and to enhance acceptable facial development. It is strongly suggested that time be spent on a careful radiographic evaluation of the size and configuration of the nasal-oral-pharyngeal cavity spaces and the soft tissue relationships within these cavities. These observations should be interpreted in conjunction with clinical examinations. Treatment procedures could be undertaken to facilitate more acceptable postural relationships of the soft tissues within these cavities, which may enhance facial development.

ROENTGENCEPHALOMETRIC STUDIES OF TONSILS AND ADENOIDS IN NORMAL AND PATHOLOGIC STATES

SAMUEL PRUZANSKY, D.D.S.
CHICAGO, ILLINOIS

Orthodontists have an abiding interest in the interrelations between nasopharyngeal lymphoid tissue and the development of dental occlusion and facial morphology. This interest expanded as orthodontists became involved in multidisciplinary enterprises such as cleft palate teams, wherein professional contact with speech scientists, audiologists, otolaryngologists, and pediatricians led to collaborative problem solving exercises. For example, removal of adenoid, though justified for medical reasons, may jeopardize velopharyngeal valving in the patient with a cleft. As a result, orthodontists were recruited to participate in studies on the structural and functional components of the nasopharyngeal region, utilizing roentgencephalometry.

With increasing interest in birth defects and in particular, craniofacial anomalies, a wide variety of experiments of nature have come to the attention of orthodontic investigators. Such anomalies range from the immunologic deficiency diseases in which lymphoid tissue is poorly developed to structural aberrations of the nasopharyngeal space.

Following is some material from three ongoing studies at our Center.* First, some comment on the natural history of tonsils and adenoids in subjects that do not present with upper respiratory tract disease. Second, to emphasize that adenoidectomy can unmask congenital palatopharyngeal incompetence and produce hypernasal speech in the absence of an overt cleft palate. Finally, to present some experiments of nature which can add to our understanding of tonsils and adenoids as part of a developmentally and functionally coupled aural-oral facial-laryngeal-pulmonary-cardiac system.

J. M. Tanner,[1] a distinguished authority on child growth and development, in discussing growth curves of different tissues and different parts of the body, wrote as follows: "The lymphoid tissue, of tonsils, adenoids, appendix, intestine, and spleen, has quite another growth curve. It reaches its maximum amount before adolescence, and then, probably under the direct influence of the sex hormones, declines to its adult value." As his source of reference, he quoted the classic growth curves published by Scammon et al[2] in 1930.

These widely reproduced growth curves have led to indiscriminate attributions to Scammon's data in the belief that his lymphoid growth curve applied to tonsils and adenoids. A closer look at the Scammon data indicates that they were based on postmortem data collected about 50 years ago. These data did not include measurements of the tonsils and adenoids. His lymphoid growth curve was based on weight of the thymus, number of Peyer's patches, number of lymphoid follicles in the appendix and weight of the mesenteric lymph nodes. It was shown that the white pulp of the spleen also followed the lymphoid curve.

---

*Center for Craniofacial Anomalies. Abraham Lincoln School of Medicine, University of Illinois Medical Center.

This investigation was supported in part by grants from the National Institutes of Health (DE 02872) and Maternal and Child Health Services, Department of Health, Education and Welfare.

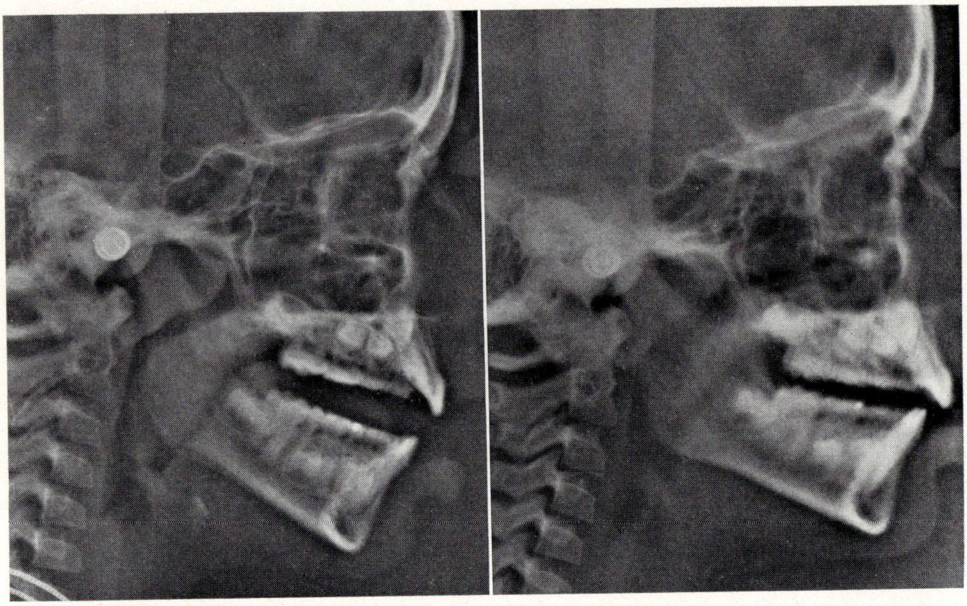

Fig. 1. A) Nine-year-old female with mandible at rest position. Note open-mouth posture, wide freeway space between dental arches, downward and forward displacement of the tongue, and distal extension of the soft palate which rests on the upper pole of a large tonsil. B) The same patient, nine months later and following tonsillectomy. Note that the soft palate now rests on the dorsum of the tongue, the tongue is elevated to rest against the palatal vault, and the freeway space is reduced.

It should be recognized that Scammon sampled a population subject to infectious diseases that for all practical purposes are now eradicated in the developed countries of the world. Thus Scammon's subjects reflected stresses of infection and other environmental factors quite different from those that prevail today. The facts are that we know very little about the variation in the size and growth pattern of tonsils and adenoids.

ROENTGENCEPHALOMETRY

At this point, it seems appropriate to discuss the utility of roentgencephalometry as an investigative tool for the study of tonsils and adenoid. In the lateral projection of the skull, it is possible to delineate a two-dimensional view of these structures as well as visualize their spatial relationship within the nasal and oral pharynx, their relationship to the tongue and soft palate, and their influence on the posture of the mandible. For example, the effect of an enlarged faucial tonsil can be illustrated in a lateral cephalometric radiograph taken at rest and during the sustained phonation of the vowel (u) as in "boom" (Figs. 1A and 1B). At rest, the soft palate is extended to lay on the upper pole of the tonsil instead of being pendant and resting on the dorsum of the tongue. The mandible is depressed excessively while the oral port is open in the configuration typical of the mouth-breather. The tongue is carried low and forward. During phonation, the radiographic image of the faucial tonsil is clearly delineated. Thus, it can be readily observed that an enlarged tonsil contributes to alteration in respiratory pattern, affects the kinesiology of the tongue and circumoral musculature with potential deleterious effects on the developing dental occlusion. It also accounts for the snoring noise produced by the soft palate when the subject is asleep.

Since the cephalometric radiograph entails positioning the head in a cephalostat in fixed and standardized relationship to x-ray source and film, it becomes possible to control enlargement and dis-

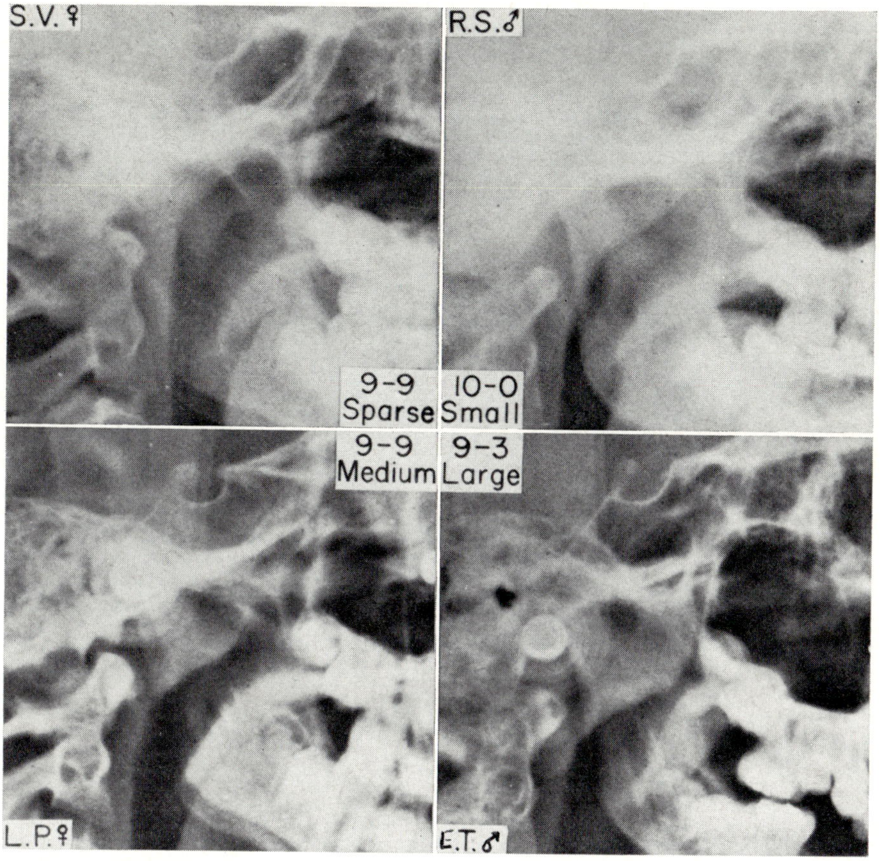

Fig. 2. Lateral cephalometric radiographs of four normal children, not subjected to tonsillectomy or adenoidectomy, and ranging in age from nine years and three months to ten years. Note range in size of adenoid from sparse to large. The size of the adenoid was not necessarily correlated with the size of the tonsil in the same child.

tortion. Such standardized films permit accurate measurement and comparison between children matched for age and sex. Seriatim measurements of single individuals through their growth period have been made by this method.

To obtain normative data on the size of the adenoid, cephalometric films were selected from the author's orthodontic practice. Admittedly, this sample is hardly representative of the universe since it was derived from an upper middle class, white, suburban population. Further, they were ascertained by their presentation for orthodontic treatment. The study was made possible because our standard history always included information on the status of the tonsils and adenoids. Children with facial clefts, other malformations, or known systemic disease were excluded from this study.

Criteria were established for coding the size of the adenoid into four groups: sparse, small, moderate, and large (Fig. 2). Since the evaluation was based on radiographic and not histologic criteria, it was considered presumptuous to state that no adenoid was present (Fig. 3). Three coders were trained to utilize the criteria and each coded the same films separately.

To determine reliability of the method, each coder was compared to the others and tested against himself by repeated measures of the same films on different occasions. The accuracy was remarkable.

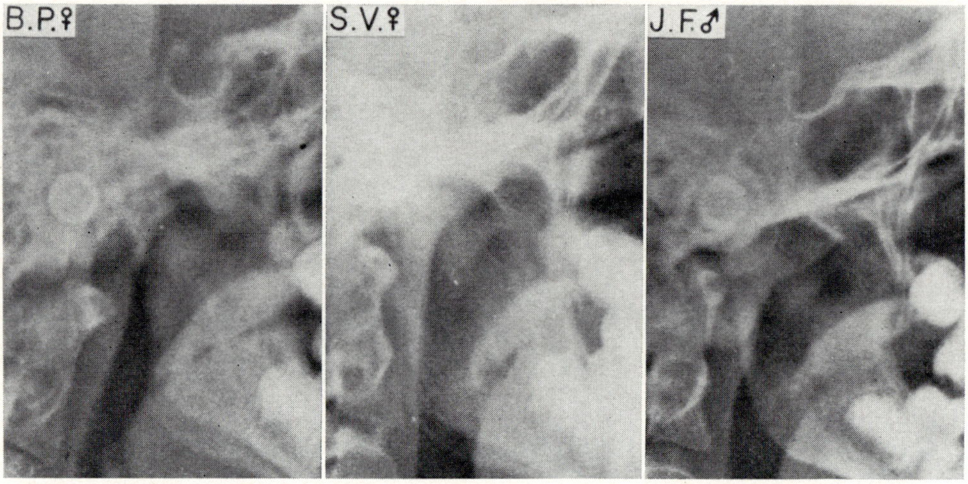

Fig. 3. Comparison of adenoid size as revealed in the radiographs of three children. Note similarity in nasopharyngeal configuration between patient with a history of adenoidectomy and unoperated patient exhibiting sparse adenoid development. A) Post adenoidectomy: 9 years, 11 months. B) Sparse: 9 years, 9 months. C) Small: 8 years, 5 months.

In several instances when a transient change in the size of the adenoid was found during the examination of serial films on a single subject, this change was confirmed by tracing and superimposing the films.

The results of our study, which was based on 460 films of 291 subjects since some had serial films (Fig. 4), are tabulated in Table I. Data on males and females were pooled when no significant differences were detected between the sexes. The results of this mixed cross-sectional and longitudinal study indicate the considerable variation in adenoid size in all of the age groups observed. Clearly, some children exhibit sparse development of adenoid tissue without any overt signs of immunologic deficiency. The findings also challenge the validity of applying Scammon's growth curve for lymphoid tissues[2] to the growth of the adenoid, as suggested by Tanner.[1]

Certain other findings emerged from this study that warrant mention. It was found that the size of the tonsils did not necessarily mimic the size of the adenoid in the same individual. That is, a large tonsil was often seen concomitant with a sparse adenoid.

TABLE I

PERCENT DISTRIBUTION OF ADENOID SIZE IN NORMAL POPULATION*

Age	*Sparse*	*Small*	*Medium*	*Large*	*Number of Readings*
4 to 6	7.7	19.2	42.3	30.7	26
6 to 8	2.9	18.9	39.6	36.6	101
8 to 10	6.8	25.0	47.7	20.5	132
10 to 12	8.7	39.6	34.9	16.6	126
12 to 14	10.1	38.9	33.8	16.9	59
14 to 16	37.5	37.5	18.7	6.2	16

*A total of 460 readings were done on 291 subjects (123 males, 168 females). Only one reading per subject for each age interval selected closest to mid point of interval.

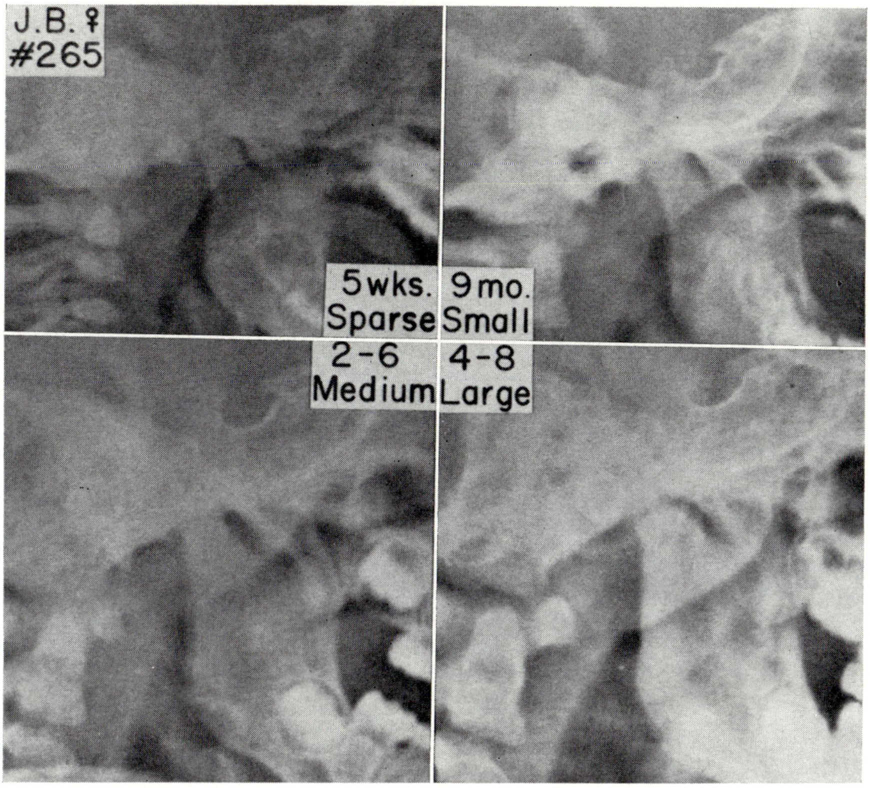

Fig. 4. Serial films of the same child from age five weeks to four years and eight months illustrate the "growth" of the adenoid.

It was also found that some children showed minimal development of the adenoid. Other children, who developed adenoids at an early age, showed involution of this structure well before puberty while the tonsil, in the same child, failed to involute (Fig. 5).

The foregoing findings lead to the following conclusions and warrant some speculation with suggestions for further study:

1. Since tonsils and adenoid are part of Waldeyer's ring, it is customary to think of them as a unitary organ. However, they have disparate embryonic origins and cytology. As the foregoing study illustrates, they do not necessarily behave similarly within the same individual. The one may be large, while the other is smaller. The one may involute early, while the other persists.

2. It is tempting to suggest that the growth curve attributed to tonsils and adenoid is not a true growth curve but rather an individualized response to variable stress influenced by the immunocompetence of the separate organs which may differ during development.

3. Extension of roentgencephalometric studies to include a wider sample of children seems warranted. It would be of interest to compare children at risk for upper respiratory infection measured at different seasons and during exacerbation and remission of upper respiratory disease.

RADIOLOGIC STUDIES BY OTHER INVESTIGATORS

It should be noted that other studies on roentgenographic visualization of the nasopharyngeal lymphoid tissue have been reported, including observations on

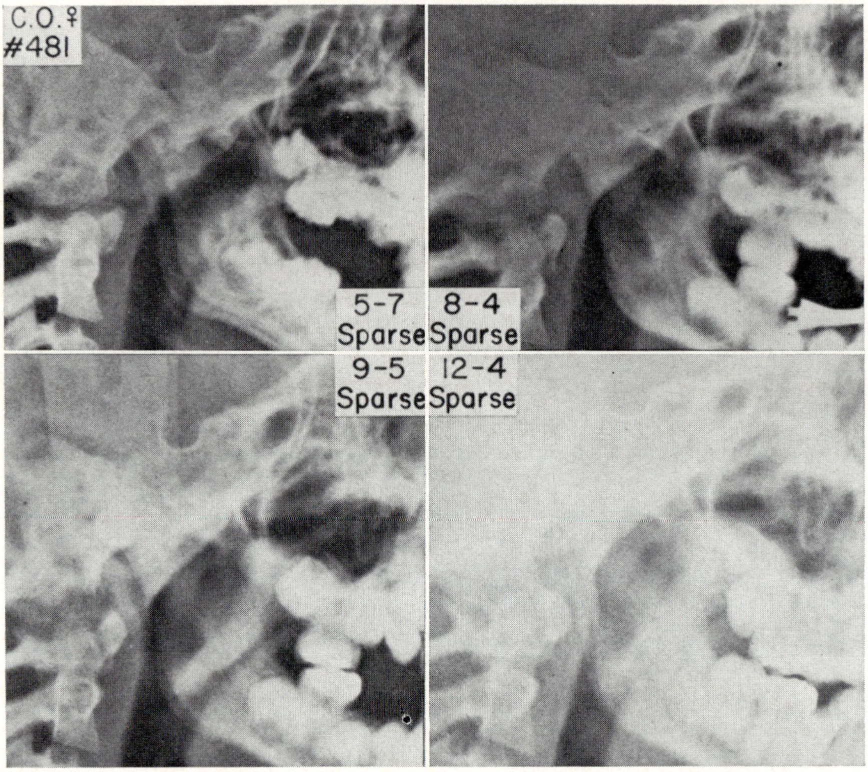

Fig. 5. Minimal development of adenoid as exhibited in serial films of the same child from age five years and seven months to 12 years and four months. Patient presented congenital palatopharyngeal incompetence. However, similar patterns were found in normal children.

257 children two years or less by Capitanio and Kirkpatrick.[3] Johannesson[4] studied 140 children, 90 boys and 50 girls in ages between three months and 15 years, examined between October 1964 and May 1965. The children were clinically free from infection of ear, nose, throat and chest. The case histories revealed no special disposition to infection or any allergic disease of the respiratory tract. No difference was observed between the values for the adenoid size for boys and girls. It was found to increase during the first two years of life and thereafter remained practically unchanged.

Eller et al[5] reported on normal nasopharyngeal soft tissue on 300 adults varying in age from 16 to 80 years with an equal number of each sex and uniform age distribution. They suggested that involution of the nasopharyngeal tissue is not complete by age 25 as previously stated by Johannesson, but continues throughout life.

Although a comprehensive review of the literature is beyond the compass of this brief report, it is clear that cross-sectional roentgencephalometric studies on a larger and varied sample would provide useful information regarding the natural history of tonsils and adenoid.

EXPERIMENTS OF NATURE

Congenital disorders of the immunologic system have refocused interest on the function of the tonsils and adenoids.[6]

Other inborn errors of metabolism leading to functional disorders of the nasopharynx have led to the association of hearing defects and cystic fibrosis. Hypobaric pressure in the middle ear,

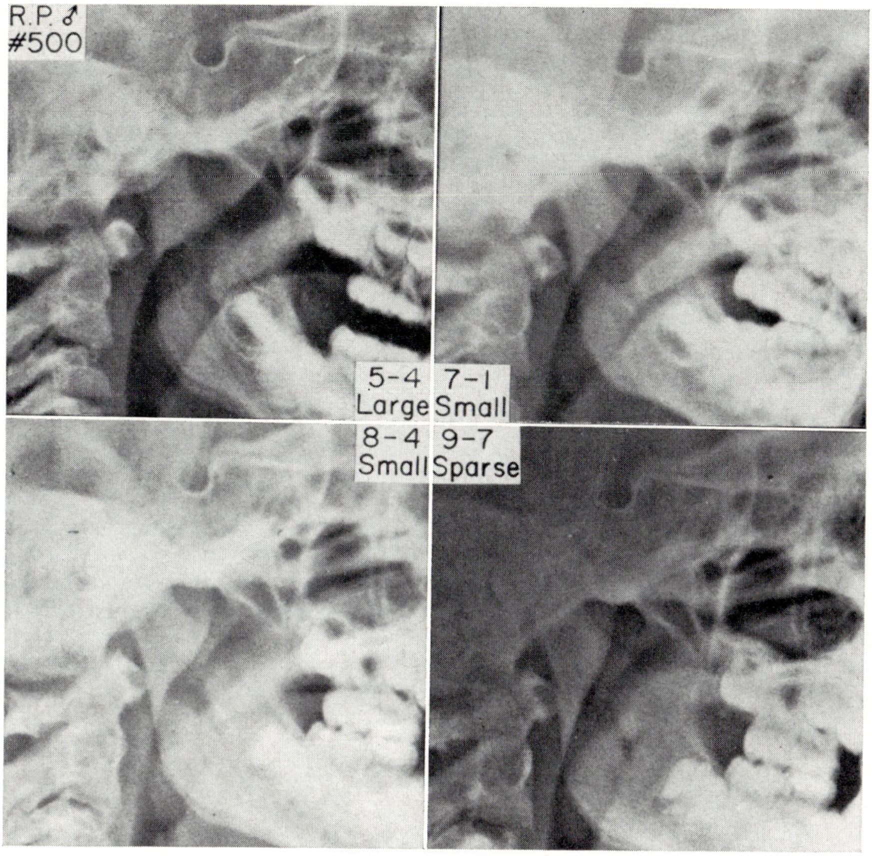

Fig. 6. Early involution of the adenoid as exhibited in serial films of the same child. At age five years and four months, the adenoid was rated as large. At nine years and seven months, the adenoid was judged as sparse. However, the tonsil is clearly visible and of moderate size. While this patient also presented congenital palatopharyngeal incompetence, similar patterns were observed in normal children.

possibly caused by pathological secretion of the mucosal glands of the Eustachian tube with resulting obstruction, has been postulated as a causative mechanism of chronic middle ear disease by Fritze et al.[7] As a test of this hypothesis, it was found that ventilation of the tube was therapeutically successful in four of our five cases and led to normalization of the audiogram.

Craniofacial dysostosis of Apert and Crouzon can produce reduction in the size of the nasopharyngeal airway and lead to cor pulmonale much as an enlarged adenoid.[8]

In contrast, anomalies of the upper cervical spine and skull base can result in increased dimensions of the nasopharyngeal port, thereby minimizing the obstructive effect of lymphoid tissues.[9]

From the increasing experience in the study of children with clefts as reported by Stool and Randall[10] Paradise et al[11] and Bluestone[12] and from the brief citation of other experiments of nature, it is clear that considerable knowledge regarding the structural and functional interaction of tonsils and adenoids with contiguous structures can be learned from the study of these special patients.

CONTRAINDICATION TO ADENOIDECTOMY

Congenital palatopharyngeal incompetence is a condition in which the patient presents hypernasality in speech, with nasal regurgitation of fluids, in the absence of an overt cleft palate. In about 25% of the cases, the velopharyngeal incompetence is "unmasked" by adenoidectomy. In a review of 110 cases in our clinic, slightly more than 80% presented visible or palpable stigmata which might have forewarned of the presence of a lanthanic state of the disorder. Such stigmata include one or more of the following: Bifid or missing uvula; zone pellucida of the soft palate or submucous defect of the muscle at the midline, and submucous cleft of the hard palate ranging from notching of the posterior nasal spine to extensive absence of the bony palatal shelves.

The presence of any one of these stigmata, readily apparent on direct peroral examination, should constitute a warning against the possibility of inducing hypernasality by adenoidectomy.

REFERENCES

1. Tanner JM: The human growth curve, in Harrison GA, Weiner JS, Tanner JM, Barnicot NA (eds): *Human Biology*. Oxford, Oxford University Press, 1964, p 310

2. Scammon RE, Harris JA, Jackson CM, et al: *The Measurement of Man*. Minneapolis, University of Minnesota Press, 1930

3. Capitanio MA, Kirkpatrick JA: Nasopharyngeal lymphoid tissue. Radiology 96: 389-391, 1970

4. Johannesson S: Roentgenologic investigation of the nasopharyngeal tonsil in children of different ages. Acta Radiol 7:299-304, 1968

5. Eller JL, Roberts MD, Ziter FMH Jr: Normal nasopharyngeal soft tissue in adults: A statistical study. Am J Roentgenol Radium Ther Nucl Med 112:537-541, 1971

6. Margulis AR, Feinberg SB, Lester RG, et al: Roentgen manifestations of congenital agammaglobulinemia. Radiology 69:354-359, 1957

7. Fritze W, Gotz M, Stur O, et al: Hearing defects in cystic fibrosis. Z Kinderheilkd 114:111-118, 1973

8. Pruzansky S: Clinical investigation of the experiments of nature, in *Orofacial Anomalies: Clinical and Research Implications*. ASHA Report No. 8. Washington, D. C., Am. Speech & Hearing Assoc., 1973

9. Osborne GS, Pruzansky S, Koepp-Baker H: Upper cervical spine anomalies and osseous nasopharyngeal depth. J Speech Hear Res 14:14-22, 1971

10. Stool SE, Randall P: Unexpected ear disease in infants with cleft palate. Cleft Palate J 4:99-103, 1967

11. Paradise JL, Bluestone CD, Felder H: The universality of otitis media in 50 infants with cleft palate. Pediatrics 44:35, 1969

12. Bluestone CD: Eustachian-tube obstruction in the infant with cleft palate. Ann Otol Rhinol Laryngol (Suppl 2) 80:1-30, 1971

THE SPEECH PATHOLOGIST LOOKS AT THE TONSILS AND THE ADENOIDS

HUGHLETT L. MORRIS, Ph.D.

IOWA CITY, IOWA

The purpose of this paper is to comment about our level of understanding of the relationships between speech production mechanics and the tonsillar/adenoidal masses and to identify some specific questions about the relationships that are currently unanswered. There are not many research findings about this matter and so the major portion of our "knowledge" is based on clinical observations, deductions made from our understanding of other aspects of the speech mechanism, and from information reported by allied health science professionals.

In general, the speech pathologist is not as interested in the tonsils/adenoids from the disease point of view as is the physician. That is because the disease state, in and of itself, does not appear to alter the communication status of the patient. There are exceptions to that generalization, of course. One is that diseased and/or enlarged lymphoid tissue in the oral and/or nasal pharynx may be associated with middle ear disease and depressed hearing levels, hence resulting in a possible impairment of *general* communication skills.

The major concern about tonsils/adenoids, however, on the part of the speech pathologist is the role that the two lymphoid masses may have in changing the size and configuration of the nasal and the oral tracts.

There is considerable evidence[1] to indicate that, for the production of normal speech, there are some restrictions on the size of the two tracts, the relationship between the sizes of the two tracts, and the relationship between the size of each tract to the amount and rate of movement required of certain articulators to open or close that tract.

Using a cephalometric view of a normal speaker as an example (Fig. 1A), note that the pharynx bifurcates, in a manner of speaking, at the level of the oral cavity (Figs. 1A and 1B). While there appear to be some exceptions to the rule, the degree of nasal-oral balance in speech depends, in general, on which tract (nasal or oral) is open, the degree to which the two tracts are open, and, possibly, the relationship between the two openings.

In the most simplified case, the oral tract is open for so-called oral speech, the nasal tract is open for so-called nasal speech, and it is the velum (the soft palate) which assumes positions determining which tract is open and which is closed. For example, when the velum is at rest (Fig. 1A), it seems to "lay" against the upper surface of the tongue, thereby opening the nasal tract and closing the oral tract. In contrast, when the velum is elevated maximally (Fig. 1B), there is contact between it and the pharyngeal walls so that, in the normal speaker, the oral tract is open and the nasal tract is closed.

It is relatively obvious from the discussion so far, that structures which serve to obstruct the posterior parts of the two tracts or which change the relationships of the structures necessary for the opening and closing mechanism may, under certain circumstances, have an effect on speech production, particularly nasal-oral balance aspects of speech production.

That, in essence, is the role the tonsils

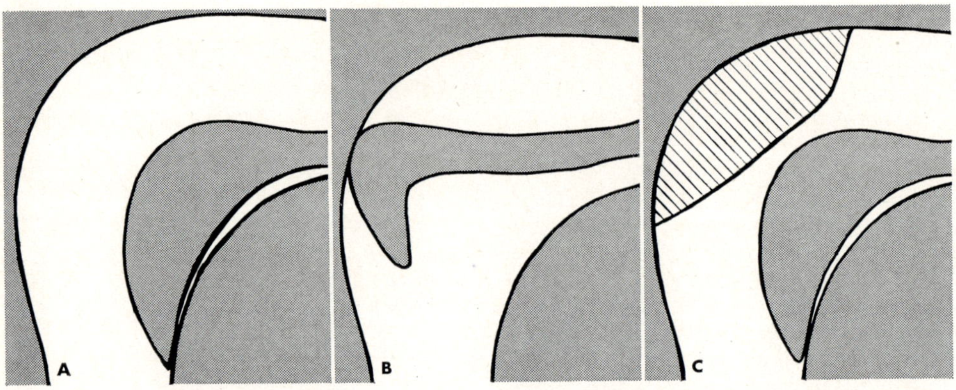

Fig. 1. A) Cephalometric view of normal speaker; velum in rest position, no adenoid pad. B) Velum elevated to maximal (/s/) position, normal speaker, no adenoid pad. C) Rest position, very large adenoid pad.

and the adenoids appear to have in speech production.

ADENOIDS

The adenoids appear in the nasopharynx at the level, approximately, at which the soft palate raises to effect velopharyngeal closure. Thus, if the adenoids have an effect on the mechanics of speech production, it will be in the direction of influencing the separation, posteriorly, of the oral and nasal tracts.

Depending on the circumstances, enlarged adenoids may either hinder or facilitate speech production.

An enlarged adenoid mass may hinder the production of normal speech if the mass is so large that it effectively occludes the posterior aspect of the nasopharynx (Fig. 1C). Since normal nasalization of speech is dependent on an open nasopharyngeal tract, the resultant speech would be denasal (or hyponasal) in quality and, if the condition is relatively extreme, listeners would judge the speech to be abnormally denasal.

In such an extreme case, there may also be a tongue carriage position that is unusually anterior in the oral cavity, which might adversely affect speech articulation patterns. This extreme circumstance is rarely observed in clinical practice, however.

Two courses of action seem possible for such problems: defer treatment, assuming that normal atrophy of the adenoidal mass will result in a more normal-sized nasopharynx; or surgical removal of the adenoidal pad. Unless the obstruction is extreme, and unless the obstruction is resulting in other kinds of health problems, the first course of action seems preferable.

If, however, surgical removal seems indicated, one of two series of events will result.

If the velopharyngeal mechanism is normal, the patient will demonstrate noticeable *hyper*nasality immediately following the adenoidectomy. That is because the patient will require a short period of time, usually only a matter of days or even hours, to accommodate to the change in dimension of the nasopharyngeal port.

If the velopharyngeal mechanism is not normal, then the adenoidectomy may reveal a physiological deficit that will cause a serious impairment of speech production. The impairment will result from physiological velopharyngeal incompetence (Figs. 2A and B) and will be characterized by nasal emission of oral air pressure/flow during consonant articulation and excessive nasal resonance (hypernasal voice quality).

This situation appears to occur with some frequency in patients who have surgically managed cleft palate. (There

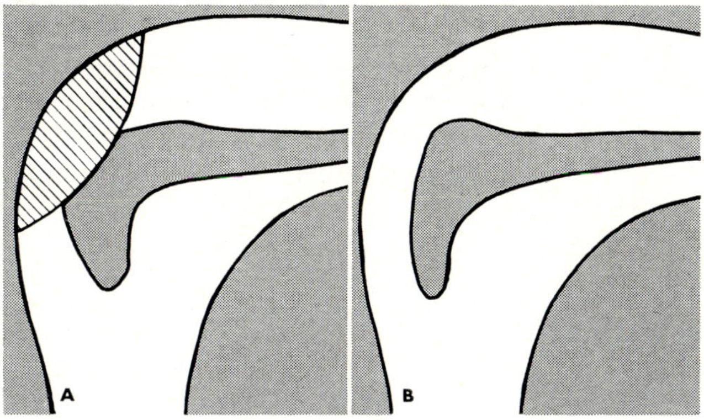

Fig. 2. A) Preadenoidectomy, congenital palatal insufficiency (CPI) patient, /s/ position. B) Postadenoidectomy, CPI patient, /s/ position.

are no data about what the frequency of occurrence is, however.) Apparently, in such cases, the surgically repaired cleft palate is too short or perhaps too restricted in superior-posterior movement to effect velopharyngeal competence against the pharyngeal walls. The adenoidal pad provides a cushion against which velar contact is achieved; when the cushion is removed, the "palatal problem" is revealed.

This postadenoidectomy disorder is also seen in another category of patients, that group with congenital palatal incompetence (CPI).[2-4] These patients demonstrate physiological deficits of the velopharyngeal mechanism (frequently along with other types of congenital anomalies) but in the absence of history of cleft palate.

It is interesting to note that, apparently, even in instances in which there is abnormal palatal length and/or mobility, velopharyngeal incompetence does not result from the normal process of adenoidal atrophy or from the increase in anterior-posterior dimensions of the nasopharynx as the child grows to adulthood. (Or at least there are no documented case reports that this author knows about.) Based on what we know about the phenomenon, the mechanism is apparently able to compensate by increased movement for the decrease in dimensions, provided that decrease occurs in very small decrements. On the other hand, when the dimensions of the nasopharynx are changed dramatically, such as following an adenoidectomy, the deficient mechanism cannot accommodate satisfactorily.

The problem of predicting preadenoidectomy which patients will demonstrate velopharyngeal incompetence postoperatively has interested many specialists,[5,6] but as yet there are few diagnostic tools which are reliable in prognostic capability.

TONSILS

Not very much is known about the effects of hypertrophied tonsils on speech production.[1,7] Clinical experience indicates that enlarged tonsils usually have no noticeable effect on speech. An exception might be the instance in which the tonsils are so large that maintaining a normal oral airway is difficult.[8] That situation would probably cause an alteration in both voice quality and speech articulation. Another exception might be the case in which velopharyngeal competence with a pharyngeal flap mechanism or an obturator is facilitated by the presence of large tonsils because they assist in reducing the size of the two ports laterally to the flap structure.[1]

Clearly, more data are needed about the relationship between tonsils and speech production.

QUESTIONS WHICH NEED ANSWERING

Questions concerning the role of tonsils/adenoids in the development of normal speech are:

1. In the normal individual, do the tonsillar and adenoidal masses appear to have a role in defining the structural requirements for normal speech?

2. If the adenoids appear to facilitate velopharyngeal closure in the normal individual, what is the result of normal patterns of adenoidal atrophy and what is the mechanism for accommodation, if any, to that atrophy?

3. Are there identifiable relationships between tonsillar/adenoidal size and tongue position for the normal individual?

Questions concerning the surgical procedures used in tonsillectomy and/or adenoidectomy are:

1. In patients with an apparently normal velopharyngeal mechanism, what is the usual postoperative sequence for speech production and voice quality following tonsillectomy; following adenoidectomy?

2. What is the postoperative sequence for patients with a deficient velopharyngeal mechanism following tonsillectomy; following adenoidectomy?

3. Can a diagnosis of deficient velopharyngeal mechanism be made preoperatively?

REFERENCES

1. Shelton RL, Morris HL, McWilliams BJ: Anatomical and physiological requirements for speech, in McWilliams BJ, Wertz T (eds): *Speech, Language, and Psychosocial Aspects of Cleft Lip and Cleft Palate: The State of the Art.* ASHA Reports Number 9. Washington, D. C., American Speech and Hearing Association, 1974, p 2-18

2. Bradley DP: Congenital and acquired palatopharyngeal insufficiency, in Grabb WC, Rosenstein SW, Bzoch KR (eds): *Cleft Lip and Palate: Surgical, Dental, and Speech Aspects.* Boston, Little, Brown, 1971, chap 42

3. Crikelair GF, Kastein S, Fowler EP, et al: Velar dysfunction in the absence of cleft palate. NY State J Med 64:263-269, 1964

4. Randall P, Bakes FP, Kennedy C: Cleft palate-type speech in the absence of cleft palate. Plast Reconstr Surg 25:484-495, 1960

5. Lubit EC: Before an adenoidectomy, stop! look! and listen! NY State J Med 67: 681-685, 1967

6. Mason RM: Preventing speech disorders following adenoidectomy by preoperative examination. Clin Pediatr (Phila) 12:405-414, 1973

7. Cole RM: Speech, in Morris HL (ed): *Patterns of Orofacial Growth and Development; Proceedings of the Conference.* ASHA Reports Number 6. Washington, D. C., American Speech and Hearing Association, 1971, p 79-95

8. Subtelny JD, Sakuda M: Open-bite: diagnosis and treatment. Am J Orthod 50:337-358, 1964

NATURAL HISTORY OF OTITIS MEDIA

VIRGIL M. HOWIE, M.D.

HUNTSVILLE, ALABAMA

The title of this presentation implys that there is some place in the world where the uninterrupted course of otitis media has been observed and a typical "Natural History of Otitis Media" chronicled. Of course there is no such place in the world, so the history of otitis media must be told in terms of different patients who are all treated in different ways or with different mechanical procedures performed on them.

Incidence of Otitis Media. The most completely studied group of otitis media patients in whom the "natural" course of the disease underwent minimal therapeutic interference is comprised of 503 children surveyed periodically in remote Eskimo villages by Kaplan et al.[1] Thirty-two percent of the Eskimo children studied displayed visible permanent structural changes manifested by perforation or significant scarring of the tympani. In addition, it was found that, overall, 76% of all Eskimo children have at least one bout of otitis media as defined by a history of presenting with a draining ear. Kaplan et al[1] further recorded a significant lowering of verbal intelligence in children whose ears began draining before they were two years of age. Loss of verbal intelligence has also been reported by Holm and Kunze in a group of Baltimore children with a history of serous otitis media accompanied by intermittent hearing loss.[2]

There have been few studies done of the incidence of otitis media in patients under adequate medical care. One such study was that reported by Brownlee et al in South Carolina.[3] These investigators selected patients coming in for their preschool audiogram who had been followed in private practice since birth or early infancy. Using a two-thirds red

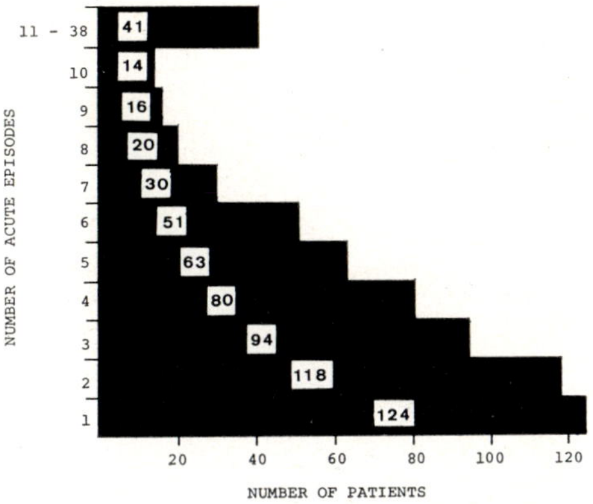

Fig. 1. Incidence of recurrent acute otitis media includes 651 patients with 2,876 episodes. (Modified from Brownlee et al.[3])

eardrum as their diagnostic criterion, Brownlee et al found that 84% of all subjects seen were noted to have had at least one bout of otitis media by the time they were five years old, and that multiple episodes were the rule rather than the exception. The incidence of otitis media in the 651 patients reported by Brownlee et al is shown in Figure 1. Fifty percent of all patients had three or more bouts of otitis and half of those went on to record six or more episodes. All of the patients were treated with antibiotics but only three myringotomies were performed throughout the 2,876 episodes of disease. The investigators did not encourage tonsillectomy and adenoidectomy but noted that of the 60 patients that were subjected to that operative procedure, no significant difference in the subsequent incidence of otitis media was seen. No patient in the series had tympanostomy tubes inserted and there was an incidence of 13% temporary hearing loss observed from random audiograms. For purposes of com-

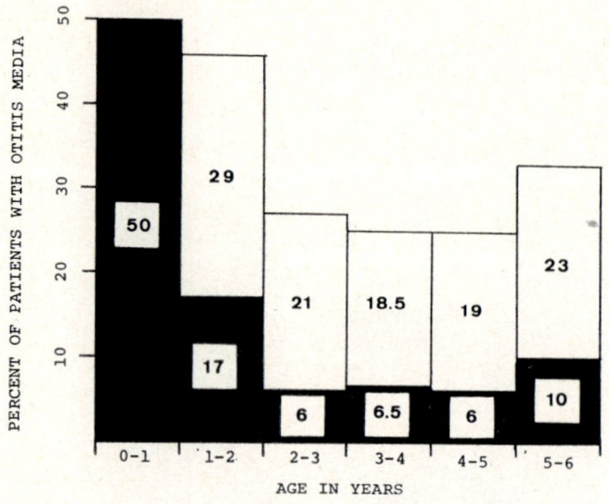

Fig. 2. Incidence of otitis media in unselected pediatric patients followed from birth. Solid area — patients presenting with first otitis episode.

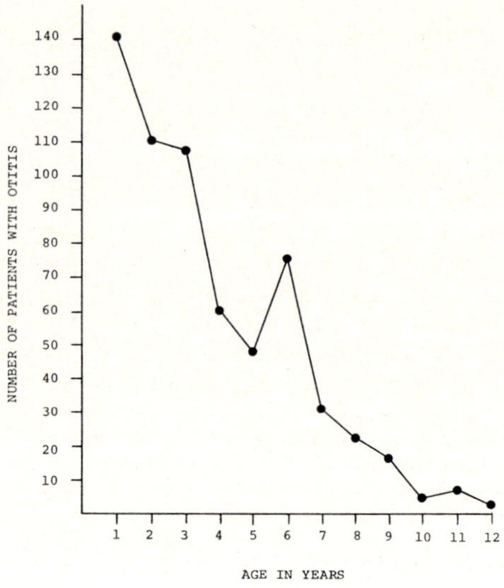

Fig. 3. Relationship of age with incidence of otitis media.

parison, if six or more episodes of acute otitis media as seen in the South Carolina study are equated with the permanent structural changes seen in Eskimo children, the percentage of children having chronic otitis media in the two populations becomes substantially the same (26 and 32%, respectively).

Figure 2 reflects our own experience with otitis media in Huntsville, Alabama. The cohort consisted of 488 patients born since January 1, 1967 and followed in private practice for at least eight months. In the Huntsville study, otitis media was defined as the presence of middle ear fluid detected by use of the pneumatic otoscope. Seventy percent of the patients were aspirated and the middle ear fluid cultured at the time of each episode. Ventilatory tubes were usually inserted at the time of the third acute episode within a year or, if middle ear fluid persisted for more than one month following an acute bout. As shown, the incidence of patients having an initial episode of otitis before two years of age was 67%, a value that corresponds closely with the 60% of Eskimo children that presented with otorrhea before age two. The overall incidence of otitis media with respect to age was derived from separate data and is shown in Figure 3. Unselected pediatric patients with otitis were plotted over a two-year period. The incidence curve showing a general decline in otitis media with age except for the small upward trend at five to six years is almost identical to the data reported by Brownlee et al in South Carolina[3] and by Niel et al in England.[4] The Huntsville study further showed that recurrent otitis was associated with early onset of the first episode. As indicated in Table I, otitis prone children (patients with six or more bouts of acute otitis media)[5] were derived entirely from a population that had their initial episode during the first year and a half of life. Only five of the 41 patients in whom the initial bout occurred after eighteen months of life had more than one additional episode at the time the data was compiled. The incidence of children showing the otitis-prone condition (14%) was lower than either of the two earlier studies[1,3] but this was thought to be a reflection of the shorter period of observation.

Bacterial Etiology of Otitis Media. Bass, et al[6] summarized the results of middle ear fluid cultures made from more than 3,000 aspirates taken by ten independent investigating groups throughout the United States and Europe. Although the incidence of *Streptococcus pneumoniae* (pneumococcus) and *Hemophilus influenzae* (H. influenzae) varies somewhat, on a single aspiration, the predominant organism was pneumo-

TABLE I

RELATIONSHIP OF THE INCIDENCE OF OTITIS MEDIA TO AGE AT THE FIRST ACUTE EPISODE

Total Episodes of Otitis	Number of Patients* First Episode at 0-18 Months	First Episode at 19-72 Months
1	98	22
2	62	14
3	34	2
4	24	2
5	26	1
6	18	0
7	9	0
8	8	0
9	2	0
10	2	0
11	1	0
12	3	0
13	1	0
14	2	0
15	1	0
16	0	0
17	1	0

*335 patients with 1,012 episodes, Howie et al.[5]

coccus (41.6%, overall). Results from studies in Huntsville bear out the particularly high incidence of pneumococcal otitis media. In Table II are summarized data from 116 patients placed on placebo treatment for a period of two to seven days.[7] The 42% incidence of pneumococcal otitis (49 of 116) on initial culture was almost identical to the overall figure compiled by Bass et al. However, when both initial and follow-up cultures were considered, there were 57 instances in which pneumococcus was implicated, giving a total incidence of 50% of otitis media due to that organism. Of particular interest is that with the exception of a single isolate of Group A Streptococcus, no other group of pathogens displayed a tendency toward increased incidence.

Clearly pneumococcus ranks as the major pathogen in otitis media. However, of the more than 80 types of *Streptococcus pneumoniae*, only a relative few are associated with the vast majority of otitis episodes. Four types (6, 14, 19, 23) are involved in approximately 50% of all pneumococcal otitis, and another three types (1, 3, 18) account for an additional 20%.[8] In an independent study, Kamme found that six of the same sero-

TABLE II

BACTERIOLOGY OF PLACEBO TREATED OTITIS MEDIA

Cultural types	Number at Initial culture	Follow-Up Cultures DP	DP:HF	HF	STA	NP	S	No Exudate*
Pneumococcus (DP)	45	36				2	5	2
Pneumococcus and *H. influenzae* (DP:HF)	4	2	1			1		
H. influenzae (HF)	21	3		12		2	1	3
Streptococcus Group A (STA)	2	0			2			
Nonpathogen (NP)	25	3				13	2	7
Sterile (S)	19	2			1	3	1	12
Total number of cultural types found on follow-up visit		46	1	12	3	21	9	24

*Middle ear fluid cleared at time of follow-up visit.

TABLE III

RELATIONSHIP OF THE NUMBER OF SUBSEQUENT EPISODES OF OTITIS MEDIA TO THE TYPE OF ORGANISM ISOLATED DURING THE INITIAL EPISODE

Organism	*Age at First Episode (months)*	*Number of Patients*	*Number of Patients Having Recurrent Otitis* — *Less than 6 Episodes*	*6 Episodes* or more*
Streptococcus pneumoniae (pneumococcus)	0-12	51	37	14 (27.5%)
All other	0-12	115	102	13 (11.3%)

*Difference between the two values significant at $p < 0.025$ by chi square ($X^2 = 5.6$).

types were responsible for 80% of pneumococcal otitis media in Lund, Sweden.[9]

The second most common single organism isolated from middle ear disease is *H. influenzae*.[6,10,11] The type-specific etiologies are less clear, however, as only 10% of the *H. influenzae* isolated from the middle ear is typable. Of the latter, most are type B.

Bacterial Priming of the Otitis Prone Condition. Recent data from patients studied in Huntsville has indicated that the specific bacterial etiology of early otitis episodes, acting in concert with the age factor discussed earlier, predisposes toward the otitis prone condition. Table III compares the otitis proneness of patients under one year of age whose first otitis episode was determined to have either a pneumococcal or nonpneumococcal etiology. Patients whose first aspirate contained pneumococcus were two and one-half times as likely to go on to have six or more episodes. Additional data indicated that subjects whose initial experience with otitis occurred during the second year of life and was *not* of pneumococcal origin were statistically no less likely to become otitis prone than if their initial episode had occurred during the first year. The common denominator predisposing to the otitis prone condition, therefore, was initial infection with pneumococcus.

Participation of the Immune Response in Otitis Media. Although the immunology of otitis media is far from understood, data from natural infections suggest a correlation between local and systemic antibody concentrations and clinical observations with respect to clearing of the middle ear fluid. To determine the presence of specific antibody in the serum and middle ear fluids, an indirect immunofluorescence test was used employing known pneumococcal serotypes or the patients' own *H. influenzae* isolates as indicator organisms.

TABLE IV

CLINICAL SIGNIFICANCE OF SPECIFIC ANTIBODY IN MIDDLE EAR FLUID (MEF) FROM PATIENTS WITH OTITIS MEDIA DUE TO HEMOPHILUS INFLUENZAE OR STREPTOCOCCUS PNEUMONIAE

Middle ear Status at 2-7 Day Follow-up Visit	*Immune Status of MEF* — *MEF with specific antibody to:* *H. influenzae*	*pneumococcus*	*MEF without specific antibody to:* *H. influenzae*	*pneumococcus*
MEF cleared*	17	6	7	2
MEF remaining	8	9	21	42

*Status of middle ear at follow-up was determined by use of the pneumatic otoscope. The presence of fluid was confirmed by aspiration.

TABLE V

RELATIONSHIP OF SPECIFIC IgM ANTIBODY RESPONSE IN BACTERIAL OTITIS MEDIA TO SUBSEQUENT HOMOLOGOUS RELAPSE

	Number of Patients	*Number of Patients Suffering Homologous Relapse**
IgM present in convalescent serum	15	0
IgM absent in convalescent serum	30	10

*Difference between values significant at $P<0.05$ by chi square (4.64).

Otitis media was observed to occur fairly often even in the presence of pathogen-specific antibody. Furthermore, antibody of all three major classes (IgG, IgM, IgA) was variably found in either serum or middle ear aspirate.

Table IV shows the correlation between the presence of specific antibody in acute middle ear fluids and the subsequent return of the middle ear to the normal state.[12] Although individual values for the two pathogens differed somewhat, the overall clearing rate of patients who had detectable specific antibody in the middle ear fluid was 58% compared to only 12.5% of those in whose middle ear fluid no specific antibody was found. It is important to note that time was not a factor in that there was no significant difference between the four experimental groups with respect to the average number of days (three) separating the initial and follow-up visit. The evidence supports the notion that local specific antibody is associated with rapid clearing of middle ear fluid.

To further evaluate the significance of host immunity in bacterial otitis media, the relationship between development of bacteria-specific IgM and subsequent relapse due to an organism of the same genus is shown in Table V. In patients followed for at least eight months after the initial episode, homologous relapse did not occur if a primary antibody response to the etiologic agent was detected.[13]

In a separate report we showed that the percentage of patients responding immunologically to pneumococcal otitis media increased with age.[8] An additional factor shown to be of increasing importance in the immune response to bacterial otitis was the antimicrobial used during the acute episode. A recent study has compared IgM antibody production in two groups of patients treated with either ampicillin or erythromycin and sulfonamide (Table VI). Only 18% of the ampicillin treated patients reacted to the infecting organism with a primary or IgM response as opposed to almost 48% of the patients given the erythromycin:sulfonamide combination therapy.[13]

These preliminary findings on the immune response in naturally occurring episodes of acute otitis media appear to be encouraging with respect to the potential for immunization procedures. The immediate goal would seem to be the development of a suitable vaccine against the target types of *Streptococcus pneumoniae*. Such a vaccine would not only prevent 70% of acute pneumococcal otitis media but also arrest the onset of the otitis prone condition. We estimate

TABLE VI

RELATIONSHIP OF ANTIBIOTIC THERAPY TO SPECIFIC IgM ANTIBODY RESPONSE IN OTITIS MEDIA

Treatment	*Number of Patients*	*Patient IgM Antibody Response*	
		*Positive**	*Negative*
Ampicillin	22	4 (18.2%)	18
Erythromycin and Sulfonamide	23	11 (47.8%)	12

*Difference between values significant at $p<0.1$ by chi square ($X^2 = 3.2$).

that the average uncomplicated episode of otitis media causes a decreased hearing for four to six weeks and costs the family twenty to thirty dollars to pay both doctor and druggist for their services. An effective octavalent vaccine could possibly prevent one-third of all episodes of acute otitia media. The elimination of approximately one to one and one-half bouts of otitis per child born seems a worthwhile goal from both a medical and economic point of view.

REFERENCES

1. Kaplan GJ, Fleshman JK, Bender TR, et al: Long-term effects of otitis media. A ten year cohort study of Alaskan Eskimo children. Pediatrics 52:577-585, 1973

2. Holm VA, Kunze LH: Effect of chronic otitis media on language and speech development. Pediatrics 43:833-839, 1969

3. Brownlee RC Jr, DeLoache WR, Cowan CC Jr, et al: Otitis media in children. J Pediatr 75:636-692, 1969

4. Neil JF, Harrison SH, Morbey RD, et al: Deafness in acute otitis media. Brit Med J 1:75-77, 1966

5. Howie VM, Ploussard JH, Sloyer J: The "otitis prone" condition. To be published

6. Bass JW, Cohen SH, Corless JD, et al: Ampicillin compared to other antimicrobials in acute otitis media. JAMA 202:697-702, 1967

7. Howie VM, Ploussard JH: Efficacy of fixed combination antibiotics versus separate components in otitis media. Clin Pediatr (Phila.) 11:205-215, 1972

8. Sloyer JL, Howie VM, Ploussard JH, et al: Immune response to acute otitis media in children. I. Serotypes isolated and serum and middle ear fluid antibody in pneumococcal otitis media. Infect Immun 9:1028-1032, 1974

9. Kamme C, Ageberg M, Lundgren K: Distribution of *Diplococcus pneumoniae* types in acute otitis media in children and influence of the types on the clinical course in penicillin V therapy. Scand J Infect Dis 2:183-190, 1970

10. Howie VM, Ploussard JH, Lester RL: Otitis media: A clinical and bacteriological correlation. Pediatrics 45:29-35, 1970

11. Kamme C, Lundgren K, Mardh PA: The aetiology of acute otitis media in children. Scand J Infect Dis 3:1-4, 1971

12. Sloyer JL, Howie VM, Ploussard JH, et al: Immune response to acute otitis media in children. III. Possible role for middle ear fluid antibody. To be published.

13. Sloyer JL, Howie VM, Ploussard JH, et al: Immune response to acute otitis media in children. IV. Effects of antimicrobial therapy. To be published

DISEASES OF THE TONSILS AND ADENOIDS IN RELATION TO RHINITIS AND SINUSITIS

SYLVAN E. STOOL, M.D.

PHILADELPHIA, PENNSYLVANIA

The importance of the relationship of tonsillectomy and adenoidectomy to rhinitis and sinusitis is aptly expressed by Fry[1] in his book *The Catarrhal Child* when he states, "A history of recurrent coughs, colds, catarrh and nasal obstruction is probably the most frequent reason for carrying out the operation. It is indeed a very large group of indefinite and vague conditions that cannot be separated off or blessed by a good diagnostic label."

Rhinitis and sinusitis are common illnesses and a frequent diagnosis. However, the etiology of these conditions is frequently not obvious as the condition may be due to numerous agents such as infection, allergy, toxic substances and even psychosomatic factors. With this high incidence of disease it is not surprising that there may be much confusion regarding the relationship of tonsillectomy and adenoidectomy in the treatment of these diseases.

A diligent search of the available literature and textbooks provides very little in the way of objective information based on well-controlled studies. A general impression is that an interrelationship does exist. This paucity of information regarding the subject seems to indicate that either no effort has been made to investigate this relationship or the efforts that have been made were not sufficiently conclusive to merit publication.

In view of the magnitude of the problem it certainly would be appropriate that a concerted interregional and interdisciplinary effort to gain insight into this aspect of the problem would be of immense value. What information should be sought and how should this be accomplished?

The incidence of rhinitis and sinusitis in patients who are evaluated for tonsillectomy and or adenoidectomy should be established. This will require careful history taking and accurate physical examination. The various social and economic factors should be documented and a search for allergic and environmental toxic substances made. It is only by establishing incidence of disease that the influence of surgery can be ascertained. Although the etiology of the patients' respiratory infections may be difficult to establish, many of the newer techniques of tissue culture and immunology may yield valuable information and make otherwise seemingly unrelated clinical observations valid. An example of this is in our own recent experience. We have seen infants with corpulmonale secondary to lymphoid hyperplasia who have profuse rhinitis and in whom study of the removed tissue reveals strong evidence they had recent infectious mononucleosis. The usual tests were not positive.

The diagnosis of sinusitis by radiographic methods poses many problems. Although the technique is noninvasive, the use of x-ray may be questioned. The risks are small and the information obtained may be significant. Much of the meaningful information may be of a negative nature. If the sinuses are normal one can exclude sinusitis. Abnormal studies will establish incidence of disease but not etiology. The correlation of the history, microbiology and radiographic information with the response to the surgical procedure may clarify some of the mystery of these interrelationships.

The influence of airway obstruction from tonsils, and especially adenoids and infection of these organs, on the physiology of taste and smell has not been studied. These senses are extremely important to the patient's well being and an orderly evaluation of these senses in the pre- and postoperative patient may be very revealing. Some of the improvement postoperatively may be due to the improved state of the chemical senses.

There are now excellent studies that emphasize the physiological effects on gas exchange secondary to hypertrophy of tonsils and adenoids. A number of techniques are now available, many of which are noninvasive, which will allow the physician to obtain objective information regarding the influence of surgery.

Other physiological and psychological factors secondary to rhinitis and sinusitis have not been studied in children and may be significant; such as the effect of chronic rhinorrhea on the individual's acceptance into society. Although difficult to evaluate, behavioral and personality tests are available and will give some insight into these factors. All physicians are aware that the child with chronic rhinorrhea is the subject of much concern to parents, grandparents and even school authorities. Many referrals for surgical therapy are initiated by these groups. The influence of pressures by these groups should be documented.

The present status of our knowledge is again stated by Fry,[1] "In view of this uncertainty of the causes of this catarrhal state we cannot be dogmatic as to the propriety of any one treatment, and use of tonsillectomy must be assessed most critically. Can we, in fact, alter the natural history of these recurrent coughs and colds by any form of treatment." This is also emphasized in a review of the past twenty years literature by Shapiro who comments on the immunologic work of Veltu et al. These papers are solid factual islands in a sea of controversial opinion.[2]

This study is too comprehensive for any one group and it is only by making a major commitment of a large interdisciplinary group that satisfactory information may be obtained.

REFERENCES

1. Fry J: *The Catarrhal Child,* Butterworths, London, 1961

2. Shapiro SL: Tonsillectomy and adenoidectomy. ENT Monthly, 52:407-411, 1973

CHAPTER IV

REPORTS OF SUBCOMMITTEES

I. A Study Design

(Drs. Paradise, [Chairman], Baumgartner, Hurst, Lamb, Oleinick, Rosner, Stearns, and Taylor)

After careful consideration, the Subcommittee favors the undertaking of a collaborative, prospective study of the effects of adenoidectomy and tonsillectomy, to be conducted at a number of clinical centers in order to achieve suitable geographic and socioeconomic representation, and employing a uniform protocol. It was agreed that the design of the Paradise study could serve as a prototype in planning such a collaborative study. Important points to emphasize in designing the study would be: 1) the need to observe patients over time in order to be certain that they actually meet criteria established for surgery; and 2) the need to extend the observation period after randomization until at least early adulthood, so that both short- and long-term effects of undertaking or withholding surgery can be considered.

The Committee felt that some of the participants in a collaborative study would be expected to be involved additionally in valuable, related studies (e.g., studies of the microbiology and epidemiology of tonsillar and related infection; the effects of surgery or nonsurgery on craniofacial development and speech), so long as such studies would not interfere with execution of the protocol of the collaborative study itself. It is to be understood that funding for such additional efforts would be required over and above the funding of the basic protocol.

The group assuming responsibility to design the study should include epidemiologists and biometricians, so that they might advise concerning the numbers and distributions of subjects necessary to show substantial differences between experimental and control groups.

II. The Microbiology

(Drs. Howie, Klein [Chairman], Ogra, Sprinkle and Weinstein)

It is clear that there are significant areas of ignorance about the pathogenesis, microbiology and immunology of the diseases of the tonsils and adenoids. The specific areas are suggested in the presentations by the members of this committee. A rational approach to the medical or surgical treatment of these diseases demands clarification of these areas. Every effort should be made to encourage funding agencies to support valid programs.

The Core Program of evaluation of medical and surgical therapies of diseases of the tonsils and adenoids should include:

1. Cultures of the throat and nasopharynx for isolation of bacteria in cases of acute sore throat or tonsillopharyngitis.

2. Cultures of the nasopharynx for isolation of bacteria in cases of acute otitis media. Middle ear fluid should be examined whenever possible to further define the immunology and microbiology of these effusions.

The Committee noted that virus and immunologic studies were not necessary for all patients but should include selected patients in the Core Study. The materials should be sent to designated study groups chosen on the basis of their technical competence. Tissues, serums and body fluids should be studied intensively by sophisticated microbiologic, histologic and immunologic techniques.

III. Physiologic Aspects of Diseases of T & A

(Drs. Bluestone [Chairman], Jako, Mead, Morris, Ogura, Proctor, Pruzansky, and Shapiro)

The members of the subcommittee on physiologic aspects of the diseases of the tonsils and adenoids identified the following questions thought to warrant further study with suggested methods of evaluation. They stressed the need for noninvasive methods of study.

What is the Effect of Upper Airway Obstructive Disease on the Lower Respiratory Tract and Cardiovascular System? Since the tonsils and adenoids can obstruct the upper airway sufficiently to cause cor pulmonale in children, it seems desirable to evaluate children with obstructive tonsils and adenoids who might be in a less severe stage but whose respiratory problems might be detrimental to their health. The following methods might be helpful in evaluating such an obstruction.

1. The recording of pressures from an *esophageal balloon or transducer* both immediately before and after an adenoidectomy or tonsillectomy, or both, while a child is anesthetized for the operative procedures.

2. Determination of *lung volume* employing a plethysmograph.

3. *Sound recordings* of the oro- and nasopharynx employing frequency and spectrum analysis.

4. Recording sound reflections employing *ultrasound.*

5. Studies of the *anterior-posterior diameter of the chest* to look for paradoxical movements of the chest.

6. Studies of *respiratory exercise tolerances* and determine the maximum volume ventilation (MVV).

What is the Effect of Obstructive Adenoids on Nasal Breathing?

1. Determination of *nasal resistance* employing rhinomanometry.

2. *Roentgenographic studies* employing lateral cephalometric studies and tele- or cinefluorography employing contrast media.

3. *Rhinoadmittance* studies to determine nasal and nasopharyngeal volume.

What is the Effect of Obstructive Diseases of the Tonsils and Adenoids on Swallowing?

1. *Cine-* or *telefluorography* with *simultaneous manometric* recordings before and after adenoidectomy or tonsillectomy or both.

What are the Orthodontic Changes?

1. Preparation of *dental casts.*

2. Lateral and basal *cephalometric roentgenograms* for *tongue posture.*

3. Determination of orthodontic changes employing *ultrasound* techniques.

What are the Effects on Speech?

1. The employment of "*psychological scaling*" might be helpful.

2. *Cephalometric roentgenograms* taken during the formation of the letter "s."

3. *Short tape recordings* of connected speech.

4. *Airflow studies.*

5. *Motion picture studies* of posture during speech.

What is the Effect of Obstructive Adenoids on the Eustachian Tube? Studies of the nose, nasopharynx, Eustachian tube, middle ear-mastoid system employing the following:

1. Cine- or telefluoroscopic *roentgenographic studies* utilizing contrast media.

2. *Pneumophone* technique.

3. *Electroacoustic impedance* bridge and a pressure chamber.

4. Inflation-deflation *airflow studies* through a nonintact tympanic membrane with simultaneous recordings of nasopharyngeal pressures.

5. *Improved* methods of otoscopy employing objective techniques.

The Subcommittee concluded that these studies would be important to objectively assess the physiologic aspects of obstructive disease of the tonsils and adenoids.

CHAPTER V

CONCLUSIONS AND RECOMMENDATIONS

I. Nationwide Collaborative Prospective Study

A nationwide collaborative, prospective study of the effects of tonsillectomy and adenoidectomy is indicated. This should be conducted at a number of clinical centers in order to achieve suitable geographic and socioeconomic representation and employ a uniform protocol. The design of the Paradise study could serve as a prototype in planning such a study. Important points to emphasize in designing the study would be: 1) the need to observe patients over time in order to be certain that they actually meet criteria established for surgery; 2) the need to extend the observation period after randomization until at least early adulthood, so that both short- and long-term effects of undertaking or withholding surgery can be considered.

The primary purpose of the prospective study would be to answer the two most important questions related to the tonsil and adenoid problem:

What is the Effect of Adenoidectomy or Adenotonsillectomy on the Outcome of Otitis Media? The patients would be randomly divided into three groups, 1) control (medical management), 2) adenoidectomy, and 3) adenotonsillectomy.

What is the Effect of Tonsillectomy or Adenotonsillectomy on Patients with Tonsillitis or Pharyngotonsillitis? The subjects would be randomly divided into, 1) control (medical management), 2) tonsillectomy, and 3) adenotonsillectomy.

By attempting to answer these two most important questions, the Committee felt a satisfactory answer could be obtained, rather than attempting to answer all the questions identified by the Workshop participants.

II. Related Studies

Some of the participants in the collaborative study would be expected to be involved additionally in valuable, related studies that would not interfere with the execution of the protocol of the collaborative study itself. The following studies were suggested:

Immunology and Microbiology. Cultures of the throat and nasopharynx for isolation of bacteria in cases of acute sore throat or tonsillopharyngitis. Cultures of the nasopharynx for isolation of bacteria in cases of acute otitis media. Middle ear fluid should be examined whenever possible to further define the immunology and microbiology of these effusions. Virus and immunologic studies would not be necessary for all patients but should include selected patients in the core study. The material should be sent to designated study groups chosen on the basis of their technical competence.

Physiologic Studies. Selected centers would study the physiologic effects of the diseases of the tonsils and adenoids. Selection of centers would depend upon their technical competence. These studies would assess the effect of adenoidectomy and tonsillectomy, or both on the 1) lower respiratory tract and cardiovascular system, 2) nasal breathing, 3) swallowing function, 4) speech, 5) dental-facial morphology, and 6) the nose, nasopharynx, Eustachian tube, middle ear-mastoid system.

III. Concurrent Studies

The following studies appear indicated but would not be part of the collaborative prospective study.

Epidemiology. Studies of the population characteristics of those affected by the diseases of the tonsils and adenoids and related conditions, e.g., otitis media. An ideal setting for such a study would be a prepaid health care program.

Microbiology and Immunology. Concurrent studies of the etiology of pharyngotonsillitis as well as otitis media would appear indicated. Although we are accustomed to consider an infectious disease as caused by a single microorganism, it is possible that disease may result from the interaction of two or more agents or the combined effect of a noninfectious condition (allergy, smoking, environmental pollution) with an infectious agent.

Studies of the state of the host defense and nasopharyngeal immunity in patients who suffer from recurrent sore throat and who eventually undergo tonsillectomy, would appear to be indicated. The role of the tonsils in the protection or pathogenesis of allergic disorders would also be important.

Physiologic Aspects. Concurrent studies of the physiologic aspects of obstructive tonsils and adenoids should be instituted. These should include the following:

1. Effect of upper airway obstructive disease on the lower respiratory tract and cardiovascular system.

2. Effect of obstructive adenoids on nasal breathing.

3. Effect of obstructive tonsils and adenoids on swallowing.

4. Effect of tonsils and adenoids on dental-facial morphology.

5. Effect of tonsils and adenoids on speech.

6. Effect of obstructive adenoids on the Eustachian tube.

IV. Course of Action

The participants of the Workshop on Tonsillectomy and Adenoidectomy recommended the following course of action.

Collaborative Prospective Study. All of the Workshop participants agreed that a nationwide collaborative, prospective study of tonsillectomy and adenoidectomy is indicated. They recommended that a small group of interested investigators should submit a *planning grant* to the National Institutes of Health. The mission of those involved in the planning phase of the study would be to carefully plan a collaborative study. The planning committee should include the following areas of expertise; pediatrics, otorhinolaryngology, epidemiology-biostatistics, and a specialist in infectious diseases. In accordance with the guidelines for organization and administration of National Institutes of Neurological Diseases and Stroke grant supported fixed protocol cooperative studies, they suggested that the advisory committee of the cooperative study should include investigators in the same disciplines as suggested for the planning grant, but should also include a physician in family practice. They also suggested an additional "consultant group" to the advisory committee composed of experts in the field of public health, orthodontia, speech pathology, audiology, immunology and pathology.

Concurrent Studies. The participants of the Workshop strongly suggested that both investigators and funding agencies should consider studies of the epidemiology, pathogenesis and pathophysiology of the diseases of the tonsils and adenoids and its related conditions, e.g., otitis media, receive high priority consideration in the future.

Workshop on Tonsillectomy and Adenoidectomy Report. The participants suggested that the findings of the Workshop should be published as a supplement in either the pediatric or otolaryngology literature as soon as possible to inform the medical community of the state of our knowledge and to stimulate further investigation. Editorials should be written in appropriate Journals (e.g., Journal of American Medical Association, Journal of Infectious Diseases, Journal of American Speech and Hearing Society) by various Workshop participants who would direct the interested reader to the supplement.

SECRETORY IMMUNOGLOBULIN A IN ORAL AND RESPIRATORY PASSAGES IN MAN

Goro Mogi, M.D.

Ube, Japan

From the Department of Otolaryngology, Yamaguchi University School of Medicine, Ube, Japan.

This work was supported by grant number 848193 from the Ministry of Education, Japan.

SECRETORY IMMUNOGLOBULIN A IN ORAL AND RESPIRATORY PASSAGES IN MAN

GORO MOGI, M.D.

UBE, JAPAN

SUMMARY – Secretory IgA (SIgA) is the predominant immunoglobulin in certain external secretions and may have an important role in immunological mucosal resistance. SIgA differs in chemical and immunological properties from serum IgA. The present study was undertaken to investigate the antigenic relationship between SIgA, free secretory component (FSC) and serum IgA and the localization of SIgA as well as other immunological classes in tissues of oral and respiratory passages by use of immunofluorescence technique. SIgA and FSC were highly purified from human colostrum and rabbit anti-SIgA and anti-SC antisera were prepared. On the basis of antigenic relationships between SIgA, FSC and serum IgA, it was emphasized that individual specific antisera for SC and IgA and/or SIgA should be used in immunochemical or immunohistological investigations for SIgA. The present study failed to detect SC determinants in palatine and lingual tonsils. However, it was evident that cells present in the pharyngeal tonsillar epithelium contain SC determinants. SC molecules may be synthesized in certain secretory cells of mucous membrane and glandular epithelium and the combining of SC with IgA could occur in the cytoplasm of epithelial cells, the intercellular spaces and/or in the lumens of glandular acini and ductules.

In 1959, Heremans et al[1] first reported the existence of immunoglobulin A (IgA) in normal human serum. Subsequent studies[2-4] have demonstrated that IgA is the predominant type of immunoglobulin in various external secretions, such as parotid saliva, colostrum, lacrimal secretions, nasal secretions, and bronchial fluids. Moreover, it has been elucidated by Tomasi et al[5] that IgA present in these external secretions differs in chemical and immunological properties from IgA of serum. At present, it is known that IgA in external secretions is predominantly 11 S in sedimentation whereas IgA in serum is 7 S and that exocrine IgA possesses an extra antigenic determinant not present in serum IgA, called secretory component (SC).[6,7] IgA associated with SC is now called secretory IgA (SIgA). SC is a nonimmunoglobulin glycoprotein, existing as bound SC (associated with IgA) and/or free SC (unassociated with IgA) in colostrum[8,9] and saliva.[6,10] Although the exact biologic behavior of free secretory component (FSC) is not known, it has been suggested that SC facilitates the transport of IgA to the epithelial surface and that SIgA is more resistant to proteolysis than serum IgA lacking SC.[6,7,11,12]

SIgA is synthesized locally in the mucous membrane or glandular epithelium[7] and this class of antibody contributes significantly to the immunological mucosal resistance mechanism, since viral and bacterial antibody activities have been demonstrated in SIgA antibodies.[6,13-15] It is conceivable that SIgA plays an important role in local immunity, which is independent from systemic immunity, on the basis of its chemical structure, local synthesis in epithelial cells, and production along the invading route of organisms. South et al[16,17] reported that persons who lack or have low concentrations of SIgA are predisposed to chronic respiratory infections. This evidence supported the important role of SIgA in the local immunologic defense system. Several immunofluorescence studies[5,18,19] found localization of SIgA in the mucosal membrane epithelium of the respiratory tract and in the salivary gland, emphasizing the local synthesis of this immunoglobulin in the epithelium of these tissues. However, incompatible data have appeared concerning the existence of SC determinants in tonsils. Rossen et al[18] reported the presence of SIgA in the membrane lining the crypts of the pharyngeal and palatine tonsils, whereas no SC determinants were found in palatine tonsil by studies of Schmedtje and Batts.[20]

In previous studies[21-24] we have isolated SIgA from saliva, nasal discharge and colostrum to investigate SIgA immunochemically in middle ear effusions. Although there was no interference with our results, the isolated SIgA by the method employed previously was not completely pure. Lactoferrin, one of the locally synthesized proteins, contaminated the final product of SIgA occasionally. The present study was undertaken to isolate SIgA and FSC by a modified technique for obtaining an increasingly more purified state in order to study SC determinants immunochemically and immunohistologically in the oral and respiratory passages.

METHODS AND MATERIALS

Collection of Secretion Samples. Colostrum provided from the Department of Gynecology and Obstetrics, Yamaguchi University School of Medicine, was collected up to three days postpartum and pooled. Parotid secretions were collected and pooled from normal adult humans as described in a previous paper.[22] Tracheobronchial secretions were obtained from patients who had undergone endotracheal anesthesia for various diseases, but all were free from recent lower respiratory disease. The method of collection was nearly the same as that reported by Keimowitz.[4] The fluids aspirated were centrifuged at 11,180 g for 30 minutes at 4 C. The supernatants were concentrated approximately tenfold by means of an ultrafiltrator* using DIAFLO membrane** (PM-10, 76 mm in diameter). Individual nasal secretions were collected from normal subjects and patients with various nasal and paranasal diseases as reported previously.[25] Two laryngeal secretions were obtained by a method to be reported in a separate paper.[26] Nasal discharges and laryngeal secretions which were absorbed into filter papers were eluted by 0.2 M phosphate buffer at pH 6.5. The eluates were used for disc electrophoresis.

Collection of Tissue Specimens. Specimens of pharyngeal, palatine and lingual tonsils, nasal and paranasal sinus mucosae, nasal polyps, postoperative cheek cysts, submaxillary salivary glands, laryngeal and tracheobronchial mucosa were obtained at the time of surgery and bronchoscopic examination. The sources and numbers of tissue specimens examined are listed in Table I. Specimens of laryngeal and tracheal mucosa and submaxillary salivary glands removed surgically for cancer lesions were judged "not invaded by the carcinoma" macroscopically as well as microscopically.

Serum Samples. In order to evaluate effects of adenotonsillectomy (T and A) or tonsillectomy (T) on serum SIgA levels, blood samples were drawn prior to surgery from 25 patients who had undergone T and A or T and on the sixth and 30th day postoperatively. The sex, age, diagnosis and operation method of patients selected for this investigation are given in Table II.

Preparation of Tissue Extracts. For examining the concentration of SC determinants in palatine tonsils, tissue extracts were made from 50 palatine tonsils as follows. Palatine tonsils were washed with cold saline immediately after removal to eliminate blood. Connective tissue and clotted blood were removed as well as possible. The tonsils were cut into small fragments and homogenized in a threefold volume of phosphate buffer saline (PBS) at pH 7.2 in an electric juicer*** at 15,000 rpm for one minute. This homogenizing was performed in an ice bath and repeated twice. The resulting suspension did not contain any single cells. The homogenates were left in a cold chamber overnight and then centrifuged at 16,100 g for one hour. The supernatants, however, were contaminated with a small amount of blood elements.

Isolation of SIgA and FSC. The fractionation of SIgA and FSC from colostrum was carried out by the method of Kobayashi[27] with slight modification. The outline of the isolation is illustrated in Figure 1. The pooled colostrum was centrifuged at 16,100 g for one hour to remove fat and then acidified to pH 4.2 with 2% acetic acid to precipitate casein. After the centrifugation to remove casein the supernatant was then readjusted to pH 7.0 with 1 N NaOH solution. The colostral whey was treated with saturated ammonium sulfate at 50% final saturation. The precipitate was redissolved and dialyzed against 0.01 M phosphate buffer at pH 7.6. The solution was applied to a column, 2.5 x 45 cm in size, packed

* Nippon Shinku Gizutsu Co., Tokyo, Japan.
** Amicon Corporation, Lexington, Massachusetts.
*** Nihon Seiki Ltd., Tokyo, Japan.

TABLE I

SOURCES AND NUMBERS OF SPECIMENS

Tissue	*Number of Sample*	*Patient's Age*	*Reason for Excision*	
Palatine tonsil	50	5 - 25	Hypertrophy Chronic tonsillitis Habitual angina	28 14 8
Lingual tonsil	4	31 - 43	Hypertrophy	
Pharyngeal tonsil	36	2 - 12	Hypertrophy	
Inferior turbinate	6	18 - 26	Hypertrophic rhinitis Chronic sinus infection	3 3
Maxillary and ethmoidal sinus mucosa	18	15 - 58	Chronic infection	
Nasal polyp	8	8 - 63	Chronic sinus infection	
Cyst	4	37 - 56	Postoperative cheek cyst	
Submaxillary salival gland	8	22 - 51	Neck dissection for head and neck cancer Calculi	5 3
Larynx	5	48 - 67	Cancer	
Bronchial mucosa (biopsy specimen)	10	26 - 68	Various reasons excluding cancer and severe infection	

TABLE II

PATIENTS SELECTED FOR T & A OR T FOR INVESTIGATING SERUM SIgA LEVELS

Sex:	Male	9
	Female	16
		25 cases
Age:	5 - 10	18
	11 - 15	3
	16 - 25	4
		25 cases
Diagnosis:		
	Enlarged tonsil and adenoid	14
	Chronic tonsillitis	7
	Habitual antina	4
		25 cases
Operation Method:		
	Adenotonsillectomy	14
	Tonsillectomy	11
		25 cases

with diethylamino-ethyl (DEAE)-cellulose, saturated with 0.01 M phosphate buffer at pH 7.6. DEAE-cellulose column chromatography was performed by a stepwise gradient procedure as outlined by Sober and Peterson.[28] The elution was done first by 0.01 M phosphate buffer at pH 7.6 and then succeeded by 0.02 M buffer at pH 7.6 and 0.1 M buffer at pH 6.4. Eluates of 0.01 M and 0.02 M buffers were collected and submitted to carboxymethyl (CM)-cellulose chromatography for fractionating FSC. The fraction eluted by 0.1 M buffer at pH 6.4 was further chromatographed on a CM-cellulose column (2.5 x 45 cm) using linear gradient between 0.01 M (500 ml) and 0.5 M (1000 ml) sodium acetate buffers, pH 5.0. The fraction containing IgA, checked by immunodiffusion analysis using rabbit anti-human α-chain antiserum, was concentrated and passed through Sepharose 6B®* gel packed in a 1.5 x 100 cm column using borate buffer saline (BBS) at pH 7.8. The second peak was further fractionated by G-150 Sephadex®* gel filtration in a 2.5 x 100 cm column with BBS. The first excluded fraction contained pure SIgA. For isolating FSC, eluates of 0.01 M and 0.02 M phosphate buffers were concentrated and applied for CM-cellulose chromatographic separation. The procedure was the same as employed in the isolation of SIgA. Three peaks appeared, the third rich in FSC. This fraction was further fractionated by G-150 Sephadex® gel filtration.

Preparation of 7 S IgA (Serum IgA). Serum IgA was purified from the serum of an IgA myeloma patient. The procedure was done as previously described.[23]

Affinity Chromatography (Immunoadsorbents). Affinity chromatography was adopted to isolate SC determinants from parotid saliva and tracheobronchial secretions. This technique was carried out as reported previously.[23]

Disc Electrophoresis. This method was used for analyzing protein components of various body fluids and for testing the purity of isolated SIgA, FSC and serum IgA. The procedure was carried out as described in a previous paper.[29]

Immunodiffusion and Immunoelectrophoresis. These techniques were done according to the method of Ouchterlony.[30] Immunodiffusion analysis was carried out in 1% agar gel containing 1% NaCl. The gel used for im-

* Pharmacia Fine Chemicals AB, Uppsala, Sweden.

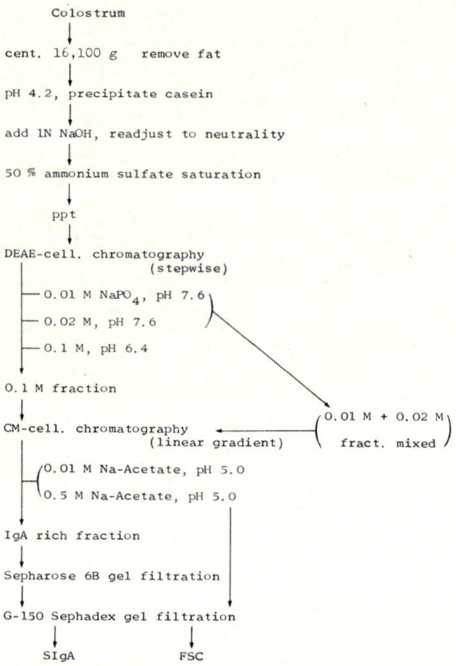

Fig. 1. Isolation of SIgA and FSC from human colostrum. SIgA—Secretory IgA. FSC—Free secretory component.

munoelectrophoresis was 1.2% of equal volumes of agar and agarose in veronal buffer (pH 8.6, $\mu = 0.05$).

Antisera. Antiserum against human SIgA was prepared by immunizing rabbits subcutaneously with colostral IgA preparation described above in complete Freunds adjuvant at seven-day intervals over a period of one month. The rabbit anti-SIgA antiserum was absorbed with cordal serum in order to make monospecific antiserum. Anti-SC antiserum was made by immunizing rabbits with FSC isolated from colostrum. Anti-lactoferrin antiserum was prepared by immunizing rabbits with lactoferrin purified from human colostrum by the method of Kobayashi.[27] Rabbit antiserum against the α chain was obtained from a commercial source.*

Fluoresceinated Antisera. The IgG fraction purified from the rabbit anti-SC antiserum by QAE-Sephadex® chromatography[31] was conjugated with fluorescein isothiocyanate (FITC) by the method of Hamashima and Kyogoku.[32] The 7 S gamma globulin, which was obtained from sheep anti-human IgE antiserum** by salting out with 40% saturated ammonium sulfate, followed by G-200 Sephadex® gel filtration, was labeled with FITC. Fluorescein conjugated rabbit anti-human IgG, IgA and IgM antisera were purchased from a commercial source.* These five antisera were absorbed with human liver powders in order to remove nonspecific staining for connective tissue.

Quantitative Analysis of SC Determinants. The concentration of SC determinants was measured in tonsillar extracts and serum samples from 25 patients who had undergone T and A or T by radioactive single radial diffusion as reported previously.[24]

Preparation of Tissues and Immunofluorescence Studies. Specimens of the fresh tissues were fixed in cold ethanol (95%) for paraffin sectioning according to the method described by Hamashima and Kyogoku.[32] Consecutive sections approximately 4 μ thick were obtained from each tissue. The sections were air dried, deparaffinated, and incubated immediately with these five FITC antisera respectively overnight in a cold and moist chamber. The sections were rinsed in PBS, washed for one hour with three changes of PBS, and mounted with nonfluorescein glycerin. The specimens were immediately examined with a Leitz incident-light fluorescence microscope (Dialux)*** using 1 mm UG and BG 38 excitation filters and a dichroic beam splitting mirror (TK 510) and suppression filter (K 515). Control experiments included incubation of tissue sections with fluoresceinated normal rabbit IgG. Blocking tests were also performed by applying the appropriate unconjugated antiserum to the consecutive tissue sections prior to staining with FITC antiserum. Paraffin sections from each block were stained with H. and E. for light microscopy.

RESULTS

Protein Components of Body Fluids. Figure 2 shows disc electrophoretic patterns of various external secretions and serum. Protein concentrations, pH and loading volumes of each fluid are listed as follows: The concentration of serum sample was 74 mg/ml, pH 7.4 and loading volume 3 μl; colostrum, 16.6 mg/ml, pH 7.0, 12 μl; nasal discharge (ND), 1.4 mg/ml, pH 6.5, 140 μl; parotid saliva, 8.4 mg/ml, pH 7.2, 25 μl; laryngeal secretion (LS), 1.01 mg/ml, pH 6.5, 200 μl; and tracheobronchial secretion, 7.05 mg/ml, pH 6.8, 25 μl. The gels were stained with Amido Black 10B®.**** The number of protein bands appearing in the patterns of each exocrine secretion was less than that of

* Behringwerke, Marburg, Lahn, Germany.
** Pharmacia Fine Chemicals AB, Uppsala, Sweden.
*** Leitz, Wetzlar, Germany.
**** E. Merck AD, Darmstadt, Germany.

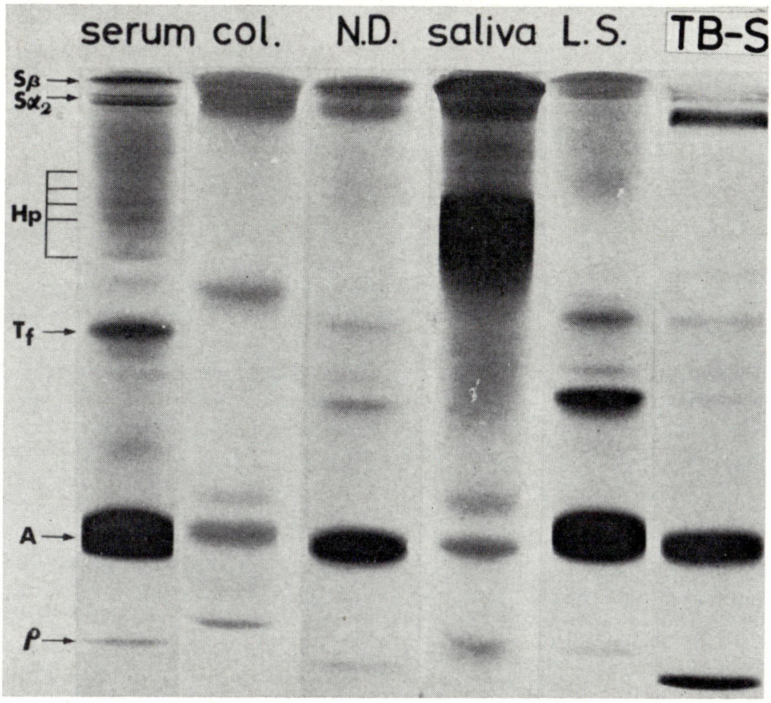

Fig. 2. Disc electrophoretic patterns of various body fluids. In the pattern of each external secretion a few fractions appear just beneath the separation gel, suggesting the existence of SIgA. Col—Colostrum. N.D.—Nasal discharge. L.S.—Laryngeal secretion. TB-S—Tracheobronchial secretion. Sβ—Slow beta lipoprotein. $S\alpha_2$—Slow alpha 2 macroglobulin. Hp—Haptoglobin. Tf—Transferrin. A—Albumin. ρ—Prealbumin.

serum. While albumin was the main fraction in nasal discharge, laryngeal secretion, tracheobronchial secretion, and colostrum and in serum, the albumin band showed only a trace in the pattern of parotid secretion. Each exocrine secretion had distinct bands near the origin which were the same as the isolated SIgA in electrophoretic mobility. The serum pattern also showed two distinct bands at the origin and just within the separation gel, but these have been identified as beta-lipoprotein and slow alpha-macroglobulin.[33]

Isolated SIgA and FSC. As shown in Figure 3, the isolated SIgA migrates near the origin and produces two distinct bands in disc electrophoresis, while the FSC preparation gives a single homogeneous band migrating faster than SIgA. In the pattern of isolated SIgA, the fast band is 11 S SIgA and the slow one is probably a more polymeric SIgA. The purified serum IgA was separated into four or five moving bands in which the fastest fraction was 7 S IgA. The slower bands were polymeric types of serum IgA. In immunoelectrophoretic analysis using anti-whole human colostrum the isolated SIgA and FSC produce a single precipitation line as shown in Figure 4B. This finding indicates the high purity of both preparations.

Immunodiffusion and Immunoelectrophoretic Studies of SIgA, FSC and Serum IgA. The isolated SIgA and FSC reacted to both anti-SIgA and anti-SC antisera in an agar gel (Fig. 4A). The precipitation line developing between SIgA and anti-SIgA antiserum fused with the precipitation line between SIgA and anti-SC antiserum. The line of FSC against anti-SIgA antiserum also fused with the line between FSC and anti-SC antiserum. This phenomenon indicates the presence of the com-

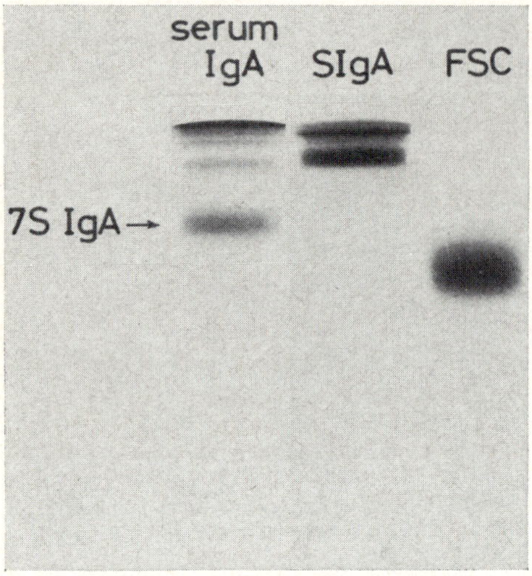

Fig. 3. Disc electrophoresis of the isolated SIgA, FSC, and serum IgA. The isolated SIgA migrates near the origin, producing two distinct bands. The faster band is 11 S SIgA and the slower is probably a more polymeric SIgA. The FSC preparation gives a homogeneous band which migrates faster than the SIgA fraction. Purified serum IgA is separated into four or five moving bands in which the fastest fraction is 7 S monomer IgA. The slower bands are polymeric types of serum IgA.

mon antigenic determinant, SC, in SIgA and FSC molecules. In the patterns of gel diffusion analysis as illustrated in Figure 5, the precipitation line of SIgA against anti-SIgA antiserum makes a spur over the line of FSC, demonstrating the existence of an antigenic determinant not found in FSC, that is, IgA molecule. The line of FSC crossed over that of serum IgA. This finding shows no antigenic relation between FSC and serum IgA. Gel diffusion analysis demonstrated that colostrum, tracheobronchial secretions and parotid saliva possess both SIgA and FSC. Serum IgA did not react to anti-SC antiserum. Figure 6 shows immunoelectrophoretic patterns of the isolated SIgA, FSC, serum IgA and various external secretions. The SIgA reacted to both anti-SIgA and anti-SC antisera to produce a single precipitation arch in the cathodal area, whereas the major part of the FSC arch against both anti-SIgA and anti-SC antisera occurred in the anodal area. The serum IgA reacted to anti-SIgA antiserum in the cathodal area but did not respond to anti-SC antiserum. Colostrum, tracheobronchial secretions and parotid saliva responded to both anti-SIgA and anti-SC antisera, producing two precipitation lines which fused with each other. One of the two lines corresponded to the line of SIgA and the other to that of FSC in electrophoretic mobility. This observation confirmed the existence of both SIgA and FSC in these secretions. Figure 7 is a picture showing patterns of gel diffusion and immunoelectrophoresis of individual nasal discharges. A spur of SIgA line against anti-SIgA antiserum over that of serum IgA was observed. A faint spur was also seen on the line of nasal dis-

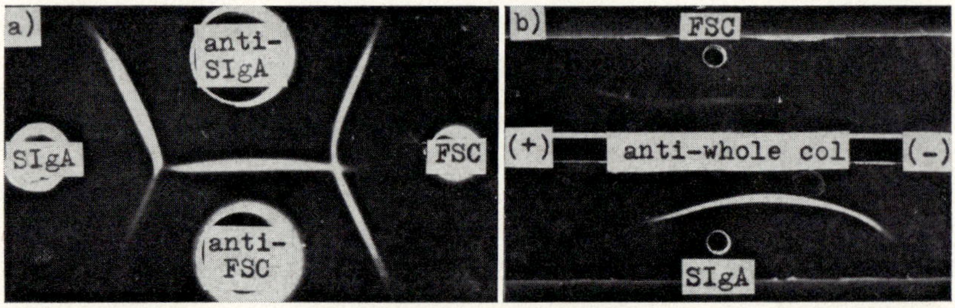

Fig. 4. Immunodiffusion and immunoelectrophoretic analysis of the isolated SIgA and FSC. a) Immunodiffusion. The precipitation line of SIgA against anti-SIgA fuses with the line developing between SIgA and anti-SC. The line of FSC against anti-SIgA also fuses with the line of FSC against anti-SC. This evidence indicates the presence of the common antigenic determinant, SC, in SIgA and FSC molecules. b) Immunoelectrophoresis. SIgA and FSC produce a single precipitation arch with anti-whole human colostrum. This finding indicates high purity of both preparations.

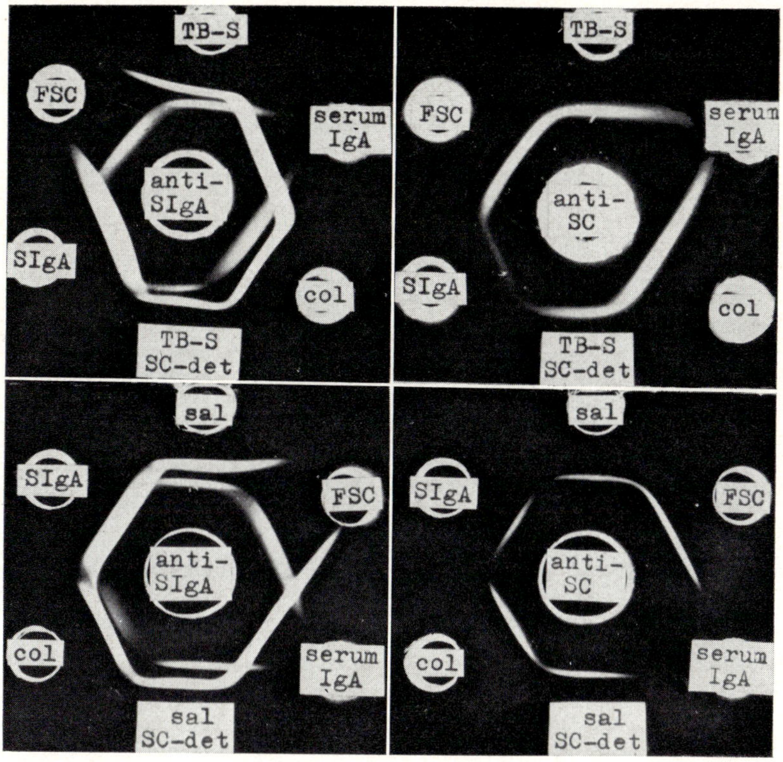

Fig. 5. Gel diffusion analysis of the SIgA, FSC, serum IgA and exocrine secretions. The precipitation line of SIgA against anti-SIgA forms a spur over the line of FSC, demonstrating the existence of an antigenic determinant not found in FSC, that is, the IgA (α chain) molecule. The line of FSC crosses over the line of serum IgA. This finding exhibits no antigenic relation between FSC and serum IgA. Tracheobronchial secretions, saliva and colostrum develop two precipitation lines against anti-SIgA antiserum. Serum IgA causes no precipitation line against anti-SC antiserum.

charge over the serum IgA line (Fig. 7A). This spur formation demonstrates the presence in SIgA of an antigenic determinant not found in serum IgA, that is, SC. The spur formation on the line of nasal discharge points out the presence of SIgA in nasal discharges. While ND (101) produces a line in the cathodal area, ND (102) forms an additional line in the anodal area as shown in Figure 7B. This additional line was FSC.

Concentration of SC Determinants in Tonsillar Extracts. The concentration of SC determinants in tonsillar extracts is exhibited in Figure 8. The mean value of 50 extracts was 3.2 ± 0.9 μg/g tissue. This value was much lower than that of sera from these patients.

Effects of T and A or T on the Serum Levels of SC Determinants. Figure 8 demonstrates serum levels of SC determinants pre- and postoperatively. The mean value of SC determinant concentrations in sera of preoperative state was 20.5 ± 8.4 μg/ml, while that at six days post surgery was 19.3 ± 6.9 μg/ml and that at 30 days post surgery 19.8 ± 8.0 μg/ml. There was no statistically significant difference between these values. In only a few cases remarkable change was observed in the postoperative samples.

Immunofluorescent Studies. Pharyngeal, Palatine and Lingual Tonsils: FITC labeled anti-SC antiserum caused no fluorescence in any area of the tissue section of palatine and lingual tonsils examined. Weber's glands were ob-

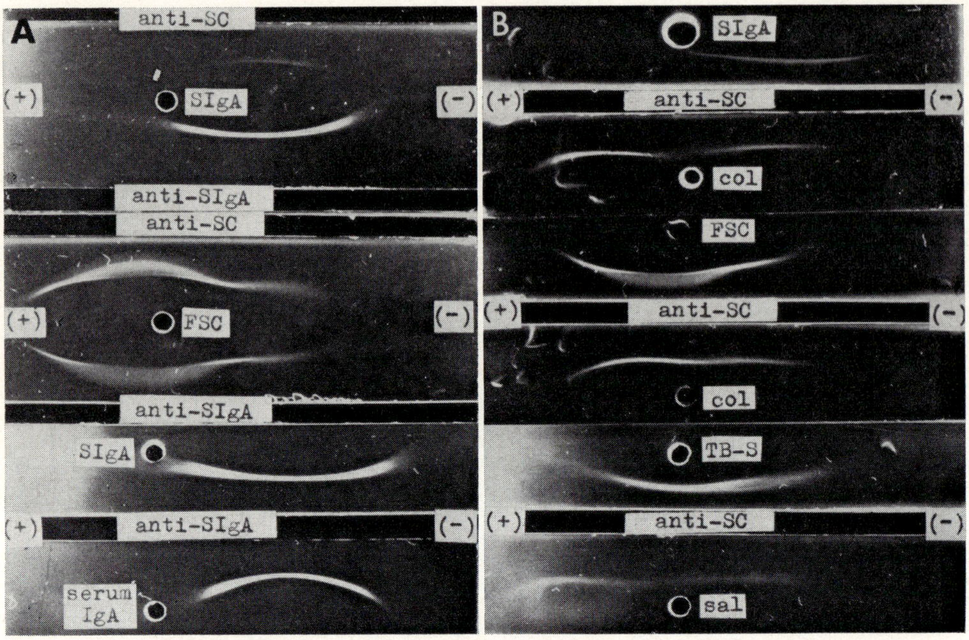

Fig. 6. Immunoelectrophoretic analysis of isolated SIgA, FSC, and serum IgA, and of external secretions. SIgA reacts to both anti-SIgA and anti-SC antisera to produce a single precipitation arch in the cathodal area, whereas the major part of the FSC arch against both anti-SIgA and anti-SC antisera occurs in the anodal area. Serum IgA reacts with anti-SIgA producing an arch at the same portion in the anodal area as that of SIgA. Two precipitation lines develop between colostrum, tracheobronchial secretions and saliva, and anti-SIgA. One of the two lines accords to the line of SIgA and the other to that of FSC in electrophoretic mobility.

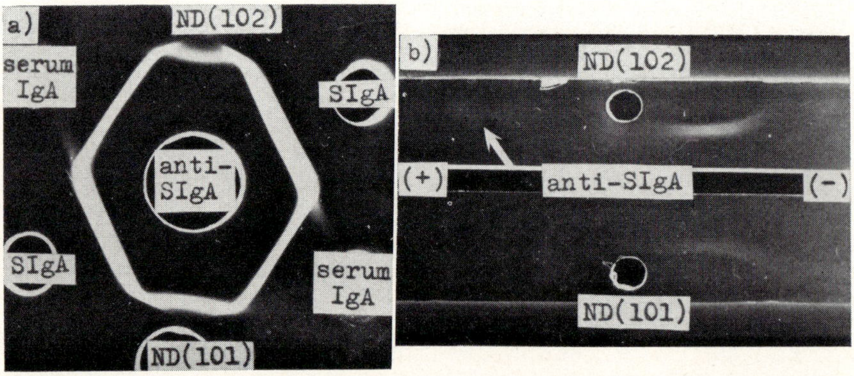

Fig. 7. Gel diffusion and immunoelectrophoretic analysis of individual nasal discharges. a) Immunodiffusion. Note the spur of SIgA line against anti-SIgA over the line of serum IgA. A faint spur is also seen on the line of nasal discharge over the serum IgA line. This observation indicates the presence of SIgA in nasal discharges. b) Immunoelectrophoresis. ND (101) produces a line in the cathodal area, whereas ND (102) forms an additional arch in the anodal area. The additional line is for FSC.

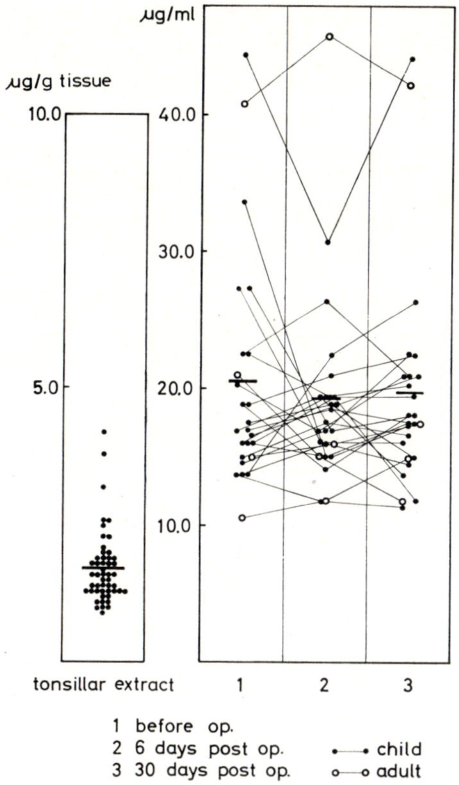

Fig. 8. The concentration of SC determinants in tonsillar extracts and sera from patients who had undergone tonsillectomy and adenotonsillectomy. The mean value of extracts is extremely low as compared to that in sera.

served in the ten palatine tonsil specimens, but these glands did not react to anti-SC conjugate. In pharyngeal tonsils, however, cytoplasmic staining of epithelial cells with anti-SC conjugate was clearly seen (Fig. 9A,B). Adjacent sections stained with H. and E. revealed that epithelium stained with anti-SC was columnar epithelium on many occasions. Epithelial layers of pharyngeal tonsils, which were metaplastic to squamous type, did not react to anti-SC. No SC-staining was seen in the basement membrane, subepithelial area, medullary portion, germinal center, or fibrous septum of pharyngeal tonsils, as well as palatine and lingual tonsils. Figure 9 shows positive staining with both anti-SC and anti-IgA conjugates in epithelial cells of adjacent sections of pharyngeal tonsil. Bright, granular fluorescent staining for SC and IgA was seen in the cytoplasm of cells present in the pharyngeal tonsillar epithelium (Fig. 9B,D). As shown in Figure 10A, IgA-forming cells accumulate close to the basement membrane and IgA deposits are observed in intercellular spaces between columnar epithelial cells of pharyngeal tonsils. Neither cytoplasmic nor luminal staining of Weber's glands occurred except for a very faint staining with anti-IgA in intercellular spaces of glandular epithelial cells (Fig. 10B) when all five specific antisera were employed, whereas heavy staining for IgA was obviously seen in interstitial connective tissues of glands (Fig. 10B). Patterns of the distribution of all immunoglobulin-forming cells were consistent in specimens of pharyngeal, palatine and lingual tonsils. The most abundant cells observed were IgG-forming cells, followed in predominance by IgA-forming cells. Aggregations of IgG-forming cells were detected frequently in the medullary portion and subepithelial area (Fig. 10C,D). Germinal centers contained lesser numbers of IgG-forming cells (Fig. 10C). IgA-forming cells formed aggregations mainly in the subepithelial area close to the basement membrane (Fig. 10A,E.F). Fewer IgA-forming cells were seen further from the tonsillar epithelium and the membrane lining crypts. There were few cells stained with anti-IgA in germinal centers (Fig. 10E). A few IgM-forming cells were observed in every ten fields (at x 312 magnification), and seemed to have no privileged site of localization (Fig. 10G,H). The number of IgE-forming cells was quite small. A part of the epithelial layer, basement membrane and medullary portion reacted to both anti-IgG and anti-IgA conjugates (Fig. 10C). A lesser staining for IgM was seen in these areas. Cryptal masses were usually positive for IgA and IgG but not for SC.

Inferior Turbinates, Nasal Polyps, Mucosae of Maxillary and Ethmoidal Sinuses, and Postoperative Cheek Cysts: Staining patterns obtained with the five

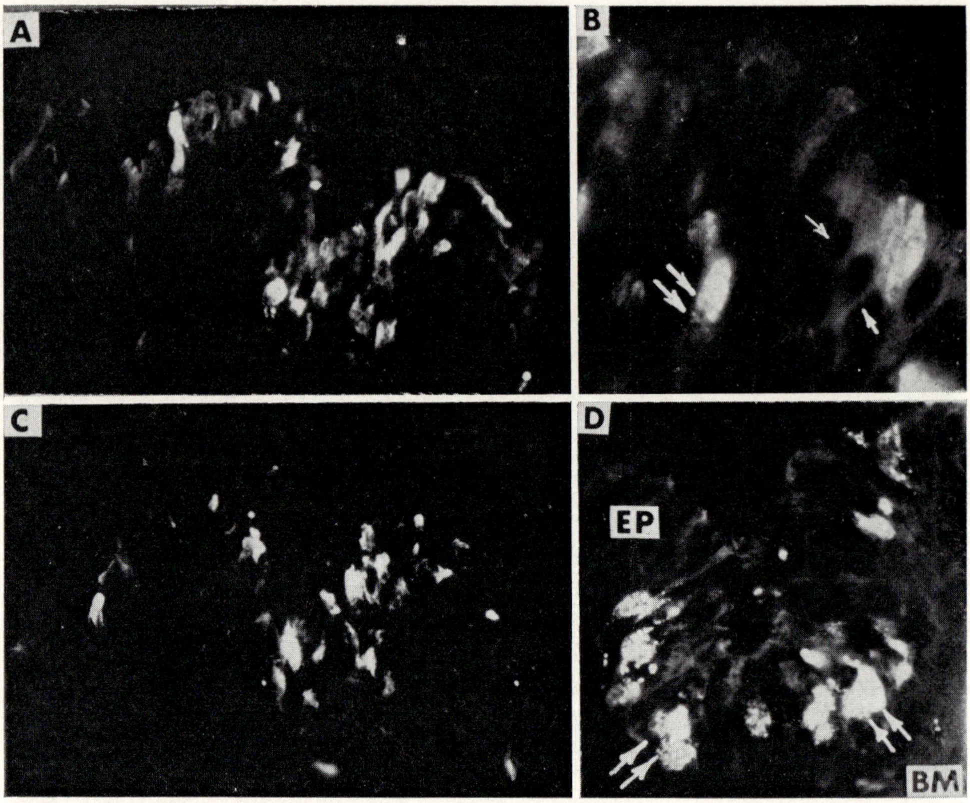

Fig. 9. Immunofluorescence localization of SC and IgA in the epithelium of pharyngeal tonsil. A) Tissue section treated with anti-SC (x 312). B) Tissue section treated with anti-SC (x 675). Note cytoplasmic fluorescence (double arrows) and intercellular staining (single arrow) of epithelial cells. C) Adjacent section of the same tissue specimen as in section A stained with anti-IgA (x 312). D) Tissue section incubated with anti-IgA (x 675). Bright and granular fluorescence is seen in the cytoplasm (double arrows) and intercellular space (single arrow) of epithelial cells. EP–Epithelium. BM–Basement membrane.

specific antisera were similar in these nasal and paranasal sinus specimens. Adjacent sections treated with anti-SC and anti-IgA conjugates respectively, produced brilliant fluorescence at nearly the same sites of the epithelial layers, submucosal acini and lumens of glandular acini and ductules (Fig. 11A,B,C,D). Cytoplasmic and intercellular staining in cells of the epithelial layer and of glandular acinar cells was obtained when tissue sections were incubated with anti-SC or anti-IgA antiserum (Fig. 12). As demonstrated in Figure 12, SC staining is much more pronounced in the cytoplasm of glandular acinar cells, whereas anti-IgA caused brilliant fluorescence predominantly in the intercellular space between epithelial cells and on the epithelial surface and cavity of the glandular acini and ductules. IgA-conjugate caused additional deposits in the basement membrane (Fig. 11B), subepithelial connective tissue (Fig. 11D), and interstitial connective tissue between acini (Fig. 12B). In some simple acini or ductules neither cytoplasmic nor intercellular staining occurred when tissue sections were treated with anti-SC or anti-IgA antiserum. Figure 11E exhibits a staining pattern of ductules with anti-SC, in which positive reaction is only seen in the cavity of the ductules. Perhaps, SC or SIgA synthesized at some other place is passing through the duct. The intensity of fluorescent staining with anti-SC and anti-IgA antisera varied considerably between acini in the same section as well as different samples. The acinar cells of inferior turbinate mucosae appeared to have the most intense staining. IgA-forming cells were infrequently seen beneath the epithelial basement membrane, although the adjacent section stained with H. and E. showed many plasma cells in the same portion (Fig. 13A,B). In the specimen of postoperative cheek cysts there were many acinar cells in the submucosa. However, many of these acinar cells were negative for SC or IgA. IgA deposits were found on the surface of glandular epithelia and in the lumens of a few acini. A few acinar cells produced a very faint fluorescence when stained with anti-SC. Little or no epithelial cells or luminal staining occurred, when IgG, IgM and IgE specific antisera were used for the section of various nasal and paranasal sinus samples. In some instances, however, heavily diffuse staining for IgG was evident all through the section as shown in Figure 11H. Figure 11F illustrates a very faint anti-IgG fluorescence in the intercellular space of acinar cells. Anti-IgG and IgM conjugates caused diffuse staining in the connective tissues (Fig. 11G). Figure 13C exhibits a cell stained with anti-IgE antiserum in a section of an ethmoidal sinus mucosa. In other sections of this sample a few IgE-staining cells were detected. However, the presence of IgE-forming cells was very rare in nasal tissue specimens.

Submaxillary Salivary Glands: Anti-SC localized in the cytoplasm of glandular acinar cells and in their intercellular spaces (Fig. 14). Heavy concentrations of anti-SC fluorescence were usually observed in the portion of cytoplasm which bordered the acinar lumen and in the cavity (Fig. 14C). Anti-IgA conjugate produced similar staining patterns at that of anti-SC (Fig. 14D). In many sections some acini were positive for SC or IgA, while others did not react. Moreover, in one or more cells forming an acinus, positive staining for SC or IgA was seen, but remaining cells were not stained. The intensity of fluorescence with anti-SC and anti-IgA varied between acini on many occasions. The number of acini positive for SC was greater than those positive for IgA. Only a few interstitial plasma cells stained for IgA. Adjacent sections stained with H. and E. revealed that submaxillary gland tissue specimens tested were composed mainly of serous glands while mucous type glandular cells were scanty. Perhaps submaxillary epithelial cells positive for SC and IgA belonged to serous type. When tissue sections were incubated with IgG, IgM and IgE specific antisera, no staining or very weak reaction in a few sections was observed in the cytoplasm and intercellular space of glandular acinar cells and in the lumen. Anti-IgG and anti-IgM antisera caused positive staining only in interstitial connective tissues. None or few IgG and no IgM or IgE-forming cells were detected.

Laryngeal and Tracheobronchial Mucosae: SC and IgA staining of laryngeal and tracheobronchial mucosal specimens revealed patterns similar to those obtained with nasal tissues. Brilliant cytoplasmic staining was observed in cells present in the epithelial layer and glandular acinar cells in the submucosa. Figure 15 shows typical staining with anti-SC in the glandular epithelium of the tracheal mucosa. A linear surface staining of the epithelium with anti-IgA was seen in a biopsy specimen taken from the carina (Fig. 15A). In specimens of the larynx acinar cells positive for SC or IgA were distributed predominantly in the area of subglottis. Staining with anti-IgA conjugate produced very faint fluorescence in the epithelial cells covering the vocal cord and epiglottis, which were squamous cell type. No SC staining occurred in the cytoplasm of these epithelial cells. A few IgA-forming cells were found scattered in the submucosa of tracheobronchial tissues. Lesser numbers of IgG-forming cells than IgA-forming cells

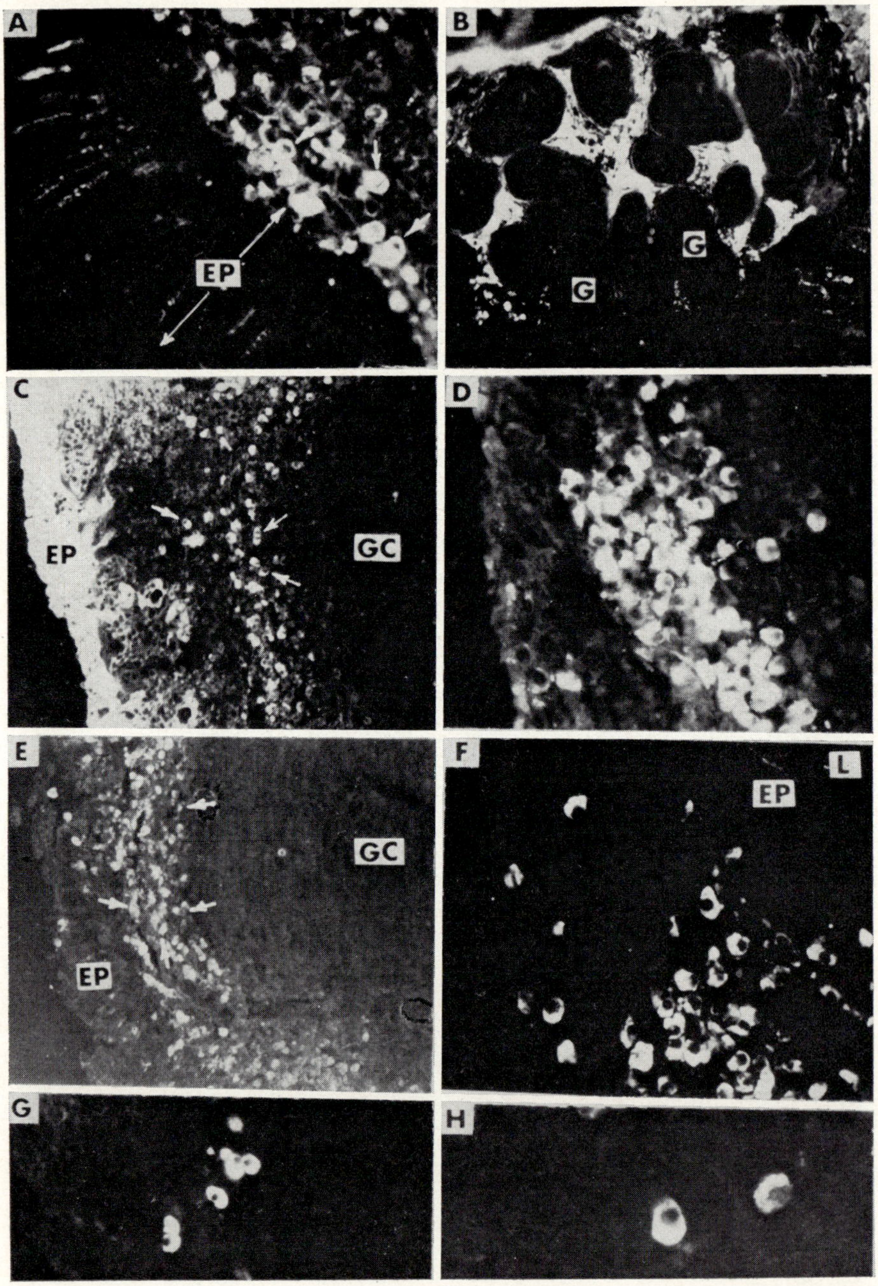
A
B
EP
G
G
C
D
EP
GC
E
F
GC
L
EP
EP
G
H

were detected. IgM or IgE-forming cells could not be seen in any sections of the specimens examined.

DISCUSSION

In our previous study[23] a comparison of the electrophoretic mobility and molecular weight was done between subunits of SIgA isolated from various external secretions, such as nasal discharge, parotid saliva, middle ear effusion, and colostrum. The isolated SIgA was divided by SDS-polyacrylamide gel electrophoresis into three fractions, L-chain, H-chain and SC. There was little difference of the electrophoretic mobility and molecular weight between the subunits of SIgA derived from these external secretions. In addition to these three types of polypeptides a fourth subunit, termed J chain, was recently identified in SIgA molecules of rabbit by Halpern and Koshland.[34] It is now known that 11 S SIgA molecule is composed of four H-chains (α chain), four L-chains, one J chain and one SC. These subunits possess their own antigenecity respectively. However, anti-J chain antiserum failed to precipitate with J chains on the untreated molecules of SIgA,[35] probably because the antigenic determinants of J chain are hidden by SC molecules.

Anti-SIgA antiserum can react with serum IgA, SIgA and FSC, while anti-IgA antiserum responds to SIgA and serum IgA but not to FSC. Antiserum against SC reacts with both SIgA and FSC, but fails to precipitate with serum IgA. These antigenic relationships were confirmed in the present study. It is necessary when analyzing SIgA immunochemically or immunohistologically that individual antisera specific for α chain, SC and/or SIgA be used. Since various external secretions contain SIgA, FSC, and serum type IgA in varying proportions,[6-10,36] it seems difficult to determine accurate SIgA concentrations in secretions. Many investigators have employed single radial immunodiffusion technique for quantitation of IgA in secretions. However, it should be cautioned that proteins of larger molecular weight produce smaller precipitation rings in single radial immunodiffusion. According to Tomasi et al,[6] if a 7 S serum IgA standard is used in single radial immunodiffusion analysis of SIgA, it underestimates the level of SIgA (11 S) approximately three times.

Formerly it had been suggested that SIgA is synthesized in such a way that the locally produced IgA which is probably identical to 7 S serum IgA transverses the mucous membrane or glandular epithelium, where SC is produced, and complexes with SC.[6] However, since evidence from recent studies[27,37,38] shows that FSC combines *in vitro* with serum IgA (10 S IgA having J chain but not monomer type) producing 11 S IgA indistinguishable from native SIgA, and since J chain and IgA were found in the same plasma cells of lamina propria,[39,40] it is probable that 10 S IgA molecule formed by plasma cells in the submucosa is transported to the epithelial cell layer and secreted to the luminal secretions. SC might facilitate this transport

---

Fig. 10. Immunofluorescent studies of tonsil. A) Section of pharyngeal tonsil stained with anti-IgA (x 312). IgA forming cells (single arrow) accumulate close to the basement membrane. IgA deposits are present in the intercellular space between columnar epithelial cells. B) Weber's glands of palatine tonsil treated with anti-IgA (x 312). Note that little or very faint positive staining is observed in the intercellular space of glandular epithelial cells, whereas heavy concentrations of fluorescence are evident in the interstitial connective tissue of glands. C) Section of palatine tonsil incubated with anti-IgG (x 125). There are many IgG-forming cells (single arrow) in the subepithelial portion. However, the germinal center contains few positive cells. The epithelial layer is heavily stained by anti-IgG fluorescence. D) Aggregation of IgG-forming cells in the subepithelial area of palatine tonsil (x 312). E) Section of pharyngeal tonsil stained with anti-IgA (x 125). IgA-forming cells (single arrow) accumulate in the subepithelial portion close to the basement membrane. In the epithelial layer a few IgA-forming cells are detected. No IgA-forming cells are present in the germinal center. F) Aggregation of IgA-forming cells just beneath the epithelium of pharyngeal tonsil (x 312). G) IgM-forming cells in palatine tonsil (x 312). H) IgM-forming cells in a section of pharyngeal tonsil (x 675). EP—Epithelium. G—Gland. GC—Germinal center. L—Lumen.

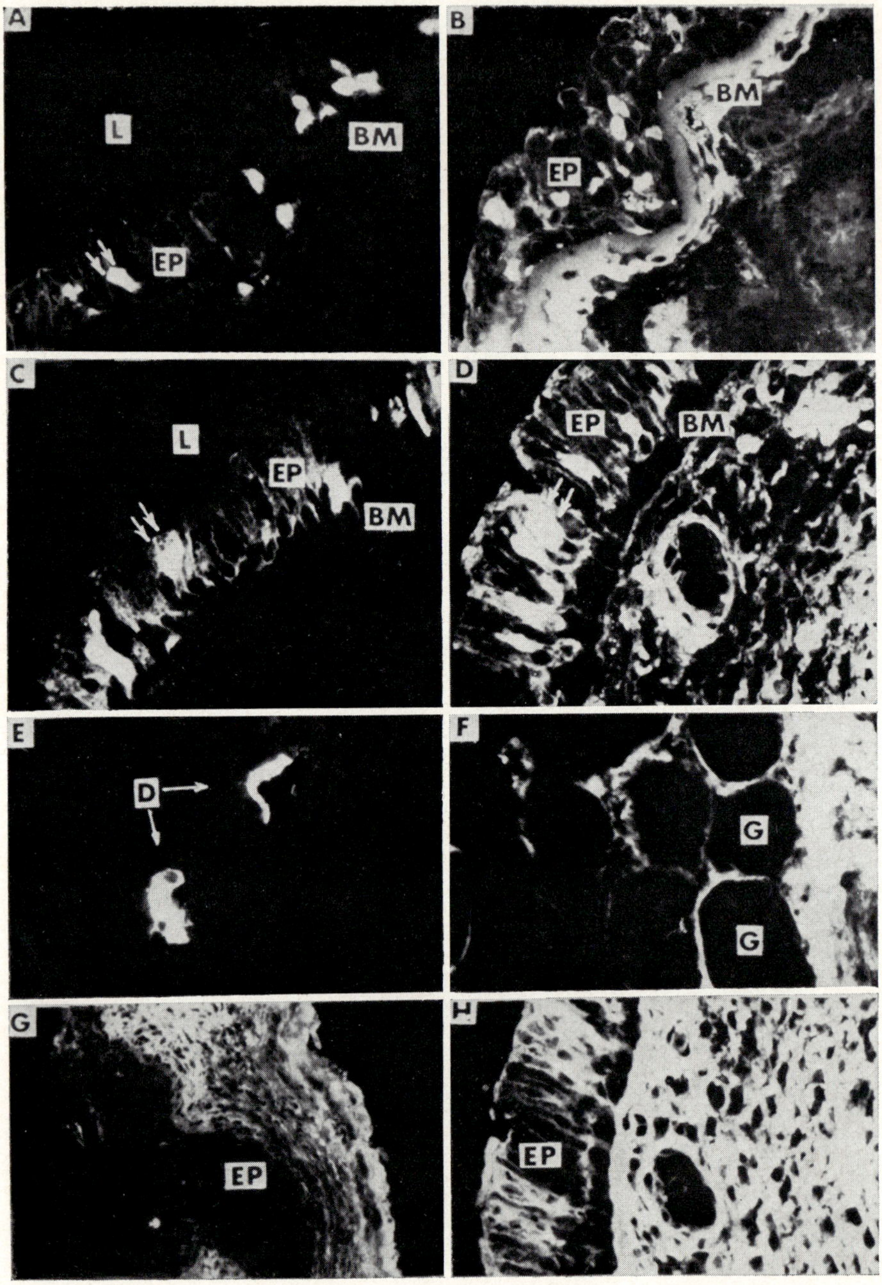
A
L
BM
EP
B
BM
EP
C
L
EP
BM
D
EP
BM
E
D
F
G
G
G
EP
H
EP

and protect SIgA from intracellular degradation during its transport through the epithelial cell cytoplasm.[7] The exact location where complexing of SC with IgA molecules occurs is still unsettled. The immunofluorescent investigation in the present study as well as others[5,19] revealed that SC is localized only in the mucous membrane, acinar and ductular epithelium, and in the lumen, although conflicting data suggesting the existence of SC in lymphoid plasma cells present beneath the basement membrane was reported by Rossen et al.[18] They suggested that SC and IgA molecules are synthesized within the same plasma-like cell. The reason for this discrepancy is not clear but fluorescent antibody technique is very sensitive and requires highly specific antibody. In addition to the problem of specificity, Tourville et al[19] emphasized that epithelial cells often break off from the acini, particularly in diseased tissue and are difficult to identify as epithelial cells by fluorescent microscopy. Results of this study demonstrated fluorescent staining for IgA in the cytoplasm, intercellular space and lumen of the glandular epithelium and mucosa. IgA-forming cells were found in the lamina propria and IgA deposits were also seen in the basement membrane and submucosa. Tourville et al[19] have previously reported similar observations. They suggested that IgA produced by plasma cells present in the lamina propria is transported through the basement membrane into the intercellular space between the epithelial cells until it reaches the apical end, where the tight junction of adjacent epithelial cells prevents it from directly reaching the lumen via the intercellular route. This hypothesis was based on findings showing heavy concentrations of anti-IgA fluorescence in a portion of cytoplasm which bordered the acinar lumen. This staining pattern was also obtained in this study. The presence of SC in the cytoplasm and intercellular space of epithelial cells and in the lumen, was a conclusive finding of the present investigation. Therefore complexing between SC and IgA could occur in the epithelial layer, either in the cytoplasm or intercellular space, unless some inhibitor to this conjugation is present in the epithelium. The finding of this study that adjacent sections treated respectively with anti-SC and anti-IgA antisera produced brilliant fluorescence in nearly the same site of the epithelial layers and glandular acinar cells, suggests to us the local synthesis of SIgA in these epithelial cells. It was another finding of our study that some mucosal or glandular acinar cells were positive for SC but not for IgA. This evidence suggests the secretion of SC to the lumen. This supposition was supported by the immunochemical identification of FSC in various external secretions in the present work. If IgA molecule is transported to the lumen without complexing with SC, the conjugation between SC and IgA could oc-

---

Fig. 11. Immunofluorescent studies of nasal tissues. A) Tissue section of inferior turbinate stained with anti-SC conjugate (x 312). Fluorescence localizes in the cytoplasm (double arrows) of cells present in the epithelial layer and intercellular space between mucosal cells. Note no fluorescence staining in the basement membrane and submucosal area. B) Adjacent section of the same tissue specimen as in A, treated with anti-IgA (x 312). Cytoplasmic staining and intercellular space deposit between epithelial cells are evident. Note IgA deposit in the basement membrane and submucosal area. C) Section of nasal polyp incubated with anti-SC conjugate (x 312). Cytoplasmic and intercellular staining is demonstrated in the epithelial cells. D) Adjacent section of the same tissue specimen as in A, treated with anti-IgA (x 312). In addition to cytoplasmic and intercellular staining of the epithelial cells, IgA deposit is also seen in the submucosal connective tissue. E) Luminal staining for SC of the ductule of maxillary sinus mucosa (x 312). F) Tissue section of inferior turbinate treated with anti-IgG conjugate (x 312). Positive staining is observed in the connective tissue and basement membrane of glandular epithelium. Note no cytoplasmic or luminal staining of glandular cells. G) Tissue section of ethmoidal sinus mucosa treated with anti-IgG antiserum (x 125). Note that diffuse IgG deposits are obvious in the submucosal area while the epithelial layer is not stained. H) Section of nasal polyp stained with anti-IgG (x 312). Heavily diffuse staining is evidently seen all over the section. This finding suggests exudation of blood elements. L—Lumen. EP—Epithelium. BM—Basement membrane. D—Ductule. G—Gland.

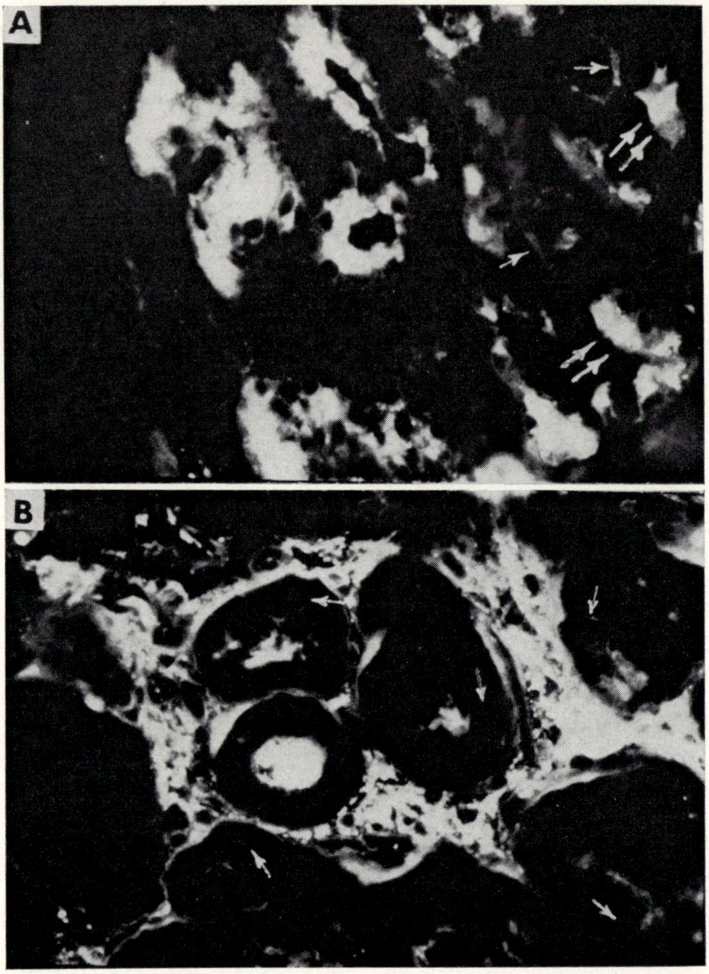

Fig. 12. Immunofluorescence localization of SC and IgA in compound alveolar glands of inferior turbinate. A) Stained with anti-SC conjugate (x 312). Note heavy concentrations of anti-SC fluorescence in the portion of cytoplasm which borders the acinar lumen (double arrows). B) Staining with anti-IgA conjugate of a section of the inferior turbinate from the same individual as in A (x 312). Luminal, cytoplasmic (double arrows) and intercellular (single arrow) fluorescences are observed. The basement membrane of the glandular epithelial layer and connective tissue between acini are also stained.

cur in the lumen. It is probable that SC and IgA molecules are independently synthesized and that they are under independent control. Since recent studies[27,37,38] demonstrated the *in vitro* association of FSC with 10 S serum IgA, it is conceivable that conjugation could occur wherever they meet unless some inhibitor exists.

In general IgG and IgM deposits were observed in connective tissue beneath the basement membrane but not in the cytoplasm and intercellular space of epithelial cells. As demonstrated in Figure 11H, heavily diffuse staining with anti-IgG occurred through the whole tissue section in some instances, particularly when inflammation was dominant. This observation suggests that blood elements passed through disrupted capillaries and reached the secretion by going through the basement membrane via the tight junction of epithelial cells. In this situation the secre-

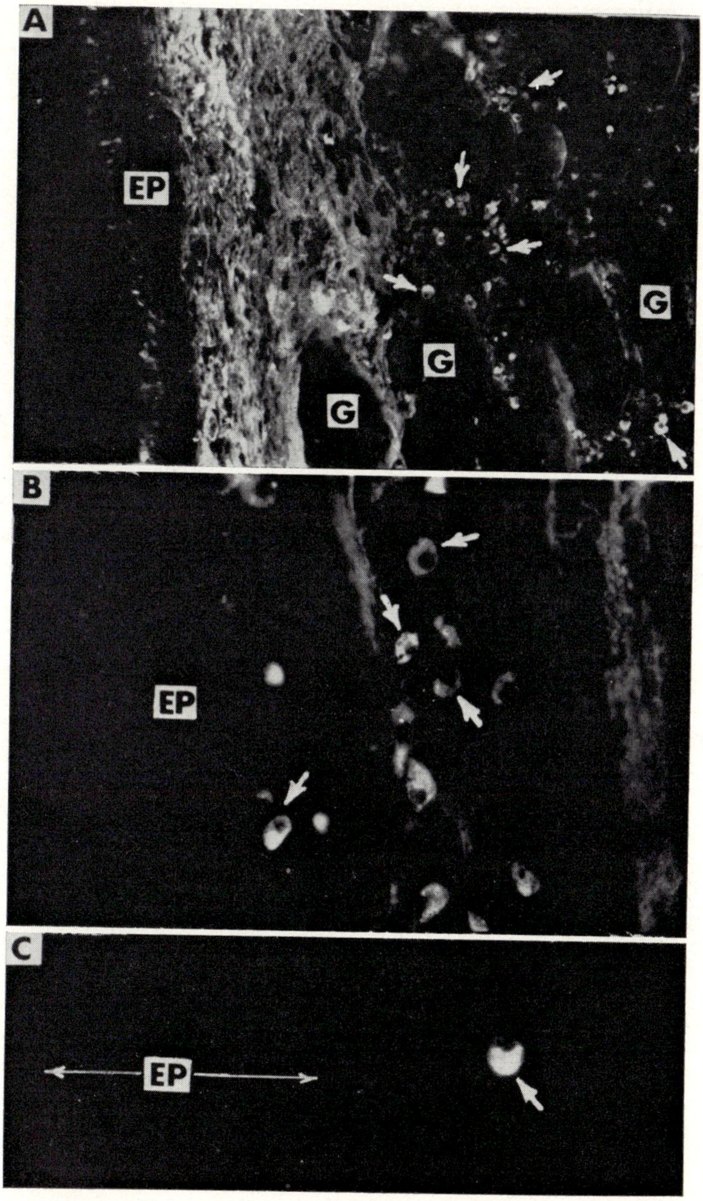

Fig. 13. Localization of immunoglobulin-forming cells in nasal tissue specimens. A) Section of nasal polyp stained with anti-IgA (x 125). Note that plasma-like cells (single arrow) positive for IgA are found scattered in the connective tissue between glandular acini. In this section glandular acinar cells do not react to anti-IgA conjugate. B) Section of maxillary sinus mucosa treated with anti-IgA (x 312). Occasional IgA-forming cells (single arrow) exist in the submucosal area. C) A single cell stained with anti-IgE antiserum in the subepithelial area of ethmoidal sinus mucosa (x 675). EP—Epithelium. G—Glandular acinus.

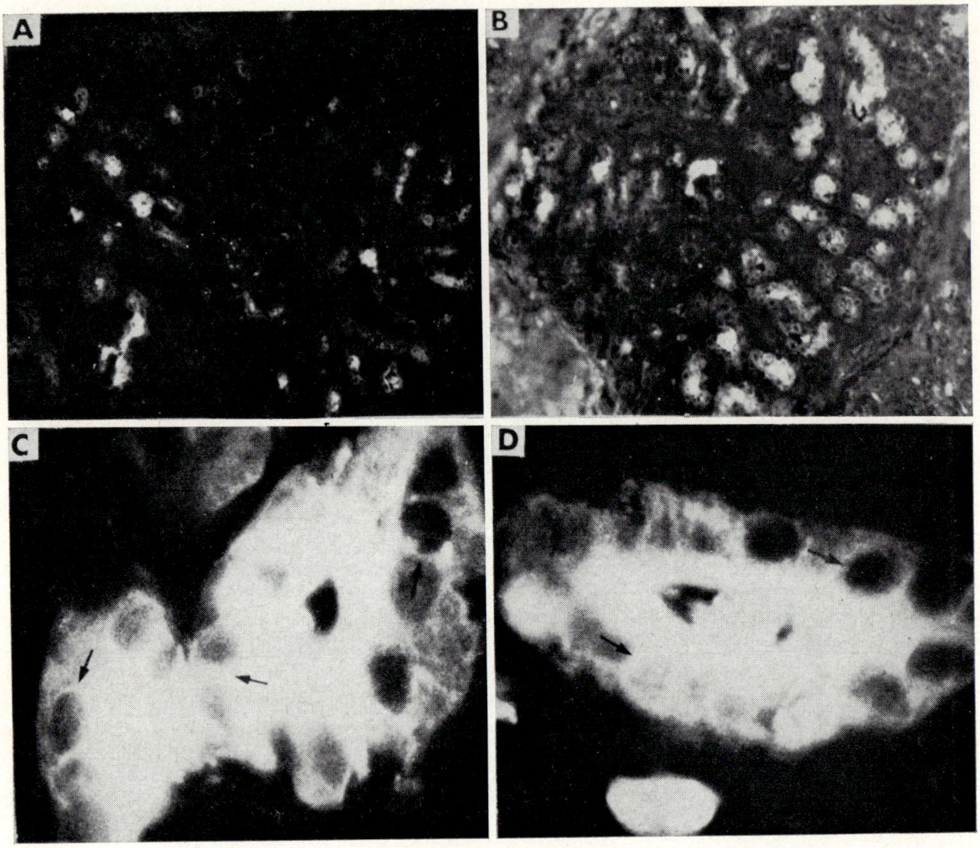

Fig. 14. Immunofluorescence staining with anti-SC and anti-IgA conjugates of submaxillary salival gland. A) Stained with anti-SC (x 125). Note SC fluorescence in the lumen and acinar cells of compound glands. B) Adjacent section of the same specimen as in A, stained with anti-IgA (x 125). The staining pattern is similar to that of anti-SC. C) Stained with anti-SC (x 675). D) Heavy fluorescence is seen in both C and D in the portion of cytoplasm which borders the acinar lumen. Single arrow indicates fluorescence of intercellular space.

tion could be contaminated with large amounts of blood elements. The basement membrane may act as a barrier to permit selective transport and the tight junction prevent large molecules from passing directly to the lumen via the intercellular space in normal condition.

This immunofluorescence study failed to find SC determinants in any portions of palatine and lingual tonsils including Weber's glands. Rossen et al[18] in their immunofluorescent studies, reported the presence in tonsil of SC in the cytoplasm of cells: 1) lining the tonsillar crypts, 2) scattered beneath the epithelial surface, and 3) in the fibrous septum. Schmedtje et al[20] could not detect SC or SIgA in cells of the tonsillar epithelium or infiltrated plasma cells. They postulated that the positive results of Rossen's investigation were caused by nonspecific reactivity of their anti-SC with lactoferrin. Results in this study of the quantitative analysis of SC determinants in tonsillar extracts and sera would deny the production of SIgA in palatine tonsils. Very small amounts (3.2 ± 0.9 $\mu g/g$ tissue) of SC-determinants in tonsillar extracts probably come from the contaminating blood.

In contrast to the absence of SC or SIgA in palatine and lingual tonsils, it was evidently detected that some columnar epithelial cells of the pharyngeal

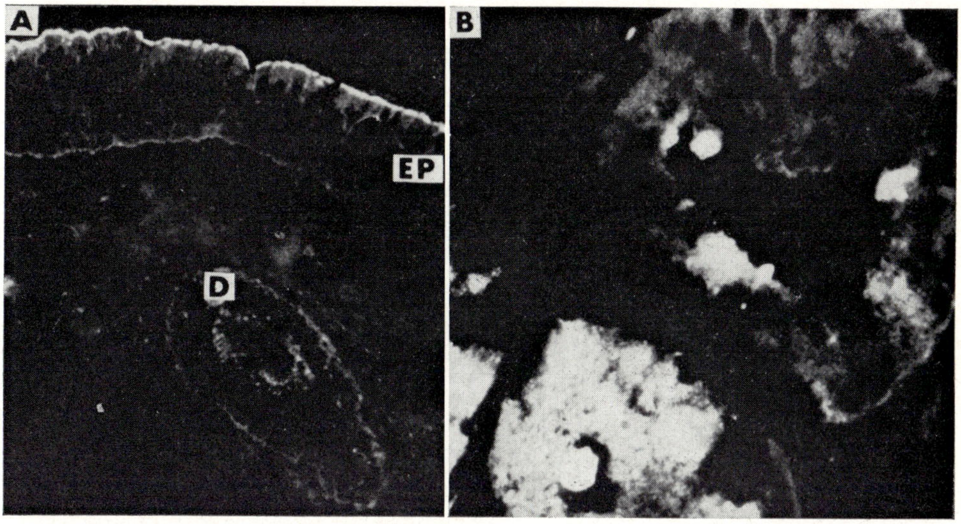

Fig. 15. Immunofluorescence studies of tracheobronchial mucosa. A) Section of a biopsy specimen taken from the carina, treated with anti-IgA (x 312). A linear surface staining is seen. EP—Epithelium. D—Glandular acinus. B) Section of tracheal mucosa stained with anti-SC, showing brilliant fluorescence in the cytoplasm of glandular acinar cells (x 675).

tonsil contain SC determinants. Local synthesis of SIgA in the pharyngeal tonsillar epithelium is suggested by the fact that adjacent sections treated respectively with anti-SC and anti-IgA caused brilliant fluorescence at nearly the same site of the epithelium. The epithelium of pharyngeal tonsil is respiratory type while that of palatine tonsil is squamous type. Results of many investigators[5,19] as well as the present work indicate that SC is localized in secretory cells. However, not all secretory cells contain SC. Although Tourville et al[19] reported that SC was found in goblet cells of the intestinal and bronchial mucosae and that SC staining was much more intense in the mucous secretory cells rather than the serous type, it is yet to be proven with certainty what type of secretory cells synthesize SC molecules. The striking difference of SC or SIgA production between pharyngeal tonsils and palatine tonsils could be accounted for by the different types of epithelium. Ogra[41] reported a significant fall of poliovirus antibody levels in nasopharyngeal secretions after tonsillectomy and adenoidectomy. Antibodies against poliovirus in secretions belonged to IgA type. Although he speculated that pharyngeal tonsils produce secretory IgA antibodies against poliovirus, which may act as local immunologic resistance against this virus invasion, there has been no reported data to demonstrate SIgA synthesis in pharyngeal tonsils. It has been found that tonsils have cells producing immunoglobulins of all five classes.[42,43] This was confirmed by the present study. Accumulations of IgA-forming cells were detected close to the basement membrane of both pharyngeal and palatine tonsils. In pharyngeal tonsils IgA produced by these accumulated cells may be transversed to the epithelium and may complex with SC. However, it is not known whether IgA-forming cells accumulating to the basement membrane of palatine tonsil produce 10 S IgA or not. On the basis of immunologic functions of tonsil, such as antibody production organ, lymphopoiesis,[44,45] and immune memory,[46] it is suggested that tonsils serve in immunologic development of the host in such a way that tonsils are adjacent to the outside with wide epithelial surfaces and receive constant antigenic stimulations.

Even though SIgA is the predominant

immunoglobulin in external secretions, this immunoglobulin was detected in normal sera as well as those from patients with various disorders.[24,47-49] The amount in sera of SIgA is extremely small. The reported average concentrations of SIgA in sera were between 0.025 and 0.04 mg/ml.[24,28,48] These values appeared to be approximately 1% of the total IgA in serum. The exact mechanism for the appearance of SIgA in serum is not known. However, Brandtzaeg[48] suggested that any condition that increases the permeability of glandular and mucosal tissues may raise the "spill-over" or absorption of secretory IgA into the circulation. An increased production of SIgA would account for the elevation of serum SIgA due to the fact that the highest SIgA levels in sera were seen in lactating women.[47] Waldman et al[47] also reported an elevated serum SIgA level in patients with a variety of disorders involving secretory surfaces: e.g., acute bacterial enterocolitis or respiratory tract carcinoma. It is speculated that SIgA is directly absorbed from the sections in individuals with widespread inflammation of epithelial surfaces. In this study serum SIgA levels were observed before and after tonsillectomy or adenotonsillectomy. However, no remarkable changes of values were detected. This evidence suggests that direct absorption of SIgA into circulation from the surgical wound may not occur or, if it does, it may be trivial.

DEPARTMENT OF OTOLARYNGOLOGY, YAMAGUCHI UNIVERSITY, SCHOOL OF MEDICINE, UBE-CITY, JAPAN.

REFERENCES

1. Heremans JF, Heremans MT, Schultze HE: Isolation and description of a few properties of the β-2A globulin of human serum. Clin Chim Acta 4:96-102, 1959

2. Chodirker WB, Tomasi TB: Gamma globulins: Quantitative relationship in human serum and nonvascular fluids. Science 142: 1080, 1963

3. Remington JS, Vosti KL, Lietze A, et al: Serum proteins and antibody activity in human nasal secretions. J Clin Invest 43:1613-1624, 1964

4. Keimowitz RI: Immunoglobulins in normal human tracheobronchial washings. A qualitative and quantitative study. J Lab Clin Med 63:54-59, 1964

5. Tomasi TB Jr, Tan EM, Solomon A, et al: Characteristics of an immune system common to certain external secretions. J Exp Med 121:101-124, 1965

6. Tomasi TB Jr, Bienenstock J: Secretory immunoglobulins. Adv Immunol 9:1-96, 1968

7. Tomasi TB Jr: Secretory immunoglobulins. N Engl J Med 287:500-506, 1972

8. Newcomb RW, Normansell D, Stanworth DR: A structural study of human exocrine IgA globulin. J Immunol 101:905-914, 1968

9. Kobayashi K: Studies on human secretory IgA. Comparative studies of the IgA-bound secretory piece and the free secretory piece protein. Immunochemistry 8:785-800, 1971

10. South MA, Cooper MD, Wollheim FA, et al: The IgA system. I. Studies of the transport and immunochemistry of IgA in the saliva. J Exp Med 123:615-627, 1968

11. Brown WR, Newcomb RW, Ishizaka K: Proteolytic degradation of exocrine and serum immunoglobulins. J Clin Invest 49:1374-1380, 1970

12. Shuster J: Pepsin hydrolysis of IgA-delineation of two populations of molecules. Immunochemistry 8:405-411, 1971

13. Adinolfi M, Glynn AA, Lindsay M, et al: Serological properties of γ A to *Escherichia coli* present in human colostrum. Immunology 10:517-526, 1966

14. Douglas RG Jr, Rossen RD, Butler WT, et al: Rhinovirus neutralizing antibody in tears, parotid saliva, nasal secretions and serum. J Immunol 99:297-303, 1967

15. Waldman RH, Jurgensen PF, Olsen GN, et al: Immune response of the human respiratory tract. I. Immunoglobulin levels and influenza virus vaccine antibody response. J Immunol 111:38-41, 1973

16. South MA, Wollheim FA, Warwick WJ, et al: Local deficiency in immunoglobulin A in the saliva of patients with chronic sinopulmonary disease. J Pediatr 67:940-941, 1965

17. South MA, Cooper MD, Wollheim FA, et al: The IgA system. II. Clinical significance of IgA deficiency: Studies in patients with agammaglobulinemia and ataxia telangiectasia. Am J Med 44:168-178, 1968

18. Rossen RD, Morgan C, Hsu KC, et al: Localization of 11 S external secretory IgA by immunofluorescence in tissues lining the oral and respiratory passages in man. J Immunol 100:706-717, 1968

19. Tourville DR, Adler RH, Bienenstock J, et al: The human secretory immunoglobulin system: Immunohistological localization of γ A, secretory "piece" and lactoferrin in normal human tissues. J Exp Med 129:411-429, 1969

20. Schmedtje JF, Batts AF: Immunoglobulins and blood vessels in the tonsillar cryps epithelium. Ann Otol Rhinol Laryngol 82:359-369, 1973

21. Mogi G, Yoshida T, Honjo S, et al: Middle ear effusions. Quantitative analysis of immunoglobulins. Ann Otol Rhinol Laryngol 82:196-202, 1973

22. Mogi G, Honjo S, Maeda S, et al: Secretory immunoglobulin A (SIgA) in middle ear effusions. Observation of 160 specimens. Ann Otol Rhinol Laryngol 82:302-310, 1973

23. Mogi G, Honjo S, Maeda S, et al: Secretory immunoglobulin A (SIgA) in middle ear effusions. A further report. Ann Otol Rhinol Laryngol 83:92-101, 1974

24. Mogi G, Honjo S, Maeda S, et al: Quantitative determination of secretory immunoglobulin A (SIgA) in middle ear effusions. Ann Otol Rhinol Laryngol 83:239-246, 1974

25. Mogi G: Immunochemical studies of nasal secretions. To be published

26. Mogi G: Biochemical properties of laryngeal secretions. Unpublished data

27. Kobayashi K: Secretory IgA. The Physico-Chemical Biology (Japan) 18:107-110, 1974

28. Sober HA, Peterson EA: Protein chromatography on ion exchange cellulose. Fed Proc 17:1116-1126, 1958

29. Mogi G, Honjo S: Middle ear effusion. Analysis of protein components. Ann Otol Rhinol Laryngol 81:99-105, 1972

30. Ouchterlony O: In: *Handbook of Immunodiffusion and Immunoelectrophoresis.* Ann Arbor, Michigan, Ann Arbor Science Publication, Inc, 1968

31. Joustra M, Lundgren H: Preparation of freeze-dried monomeric and immunochemically pure IgG by a rapid and reproducible chromatographic technique, in Peeters H (ed): *Protides of the Biological Fluids.* (Proc. 17th Colloquium, Bruges, 1969) Oxford and New York, Pergamon Press, 1970, pp 511-515

32. Hamashima Y, Kyogoku M: *Immunohistology. Immunofluorescent Technique, Immuno-electron Microscopic Technique, Radioisotope Labeled Antibody Technique,* ed 2. Tokyo, Japan, Igaku Shoin Ltd, 1968

33. Davis BJ: Disc electrophoresis: Method and application to human serum proteins. Ann NY Acad Sci 121:404-427, 1964

34. Halpern MS, Koshland ME: Novel subunit in secretory IgA. Nature 228:1276-1278, 1970

35. Mestecky J, Zikan J, Butler WT, et al: Studies on human secretory immunoglobulin A. III. J chain. Immunochemistry 9:883-890, 1972

36. Bull DM, Bienenstock J, Tomasi TB Jr: Studies on human intestinal immunoglobulin A. Gastroenterology 60:370-380, 1971

37. Mach JP: In vitro combination of human and bovine free secretory component with IgA of various species. Nature (New Biol) 228: 1278-1282, 1970

38. Brandtzaeg P: Human secretory immunoglobulins. IV. Association of free secretory piece with serum IgA in vitro. Immunology 29:323-332, 1971

39. O'Daly JA, Cebra JJ: Rabbit secretory IgA. I. Isolation of secretory component after selective dissociation of the immunoglobulin. J Immunol 107:436-448, 1971

40. Parkhouse RME: Biosynthesis of J-chain in mouse IgA and IgM. Nature (New Biol) 236:9-11, 1972

41. Ogra PL: Effect of tonsillectomy and adenoidectomy on nasopharyngeal antibody response to poliovirus. N Engl J Med 284:59-64, 1971

42. Tada T, Ishizaka K: Distribution of γE-forming cells in lymphoid tissues of human and monkey. J Immunol 104:377-387, 1970

43. Ishikawa T, Wicher K, Arbesman CE: Distribution of immunoglobulins in palatine and pharyngeal tonsils. Int Arch Allergy Appl Immunol 43:801-812, 1972

44. Lennert K, Caesar R, Müller HK: Electron microscopic studies of germinal centers in man, in Cottier H, Odartchenko N, Schindler R, et al (eds): *Germinal Centers in Immune Responses.* Berlin, Heidelberg, New York, Springer-Verlag, 1967, pp 49-59

45. Tazima K: Age changes in the human palatine tonsils, with remarks on the histology of the secondary nodules. Arch Histol Jap 28: 63-78, 1967

46. Surján L Jr, Surfán M: Immunological role of human tonsils. Acta Otolaryngol 71: 190-193, 1971

47. Waldman RH, Mach JP, Stella MM, et al: Secretory IgA in human serum. J Immunol 105:43-47, 1970

48. Brandtzaeg P: Human secretory immunoglobulins. V. Occurrence of secretory piece in human serum. J Immunol 106:318-323, 1971

49. Waldman RH, Rowe DS, Mach JP: Secretory IgA levels in serum of patients with various disease. Clin Med 80:11-13, 1973

TEMPORAL BONE HISTOPATHOLOGICAL FINDINGS IN TRISOMY 13 SYNDROME

ISAMU SANDO, M.D.

ALBERTO LEIBERMAN, M.D. LAVONNE BERGSTROM, M.D.

DENVER, COLORADO

SOJI IZUMI, M.D.
YOKOHAMA, JAPAN

RAYMOND P. WOOD II, M.D.
DENVER, COLORADO

From the Department of Otolaryngology, University of Colorado School of Medicine, 4200 East Ninth Avenue, Denver, Colorado.

This study was supported by the NIH Research Grant 2 R01 NS09293-041A CMS, Training Grant NIH 5T01 NS05504-09 and Dr. Wood's Contract HSM 77-72-171.

Presented at the meeting of the American Otological Society, Atlanta, Georgia, April 11-12, 1975.

TEMPORAL BONE HISTOPATHOLOGICAL FINDINGS IN TRISOMY 13 SYNDROME

ISAMU SANDO, M.D.

ALBERTO LEIBERMAN, M.D. LAVONNE BERGSTROM, M.D.

DENVER, COLORADO

SOJI IZUMI, M.D. RAYMOND P. WOOD II, M.D.

YOKOHAMA, JAPAN DENVER, COLORADO

SUMMARY — This study reports the histopathological findings of 14 temporal bones from infants with trisomy 13 syndrome. The most primitive anomalies in the structures of the inner and middle ears in the present series are those of the semicircular canals, particularly of the horizontal canals: flattened horizontal canal cristae, absence or opening of the utricular endolymphatic valve, small facial nerve, and obtuse angle of the geniculate area of the facial nerve. Each ear demonstrated more than one of those anomalies. The anomalies present features similar to those found in the structures of the normal six to ten-week fetus. Many other mild anomalies observed appear to demonstrate features similar to those seen in the same structures in later fetal life. Reviewing these findings, most of the anomalies that were found in the inner and middle ears appear to be the result of poor development of the structures for reasons which are now unclear. In addition, middle ear infection was found in all cases.

The association of multiple congenital anomalies with trisomy 13 was first described by Patau *et al*[1] in 1960. This syndrome was characterized by the presence of an extra chromosome (trisomy) in the D group of autosomes. Originally it was not certain which D chromosome was responsible for this syndrome and it was referred to as trisomy 13-15. Present methods of identification, utilizing autoradiography and banding, have shown the chromosome responsible for this group of anomalies to be chromosome 13.[2] The morphological abnormality noted in the karyotype may be due to a genuine trisomy or to a translocation defect. The most common clinical and pathological findings[3] are: apneic spells, mental retardation, muscular hypertonia or hypotonia, microcephalia, eye defects (microphthalmia, iris colobomas, cataracts), small, low-set, and malformed ears, cleft palate and lip, polydactylia, heart defects (septal defects or patent ductus arteriosus), polycystic kidney, inguinal and umbilical hernia, undescended testes, biseptate uterus and capillary hemangioma of the skin. The first histopathological study of the temporal bone in trisomy D syndrome was reported by Mottet and Jensen,[4] who found no abnormalities. Since then, eight additional temporal bone cases have been reported.[5-11] The purpose of this study is to present a series of 14 temporal bones (seven cases) obtained from trisomy D patients, including three cases reported earlier,[8-10] with the object of demonstrating the common findings in this disorder and discussing the embryological impairment. These patients all fit the clinical and pathological criteria for the trisomy 13 syndrome.

CASE REPORTS

CASE 1

A full-term Caucasian male, weighing 2850 g, was born to a 27-year-old, gravida four, para four mother. The pregnancy had been uncomplicated by drugs or recognized illness. The infant had multiple anomalies consisting of microcephalia, bilateral cleft palate and lip, polydactylia in both hands and left foot, and capillary hemangioma of the neck. After birth the infant developed cyanosis, jaundice, bradycardia, and apneic spells. Chromosomal studies confirmed the clinically suspected D trisomy. Audiometric studies could not be performed satisfactorily upon the terminally ill infant. He died 24 days after birth. At autopsy, a number of additional pathological findings were discovered: arrhinencephalia, microphthalmia, heart defects (patent foramen ovale with maldevelopment of septum secundum), hydronephrosis of the right kidney, and bronchopneumonia. Temporal bones were obtained 24 hours after death from the refrigerated cadaver. They were placed in 10% formalin, decalcified, imbedded in celloidin, and sectioned horizontally at 20 μ intervals. Every tenth section was stained with H. and E. and carefully studied. A graphic cochlear reconstruction of each ear was made for measurement of the cochlear length.[12,13]

HISTOPATHOLOGICAL FINDINGS

LEFT TEMPORAL BONE

External and Middle Ear. The external auditory canal and the tympanic membrane were normal. The tympanic cavity was partly filled with mesenchymal tissue. The antrum and mastoid air cells were absent; instead, the mastoid bone was filled with the bone marrow. Pus was present in the tympanic cavity and the mucosa was infiltrated with inflammatory cells.

Inner Ear – Cochlea. The cochlea had 2½ turns and was 24 mm long. The organ of Corti appeared to be well-developed. The hair cells were present; however, their histological analysis was difficult due to some postmortem changes. The tectorial membrane was normal. There were mild endolymphatic hydrops in all turns, malformed scala vestibuli with moderately small space in the basal turn, and absence of the bony interscalar septum between the middle and apical turns.

Inner Ear – Vestibule. The bony, horizontal semicircular canal demonstrated a large canal. The posterior semicircular canal was a mere outpouching of the vestibule. The sensory and supporting epithelial lining of the vestibular maculae and cristae was well developed.

RIGHT TEMPORAL BONE

Pathological findings were similar to those described for the left ear with the following exceptions: the mastoid antrum was extremely small; the cochlea was 24.5 mm long and consisted of 2½ turns, with no other particular pathological findings in the cochlea. The bony interscalar septum was present.

CASE 2

A full-term Caucasian female, weighing 1760 g, was born to a 34-year-old, gravida two, para two mother. The mother had been taking contraceptive pills for two to three years until six to eight months prior to pregnancy. During the neonatal physical examination several anomalies were noted: confluent anterior and posterior fontanelles, low-set ears, cleft soft palate, polydactylia of both hands, bilateral club feet, a single umbilical artery, and vascular nevi. After birth, the infant developed respiratory distress with apneic spells and seizures. The clinical appearance suggested trisomy D, which was confirmed by chromosomal studies. Audiometric studies could not be performed satisfactorily. The infant died 16 days after birth. A number of additional pathological findings were discovered during the autopsy, which included: congenital heart diseases (atrial septal defects and ventricular septal defect), ileal diverticulum, uterus septus duplex with double vagina, bilateral hydronephrosis, and bronchopneumonia. Both

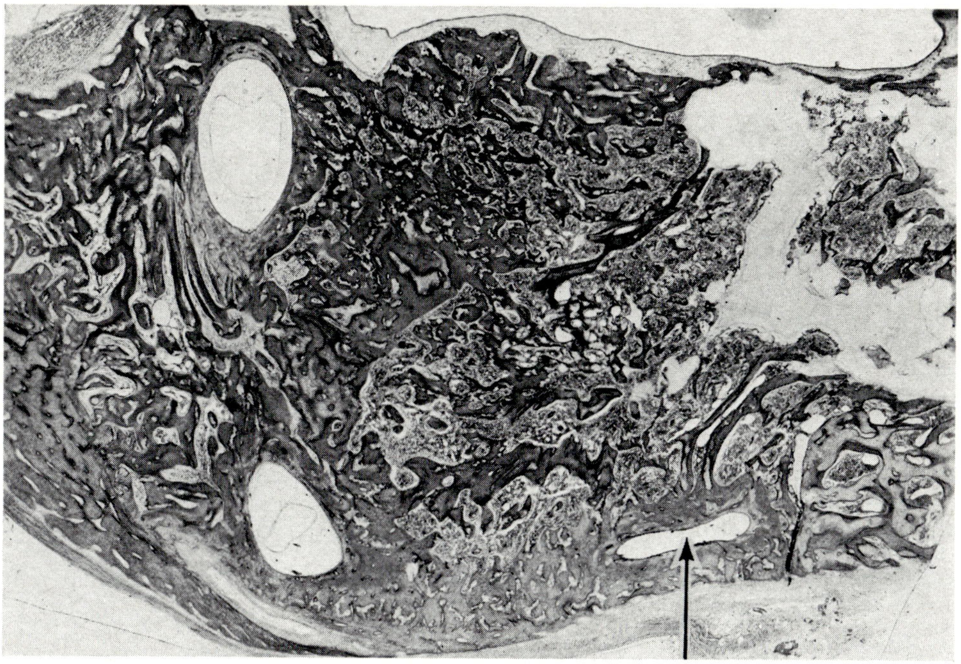

Fig. 1. Case 2) Right Ear. The posterior bony semicircular canal (arrow) has an extremely narrow lumen. X13

temporal bones were obtained 12 hours after death.

HISTOPATHOLOGICAL FINDINGS

LEFT TEMPORAL BONE

External and Middle Ear. The external auditory canal was normal. The epitympanum contained mesenchymal tissue. The mucosa of the middle ear was thick and pseudopolypoid, with lymphocytic and plasma cell infiltrates. The stapes had a bulky fetal form. The incudostapedial joint contained a space surrounded by cartilaginous tissue, except laterally where there was fibrous mesenchymal tissue. The malleus and incus had persistent, large marrow cavities. At the second genu of the facial nerve, the facial canal was widely dehiscent. The mastoid antrum could not be fully evaluated because of technical artifact.

Inner Ear – Cochlea. The cochlea was only 23.5 mm long and consisted of 2¼ turns. However, the organ of Corti appeared to be well developed. The hair cells were present but affected by some postmortem autolysis. Reissner's membrane and the tectorial membrane were within normal limits. The stria vascularis contained cystic structures in the lower half of the basal turn. Some cochlear vessels appeared to run obliquely in the scala tympani. The cochlear aqueduct was wide, measuring 350 μ in its narrowest portion. The inferior cochlear vein was present in a separate bony channel.

Inner Ear – Vestibule. The saccular membrane was partially collapsed and adherent to the macula, where there were disintegrated hair cells and conglomerated otoconia. All bony semicircular canals were malformed and both superior and posterior canals demonstrated extremely narrow lumina (Fig. 1). The horizontal canal consisted only of an outpouching of the vestibule. The horizontal canal had a nearly flat crista. The sensory and supporting epithelial lining of the utricular macula and the canal cristae appeared to be well developed and visualized.

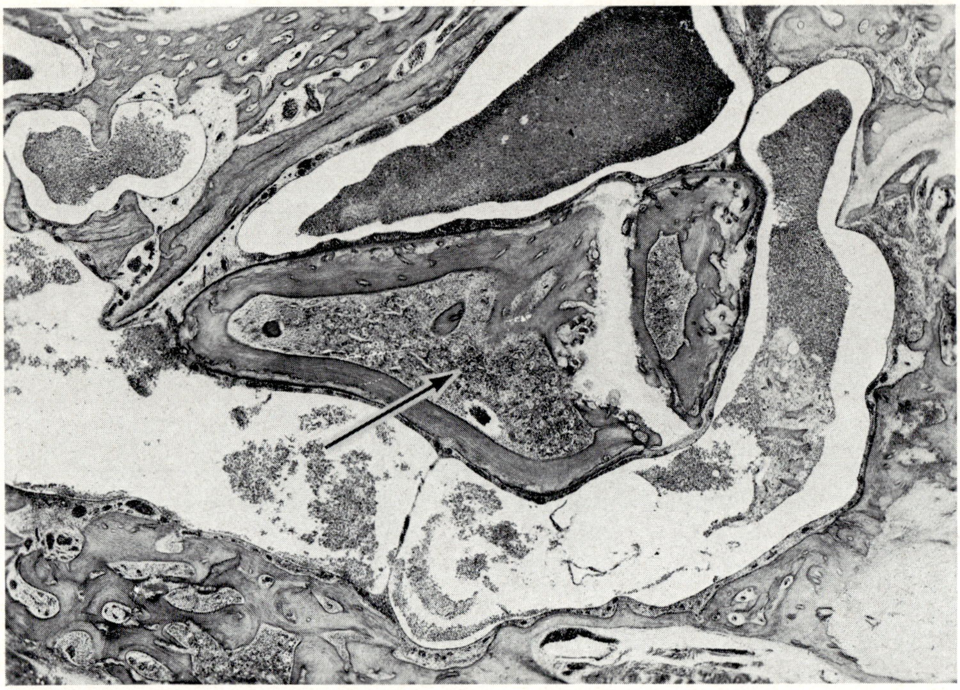

Fig. 2. Case 3) Left Ear. The incus contains a large bone marrow cavity (arrow). Note the infiltration of the inflammatory cells in the middle ear cavity. X25

Other. The internal auditory canal was shallow, measuring only 5 mm in depth.

RIGHT TEMPORAL BONE

Pathological findings were similar to those in the left ear, with the following exceptions: the mastoid antrum was extremely small; the cochlea was 24.8 mm in length, with 2¼ turns and with the hook portion absent. The epitympanum, the facial canal, the cochlear vessels and the cochlear aqueduct were normal.

CASE 3

Full-term Caucasian female, weighing 1980 g, was born to an 18-year-old, gravida two, para two mother. The pregnancy was uncomplicated. After birth, multiple anomalies were noted: microcephalia, corneal opacity, coloboma of the ciliary body, aplasia of facial bones and face, aplasia of the hard and soft palate, absence of external nares, hypoplasia of the upper lip, "rocker bottom" feet, and contraction of the thumbs bilaterally. The karyotype study was unsuccessful. The infant died four days after birth. A number of pathological findings were discovered during the autopsy: arrhinencephalia, absence of the sylvian and temporal fissures, retinal dysplasia, congenital heart disease (cor triloculare, biventriculare, ventricular septal defect, patent ductus arteriosus), omphalocele, bicornuate uterus, and pneumonia. The clinical appearance and the anatomical pattern of the various abnormalities observed during the autopsy strongly suggest a trisomy 13 abnormality, although, in this case, the diagnosis was not proved by a karyotype. The temporal bones were obtained from the refrigerated cadaver four hours after death.

HISTOPATHOLOGICAL FINDINGS

LEFT TEMPORAL BONE

External and Middle Ear. The external auditory canal was stenotic. The tympanic membrane was small. The middle ear mucosa was polypoid and

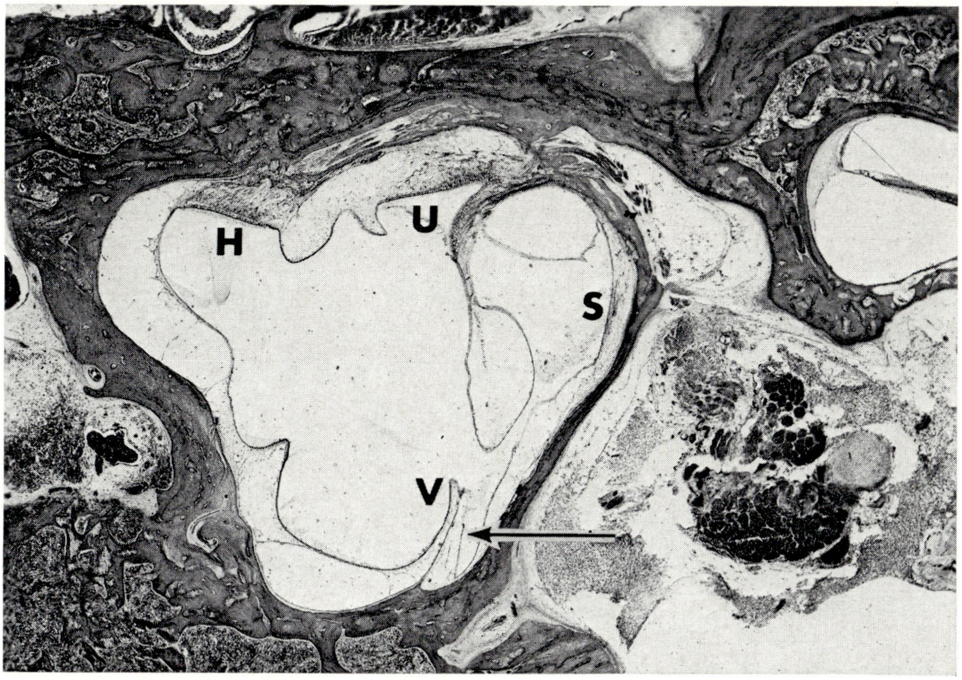

Fig. 3. Case 3) Left Ear. Broad outpouching containing a flat crista (H), probably representing a vestigial horizontal semicircular canal. The sensory and supporting epithelial lining were well-developed and preserved. Peculiar shape of the utricular macula (U) with acute angle. The sensory and supporting epithelial lining were well-developed and preserved. Shortened endolymphatic valve (V) resulting in free communication between utricle, saccular duct, and endolymphatic duct. Arrow - Endolymphatic duct. S - Saccule. X16

was infiltrated by inflammatory cells. The crura, particularly the anterior crus, as well as the footplate of the stapes, were thick. The malleus and incus contained large marrow cavities (Fig. 2). The manubrium of the malleus was thick. The first external genu of the facial nerve formed an obtuse angle of approximately 110°. In the mastoid the antrum was small and surrounded by bone marrow. There were no mastoid cells.

Inner Ear — Cochlea. The cochlea was 25.9 mm in length, with 2½ turns. The organ of Corti appeared to be well-developed. The hair cells were present with slight postmortem change. The stria vascularis contained some cystic structures in a portion of the basal turn. Reissner's membrane and the tectorial membrane were normal. The cochlear aqueduct was wide for most of its length; however, it showed no communication with the cochlea. A microvascular channel lay between the end of the cochlear aqueduct and the scala tympani. However, a well-developed, inferior cochlear vein was clearly observed, running in a separate bony channel.

Inner Ear — Vestibule. The vestibular maculae and cristae appeared to be fully developed. The hair cells in the end-organ were present. However, the following findings were observed: the utricular macula showed a peculiar shape, forming almost a right angle. The bony as well as the membranous labyrinth of the superior canal were partially absent at the lateral-superior limb. The bony, horizontal semicircular canal was extremely small, with large communication with the vestibule. The horizontal canal crista was flattened.

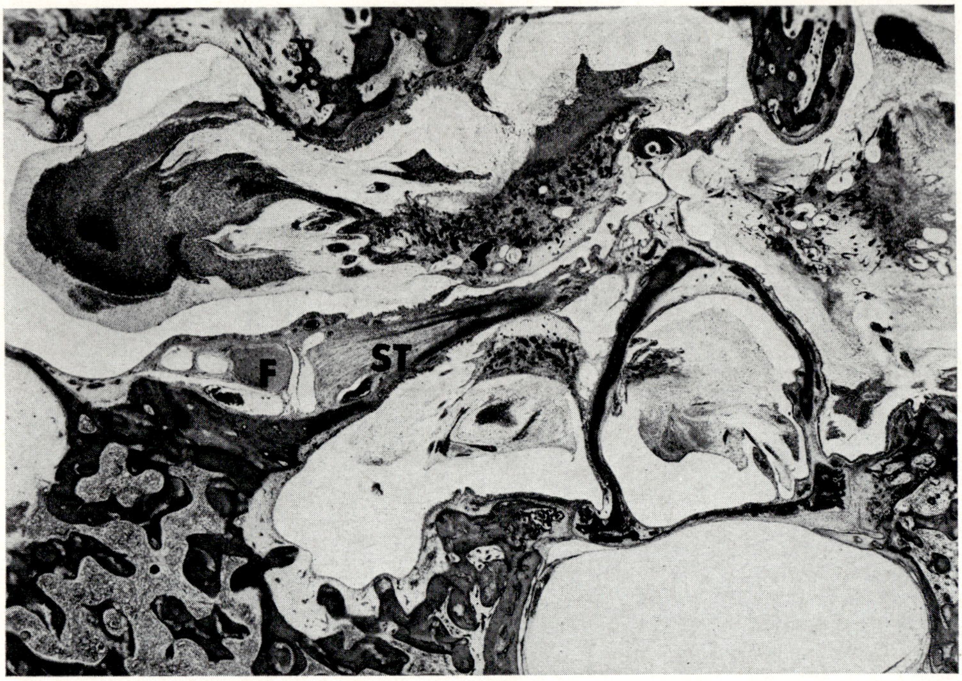

Fig. 4. Case 4) Left Ear. Absence of the pyramidal eminence and the facial canal result in wide exposure of the tendon of the stapedial muscle (ST) and the facial nerve (F) to the middle ear space. X19

The utriculoendolymphatic valve was shortened, allowing a free communication between the utricular endolymphatic space and the endolymphatic duct (Fig. 3). The endolymphatic duct was short and almost straight, and the sac ended blindly in the otic capsule without reaching the subarachnoid space.

Other. The internal auditory meatus was wide and shallow. A huge vessel was present in the subarcuate fossa.

RIGHT TEMPORAL BONE

Pathological findings were similar to those in the left ear, with the following exceptions: the external auditory canal and the tympanic membrane were normal. The incus and the malleus could not be evaluated due to artifact. The facial nerve was small in its tympanic portion. The course of the facial nerve was normal. The mastoid antrum was absent. The cochlea was 27.5 mm long and consisted of 2½ turns. The cochlear modiolus was malformed. The saccular membrane was partially collapsed and adherent to conglomerated otoconia and disintegrated sensoriepithelial lining. The membranous superior canal was partially absent. The utricular macula and the horizontal crista were normal.

CASE 4

A 38-week-gestation, Caucasian female, weighing 2280 g, was born to a 21-year-old, gravida four, para zero mother with a history of previous first-trimester, spontaneous abortions. This gestation was complicated by three episodes of upper respiratory infections. This infant was transferred from another hospital because of increasing jaundice, lethargy, and apneic spells. Multiple anomalies noted during the physical examination were: prominent, atrophic middle scalp defect, bilateral microphthalmus, low-set, abnormally shaped pinnae, cleft lip and palate, polydactylia in both hands, and transverse midpalmar crease. Chromosomal studies confirmed the clinical impres-

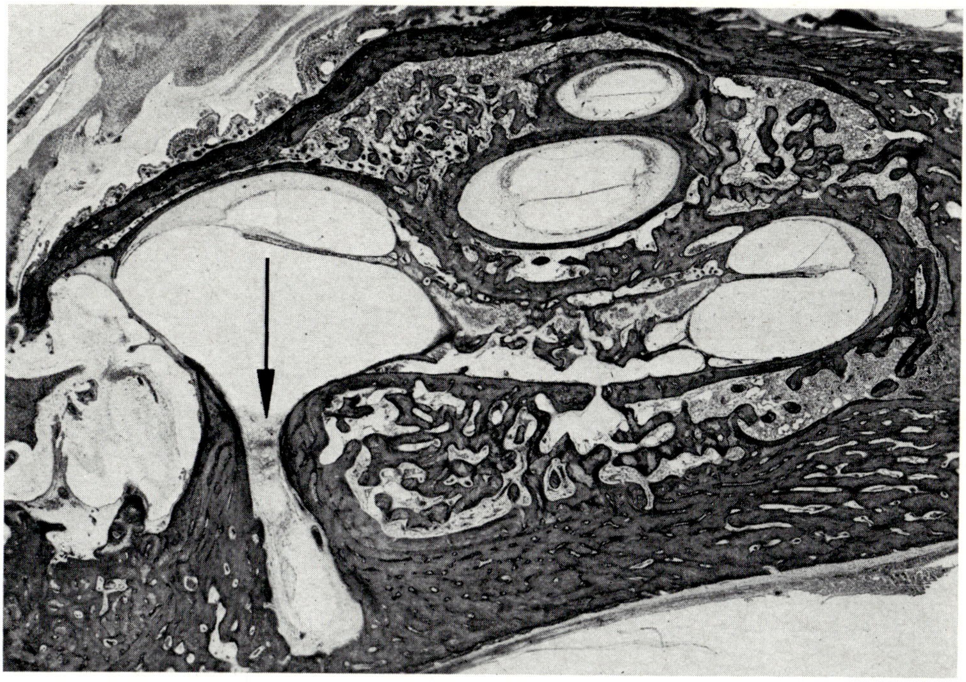

Fig. 5. Case 4) Left Ear. Widely opened cochlear aqueduct, 500 μ in diameter at the narrowest portion (arrow). X14

sion of trisomy D. The infant died 21 days after birth. At autopsy, polycystic kidneys (adult type) and pneumonia were discovered. The temporal bones were obtained 18 hours after death.

HISTOPATHOLOGICAL FINDINGS

LEFT TEMPORAL BONE

External and Middle Ear. The external auditory canal appeared normal. The tympanic membrane (pars tensa) was moderately thick (0.3 mm). The mucosa was polypoid, infiltrated with inflammatory cells (leukocytes, plasma cells, and lymphocytes). Pus occupied the air space. The incus and malleus had huge, bone marrow cavities. There was no bony pyramidal eminence to cover the stapedius tendon. The facial nerve was widely exposed in its tympanic and mastoid portions (Fig. 4). The geniculate turn of the facial nerve formed an obtuse angle of approximately 120°. The mastoid was extremely small, was occupied by bone marrow, and contained no air cells.

Inner Ear – Cochlea. The cochlea, which measured 29.8 mm, consisted of 2½ turns. The organ of Corti, the limbus, the tectorial membrane, and the stria vascularis were well-developed and preserved. The hair cell population was normal, but the cells were moderately disintegrated by postmortem autolysis. Reissner's membrane extended slightly into the scala vestibuli of the apical turn. The cochlear aqueduct was widely open to the posterior cranial fossa, measuring in its narrowest portion 500 μ (Fig. 5).

Inner Ear – Vestibule. The vestibular maculae and cristae appeared to be well-developed. The hair cells of the end-organs were present with some postmortem autolysis. The horizontal semicircular canal was present as an outpouching of the vestibule and had a flattened crista. The superior division of the vestibular nerve in the cribriform area of the otic capsule lacked a bony covering laterally.

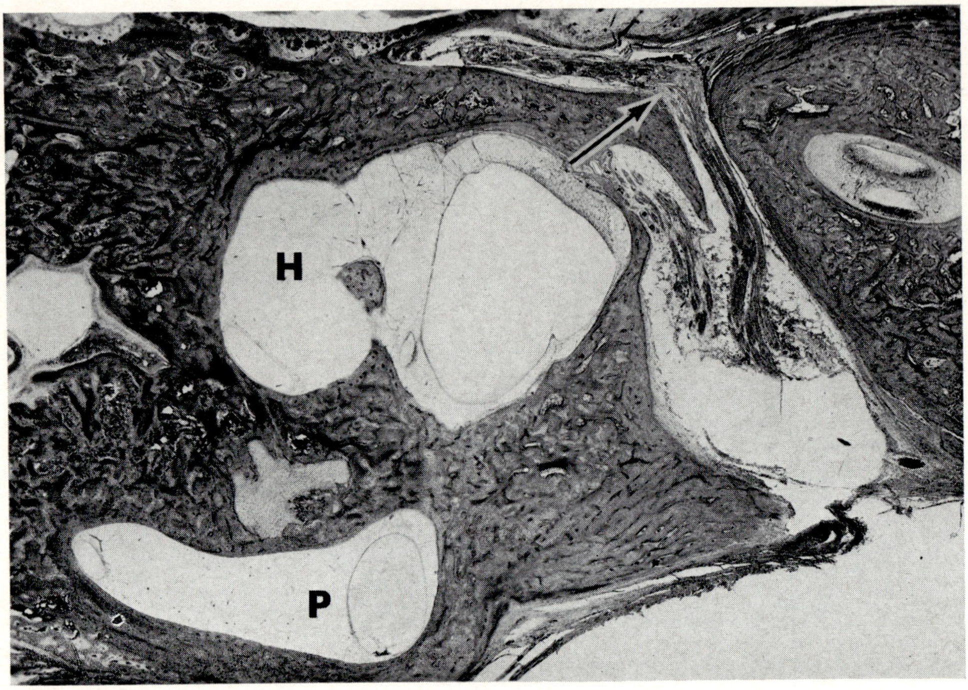

Fig. 6. Case 5) Left Ear. The facial nerve demonstrating obtuse angle at its geniculate ganglion area (arrow). Note poorly-developed horizontal canal (H) and compare with normally-developed posterior semicircular canal (P). X11.5

Other. The internal auditory canal was extremely shallow.

RIGHT TEMPORAL BONE

Pathological findings were similar to those in the left ear except for the following: the antrum was absent. The course of the facial nerve was normal. The pyramidal eminence was normal. There was no endolymphatic hydrops in the cochlea. There were technical artifacts that made it impossible to render a graphic reconstruction of the cochlea and to visualize the structure of the end-organ. The cochlear aqueduct was wide (400 μ), and contained the cranial nerve, ganglion cells, possibly those of the IX nerve. The utricle had an anomalous shape with a septum in the macula. The horizontal semicircular canal was a pedunculated, cyst-like outgrowth of the vestibule. The posterior semicircular canal was extremely narrow. The otic capsule covering over the superior division of the vestibular nerve was intact.

CASE 5

A full-term, Caucasian female, weighing 2550 g, was born to a 22-year-old, gravida three, para two mother who had been treated with sulfisoxazole for a bladder infection during pregnancy. She had taken contraceptive pills for three years until just before the pregnancy. During physical examination multiple anomalies were noted, including: microcephalia, severe microphthalmia, dense bilateral cataracts, abnormally shaped pinnae, hypoplastic nasal septum, midline cleft lip and palate, polydactylia of both hands, "rocker bottom" feet, an enlarged kidney, a grade 3-4 pansystolic murmur, and a generalized increase in motor tone. The hospital course was complicated by aspiration and many apneic spells. Chromosomal studies revealed trisomy

D. Auditory testing* showed a definite response to 90 dB at 3 kHz and the hearing threshold was considered to be at least 40 dB or better. Normal range was estimated. The infant was discharged to a custodial care facility. During the infant's stay there, tube feeding was required. A fatal aspiration occurred and the infant died 41 days after birth. A number of additional pathological findings were discovered during the autopsy, including: aplasia of the olfactory bulbs, tracts, and fornices of the brain, aplasia of anterior horns of lateral ventricles and of the anterior portion of corpus callosum, cardiac anomalies (ventricular septal defect and patent foramen ovale), polycystic kidney, and pneumonitis. The temporal bones were obtained from the refrigerated cadaver 26 hours after death.

HISTOPATHOLOGICAL FINDINGS

LEFT TEMPORAL BONE

External and Middle Ear. The external auditory canal was normal. The tympanic cavity contained pus. The mucosa of the middle ear cavity was thick and infiltrated with inflammatory cells, particularly with polymorphonuclear leukocytes. The facial nerve appeared normal except that the first genu of the nerve formed an obtuse angle (115°) (Fig. 6). The facial canal in the vertical portion had a large pocket posteriorly which communicated with the facial recess. The stapes was bulky. The malleus handle lay in a niche of the otic capsule. The mastoid antrum was absent, and the mastoid was completely filled by bone marrow.

Inner Ear — Cochlea. The cochlea measured 28 mm in length and had 2⅜ turns. The organ of Corti appeared to be well-developed. The hair cells were present; however, because of postmortem autolysis, histological analysis of fine structures was difficult.

Inner Ear — Vestibule. The vestibular maculae and cristae appeared to be fully developed. The hair cells were present. The horizontal semicircular canal was extremely small (Fig. 6), with a flat crista.

RIGHT TEMPORAL BONE

Pathological findings were similar to those in the left ear with these following exceptions: the facial nerve was relatively small; the stapes was normal; the incus and the malleus had huge bone marrow cavities; the cochlear aqueduct was wide, measuring 400 μ in its narrowest portion; the ampulla of the horizontal semicircular canal was huge, with the rest of the semicircular canal being part of the vestibule; the macula of the utricle had an unusual shape, forming a right angle.

CASE 6

A full-term, Caucasian male, weighing 2721 g, was born to a gravida two, para two mother who had previously undergone a thyroidectomy and taken thyroid medication for hypothyroidism throughout her pregnancy. At 6½ weeks of age the infant was admitted to Colorado General Hospital because of dyspnea, cyanosis, and rhinorrhea. At physical examination multiple anomalies were noted, including posterior, sloping forehead, bilateral microphthalmus, colobomas of the irides, low-set, abnormally shaped pinnae, bilateral cleft lip, complete cleft of the hard and soft palate, flexion deformities of fingers, and polydactylia on each hand. Chromosomal studies confirmed the clinical impression of trisomy D. Audiometric testing detected no responses to loud noise until the 100 dB level was reached. The infant died one day after admission to the hospital. A number of pathological findings were discovered during the autopsy. They were: arrhinencephalia, multiple cardiac anomalies (atrial septal defect, interventricular septal defect, patent foramen ovale, and patent ductus arteriosus), umbilical hernia, postanal cleft, didelphic uterus, and acute bronchopneumonia. The temporal bones were obtained from the refrigerated cadaver 12 hours after death.

* The auditory test was performed by Marion Downs, M.A., audiologist, University of Colorado Medical Center, using her newborn-hearing testing method.

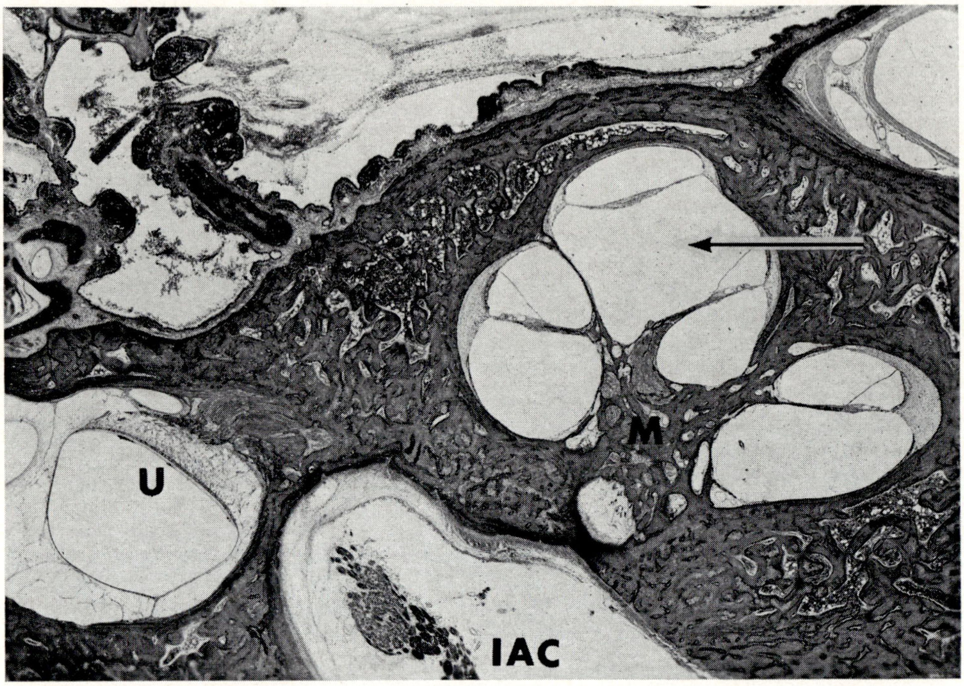

Fig. 7. Case 6) Right Ear. The cochlea with its shortened length, absence of the bony interscalar septum (arrow), and malformed modiolus (M). Note well-developed organ of Corti. U - Normal utricular macula. IAC - Internal auditory canal. X14. (Reproduced from Sando I, Baker D, Black FO, *et al*: Persistence of stapedial artery in trisomy 13-15 syndrome. Arch Otolaryngol 96:441-447, 1972, with permission.)

HISTOPATHOLOGICAL FINDINGS

LEFT TEMPORAL BONE

External and Middle Ear. The medial portion of the external auditory canal space was tortuous, extremely narrowed, and partially filled with desquamated material. The tympanic cavity contained pus, and its mucosa was thickened by inflammatory cells and granulation tissue. Mesenchymal tissue was present in the epitympanum. Both anterior and posterior crura of the stapes were attached to the foot-plate more centrally than usual. There was approximately 1 mm of thick connective tissue between the tympanic membrane and the manubrium of the malleus down to the level of the umbo. The stapedius tendon was absent. The stapedius muscle was observed only in the lower, vertical portion of the facial canal. The persistence of the stapedial artery was observed in the obturator foramen. The geniculate turn of the facial nerve formed an obtuse angle of approximately 120°. At the area of the second genu of the facial nerve, the facial canal was quite large and dehiscent, with much of the nerve presenting in the middle ear space. The other middle ear structure appeared to be normal.

Inner Ear — Cochlea. The cochlea measured 23.1 mm in length, with 2½ turns (Fig. 7). The organ of Corti, the limbus, and the tectorial membrane appeared to well-developed and preserved. The hair cells were present in normal numbers although they showed slight postmortem autolysis, pyknotic changes, and abnormal position of the nuclei. The stria vascularis appeared to be cystic in part of the basal turn. A malformed modiolus demonstrated absence of the bony interscalar septum between the second and third turns of the cochlea. In the lower half of the basal turn of the cochlea, most of the osseous spiral lamina did not contain a lumen for the cochlear nerve fibers. Rosenthal's canal was almost absent in this particular area (Fig. 7). The cochlear aqueduct was wide, measuring 400 μ in its narrowest portion.

Inner Ear – Vestibule. The ductus reuniens was obstructed. The nerve to the posterior semicircular canal crista left the posterior cranial fossa directly via its own bony canal rather than via the internal auditory meatus and singular canal.

Other. At the fundus of the internal auditory canal, spiral ganglion cells were present. Abnormal neural tissue, closely resembling central nervous system (CNS) tissue, was observed in the internal auditory canal. This tissue appeared to be associated with the vestibular nerve whose ganglion cells were both in the central neural tissue and the peripheral nerve tissue.

RIGHT TEMPORAL BONE

Pathological findings were similar to those described for the left temporal bone with the following exceptions: the anterior crus of the stapes was hollow but thickened; the posterior crus attached in part to the center and in part to the posterior inferior margin of the foot-plate; the stapedial tendon, muscle, and pyramidal eminence were normal. There was no abnormal neural tissue in the internal auditory canal.

CASE 7

A full-term, Caucasian male, weighing 3300 g, was born to a 28-year-old gravida one, para one mother. The pregnancy had been uncomplicated. Delivery was complicated by a long period of neonatal apnea. The infant did poorly with frequent apneic episodes. At the age of one week, the patient was transferred to Colorado General Hospital because of cardiovascular distress. During the physical examination several pathological findings were noted. Those were: frontal hemangioma, arrhinencephalic profile, bilateral cleft palate, low-set pinnae, loud systolic cardiac murmur, bilaterally undescended testes, polydactylia in both hands, and bilateral simian palmar creases. Behavioral responses to noise makers were absent. Other audiometric studies could not be performed satisfactorily on the terminally ill infant. Karyotype determination confirmed the clinically suspected trisomy D. The infant died one day following admission. A number of additional pathological findings were discovered during the autopsy. They were: absence of olfactory tract and bulb, cardiac anomalies (patent foramen ovale and patent ductus arteriosus), polycystic kidney (adult type), accessory spleen, patent urachus, and pneumonia. Both temporal bones were obtained one hour after death from the refrigerated cadaver.

HISTOPATHOLOGICAL FINDINGS

LEFT TEMPORAL BONE

External and Middle Ear. The bony external auditory canal was normal. Granulation tissue and thick, polypoid mucosa, infiltrated with inflammatory cells (polymorphonuclear leukocytes, plasma cells, and lymphocytes), protruded into the middle ear cavity. Through a dehiscence in the periosteal layer, the middle ear space communicated with the enchondral layer of the otic capsule. The posterior stapedial crus was attached near the center of the foot-plate. The anterior part of the foot-plate was thickened. The incudostapedial joint was located in an abnormally medial position. The geniculate turn of the facial nerve formed an obtuse angle of approximately 120°.

Inner Ear – Cochlea. The cochlea measured 24.1 mm in length with 2⅛ turns. The organ of Corti was well-developed. Hair cells were present although some postmortem autolysis was observed. Blood vessels crossed the perilymphatic spaces in all turns. A secondary osseous spiral lamina was present throughout the basal turn and a portion of the middle turn. A maldeveloped Rosenthal's canal consisted of approximately 1½ turns. The cochlear aqueduct was widened, being 400 μ

in diameter in its narrowest portion.

Inner Ear – Vestibule. The vestibular maculae and cristae appeared to be fully developed. The endolymphatic valve was shortened, allowing a direct communication between the utricle and saccule.

RIGHT TEMPORAL BONE

Pathological findings were similar to those described above for the left ear with the following exceptions: the anterior crus of the stapes formed a widened attachment to an otherwise normal foot-plate; the cochlear aqueduct was 500 μ in its narrowest portion close to the scala tympani; the utriculoendolymphatic valve was normal. The singular nerve was divided into two portions: one branch entered the otic capsule from the posterior fossa via a separate canal; the anterior branch followed the normal course of the nerve.

DISCUSSION

A review of the histopathological findings in the temporal bones of patients with trisomy 13 reveals some of the following findings: the first histopathological study of the temporal bone from a trisomy 13 syndrome case was reported in 1965 by Mottet and Jensen,[4] who found no abnormalities. In the following year, Kos *et al*[5] reported two cases which demonstrated inner ear morphology consistent with cochleosaccular degeneration. In 1968, Kelemen *et al*[6] reported no temporal bone abnormalities in their case. In 1970, Maniglia *et al*[7] reported histopathological changes of the Mondini or Mondini-Alexander type. In their case, the organ of Corti was "disintegrated throughout the cochlea." In 1971, Black *et al*[8] first reported involvement of organs related to second branchial arch anomalies. They also found anomalies in the cochlea and the vestibule. In 1972, Sando *et al*[9] first described the persistence of the stapedial artery in a case which included anomalies in the cochlea and the internal auditory canal. Bergstrom *et al*[10] reported a case in 1972 which had a preponderance of vestibular anomalies. In 1974, one case with anomalies in the middle ear and the inferior part of the inner ear was added by Saito *et al.*[11]

A careful analysis of the temporal bones of our seven cases (14 ears) of trisomy 13 syndrome (including the three cases reported earlier)[8-10] reveals the following histopathological findings in the middle and inner ears. The vestibular anomalies include: 1) anomalies of the horizontal semicircular canal (ten ears); 2) presence of a flat, horizontal canal crista (seven ears); 3) anomaly of the posterior semicircular canal (four ears); 4) anomaly of the superior semicircular canal (three ears); 5) absence or shortening of utriculoendolymphatic valve (three ears); 6) peculiar shape of utricular macula (three ears); 7) saccular abnormalities (three ears); 8) partial absence of superior membranous canal (one ear); 9) dislocation of nervus singulare (two ears); and 10) short, straight course of the endolymphatic duct and sac ending blindly in the otic capsule (one ear). In all cases, the hair cell development and condition in the vestibular end-organs, except for saccular abnormalities in three ears mentioned above, appeared to be normal.

As described by Bast and Anson,[14] the embryology of the vestibular structures mentioned above is as follows: At 4½ weeks of fetal life, an infolding (Fold I) of the wall of the otic vesicle appears, the top portion of which is destined to be the utriculoendolymphatic valve which separates the endolymphatic duct from the rest of the otic vesicle, although there is still a wide opening between those two endolymphatic spaces. In the five-week fetus, the semicircular ducts appear as compressed outpouching from the dorsolateral portion of the otic vesicle. At six weeks gestation the primordium of the superior semicircular duct is formed, then the posterior, and the horizontal semicircular ducts follow in that order. At seven to eight weeks of fetal life, the maculae of the utriculus and sacculus begin to differentiate. At eight weeks of development, two other infoldings (Fold II & III) of the wall of the otic vesicle appear. In the same period, the crista ampularis of the canals develops as a ridge. At the nine-week stage, an infolding (Fold III) of the wall of the otic vesicle first separates the sacculus from the utriculus, leaving only a narrow channel, the utriculosaccular duct, between them. As this infolding (Fold III) becomes deeper, the utriculosaccular duct is bent at the midportion so that the utricular and saccular ducts are formed. At this fetal age of nine weeks another infolding (Fold I) first is seen as the utriculo-endolymphatic valve. At 10 to 12 weeks of gestation, the cells of the maculae and the otolithic membrane are being formed. At 10½ weeks, the ampulla of the canal has low mounded or flattened crista. In the fetus of 14 to 16 weeks, the maculae of the utriculus and the sacculus appear to be well-differentiated and are similar to those seen in the adult. In the 20-week fetus, the superior duct reaches its maximum growth as does the posterior duct (5.5 to 6.0 mm in diameter) at 21 weeks. The superior duct is slightly smaller than the posterior. The horizontal duct (4.5 mm) is full size in the fetus of 23 weeks. At 23 weeks of gestation, the adult structures and size of the cristae are present. The course of the endolymphatic duct and sac is straight in early fetal life (up to midterm) whereas, in the latter half of fetal life, the course begins to curve.

Anomalies of the vestibular system occurred in a majority of our cases in the form of poor development of the semicircular canals. Among those anomalies, the horizontal canal anomaly is the most common (ten ears). Most of the ears (seven) showed a compressed outpouching (Fig. 3) of the otic vesicle as seen at six weeks of fetal development; whereas other cases showed either a large bony canal in diameter (two ears) or a primitive small canal (one ear) (Fig. 6). It is interesting that the canals which develop earlier in embryonic life (superior and posterior canals) show fewer anomalies; whereas the canal which is formed later, the horizontal canal, demonstrates more anomalies. The flattened horizontal canal cristae probably indicate underdevelopment; findings similar to this may be seen in the crista of the fetus at 10½ weeks of age. Another interesting anomaly observed is the absence or shortening of the utriculoendolymphatic valve. This particular feature also probably indicates failure to develop in early fetal life; features similar to this may be seen in the fetus at eight weeks which indicate a direct communication between the utriculus and the sacculus, the "utriculosaccular duct." The straight course of the endolymphatic duct and sac probably represents another anomaly associated with poor development, resembling those structures as they are seen in the earlier half of the fetal life.

The cochlear findings in 14 ears consist mainly of a shortening of the length. The mean length was 25.78 mm with range of 23.1 mm to 29.8 mm in 2⅛ to 2½ turns as shown in the graphic cochlear reconstruction method[12,13] which is currently used in our laboratory. Associated anomalies in the cochlea were: 1) a wide cochlear aqueduct with its narrowest part measuring 350 μ to 600 μ in diameter (eight ears); 2) anomaly of the modiolus (three ears); 3) absence of bony interscalar septum in the upper cochlear turns (three ears); 4) vessels running through the perilymphatic spaces (three ears); 5) lack of communication of the cochlear aqueduct with the scala tympani (two ears); 6) cystic stria vascularis in part of the basal turns (six ears); 7) endolymphatic hydrops in the upper cochlear turns (two ears); and 8) maldeveloped scala vestibuli in the basal turn of the cochlea (one ear). However, in all cases, the organ of Corti appeared to be well-developed. Also, even though some postmortem autolysis was present, the hair cells appeared to be well-developed. The tectorial membrane, Reissner's membrane, cochlear nerve in the cochlea, and the internal auditory canal were normal.

According to Bast and Anson,[14] development of the organ of Corti, the cochlea itself, and the cochlear aqueduct in fetal life is as follows: in the fetus at six weeks, the cochlear duct is a curved tube which develops as an outgrowth from the anteromedial end of the saccular portion of the otic vesicle. At seven weeks of fetal life, one turn of the cochlear duct is completed. At eight weeks, the otic capsule is changing from precartilage into cartilage, and dedifferentiation of precartilage around the otic labyrinth is initiated. At nine weeks this newly-formed mesenchymal tissue is clearly distinguishable from the surrounding cartilaginous otic capsule. The mesenchyme is present in the area of the future cochlear aqueduct from the cochlear duct to the cranial cavity. The mesenchymal tissue in this area, containing the cochlear vein and the glossopharyngeal nerve, fills the future fenestra cochleae. At ten weeks, the periotic duct is visible. At the fetal age of 10 to 11 weeks, the full 2½ to 2¾ turns of the cochlea are completed. At 11 weeks, the organ of Corti starts to differentiate in the middle of the basal turn of the cochlear duct. At 13 weeks, the periotic duct is separated from the glossopharyngeal nerve by the cartilage. At 15 weeks of fetal age, this primitive cochlear aqueduct is separated from the fossula fenestrae by a cartilaginous bar. The periotic duct and the cochlear vein still lie in the same connective tissue. At the same fetal stage, the outer hair cells in the organ of Corti of the basal turn appear more definite and, therefore, more advanced in development than those in the middle and apical turns. In contrast, the pillar cells are not yet clearly differentiated. During the period of 15 weeks to 21 weeks of gestation, the organ of Corti progressively develops toward the apical end so that, by the end of the period, the tunnel of Corti is present in all turns. In the fetus at 16½ weeks, small vessels are present in the periotic duct but later disappear. A short distance medial to the scala tympani orifice, the cochlear aqueduct is narrowest. Its maximum width, 250 μ, is attained at 20 weeks of fetal life and becomes narrower after that time. At the same age (20 weeks), the connective tissue of the primitive cochlear aqueduct begins to be transformed into bone. At 21 weeks, this process is largely complete. As a result, the cochlear vein and the periotic duct lie within separate bone channels. At 21 to 25 weeks, the cochlea attains its maximum size and becomes completely encased in a bony capsule.

Igarashi and Yoshinobu[15] found the mean length of the cochlea of 17 human adults to be 32.3 mm with a range of 29.8 mm to 33.5 mm. Sando[16] found in six newborn infant temporal bones that the mean length was 31.73 mm, with a range of 30.0 to 33.3 mm, in 2⅝ to 2⅞ turns. It would appear, therefore, that the length and turns of the cochlea in the fetus at 25 weeks should approximate those seen in newborn and adult temporal bones.

It is of interest to note that the shortened cochleae, with their well-developed organs of Corti and the normal number of cochlear turns (2½ - 2¾) observed in all cases in the present study appear to be due to underdevelopment of unknown etiology, and they resemble features seen in the fetus at 21 to 25 weeks.

The widely-open cochlear aqueduct (over 350 μ at the narrowest portion of the duct) appears to be a common finding in these cases. Regarding the cochlear aqueduct in the newborn, Palva[17] reported that in six ears (three cases) between 36 hours and 15 days of age, the range of width in the ducts was 150 to 300 μ at their narrowest points, located 0.5 to 1.0 mm from the scala tympani. Reviewing these data in view of the embryology[14] and neonatology[17] described above, it appears that the cochlear aqueducts observed in our cases are larger than normal. These features probably are a consequence of the poor development of the cochlear aqueduct and result in a wider duct than that seen at its widest point in fetal life at the 20-week stage.

The anomalies in the vestibular and the cochlear systems may be summarized as follows: in all cases, a number of vestibular and cochlear anomalies were observed. Most of the anomalies appear to be the result of poor development in fetal life of the structures within the otic and periotic labyrinth, for reasons which are as yet unclear. It is interesting that the most severe and/or primitive anomalies appear to be in the vestibular system. They resemble features seen in the embryo at six to ten weeks. This finding agrees with the results of radiologic examinations reported by Valvassori *et al*:[18] 40% of their series (76 ears) of abnormal inner ears demonstrated anomalies limited to the vestibular system. Other less severe anomalies are present in both the vestibule and cochlea and have features similar to those in the structures in later fetal life.

Except for partial saccular dysplasia in three ears, the inner ears in our series demonstrated the presence of the hair cells in well-developed vestibular and cochlear end-organs despite some postmortem autolysis. However, there were macroscopic anomalies of the membranous labyrinth, such as absence of the horizontal canal duct, resulting in the presence of a huge lateral outpouching of the utricular space. This type of anomaly seems not to correspond entirely with anomalies previously described, such as: 1) complete failure of the development of the inner ear (Michel);[19] 2) incomplete failure of the development of bony and membranous labyrinth (Mondini*[20] and others);[21-23] 3) incomplete development of membranous labyrinth (Siebenmann and Bing);[24] 4) membranous cochleosaccular aplasia (Scheibe);[25] and 5) membranous cochlear aplasia (Alexander).[26]

There were some findings which are not considered to be due to incomplete development of the structures in the inner ear, such as endolymphatic hydrops in the cochlea. Further study of those pathological findings should be done.

The findings in the middle ear and its accessory structures are summarized. Ossicular abnormalities found in 12 ears were: 1) bulky or thick stapes, resembling the fetal form (five ears); 2) incus containing a huge bone marrow space (six ears); 3) malleus containing a huge bone marrow space (six ears); and 4) abnormal stapes (four ears). Abnormalities associated with the facial nerve were: 1) an obtuse geniculate turn of the facial nerve (eight ears); and 2) a small facial nerve (two ears). Other anomalies observed in the middle ear cavity were: 1) wide dehiscence of the facial canal (seven ears); 2) persistence of the stapedial artery (two ears); 3) the manubrium of the malleus indenting the otic capsule (two ears); and 4) absence of the pyramidal eminence (one ear). In addition, anomalies of the mastoid antrum seen in nine ears were: 1) absence of the antrum (five ears); and 2) small antrum (four ears). In one ear, absence of the antrum was associated with a huge facial canal which, in its mastoid portion, communicated laterally with the tympanic cavity via the facial recess. Infections of the middle ear were present in all cases.

A review of middle ear embryology[14,27-32] and its stages of development may shed some light on the anomalies seen in our cases. At six weeks of fetal life, as a part of facioacoustic primordium, the facial nerve arises in common with the acoustic nerve, but neither branch nor the geniculate ganglion can be identified.[30] At 6½ weeks to seven weeks of fetal age, the geniculate ganglion begins to develop; however, no particular "geniculate" angle for this area seems to be present. During this period, the facial nerve separates into two almost equal parts, with the caudal part becoming the main trunk of the facial nerve and the rostral nerve becoming the chorda tympani.[30] At about seven weeks, the stapedial artery which develops from the hyoid artery becomes interrupted at the stapes.[32] In the fetus at eight weeks, the geniculate ganglion is well defined. According to the graphic reconstruction of the facial nerve's

* The original spelling in 1791 was Mundini; now referred to as Mondini.

course in the human embryo described by Gasser,[30] this particular area first appears with an angle which is obtuse and forms approximately a straight line. At the 8½ weeks of development, the geniculate ganglion area shows a narrower angle than that in the fetus of eight weeks but is still much greater than a right angle. The chorda tympani nerve, at this time, is considerably smaller than the motor root of the facial nerve.[30] At nine weeks, the angle of the geniculate ganglion approximates a right angle.[30] Ossicular primordia arise mainly from mesodermal tissue of the first and second branchial arches, in which Meckel's and Reichert's cartilages will be formed. The ossicles attain the general configuration that characterizes their appearance in the adult.[29] During the period from 9 to 12 weeks of gestation, the stapedial artery normally disappears, although a portion of the artery appears to persist as part of the middle meningeal artery.[32] At 15 weeks, the stapedial muscle and tendon contact the neck portion of the stapes in its fetal form.[29] In the 16-week fetus, ossification of the ossicles begins in the incus and the malleus; whereas, this process will start in the stapes at about the 19-week stage.[29] The malleus and the incus retain their general form,[28] while the stapes will change its bulky embryological form to a much thinner ossicle. In the period between 20 and 24 weeks of fetal life, the malleus and the incus contain moderately large central bone marrow cavities surrounded by periosteal bone which is later replaced by endosteal bone. At this stage, the endosteal bone in the incus appears chiefly in the form of interconnected spicules, whereas its true location is internal to the periosteal layer in the malleus.[29] During the period between 24 and 28 weeks of fetal life, the bone of the inner wall of the stapedial crura is removed. The scattered "spicules" of endosteal bone and the bone marrow in the stapes are being resorbed.[29] At 26 weeks, the periosteal bone of the otic capsule begins to enclose the facial nerve to form the tympanic portion of the facial canal.[29] In the fetus at 22 weeks, the mastoid antrum begins to form.[14] In the 29 weeks fetus, the antrum is still part of the epitympanum without any pneumatization.[14] At 31 weeks, except for the persistence of bone marrow and the presence of a remnant of the obturator wall, the stapes is now an adult ossicle.[27] In the 34-week specimens, the antrum is much larger than that seen at 29 weeks, and about one-half of it is pneumatized.[14] In the 38-week fetus, the stapes, as well as the malleus and the incus, assume adult form.[14] Enlargement of the antrum and formation of the antral and mastoid air cells begin late in fetal life.[14] Near birth, the pyramidal eminence which arises from the laterohyale of the second branchial arch[31] is identifiable. At this point, the facial canal is fully formed,[29] from which the pyramidal eminence develops.[29] Enlargement of the antrum and the formation of the mastoid air cells progress during infancy and childhood.[14]

Among all of these anomalies in the middle ear, the most primitive anomalies observed in our cases were an obtuse angle of the geniculate ganglion and an anomalously small facial nerve, both of which seem to be features similar to those seen in embryos at 8½ to 9 weeks of fetal development. Histologically, these structures appear to be normal. Other anomalies seen in the middle ear have features similar to those seen in later fetal life. It may be that both groups of anomalies mentioned above are manifestations of poor development of those structures in the middle ear for reasons which are unclear.

It is interesting to note that only two previous histopathological reports of the temporal bones of infants with trisomy 13 syndrome describe middle ear anomalies. We feel that our cases confirm the presence of middle ear anomalies as a common finding in full-term infants suffering from trisomy 13 syndrome.

All our cases showed inflammation in the middle ear cavity, but the degree of inflammation varied. Some ears showed only signs of acute and chronic inflammation, manifested by polypoid mucosa, granulation tissue, and infiltration of chronic inflammatory cells. Similar findings were reported earlier by Maniglia *et al.*[7] Such infection may be secondary to upper respiratory infection in the presence of a cleft palate, which was seen in all cases.

Request for reprints should be sent to Isamu Sando, M.D., Dept. of Otolaryngology, Univ. of Colorado School of Medicine, 4200 East Ninth Ave., Denver, Colo. 80220.

At the present time, Dr. Izumi is Assistant, Department of Otolaryngology, Yokohama Municipal University School of Medicine, Yokohama, Japan.

ACKNOWLEDGMENT—We gratefully acknowledge the assistance of Dr. Steven G. Silverberg, Department of Pathology, University of Colorado Medical Center, for his help in the interpretation of some of the pathological findings and the advice of Dr. Vincent M. Riccardi, Department of Biophysics and Genetics, for genetic interpretation of trisomy 13 syndrome.

REFERENCES

1. Patau K, Smith DW, Therman E, *et al*: Multiple congenital anomaly caused by an extra autosome. Lancet 1:790-793, 1960

2. Miller DA, Allderdice PW, Miller OJ, *et al*: Quinacrine fluorescence patterns of human D group chromosomes. Nature 232:24-27, 1971

3. Holmes LB: *Mental Retardation: An Atlas of Diseases with Associated Physical Abnormalities.* New York, MacMillan Co, 1972, pp 164-167

4. Mottet NK, Jensen H: The anomalous embryonic development associated with trisomy 13-15. Am J Clin Pathol 43:334-346, 1965

5. Kos A, Schuknecht HF, Singer JD: Temporal bone studies in 13-15 and 18 trisomy syndromes. Arch Otolaryngol 83:439-445, 1966

6. Kelemen GR, Hooft C, Kluyskens P: The inner ear in autosomal trisomy. Pract Otorhinolaryngol (Basel) 30:251-258, 1968

7. Maniglia AJ, Wolff D, Herques AJ: Congenital deafness in 13-15 trisomy syndrome. Arch Otolaryngol 92:181-188, 1970

8. Black FO, Sando I, Wagner JA, *et al*: Middle and inner ear abnormalities. Arch Otolaryngol 93:615-619, 1971

9. Sando I, Baker D, Black FO, *et al*: Persistence of stapedial artery in trisomy 13-15 syndrome. Arch Otolaryngol 96:441-447, 1972

10. Bergstrom L, Hemenway WG, Sando I: Pathological changes in congenital deafness. Laryngoscope 82:1777-1792, 1972

11. Saito H, Okano Y, Furuta M, *et al*: Temporal bone findings in trisomy D. Arch Otolaryngol 100:386-389, 1974

12. Guild SR: A graphic reconstruction method for the study of the organ of Corti. Anat Rec 22:141-159, 1921

13. Schuknecht HF: Techniques for study of cochlear function and pathology in experimental animals. Arch Otolaryngol 58:377-397, 1953

14. Bast TH, Anson BJ: *Temporal Bone and the Ear.* Springfield, Illinois, Charles C Thomas, 1949, pp 30-374

15. Igarashi M: Personal data

16. Sando I: Personal data

17. Palva T: Cochlear aqueduct in infants. Acta Otolaryngol (Stockh) 70:83-94, 1970

18. Valvassori GE, Naunton RF, Lindsay JR: Inner ear anomalies, clinical and histopathological consideration. Ann Otol Rhinol Laryngol 78:929-938, 1969

19. Michel EM: Memoire sur les anomalies congenitales de l'oreille interne. Gaz Med Strasb 3:55-58, 1863

20. Mundini C: Anatomia surdi nedi sectio. De Bononiensi Scientiarum et Artium Instituto Atque Academi Commentarii, Bologna 7:28-29, 419-431, 1791

21. Siebenmann F: *Grundzüge der Anatomie und Pathogenese der Taubstummheit.* Wiesbaden, Germany, JF Bergman, 1904

22. Alexander G: Zur Pathologie und pathologischen Anatomie der knogenitalen Taubheit. Arch Ohrenheilk 61:183, 1904

23. Paparella MM, ElFiky FM: Mondini's deafness. Arch Otolaryngol 95:134-140, 1972

24. Siebenmann F, Bing R: Über den Labyrinth und Hirnbefund bei einem an Retinitis pigmentosa erbindeten Angeboren-Taubstummen. Z Ohrenheilk 54:265-280, 1907

25. Scheibe A: Ein Fall von Taubstummheit mit Acusticusatrophie und Bildungsanomalien im häutigen Labyrinth beiderseits. Z Ohrenheilk 22:11-23, 1891-1892

26. Alexander, quoted by Schuknecht HF: Pathology of sensorineural deafness of genetic origin in *Deafness in Childhood,* Nashville, Tennessee, Vanderbilt University Press, 1967, pp 75-76

27. Anson BJ, Bast TH: Development of the stapes of the human ear. Q Bull Northwestern U Med Sch 33:44-59, 1959

28. Anson BJ, Bast TH: Development of the incus of the human ear. Q Bull Northwestern U Med Sch 33:110-119, 1959

29. Anson BJ, Donaldson JA: *Surgical Anatomy of the Temporal Bone.* Philadelphia, Pennsylvania, WB Saunders Co, 1973, Part II. The ear: development anatomy, pp 17-87

30. Gasser RF: The development of the facial nerve in man. Ann Otol Rhinol Laryngol 76:37-57, 1967

31. Pearson AA, Jacobson AD, Van Calcar RJ *et al*: The development of the middle ear. in *The Development of the Ear.* A manual prepared for use of graduates in medicine, Rochester, Minnesota, by the American Academy of Ophthalmology and Otolaryngology, 1973, p 28

32. Steffen TN: Vascular anomalies of the middle ear. Laryngoscope 78:171-197, 1968

PAGET'S DISEASE OF THE TEMPORAL BONE

GEORGE T. NAGER, M.D.

BALTIMORE, MARYLAND

SUMMARY – Osteitis deformans Paget is a fairly common, heritable, sometimes progressive disease of bone which affects primarily the axial skeleton and may lead to deformity and weakness. It affects 3% of the population over forty years of age and males more frequently than females. The skull and temporal bones become involved in about two-thirds of the patients. Progressive involvement of the temporal bones may lead to alteration of position, increase in size and change of architecture of the petrous pyramid, external canal, middle ear and inner ear capsule. These changes in turn may produce impairment of hearing (about 30-50% of cases) and vestibular function (20-25%). The clinical, radiological, and pathological manifestations of Paget's disease of the temporal bone are discussed in detail and explained with photomicrographs. Examples of tumor formations and vascular changes are presented.

DEFINITION

Osteitis deformans Paget is a fairly common, heritable, chronic, sometimes progressive disease of bone of so far undetermined etiology, in which recurrent episodes of bone resorption, followed by exaggerated attempts at repair, result in a structurally weakened, deformed skeleton of increased bone mass. It may legitimately be considered as a heritable abiatrophy, most likely of the collagen matrix of bone,[1] inherited either as an incomplete dominant gene, carried on an X-chromosome,[2] or as a simple autosomal Mendelian dominant gene.[1] The disease may present itself as a solitary, monostotic form, remaining asymptomatic forever, only to be discovered as an incidental finding. Or, it may evolve into a clinically manifest and obvious expression of Paget's disease. In its disseminated, polyostotic form, many bones in different regions of the skeleton may be affected. However, in no instance are all bones involved as in a generalized bone disorder, such as hyperparathyroidism. Cylindrical and flat bones are affected with equal frequency.

INCIDENCE, AGE AND SEX DISTRIBUTION

The incidence of osteitis deformans in the general population is estimated at around 0.013%.[3] Autopsy studies of unselected patients, older than 40 years, reveal an overall incidence of 3 to 3.7%, steadily increasing from 1% in the fifth decade to 5 to 10% in the ninth.[4,5] The disease is seldom encounterd under the age of 30 to 40. The actual incidence may well be higher, as asymptomatic and small lesions may never be detected. The disease appears to be more common in England, Australia and New Zealand, whereas it is less frequently encountered in North America and rarely in Switzerland, South America, Japan, China, India, and Africa.[6] It has been generally accepted that men are more often affected than women. The difference is slight. The actual proportion is probably about five to four.

From the Otological Research Laboratory, Department of Laryngology and Otology, the Johns Hopkins University School of Medicine and Hospital.

This study was supported by Grant Number 5 RO1-NS 02182-16 from the National Institute of Neurological and Communicative Disorders and Stroke, U.S.P.H.S.

Presented at the meeting of the American Otological Society, Atlanta, Georgia, April 11-12, 1975.

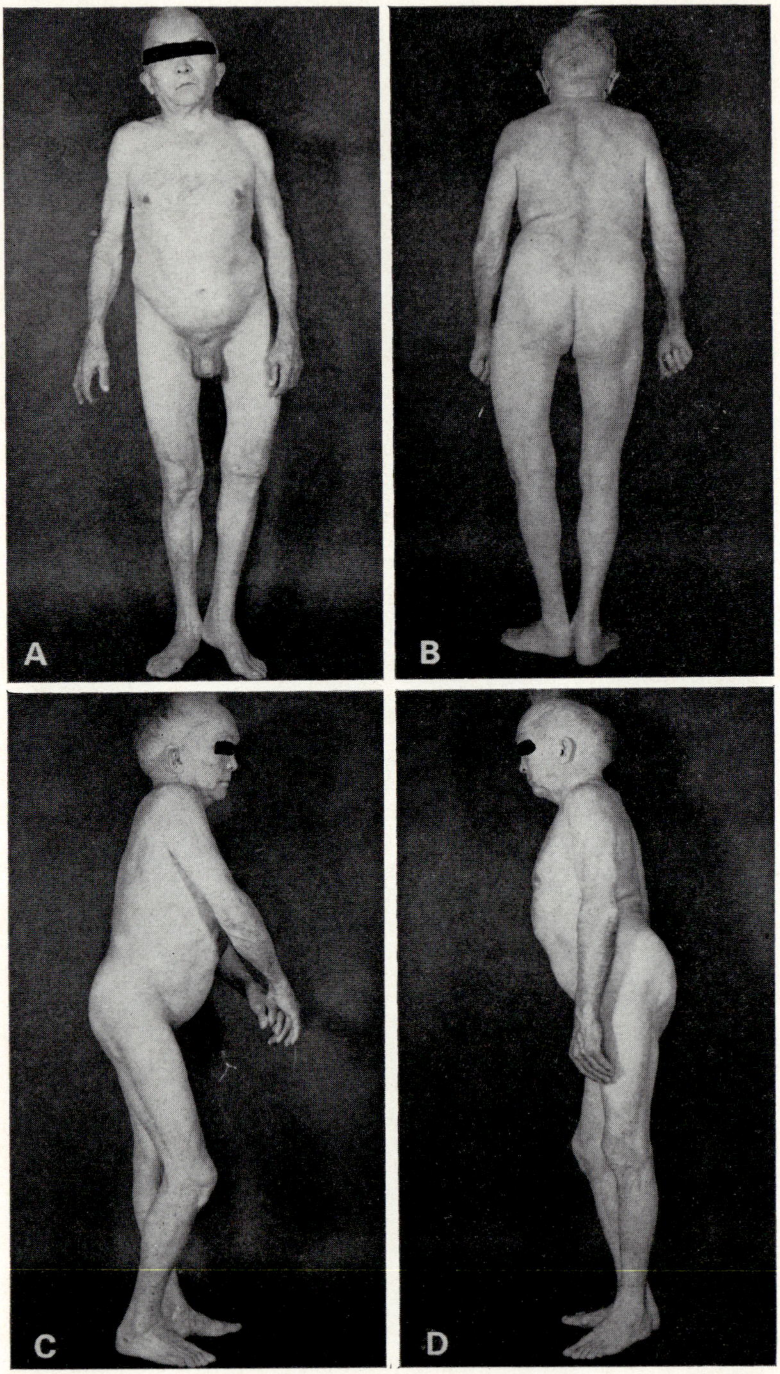

Fig. 1. K.H., a 78-year-old male with polyostotic Paget's disease involving the entire skull, spine, sacrum, (L) femur and tibia. The anterior bowing of the (L) femur and the shortening of stature (A-C), the kyphosis of the thoracic spine with the forward thrust of the head (B and D), and the enlargement of the skull are well recognized.

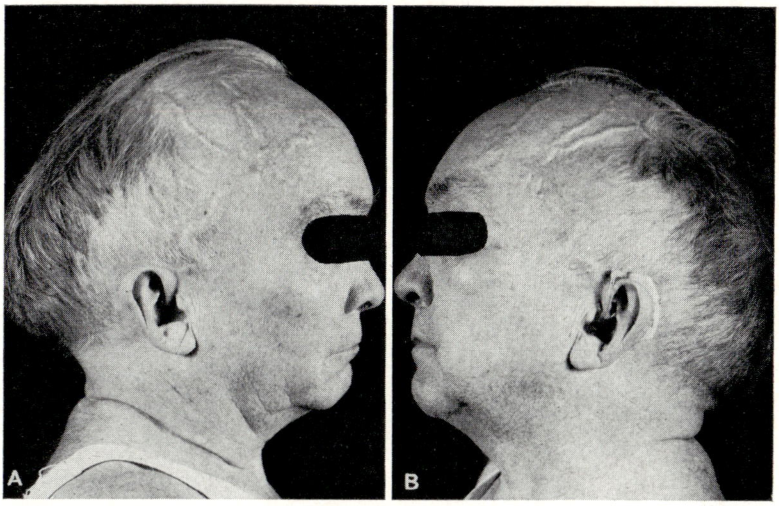

Fig. 2. Patient K.H. The enlargement of the neurocranium, the basilar impression and the enlargement and tortuosity of the superficial temporal artery and its parietal and frontal branches are well recognized.

LOCALIZATION

Osteitis deformans is principally a disease of the axial skeleton. Bones under particular mechanical stress usally are affected more often. The bones of the leg are involved more often than those of the arm. The bones most frequently affected are the sacrum (57% of cases), followed by the spine (50%), pelvis (43%), and femur (35%). The incidence of vertebral involvement decreases steadily from the sacral (76%), to the lumbar (26%), thoracic (17%), and cervical (7%) region of the spine. The right femur is about twice as often involved as the left (31% as against 15%).[4] A similar observation was made of a brother and sister with Paget's disease, both with unilateral involvement of the radius. In the left-handed individual the left radius was involved, whereas in the right-handed sibling, the right radius was affected.[7] The structural changes tend to be most pronounced at the attachments of tendons and ligaments.[4] Although the involvement of the skeleton generally follows a pattern of localization consistent with the concept of stress and weight bearing, or "wear and tear," it should be remembered that this involvement probably represents only a contributing factor to localization and development of a lesion and that a hereditary weakness possibly represents the primary factor.

CLINICAL MANIFESTATIONS

Osteitis deformans appears in hospital practice more often as an incidental or subsidiary finding than as a principal cause of admission. Only about 15% of patients exhibit an advanced form of the disease with the well-recognized skeletal changes, the striking deformities of the long bones, the progressive kyphosis with shortening of stature, and the enlargement of the skull (Fig. 1). Thus, a large percentage escape clinical detection. The skull becomes involved in about 65 to 70% of patients[5] (Fig. 2). In the majority of instances (about 70%), the skull shows evidence of an advanced stage of the disease. However, in only one-third does the disease process eventually lead to deformity and enlargement. The neurocranium is more often the site of involvement than the facial cranium, and of the facial bones the mandible is more frequently affected than the

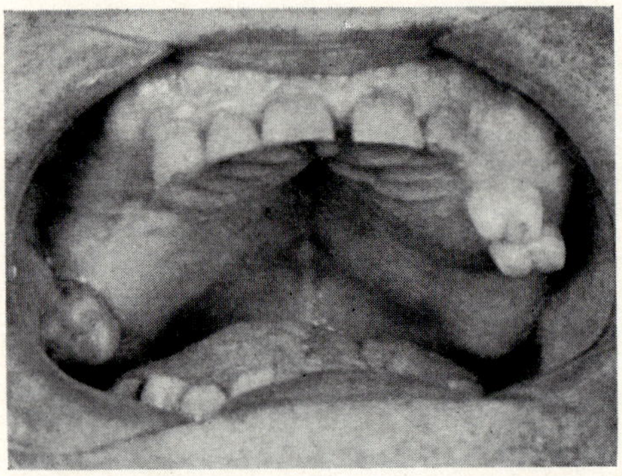

Fig. 3. Patient K.H. Reveals the enlargement and deformity of the alveolar process of the maxilla caused by Paget's disease.

maxilla[4] (Fig. 3). The calvaria is in most instances involved in a diffuse and even manner, with the thickening and deformity varying greatly in different regions. Occasionally, only a portion or only one-half of the calvaria is affected. At times, well-circumscribed lesions are scattered throughout the calvaria. In about 10% of the cases, the disease does present itself in the form of a sharply outlined, predominantly resorptive lesion, recognized as osteoporosis circumscripta cranii.[8,9] The weight of the brain and enlarged skull may cause flattening of the softened bones at the base. Dorsal inclination of the plane of the foramen magnum and projection of the odontoid process into the posterior fossa lead to a bending of the brain stem over the odontoid and ventral margin of the foramen magnum; to a protrusion of the olivary processes of the cerebellum into the cervical canal; to tension on the nerve roots; and compression of the basilar vessels. Reduction in volume of the neurocranium, invagination of the occipital condyle and advanced changes in the cervical spine can produce cerebral and cerebellar dysfunction and result in vertebrobasilar ischemia. Impingement upon cranial and spinal nerves in their foramina of exit by periosteal new bone formation can result in impairment of hearing, equilibrium and vision, and produce motor and sensory disturbances. Impairment of hearing is the most common manifestation of cranial nerve involvement. It is present in 30 to 50% of patients with skull involvement. It is sensorineural in nature, and of cochlear origin, and it is often associated with a low frequency conductive loss with a peak of the air-bone gap at 500 cycles. Tinnitus is observed in 20% of these patients and vertigo and unsteadiness occur in about 20 to 25%.[10,11] A decreased response to caloric stimulation is frequently observed in these individuals.[11] Once the skull becomes obviously involved, headaches become a prominent and constant symptom. Patients with extensive involvement of the calvaria often display marked enlargement and tortuosity of the superficial temporal artery and its branches. The enlargement of this vessel, when associated with a mixed hearing loss, should arouse suspicion of Paget's disease.[11]

MICROSCOPIC APPEARANCE

The osseous lesions of advanced osteitis deformans reflect a long-standing and involved sequence of pathological changes affecting both the osseous tissue and the marrow (Fig. 4). The first appearance of the disease is osteoclastic resorption of bone. The original bone is dismantled by osteoclastic activity and replaced by densely packed, narrow trabeculae of coarse-fibered bone, which in turn may undergo resorption. The marrow is entirely replaced by a cellular fibrovascular tissue. Waves of resorption and regeneration may ebb and flow over the same territory. The variation of osteoclastic and osteoblastic activity and the frequency of local exacerbations and remissions leads to simultaneous occurrence of different stages of bone formation in closely adjacent areas.

Areas of active bone transformation (Fig. 5) are recognized by the presence of a large number of osteoclasts and osteoblasts, often side by side and lining the same trabecula, and by a highly vascular, cellular, fibrous bone marrow. During the phase of remission,

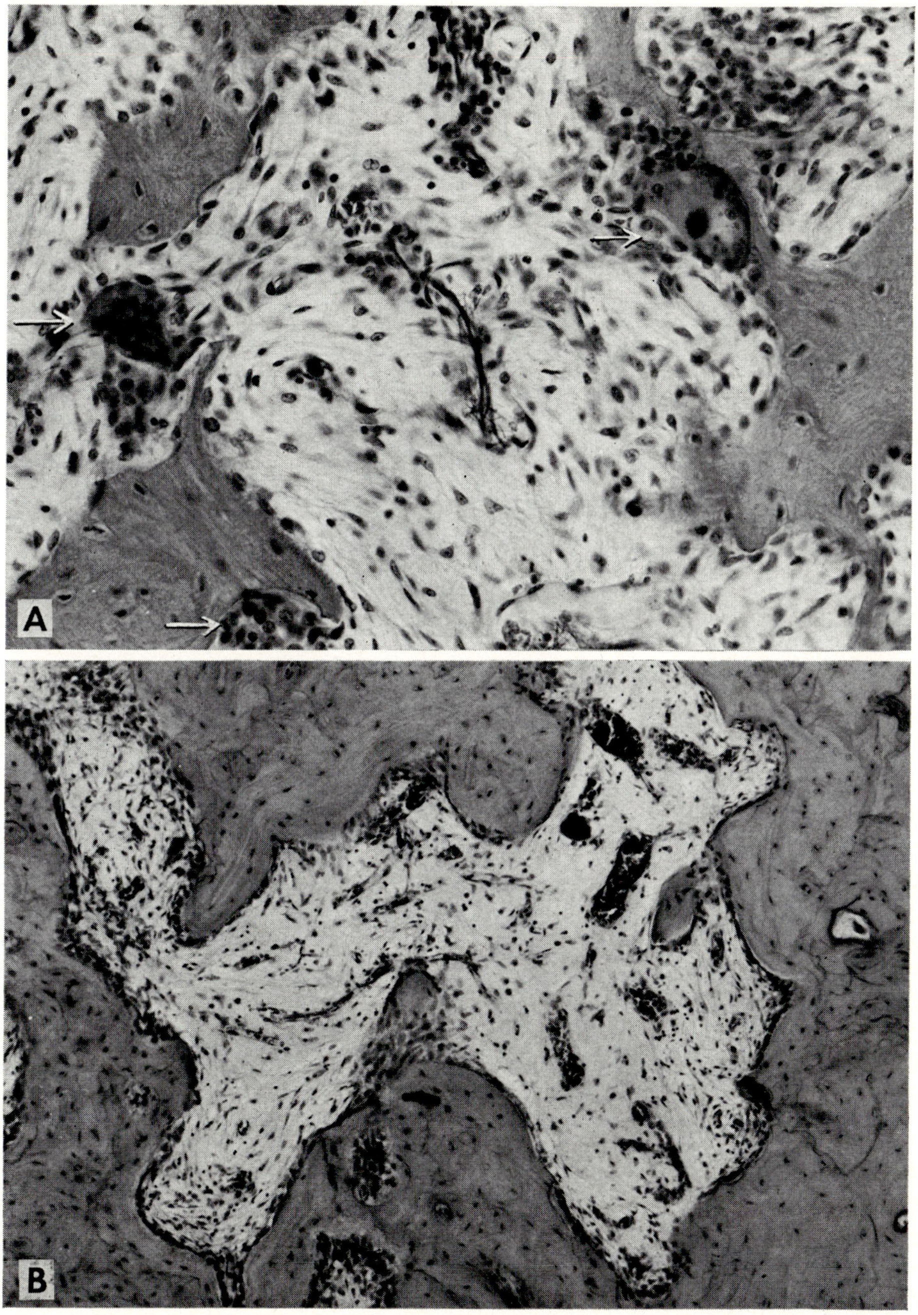

Fig. 4. A) Destruction of the original bone begins in adjacent marrow spaces with lacunar erosion by osteoclasts (arrows). (H. and E. stain; X350.) B) The marrow is replaced by a vascular, cellular, fibrous tissue. (H. and E. stain; X135.)

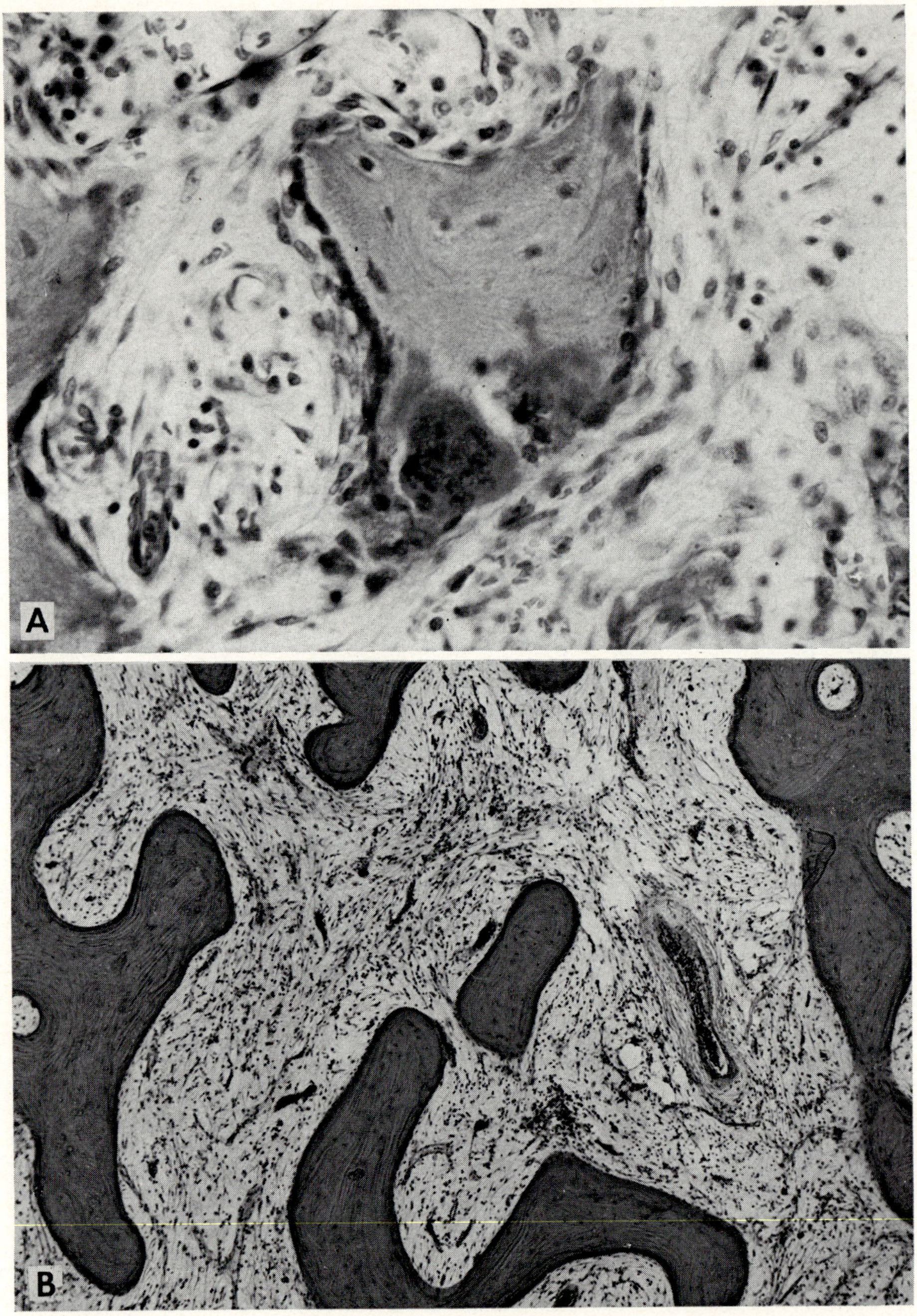

Fig. 5. A) In areas of active bone transformation, osteoclasts and osteoblasts are seen lining the same trabecula. (H. and E. stain; X500.) B) During a remission, the bone marrow becomes aplastic, lacks osteoclastic and osteoblastic activity, and the trabeculae are surrounded by aplastic resting lines. (H. and E. stain; X70.)

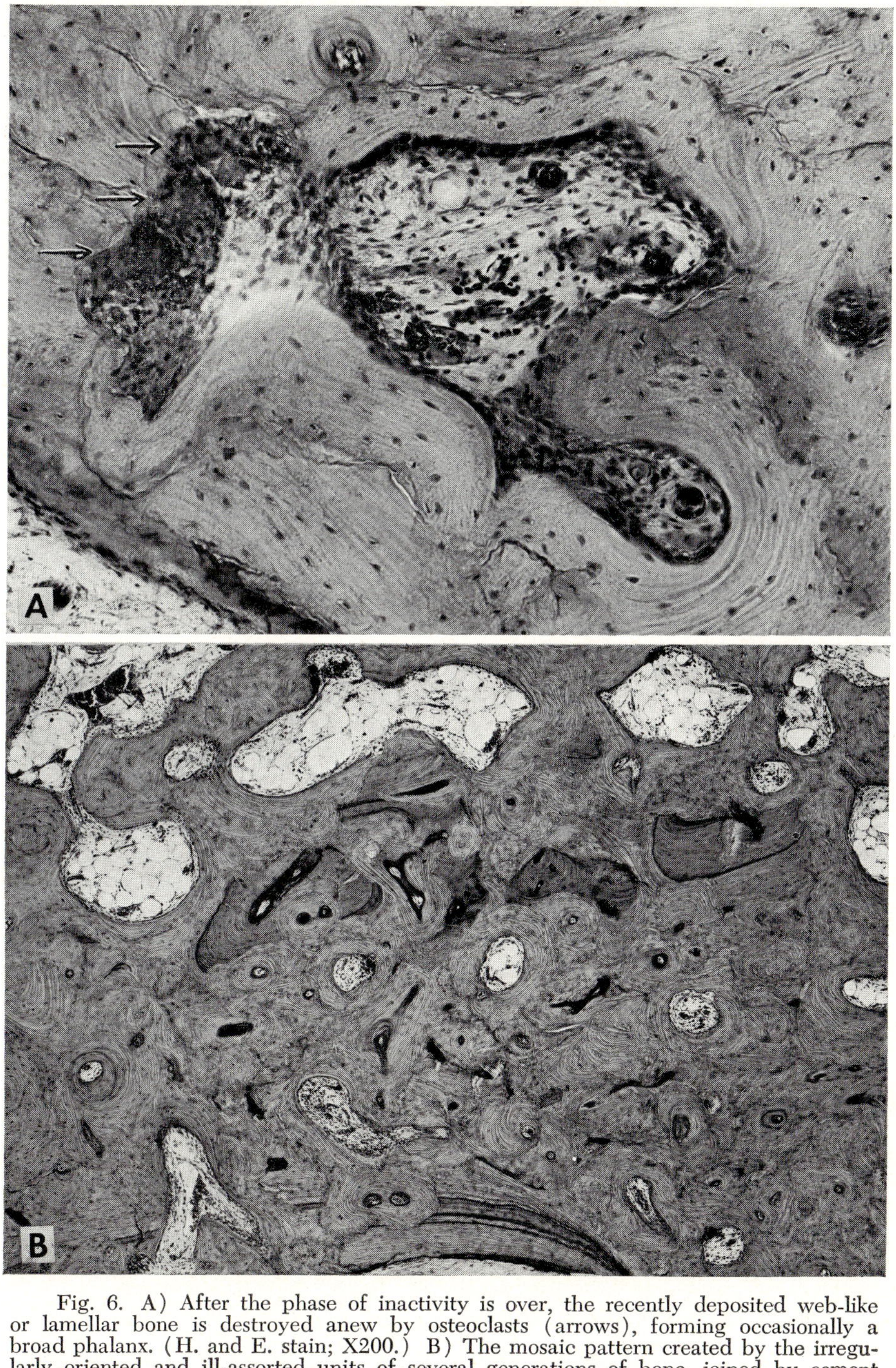

Fig. 6. A) After the phase of inactivity is over, the recently deposited web-like or lamellar bone is destroyed anew by osteoclasts (arrows), forming occasionally a broad phalanx. (H. and E. stain; X200.) B) The mosaic pattern created by the irregularly oriented and ill-assorted units of several generations of bone, joined by cement lines, identifies the arrested, final phase of osteitis deformans. (H. and E. stain; X50.)

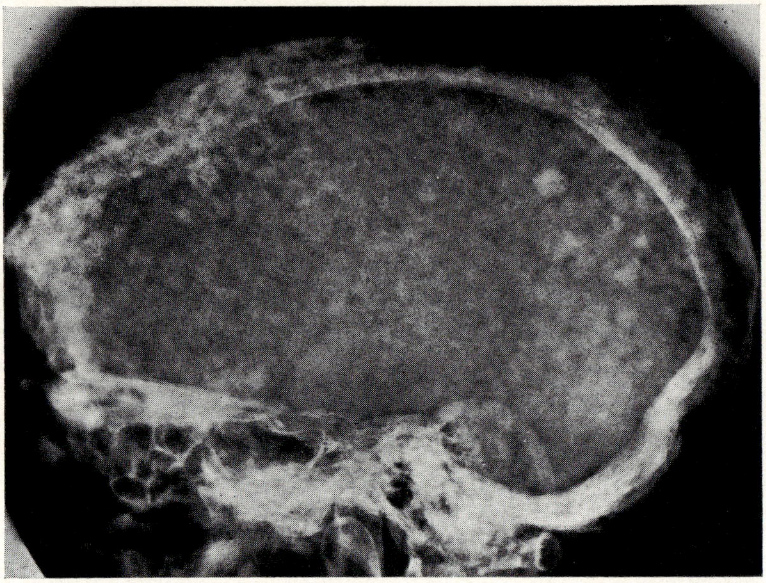

Fig. 7. Lateral skull. C.G., a 78-year-old male. Enlargement and change in configuration are the result of thickening of the diploë and outer table. The close association of areas of radiolucency (osteoporosis) and increased density (osteosclerosis) produces a "cotton-wool" pattern, most prominent in the frontal and parietal region. The alteration of the hypophyseal fossa and the bulging of the base of the skull into the cranial cavity are apparent.

there is neither osteoclastic nor osteoblastic activity. The trabeculae are surrounded by aplastic resting lines. The marrow has become aplastic and may revert to the adipose type. The process of bone transformation temporarily has come to a standstill. After a while, the phase of inactivity is over and resorption of the resting bone begins again (Fig. 6).

The arrangement of fragments of newer bone, laid down on partially destroyed segments of older bone (which in turn may contain fragments of yet older bone, partially destroyed), all without recognizable orientation, constitutes the mosaic-like pattern of osteitis deformans.

ROENTGENOLOGICAL MANIFESTATIONS

The roentgenological appearance reflects bone resorption and excessive repair singly or in combination. The initial phase is predominantly osteolytic. Sharply defined areas of demineralization, generally confined to the vault and in close proximity to the base, are frequently encountered in the occipital bone and in the area about the pterion. This phase of circumscribed osteoporosis then progresses to a more often observed stage in which bone resorption and formation of new bone occur simultaneously. The coexistence of osteolysis with circular areas of sclerosis creates irregular shadows of varying density which lend the calvaria the characteristic "cotton-wool" appearance, a pattern most frequently encountered in the fronto- and fronto-parietal regions (Figs. 7 and 8). As these areas of radiolucency and density increase and coalesce, the calvaria assumes the classic mottled appearance. The outer table and the diploë of the skull are generally the first to become involved. The characteristic features of the skull involvement are enlargement and deformity of the calvaria, invagination of the base, distortion of the foramen magnum, and outward rotation of the petrous pyramids with upward tilting of the petrous apices.

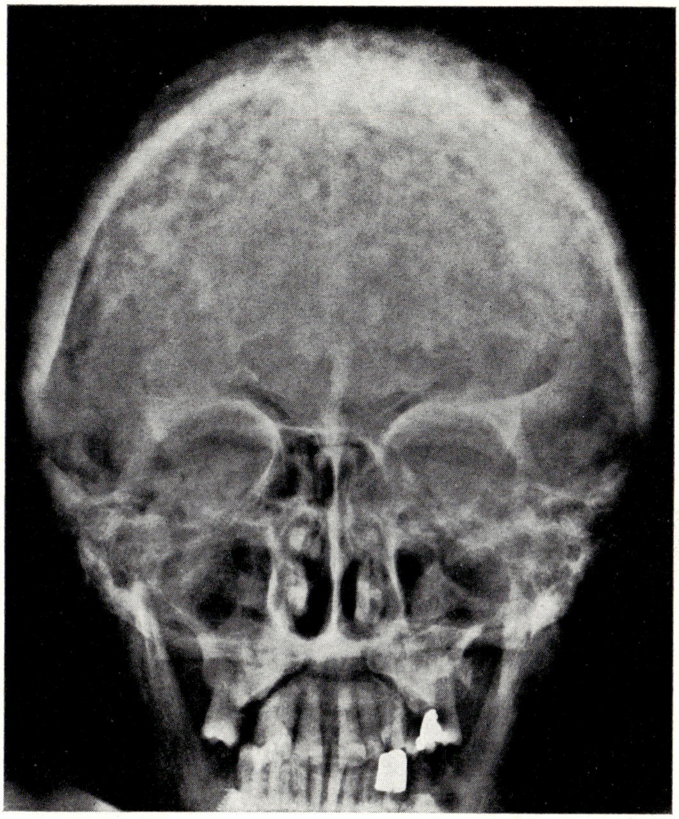

Fig. 8. P-A skull. F.Ch., a 63-year-old male. The involvement and enlargement of the calvaria are symmetrical. The outer table and diploë exhibit the most characteristic changes. Progressive softening of the base resulted in platy- and convexobasia with elevation of the petrous apices and a downward slanting of the petrous crests. Note the partial obliteration of the frontal sinuses.

Whenever osteitis deformans affects the skull, in general both temporal bones also are involved. The initial osteolytic phase is often characterized by an increased distinctness of the otic and labyrinthine capsule with unusually clear identification of the cochlea and semicircular canals. However, with progressive Pagetoid involvement the recognition of the inner ear capsule decreases. In the advanced stage of the disease (Fig. 9), there is complete obliteration of the cochlear and vestibular capsule and it becomes impossible to assess size and configuration of the internal acoustic meatus. Since there has to be a considerable change (30-50%) in the amount of bone calcium in a given area before radiological alterations become discernible, it is possible for a patient to have Paget's disease without any roentgenological evidence.

The long bones may be thick and opaque, but pseudo-fractures and lateral bowing of the femur and anterior bowing of the tibia, under the influence of weight bearing, reflect their diminished strength. Vertebral bodies affected by the disease may exhibit coarse trabeculation in a horizontal distribution, accentuating the margins of the bodies, or they may simply reveal a homogeneous opacification. Compression fractures are not uncommon, resulting in an anterior narrowing of the vertebral body. Pagetoid involvement of the maxilla and mandible is most prominent in areas adjacent to the tooth sockets.

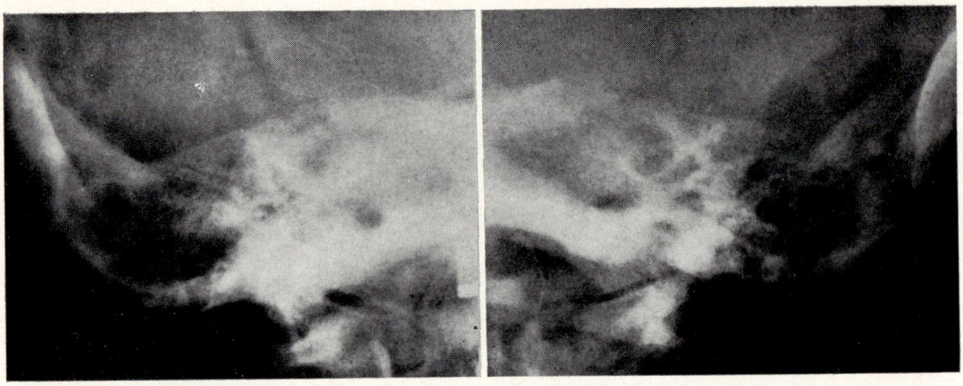

Fig. 9. Longitudinal (Stenvers) position of the temporal bones of a 63-year-old male (F. Ch.) with Paget's disease. Extensive osteosclerosis of the perilabyrinthine bone, characteristic in the advanced stage of the disease, renders visualization of the vestibular labyrinth and cochlea more difficult. Note the elevation of the petrous apices.

MORPHOLOGICAL CHANGES INVOLVING THE TEMPORAL BONE

In all of our eight patients, both temporal bones are involved by the disease. Whereas the extent of involvement varies to a certain degree with each case, the structural changes within a given pair of temporal bones are very similar (Fig. 10). In some instances, the periosteal and only part of the endochondral capsule layer are involved. In other instances, almost the entire endochondral and a considerable portion of the endosteal layer of the cochlear and vestibular capsule have been replaced by Pagetoid bone. As the bone transformation steadily progresses, it may cause alteration of position, increase in size, and change in the architecture of the petrous pyramid and other areas of the temporal bone. The petrous pyramid may undergo an outward rotation around its long axis to the extent that the posterior, cerebellar aspect, finally becomes the upper surface of the pyramid.

In instances of wide-spread involvement of the petrous pyramid, some distortion and narrowing of the internal acoustic meatus can be observed. This narrowing in general is not severe enough to exert pressure on the cranial nerves and blood vessels which it contains. Occasionally, the tractus spiralis foraminosus, the cochlear modiolus, and the macula cribrosa of the inferior and superior vestibular area are involved in the bone disease (Fig. 11). The foramina and longitudinal canals of the modiolus and vestibular areas are lined with seams of hyalin and osteoid tissue. The nerve fibers in these areas appear crowded and even strangulated. The foramina and neural canals can also be invaded by connective tissue after preceding osteoclastic resorption of the endosteal bone. This process, which begins in an adjacent marrow space, can lead to a separation and even destruction of nerve bundles. Separation of nerve bundles occasionally can enhance the formation of neuromas.[12]

Remodeling of bone in the walls of the middle ear frequently leads to obvious constriction of the tympanic cavity and its recesses (Fig. 12). Marked thickening of the tegmen tympani can cause impingement upon malleus and incus. Similarly, new bone formation in the lateral or medial wall of the epitympanic recess may produce a jamming of the two outer ear ossicles, and occasionally lead to a fibrous or osseous union.

Concentric growth of the tympanic bone can cause a considerable decrease in diameter of the tympanic annulus with relaxation of the tympanic membrane (Figs. 13 and 14). It can also produce narrowing and tortuosity of

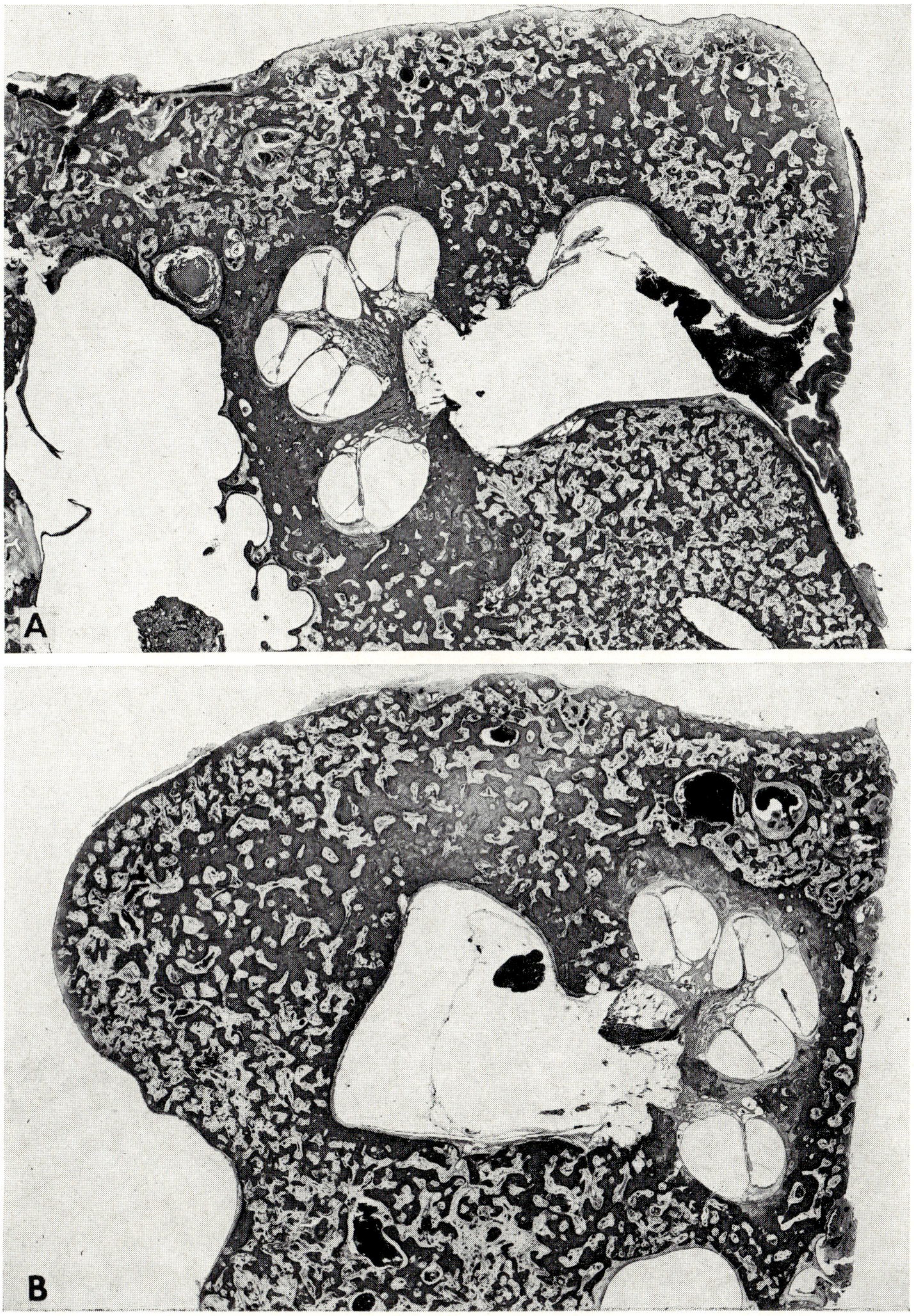

Fig. 10. Vertical, midmodiolar section through the right and left petrous pyramid in an 80-year-old female (H.V.). The increase in size and change of configuration of the pyramid, and the narrowing of the entrance to the right (A) and the irregular contours of the left internal acoustic meatus (B) are well recognized. (H. and E. stain; X8.)

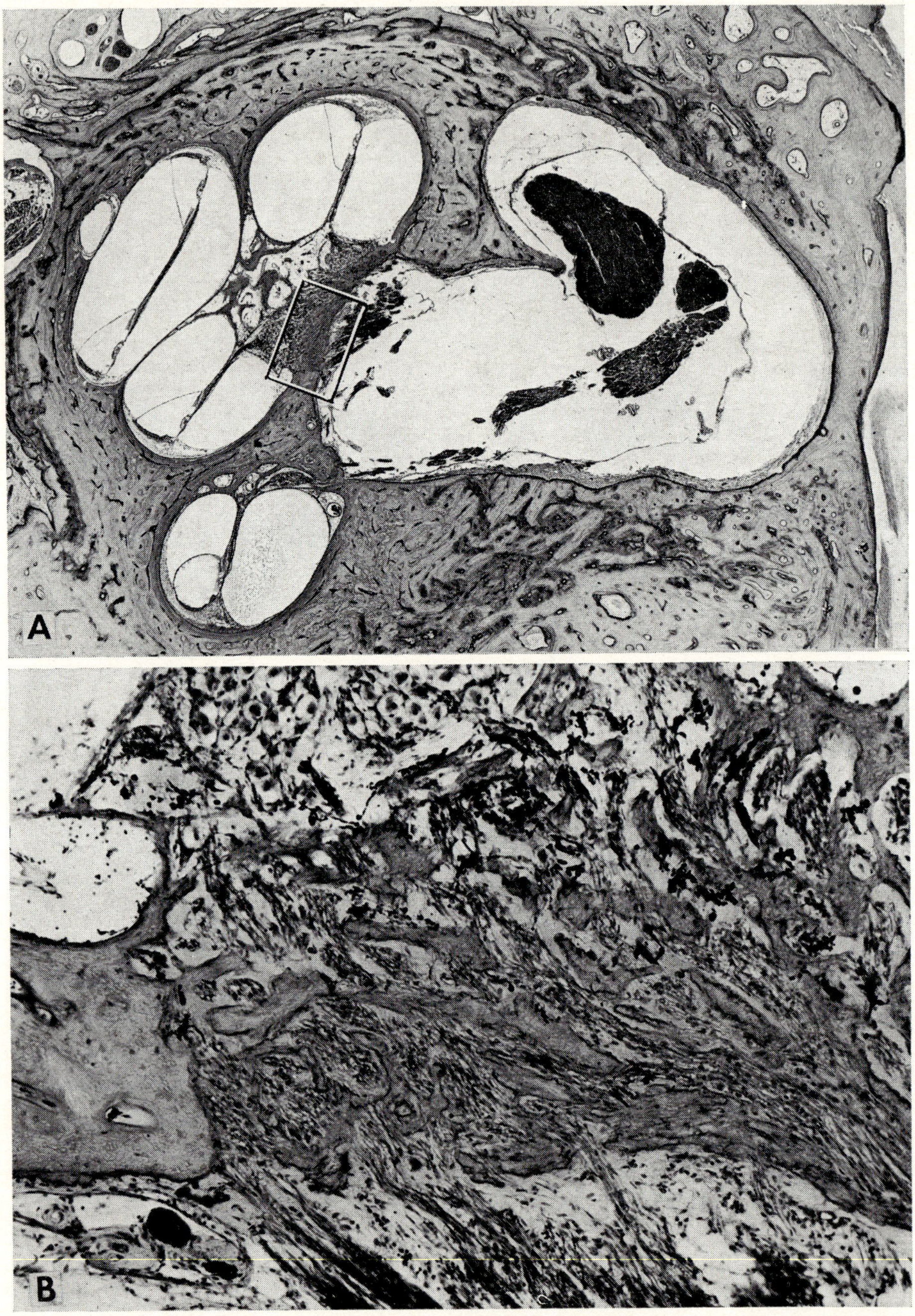

Fig. 11. A) Vertical, paramodiolar section through the right petrous pyramid in a 66-year-old male (K.W.) with partial Pagetoid involvement of the periosteal and endochondral layer of the otic capsule and of the tractus spiralis foraminosus. (H. and E. stain; X14). B) Same section; X135. The foramina and longitudinal canals of the modiolus are lined with seams of hyaline and osteoid tissue, and the nerve fibers appear crowded and in some areas constricted.

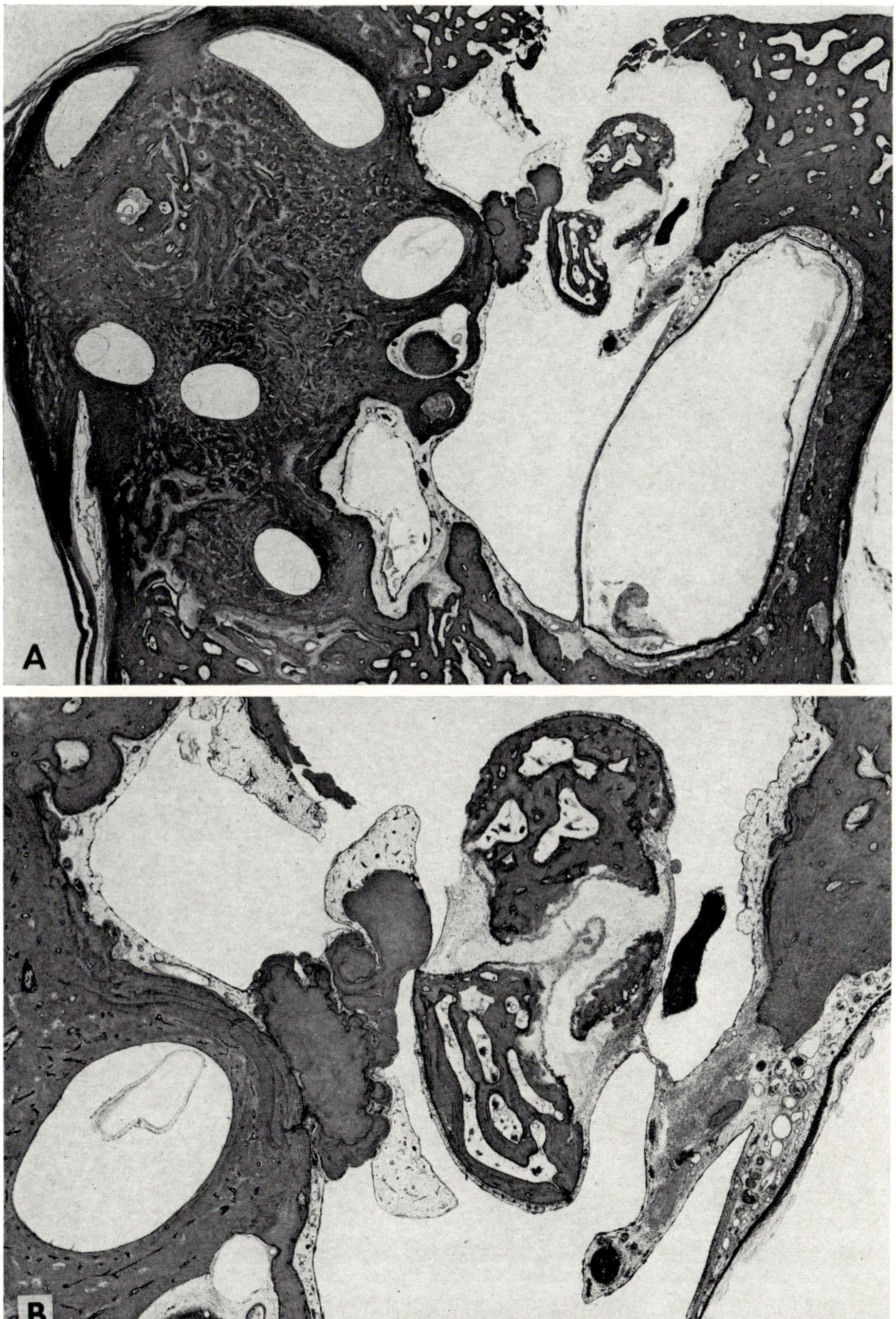

Fig. 12. A) Vertical section through the left petrous pyramid at the level of the incudo-malleolar articulation in the 66-year-old male (K.W.) with an irregular new bone formation attached to the wall of the lateral semi-circular canal. (H. and E. stain; X8½.) B) Same section; X20. The exostosis, which appears to have arisen in the mucoperiosteum over the lateral canal, impinges upon the body of the incus.

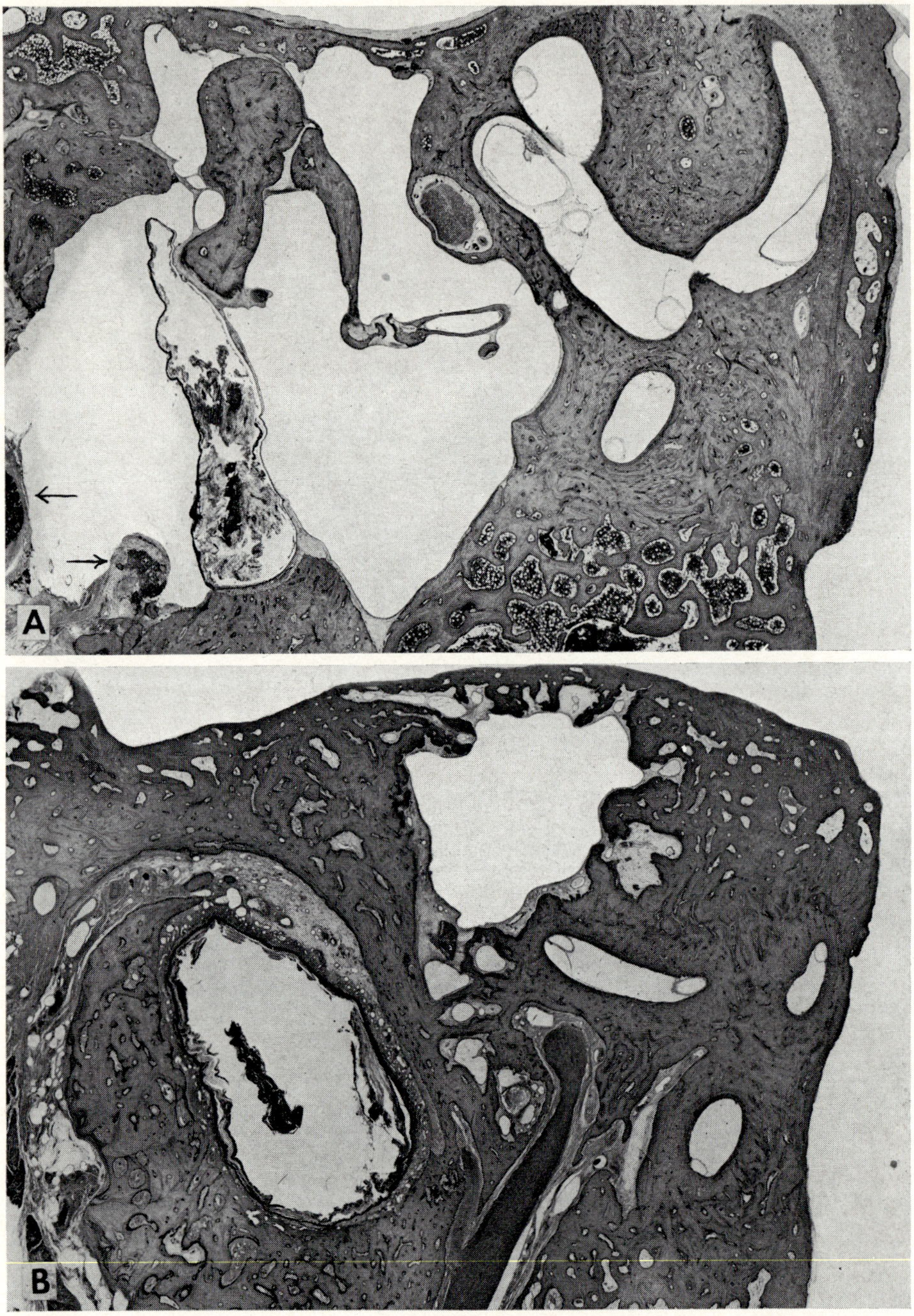

Fig. 13. A) Vertical section through the right petrous pyramid at the level of the incudo-stapedial articulation in a 75-year-old male (Q.Ch.) Note the irregular narrowing of the external auditory canal, the formation of exostoses (arrows), and the presence of an external cholesteatoma. (H. and E. stain; X8½.) B) Vertical section through the right petrous pyramid at the level of the descending portion of the Fallopian canal in the 66-year-old male (K.W.). The concentric narrowing of the outer ear canal and the chronic external otitis are well recognized. (H. and E. stain; X7.)

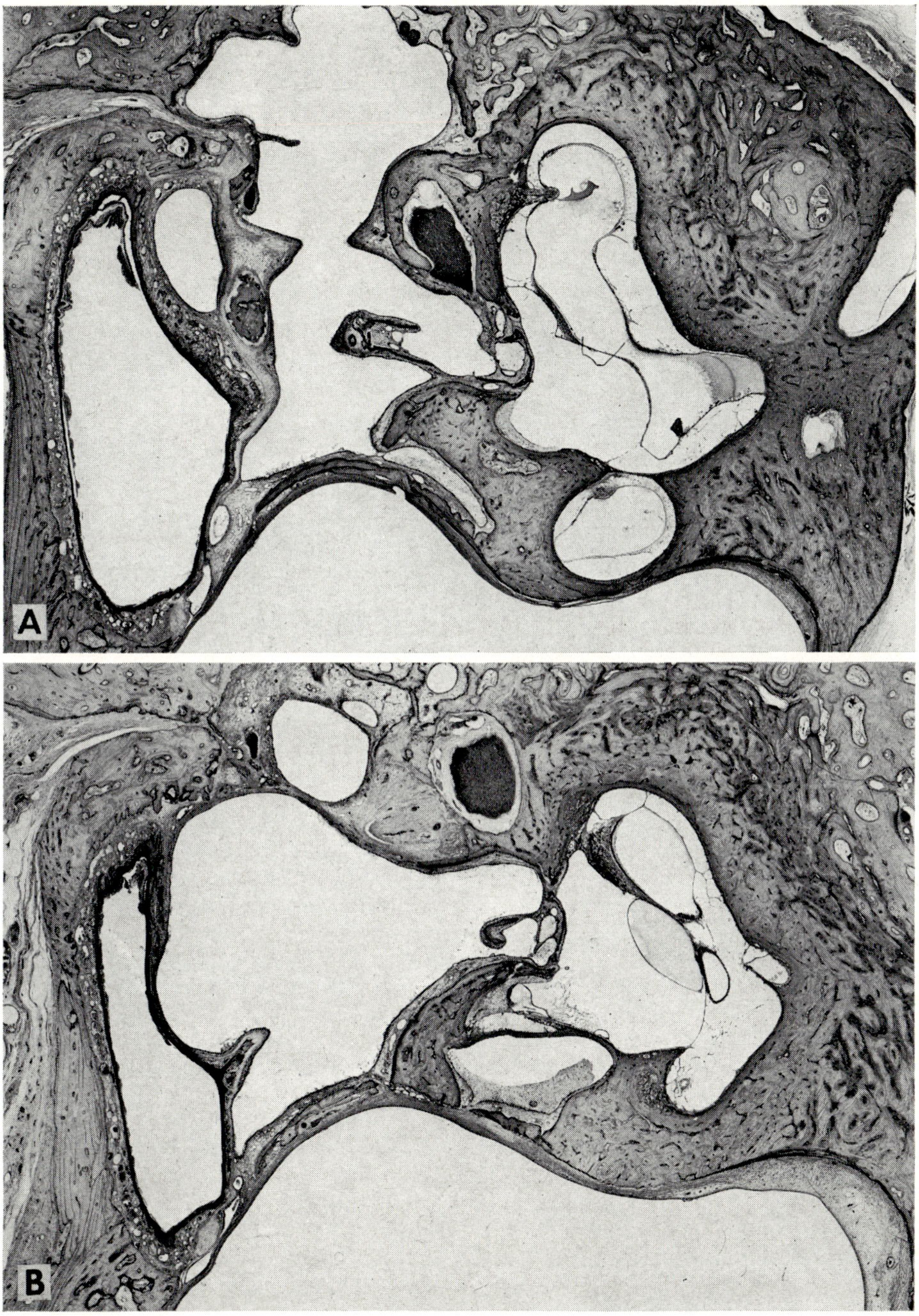

Fig. 14. Vertical section through the right petrous pyramid near the posterior (A) and anterior end (B) of the oval window in the 66-year-old male (K.W.). Concentric growth of the tympanic bone with decrease in diameter of the tympanic annulus led to relaxation of the tympanic membrane. New bone formation within the promontory caused an upward tilt of the promontory with narrowing of the oval window niche and jamming of the stapes (A). The enormous enlargement of the jugular bulb caused marked elevation of the floor of the hypotympanum to almost the level of the umbo, and total obliteration of the round window niche (B). (H. and E. stain; X9½ and 10.)

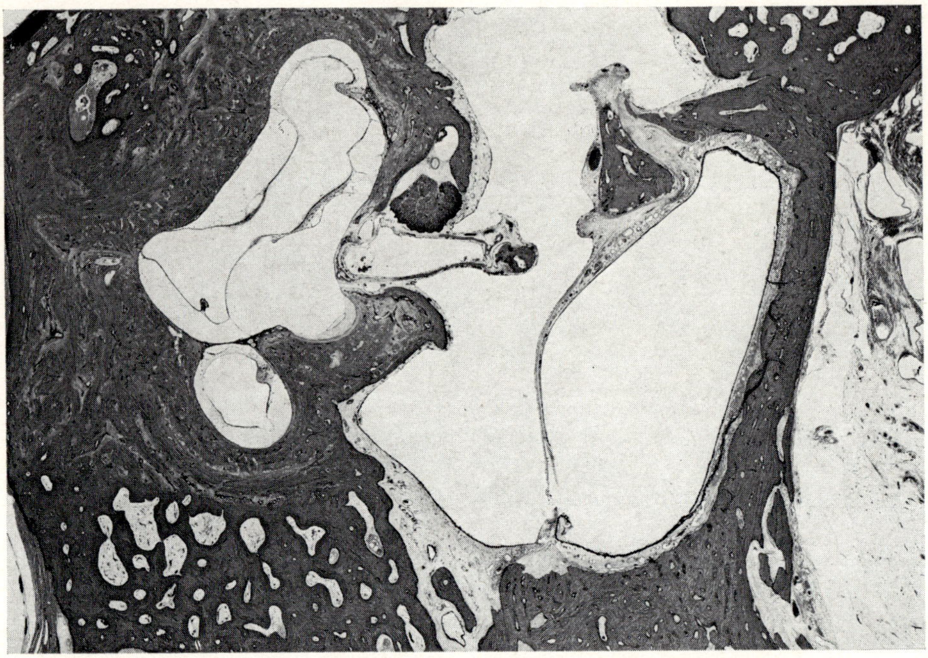

Fig. 15. Vertical section through the left petrous pyramid at the level of the oval window in the 66-year-old male (K.W.). Intrinsic narrowing of the Fallopian canal produced a partial extrusion of the facial nerve through a dehiscence in the floor, impingement upon, and partial destruction of the posterior crus of the stapes. (H. and E. stain; X8½.)

the external auditory canal, formation of exostoses, induce chronic external otitis and lead to the development of an external cholesteatoma.

Involvement of the oval window may give rise to marked distortion of its architecture (Fig. 14). This, in turn, will produce jamming and immobilization of the stapes. New bone formation in the region of the promontory can produce an upward tilt of the promontory with protrusion of the inferior, oval window margin into the vestibule.

The tympanic section of the Fallopian canal can be severely affected by the bone disease (Fig. 15). Concentric narrowing of the bony canal can result in partial extrusion of the facial nerve through a dehiscence in the floor of the canal. Such a displaced facial nerve can impinge upon the posterior crus of the stapes and, by constant pressure, cause its partial destruction.

Ankylosis of the stapes does occur but has not been observed in our material. The mechanisms are as follows: Pagetoid bone in the oval window margin may grow across the annular ligament in the form of an osseous bridge and substitute an adjacent portion of the foot-plate; or, the cartilaginous rim and the underlying bone of the stapedial foot-plate can be resorbed in a localized area. This area subsequently is replaced by Pagetoid bone which, in turn, becomes connected with Pagetoid bone in the adjacent oval window margin. A predisposing factor to the development of stapedial ankylosis is the jamming of the stapes in the distorted oval window which results in direct contact of two bony surfaces. Ossification of the annular ligament is another mechanism which can lead to stapedial ankylosis.[12,13]

Involvement of the round window niche can result in marked distortion of its architecture with constriction or even total obliteration of the niche. On the other hand, progressive enlargement of the jugular bulb with elevation of the floor of the hypotympanum can cause narrowing or total occlusion of the round window niche from below. Occasionally the floor of the hypotympanum can rise to the level of the umbo whereby the jugular bulb may become widely exposed and covered only by mucosa of the middle ear. Similarly, an enlargement of the jugular bulb in a more medial direction can lead to distension of this vessel until it reaches the dura lining the floor of the internal acoustic meatus. In all instances of wide-spread Pagetoid bone transformation, the contributing arteries and arterioles and the corresponding venous blood vessels are markedly increased in size and number (Figs. 16 and 17). In addition to an enormous increase in blood flow, there is also ample evidence of arteriovenous shunting, often across large venous lakes. All temporal bones with extensive, active bone transformation display an enormous enlargement of the jugular bulb (Figs. 14 and 18).

Pagetoid changes, although to a lesser degree, are also encountered in all auditory ossicles. Malleus and incus may show extensive areas of bone resorption and remodeling (Fig. 19 A and B and Fig. 19 C). Involvement of the osseous portion of the Eustachian tube can lead to narrowing or collapse of its lumen.

An interesting observation is the occurrence of clefts or microfractures (Figs. 20 and 21). Some are filled with newly formed bone, others contain connective tissue. They are encountered in certain regions of the labyrinth capsule and in areas where Pagetoid bone borders on old endosteal bone. They may be seen in the fundus of the internal acoustic meatus near the tractus spiralis foraminosus, in the wall of the cochlea, frequently in a radial distribution, in the vestibular capsule connecting the macula cribosa of the superior vestibular area with the superior semicircular canal, or coursing across remnants of endosteal bone. In the endosteal bone, these clefts are usually sharp-edged, straight and may show a considerable diastasis. In the endochondral capsule layer, they have irregularly fringed margins. These clefts and fissures develop during the remodeling, slanting, and outward rotation of the petrous pyramid, a process which unquestionably produces tearing of bone in areas of least resistance.

The morphological changes encountered in the cochlea include varying degrees of atrophy of receptor cells, nerve fibers, ganglion cells, and stria vascularis throughout all turns, increasing towards the end of the lower basal turn. Similarly, the vestibular labyrinth discloses partial atrophy of its first order neurons. It appears that the morphological changes in the cochlea and labyrinth are related to the extent of the bone transformation process, whereby the actual mechanism for the sensorineural hearing loss and vestibular dysfunction requires further clarification.

Extensive Pagetoid bone transformation of the petrous pyramid and otic capsule, in a few instances, has led to an obvious distortion of the normal configuration of the cochlea (Fig. 22). The change in architecture, in turn, caused axial and minor radial distortion of the modiolus with spontaneous fractures of the osseous partition between the basal and middle cochlear turn (Figs. 23 and 24).

Benign and malignant tumor formations were observed in several of our eight patients. In one, a localized proliferation of densely populated spindle cells was regarded as a fibroma. In two patients, a circumscribed proliferation of myelinated nerve fibers and Schwann cells arranged in interlacing fascicles were interpreted as neuromas (Fig. 25). These neuromas had developed in identical locations. One patient revealed a poorly differentiated spindle cell sarcoma originating in the hematopoietic marrow at the entrance to the left internal auditory meatus (Fig. 26). This tumor gave the impression of having a multicentric origin. Another patient disclosed multiple metastases in both tem-

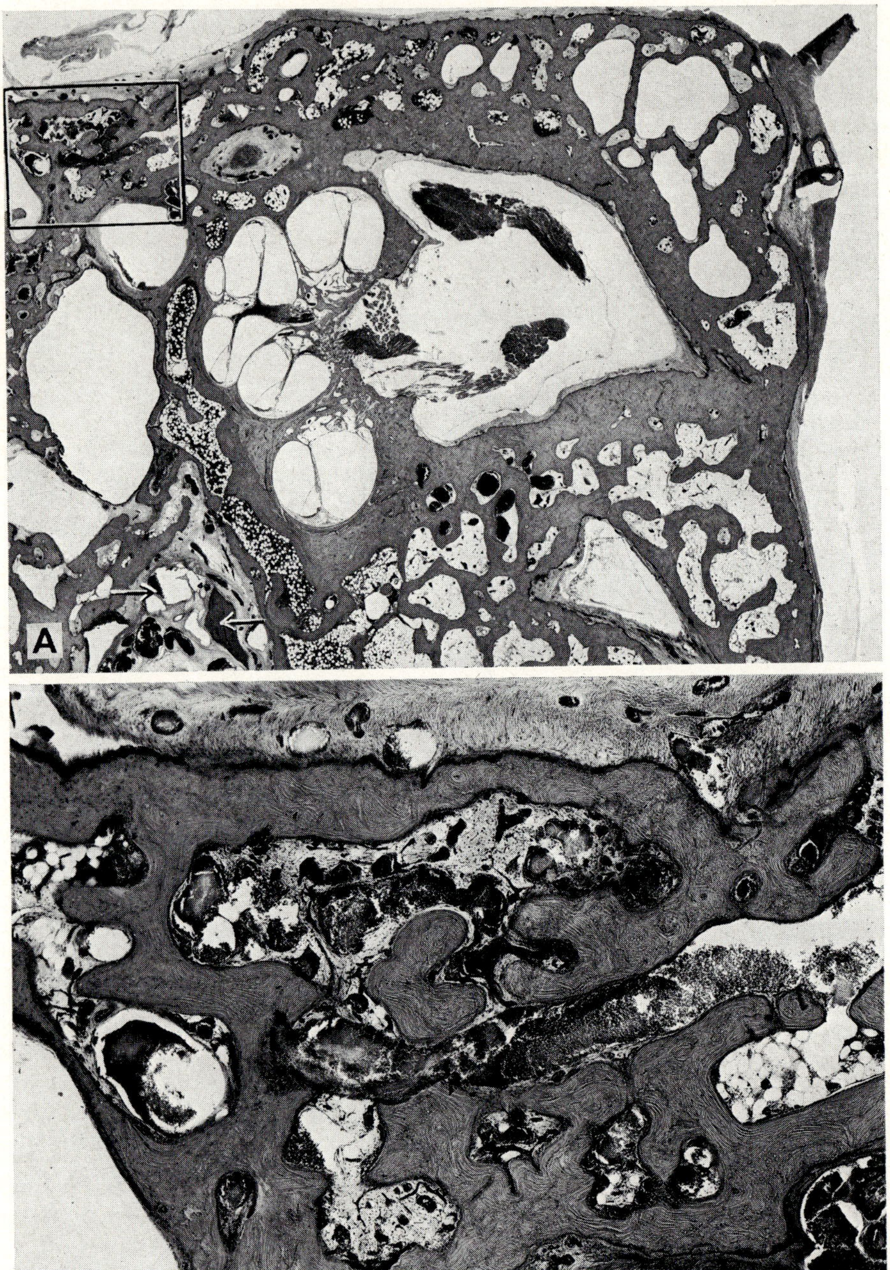

Fig. 16. A) Vertical, midmodiolar section through the right pyramid of the 78-year-old male (B.M.), displaying an increased blood flow and arteriovenous shunting in localized areas. (H. and E. stain; X8.) B) Same section; X40. Numerous arteries of varying caliber from the dura covering the tegmen near the tympanic orifice of the Eustachian tube enter the underlying bone, subdivide into smaller branches and contribute to a large venous lake, which eventually drains into the pericarotid venous plexus (arrows).

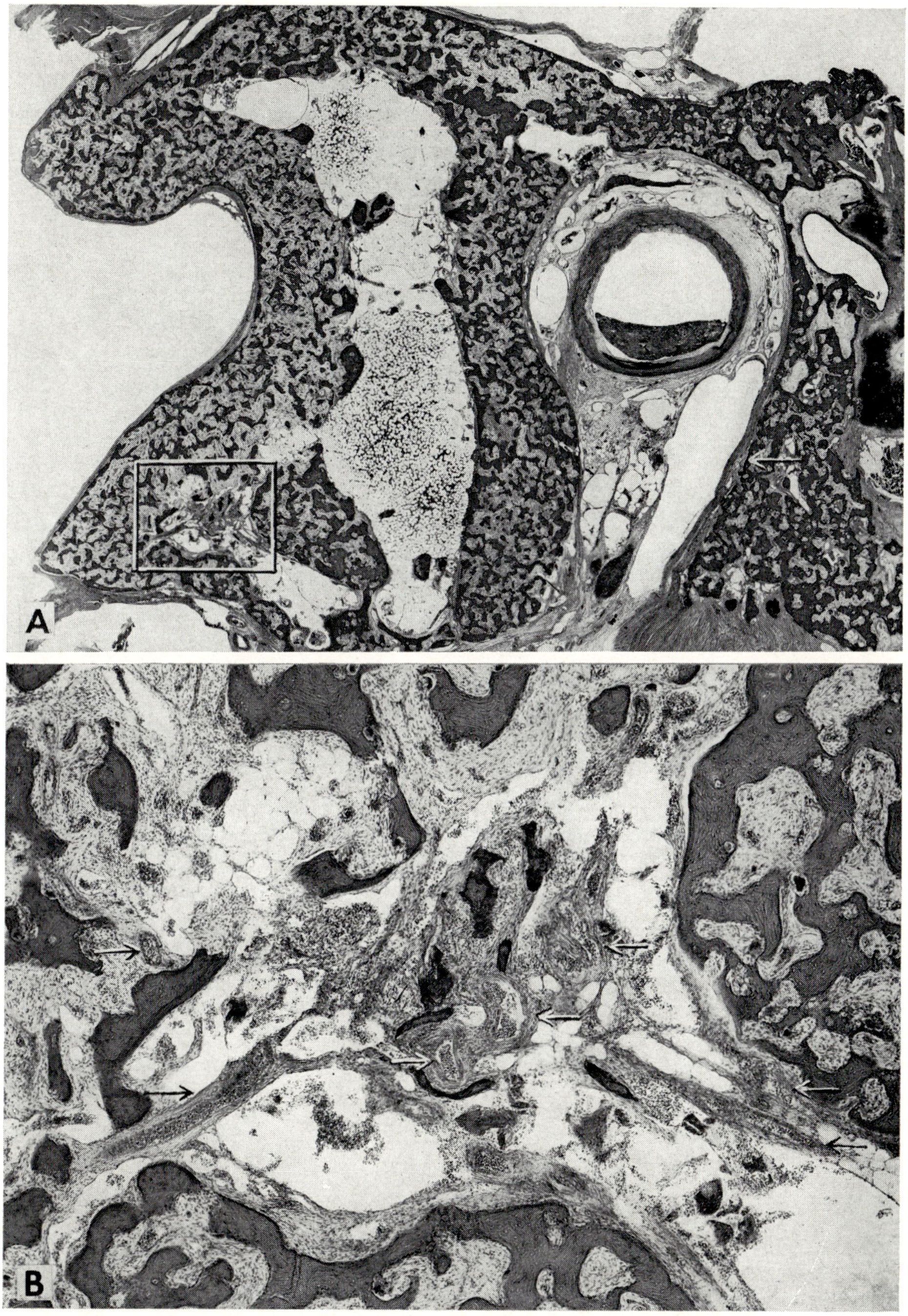

Fig. 17. A) Vertical section through the left pyramid near the anterior wall of the internal acoustic meatus of the 74-year-old female (S.M.) with extensive, active Pagetoid bone transformation. It reveals a vast area of former bone resorption, partially filled with adipose marrow and containing large venous channels and lakes. Note the enlargement of the pericarotid venous plexus (arrow). (H. and E. stain; X8.) B) Same section; X50. Numerous arteries of varying size (arrows), mainly from the dura, lining the neural compartment of the jugular foramen, enter the overlying petrous bone, ramify and shunt arterial blood across venous lakes into the pericarotid venous plexus.

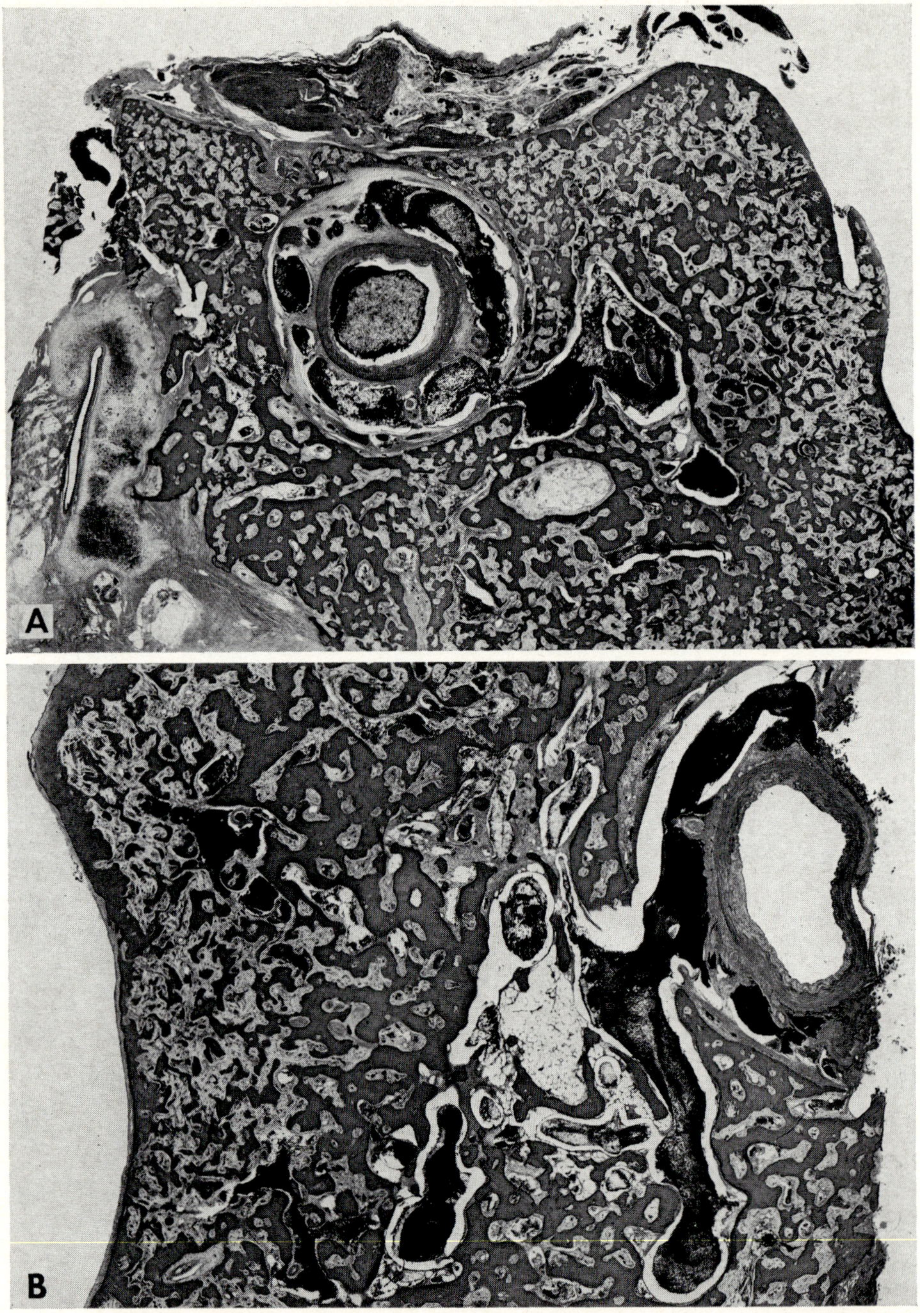

Fig. 18. A and B. Vertical sections through the right and left petrous apex of the 80-year-old female (M.V.) with extensive active Pagetoid remodeling. Large venous channels and lakes collecting blood from many areas of the pyramid are seen emptying into a markedly distended pericarotid venous plexus which in turn drains into an enormously enlarged internal jugular vein bilaterally. (H. and E. stain; X8 and 12.)

poral bones from an anaplastic carcinoma in the nasopharynx.

LITERATURE

The first and most comprehensive description of the morphological changes in the temporal bones of patients with osteitis deformans was provided by Mayer[12] in 1917. Nager and Meyer[13] confirmed many of the earlier observations in 1932. In subsequent decades, a vast literature has accumulated. It is well summarized in Davis's[11] excellent clinical and pathological review of 1968 on Paget's disease of the temporal bone. To this Lindsay and Lehman[14] added another valuable contribution.

Rüedi[15] in 1964, drew attention to the existence of shunts between the vascular network of an ostosclerotic process and the vessels in the adjoining spiral ligament. Such shunting was also observed between an otosclerotic lesion in the basal turn and the posterior spiral vein. He feels that these shunts cause venous congestion, and that persistent venous congestion may produce increasing damage to the inner ear. The sensorineural hearing loss in otosclerosis, in Rüedi's opinion, probably is the result of venous congestion produced by these shunts.

The striking morphological similarity between otosclerosis and osteitis deformans has long been recognized and was first described by Mayer[16] in 1913. In the search for an analogous phenomenon in Paget's disease, Rüedi[17] found the same shunts between the vascular network in Pagetoid bone and vessels in the adjacent cochlear modiolus and internal auditory canal. He postulates that these vascular connections may be responsible for the sensorineural hearing loss in Paget's disease.

Our communication is primarily concerned with the description of the morphological changes in Paget's disease. In so doing, it mentions a number of structural alterations, of which some can account for the conductive, and others for the sensorineural component of the hearing loss in osteitis deformans. However, it would be beyond the scope of this paper to elaborate or speculate on the actual mechanisms responsible for the sensorineural element which, in our opinion, still requires further clarification.

COMPLICATIONS

Cardiovascular disease ranks as the most common cause of death in advanced, wide-spread Paget's disease with several factors playing a contributing role. Limited ventilatory capacity resulting from the deformity of the thorax may increase cardiac output leading to right-sided hypertrophy and ultimately to right heart failure. In Paget's disease the incidence of arteriosclerosis, valvular disease and hypertension is increased. The augmentation of blood flow, the amount of arteriovenous shunting and the large venous sinuses alone can account for the rise in cardiac output.[18,19] The high level of serum alkaline phosphatase is a reflection of the ubiquitous osteoblastic activity.

One of the most tragic complications of osteitis deformans is the superimposition of a sarcoma, usually osteosarcoma, although in some instances fibrosarcomas, chondrosarcomas, and giant cell tumors have been reported. The reasons for this malignant transformation are not clear. The suggestion has been made that the exaggerated stromal and osseous activity encountered in Paget's disease might serve as the precursor of this malignant group of mesenchymal neoplasms.[20] In patients with advanced polyostotic disease the incidence of osteosarcoma may be about 10%. If all forms of Paget's disease are included, the frequency rate drops to .9%.[21] Although sarcoma is usually encountered in patients beyond the age of 50 and with polyostotic disease, it can occur in the monostotic form as well. The sites of sarcoma in patients with osteitis deformans, based on 250 observations, in decreasing frequency are: 1) the femur (31%); 2) the humerus (20%); 3) the pelvis (15%); 4) the tibia (11.2%); and 5) the skull and facial

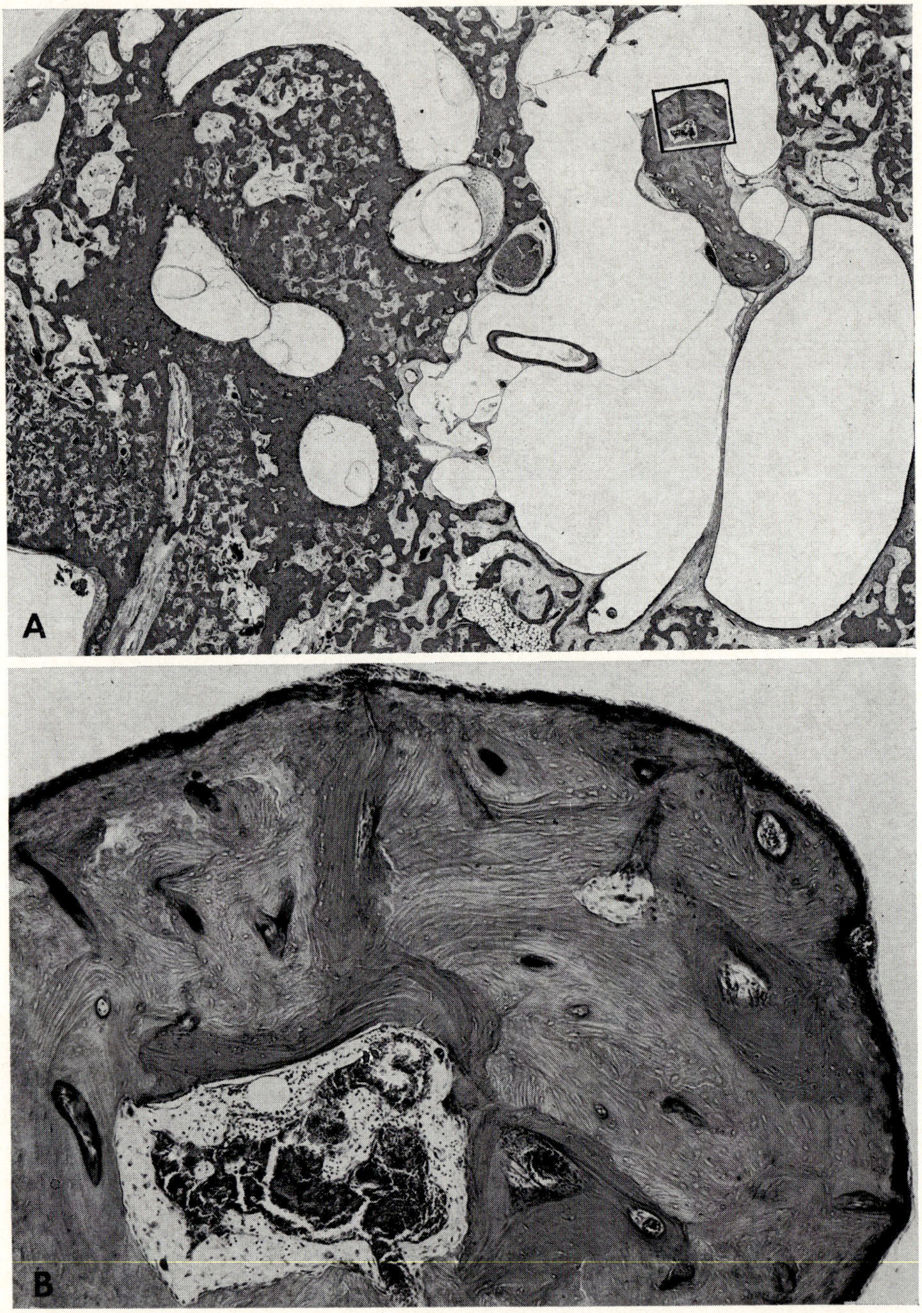

Fig. 19. A) Vertical section through the left petrous pyramid at the level of the head and neck of the malleus in a 74-year-old female (S.M.). The original bone of the pyramid and tympanic bone has been replaced by densely packed, narrow trabeculae of coarse-fibered Pagetoid bone. H. and E. stain; X9.). B) Same section; X110. The malleus reveals a characteristic mosaic pattern of osteitis deformans and a highly vascular fibrous bone marrow.

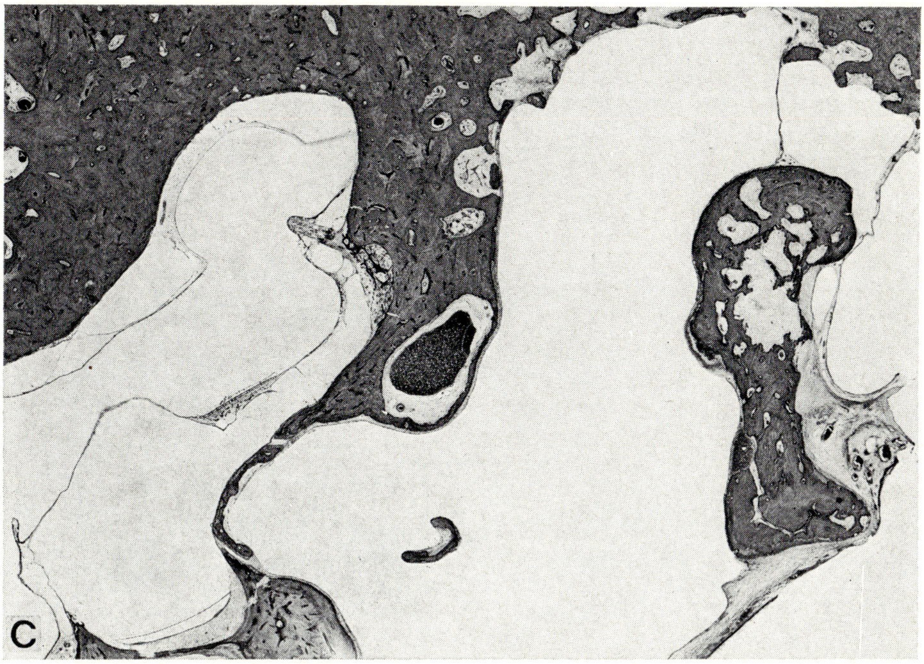

Fig. 19. C) Vertical sections through the left pyramid at the level of the malleus in the 80-year-old male (D-G. V.). The malleus head has been involved in recent bone resorption. An occasional osteoclast bears witness of still on-going bone destruction (H. and E. stain; X14.).

bones (10.8%), etc.[22] It is estimated that about 30% of patients eventually have sarcomatous involvement of multiple bones. Some investigators interpret these as metastases rather than multiple primary tumors. The prognosis of sarcoma arising in Paget's disease is very poor, with most patients dying within two years.[22]

ETIOLOGY AND HEREDITY

Little progress has been made in the search for an etiological factor since Sir James Paget's description of the disease in 1877.[23] Theories and hypotheses have been advanced describing osteitis deformans as a chronic, inflammatory, connective tissue, autoimmune, endocrine and metabolic, vascular, hereditary, and neoplastic disease. The hereditary nature of the disease appears to be established. The malady has been reported repeatedly in identical twins, in several siblings, and in several generations of numerous families.[1] While some investigators wonder whether or not heredity plays a significant role in osteitis deformans,[10] others are convinced that the disease is inherited either as a sex-linked recessive,[2] or, more likely, as a simple autosomal Mendelian dominant gene.[1] Pseudoxanthoma Elasticum (PXE), a definite disorder of connective tissue, is regularly associated with angioid streaks of the retina. The fact that PXE and angioid streaks, singly or in combination, are occasionally observed in patients with osteitis deformans, suggests the possibility that Paget's disease may be a more or less generalized abiotrophy of connective tissue.[1]

SUMMARY

1. Osteitis deformans Paget is a fairly common, sometimes progressive disease of bone, which affects primarily the axial skeleton and may lead to weakness and deformity. It may be considered as a heritable abiotrophy of the collagen matrix of bone.

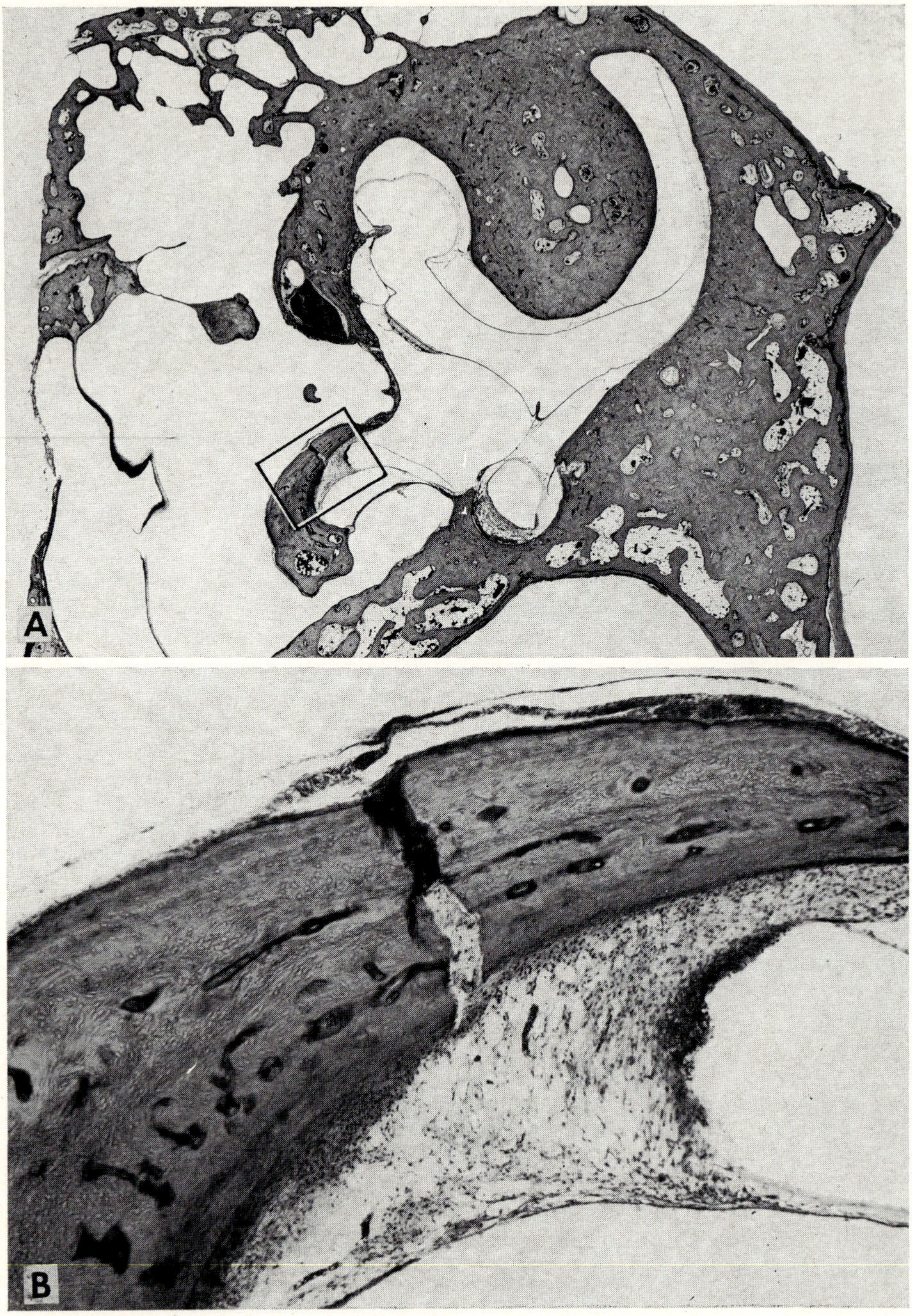

Fig. 20. A) Vertical section through the right pyramid at the level of the oval and round window in a 78-year-old male (B.W.). An older radial microfracture traverses the promontory. It extends from the middle ear surface to the base of the spiral ligament of the lower basal turn. (H. and E. stain; X8.). B) Same section; X80. The medial portion of the cleft is filled with connective tissue. In the lateral portion a callus of calcified connective tissue unites the two bony surfaces.

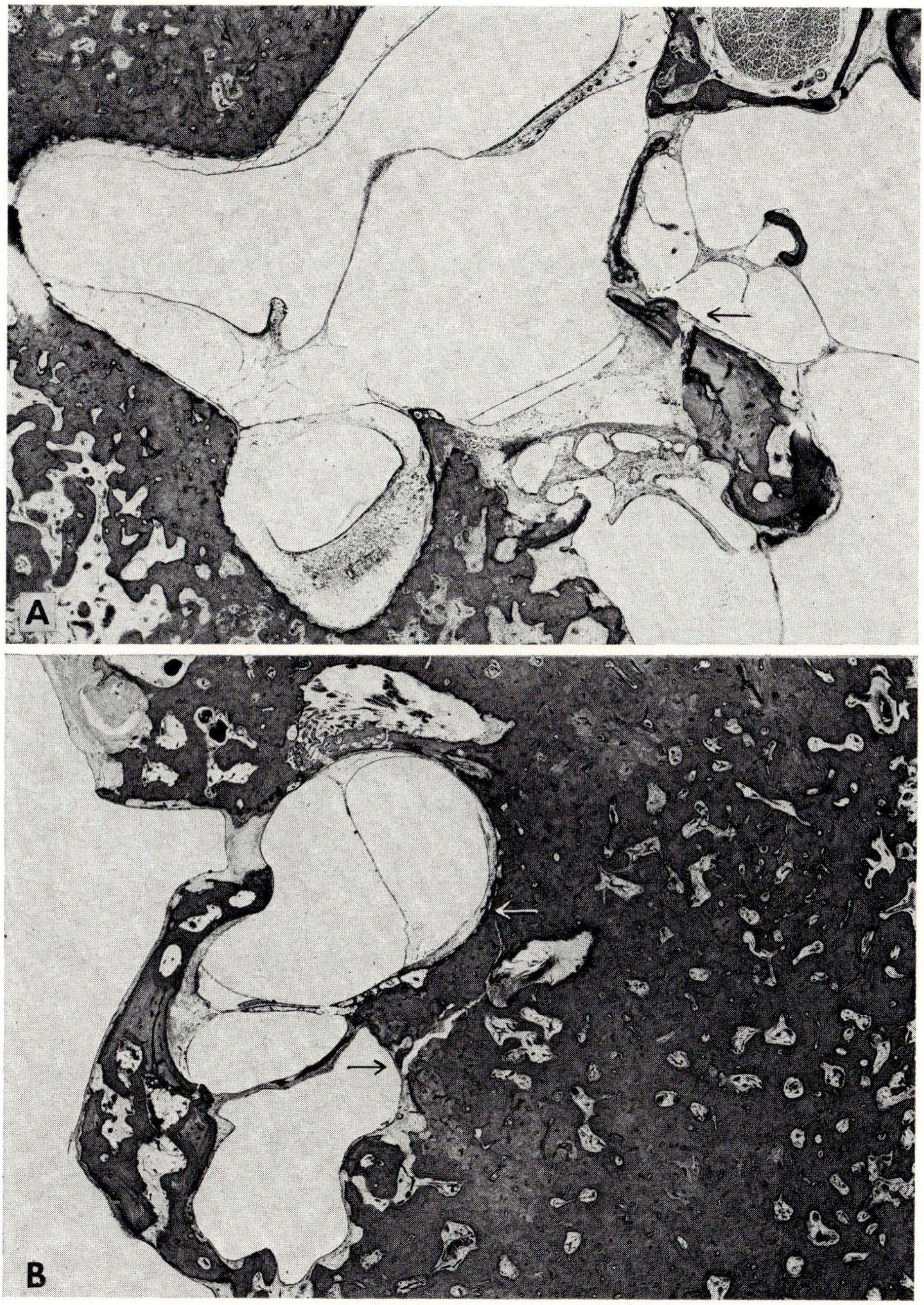

Fig. 21. A) Vertical section through the left pyramid at the level of the oval and round window in the 74-year-old female (S.M.). The radial microfracture below the inferior oval window margin is well recognized (arrow). (H. and E. stain; X20.) B) Vertical section through the right pyramid at the anterior end of the oval window in the 80-year-old male (D-G. V.). A microfracture extends from the medial wall of the round window niche, to the macula cribrosa of the saccule, and to the anterior medial wall of the vestibule (arrows). (H. and E. stain; X14.)

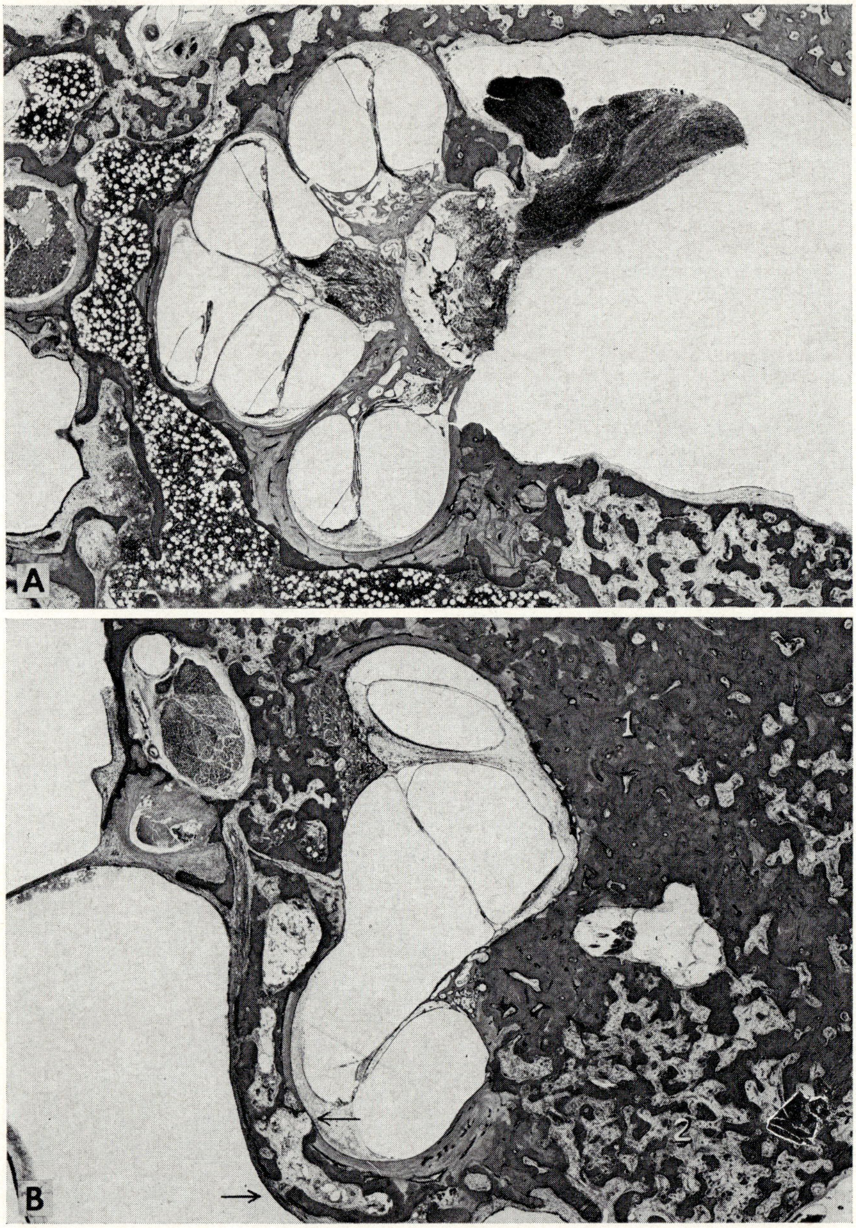

Fig. 22. A) Vertical midmodiolar section through the right pyramid of the 74-year-old female (S.M.). In the cochlear capsule, bone resorption predominated over new bone formation. As a result, almost the entire endochondral capsule layer has been destroyed and replaced by hematopoietic marrow. (H. and E. stain; X15.) B) Vertical section through the same temporal bone at the level of the fissura ante fenestram; X16. Areas of osteosclerosis, made of a dense, more regular and mature lamellar bone (1), and areas of osteoporosis, consisting of a loose newtork of irregular trabeculae of web-like and lamellar bone (2), are seen side by side. With bone resorption predominating in the cochlear capsule, the osteoclastic marrow extends in some areas from the mucoperiosteum of the middle ear to the base of the spiral ligament (arrows).

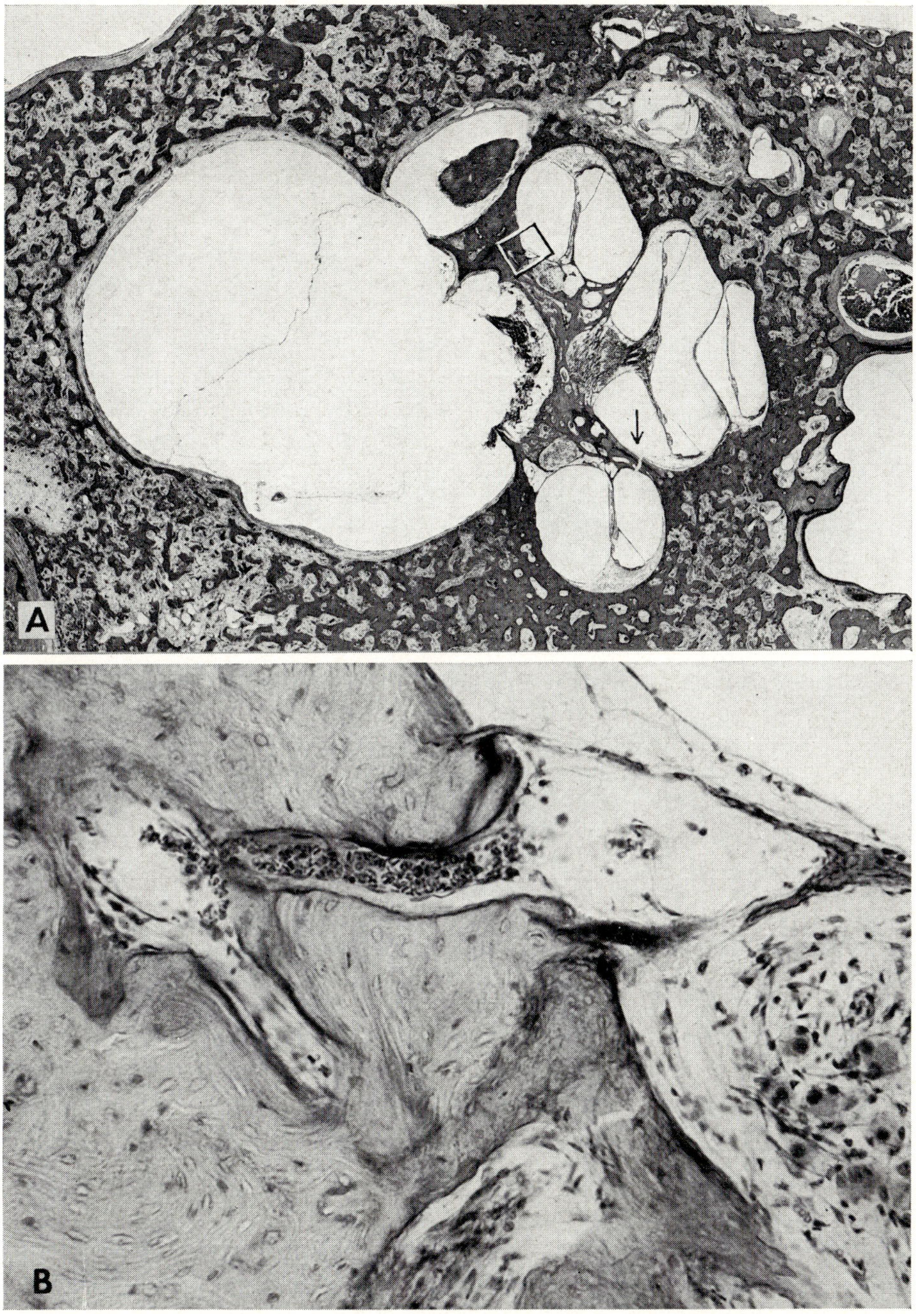

Fig. 23. A) Vertical, midmodiolar section through the left pyramid of the 74-year-old female (S.M.). Extensive Pagetoid remodeling caused obvious axial and radial distortion of the cochlear capsule, and a fracture of the osseous partition between the lower basal and the middle cochlear turn (arrow). (H. and E. stain; X12.) B) Same section; X300. Vascular shunt between the posterior spiral vein of the upper basal turn and a vein in the adjacent Pagetoid bone of the cochlear capsule.

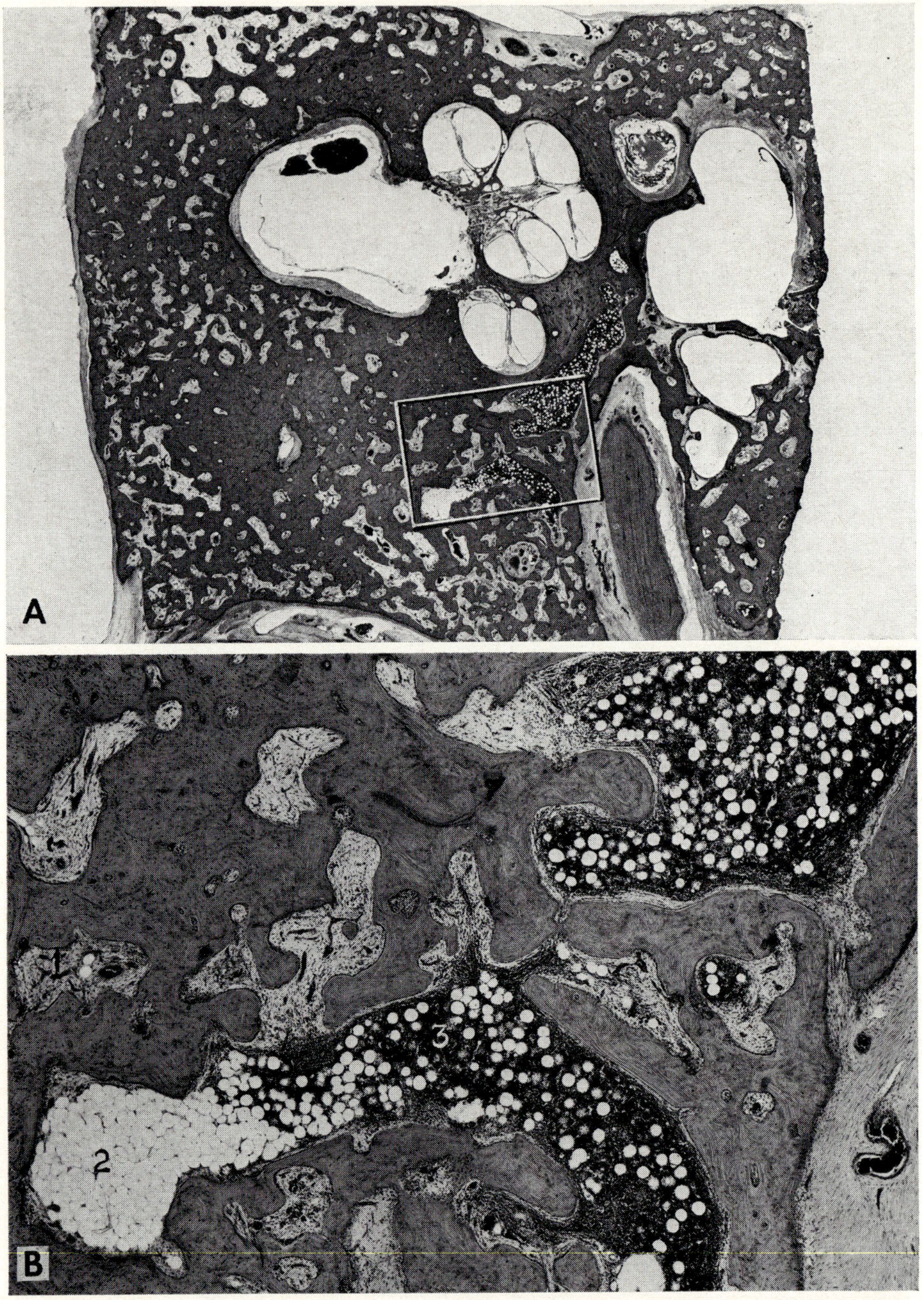

Fig. 24. A) Vertical, midmodiolar section through the left pyramid of the 80-year-old male (D-G. V.). It shows the different types of bone marrow encountered with the respective phases of Pagetoid bone transformation. (H. and E. stain; X7.) B) Same section; X35. In areas of active bone transformation, the marrow is made of a loose reticular, vascular connective tissue with a varying number of osteoclasts and osteoblasts (1). In areas where the remodeling process has come to a stand-still, the marrow has become adipose (2) or hematopoietic (3).

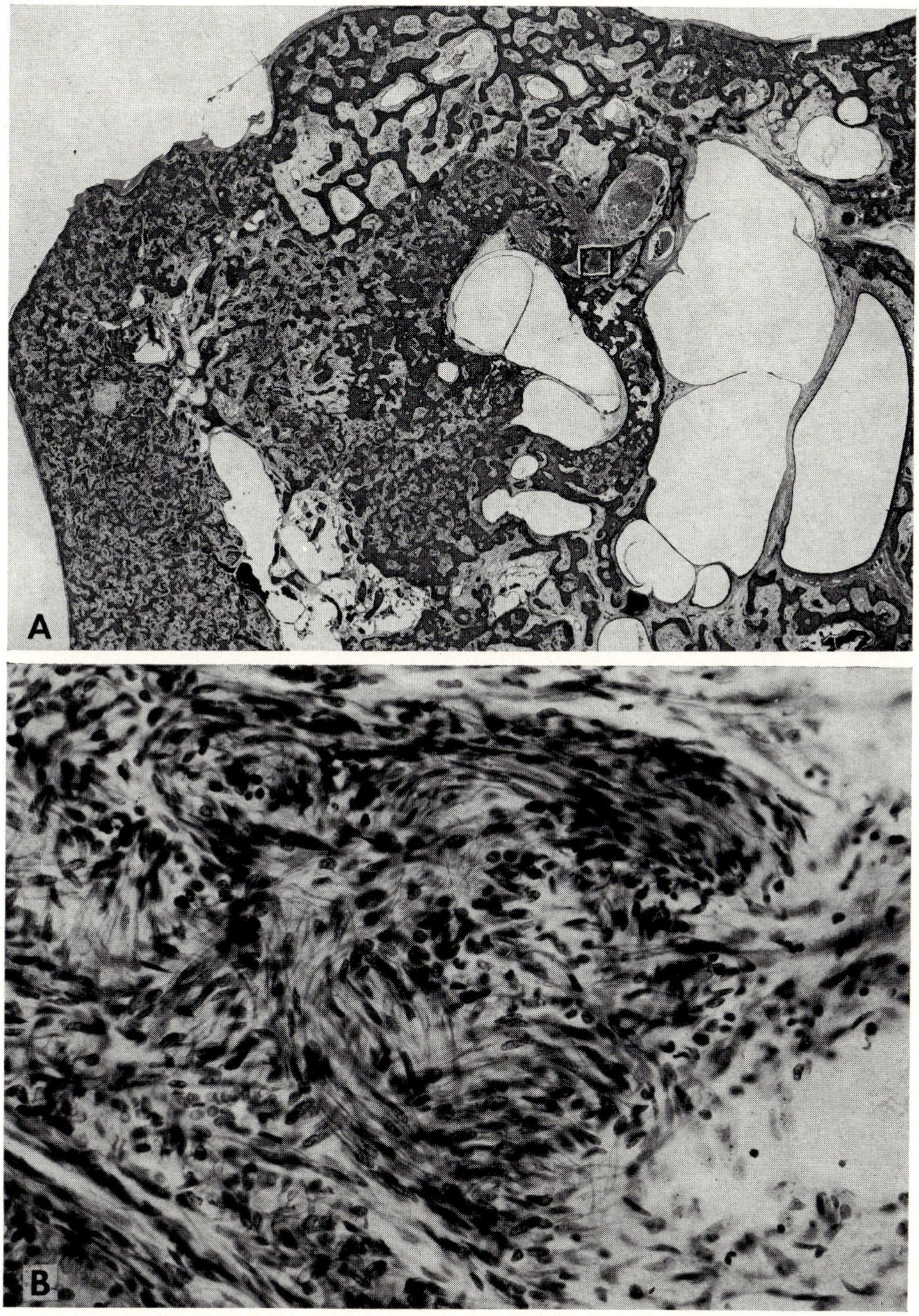

Fig. 25. A) Vertical section through the left pyramid near the anterior margin of the oval window to show the location of a neuroma in the 74-year-old female (S.M.). It is situated between the macula cribrosa of the utricle and the Fallopian canal. (H. and E. stain; X8.) B) Same section; X400. The tumor cells form interlacing bundles of long bipolar spindle cells with ovoid, rod-shaped, central nuclei containing variable amounts of chromatin and delicate fibers in parallel arrangement.

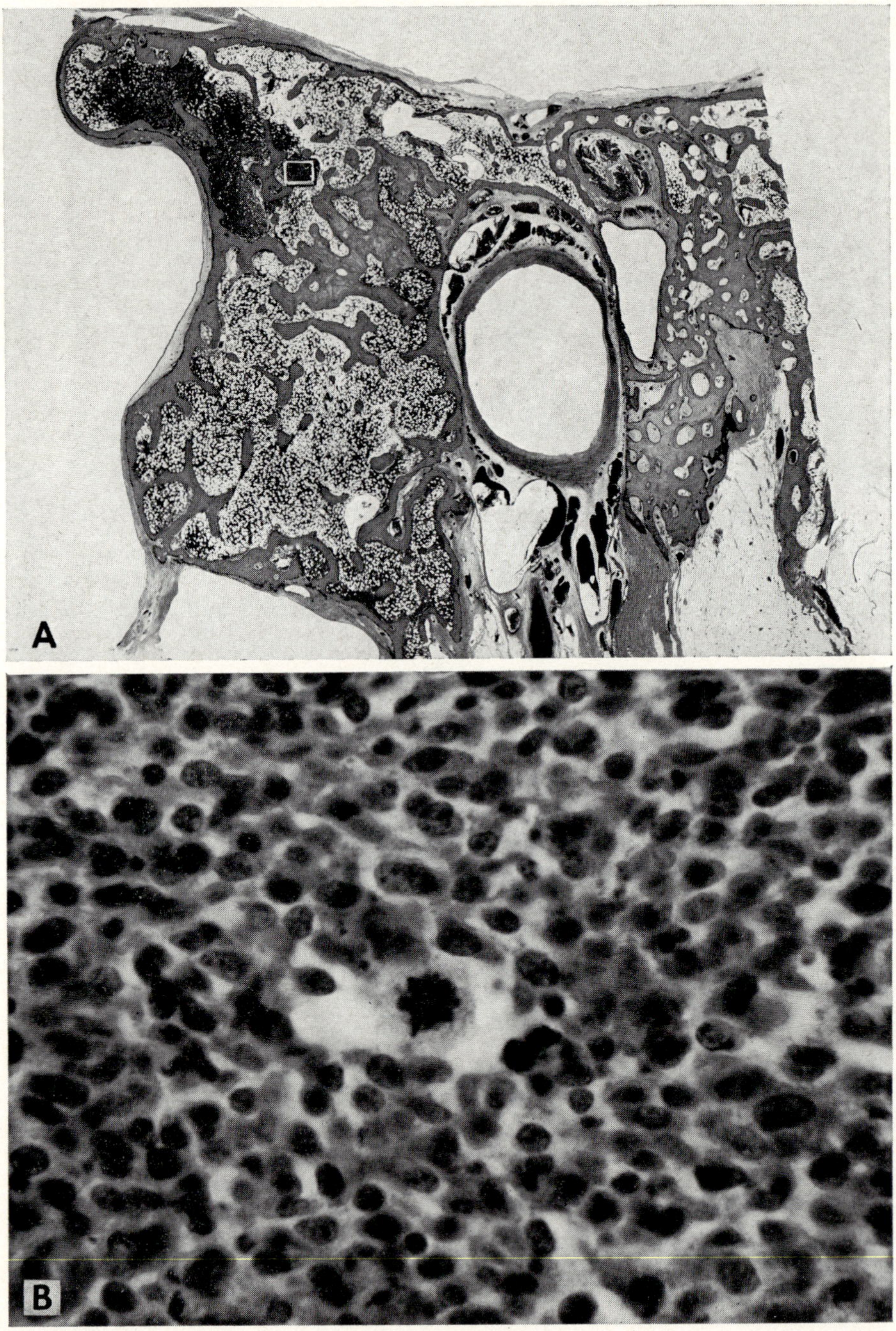

Fig. 26. A) Vertical section through the left petrous pyramid near the anterior wall of the internal acoustic meatus of the 78-year-old male (B.W.). A neoplasm which arises in the hematopoietic marrow is recognized near the porus acousticus. (H. and E. stain; X6½.) B) Same section; X750. The neoplasm has the features of a poorly differentiated spindle cell sarcoma.

2. It affects 3% of the population over forty years, and males more frequently than females.

3. Since it is more often an incidental finding, the large majority escapes clinical detection. Only 15% exhibit the advanced stage with deformity of the long bones, progressive kyphosis with shortening of stature, and enlargement of the skull.

4. Three phases may be recognized histologically: 1) an initial phase of osteoclastic resorption of existing bone; 2) a subsequent phase of osteoblastic regeneration of primitive bone; and 3) a final phase of "mosaic" bone replacing the original structure.

5. Progressive involvement of the temporal bone results in alteration of position, increase in size and change of architecture of the petrous pyramid, external canal, middle ear, and inner ear capsule. These structural changes in turn may produce impairment of hearing and vestibular disturbances.

6. Increase in size and number of blood vessels and extensive arteriovenous shunting are frequently encountered.

7. In Pagetoid bone remodeling, the exaggerated stromal and osseous activity may account for the development of benign and malignant neoplasms of mesenchymal and neural origin.

Request for reprints should be sent to George T. Nager, M.D., Department of Laryngology and Otology, The Johns Hopkins Hospital, 601 North Broadway, Baltimore, Maryland 21205.

ACKNOWLEDGMENT—Mr. Chester S. Reather, R.B.P., Director of the Photomicrography Laboratory, prepared the photographs.

REFERENCES

1. McKusick VA: *Heritable Disorders of Connective Tissues.* St. Louis, C.V. Mosby, 1972, pp 718-723

2. Ashley-Mongtague MF: Paget's disease (osteitis deformans) and heredity. Am J Hum Genet 1:94-95, 1947

3. Koller F: Über die Heredität der Ostitis deformans Paget. Helv Med Acta 13:389-400, 1946

4. Schmorl G: Üeber Ostitis deformans Paget. Virchows Arch 283:694-751, 1932

5. Collins DH: Paget's disease of bone. Incidence and subclinical forms. Lancet 2: 51-57, 1956

6. Hsu T-H: Personal communictaion

7. Kay HD, Simpson SL, Riddock G: Osteitis deformans. Arch Intern Med 53:208-247, 1934

8. Schüller A: Üeber circumscripte Osteoporosis des Schädels. Med Klin 25:631-632, 1929

9. Collins DH, Winn JM: Focal Paget's disease of the skull. (Osteoporosis circumscripta). J Pathol 69:1-9, 1955

10. Gutman AB, Kasabach H: Paget's disease (Osteitis deformans). Analysis of 116 cases. Am J Med Sci 191:361-380, 1936

11. Davis DG: Paget's disease of the temporal bone. Acta Otolaryngol [Suppl] (Stockh) 242:1-47, 1968

12. Mayer O: Untersuchungen über die Otosklerose. Wien, Alfred Hödler, 1917, pp 74-113

13. Nager FR, Meyer M: Die Erkrankung des Knochensystems und ihre Erscheinungen an der Innenhorkapsel des Menschen. Berlin, A.G. Karger, 1932, p 124

14. Lindsay JR, Lehman RH: Histopathology of the temporal bone in advanced Paget's disease. Laryngoscope 79:213-227, 1969

15. Rüedi L: Weitere histo-pathologische Veränderungen des Innenohres bei Otosklerose. Acta Otolaryngol (Stockh) 57: 236-245, 1964

16. Mayer O: (Wien) demonstriert die Mikrophotogramme von zwei Fällen von Otosklerose mit vier Schläfenbeinen. ZBL Ohrenheilk 11:530-531, 1913

17. Rüedi L: Are there cochlear shunts in Paget's Disease and von Recklinghausen's Disease? Acta Otolaryngol (Stockh) 65: 13-24, 1968

18. Edholm OG, Horwarth S, McMichael J: Heart failure and blood flow in osteitis deformans. Clin Sci 5:249-260, 1945

19. Edholm OG, Horwarth S: Studies on the peripheral circulation in osteitis deformans. Clin Sci 12:277-285, 1953

20. Spjut HJ, Dorfman HD, Fechner RE, *et al*: *Tumors of Bone and Cartilage.* Fasc.

5, Armed Forces Institute of Pathology, Washington, D.C., 1972

21. Porretta CA, Dahlin DC, James JM: Sarcoma in Paget's disease of bone. J Bone Joint Surg (Am) 39A:1314-1329, 1957

22. McKinna RJ, Schwinn CP, Soong KY, *et al*: Osteogenic sarcoma arising in Paget's disease. Cancer 17:42-66, 1964

23. Paget J: On a form of chronic inflammation of bones (Ostitis deformans). Med Chir Trans 60:37-63, 1877

FREQUENCY RESPONSES OF HEARING AIDS AND THEIR EFFECTS ON THE SPEECH PERCEPTION OF HEARING-IMPAIRED SUBJECTS

David Pedro Pascoe, Ph.D.

St. Louis, Missouri

From the Central Institute for the Deaf, 818 South Euclid Ave., St. Louis, Missouri.

This Supplement is an edited reproduction of the author's doctoral dissertation (Washington University, Saint Louis, Missouri, 1974) which was supported by Mr. G. H. Packwood, Jr., of Glencoe, Missouri, and by grant NS 03856 from the National Institute of Neurological Diseases and Stroke to Central Institute for the Deaf.

TABLE OF CONTENTS

Page

SECTION I. HEARING AID DESIGN – RATIONALE 5

SECTION II. DESCRIPTION OF SUBJECTS 9

Normally Hearing 9

Hard of Hearing 9

SECTION III. FIELD AUDIOMETRY 10

Unaided Field Thresholds 10

Aided Field Thresholds 14

SECTION IV. MEASUREMENTS OF WORD DISCRIMINATION 18

Word Lists 18

Preliminary Tests: Unaided Listening 19

First Experiment 20

Second Experiment 26

Supplementary Tests: Listening Through Commercial Hearing Aids 30

SECTION V. GENERAL DISCUSSION 31

Functional vs Coupler Gains 31

Relations Between Frequency Response and Discrimination Scores 31

Effects of Word List Type (HF vs PB) 34

Relations Between Hearing Levels and Discrimination Scores 34

SECTION VI. SUMMARY 36

SECTION VII. RECOMMENDATIONS 38

APPENDIX A. High-Frequency Word List (HF) 39

FREQUENCY RESPONSES OF HEARING AIDS AND THEIR EFFECTS ON THE SPEECH PERCEPTION OF HEARING-IMPAIRED SUBJECTS

DAVID PEDRO PASCOE, PH.D.

ST. LOUIS, MISSOURI

SUMMARY – Eight hearing-impaired subjects were tested with a binaural master hearing aid. This aid has "on-the-head" miniature transducers and has an adjustable frequency response. Five frequency responses were used, two of them were defined by their response in a 2-cm^3 coupler: 1) uniform coupler gain (UCG), and 2) 6 dB per octave rise (6 dB). The other responses were defined in terms of functional gain (difference between unaided and aided thresholds): 3) uniform functional gain (UFG); 4) uniform hearing level (UHL); and 5) a simulation of a commercial hearing aid (AS). A significant difference between coupler and functional gain was seen. Discrimination was tested with a special closed-set word list which includes fifty monosyllabic words with a high percentage of voiceless phonemes. Discrimination scores were consistently better with the UHL response. The lowest scores were obtained with the AS response. The average difference in scores between these two responses was 18.4%. Further testing replicated these results and also compared the effects of a different type of word list phonetically balanced (PB); with these lists, the above-mentioned difference in scores was smaller in quiet (5.9%) but larger in noise (20.9%).

SECTION I

HEARING AID DESIGN – RATIONALE

Recent research has shown that an experimental hearing aid can be assembled that is significantly superior to standard hearing aids when tested under laboratory conditions. This superiority is defined in terms of improvement in the listener's word-discrimination scores.[1] The experimental aid has on-the-head miniature transducers and a frequency response that compensates for: 1) the loss, resulting from the use of earmolds, of external-ear resonances and normal head diffraction; 2) head-diffraction effects related to the position of the hearing-aid microphone; and 3) the subject's high-frequency hearing loss.

The investigation that led to the development of the aid used a master hearing aid with a variable frequency response. Many alternative responses were tested to search for optimum discrimination scores. The response that consistently accompanied the highest scores had characteristics which simulated the normal field-to-eardrum transfer function,[2] and gave an extra boost (10 to 15 dB) to the frequencies above 4 kHz. The alterations to this response that were most effective in reducing the word-discrimination scores were concentrated within the frequency range from 2.5 to 6.3 kHz. Gain reductions of 20 dB at either end of this band (2.5 to 3.1 kHz and 5.0 to 6.3 kHz) lowered the discrimination scores by 12%, while a similar reduction of the entire band (2.5 to 6.3 kHz) lowered the scores by 24%.

That investigation was guided by the notion that the normal field-to-eardrum transfer function plays an important role in speech reception.[3] The results, in spite of representing only one subject, supported this idea. Furthermore, they showed that important information could be given to this particular listener by boosting the frequencies between 4.0 and 6.3 kHz.

The capacity to receive valuable information from speech frequencies higher than 4.0 kHz is a challenge to a long-standing premise in hearing-aid design and manufacture. Both the Harvard Report[4] and the British Report[5] stated that frequencies above 4.0 kHz were unimportant because they did not contribute enough to the word discrimination of hard-of-hearing subjects to warrant the expense of including them within the frequency response of hearing aids.

Both the Harvard and the British reports described research done with equipment and under conditions that do not relate to the use of modern hearing aids. They used over-the-ear phones which preserved some of the resonances of the external ear while hearing aids usually require earmolds that eliminate these resonances. Furthermore, they placed their microphones close to the talkers, a factor which differs greatly from the on-the-head configuration of today's aids. In spite of these differences, their results regarding the relative unimportance of the higher frequencies have not been adequately reinvestigated.

The effects of frequency-response variations in hearing aids have been tested.[6-8] These studies confirmed the idea that changes in frequency response produce unimportant or unmeasurable differences in word discrimination, thus partially supporting the previous findings. Others have concluded that although only minor improvements in discrimination can be measured, the listener's preference is sufficient to establish the importance of frequency-response alterations,[9] while still others have shown that bandwidth is correlated with speech discrimination.[10] However, in all of these studies, bandwidths were limited to those of the available commercial aids. The possibility that frequencies above 4 kHz can give important information to the hard-of-hearing listener was not tested.

This review suggests three important questions: 1) Does the restoration of the normal field-to-eardrum transfer function improve word discrimination? 2) Is the restoration of the normal shape of the audibility curve (uniform hearing level at all frequencies) beneficial to hard-of-hearing listeners? 3) Can speech discrimination be improved by an extension of the present narrow-band response in hearing aids when the above-mentioned compensations are included?

These questions are all related to the effects that frequency characteristics of hearing aids have on the word discrimination of hard-of-hearing listeners, and the answers to these questions are the main objectives of this investigation.

Since commercial hearing aids are limited in their high-frequency response, the master aid mentioned previously was used again on a larger group of subjects. Although this aid has a variable response and considerable gain in frequencies as high as 6.3 kHz, it retains some of the features of commercial aids in that its receivers (earphones) are of the insert type and require earmolds. Its miniature microphones are worn on the head and they, as well as the receivers, are components designed for commercial hearing aids.

Five frequency responses were selected that would be useful in the search for answers to the stated questions. These responses will be described later.

Evaluation of the value of high-frequency sounds to hearing-aid users requires determining whether the energy at those frequencies is really being heard. It is not sufficient to base assumptions of presumed sensation on standard measurements of frequency response made in 2-cm^3 couplers because these measurements are known to differ significantly from functional measurements made in human ears.[11-15]

For 30 years, coupler measurements have been preferred in defining hearing-aid response over other procedures, such as probe-tube measurements and subjective comparisons of loudness, because coupler measurements have been considered easier and more reliable, and because the acoustic factors responsible for their lack of "reality" have been considered "extrinsic" to the hearing aid.[16,17]

These extrinsic acoustic factors are well known and have been studied extensively: 1) the effects of outer-ear resonances and normal head diffraction have been shown to amplify the high-frequency region[2,11] and thus alter the long-term average spectrum of speech when measured at the eardrum;[18] 2) the difference in impedance between the 2-cm^3 coupler and the human ear has been measured repeatedly but with conflicting results;[11,14,19-24] 3) the effects of head diffraction and microphone placement have been explored diligently but without definitive answers;[25-28] and finally, 4) earmold parameters have been shown to be important variables controlling the sound delivered to the eardrum.[19,29-32]

The combined effect of all these hard-to-measure variables has to be determined in order to know whether a variation in frequency emphasis or in bandwidth significantly alters the listener's ability to detect sounds. This was accomplished by measuring the total effect, as revealed by the difference in decibels between unaided and aided thresholds. This difference is referred to as "functional gain."

Since the principal purpose of this investigation is to describe the relations between frequency response and word-discrimination performance, each of these elements must be clearly defined and carefully measured.

Definition and Measurement of Frequency Response. All frequency responses were measured both in a type HA-2, 2-cm^3 coupler (ANSI, S 3.3-1960) and by the functional gain they produced. Five frequency responses were selected for testing. Of these, two were based on coupler definitions: a uniform (flat) response and one rising at 6 dB per octave increase in frequency. Two more were individually adjusted to produce specific types of aided thresholds: an aided threshold curve which is parallel to the unaided one (equal functional gain at all frequencies or "uniform functional gain"), and an aided threshold curve which is parallel to the normal audibility curve ("uniform hearing level"). These four responses have wide bandwidths when defined by the bandwidth of the master aid (0.1 to 6.3 kHz). A fifth response was chosen to simulate the functional gain given by a typical commercial hearing aid ("aid simulation") and it was identical for all eight subjects.

Measurement of Word-discrimination Performance. A basic feature of this investigation was the use of a procedure suggested by J. D. Miller.[33] Different randomizations of the same fifty words were assigned to various listening conditions, each of which included a frequency response, a talker, and a signal-to-noise ratio. Only ten words were heard in each listening condition per session, thus requiring five sessions to complete each test. The sequence of conditions was changed after every session, following a modified latin-square rotation, so that no listening condition was fully tested before any other one. In this manner, the possibility that effects related to list difficulty or to sequence (fatigue, learning, session variability) could be confounded with other variables of interest was greatly diminished.

More specific descriptions of these procedures, the equipment, and the results are presented in the following sections.

Section II is a short description of the subjects.

In Section III the field audiometry done to measure the subjects' hearing is described. The first part of this section deals with the unaided thresholds. The second part presents the results of aided tests, describes the functional gains obtained with each frequency response, and compares these functional gains to the 2-cm^3 coupler measurements.

Section IV deals with word discrimination tests. Here the scores obtained by each subject and the group means are compared to evaluate the effectiveness of the frequency responses. Comparisons are also made of the score differences related to the talker, the signal-to-noise ratio, and the type of word list used.

Section V is a general discussion in which the interrelations and implications of the various measurements and findings are presented.

The findings, conclusions, and recommendations flowing from this investigation are summarized in Sections VI and VII.

SECTION II

DESCRIPTION OF SUBJECTS

NORMALLY HEARING

Twenty young adults (19 to 24 years of age) with pure-tone thresholds between 0 and 10 dB HL (ANSI, S 3.6-1969) were tested to provide normal reference levels.

HARD OF HEARING

Eight adult hard-of-hearing subjects (55 to 75 years of age) were selected from the Central Institute for the Deaf (C.I.D.) Hearing Clinic files. Their average hearing levels at 0.5, 1, and 2 kHz were between 30 and 60 dB and the average slope of their audiometric curves (0.25 to 6.0 kHz) did not exceed +10 dB per octave. Their discrimination scores on the Rush-Hughes version of the PB-50 test* ranged from 48 to 78%, with a mean score of 57.6%. Except for one subject, they had similar hearing in both ears.

These subjects had all been seen by otolaryngologists and had been told that there was no medical treatment or surgery that would improve their hearing. All of them had normal hearing in their youth and had experienced a gradual change in hearing acuity.

All but one had used hearing aids for at least three years. All the aid users reported some degree of satisfaction when they used their aids in quiet conditions. However, in noisy conditions their aids seemed to add only to the confusion. Their greatest difficulty, as far as hearing is concerned, was the lack of clarity in the speech they hear.

These subjects were chosen because their hearing and age characteristics were similar to those of the one subject tested previously.[1]

---

*Technisonic Studios, St. Louis, Mo.

SECTION III

FIELD AUDIOMETRY

UNAIDED FIELD THRESHOLDS

STIMULUS AND CALIBRATION

The output of a noise generator* was fed into a multifilter** with independently controlled gains in contiguous third-octave bands at center frequencies from 0.2 to 6.3 kHz. These bands were used as external inputs to a Békésy audiometer.*** With this audiometer set on its discrete-frequency mode, with a pulsed-signal output, and with the +20 dB setting, the output (appropriately loaded) was fed into a power amplifier**** and finally into a loudspeaker.***** A block diagram of this equipment is given in Figure 1.

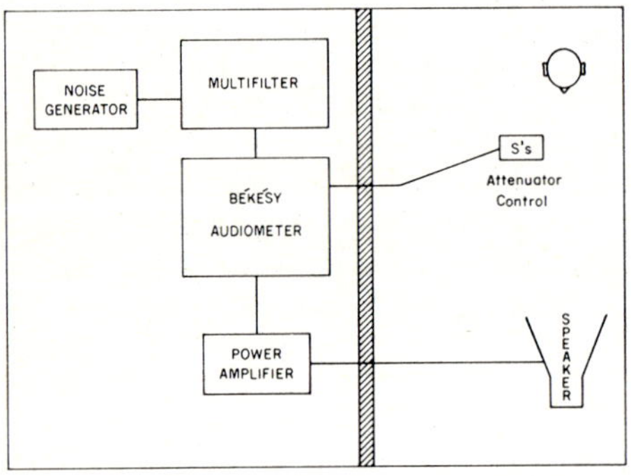

Fig. 1. Block diagram of the equipment used for the field-threshold tests.

Calibration of the noise bands was as follows. A condenser microphone****** was placed at the presumed center of the listener's head (listener absent), facing the loudspeaker, and an audio spectrometer†††**** was used to measure the root mean square (RMS) band levels. With the audiometer's automatic attenuator set at 70 dB sound pressure level (SPL) on its paper chart, the band levels were equalized to 70 dB SPL (±0.5 dB) by adjusting the multifilter. The calibration of the attenuator in the Békésy audiometer was verified acoustically down to 20 dB SPL and electrically down to the equivalent of 0 dB SPL.

TESTING ROOM

Field tests were carried out in a 4 x 4 m sound treated room (C.I.D. Hearing Clinics, Lab II). The ambient noise levels in this room were lower than 30 dB(A) and about 40 dB(C).

PROCEDURES

A subject sat approximately 2.5 m away from a loudspeaker and directly facing it, as shown in Figure 1. He was given typical Békésy-test instructions, and he controlled the level of the pulsed-noise signals until six relatively stable threshold crossings were completed for each third-octave band. The mean of the midpoints between each peak-to-peak tracing was designated as his threshold. The presentation of the noise bands was always started with the band centered at 0.2 kHz and followed progressively with each subsequent third-octave band until sixteen bands were tested (0.2 to 6.3 kHz). The sequence of the tests (binaural, monaural right, and monaural left) was changed from subject to subject. The monaural con-

----

*Model 455-C, Grason-Stadler Co., Inc., Concord, Mass.

**Type 1925, General Radio Co., Concord, Mass.

***Type E-800, Grason-Stadler Co., Inc., Concord, Mass.

****Dynakit Mark III, Dyna Co., Philadelphia, Pa.

*****Model KLH-6, Research Development Corp., Cambridge, Mass.

******Model 4131, B and K Instruments, Inc., Cleveland, Ohio.

†††****Type 2112, B and K Instruments, Inc., Cleveland, Ohio.

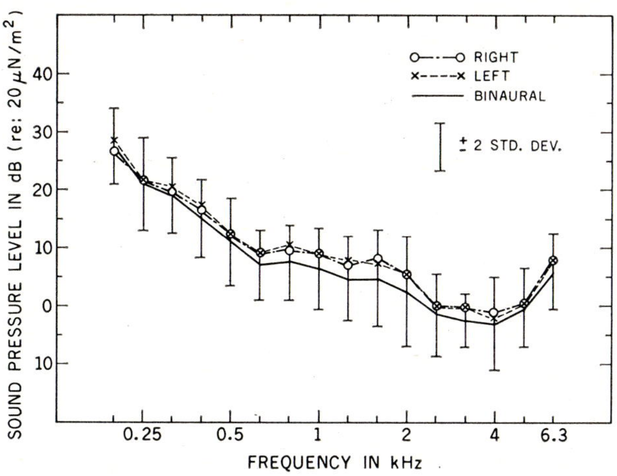

Fig. 2. Monaural and binaural minimum audible fields, means of twenty normally-hearing subjects. (Stimulus: Third octave bands of noise, centered at stated frequencies.)

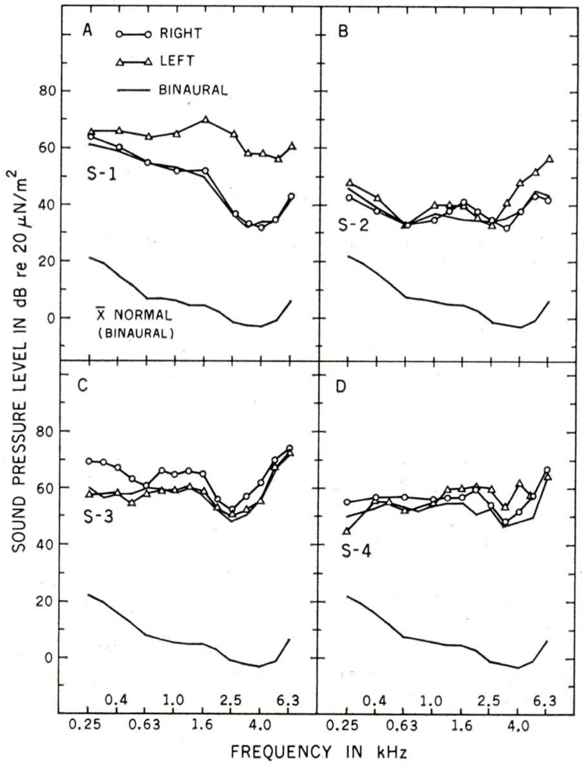

Fig. 3. Monaural and binaural minimum audible fields, individual results of four hard-of-hearing subjects. (Stimulus: Third octave bands of noise, centered at stated frequencies.)

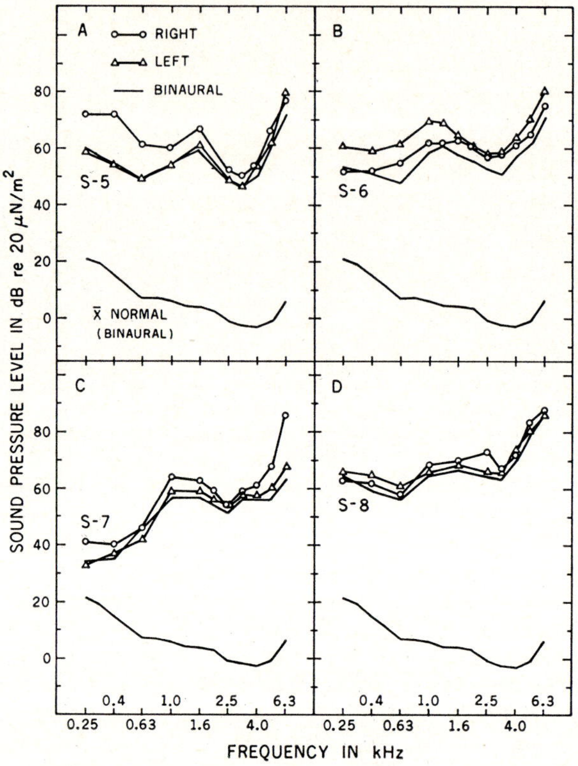

Fig. 4. Monaural and binaural minimum audible fields, individual results of four hard-of-hearing subjects. (Stimulus: Third octave bands of noise, centered at stated frequencies.)

dition was achieved by placing an earplug and an earmuff on the untested ear.

RESULTS

Normally-hearing Subjects. The average third-octave band levels at threshold for right, left, and binaural conditions are shown in Figure 2. The two sets of monaural thresholds are practically identical, while the binaural thresholds are lower by about 3 dB at most frequencies. The mean standard deviation for the binaural thresholds was 3.5 dB, ranging from 4.7 dB at 2 kHz to 2.2 dB at 3.15 kHz.

When these thresholds were compared to Sivian and White's[34] binaural minimum audible fields (MAFs) for pure tones at 0° incidence, they were found to be in good agreement (± 3 dB for frequencies above 0.5 kHz) when the difference between third-octave bandwidth and critical bandwidth[35] was taken into account. At frequencies below 0.5 kHz the difference was greater, reaching 9 dB at 0.2 kHz, probably due to greater ambient noise levels in this testing environment.

The average binaural levels were used as the 0 dB hearing-level reference in plotting the "field audiograms" of the hard-of-hearing subjects.

Hard-of-hearing Subjects. The field thresholds of the individual hearing-impaired subjects are shown in Figures 3 and 4. Each graph includes the normal reference as well as the monaural and binaural thresholds of each subject. The subjects are numbered in the order of their "adjusted hearing levels." This will be defined later.

The binaural unaided thresholds, plotted in terms of hearing level (re:

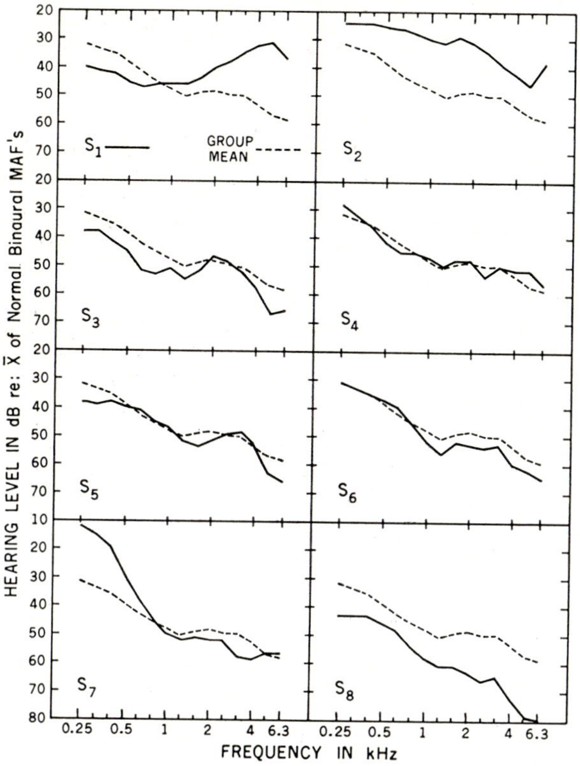

Fig. 5. Binaural field audiograms of eight hard-of-hearing subjects. (Stimulus: Third octave bands of noise, centered at stated frequencies.)

average of normal binaural thresholds) are shown in Figure 5. These binaural audiograms are shown again in Figure 6, where they appear superimposed. These curves match the subjects' clinical pure-tone audiograms (re: ANSI, 1969), with deviations no greater than 10 dB.

The width of the Békésy tracings produced by the subjects during these tests varied from session to session. At no time, however, did any of the subjects display abnormally narrow tracings, such as may appear when recruitment is present.[36]

Adjusted Hearing Levels. In order to describe these audibility curves in terms of average hearing levels, and since the usual hearing-level average ($\bar{X}$HL of 0.5, 1, and 2 kHz) did not differentiate adequately among curves of different slope, a system that includes the slope factor was devised. This adjusted hearing level (AHL), was defined as the average of binaural field thresholds at 2, 2.5, 3.1 and 4 kHz, plus the difference between this average and that of thresholds at 0.5, 0.63, 0.8 and 1 kHz. Thus, the average level of the high band was taken as the main descriptor, and the difference between the high and low bands as a correction for slope. This definition can be formulated in this manner:

$$\text{AHL} = 2\,\bar{X}_{\text{high band}} - \bar{X}_{\text{low band}}$$

It is evident that when the two band averages are equal, as in a "flat" audiogram, the AHL is simply the mean of the high band. An exception was made for the "rising" audiograms, such as S-1 in Figure 5: the difference in band levels was disregarded and this curve was treated as though it were "flat." These are the dB values given by both systems:

Subjects:	1	2	3	4	5	6	7	8
$\bar{X}$ HL:	43.6	28.6	48.0	45.6	46.3	47.3	43.6	55.6 dB
A HL:	36.3	46.2	52.5	57.7	58.8	65.3	67.9	81.7 dB

Notice that under the average HL system, curves 1 and 7 have identical dB values, while under the AHL system they are shown to be very different. Figure 5 shows how different these two curves really are. The measurements of correlation between AHL and discrimination will be shown later.

AIDED FIELD THRESHOLDS

EQUIPMENT

The hard-of-hearing subjects were tested under several aided conditions. Both the equipment and the procedures were identical to those used for the unaided tests, except for the use of two types of hearing aids.

Commercial Hearing Aids. Aided thresholds were obtained with the subjects' own hearing aids. Seven of these subjects had used hearing aids for at least three years. The eighth subject was tested with a commercial loaner aid. All of the aids were worn on the head, three being "eye-glass" aids, one a "within-the-ear" aid, and four "behind-the-ear" units. Three of the latter were "directional," that is, they had double-entry-port, phase-cancelling microphones. All of the aids were in good condition and functioning to published specifications.

The earmolds used with the aids were of various types, none of them being full standard size. Three subjects used vented molds. In general, it can be said that the molds were representative of those that are presently being prescribed by hearing-aid dealers.

The threshold tests made with these aids were used to derive a "typical" functional gain given by commercial on-the-head aids which could then be simulated by the master aid.

Master Hearing Aid. A block diagram of the previously described master aid[1] is shown in Figure 7. Two miniature mi-

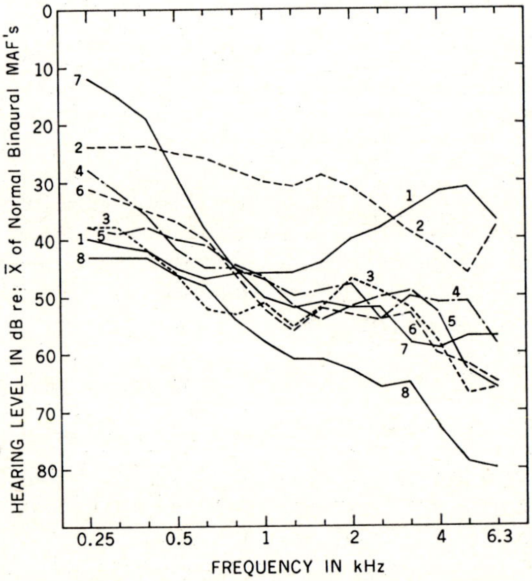

Fig. 6. Superimposed binaural field audiograms of eight hard-of-hearing subjects. (Stimulus: Third octave bands of noise, centered at stated frequencies.)

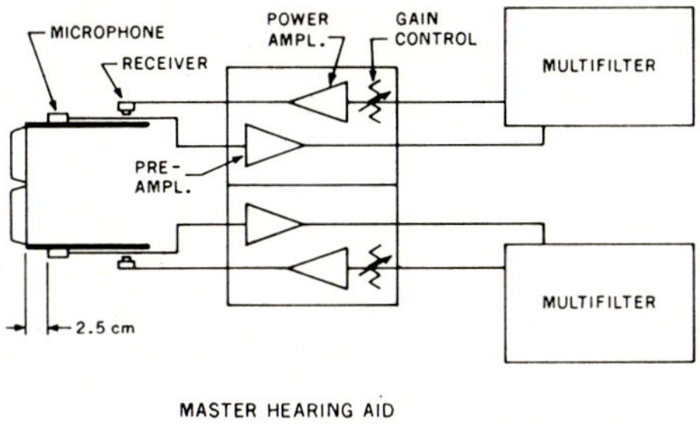

Fig. 7. Block diagram of the master hearing aid.

crophones* were mounted on the bows of safety eye glasses, 2.5 cm back from the hinges. Their independent outputs were fed into AC-powered preamplifiers and then into GR multifilters. These two multifilters serve to vary the frequency response of each channel. Their outputs, after further amplification, are finally fed into insert receivers.** The receivers are plugged into standard size, unvented earmolds, made for each subject.

The maximum output of this aid, limited by peak clipping, does not exceed 124 dB SPL at any one frequency. It is capable of providing a flat response from 0.1 to 6.3 kHz in the 2-cm^3 coupler without any subjectively detectable distortion. Within this frequency range, the multifilters can vary the frequency response within a ± 25 dB range at any third-octave band, except for the limitations imposed by the filter skirts. Over the range of settings of the volume control used in these experiments, with speech-noise input the signal-to-noise ratio at the aid's output was 36 dB.

FREQUENCY RESPONSES

Five frequency responses on the master aid were used to establish aided thresholds for each ear. These responses were: 1) uniform in the coupler (UCG); 2) rising at a 6 dB/octave slope in the coupler (6 dB); 3) adjusted individually to provide equal or uniform functional gain (UFG); 4) adjusted individually to produce a uniform hearing level (UHL), that is, an aided audibility curve which is parallel to normal; and 5) a single simulation of a commercial aid, selected to provide functional gains similar to those obtained by the subjects with their own aids (AS). All of these responses used the entire frequency range allowed by the master aid, except for the AS response. For this response, the multifilters were set so that the bands below 0.4 kHz and above 4.0 kHz were at their minimum possible gain.

TEST PROCEDURES

All of the threshold measurements were referred to the level of the undisturbed signal at the presumed center of the listener's head. Functional gain was measured by the reduction of the signal level from the unaided threshold to the aided one. The aid's gain was set at the listener's most comfortable level for live conversational speech (65 to 70 dB SPL).

A secondary technique[37] was used to check the possibility of ambient noise and/or internal noise interference in aided-threshold estimation. Instead of reducing the level of the signal needed for unaided threshold, it was kept constant and the aid's gain was reduced until threshold was reached again. This was done by placing an adequately matched attenuator between the amplifier output and the receiver. Since this technique gave identical results but was more difficult to administer, it was discontinued after three replications. With minor changes in the configuration of the equipment, this procedure may be a better way of measuring aided thresholds and therefore warrants further investigation.

RESULTS

The top panels of Figure 8 are examples of the aided thresholds obtained by one subject (right ear of S-6) with various frequency responses of the master aid. The left panel shows the aided thresholds for the uniform response in

*Model BT-1754, Knowles Electronics, Franklin Park, Ill.
**Type 9-C, Audivox, Inc., Newton, Mass.

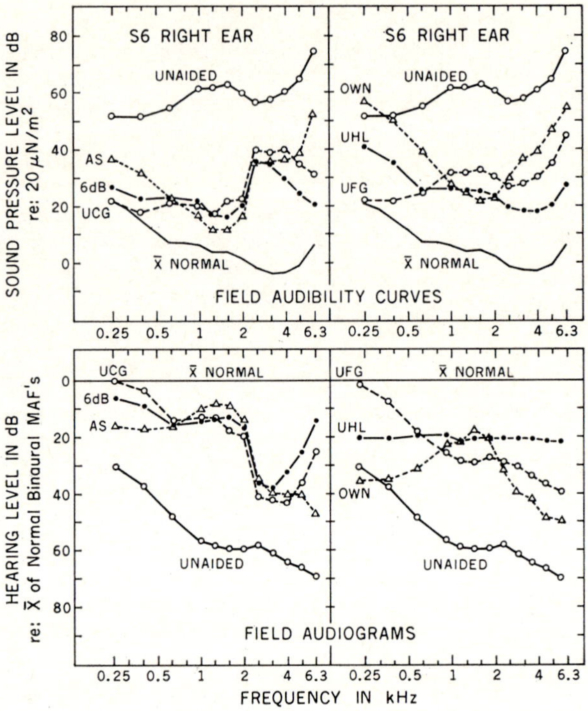

Fig. 8. Aided monaural minimum audible fields and field audiograms of one hard-of-hearing subject. Right ear tested with six frequency responses.

the coupler (UCG), for the 6 dB/octave rise in the coupler (6 dB), and for the aid simulation (AS), while the panel on the right shows the aided thresholds produced by a uniform functional gain (UFG), by the uniform hearing level response (UHL), and by a commercial hearing aid (CA). These same thresholds are shown in the lower two panels in terms of hearing level. In the lower right panel, the parallel relationships between UHL and normal hearing (0 dB HL) and between UFG and the unaided thresholds are clearly shown.

The mean responses defined as coupler gains and as functional gains can be seen in Figure 9. The difference in decibels between these measurements was relatively constant within subjects and frequency responses. It is important to remember that the mean differences shown in Figure 9 represent the coupler vs eardrum differences that result from the acoustical configuration of this master aid. This configuration includes a receiver attached to a standard earmold, and a microphone placed farther forward on the head than is customary. The exact relationship for other specific hearing aids can only be known by the results of field measurements and the comparison of functional gain vs coupler gain. Nevertheless, examination of Panel F of Figure 9 reveals that coupler descriptions of hearing-aid gain seriously overestimate functional gain in the 2 to 4 kHz region and that they underestimate functional gain in the 1 to 2 kHz region. These opposite effects do not cancel each other; their total effect results in a discrepancy greater than 20 dB.

The mean functional gain required to achieve uniform hearing level, or in other words, to correctly "mirror" the audiogram, is an approximately 6 dB/octave rising functional gain. This is, of course, the inverse of the mean audio-

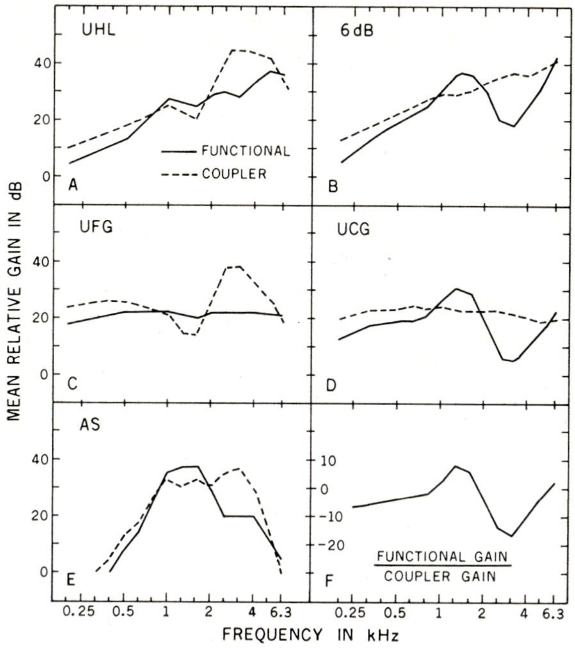

Fig. 9. Mean functional gains and associated coupler measurements of five frequency responses. Mean difference between functional and coupler gains.

gram for this group of subjects, which shows about a 6 dB/octave falling slope. The individual UHL response represents the true mirroring of each audiogram. This relation is "true" only when all the measurements have the same reference, that is, when the aided, the unaided, and the normal threshold reference are field measurements calibrated to the undisturbed free field.

Having thus defined five frequency responses both by their functional gains and by their associated coupler measurements, we can proceed to examine their effects on the speech perception of eight hard-of-hearing subjects.

SECTION IV

MEASUREMENTS OF WORD DISCRIMINATION

WORD LISTS

MATERIALS

A word list (referred to as the "high-frequency" list (HF); see Appendix A) was assembled to include fifty monosyllabic words that emphasize phonemes that are difficult for hard-of-hearing subjects.[38] Only three vocalic nuclei are used (/I/, /ai/, /Ou/) in order to increase the weight of consonants in the correct identification of words. Voiceless fricatives and voiceless plosives form 63% of the number of consonant sounds; the rest are nasals, laterals, and voiced plosives. Phonetic balance had to be neglected because every word was chosen so that it would have at least six very similar words also present in the list. This multiplicity of easily-confused groups of words is necessary so that various randomizations of the same list can be used without too much learning. The words were shown to the subjects before testing and sufficient pretest practice was given so that the list could be considered a closed set.

RECORDING PROCEDURES

The words were recorded by one male and one female talker who sat in an anechoic chamber. They faced a B. and K. condenser microphone and controlled their voice levels by watching a sound level meter.* Each word was recorded within the frame: "write ______, please," and the level of the word "write" was used for calibration. Test words were recorded within equal sound levels (±1 dB). The female talker's level was amplified to the level of the male talker. These initial recordings were done in a professional-grade, magnetic-tape recorder.**

The initial recordings were then re-recorded into Random-Access Programmable Recorder (RAP),[39] and various sets of randomized sequences were arranged with paper tapes punched by a PDP-8S computer. These final sequences were then taped on a recorder.*** This recorder was used for the play-back procedure, along with a power amplifier**** and a loudspeaker.*****

The final fidelity of these recordings was measured with third-octave bands of noise of known acoustic intensity. These bands were recorded and processed in the same manner as the words. A comparison of their levels from initial input to final acoustic output at the location of the listener's head revealed a slight loss in the high frequency region (above 5 kHz), which was compensated by a combination of amplifier and speaker treble-control settings. The final measurements showed a preservation of the original band levels within ± 3 dB, from 0.2 to 6.3 kHz.

PRESENTATION PROCEDURES

One sequence of the list was assigned to each listening condition (e.g., combination of talker, frequency response of the master aid, and signal-to-noise ratio). Each sequence was divided into five ten-word sections and each section was presented separately. The listening conditions were changed every ten words and their order of presentation was counterbalanced to minimize the effects of

---

*Model 1560, General Radio Co., Concord, Mass.

**Model 300, Ampex Corp., Redwood City, Calif.

***Series 3000-X, Tandberg's Radiofabrikk A/S, Norway.

****Model A-245, Superscope, Sun Valley, Calif.

*****Model ST-465, Fisher Radio, New York, N. Y.

TABLE I

DISCRIMINATION SCORES FOR UNAIDED LISTENING

	Female Talker				*Male Talker*				$\overline{X}$ *of Both*			
	List:				*List:*				*List:*			
S	*1*	*2*	*3*	$\overline{X}$	*1*	*2*	*3*	$\overline{X}$	*1*	*2*	*3*	$\overline{X}$
1	80	86	84	83.3	96	94	94	94.7	88	90	89	89.0
2	82	86	84	84.0	94	90	92	92.0	88	88	88	88.0
3	66	68	68	67.3	76	78	72	75.3	71	73	70	71.3
4	44	46	52	47.3	76	72	70	72.7	60	59	61	60.0
5	42	48	52	47.3	72	68	76	72.0	57	58	64	59.7
6	54	60	64	59.3	82	86	84	84.0	68	73	74	71.7
7	40	50	42	44.0	68	68	68	68.0	54	59	55	56.0
8	36	30	36	34.0	50	48	52	50.0	43	39	44	42.0
Group $\overline{X}$	55.5	59.3	60.3	58.4	76.8	75.5	76.0	76.1	66.1	67.3	68.1	67.2

S — Subject.

fatigue, learning, or any other sequence-related factors.

Every ten-word section was introduced by the words: "list ______, word ______." Every word was presented within the frame: "write ______, please." These were not the original frame words spoken with each word in the initial recordings, since the time limitations of RAP did not allow the recording of repetitions of the frame. Only one token of each word spoken by each talker was used. The words and their frames were assembled by the programming procedures.

Five-second pauses separated each word frame to allow time for writing the response. This pause was too long for some of the subjects and barely enough for others. When necessary, the pause was increased by stopping the recorder.

A written form of the list was mailed to each subject, who was instructed to read it and become familiar with it. The list was also read to each of them in a face-to-face situation before the actual tests began. The similarity of various sets of words and the use of only three vowels was emphasized.

Word-recognition tests were conducted in a relatively quiet but partially hard-walled room in which the ambient noise level varied from 28 to 32 dB(A), and from 52 to 57 dB(C).

PRELIMINARY TESTS: UNAIDED LISTENING

PROCEDURES

The purpose of these initial tests was to estimate the range of score variability within identical listening conditions, as well as to provide test experience.

Each subject heard six randomizations of the word list, three spoken by each talker. The subjects faced the loudspeaker and chose their most comfortable levels for listening. The chosen levels ranged from 75 to 90 dB SPL, measured at the presumed center of the subject's head. The linear RMS-slow level reached by the vowel in the word "write" was used as the calibration reference. Male and female ten-word sections were alternated and a rest was given after each sequence of two sections. An average of two hours was needed to complete the six randomizations.

RESULTS

Individual scores are shown in Table I. Lists 1, 2, and 3, under each talker, represent different randomizations of the same fifty words heard in a quiet background. The subjects are listed in the rank order of their adjusted hearing levels.

These scores give information in the following areas: 1) they are estimates of optimum hearing in high-fidelity reproduction conditions; 2) they describe the group's range and each subject's standing in the dimension of word discrimination; 3) they reveal consistent differences in talker discriminability; 4) they serve as comparison for the UFG-response scores (since this response attempts to be an aided simulation of unaided listening); and 5) they give an estimate of possible variations in score within identical listening conditions.

All subjects had higher scores with the male-talker recordings. The individual scores ranged from 30% to 86% with the female talker, and from 48% to 96% with the male. The group average with the female talker was 17.7% lower than with the corresponding average for the male talker. Individual average differences ranged from 8% to 25.4%. The coefficient of correlation between scores on both talkers is 0.95.

The correlation between adjusted hearing levels and grand means of these discrimination scores is -0.91.

The individual scores for identical listening conditions differed from 0% to 10%, with a mean difference of 7% for the female talker and 4.3% for the male.

The group mean scores had maximum variations of 4.8% for the female, 1.3% for the male, and 2.0% for the average of both talkers. Scores on lists 1 and 3 of the female talker were shown to be significantly different ($p < .05$, t tests for related samples).[40] All other list-score comparisons are not significantly different.

FIRST EXPERIMENT

Word discrimination was compared through five frequency responses: UHL, 6 dB, UFG, UCG, and AS.

PROCEDURES AND EQUIPMENT

All aided discrimination tests were administered binaurally. The five frequency responses previously described were tested in four different listening conditions: male and female talkers, in quiet and in noise (6 dB S/N). These twenty listening conditions (five frequency responses x two talkers x two noise ratios) were tested in five sessions. Each session included a ten-word section from each listening condition for a total of 200 words. A frequency response was selected in the master aid and its four listening conditions were presented contiguously (e.g., UHL: male in quiet, male in noise, female in quiet, female in noise). The talkers' sequence was alternated between frequency responses, and the quiet conditions always preceded the noise ones. The sequences of frequency responses were arranged so that after the five sessions, each of the responses had been presented in every ordinal position.

The master aid's gain was adjusted for each ear to achieve binaural balance, as evidenced by correct localization of the experimenter's voice, without visual contact.

The overall level of gain was chosen by each subject at his most comfortable level. Choice of level was made by listening to the recorded list's introduction, repeated as many times as necessary. This procedure was repeated each time the frequency response was changed. The levels chosen were found to vary within a 5 dB range.

The background noise was filtered to approximate the long-term average spectrum of speech as described by Benson and Hirsh.[41] The half-power points of the speech-noise filters used were located at 0.2 and 0.8 kHz, with a 12 dB/octave slope. The noise was diffuse, in the sense that it came from three independent channels: noise sources, filters, amplifiers, and speakers. These speakers were placed at 60°, 180°, and 300° around the listener. Words came from a fourth speaker situated at 0° incidence (Fig. 10).

The overall level of the combined

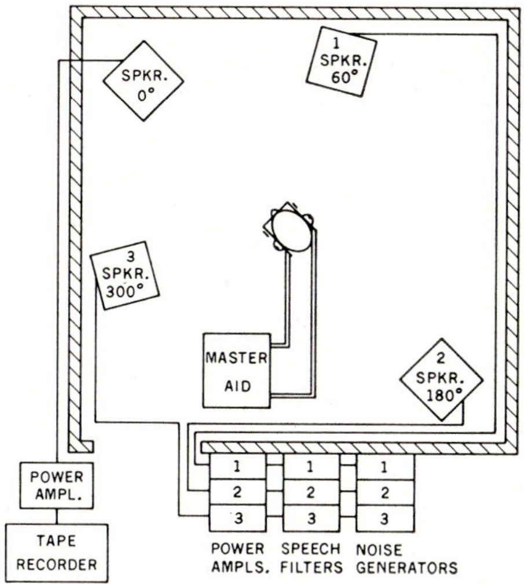

Fig. 10. Block diagram of the equipment and room distribution used for the word-discrimination tests.

noise was measured in the absence of the listener, at the presumed center of his head. The noise level was set at 64 dB SPL while that of the calibrating vowel was set at 70 dB SPL (RMS, slow) to achieve the 6 dB signal-to-noise condition.

The tape recorder was stopped and words were repeated whenever a subject requested it. Rests were provided after every forty words, while the frequency responses of the master aid were being changed.

RESULTS

Differences in Discrimination Scores Between Frequency Responses. Scores for each subject and for the group means are shown in Table II and in Figure 11. Each of these scores is the mean of four listening conditions (two talkers, in quiet and in noise). Also shown in this table are the correlation coefficients between discrimination scores and adjusted hearing levels. Like the unaided-listening scores, these scores are highly correlated with the adjusted hearing levels (-.94 to -.99). Table III shows the group mean scores for each listening condition.

The frequency responses are ranked consistently by the subjects' scores (Ta-

TABLE II

CORRELATIONS BETWEEN AIDED DISCRIMINATION SCORES* AND ADJUSTED HEARING LEVELS (AHL)**

S	*AHL (dB)*	*UHL*	*6 dB*	*UFG*	*UCG*	*AS*	*Mean*
1	36.3	89.5	87.5	92.0	82.0	82.0	86.6
2	46.2	87.0	78.5	79.5	67.5	63.5	75.2
3	52.5	76.5	69.5	74.0	62.5	57.5	68.0
4	57.7	74.5	76.0	55.5	57.0	57.5	64.1
5	58.8	70.0	64.5	59.0	52.0	54.5	60.0
6	65.3	66.5	61.5	61.0	52.5	49.0	58.1
7	67.9	68.0	54.5	39.0	39.5	48.0	49.7
8	81.7	52.5	38.5	36.5	34.5	25.5	37.5
Group means		73.1	66.3	62.1	55.9	54.7	62.4
Coefficients of correlation: (AHL vs disc.)		-.98	-.96	-.94	-.97	-.98	-.99

*Each discrimination score is the mean of four listening conditions: two talkers, in quiet and in noise (in percent).

**AHL is derived from the mean of the subjects' binaural thresholds at 2.0, 2.5, 3.1, and 4.0 kHz plus the difference between it and the mean of their thresholds at 0.5, 0.63, 0.8, and 1.0 kHz.

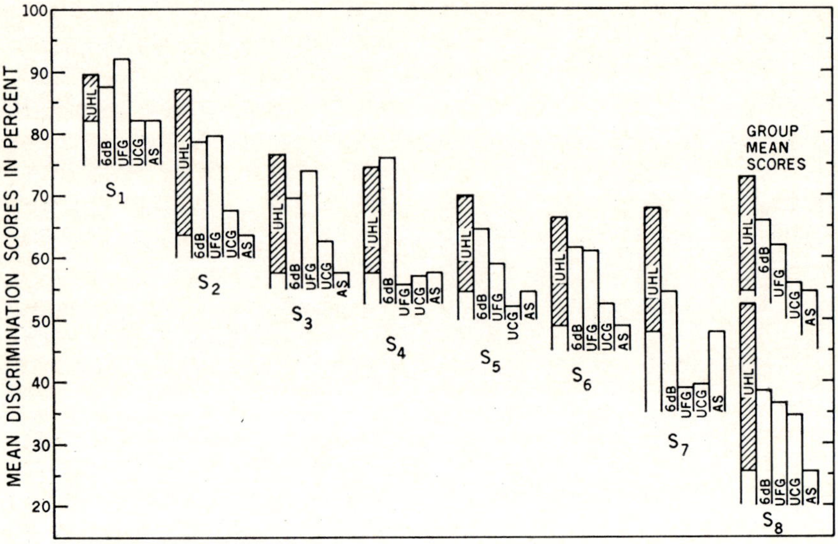

Fig. 11. Individual and group mean word-discrimination scores for five frequency responses. Shaded areas represent UHL advantage over AS.

ble IV). The scores with UHL were highest for six out of eight subjects, and were second by only 2.5% and 1.5% in the remaining two. With the AS, the scores were either fourth or fifth in six cases, and third in two. There was no overlapping between the ranks of these two responses (UHL vs AS). The UFG response, reflecting the subjects' unaided thresholds, was rated high by the scores of those subjects whose hearing curve is flat or mildly sloped. It was rated lowest by the subjects with the steepest hearing curves. Figure 12 shows the distribution of ranks clearly. The coefficients of correlation between the discrimination scores for the various pairs of frequency responses are high (.88 to .96), as shown in Table V.

The mean differences in discrimination scores between frequency responses appear in Table VI and in Figure 13. That UHL is significantly superior to all the other responses is evidenced by the t-ratios shown in Table VII. Both UHL and 6 dB are clearly better than either UCG or AS. These last two, in spite of their gross differences in coupler frequency response, are not significantly different from each other in discrimination scores.

The relations among the first four responses (UHL, 6 dB, UFG, and UCG)

TABLE III

MEAN DISCRIMINATION SCORES FOR EIGHT SUBJECTS

	Female Talker			*Male Talker*			$\overline{X}$
Resp.	*Quiet*	*Noise*	*Av*	*Quiet*	*Noise*	*Av*	*Total*
UHL	71.3	67.5	69.4	80.0	73.5	76.8	73.1
6 dB	60.3	57.8	59.1	76.0	71.3	73.7	66.4
UFG	57.3	49.3	53.3	74.5	67.3	70.9	62.1
UCG	47.5	41.3	44.4	71.5	63.5	67.5	55.9
AS	48.5	42.8	45.7	64.8	62.8	63.8	54.7

Resp. — Response.

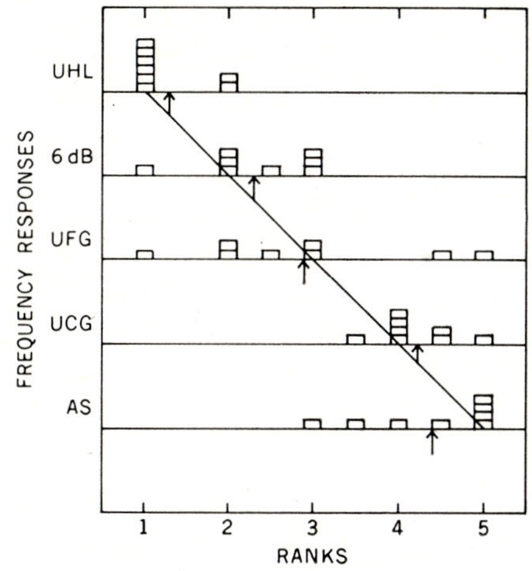

Fig. 12. Distribution of ranks assigned to each frequency response by the individual word-discrimination scores.

TABLE IV

RANKS ASSIGNED TO THE FREQUENCY RESPONSES

	Frequency Responses				
S	*UHL*	*6 dB*	*UFG*	*UCG*	*AS*
1	2	3	1	4.5	4.5
2	1	3	2	4	5
3	1	3	2	4	5
4	2	1	5	3.5	3.5
5	1	2	3	5	4
6	1	2.5	2.5	4	5
7	1	2	4.5	4.5	3
8	1	2	3	4	5
$\overline{X}$ rank	1.3	2.3	2.9	4.2	4.4

are shown in Figure 14. The differences between UHL and 6 dB are exactly proportional to the differences between UFG and UCG. These two pairs represent the difference between functional and coupler measurements. On the other hand, the differences between UHL and UFG are also proportional to those between 6 dB and UCG. These are differences in slope. It is interesting to note that proportional changes in frequency response produced approximately equal changes in discrimination scores.

The first set of differences of about 6.5% in discrimination scores (UHL-6 dB, and UFG-UCG) can be seen as the result of compensation for outer-ear resonances and head-diffraction effects. The second set of differences of about 10.7% (UHL-UFG, and 6 dB-UCG) are related to the compensation for the slope in the subjects' hearing-level curves. The

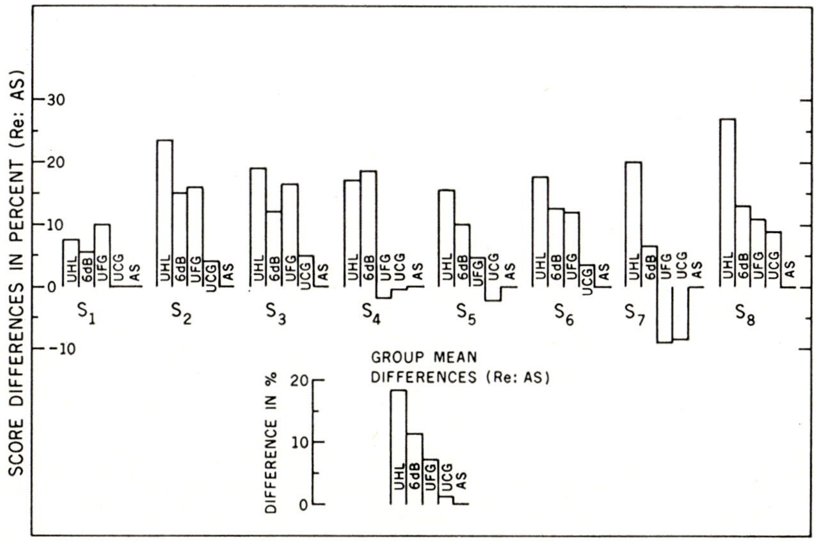

Fig. 13. Differences in percent between the word-discrimination scores obtained with the AS response and those obtained with the other responses.

TABLE V

CORRELATION BETWEEN DISCRIMINATION SCORES

	Frequency Responses			
	6 dB	UFG	UCG	AS
UHL	.96	.90	.93	.96
6 dB		.88	.95	.96
UFG			.98	.89
UCG				.94

TABLE VI

MEAN DIFFERENCES BETWEEN DISCRIMINATION SCORES*

	Frequency Responses			
	6 dB	UFG	UCG	AS
UHL	6.8	11.0	17.2	18.4
6 dB		4.2	10.4	11.6
UFG			6.2	7.4
UCG				1.2

*Each number (percent) represents the superiority of the responses listed on the left over those listed above.

sum of these two effects appears in the difference of 17.2% between UHL and UCG.

Figure 15 shows the distribution of scores obtained in the UHL and the AS responses, plotted in relation to the subjects' adjusted hearing levels. As has been shown, the discrimination scores obtained with these two responses are highly correlated with the subjects' adjusted hearing levels (-.98); these scores are highly correlated with each other (.96); and they are very significantly different ($p < .001$). The difference in the slopes of their regression lines (-.83 and -1.12) implies that the difference between UHL and AS diminishes as the absolute scores get higher, or inversely, that the advantage given by UHL is greater when the absolute scores are lower. It is more likely however, that differences in the quality of sound are still present but cannot be adequately measured in the better discrimination-score levels, unless listening is done under more adverse conditions. This possibility merits further attention.

Differences in Discrimination Related to the Talkers. As in the unaided listening condition, the scores obtained with the male talker were higher than those with the female talker for every subject and in every frequency response (ex-

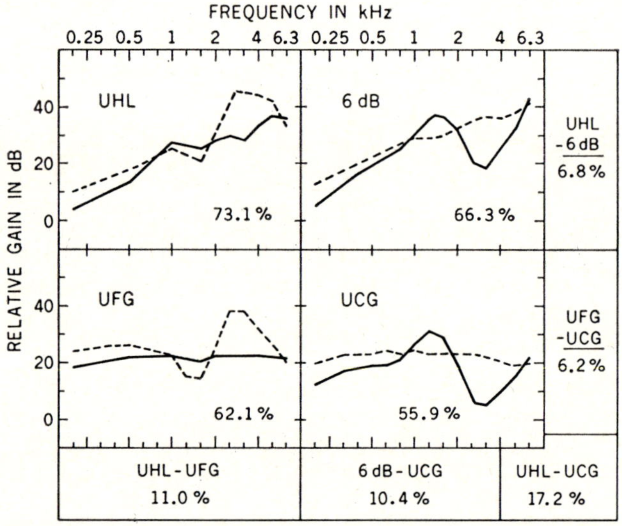

Fig. 14. Functional and coupler measurements of four frequency responses and their associated mean discrimination scores.

TABLE VII

DIFFERENCES BETWEEN DISCRIMINATION SCORES*

	Frequency Responses			
	6 dB	*UFG*	*UCG*	*AS*
UHL	3.6	3.1	11.5	9.2
6 dB		1.3	5.8	7.8
UFG			3.2	2.3
UCG				0.7

Levels of significance with 7 d.f.:

p< .05, t = 2.4
.02, t = 3.0
.01, t = 3.5
.001, t = 5.4

*Expressed as t-ratios for related samples.

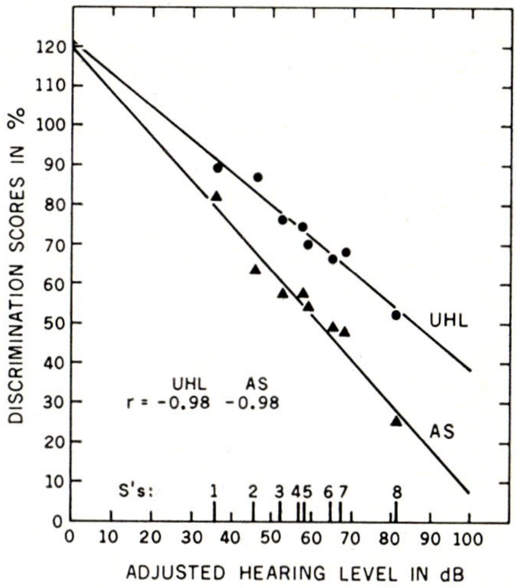

Fig. 15. Correlation between the subjects' adjusted hearing levels and their discrimination scores on the UHL and the AS responses of the first experiment.

cept S-8, in UHL). Table VIII shows these differences in terms of male-talker superiority. The mean differences per frequency response show that UHL was least affected by the talker difference. The subjects' means suggest that the better-hearing subjects (1, 2, and 3) were less affected than the rest of the group. This distribution was also present in the unaided results. Talker effects in the quiet (16.4%) were similar to those in the noise (15.9%).

In spite of the fact that these two talkers have been referred to as female and male, their difference in scores cannot be generalized as a sex difference since there is only one of each. Both of them would be described as extremely clear and precise talkers by normally hearing listeners. In this respect, it is interesting to note that the UHL response reduced the talker difference down to 7.4%, while the mean difference of the other four responses was 18.3%.

Differences in Discrimination Scores Between Quiet and Noise Conditions. Table IX shows individual differences

TABLE VIII

DIFFERENCES IN DISCRIMINATION SCORES BETWEEN TALKERS*

	Aided						*Unaided*
S	*UHL*	*6 dB*	*UFG*	*UCG*	*AS*	$\overline{X}$	$\overline{X}$
1	9	15	4	16	10	10.8	11.4
2	0	13	21	19	19	14.4	8.0
3	7	9	4	19	11	10.0	8.0
4	15	10	19	30	29	20.6	25.4
5	8	17	18	30	29	20.4	24.7
6	15	23	24	21	18	20.2	24.7
7	10	21	26	31	16	20.8	24.0
8	-5	9	25	19	13	12.2	16.0
$\overline{X}$	7.4	14.6	17.6	23.1	18.1	16.2	17.8

*Results represent male minus female scores in percent and include quiet and noise conditions.

TABLE IX

DIFFERENCES IN DISCRIMINATION SCORES BETWEEN QUIET AND NOISE*

	Frequency Responses					
S	*UHL*	*6 dB*	*UFG*	*UCG*	*AS*	$\overline{X}$
1	7	7	10	6	10	8.0
2	6	11	7	17	7	9.6
3	3	- 3	2	15	5	4.4
4	7	14	7	8	1	7.4
5	4	- 1	10	- 4	5	2.8
6	7	- 3	8	7	4	4.6
7	4	7	8	5	- 6	3.6
8	3	- 3	9	3	5	3.4
$\overline{X}$	5.1%	3.6%	7.6%	7.1%	3.9%	5.5%

*Discrimination scores include male and female-talker results.

related to the signal-to-noise ratio, including the averaged scores of male and female conditions. Although there are no significant differences related to how each frequency response handled the noise factor, it would appear that listening through the two responses which have the greatest amount of gain in the low frequencies (UFG and UCG) was more difficult in the noise. The better-hearing subjects, if judged by the mean of the best four (7.4%) against the mean of the lowest four (3.6%), appear to have suffered more from the interference of noise.

Similarity Between UFG and Unaided Listening. Since UFG is an attempt to reproduce unaided sensation levels without frequency distortion, a good test of the procedures is the comparison of discrimination scores between these two conditions. When the unaided and the UFG (in quiet) score distributions are compared, they are found to be insignificantly different: mean of unaided scores = 67.1%, mean of UFG (quiet) scores = 65.9% (t-ratio = 0.5). They are also highly correlated (0.94) (Fig. 16).

SECOND EXPERIMENT

Aided listening was compared through two frequency responses (UHL and AS).

PROCEDURES

UHL and AS were used again so that some of the results obtained in the previous experiment (both talkers in the quiet condition) could be replicated. Other listening conditions were changed or added as follows:

The Signal-to-noise Ratio of the Noise Condition was Changed to 0 dB. To achieve this, the noise level was raised to 67 dB (linear) SPL while the voice was lowered to the same level.

A Second Type of Word List was Added. (PB lists 9-B, 10-B, 11-B, and 12-B which are used in the Rush-Hughes recordings, Technisonic Studios, a commonly used clinical test). These lists were recorded in exactly the same manner as the previous one (HF) and by the same talkers. Lists 9-B and 11-B were recorded by the male talker, while 10-B and 12-B were recorded by the female talker.

The assignment of these lists to the listening conditions was different for each half of the group, in an attempt to eliminate the effects of list-difficulty differences from the group average scores.

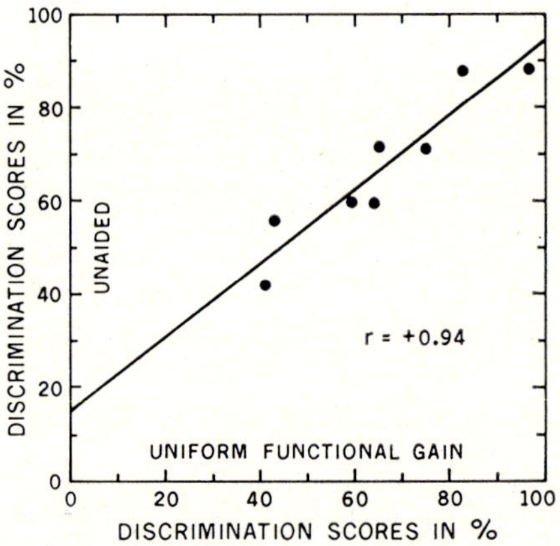

Fig. 16. Correlation between the discrimination scores of the unaided and of the aided tests using the UFG response under quiet conditions.

The sixteen listening conditions (two frequency responses x two types of list x two talkers x two S/N conditions) were presented in the same subdivided and shuffled procedure mentioned previously. All other procedures and conditions were identical to those of the previous experiment.

RESULTS

Comparison of the Results in Quiet Between the First and Second Experiments (UHL vs AS). The coefficients of correlation between Exp. 1 and Exp. 2 are high (0.98 for UHL, and 0.97 for AS), as shown in Figure 17. However, while the UHL response produced almost identical results in both experiments ($\bar{X}_1$ = 75.6%, $\bar{X}_2$ = 75.5%), as can be seen in Table X, the AS response was significantly better in the second experiment

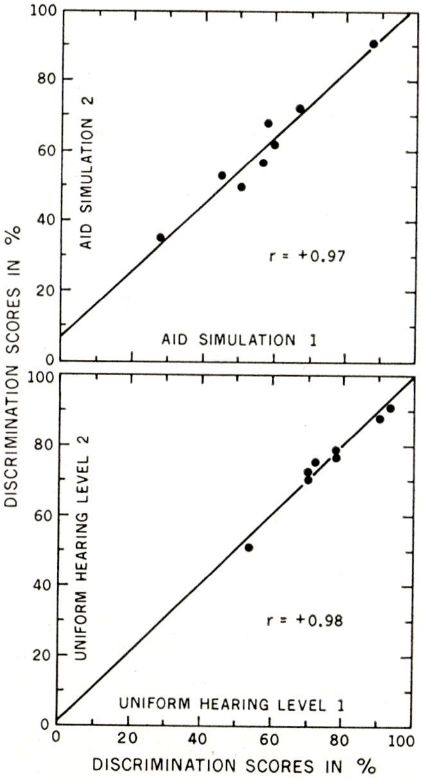

Fig. 17. Correlations between the discrimination scores of the first and second experiments using the UHL and the AS responses under quiet conditions.

TABLE X

DISCRIMINATION SCORES WITH UHL AND AS*

Freq. Resp.	*Exp.*	*Female*	*Male*	*Av*
UHL	1	71.3	80.0	75.6
	2	70.5	80.5	75.5
	Diff. =	- 0.8	0.5	- 0.1
AS	1	48.5	64.8	56.6
	2	52.5	69.5	61.0
	Diff. =	4.0	4.7	4.4
UHL-AS	1	22.8	15.2	19.0
	2	18.0	11.0	14.5

*In quiet for first and second experiments (HF lists).

($\bar{X}_1$ = 56.6%, $\bar{X}_2$ = 61.0%; $p = <.05$). The difference in group means is only 4.4%, but the small improvement was consistent for all subjects. Because of this change, the UHL advantage over AS went from 19% (in quiet) in the first experiment to 14.5% in the second.

Effects of the Reduction in Signal-to-Noise Ratio. The group-mean scores of the noise condition (first experiment S/N = 6 dB, second experiment S/N = 0 dB) can be seen in Table XI. In general, the increase in noise had similar effects for both frequency responses and with either talker. With this change in S/N, the UHL scores dropped 9.8%, while the AS scores dropped 10.7%.

The UHL advantage over AS did

TABLE XI

DISCRIMINATION SCORES WITH UHL AND AS IN NOISE*

Freq. Resp.	*Exp.*	*Female*	*Male*	*Av*
UHL	1	67.5	73.5	70.5
	2	57.3	64.0	60.7
	Diff.:	10.2	9.5	9.8
AS	1	42.8	62.8	52.8
	2	33.8	50.3	42.1
	Diff.:	9.0	12.5	10.7
UHL-AS	1	24.7	10.7	17.7
	2	23.5	13.7	18.6

*S/N in first experiment was 6 dB, S/N in second experiment was 0 dB (HF lists).

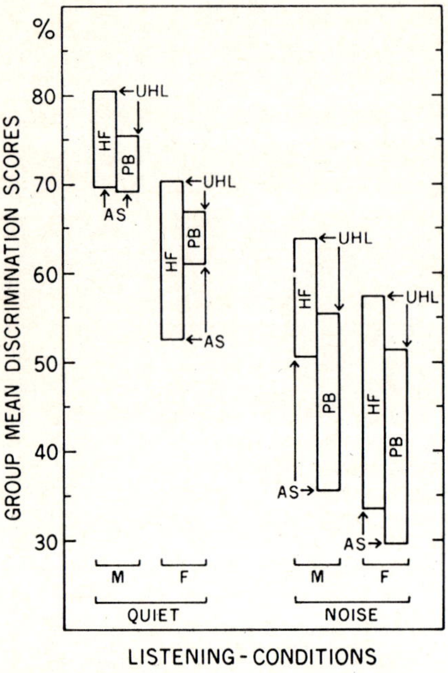

Fig. 18. Mean discrimination scores of UHL and of AS in the second experiment, using two types of word lists.

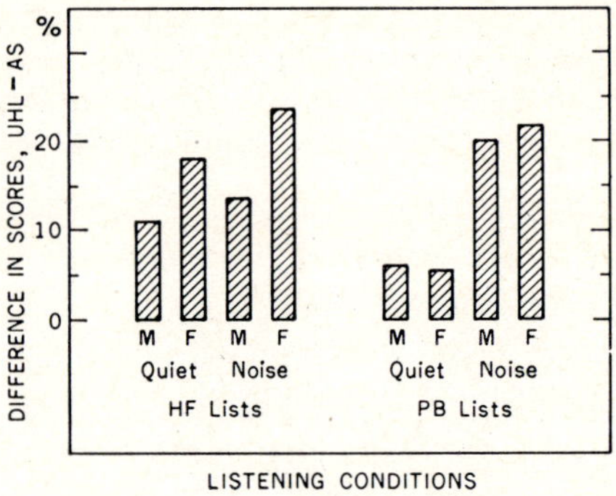

Fig. 19. A comparison of the discrimination-score advantages given by UHL over AS, in the second experiment.

not change therefore with increased noise (17.7% advantage in first experiment, and 18.6% in the second). Table XI shows these advantages in noise. As with the first experiment, the UHL advantage with the female voice was considerably greater than with the male voice (23.5% vs 13.7%).

The improvement which was seen in the quiet condition for the AS response was either not there in the noise or was counterbalanced by an increased noise effect.

Comparison Between the Results Obtained with Two Types of Word Lists (HF vs. PB). Table XII and Figure 18 show the group-mean scores obtained with the "high-frequency" word list (HF) designed for these experiments, and the PB lists included in the second experiment.

If we look at the total average scores we see that they were only slightly higher with the HF lists than with the PB lists (5.7% higher for the UHL, and 2.5% higher for the AS, or a mean difference of 4.1%). However, there are important differences that can be seen in the subscores.

With the HF lists, the advantage of UHL over AS is greater on the female voice (20.8%) than on the male voice

TABLE XII

MEAN DISCRIMINATION SCORES IN THE SECOND EXPERIMENT*

Freq.		*Female Voice*			*Male Voice*			*Total*
Resp.	*List*	*Quiet*	*Noise*	*Mean*	*Quiet*	*Noise*	*Mean*	*Av*
UHL	HF	70.5	57.3	63.9	80.5	64.0	72.5	68.1
	PB	67.0	51.5	59.3	75.3	55.8	65.5	62.4
AS	HF	52.5	33.8	43.1	69.5	50.3	59.9	51.5
	PB	61.3	29.8	45.5	69.3	35.8	52.5	49.0
UHL-AS	HF	18.0	23.5	20.8	11.0	13.7	12.4	16.6
	PB	5.7	21.7	13.8	6.0	20.0	13.0	13.4

*HF and PB word lists.

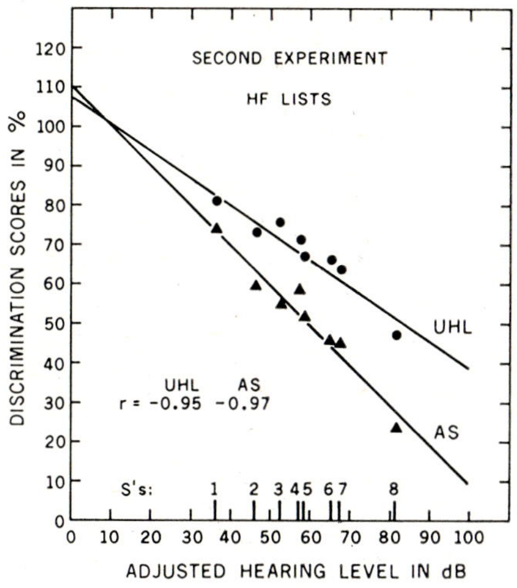

Fig. 20. Correlation between the subjects' adjusted hearing levels and their discrimination scores on the UHL and AS responses, using the HF list.

(12.4%); this advantage is only slightly greater in noise (18.6%) than in quiet (14.5%).

With the PB lists, these relationships are almost exactly the opposite: the UHL advantage on the female voice (13.8%) is almost the same as on the male voice (13.0%), while the advantage

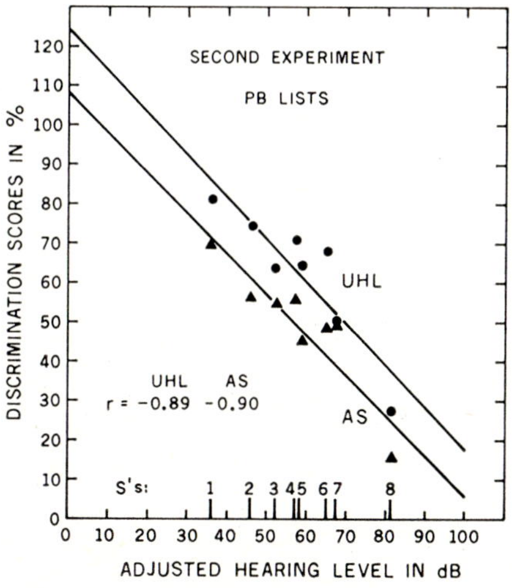

Fig. 21. Correlation between the subjects' adjusted hearing levels and their discrimination scores on the UHL and AS responses, using the PB lists.

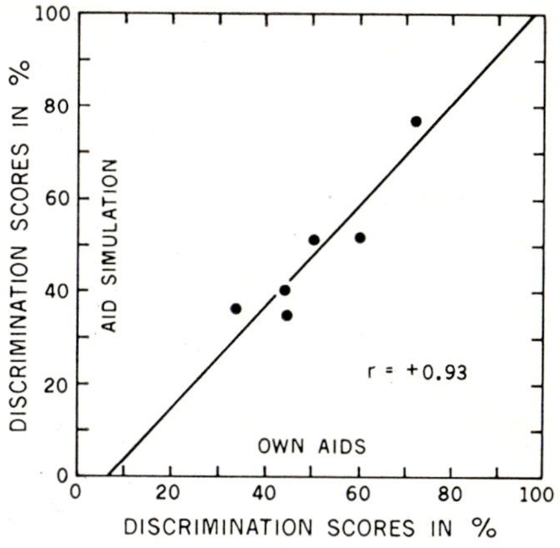

Fig. 22. Correlation between the discrimination scores made with the subjects' own hearing aids and the scores made with the AS response.

in the noise (20.9%) is much greater than in the quiet (5.9%).

Figure 19 displays these UHL vs AS differences in score and shows the patterns of interaction between lists and listening conditions. The talker effect is

TABLE XIII

DISCRIMINATION SCORES WITH AS AND COMMERCIAL AIDS*

S	*Aids*	*Quiet*	*Noise*	*Av*
	With female talker:			
1	AS	80	74	77
	Own	84	62	72
3	AS	58	46	52
	Own	66	54	60
4	AS	72	30	51
	Own	68	32	50
5	AS	54	26	40
	Own	56	32	44
7	AS	44	26	35
	Own	56	34	45
	With male talker:			
8	AS	39	33	36
	Own	38	30	34
$\overline{X}$	AS	57.8	39.1	48.5
	Own	61.3	40.6	50.9
	Diff. =	3.5	1.5	2.4

*Separate tests with HF lists.

evident on the HF lists, while the noise effect is obvious on the PB lists.

Another important difference is shown in Figures 20 and 21. Here, the correlations between discrimination scores and the subjects' adjusted HL's on each list type display different slope relationships in their regression lines. On the HF lists, as in the first experiment, the UHL vs AS difference in scores tends to increase as the adjusted HL increases. On the PB lists, the UHL vs AS difference does not show this tendency: their regression lines are virtually parallel.

SUPPLEMENTARY TESTS: LISTENING THROUGH COMMERCIAL HEARING AIDS

Six subjects were tested with the HF word lists and wearing their own hearing aids. Five of them were tested with the female voice and one with the male. All of them were tested in quiet and in noise (6 dB S/N). The quiet and noise conditions were alternated every ten words.

In every case, the aid's gain was set by each subject at his own comfort level. Three subjects wore binaural aids and three wore only one aid.

Although these tests were not done in direct conjunction with the AS tests, their results indicate that the AS response, as heard through the master aid, was a good simulation of commercial aids. Table XIII and Figure 22 show these results and their correlation. AS scores and those made with the subjects' own aids do not differ significantly from each other ($p < .05$, t-test for related samples).[40] The commercial aid scores were higher by 3.5% in the quiet and by 1.5% in the noise, for a total mean difference of 2.4%. The quiet-noise mean difference for these aids was 20.7%, while in the corresponding AS results the difference was 18.7%.

SECTION V

GENERAL DISCUSSION

FUNCTIONAL VS COUPLER GAINS

Functional gains can be reliably measured in clinical conditions. Reliability will depend on: 1) careful control of the signal levels and of the subject's head position; 2) appropriate settings (usually low) of the aid's gain in order to avoid both the masking produced by the aid's internal noise and the interference of ambient noise in the room; and 3) careful blocking of the untested ear either through the use of earplugs, earmuffs, or preferably both.

When adequate precautions are taken, functional gain reveals the summed effect of all acoustical changes produced by the aid and its earmold. These changes may be considered extrinsic to the aid itself, but this attitude is wrong, because they are inseparable and therefore real components of the total configuration.

Coupler measurements seriously misrepresent functional gain. They underestimate gain in the 1 to 2 kHz region and they overestimate it from 2 to 5 kHz. These differences are the result of altered head diffraction and outer-ear resonance characteristics as well as of the coupler's inexact replication of real-ear impedance. These factors do not cancel each other; they are, in fact, additive. The combined effect of these misrepresentations is a greatly reduced functional frequency range compared to that inferred from coupler calibrations. Aids which are said to reach frequencies as high as 4 kHz (based on coupler measurements and HAIC definitions) are probably not giving any significant help above 2.5 kHz. This combined effect can mean a 24 dB drop in gain from 1.5 to 3 kHz. When this deficit is added to the negative slope of a hard-of-hearing person's threshold and to the spectrum of speech, the resulting sensation levels for speech signals in that region of frequency cannot be positive.

In spite of their limitations, coupler measurements are necessary as common points of reference between individual functional measurements. These measurements cannot be used alone because it is not possible to apply standard or fixed corrections. This is not possible because the acoustic factors present in each case are specific to the aid, the user, and his earmold.

The careful estimation of functional gain is indispensable in research definitions of hearing-aid frequency response. Similar measurements should be carried out clinically in order to estimate the true frequency range of a specific aid configuration, the effects of earmold parameters, and the possible changes in frequency response that may be suggested to the manufacturer.

This investigation has shown that the gain deficit inherent in coupler measurements is accompanied by a proportional and significant loss in discrimination scores (6 to 7%). These data support the concept that hearing aids must be tested on people and that their frequency response must be defined in terms of functional gain.

RELATIONS BETWEEN FREQUENCY RESPONSE AND DISCRIMINATION SCORES

It has been said that a peculiarity of hearing aids is that they show a "small effect of marked changes of frequency response on articulation efficiency."[8] This statement would be confirmed by a comparison between the results of the UCG and the AS responses as well as between 6 dB and UFG. These two pairs of markedly different frequency responses produced insignificantly different discrimination scores. Yet a comparison of other sets of responses showed the opposite effect: changes in frequency response had significant effects on "articulation efficiency" or word-discrimination scores, and furthermore, these effects were proportional to the changes in response.

The UHL response was significantly better for this group of listeners. The achievement of uniform hearing levels requires a "true" mirroring of the audiogram, based on functional measurements. In this investigation, mirroring was achieved with a ± 6 dB degree of approximation in the worst of cases, and with a ± 1 dB in the best.

A good way of summarizing the differences related to hearing-aid frequency

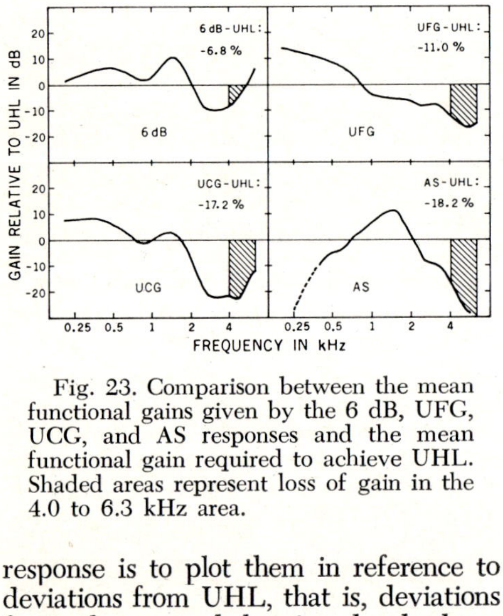

Fig. 23. Comparison between the mean functional gains given by the 6 dB, UFG, UCG, and AS responses and the mean functional gain required to achieve UHL. Shaded areas represent loss of gain in the 4.0 to 6.3 kHz area.

response is to plot them in reference to deviations from UHL, that is, deviations from the normal hearing level slope. This is done in Figure 23. The shaded areas in these graphs show the mean deficit in gain in the higher frequencies (4.0 to 6.3 kHz) of the 6 dB, UFG, UCG, and AS responses when they are compared to UHL. The corresponding discrimination-score deficits are included. It is clear that as the gain deficit increases, the discrimination scores diminish in a proportional manner.

These data are not sufficient to support the concept that the "mirroring" of the audiogram is indispensable, but they certainly suggest that it is a good aided condition to approximate for these subjects.

Mirroring the audiogram as a means for selecting an optimum frequency response has been considered objectionable because listening is usually done at supra-threshold levels.[12,42,43] Accordingly, an equal-loudness contour at the level of comfortable listening has been suggested as a more practical fitting alternative.[42,43] But even this alternative has been rejected by some investigators as unreliable and unnecessary because listeners' estimates of equal loudness are time consuming and inconsistent, while one frequency response (either flat or rising at 6 dB per octave) can serve most hearing-impaired listeners equally well.[4] Recently however, one investigator has shown that frequency-selective compression ratios added to frequency-selective amplification can improve the recognition of speech for six perceptively deaf subjects.[44] He concluded that frequency-selective compression made feasible both the necessary treble boost and the extension of usable frequencies above 4 kHz (to 6.5 kHz). His frequency-selective amplification was based primarily on an approximation to the relative loudness of normal speech reception, which is a variation of the equal-loudness concept.

The differences shown here between functional and coupler gains do not seem to have been adequately taken into account in previous research in this area. Because of this it is doubtful if the various attempts to "fit the audiogram," either with threshold or equal-loudness approximations, have truly tested the stated hypothesis.

Given the relatively mild mean hearing-level slope (+ 6 dB/octave) shown by the group of subjects tested in this investigation, it is evident that an equal-loudness-contour fitting could not be very different from the uniform-hearing-level fitting. Fitting for an equal-loudness contour would have required a functional gain with a slope greater than

0 dB and smaller than a 6 dB/octave rise. In other words, it would have required a functional-gain response somewhere between uniform functional gain and uniform hearing level.

Considering the clear superiority of UHL over UFG, it is unlikely that a frequency response that would fit between them would produce a greater advantage. Nevertheless, this possibility was not tested and merits further investigation.

Since a procedure based on aided-threshold measurements is easier and more reliable than one based on equal-

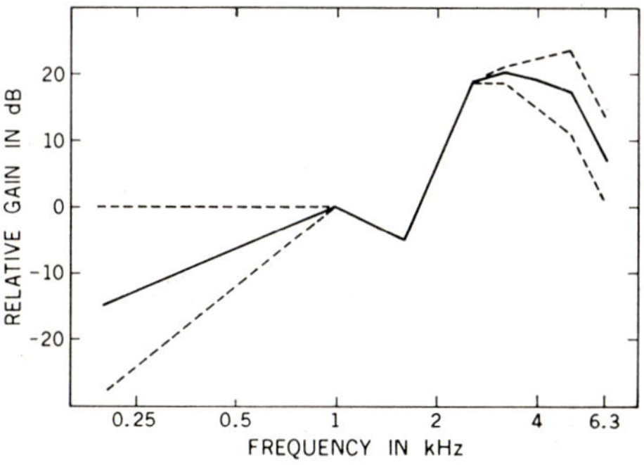

Fig. 24. Idealized coupler response needed to achieve the mean UHL with the master hearing aid, and variations needed to include the specific responses required for each subject.

loudness estimates, it can be expected to be more clinically feasible. Whether or not the UHL correction is applicable to hearing losses of greater slope than those tested here, the aided-threshold procedure can still be used to establish the functional gain required to produce either UHL or UFG with a specific hearing-aid configuration. From a given frequency response derived in this manner, the effectiveness of minor alterations in slope can be easily determined.

Figure 24 shows the mean coupler response needed to achieve UHL in this investigation. It also shows the variations which would be necessary in order to cover the individual variations within this group. It can be seen that the frequency response is divided into three areas. The central portion (1 to 2.5 kHz) has to retain its configuration in order to adjust to the aid's external acoustical elements. (It must be remembered that this coupler curve is only valid for the master aid used.) The low-frequency area (below 1 kHz) would require changes in slope from 0 to about -12 dB per octave. The high-frequency area (2.5 to 6.3 kHz) would need a ± 6 dB range of relative gain centered at 5 kHz. The overall gain level required for this group varied from 10 to 40 dB at 1 kHz. A master aid capable of these adjustments has been assembled by the C.I.D. Electroacoustics Lab and will be used for further clinical research.

As can be seen in Figure 24, the master aid emphasizes two main frequency bands: a low one (0.5 to 1.25 kHz) and a high one (2 to 6.3 kHz). At present, hearing aids emphasize the central portion of the spectrum. Support for central emphasis has been based, in part, on interpretations of the research done by French and Steinberg,[45] which was clearly described in the classic graph published by G. A. Miller.[46] This graph can be interpreted to indicate that there are two apparently redundant areas of frequency which contribute equally well to word discrimination. This redundancy, however, becomes indispensable when the low area is masked by the presence of noise. This is a common listening condition and is the condition which most heavily punishes the hard-of-hearing listener.

A conclusion that may be derived from these results is that in order for changes in frequency response to have an effect on word discrimination, these changes must occur in specific frequency areas, at specific levels, and in specific directions. The critical range of frequencies where even minor changes in response may have significant effects on word discrimination includes frequencies between 2.5 and 6.3 kHz (when these changes are relative to the low and the central frequency areas). Most of the critical high frequencies lie beyond the reach of today's hearing aids, if their response is measured in terms of functional gain.

EFFECTS OF WORD-LIST TYPE (*HF vs PB*)

The two types of word list used in this investigation differ in several dimensions. The HF lists were presented as a closed or known set, they are phonetically unbalanced in favor of high-frequency phonemes, and every repetition of the list is identical to the others, except for differences in word order. On the other hand, the PB lists, besides being phonetically balanced, are an open set with a different set of words in each list.

The average results on the two types of list were surprisingly similar. Furthermore, their correlation is very high (with the UHL response it is 0.94, and with the AS response it is 0.96). But the different results with each list in the various listening conditions are of greater interest and deserve further exploration.

Figure 25 summarizes the UHL and the AS scores on experiments I and II.

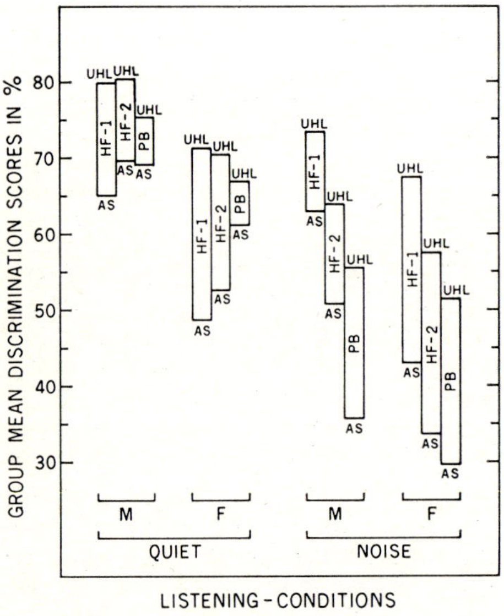

Fig. 25. Summary of group mean discrimination scores with UHL and AS frequency responses. Experiments 1 (HF lists) and 2 (HF and PB lists).

Comparing the results with the HF lists in both experiments, the effect of increased noise is apparent. When the results on the PB lists are compared to them, it appears that the two types of lists functioned in parallel form under the UHL response, with either talker and both in quiet or in noise. The HF lists yielded higher scores (in Experiment II the mean difference is 5.7%) on all the listening conditions of the UHL response. Both lists showed talker and noise effects in that the scores for the male talker in the quiet were always higher than for the other, counterpart conditions. However, for the AS response the interactions were more complex. No attempt is made here to list the factors that may participate in these results. A more specific experimental design is required in order to clarify the situation. Nevertheless, it can be said that the choice of word list and listening conditions will determine the probability of finding discrimination-score differences between frequency responses in any investigation. Evidently, the PB lists in quiet are not very useful in this respect.

Hard-of-hearing patients typically complain that although their hearing aids are acceptable in quiet surroundings, they are practically useless in noise. The PB lists appear to reflect this situation. Another typical complaint is that both women and children are more difficult to understand than men. The HF lists back this belief. Whether or not either of these lists is "life-like" in nature, both seem useful in comparing the clarity of speech received through various frequency-response conditions if the right listening conditions are chosen.

RELATIONS BETWEEN HEARING LEVELS AND DISCRIMINATION SCORES

The use of high-frequency thresholds as better predictors of word discrimination has been suggested by several investigators.[47,48] These investigators have found correlations between thresholds above 1 kHz and PB-list scores as high as -0.80.

In Experiment I of this investigation (Table II) the correlation between the subjects' adjusted hearing levels (which use a high-frequency band) and the discrimination scores on a non-PB list are shown to be very high. In fact, when the summed scores are used, the correlation reaches -0.99 (summed scores include the results of twenty word lists for each subject, or 1,000 words each). If the high-frequency band is used alone (without the slope correction) the correlation remains high (-0.95). When these same summed scores are correlated with the usual HL index (mean of .5, 1, and 2 kHz), the correlation drops to -0.61.

Experiment II showed that this type of correlation was higher on the HF lists than on the PB lists, but even for the PB lists the correlation was high (-0.89 on the UHL, and -0.90 on the AS). When only the high hand was used, the change was small (-0.87 on the UHL, and -0.86 on the AS). Again, when the correlation was made to the usual HL index, the coefficients dropped to -0.64 on the UHL, and to -0.61 on the AS.

The value of using a slope adjustment in the definition of a hearing level index is not clearly demonstrated, but that of using the high-frequency thresholds certainly is. Nevertheless, the adjustment did improve the correlations for these data and merits further investigation.

It seems evident that if the discrimination scores can be stabilized by extended and improved procedures, high correlations can be shown between them and the clinically easier-to-obtain measurements of threshold. Thus, if a discrimination-score range can be predicted on the basis of experimental evidence, clinical deviations from the expected range for a particular subject would be signals for further investigation. These deviations would point either to faulty sampling of the patient's capacities, or to true deviations with important diagnostic value.

SECTION VI

SUMMARY

1. Measurements of minimum audible fields for third-octave bands of noise were made on twenty normally-hearing young people. The means of their binaural field thresholds were used as 0 dB reference for estimating the hearing levels of eight hard-of-hearing subjects.

2. Unaided and aided measurements of minimum audibility were made on the hard-of-hearing subjects. The differences between the unaided and the aided thresholds were taken as the functional gain of the aiding system.

3. Two frequency responses of a master aid (uniform or flat and 6 dB/octave rise, defined in the 2-cm^3 coupler) were used for the aided measurements. Three other frequency responses were adjusted to produce specific types of aided audibility curves. One reproduced each individual's unaided curve with equal functional gain at each frequency: it gave a uniform functional gain (UFG). A second one gave sufficient gain at each frequency and to each subject so that the resulting aided threshold curves were parallel to the normal ones or had uniform hearing levels (UHL). The gains of the third response were adjusted to be similar to those given by a "typical" hearing aid, in other words, to be an "aid simulation" (AS).

4. The functional gain was compared to the 2-cm^3 coupler gain of each response. The coupler measurements seriously misrepresented functional gains. The coupler underestimated functional gain in the 1 to 2 kHz region and it overestimated it between 2 and 4 kHz.

5. These five frequency responses were used to test discrimination on the hard-of-hearing subjects. A special word list, heavily loaded with high-frequency consonants, was recorded by two talkers (male and female) and presented both in quiet and in noise (6 dB S/N). Different randomizations of the same set of words were assigned to each listening condition (frequency response, talker, and S/N combination). These conditions were presented in a subdivided and interwoven design that effectively counterbalanced sequential effects.

6. The discrimination scores made with the UHL response were significantly higher than the scores made with any of the other responses. The mean advantages of UHL over the other responses were as follows: 6.8% over 6 dB, 11.0% over UFG, 17.2% over UCG, and 18.4% over AS. These differences were consistent within individuals. The UHL advantage over AS was greater with the female talker (23.8%) than with the male (13.0%), and it was almost the same in quiet (19.0%) as in noise (17.7%).

7. The discrimination scores made on the UFG response (in quiet) were insignificantly different from the scores made in the unaided field (when the field was raised to most comfortable levels). In other words, UFG was an adequate replication of the unaided listening.

8. The discrimination scores made on the AS response were insignificantly different from the scores made with the subjects' own hearing aids. In other words, the AS was an adequate aid simulation.

9. A second experiment replicated successfully the discrimination scores obtained with the UHL and with the AS. The correlation between scores in the first and in the second experiments was high (+0.98 with UHL, and +0.97 with AS).

10. Although the individual scores on the HF word lists were highly correlated with the scores on the PB lists (0.94 on

UHL, and 0.96 on AS), the HF lists helped reveal UHL advantages over AS equally well in quiet (16.7%) as in noise (18.0%) while the PB lists showed only a small advantage in quiet (5.9%) but a greater one in noise (20.9%).

11. A high negative correlation was found between discrimination scores and adjusted hearing levels (-0.94 to -0.99 with the HF lists, and -0.89 to -0.90 with the PB lists).

12. The regression lines of the above correlations on the HF lists show that the UHL advantage is greater the poorer the hearing of the subject. This effect does not appear when PB lists are used.

SECTION VII
RECOMMENDATIONS

1. Broad-band hearing aids, with frequency responses that compensate for the external-ear effects altered by the aid's presence and also compensate for individual deviations from the normal-hearing slope, can greatly improve the clarity of speech for many hard-of-hearing persons. This improvement is significant in quiet backgrounds and even more so in the presence of noise. A limited number of these aids should be manufactured and tested in real-life conditions. Problems may be revealed in actual use that cannot be seen in the laboratory and which either annul or diminish the advantages shown in this investigation.

2. Whether or not this type of aid is useful for a specific person may have to be decided through clinical testing. The results of this investigation were clear for a group of older listeners, a group that typically has difficulty in using hearing aids. Individuals with similar hearing levels can be considered likely to profit from this type of aid. Further investigation must ascertain how far the advantage of truly broad-band hearing aids can be extended to other clinical groups. Individuals with extreme recruitment, as well as those with noise-induced hearing losses, will most likely not be able to use or show any improvement through such aids. All of the individuals tested in this investigation have useful hearing in the high frequencies, with hearing levels not exceeding 80 dB HL in the 4 to 6 kHz region. None of them show abrupt changes in hearing level between 1 and 6 kHz.

3. Since hearing aids have not been stimulating the higher frequency regions of hearing, there is no evidence regarding the possibility that the introduction of broad-band hearing aids may have deleterious effects on the user's hearing. However, it is conceivable that hearing loss may be accentuated by the greater exposure to sound which this type of amplification implies. It is therefore extremely important that several precautions be taken to guard against this danger:

a. The subject's hearing levels must be carefully measured in the field, and the functional gains and maximum output of the aid should be well matched to those measurements to insure adequate but not excessive high-frequency gain.

b. The maximum output in the extended high-frequency range must be kept as low as it is practical and possible.

c. Frequent retesting of the subject's hearing is indispensable, at least until more knowledge accrues in this area.

4. Although no testing was done to explore the advantages of binaural vs monaural listening in terms of word discrimination, informal tests of localization resulted in an overwhelming preference for the binaural configuration. This area requires further investigation.

5. The frequency responses of hearing aids should be determined by the functional gains they provide. This type of evaluation should include the final configuration in which the aid is used, that is, the earmold and tubing selected. Deficits or suggested changes in any area of the frequency response can be plotted on the coupler-derived curve and thus communicated to the manufacturer.

Request for reprints should be sent to the Research Department, Central Institute for the Deaf, 818 South Euclid Ave., St. Louis, Mo. 63110.

ACKNOWLEDGMENT — The author acknowledges the indispensable participation of the members of his dissertation committee: Drs. James D. Miller, (Chairman), Ira J. Hirsh, Arthur F. Niemoeller, and S. Richard Silverman, and thanks them for their advice, criticism, and encouragement.

APPENDIX A

HIGH-FREQUENCY WORD LIST (HF)

1. Chick	11. Sick	21. Boat	31. Oat	41. Grime
2. Chip	12. Sift	22. Coke	32. Poke	42. Grind
3. Hick	13. Sip	23. Coat	33. Pope	43. Lime
4. Hip	14. Sipped	24. Folk	34. Road	44. Line
5. Hiss	15. Sis	25. Goad	35. Robe	45. Mime
6. Hit	16. Sit	26. Goat	36. Rope	46. Mine
7. Hits	17. Skip	27. Hope	37. Row	47. Nine
8. Pip	18. Skit	28. Load	38. Soak	48. Rhine
9. Pit	19. Thick	29. Low	39. Soap	49. Rhyme
10. Ship	20. Tip	30. Oak	40. Wrote	50. Wine

REFERENCES

1. Pascoe DP, Niemoeller AF, Miller JD: Hearing-aid design and evaluation for a presbycusic patient. J Acoustic Soc Am 55: 461(A), 1974

2. Wiener FM, Ross DA: The pressure distribution in the auditory canal in a progressive sound field. J Acoust Soc Am 18:401-408, 1946

3. Miller JD: Possible importance of head-diffraction and ear canal resonance for speech perception and hearing-aid design. J Acoust Soc Am 55:462(A), 1974

4. Davis H, Stevens SS, Nichols RH Jr, et al: *Hearing Aids: An Experimental Study of Design Objectives.* Cambridge. Mass., Harvard Univ Press, 1947

5. Committee on Electro-acoustics: Hearing aids and audiometers. London, Medical Research Council, Special Report Series No. 261, HMS Office, 1947

6. Sheets BV: A comparative study of a flat frequency response pattern and high tone emphasis patterns in a commercial hearing aid. Unpublished PhD dissertation, Univ of Minnesota. Cited by Watson LA and Tolan T, 1949. *Hearing Tests and Hearing Instruments,* Baltimore, Williams and Wilkins, 1948, p. 385

7. Shore I, Bilger RC, Hirsh IJ: Hearing aid evaluation: reliability of repeated measurements. J Speech Hearing Dis 25:152-170, 1960

8. Knight JJ: Redetermination of optimum characteristics for a hearing aid with insert earphone. International Audiol 6:322-326, 1967

9. Redell RC, Calvert DR: Selecting a hearing aid by interpreting audiologic data. J Aud Res 6:445-452, 1966

10. Carhart R, Olsen WO: Performance features and their psychological correlates. *Sixth Annual Report* of the Auditory Research Laboratories, Northwestern Univ, 1971, pp 10-14

11. Nichols Jr RH, Marquis RJ, Wiklund WG, et al: Electroacoustical characteristics of hearing aids. OSRD Report No. 4666, Section I: 1-94, 1945

12. Davis H, Hudgins CV, Marquis RJ, et al: The selection of hearing aids. Laryngoscope 56:85-115, 135-163, 1946

13. Green DS, Ross M: The effect of a conventional versus a nonoccluding (cross-type) earmold upon the frequency response of a hearing aid. J Speech Hearing Res 11: 638-647, 1968

14. Martin MC: Are frequency characteristics important? Scand Audio Suppl I:93-98, 1971

15. König E: Some technical and audiological aspects of hearing aid fitting. Scand Audio Suppl I:72-78, 1971

16. Romanow FF: Methods for measuring the performance of hearing aids. J Acoust Soc Am 13:294-304, 1942

17. Sabine PE: Acoustical amplification by hearing aids. J Acoust Soc Am 16:38-44, 1944

18. Niemoeller AF, McCormick L, Miller JD: On the spectrum of spoken English. J Acoust Soc Am 55:461(A), 1974

19. Ewertsen HW, Ipsen JB, Nielsen SS: On acoustical characteristics of the earmould. Acta Otolaryngol (Stockh) 47:312-317, 1957

20. van Eysbergen HC, Groen JJ: The 2-ml coupler and the high frequency performance of hearing aids. Acustica 9:381-386, 1959

21. Briskey RJ, Greenbaum WH, Sinclair JC: Pitfalls in hearing aid response curves. J Audio Eng Soc 14:317-323, 1966

22. Sandberg LE, Nielsen SS: Acoustic characteristics of insert-earphone versus external earphone. Acta Otolaryngol (Stockh) 64:179-186, 1967

23. Dalsgaard SC: Discussion on frequency response characteristics. Scand Audio Suppl I: 145-146, 1971

24. Sachs RM, Burkhard MD: Insert earphone pressure response in real ears and couplers. J Acoust Soc Am 52:183(A), 1972

25. Wansdronk C: On the influence of the diffraction of sound waves around the human head on the characteristics of hearing aids. J Acoust Soc Am 31:1609-1612, 1959

26. Temby AC: Sound diffraction in the vicinity of the human ear. Acustica 15:219-222, 1965.

27. Lybarger SF, Barron FE: Head-baffle effect for different hearing aid microphone locations. J Acoust Soc Am 38:922(A), 1965

28. Kasten RN, Lotterman SH, Hinchman MJ: Head shadow and head baffle effects in ear level hearing aids. Acustica 19:154-160, 1967

29. Lybarger SF: Earmold acustics. Audecibel 16:9-19, 1967

30. McDonald FD, Studebaker GA: Earmold alteration effects as measured in the human auditory meatus. J Acoust Soc Am 48: 1366-1372, 1970

31. Northern JL, Hattler KW: Earmold influence on aided speech identification tasks. J Speech Hearing Res 13:162-172, 1970

32. Konkle DF, Bess FH: Custom-made vs stock earmolds in hearing aid evaluations. Arch Otolaryngol 99:140-144, 1974

33. Miller JD: Personal communication, 1972.

34. Sivian LJ, White SD: On minimum audible fields. J Acoust Soc Am 4:288-321, 1933

35. Hawkins Jr JE, Stevens SS: The masking of pure tones and of speech by white noise. J Acoustic Soc Am 22:6-13, 1950

36. Palva T: Recruitment tests at low sensation levels. Laryngoscope 66:1519-1540, 1956

37. Niemoeller AF: Personal communication, 1974

38. Pickett JM, Martin ES, Johnson D, et al: On patterns of speech feature reception by deaf listeners, in Fant G (ed): Paper 12 in *International Symposium on Speech Communication Ability and Profound Deafness.* Washington DC, Alexander Graham Bell Assoc, 1970

39. Spenner BF, Engebretson AM, Miller JD, et al: Random-access programmable recorder of complex sounds (RAP): a digital instrument for auditory research. J Acoust Soc Am 55:427(A), 1974

40. Friedman H. *Introduction to Statistics.* New York, Random House, 1972

41. Benson RW, Hirsh IJ: Some variables in audio spectrometry. J Acoust Soc Am 25: 499-505, 1953

42. Watson NA, Knudsen VO: Selective amplification in hearing aids. J Acoust Soc Am 11:406-419, 1940

43. Victoreen JA: *Hearing Enhancement.* Springfield, Ill., CC Thomas, 1960

44. Villchur E: Signal processing to improve speech intelligibility in perceptive deafness. J Acoust Soc Am 53:1646-1657, 1973

45. French NR, Steinberg JC: Factors governing the intelligibility of speech sounds. J Acoust Soc Am 19:90-119, 1947

46. Miller GA: *Language and Communication.* New York, McGraw-Hill, 1951

47. Mullins CJ, Bangs JL: Relationships between speech discrimination and other audiometric data. Acta Otolaryngol (Stockh) 47:149-157, 1957

48. Kryter KD, Williams C, Green DM: Auditory acuity and the perception of speech. J Acoust Soc Am 34:1217-1223, 1962